Volume 62

2013

Instructional Course Lectures

AAOS

American Academy of Orthopaedic Surgeons

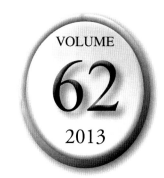

VOLUME 62 2013

Instructional Course Lectures

Edited by
Mark W. Pagnano, MD
Professor of Orthopedics
Department of Orthopedic Surgery
Mayo Clinic College of Medicine
Rochester, Minnesota

Robert A. Hart, MD
Professor of Orthopedics
Program Director, Adult Spine Fellowship
Oregon Health and Science University
Portland, Oregon

Published 2013 by the
American Academy of
Orthopaedic Surgeons
6300 North River Road
Rosemont, IL 60018

AAOS
American Academy of Orthopaedic Surgeons

AAOS

AMERICAN ACADEMY OF ORTHOPAEDIC SURGEONS

Staff

Constance M. Filling, *Chief Education Officer*

Hans Koelsch, PhD, *Director, Department of Publications*

Lisa Claxton Moore, *Managing Editor*

Kathleen A. Anderson, *Senior Editor*

Mary Steermann Bishop, *Senior Manager, Production and Archives*

Courtney Astle, *Editorial Production Manager*

Abram Fassler, *Publishing Systems Manager*

Suzanne O'Reilly, *Graphic Designer*

Karen Danca, *Permissions Coordinator*

Charlie Baldwin, *Production Database Associate*

Hollie Muir, *Production Database Associate*

Emily Nickel, *Page Production Assistant*

Michelle Bruno, *Editorial Coordinator*

Instructional Course Lectures Volume 62
American Academy of Orthopaedic Surgeons

The material presented in *Instructional Course Lectures, Volume 62* has been made available by the American Academy of Orthopaedic Surgeons for educational purposes only. This material is not intended to present the only, or necessarily best, methods or procedures for the medical situations discussed, but rather is intended to represent an approach, view, statement, or opinion of the author(s) or producer(s), which may be helpful to others who face similar situations.

Some drugs or medical devices demonstrated in Academy courses or described in Academy print or electronic publications have not been cleared by the Food and Drug Administration (FDA) or have been cleared for specific uses only. The FDA has stated that it is the responsibility of the physician to determine the FDA clearance status of each drug or device he or she wishes to use in clinical practice.

Furthermore, any statements about commercial products are solely the opinion(s) of the author(s) and do not represent an Academy endorsement or evaluation of these products. These statements may not be used in advertising or for any commercial purpose.

ISSN 0065-6895
ISBN 978-0-89203-967-8
Printed in the USA

Bone and Joint Initiative USA

Contributors

Daniel Aaron, MD
Shoulder and Elbow Fellow, Department of Orthopaedic Surgery, Mount Sinai School of Medicine, New York, New York

Benjamin A. Alman, MD
A.J. Latner Professor and Chair, Department of Orthopaedics, University of Toronto, Toronto, Ontario, Canada

Sarah A. Anderson, MD
Assistant Professor, University of Minnesota, Orthopaedic Surgeon, Department of Orthopaedic Surgery, Regions Hospital, St. Paul, Minnesota

Robert A. Arciero, MD
Professor of Orthopaedics, Department of Orthopaedic Surgery, University of Connecticut Health Center, Farmington, Connecticut

April D. Armstrong, MD, FRCSC
Associate Professor, Shoulder and Elbow, Department of Orthopaedics, Penn State, Milton S. Hershey Medical Center, Hershey, Pennsylvania

Keith D. Baldwin, MD, MPH
Orthopedic Surgeon, Department of Orthopedic Surgery, Children's Hospital of Philadelphia, Philadelphia, Pennsylvania

Paul E. Beaulé, MD, FRCSC
Associate Professor, Division of Orthopedic Surgery, University of Ottawa, Ottawa, Ontario, Canada

Asheesh Bedi, MD
Assistant Professor, Department of Orthopaedic Surgery, University of Michigan, Ann Arbor, Michigan

Jeff Belkora, PhD
Assistant Professor, Department of Surgery, Philip R. Lee Institute for Health Policy Studies, University of California, San Francisco, California

Stephen K. Benirschke, MD
Professor, Department of Orthopaedics and Sports Medicine, Harborview Medical Center, University of Washington, Seattle, Washington

Keith R. Berend, MD
Clinical Assistant Professor, Department of Orthopaedics, The Ohio State University, Mount Carmel Health System, Joint Implant Surgeons, New Albany, Ohio

Richard A. Berger, MD
Assistant Professor, Department of Orthopaedic Surgery, Rush University Medical Center, Chicago, Illinois

Kevin P. Black, MD
Chairman, Department of Orthopaedics and Rehabilitation, Penn State, Milton S. Hershey Medical Center, Hershey, Pennsylvania

Aaron J. Bois, MD, FRCSC
Shoulder and Elbow Fellow, University of Texas Health Sciences Center, University of Texas, San Antonio, Texas

Martin I. Boyer, MD, FRCSC
Department of Orthopaedics, Washington University School of Medicine, St. Louis, Missouri

Kevin J. Bozic, MD, MBA
Associate Professor and Vice Chair, Department of Orthopaedic Surgery, University of California, San Francisco, California

Jacob M. Buchowski, MD
Associate Professor, Department of Orthopaedic Surgery, Washington University, St. Louis, Missouri

Wayne Z. Burkhead Jr, MD
Clinical Professor, Shoulder Service, The Carrell Clinic, Dallas, Texas

Curtis A. Bush, MD
Sports Medicine Fellow, Steadman Hawkins Clinic of the Carolinas, Greenville Hospital System, Greenville, South Carolina

Lisa K. Cannada, MD
Associate Professor, Department of Orthopaedic Surgery, Saint Louis University, St. Louis, Missouri

Henry G. Chambers, MD
Professor of Clinical Orthopedics, Department of Orthopedic Surgery, University of California at San Diego, Rady Children's Hospital, San Diego, California

Vikram Chatrath, MBBS, MS, MCh (Ortho)
Fellow, Adult Reconstruction, Department of Orthopaedic Surgery, The Ottawa Hospital, Ottawa, Ontario, Canada

Darwin Chen, MD
Clinical Fellow in Adult Reconstruction, Department of Orthopaedic Surgery, Rush University Medical Center, Chicago, Illinois

Kate E. Chenok, MBA
Executive Director, California Joint Replacement Registry, San Francisco, California

Vanessa Chiu, MPH
Project Director, Department of Orthopaedic Surgery, University of California, San Francisco, California

Michael G. Ciccotti, MD
Professor of Orthopaedic Surgery, Chief, Division of Sports Medicine, Director, Sports Medicine Fellowship and Research, Rothman Institute, Thomas Jefferson University, Philadelphia, Pennsylvania

Peter A. Cole, MD
Professor, University of Minnesota, Chief of Orthopaedic Surgery, Department of Orthopaedic Surgery, Regions Hospital, St. Paul, Minnesota

CAPT Dana C. Covey, MD, MC, USN
Clinical Professor, Department of Orthopaedic Surgery, University of California, Naval Medical Center San Diego, San Diego, California

Joseph J. Crisco, PhD
Henry Frederick Lippitt Professor of Orthopaedic Research, Director, Bioengineering Laboratory, Department of Orthopaedic Research, The Warren Alpert Medical School of Brown University and Rhode Island Hospital, Providence, Rhode Island

Brett D. Crist, MD, FACS
Associate Professor, Department of Orthopaedic Surgery, University of Missouri, Columbia, Missouri

Brian K. Daines, MD
Orthopaedic Fellow, Colorado Joint Replacement, Denver, Colorado

Douglas A. Dennis, MD
Adjunct Professor, Department of Biomedical Engineering, University of Tennessee, Adjunct Professor of Bioengineering, University of Denver, Director, Rocky Mountain Musculoskeletal Research Laboratory, Denver, Colorado

Douglas R. Dirschl, MD
Professor and Chairman, Department of Orthopaedics, University of North Carolina, Chapel Hill, North Carolina

Derek J. Donegan, MD
Orthopaedic Trauma Fellow, Department of Orthopaedic Surgery, University of Medicine and Dentistry of New Jersey, Newark, New Jersey

Paul J. Dougherty, MD
Associate Professor, Department of Orthopaedic Surgery, University of Michigan, Ann Arbor, Michigan

Kenneth A. Egol, MD
Professor and Vice Chair, New York University Hospital for Joint Diseases, New York University Langone Medical Center, New York, New York

Jill Erickson, PA-C
Physician Assistant, Orthopaedic Department, University of Utah, Salt Lake City, Utah

Peter Ferguson, MD, FRCSC
Associate Professor, Department of Orthopaedic Surgery, University of Toronto, Toronto, Ontario, Canada

Tania Ferguson, MD
Assistant Professor, Department of Orthopaedic Surgery, Trauma Service, University of California Davis Medical Center, Sacramento, California

Evan L. Flatow, MD
Lasker Professor and Chairman, Department of Orthopaedic Surgery, Mount Sinai School of Medicine, New York, New York

Corinna C. Franklin, MD
Fellow, Department of Orthopaedic Surgery, Children's Hospital of Philadelphia, Philadelphia, Pennsylvania

Emmanuel Gibon, MD
Postdoctoral Research Fellow, Department of Orthopaedic Surgery, Stanford University, Stanford, California

John G. Ginnetti, MD
Fellow, Department of Orthopaedics, University of Utah, Salt Lake City, Utah

Steven Z. Glickel, MD
Clinical Professor of Orthopaedic Surgery, Department of Orthopaedic Surgery, Columbia University, New York, New York

Stuart B. Goodman, MD, PhD, FRCSC
Robert L. and Mary Ellenburg Professor of Surgery, Department of Orthopaedic Surgery, Stanford University Medical Center, Redwood City, California

Elisabet Hagert, MD, PhD
Co-Chairman, Senior Consultant Hand Surgeon, Hand and Foot Surgery Center, Department of Clinical Sciences, Karolinska Institutet, Stockholm, Sweden

George J. Haidukewych, MD
Academic Chairman and Program Director, Orthopaedic Surgery, Level One Orthopaedics, Orlando Health, Orlando, Florida

Kathryn H. Hanna, MD, MC, USN
Staff Orthopaedic Surgeon, Department of Orthopaedic Surgery, Naval Medical Center San Diego, San Diego, California

Richard J. Hawkins, MD
Orthopaedic Surgeon, Steadman Hawkins Clinic of the Carolinas, Greenville Hospital System, Greenville, South Carolina

William Hennrikus, MD
Professor, Department of Orthopaedics, Penn State College of Medicine, Hershey, Pennsylvania

Martin J. Herman, MD
Associate Professor, Drexel University College of Medicine, Department of Orthopaedic Surgery, St. Christopher's Hospital for Children, Philadelphia, Pennsylvania

Benton E. Heyworth, MD
Staff Surgeon, Department of Orthopaedic Surgery, Children's Hospital Boston, Boston, Massachusetts

Sandra Jarvis-Selinger, PhD
Assistant Dean, Department of Faculty Development/Department of Surgery, University of British Columbia, Vancouver, British Columbia, Canada

Chunyan Jiang, MD, PhD
Professor, Shoulder Service, Beijing Jishuitan Hospital, 4th Medical Center, School of Medicine, Peking University, Beijing, People's Republic of China

Clifford B. Jones, MD, FACS
Clinical Professor, Michigan State University College of Human Medicine, Department of Orthopaedic Surgery, Orthopaedic Associates of Medicine, Grand Rapids, Michigan

Joseph J. Kavolus, BA
Medical University of South Carolina, Charleston, South Carolina

Bryan T. Kelly, MD
Co-Director, Center for Hip Preservation, Hospital for Special Surgery, New York, New York

W. Ben Kibler, MD
Medical Director, Shoulder Center of Kentucky, Lexington Clinic, Lexington, Kentucky

Han Jo Kim, MD
Spine Fellow, Department of Orthopaedic and Neurological Surgery, Washington University, St. Louis, Missouri

Mininder S. Kocher, MD, MPH
Associate Director, Division of Sports Medicine, Children's Hospital Boston, Boston, Massachusetts

Stephen A. Kottmeier, MD
Clinical Professor of Orthopedic Surgery, Director of Orthopedic Trauma Service, Department of Orthopedic Surgery, State University New York Health Sciences Center, Stony Brook, New York

William Kraemer, MD, FRCSC
Orthopaedic Surgeon, Division of Orthopaedic Surgery, Department of Surgery, University of Toronto, Toronto, Ontario, Canada

John C. Kurylo, MD
Orthopaedic Surgeon, Boston University Medical Center, Boston, Massachusetts

Amy L. Ladd, MD
Professor of Orthopaedic Surgery, Chief of Chase Hand Center, Department of Orthopaedic Surgery, Stanford University, Stanford, California

Joshua R. Langford, MD
Director, Limb Deformity Service, Orlando Health Orthopedic Residency Program, Orlando Health, Orlando, Florida

Christopher M. Larson, MD
Minnesota Orthopedic Sports Medicine Institute, Twin Cities Orthopedics, Edina, Minnesota

Cara Beth Lee, MD
Director, Center for Hip Preservation, Department of Orthopaedics, Virginia Mason Medical Center, Seattle, Washington

Joon Y. Lee, MD
Associate Professor, Department of Orthopaedics, University of Pittsburgh Medical Center, Pittsburgh, Pennsylvania

Joe Y.B. Lee, MD
Spine Surgery Fellow, Department of Orthopaedic Surgery, Rush University Medical Center, Chicago, Illinois

Mark A. Lee, MD
Associate Professor, Department of Orthopaedic Surgery, University of California Davis Medical Center, Sacramento, California

William N. Levine, MD
Vice Chairman and Professor, Department of Orthopaedic Surgery, Columbia University Medical Center, New York, New York

Valerae O. Lewis, MD
Associate Professor and Chief, Department of Orthopaedic Oncology, MD Anderson Cancer Center, Houston, Texas

Thomas M. Link, MD, PhD
Professor of Radiology, Chief of Musculoskeletal Imaging, Department of Radiology and Biomedical Imaging, University of California, San Francisco, California

David M. Lintner, MD
Chief of Sports Medicine, Methodist Center for Sports Medicine, The Methodist Hospital, Houston, Texas

Frank A. Liporace, MD
Associate Professor, Department of Orthopaedics, Director, Trauma and Reconstructive Fellowship, University of Medicine and Dentistry of New Jersey, New Jersey Medical School, Newark, New Jersey

Adolph V. Lombardi Jr, MD, FACS
President, Joint Implant Surgeons, Clinical Assistant Professor, Department of Orthopaedics and Department of Biomedical Engineering, The Ohio State University, Attending Surgeon, Mount Carmel Health System, New Albany, Ohio

Robert J. Lucking, MD
Surgery Resident, Department of Surgery, University of New Mexico, Albuquerque, New Mexico

Douglas W. Lundy, MD, FACS
Orthopaedic Trauma Surgeon, Resurgens Orthopaedics, Atlanta, Georgia

Kevin Lutsky, MD
Rothman Institute, Thomas Jefferson University Hospital, Philadelphia, Pennsylvania

Travis G. Maak, MD
Sports Fellow, Sports Medicine and Shoulder Service, Hospital for Special Surgery, New York, New York

Andrew P. Mahoney, MD
Shoulder and Elbow Fellow, Department of Orthopaedic Surgery, New York University Hospital for Joint Diseases, New York, New York

Eric G. Meinberg, MD
Assistant Clinical Professor, Department of Orthopaedic Surgery, University of California, San Francisco, California

William M. Mihalko, MD, PhD
Professor and J.R. Hyde Chair, Department of Orthopaedic Surgery and Biomedical Engineering, Campbell Clinic, University of Tennessee, Memphis, Tennessee

Michael B. Millis, MD
Adolescent and Young Adult Hip Unit, Department of Orthopaedic Surgery, Children's Hospital Boston, Boston, Massachusetts

Todd C. Moen, MD
Orthopaedic Surgeon, Shoulder Service, The Carrell Clinic, Dallas, Texas

Emmanouil Morakis, MD
Fellow, Department of Orthopaedics, Hospital for Special Surgery, New York, New York

Carol D. Morris, MD
Associate Professor of Orthopaedic Surgery, Weill Cornell School of Medicine, Attending Surgeon, Department of Orthopaedic Surgery, Memorial Sloan-Kettering Cancer Center, New York, New York

Michael J. Morris, MD
Joint Implant Surgeons, Mount Carmel Health System, New Albany, Ohio

Martin J. Morrison III, MD
Fellow, Division of Orthopaedic Surgery, Children's Hospital of Philadelphia, Perelman School of Medicine at the University of Pennsylvania, Philadelphia, Pennsylvania

Charbel D. Moussallem, MD, FEBOT
Spine Fellow, Department of Orthopedic Surgery, Mayo Clinic, Rochester, Minnesota

Stephen B. Murphy, MD
Associate Professor of Orthopedic Surgery, New England Baptist Hospital, Tufts University School of Medicine, Boston, Massachusetts

Yvonne M. Murtha, MD
Orthopaedic Traumatologist, Clinical Assistant Professor, Advanced Orthopaedic Associates, University of Kansas, Wichita, Kansas

Markku T. Nousiainen, MD, FRCSC
Associate Program Director, Department of Surgery, University of Toronto, Toronto, Ontario, Canada

Robert F. Ostrum, MD
Professor, Department of Orthopaedic Surgery, Cooper Medical School of Rowan University, Camden, New Jersey

Juan Carlos S. Paredes, MD
Institute of Orthopedics and Sports Medicine, St. Luke's Medical Center, Quezon City, Philippines

Bradford O. Parsons, MD
Assistant Professor, Department of Orthopaedic Surgery, Mount Sinai School of Medicine, New York, New York

Theodore W. Parsons III, MD, FACS
Professor and Chairman, Department of Orthopaedic Surgery, Henry Ford Hospital, Wayne State University, Detroit, Michigan

Alpesh A. Patel, MD, FACS
Associate Professor, Department of Orthopaedic Surgery, Loyola University Medical Center, Maywood, Illinois

Brian Perkinson, MD
Orthopaedic Surgery Resident, Campbell Clinic Orthopaedics, University of Tennessee, Memphis, Tennessee

Christopher L. Peters, MD
Professor, Department of Orthopaedics, University of Utah, Salt Lake City, Utah

Frank M. Phillips, MD
Professor, Department of Orthopaedic Surgery, Rush University Medical Center, Chicago, Illinois

Daniel D. Pratt, PhD
Professor and Senior Scholar, Centre for Health Education Research, University of British Columbia, Vancouver, British Columbia, Canada

Robert A. Probe, MD
Professor and Chair, Department of Orthopaedics, Scott and White Healthcare, Temple, Texas

Tamara Pylawka, MD
Chief Resident, Department of Orthopaedics, Penn State College of Medicine, Hershey, Pennsylvania

Richard K. Reznick, MD
Dean, Faculty of Health Sciences, Queen's University, Kingston, Ontario, Canada

Michael D. Ries, MD
Professor and Chief of Arthroplasty, Department of Orthopaedic Surgery, University of California, San Francisco, California

Susanne M. Roberts, MD
Resident, Department of Orthopedic Surgery, Massachusetts General Hospital, Boston, Massachusetts

Peter S. Rose, MD
Assistant Professor of Orthopedics, Division of Orthopedic Oncology, Department of Orthopedic Surgery, Mayo Clinic, Rochester, Minnesota

Glen H. Rudolph, MD
Shoulder Fellow, Shoulder Service, The Carrell Clinic, Dallas, Texas

Thomas A. Russell, MD
Professor of Orthopaedic Surgery, Department of Orthopaedics, Campbell Clinic, University of Tennessee Center for the Health Sciences, Memphis, Tennessee

Susan A. Scherl, MD
Professor, Department of Orthopaedics, The University of Nebraska, Omaha, Nebraska

Jacob F. Schulz, MD
Pediatric Orthopedic Surgery Fellow, Orthopaedic and Scoliosis Center, Rady Children's Hospital, San Diego, California

Giles R. Scuderi, MD
Director, Insall Scott Kelly Institute, New York, New York

Joshua Shatsky, MD
Chief Orthopaedic Resident, Department of Orthopaedic Surgery, Mount Sinai Hospital, New York, New York

Rafael J. Sierra, MD
Associate Professor of Orthopedics, Department of Orthopedic Surgery, College of Medicine, Mayo Clinic, Rochester, Minnesota

Ernest L. Sink, MD
Associate Professor, Department of Pediatric Orthopaedics, Hospital for Special Surgery, New York, New York

Francois Sirveaux, MD, PhD
Professor, Service de Chirurgie Orthopédique et Traumatologique, Centre Chirurgical Emile Gallé, Nancy, France

David L. Skaggs, MD
Chief of Orthopaedic Surgery, Department of Orthopaedics, Children's Hospital of Los Angeles, Los Angeles, California

Kjeld Søballe, MD, PhD
Professor, Orthopaedic Research Unit, Aarhus University Hospital, Aarhus, Denmark

John W. Sperling, MD, MBA
Consultant, Department of Orthopedic Surgery, Mayo Clinic, Rochester, Minnesota

Bryan D. Springer, MD
OrthoCarolina Hip and Knee Center, Charlotte, North Carolina

David D. Teuscher, MD
Beaumont Bone and Joint Institute, Beaumont, Texas

Paul Tornetta III, MD
Director of Orthopaedic Trauma, Department of Orthopaedic Surgery, Boston Medical Center, Boston, Massachusetts

Anders Troelsen, MD, PhD
Associate Professor, Research Fellow, Orthopaedic Research Unit, Aarhus University Hospital, Aarhus, Denmark

Rahul Vaidya, MD, FRCSC
Chief of Orthopaedic Surgery, Department of Orthopaedic Surgery, Detroit Medical Center, Detroit, Michigan

Mandeep S. Virk, MD
Orthopaedic Resident, Department of Orthopaedic Surgery, University of Connecticut Health Center, Farmington, Connecticut

Gilles Walch, MD
Surgeon, Shoulder Surgery, Hôpital Privé Jean Mermoz, Lyon, France

Torrance Walker, MD
Adult Reconstruction Fellow, Department of Orthopaedic Surgery, Campbell Clinic Orthopaedics, University of Tennessee, Memphis, Tennessee

Andrew Weiland, MD
Professor of Orthopaedics, Department of Orthopaedic Surgery, Hospital for Special Surgery, New York, New York

Arnold-Peter C. Weiss, MD
R. Scot Sellers Scholar of Hand Surgery, Professor and Associate, Dean of Medicine (Admissions), Albert Medical School of Brown University, Providence, Rhode Island

Peter G. Whang, MD
Associate Professor, Department of Orthopaedics and Rehabilitation, Yale University School of Medicine, New Haven, Connecticut

Michael A. Wirth, MD
Professor of Orthopaedics, University of Texas Health Sciences Center, University of Texas, San Antonio, Texas

Jennifer Moriatis Wolf, MD
Associate Professor, Department of Orthopaedics, University of Connecticut Health Center, Farmington, Connecticut

Jeffrey Yao, MD
Associate Professor, Department of Orthopaedic Surgery, Stanford University Medical Center, Palo Alto, California

Zhenyu Yao, MD, PhD
Research Associate, Lab Manager, Department of Orthopaedic Surgery, Stanford University, Stanford, California

Jiwon Youm, MS
Medical Student, Department of Orthopaedics, University of California, San Francisco, California

Ira Zaltz, MD
Section Head, Pediatric Orthopaedics, William Beaumont Hospital, Royal Oak, Michigan

Joseph D. Zuckerman, MD
Professor and Chair, Department of Orthopaedic Surgery, New York University Hospital for Joint Diseases, New York, New York

Preface

Instructional Course Lectures, Volume 62 contains 53 chapters that convey timely information from some of the most informative lectures presented at the 2012 Annual Meeting held in San Francisco. My sincere thanks go to the more than 135 authors who contributed to this volume. The commitment needed to write up and illustrate their lecture material and bring it to press just 1 year after the meeting presentations speaks well for their commitment to sharing orthopaedic knowledge and helping meet the educational goals of the American Academy of Orthopaedic Surgeons.

I also wish to thank Robert A. Hart, MD, the assistant editor of this volume, for his help in reviewing and editing manuscripts, and the AAOS Publications Department staff, including their retired director, Marilyn L. Fox, PhD; new director, Hans Koelsch, PhD; managing editor of the ICL series, Lisa Claxton Moore; and senior editor, Kathleen A. Anderson. Kudos also go to my colleagues and AAOS staff of the Central Instructional Course Committee who are responsible for organizing and selecting the many educational lectures and symposia presented each year at the AAOS Annual Meeting. In expressing my appreciation, I cannot leave out Reid Stanton and the AAOS Electronic Media Department for their work in preparing the DVD video supplement that accompanies ICL 62 and nicely illustrates some of the concepts and procedures described in these lectures.

It has been my privilege to serve as the editor of this 62nd volume of the Instructional Course Lectures series. All of us involved in producing this work trust that the readers will find the material helpful in enhancing their ability to provide the best possible care for patients with musculoskeletal injuries and diseases.

Mark W. Pagnano, MD
Rochester, Minnesota

Table of Contents

	Preface	xiii	

Section 1: Trauma

1	The Traumatic Lower Extremity Amputee: Surgical Challenges and Advances in Prosthetics	3	Lisa K. Cannada Rahul Vaidya CAPT Dana C. Covey LCDR Kathryn Hanna Paul Dougherty
2	Surgical Timing of Treating Injured Extremities: An Evolving Concept of Urgency	17	Brett D. Crist Tania Ferguson Yvonne M. Murtha Mark A. Lee
3	***Symposium*** Orthopaedic Trauma Mythbusters: Intra-articular Fractures	29	Robert F. Ostrum
4	***Symposium*** Orthopaedic Trauma Mythbusters: Is Limb Salvage the Preferred Method of Treatment for the Mangled Lower Extremity?	35	Robert A. Probe
5	Locked and Minimally Invasive Plating: A Paradigm Shift? Metadiaphyseal Site-Specific Concerns and Controversies	41	Stephen A. Kottmeier Clifford B. Jones Paul Tornetta III Thomas A. Russell
6	Extra-articular Proximal Tibial Fractures: Nail or Plate?	61	John C. Kurylo Paul Tornetta III
DVD 7	Fractures and Dislocations of the Midfoot: Lisfranc and Chopart Injuries	79	Stephen K. Benirschke Eric G. Meinberg Sarah A. Anderson Clifford B. Jones Peter A. Cole

Section 2: Shoulder

DVD 8	Revision Open Capsular Shift for Atraumatic and Multidirectional Instability of the Shoulder	95	Aaron J. Bois Michael A. Wirth
9	General Surgical Principles of Open Rotator Cuff Repair in the Management of Failed Arthroscopic Cuff Repairs	105	Wayne Z. Burkhead Jr Todd C. Moen Glen H. Rudolph
DVD 10	Prevention of Complications in Shoulder Arthroplasty: Understanding Options and Critical Steps	115	Curtis A. Bush Richard J. Hawkins
11	Complications in Total Shoulder Arthroplasty	135	John W. Sperling Richard J. Hawkins Gilles Walch Andrew P. Mahoney Joseph D. Zuckerman

DVD 12	Proximal Humeral Fractures: Internal Fixation	143	Daniel Aaron Joshua Shatsky Juan Carlos S. Paredes Chunyan Jiang Bradford O. Parsons Evan L. Flatow
13	Proximal Humeral Fractures: Prosthetic Replacement	155	Daniel Aaron Bradford O. Parsons Francois Sirveaux Evan L. Flatow

Section 3: Hand and Wrist

	Symposium		
DVD 14	The Thumb Carpometacarpal Joint: Anatomy, Hormones, and Biomechanics	165	Amy L. Ladd Arnold-Peter C. Weiss Joseph J. Crisco Elisabet Hagert Jennifer Moriatis Wolf Steven Z. Glickel Jeffrey Yao
15	What Every Resident Should Know About Wrist Fractures: Case-Based Learning	181	Kevin Lutsky Steven Z. Glickel Andrew Weiland Martin I. Boyer

Section 4: Adult Reconstruction: Hip

16	The Basic Science of Periprosthetic Osteolysis	201	Stuart B. Goodman Emmanuel Gibon Zhenyu Yao
17	Monitoring and Risk of Progression of Osteolysis After Total Hip Arthroplasty	207	Michael D. Ries Thomas M. Link
18	The Changing Paradigm of Revision of Total Hip Replacement in the Presence of Osteolysis	215	Vikram Chatrath Paul E. Beaulé
19	Outpatient Minimally Invasive Total Hip Arthroplasty Via a Modified Watson-Jones Approach: Technique and Results	229	Darwin Chen Richard A. Berger
DVD 20	Total Hip Arthroplasty: The Mini-Posterior Approach	237	John G. Ginnetti Jill Erickson Christopher L. Peters
21	Total Hip Arthroplasty Using the Superior Capsulotomy Technique	245	Stephen B. Murphy
22	Primary and Revision Anterior Supine Total Hip Arthroplasty: An Analysis of Complications and Reoperations	251	Keith R. Berend Joseph J. Kavolus Michael J. Morris Adolph V. Lombardi Jr

23	Patient Selection for Rotational Pelvic Osteotomy	265	Cara Beth Lee Michael B. Millis
24	Periacetabular Osteotomy: Intra-articular Work	279	John G. Ginnetti Jill Erickson Christopher L. Peters
25	Alternatives to Periacetabular Osteotomy for Adult Acetabular Dysplasia	287	Cara Beth Lee Michael B. Millis
26	Approaches and Perioperative Management in Periacetabular Osteotomy Surgery: The Minimally Invasive Transsartorial Approach	297	Kjeld Søballe Anders Troelsen
27	The Management of Acetabular Retroversion With Reverse Periacetabular Osteotomy	305	Rafael J. Sierra

Section 5: Adult Reconstruction: Knee

28	Contemporary Internal Fixation Techniques for Periprosthetic Fractures of the Hip and Knee	317	Frank A. Liporace Derek J. Donegan Joshua R. Langford George J. Haidukewych
29	Revision for Periprosthetic Fractures of the Hip and Knee	333	George J. Haidukewych Joshua R. Langford Frank A. Liporace
DVD 30	Management of Bone Defects in Revision Total Knee Arthroplasty	341	Brian K. Daines Douglas A. Dennis
31	Evaluation and Management of the Infected Total Knee Arthroplasty	349	Bryan D. Springer Giles R. Scuderi
32	Patellofemoral Arthroplasty: The Other Unicompartmental Knee Replacement	363	Torrance Walker Brian Perkinson William M. Mihalko

Section 6: Spine

33	Modern Techniques in the Treatment of Patients With Metastatic Spine Disease	375	Han Jo Kim Jacob M. Buchowski Charbel D. Moussallem Peter S. Rose, MD
34	Lumbar Spinal Stenosis	383	Joe Y.B. Lee Peter G. Whang Joon Y. Lee Frank M. Phillips Alpesh A. Patel

Section 7: Pediatrics

35	***Symposium*** Orthopaedic Aspects of Child Abuse	399	Keith D. Baldwin Susan A. Scherl

Symposium
36 Hip Septic Arthritis and Other Pediatric Musculoskeletal Infections in the Era of Methicillin-Resistant *Staphylococcus aureus* 405 Martin J. Morrison III, Martin J. Herman

Symposium
37 Advances in Hip Preservation After Slipped Capital Femoral Epiphysis 415 Emmanouil Morakis, Ernest L. Sink

Symposium
38 Approach to the Pediatric Supracondylar Humeral Fracture With Neurovascular Compromise 429 Corinna C. Franklin, David L. Skaggs

39 Shoulder Instability in the Young Athlete 435 Benton E. Heyworth, Mininder S. Kocher

40 Patellofemoral Instability in Skeletally Immature Athletes 445 William Hennrikus, Tamara Pylawka

DVD 41 Juvenile Osteochondritis Dissecans of the Knee: Current Concepts in Diagnosis and Management 455 Jacob F. Schulz, Henry G. Chambers

Section 8: Sports Medicine

42 Superior Labrum Anterior to Posterior Injuries and Impingement 471 Michael G. Ciccotti

DVD 43 What Is a Clinically Important Superior Labrum Anterior to Posterior Tear? 483 W. Ben Kibler

44 Superior Labrum Anterior to Posterior Tears in Throwing Athletes 491 David M. Lintner

45 Superior Labrum Anterior to Posterior Tears and Glenohumeral Instability 501 Mandeep S. Virk, Robert A. Arciero

DVD 46 Sports Hip Injuries: Assessment and Management 515 Bryan T. Kelly, Travis G. Maak, Christopher M. Larson, Asheesh Bedi, Ira Zaltz

Section 9: Orthopaedic Medicine

47 Malignant and Benign Bone Tumors That You Are Likely to See 535 Valerae O. Lewis, Carol D. Morris, Theodore W. Parsons III

Section 10: The Practice of Orthopaedics

48 Orthopaedic Residency Education: A Practical Guide to Selection, Training, and Education 553 Kenneth A. Egol, Douglas R. Dirschl, William N. Levine, Joseph D. Zuckerman

	Symposium		
49	Competency-Based Education: A New Model for Teaching Orthopaedics	565	Benjamin A. Alman Peter Ferguson William Kraemer Markku T. Nousiainen Richard K. Reznick
	Symposium		
50	Resident Education in the Systems-Based Practice Competency	571	Susanne M. Roberts Sandra Jarvis-Selinger Daniel D. Pratt Robert J. Lucking Kevin P. Black
	Symposium		
51	I Feel Disconnected: Learning Technologies in Resident Education	577	April D. Armstrong Sandra Jarvis-Selinger
52	The Emerging Case for Shared Decision Making in Orthopaedics	587	Jiwon Youm Kate E. Chenok Jeff Belkora Vanessa Chiu Kevin J. Bozic
53	Surviving and Winning a Professional Negligence Lawsuit	595	Douglas W. Lundy David D. Teuscher
	Index	603	

SECTION

1

Trauma

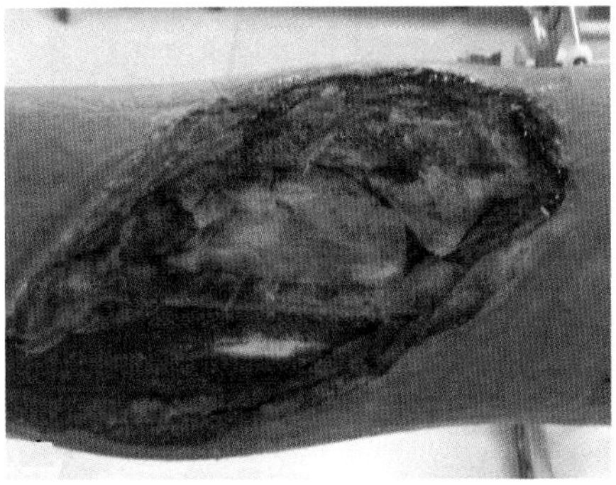

1 The Traumatic Lower Extremity Amputee: Surgical Challenges and Advances in Prosthetics

2 Surgical Timing of Treating Injured Extremities: An Evolving Concept of Urgency

Symposium

3 Orthopaedic Trauma Mythbusters: Intra-articular Fractures

Symposium

4 Orthopaedic Trauma Mythbusters: Is Limb Salvage the Preferred Method of Treatment for the Mangled Lower Extremity?

5 Locked and Minimally Invasive Plating: A Paradigm Shift? Metadiaphyseal Site-Specific Concerns and Controversies

6 Extra-articular Proximal Tibial Fractures: Nail or Plate?

DVD 7 Fractures and Dislocations of the Midfoot: Lisfranc and Chopart Injuries

1

The Traumatic Lower Extremity Amputee: Surgical Challenges and Advances in Prosthetics

Lisa K. Cannada, MD
Rahul Vaidya, MD
CAPT Dana C. Covey, MD, MC, USN
LCDR Kathryn Hanna, MD, MC, USN
Paul Dougherty, MD

Abstract

The mangled lower extremity is a challenging injury to treat. Orthopaedic surgeons treating patients with these severe injuries must have a clear understanding of contemporary advantages and disadvantages of limb salvage versus amputation. It is helpful to review the acute management of mangled extremity injuries in the civilian and military populations, to be familiar with current postoperative protocols, and to recognize recent advances in prosthetic devices.

Instr Course Lect 2013;62:3-15.

The Mangled Extremity

In some patients with a mangled extremity, the treatment plan is obvious, whereas in other patients the treatment plan evolves over time based on the extent of the soft-tissue injuries and changes in the patient's condition. When evaluating a patient with a mangled extremity, it is important to ask some basic questions: (1) What type of medical treatment can the patient tolerate? The patient's age, underlying medical comorbidities, medication usage, and support system must be considered. (2) What type of treatment is appropriate based on the condition of the injured limb? (3) What are the capabilities of the treating surgeon and the resources available at the facility where care is being administered?

Evaluation

Documentation of the injury should include an evaluation of the circulatory status of the limb, the wound size and location, the degree of contamination, the extent of degloving, and the fracture details. The extent of the soft-tissue injury will substantially affect the patient's outcome. Photographs of the injury can be helpful.

Initial Treatment

Considerations

If the patient's condition will allow surgery, a thorough débridement should be done. The débridement begins with the skin and continues through the soft tissues to the bone. It is important to note the extent of periosteal stripping and to carefully look for contamination at all levels. If vascular repair is needed, a spanning external fixator is appropriate. A vascular surgeon should be consulted so that

Dr. Cannada or an immediate family member serves as a board member, owner, officer, or committee member of the American Academy of Orthopaedic Surgeons, the Orthopaedic Trauma Association, and the Ruth Jackson Orthopaedic Society; is a member of a speakers' bureau or has made paid presentations on behalf of Smith & Nephew; serves as a paid consultant to or is an employee of Zimmer; and has received research or institutional support from Zimmer, Synthes, the Department of Defense, and the Southeast Fracture Consortium. Dr. Vaidya or an immediate family member is a member of a speakers' bureau or has made paid presentations on behalf of Synthes and Stryker; serves as a paid consultant to or is an employee of Stryker; serves as an unpaid consultant to Stryker; has received research or institutional support from Synthes; and has received nonincome support (such as equipment or services), commercially derived honoraria, or other non–research-related funding (such as paid travel) from Synthes. Dr. Covey or an immediate family member serves as a board member, owner, officer, or committee member of the American Academy of Orthopaedic Surgeons and the Society of Military Orthopaedic Surgeons. Neither of the following authors nor any immediate family member has received anything of value from or owns stock in a commercial company or institution related directly or indirectly to the subject of this chapter: Dr. Hanna and Dr. Dougherty.

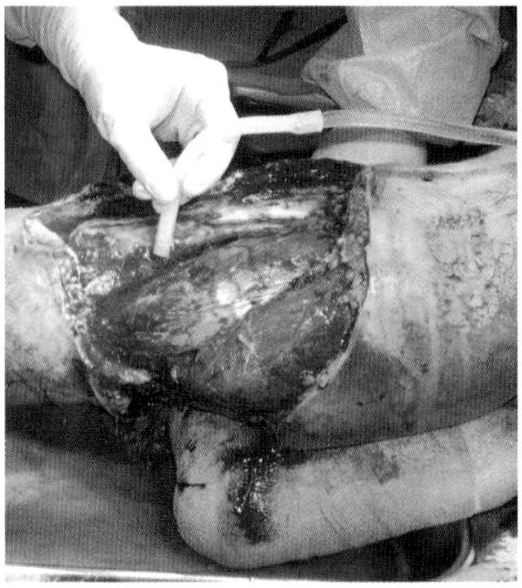

Figure 1 Intraoperative photograph of a type IIIC tibial fracture. After vascular repair, this type of fracture needs a flap. In this situation, a patient with a rotational flap is 4.3 times more likely to have an amputation than a patient with a free flap.

the spanning external fixator can be positioned to facilitate the needed vascular repair. Shunts are valuable in treating a mangled extremity because they can lower the thrombosis rate, have good overall survival, and allow stabilization of the fracture and treatment of the vascular injury in a controlled manner.[1-3]

Soft-tissue injuries are dynamic, and the initial appearance of the injury can be deceiving. The soft tissues will appear worse over time before improvement is seen. The surgeon must decide if primary closure of the wound is indicated. Reasons for delayed wound closure include a contaminated wound, a tight closure, certain mechanisms of injury (such as a crush injury), and a large zone of injury.

Débridement and Wound Contamination

Débridements should continue on a 48- to 72-hour basis until the soft-tissue injury has evolved and the wound is stable. All viable skin should be maintained at each débridement, and all devitalized and contaminated tissue should be removed.

The goals of treating a mangled extremity are to prevent infection and restore function. Infection can lead to malunion, nonunion, and amputation. In a contaminated wound, cultures may be helpful in guiding treatment and determining when closure is appropriate. A study by Lenarz et al[4] reported on the results of obtaining post débridement cultures in 346 patients with open fractures. The wounds were left open, and negative pressure wound therapy (NPWT) was applied. Wounds were closed when culture results were negative. If wound closure occurs in the presence of positive cultures, there is a substantial risk of deep infection. The authors reported an overall deep infection rate of 4.3% with their treatment protocol and a 5.7% infection rate for type III fractures; that rate was lower than previously reported for type III fractures. Antibiotic therapy should be appropriate for the identified infecting organism.

Contaminated wounds often are treated with antibiotic beads or spacers to deliver a high local concentration of antibiotics to the wound. Antibiotic beads can be threaded on a large nonabsorbable suture and changed as serial washout occurs. An antibiotic spacer is useful in fractures with bone loss, and the membrane provides a fertile environment to promote healing.[5,6] For each batch of cement, this chapter's authors use 1 g of vancomycin and a vial of tobramycin (3.6 mg) in the beads.

Soft-Tissue Coverage

If soft-tissue coverage is problematic, the plastic surgeon can consider using free flaps, rotational flaps, skin grafts, and closure by secondary intention. The appropriate coverage option depends on the wound size and location, the vascular status of the extremity, and the zone of injury. When initially examining the injury in the operating room, it is important to thoroughly evaluate the extremity. For example, an injured leg should be lifted to evaluate the posterior surface for bruising or any visible injury to the posterior soft tissues. On subsequent débridements, continued evaluation of the zone of injury should be done so that complete information can be relayed to the surgeon who will provide definitive coverage.

Pollak et al[7] reported on 190 patients in the Lower Extremity Assessment Project (LEAP; a National Institutes of Health–funded, multicenter, prospective, observational study) database who required flap coverage of the tibia. There was an overall complication rate of 27%, with most of the complications (87%) requiring some form of surgical intervention. In type IIIC tibial fractures, the authors found a rotational flap was 4.3 times more likely to have a wound complication requiring reoperation than fractures treated with a free flap (**Figure 1**). A rotational flap was acceptable for treating type IIIB tibial fractures (**Figure 2**), but a free flap was the better option if vascular repair of the extremity was required.

NPWT has revolutionized the treatment of the mangled extremity. Different sponges are available, depending on the wound size and the extent of the exposed tissue.[8-10] A continuous setting of 125 mm Hg is most often used in NPWT. It is recommended that the sponge be changed every 2 to 5 days, depending on the nature of the wound. This treatment continues until the wound has granulated or is clean. A split-thickness skin graft can then be placed, a flap can be rotated, or a free flap can be placed.

Synthetic coverage material is used for skin grafting over tendon or bone.

The Integra Dermal Regeneration Template (Integra LifeScience, Plainsboro, NJ) is currently the only FDA-approved skin regeneration system approved for this use.

Skeletal Stabilization

External fixation can be used for acute skeletal stabilization of the mangled extremity. The external fixator should provide stability and minimize fracture motion. The adaptability of an external fixator is useful in future surgeries. Pin placement should be carefully planned, and using a large number of pins should be avoided. In the femur, pin placement should avoid the knee joint, stay lateral to the quadriceps tendon, and avoid the location of a planned plate. Pins should be placed so that the patient is comfortable when lying down. In the tibia, pin placement should be avoided in locations that would make débridement difficult or would interfere with tissue transfer or the placement of NPWT dressings. Pin placement in the zone of injury should also be avoided.

Definitive skeletal stabilization should occur within the first 2 weeks after injury to decrease the risk of infection. Intramedullary nailing is commonly used for most lower extremity long-bone injuries; however, the specific characteristics of the fracture sometime dictate other fixation techniques. Fixation may include thin-wire or hybrid fixators. Combining skeletal stabilization with definitive soft-tissue coverage involves communication and teamwork among all members of the treatment team.

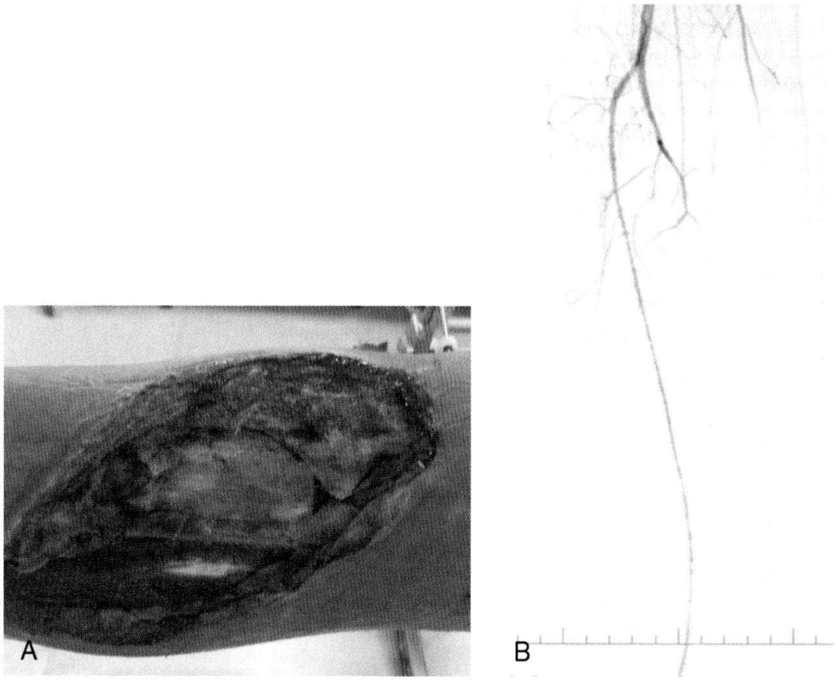

Figure 2 **A,** Photograph of a type IIIB tibial fracture. **B,** Angiogram shows a wound that cannot be covered because there is only a single vessel to the leg.

The Decision to Amputate

All mangled extremities cannot be salvaged. Absolute indications for limb amputation include a nonreconstructible soft-tissue envelope and a nonperfusable limb. Other considerations for amputation include the evaluation of life over limb, as in cases when débridements and attempts to stabilize the extremity may harm a medically unstable patient; the presence of additional injuries, including internal or traumatic brain injuries (especially those causing increased intracranial pressure), which make it difficult to return the patient to the operating room for serial débridements; a pulseless extremity that has exceeded an acceptable warm ischemia time; the presence of a severe crush injury or chronic debilitating disease; and a situation involving mass casualties with injuries requiring complex reconstructions.

The decision to perform an acute primary amputation should be fully documented with photographs of the injury (if possible) and supporting opinions by another physician. It is important to remember that the patient may have negative feelings if he or she had no input regarding this life-changing decision.

Amputation Goals

The goals of amputation surgery are to preserve limb length and provide viable soft-tissue coverage. The ideal length for transtibial amputations is 2.5 cm of bone length for each 30 cm of body height (12.5 to 17.5 cm), with posterior skin flaps of gastrocnemius and soleus muscles. For transfemoral amputations, the ideal length is 9 to 14.5 cm proximal to the knee, with posterior skin flaps. In lower extremity amputations, limb length and the need for soft-tissue padding over the residual bone must be considered. The available skin often determines the amputation level. All viable skin flaps should be preserved, including atypical flaps. Viable muscle should be saved for padding the residual limb to improve function and mechanical stability.

In the 1990s, several injury severity scoring systems were developed to evaluate mangled limbs. The LEAP study assessed whether the Mangled Extremity Severity Score; the Predictive Salvage Index; the Limb Salvage Index; the Hannover Fracture Scale-97; and the Nerve Injury, Ischemia, Soft-Tissue Injury, Skeletal Injury, Shock, and Age of Patient Score could predict the rate of early or late amputations.[11] These scoring systems used a combination of criteria, including age, shock, warm ischemia time, bone injury, muscle injury, skin injury, nerve injury, deep vein injury, soft-tissue injury, the presence of contamination, and the time to treatment to assist physicians in the decision to treat the patient with limb salvage or amputation. Sensitivity for all scores was low, and specificities were higher. A low score would be indicative of limb salvage, but a score at the cutoff or above the threshold could not be used to advocate amputation. The scores also did not predict how well a patient would function after limb salvage as measured with the Sickness Impact Profile (SIP).[12] Another study by Cannada and Cooper[13] reached the same conclusion. This chapter's authors do not recommend using these scoring systems to make a decision for limb salvage or amputation.

A 2002 LEAP study found that the absence of sensation and the severity of muscle, arterial, and vein injuries were the most influential factors for surgeons in making a decision for amputation or limb salvage.[14] In 2005, Bosse et al[15] reported no difference in sensation at 2-year follow-up between 26 insensate plantar feet that were amputated, 29 insensate feet that were salvaged, and 29 matched control sensate limbs that were salvaged. The authors concluded that the absence of plantar sensation at the time of injury did not prove to be an indication for amputation, a predictor of functional outcome, or a predictor of eventual plantar sensation. This was one of the most important findings of the LEAP study because the absence of plantar sensation had been a key variable in choosing amputation.[14] As a result of the study, plantar sensation is no longer a major variable in deciding to amputate or attempt limb salvage.

Lessons Learned From LEAP

Most surgeons choose amputation for a traumatic type IIIC tibial fracture that cannot be revascularized, or a type IIIB tibial fracture if soft-tissue coverage is not possible because of patient or injury circumstances or social situations, or if soft-tissue coverage fails. The decision to amputate or attempt limb salvage is usually more difficult in patients with vascularized limbs and bone loss, nerve injury, or limited viable soft tissue for coverage. LEAP attempted to answer many questions regarding the decision to amputate or salvage mangled extremities. Orthopaedic trauma surgeons from eight well-recognized level I trauma centers were coinvestigators in the study. They used the SIP, a validated behaviorally-based general health status instrument with 136 items in 12 categories, to prospectively evaluate 601 patients who were treated with limb salvage or amputation.[14] The data garnered from that study have proved useful in treating patients with mangled extremity injuries.

The Effect of Smoking

Castillo et al[16] reviewed a LEAP study subgroup of 268 patients with open tibial fractures who were divided into a group who had never smoked (nonsmokers), those who had quit smoking (quitters), and current smokers. The nonsmokers had the highest union rate and the lowest rates of infection and osteomyelitis. If the patient stopped smoking beginning with the day of injury, the rate of infection could be lowered to the rate of a nonsmoker. Current smokers were 37% less likely to achieve union than nonsmokers, and quitters were 32% less likely to achieve union than nonsmokers. Osteomyelitis was 2.8 times more likely to develop in quitters than nonsmokers and 3.7 times more likely to develop in current smokers compared with nonsmokers. Smoking cessation at the time of a limb-threatening injury can have a positive effect on the patient's outcome.

Infection

Infection remains a possible complication in patients treated with amputation or limb salvage. In their analysis of LEAP data, Harris et al[17] reported that patients treated with amputation had a 34.2% wound infection rate, a 14.5% stump revision rate, and a 10.5% rate of stump complications by 2-year follow-up. The limb salvage group had a 23% wound infection rate, a 31.5% rate of nonunion, a 8.6% rate of osteomyelitis, and a 3.9% late amputation rate. Patients treated with limb salvage can expect a higher rate of overall complications than those treated with amputation.

Long-Term Results

At 2 years after injury, the LEAP study found no significant difference in SIP scores for amputation versus reconstruction (12.6 versus 11.8, respectively; $P = 0.53$).[18] However, the reconstruction group was more likely to have a secondary hospitalization for a major complication than the amputation group (47.5% versus 33.9%, respectively; $P = 0.002$).[18] At 7 years after injury, 50% of patients had a SIP score of more than 10 points, which indicates severe disability. There were no significant differences in the psychosocial outcome scores between the groups. Poorer outcomes were reported for patients who were older, female, and current or previous smokers; were from a nonwhite race; had a lower educational level; lived in poverty; had low self-efficacy scores; had poor health before injury; and were involved with disability litigation.[19]

In 423 patients who were followed for 7 years, 58% returned to work. Forty-seven percent of those patients had been treated with amputation, and 62% had been treated with limb salvage. Although the difference was not statistically significant, a trend toward a higher rate of return to work was reported in the reconstruction group. On average, working patients reported limits in their ability to perform the demands of their jobs 20% to 25% of the time.[20]

Cost is also a consideration in the decision regarding limb salvage or amputation. When prosthetic costs at 2 years were included, the costs of limb salvage averaged $81,316, and amputation averaged $91,106.[21] Projected lifetime costs, however, were three times higher for the amputation group than the limb salvage group ($509,275 versus $163,282, respectively).[21] Lifetime costs were calculated by using costs incurred for up to 7 years for study patients and adding estimated annual healthcare costs along with the cost of prostheses and maintenance expenses over a lifetime. Because many trauma patients do not have medical insurance, the cost of a prosthesis is an important consideration.

The Psychological Factor

McCarthy et al[22] reported that 48% of patients with a severe injury to a lower limb tested positive for a likely psychological disorder at 3 months after injury and 42% at 2 years after injury. Only 12% and 22% of patients reported receiving mental health services 3 months and 24 months after injury, respectively. This chapter's authors recommend that surgeons consider an early psychological or psychiatric consultation for patients with severe mangled limb injuries.

Patient Expectations

In an analysis of LEAP data, five key outcome measures (the ability to return to work, the presence of depression, the SIP physical functioning score, the patient's self-selected walking speed, and the level of pain intensity) seemed to account for more than 33% of the overall variation in patient satisfaction.[15] Higher patient satisfaction was associated with the ability to work and the absence of depression. Those with higher SIP physical functioning scores generally had a higher self-selected walking speed and lower pain intensity.[23] Adequate pain control to allow function and the absence of depression were key factors in acceptable patient satisfaction ratings.

Lessons Learned From Iraq, Afghanistan, and Disaster Relief Efforts

In recent years, many US military members, Iraqi and Afghan nationals, and victims of natural disasters and third-world conflicts have sustained amputations of major limbs. Wars and natural disasters have provided important lessons in the care of a patient with a mangled extremity.

Approximately 48,000 members of the US Armed Forces have been wounded during the wars in Iraq and Afghanistan, and most had musculoskeletal injuries.[24] These injuries have resulted from explosive munitions, such as mortars, rockets, rocket-propelled grenades, and improvised explosive devices (IEDs).[25] Approximately 90% of military personnel wounded in Afghanistan survive their injuries, which translates to a 10.1% fatality rate.[26] Improved survival rates have been accompanied by a corresponding increase in the numbers of initial and late complex amputations.[27]

Injury Patterns

Amputations resulting from explosive devices are caused by the blast wave or fragmentation effects that cause mutilating bone and soft-tissue injuries. IEDs have been the most common cause of combat-related amputations in Iraq and Afghanistan.[28] During dismounted patrols, it is common for an IED to be triggered by a service member's lead leg, resulting in an upward and backward blast that passes through the extremities, groin, and buttocks (**Figure 3**). This blast pattern often necessitates an initial through- or below-knee amputation on the lead leg, and a higher above-knee amputation on the back leg. Buttock wounds are often associated with a high degree of blood loss secondary to damage to the multiple posterior arterial branches of the external iliac artery. High-velocity bullet wounds can also result in amputation of the major extremities.

In nonmilitary or humanitarian settings, blasts, falls, motor vehicle crashes, crush injuries, infections, and tumors are common etiologies resulting in major extremity amputations. A common explosive injury in nonmilitary settings occurs from landmines placed during past conflicts.[29]

Initial Treatment of the Traumatic Amputee on the Battlefield

In the immediate aftermath of a major extremity amputation resulting from trauma, treatment priorities are represented by the mnemonic CABC (catastrophic bleeding, airway, bleeding, and circulation). All US military personnel deployed to the battlefield are equipped with a personal first aid kit that includes a combat application

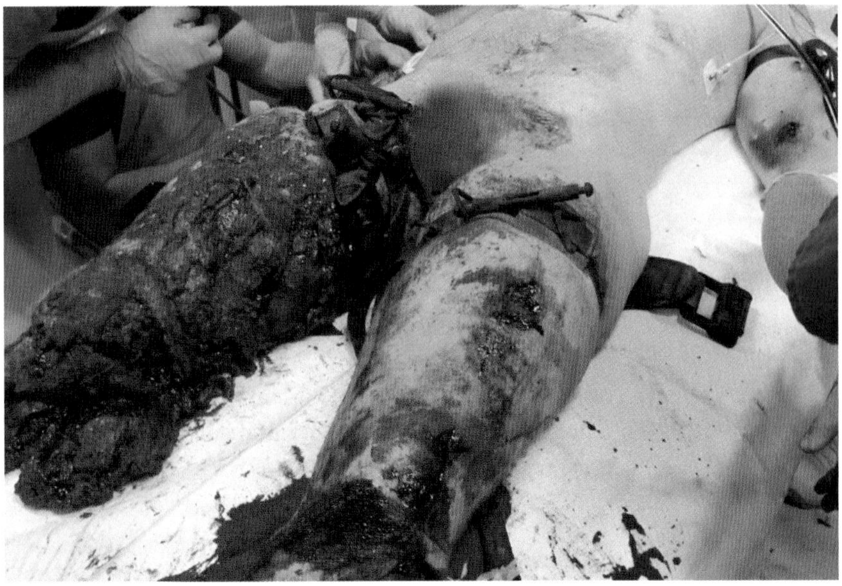

Figure 3 Bilateral combat application tourniquets on a 21-year-old Marine who required bilateral lower extremity amputations because of injuries from a dismounted IED blast in Afghanistan.

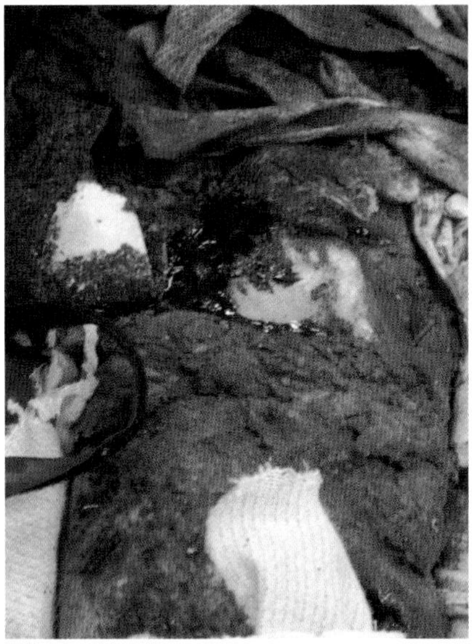

Figure 4 Photograph of a proximal thigh wound from a dismounted IED blast packed with hemostatic dressing.

tourniquet and a hemostatic dressing (QuickClot; Z-Medica, Wallingford, CT). The combat tourniquet can be applied with one hand and is very effective at controlling hemorrhage in extremity amputations. However, in very proximal amputations, there is not enough tissue available on the residual limb to hold the tourniquet. In such situations, application of hemostatic and direct pressure dressings can be an effective combination (**Figure 4**). A bandage wrapped over the shoulder instead of around the pelvis has been described as a more efficacious method of providing direct pressure over the residual limb.[30] If direct pressure over the wound does not control hemorrhage, pressure applied proximally over the femoral artery may provide control. This chapter's authors have found that the proper use of prehospital tourniquets can prevent hemorrhage and stabilize the patient for resuscitation and transport.

Hemorrhage is the main cause of preventable battlefield deaths. Combat application tourniquets can effectively manage life-threatening hemorrhage with low complication rates. Beekley et al[31] reported on 165 patients with primary traumatic extremity amputations or vascular injuries to the extremities who arrived at a combat support hospital in Iraq with and without prehospital tourniquets. Severely injured patients (Injury Severity Scale > 15) treated with combat tourniquets had substantially better bleeding control on arrival at the combat hospital than patients not treated with a prehospital tourniquet. No significant survival benefit or difference in mortality, physiologic parameters, or units of blood transfused was reported between the groups; however, the authors noted a bias toward survival of battlefield evacuation in those patients treated with a combat tourniquet. The authors reported improved hemorrhage control and no complications related to tourniquet use.

Kragh et al[32] reported on a larger cohort of patients (232 patients with 428 tourniquets applied on 309 injured limbs) treated at a combat support hospital in Iraq. Tourniquet times greater than 2 hours were associated with increased indications for fasciotomy; however, all fasciotomies were performed prophylactically without evidence of compartment syndrome. A tourniquet time greater than 3 hours was associated with the need for a higher amputation level. The authors concluded that the benefits of tourniquet use far outweighed the risks; an estimated 31 lives were saved by using prehospital tourniquets. Relatively low complication rates have been reported with prehospital tourniquet use in Iraq and Afghanistan.[32] Three complications (two compartment syndromes and one ulnar nerve palsy) occurred with the use of prehospital tourniquets in 70 patients treated at British field hospitals.

Treatment in Casualty Receiving Facilities

On arrival of patients to casualty receiving facilities, the principles of Advanced Trauma Life Support, hypotensive resuscitation, and damage control orthopaedic surgery serve as guidelines for treatment. If a major lower limb amputation is too proximal for a tourniquet, hemorrhage control is obtained via the iliac vessels.

The combat application tourniquet will often mask an underlying injury. Although the narrow width of this tourniquet makes it effective on the battlefield, it also creates increased tissue pressure over a relatively small area of tissue. Because the pressure cannot be regulated on combat application tourniquets, after resuscitation begins and the patient's blood pressure begins to normalize, there is a risk for strike-through bleeding.[31] This chapter's authors recommend that combat application tourniquets be replaced with pneumatic tourniquets with larger bandwidths and pressure control capabilities when the patient is received at the combat treatment facility. When possible, the pneumatic tourniquet should be placed proximal to the combat tourniquet over skin that has already been evaluated for injury. The pneumatic tourniquet is inflated before the combat tourniquet is released to provide a seamless transition of hemostatic control. Nonviable tissue and foreign material likely to cause infection should be excised, and rapid bony stabilization should then be performed.

Amputations caused by explosive blasts usually have extensive soft-tissue trauma and a proximal zone of injury.[33] Serial débridements are usually required (**Figure 5**). The amputation should not be closed primarily but should remain open and dressed with absorbent dressings. The knee should be splinted in extension for transtibial amputations. NPWT can be an effective adjunct in the care of battlefield amputations (**Figure 6**). Leininger et al[34] reported on the use of NPWT to treat war wounds sustained in Iraq. The authors noted a marked reduction of previous anecdotally reported infec-

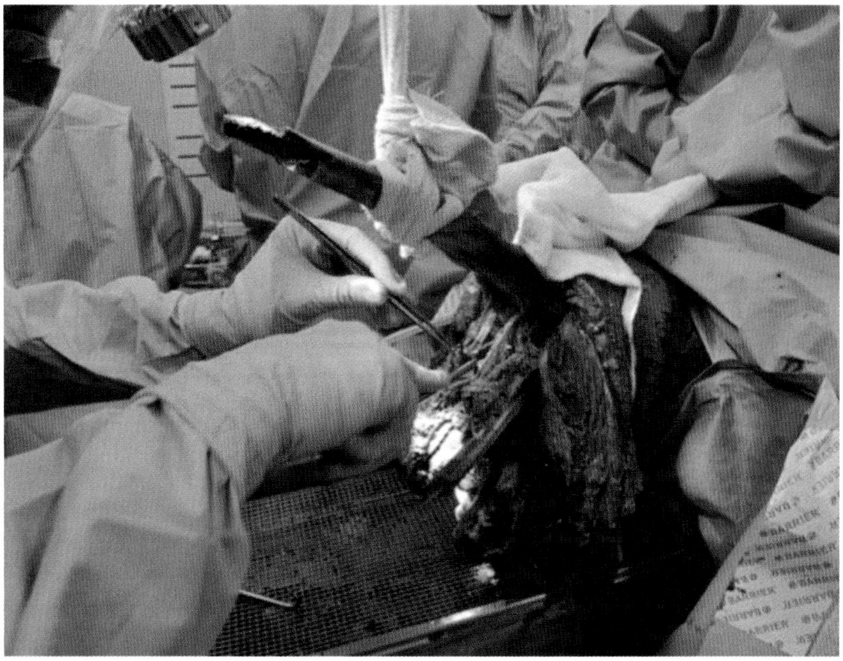

Figure 5 The femur bone is left long to help support the limb during débridement when there is a shortage of available medical personnel to assist with surgery.

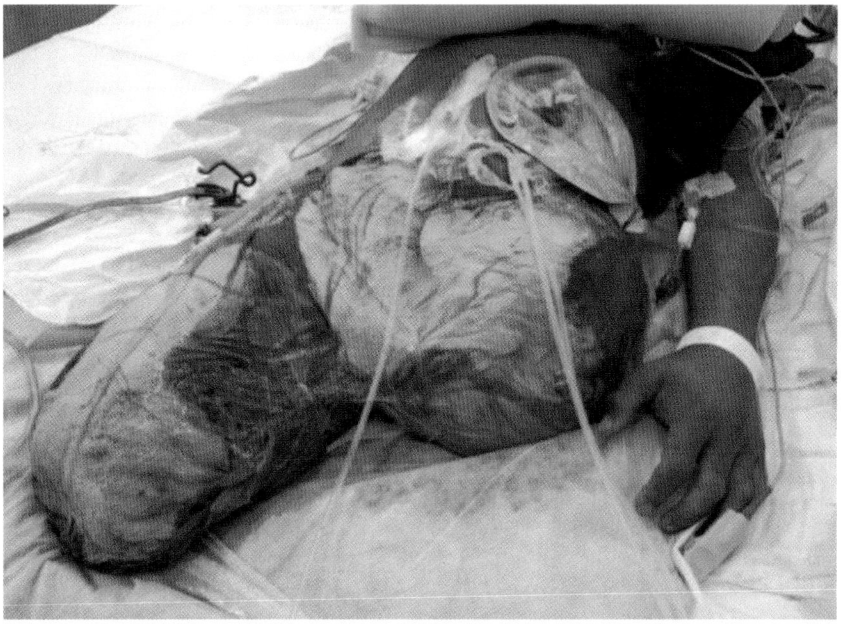

Figure 6 NPWT was used to treat open abdominal injuries in a 20-year-old military service member with abdomen and urogenital injuries and bilateral amputations.

Table 1
From Surgery to Prosthetic Fitting

Event	Goals
Wound healing	This is the period from the initial injury until a closed residual limb is achieved. The goals of surgery are to create a well-padded, functional, residual limb that is free of sores, bone protuberance, and symptomatic neuromas. Complex wounds from trauma may require nonstandard flaps and wound closure.
Preprosthetic training	Prior to fitting the initial preparatory prosthesis, conditioning exercises are used to maintain fitness and prepare the patient for the prosthesis. General conditioning is important to prepare the patient for prosthetic training and future functioning.
Preparatory provisional (temporary) prosthesis fitting	Initial fitting of the prosthesis and training for prosthetic use, including physical and occupational therapy. The socket may be changed frequently as residual limb swelling and edema subside. The prosthesis is adjusted for the patient during this period. This may be the longest period in the first year after surgery.
Definitive prosthesis fitting	When a patient has gained sufficient skill with a preparatory prosthesis, and the residual limb size has become more stable, a patient may be fitted with the definitive prosthesis. Generally, the socket is more durable and the components are consistent with those the patient will be using full time.

tion rates in a cohort of 77 patients. Whether using dressings or NPWT, closure of the amputation can be accomplished after it is clean and granulating.

Complications

Whether sustained in war or during humanitarian disasters, amputations pose challenges in initial management and in later complications that occur from the injury itself or treatment. Complications include infection, heterotopic ossification, and intractable pain. The infection rates in combat-related major limb amputations from the wars in Iraq and Afghanistan are between 20% and 40%. Heterotopic ossification is the formation of mature lamellar bone within tissues that do not normally exhibit ossification, such as muscles, tendons, ligaments, and joint capsules.[35] Potter et al[36] reported heterotopic ossification in 134 residual limbs in 213 military personnel with amputations caused by battlefield injuries (63% rate). Risk factors associated with the formation of heterotopic ossification were amputation within the zone of injury (127 of 167 limbs, 76%) and injury caused by a blast mechanism (approximately 80% of the limbs).[37] These factors, along with a concerted effort by military surgeons to preserve the length of residual limbs, can account for the high rates of heterotopic ossification in this patient population. Intractable pain in amputees with battlefield injuries is a challenging problem and often requires a multidisciplinary treatment approach.

Treatment-related complications can include knee flexion contractures and hardware failure when amputation is done along with fracture fixation. In patients requiring soft-tissue coverage, necrosis after flap placement is a possible complication.

Postoperative Care: After Surgery to the Prosthetic Fitting

The period between immediate postoperative care until the lower extremity amputee is fitted with a permanent prosthesis is critical[38,39] (**Table 1**). For orthopaedic surgeons, emphasis is usually placed on surgical techniques, but the treating surgeon should be mindful of the importance of nursing care, physical therapy, and prosthetic fitting to obtain the best patient outcomes.

The period from surgery until fitting of the permanent prosthesis is approximately 1 year. A provisional prosthetic fitting and therapy occurs during this period. As edema in the residual limb subsides, the patient's provisional prosthetic socket will be changed to accommodate the residual limb (**Figure** 7). After the residual limb size has stabilized, the permanent prosthesis can be fitted.

Ideally, patients should be cared for by a treatment team of surgeons, physical therapists, prosthetists, and nurses to provide the best outcomes. With a treatment team, wound healing, therapy, and an initial prosthetic fitting can occur simultaneously.

Lower extremity limb loss caused by trauma is more common than upper extremity loss, with the level of transtibial amputation the most common in both wartime and peacetime injuries.[19,40-42] The quality of the soft tissues of the residual limb is important for prosthetic wear and limb function. Achieving a well-padded, sensate, residual limb is the first step in providing the patient with the best function.

Postoperative care for patients with loss of a lower extremity limb may include soft dressings, rigid dressings, and an immediate postoperative prosthesis or a removable rigid dressing.[43,44] A soft dressing consists of gauze with an elastic wrap to secure the

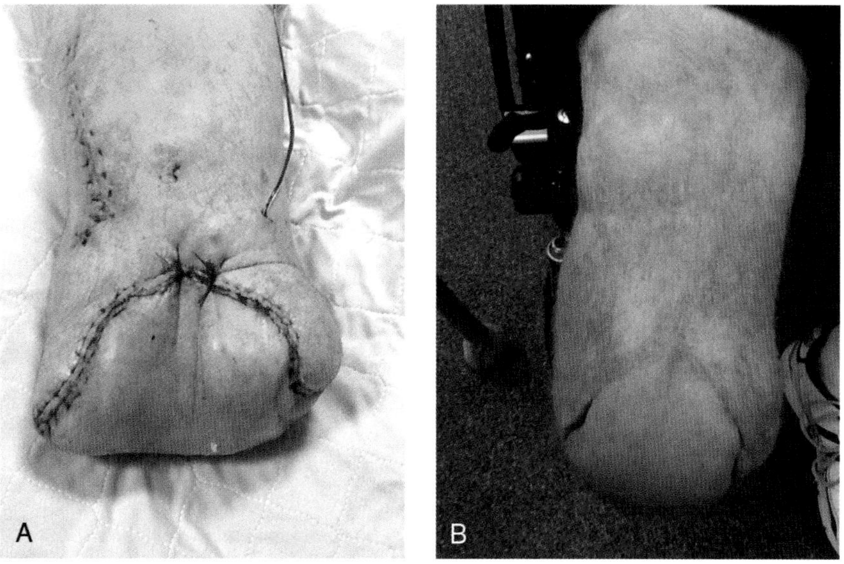

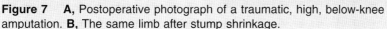

Figure 7 **A,** Postoperative photograph of a traumatic, high, below-knee amputation. **B,** The same limb after stump shrinkage.

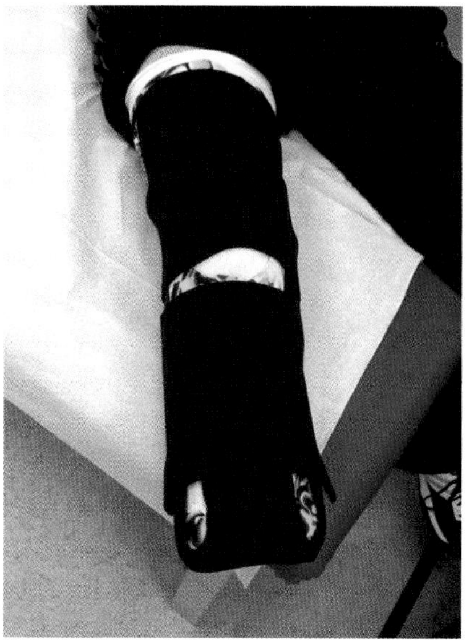

Figure 8 A rigid postoperative dressing is used in a below-knee amputation caused by trauma.

dressing and compress the residual limb. The advantages of soft dressings are ease of application and wound access. The disadvantages include a lack of soft-tissue support (with increased pain) and the potential for knee contracture in patients with a transtibial amputation. A rigid dressing is a cast that is placed around the residual limb and held in place by a suspension device (**Figure 8**). Burgess pioneered this technique for patients with transtibial limb loss. The rigid dressing is changed frequently as the size of the residual limb edema and swelling subside.[43] The rigid dressing may provide better soft-tissue support and protection for the residual limb and more consistent edema control than soft dressings. Rigid dressings, however, are more time consuming to apply, and cast complications are possible.

After amputation surgical procedures are completed, a temporary prosthesis (called an immediate postoperative prosthesis) is fitted based on a plaster cast socket.[43] The patient is encouraged to ambulate with limited weight bearing in the immediate postoperative period. The hard cast and limited weight bearing through the residual limb are believed to decrease edema. The ability to immediately ambulate may also result in improved proprioception and a better psychological outlook. A prosthetics team knowledgeable in this technique must be readily available for consultation with the patient for a successful outcome.

For patients with transtibial limb loss, a provisional prosthesis is generally fitted approximately 1 month postoperatively after some edema and swelling have subsided and the postoperative sutures have been removed. A provisional prosthesis for a transtibial level amputation often consists of a thermoplastic socket with a simple foot. The provisional prosthesis allows alignment to be changed as the patient's gait improves and the residual limb size stabilizes. The patient begins with partial weight bearing and progresses to full weight bearing. The socket is changed frequently to accommodate changes in limb size. The provisional prosthesis may be used for 6 to 12 months until the permanent prosthesis is fitted.

When the limb size becomes stable, the patient may be fitted with a permanent prosthesis. A permanent prosthesis for a transtibial amputee often consists of a thin, laminated fiberglass socket and more advanced prosthetic energy storage feet. Military patients are often fitted for several types of prostheses to accommodate sport and work activities.

In patients with transfemoral limb loss, the preparatory or provisional prosthesis may have a thermoplastic or check socket that will be changed as the residual limb size changes. The patient may frequently increase the number of stockings worn with changes in the size of the residual limb. A simpler type of prosthetic knee may be fitted, such as a stance control or a safety knee, to help the patient in learning proper gait. The permanent prosthesis will have a thin laminated socket that is reinforced in certain areas with carbon fiber. Depending on a patient's progress in rehabilitation, he or she may be fitted with more advanced knees, such as a hydraulic knee or a

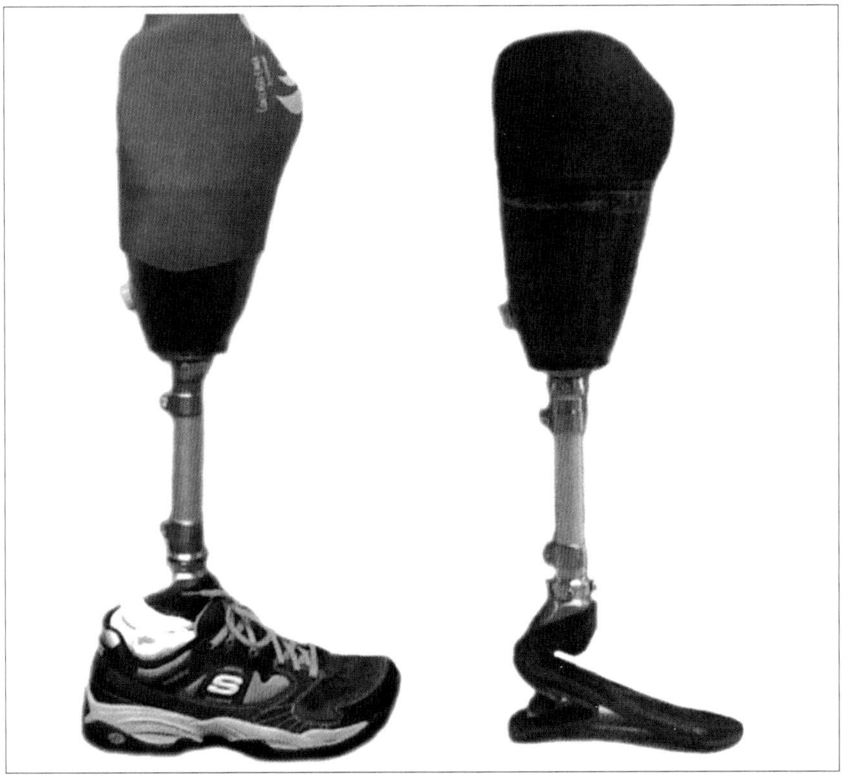

Figure 9 Example of a right adult endoskeletal prosthesis that includes a passive suction suspension and a prosthetic foot that combines multiaxial shock absorption and dynamic response capabilities. Shoe attached (left) and prosthetic foot (right).

knee with a microprocessor to control gait. A more advanced foot may also be fitted (**Figure 9**).

Outcomes

A patient with limb loss should be periodically assessed to monitor problems with the prosthesis, limb function, and the need for psychological support services. Prosthetic use by amputees often follows similar patterns. Those with a traumatic transtibial amputation report nearly 100% prosthetic use.[45] For isolated transtibial limb loss, the patient will generally wear his or her prosthesis for the entire day. Approximately 85% of patients with traumatic transfemoral limb loss wear a prosthesis, and most wear it throughout the day.[46,47] Prosthesis wear may be rejected because of medical comorbidities or very proximal limb loss, which is functionally similar to a hip disarticulation. Prosthesis wear for patients with hip disarticulation limb loss varies between 37% and 75%.[48,49] The prostheses generally are worn less than 8 hours per day and are often used only for cosmesis.

Patients may have postoperative phantom limb pain or residual limb pain. The cause of phantom limb pain is unknown.[50-52] Phantom limb pain is pain perceived as originating from the amputated limb. For example, a person with a transtibial amputation may feel burning foot pain even though the patient does not have a foot. Treatments, such as medications, biofeedback, mirror therapy, nerve blocks, early prosthetic fitting, and acupuncture have been used to reduce phantom limb pain and have achieved varying degrees of success.

Residual limb pain has been reported in 10% to 70% of patients with lower extremity limb loss.[20,47,49,53,54] Causes include sores, neuromas, bone prominence, heterotopic bone, and cysts. The evaluation of a patient with residual limb pain should include an assessment of the prosthesis, a careful physical examination, and discussion with the patient. High-quality ultrasound can detect a cyst or a neuroma. The diagnosis of a neuroma may be made by physical examination (Tinel sign or a palpable, tender mass may be present), ultrasound, and, occasionally, local anesthetic injection. For most patients with an identifiable cause, the easiest treatment is to modify the socket. Surgery should be considered only after extensive discussion with the patient with a clearly identified problem.

The use of psychological support services is variable.[19,39,46,53,55,56] Reports of the use of support services by military patients with lower extremity limb loss range from 20% to more than 50%, with those with more proximal limb loss and more severe injuries more likely to seek services.[46,53]

Employment among amputees is highly variable.[20,46,53,57] Patients who sustain isolated limb loss while in the US military have a greater than 90% employment rate after military service.[46] US military personnel who served in Iran report employment rates of 58% and 65% for those with transfemoral limb loss and transtibial limb loss, respectively.[53,54] Postamputation employment seems to be dependent on other injuries, comorbidities, and the degree of rehabilitation provided in the period after the amputation.

Nonmilitary patients in the United States have less success in obtaining work after amputations. In their study of patients with lower limb loss, Mackenzie et al[19] reported that less than 50% of the patients had returned to work at 7 years after injury. Age younger than 55 years, white race, and high self-efficacy were positive correlates for returning to work, whereas pending legal action or preinjury employment in jobs with high physical demands were negative correlates.

Summary

Musculoskeletal wounds are the most common type of injury among survivors of battlefield trauma, natural disasters, and other violent events. These injuries often require amputation of a major extremity. Methods of care are evolving, but the LEAP study and lessons learned from recent US military conflicts have provided valuable information.

Proper care between the time from surgery until the patient is fitted with a permanent prosthesis is critical for an optimal outcome. Patients benefit from care provided by a treatment team, including nurses, occupational and physical therapists, physical medicine specialists, prosthetists, and orthopaedic surgeons.

References

1. Glass GE, Pearse MF, Nanchahal J: Improving lower limb salvage following fractures with vascular injury: A systematic review and new management algorithm. *J Plast Reconstr Aesthet Surg* 2009;62(5):571-579.
2. Rozycki GS, Tremblay LN, Feliciano DV, McClelland WB: Blunt vascular trauma in the extremity: Diagnosis, management, and outcome. *J Trauma* 2003;55(5):814-824.
3. Reber PU, Patel AG, Sapio NL, Ris HB, Beck M, Kniemeyer HW: Selective use of temporary intravascular shunts in coincident vascular and orthopedic upper and lower limb trauma. *J Trauma* 1999;47(1):72-76.
4. Lenarz CJ, Watson JT, Moed BR, Israel H, Mullen JD, Macdonald JB: Timing of wound closure in open fractures based on cultures obtained after debridement. *J Bone Joint Surg Am* 2010;92(10):1921-1926.
5. Karger C, Kishi T, Schneider L, Fitoussi F, Masquelet AC; French Society of Orthopaedic Surgery and Traumatology (SoFCOT): Treatment of posttraumatic bone defects by the induced membrane technique. *Orthop Traumatol Surg Res* 2012;98(1):97-102.
6. Giannoudis PV, Faour O, Goff T, Kanakaris N, Dimitriou R: Masquelet technique for the treatment of bone defects: Tips-tricks and future directions. *Injury* 2011;42(6):591-598.
7. Pollak AN, McCarthy ML, Burgess AR; The Lower Extremity Assessment Project (LEAP) Study Group: Short-term wound complications after application of flaps for coverage of traumatic soft-tissue defects about the tibia. *J Bone Joint Surg Am* 2000;82(12):1681-1691.
8. Krug E, Berg L, Lee C, et al: Evidence-based recommendations for the use of negative pressure wound therapy in traumatic wounds and reconstructive surgery: Steps towards an international consensus. *Injury* 2011;42(suppl 1):S1-S12.
9. Stannard JP, Volgas DA, Stewart R, McGwin G Jr, Alonso JE: Negative pressure wound therapy after severe open fractures: A prospective randomized study. *J Orthop Trauma* 2009;23(8):552-557.
10. Dedmond BT, Kortesis B, Punger K, et al: The use of negative-pressure wound therapy (NPWT) in the temporary treatment of soft-tissue injuries associated with high-energy open tibial shaft fractures. *J Orthop Trauma* 2007;21(1):11-17.
11. Bosse MJ, MacKenzie EJ, Kellam JF, et al: A prospective evaluation of the clinical utility of the lower-extremity injury-severity scores. *J Bone Joint Surg Am* 2001;83(1):3-14.
12. Ly TV, Travison TG, Castillo RC, Bosse MJ, MacKenzie EJ; LEAP Study Group: Ability of lower-extremity injury severity scores to predict functional outcome after limb salvage. *J Bone Joint Surg Am* 2008;90(8):1738-1743.
13. Cannada LK, Cooper C: The mangled extremity: Limb salvage versus amputation. *Curr Surg* 2005;62(6):563-576.
14. MacKenzie EJ, Bosse MJ, Kellam JF, et al: Factors influencing the decision to amputate or reconstruct after high-energy lower extremity trauma. *J Trauma* 2002;52(4):641-649.
15. Bosse MJ, McCarthy ML, Jones AL, et al: The insensate foot following severe lower extremity trauma: An indication for amputation? *J Bone Joint Surg Am* 2005;87(12):2601-2608.
16. Castillo RC, Bosse MJ, MacKenzie EJ, Patterson BM; LEAP Study Group: Impact of smoking on fracture healing and risk of complications in limb-threatening open tibia fractures. *J Orthop Trauma* 2005;19(3):151-157.
17. Harris AM, Althausen PL, Kellam J, et al: Complications following limb-threatening lower extremity trauma. *J Orthop Trauma* 2009;23(1):1-6.
18. Bosse MJ, MacKenzie EJ, Kellam JF, et al: An analysis of outcomes of reconstruction or amputation after leg-threatening injuries. *N Engl J Med* 2002;347(24):1924-1931.
19. MacKenzie EJ, Bosse MJ, Pollak AN, et al: Long-term persistence of disability following severe lower-limb trauma: Results of a seven-year follow-up. *J Bone Joint Surg Am* 2005;87(8):1801-1809.
20. MacKenzie EJ, Bosse MJ, Kellam JF, et al: Early predictors of long-

term work disability after major limb trauma. *J Trauma* 2006; 61(3):688-694.

21. MacKenzie EJ, Jones AS, Bosse MJ, et al: Health-care costs associated with amputation or reconstruction of a limb-threatening injury. *J Bone Joint Surg Am* 2007; 89(8):1685-1692.
22. McCarthy ML, MacKenzie EJ, Edwin D, et al: Psychological distress associated with severe lower-limb injury. *J Bone Joint Surg Am* 2003;85(9):1689-1697.
23. O'Toole RV, Castillo RC, Pollak AN, MacKenzie EJ, Bosse MJ; LEAP Study Group: Determinants of patient satisfaction after severe lower-extremity injuries. *J Bone Joint Surg Am* 2008; 90(6):1206-1211.
24. Department of Defense: US Casualty Status, Fatalities as of May 15, 2009. http://www.defenselink.mil/news/casualty.pdf. Accessed April 25, 2012.
25. Department of Defense: Global War on Terrorism by Reason: October 7, 2001 through April 2, 2012. http://siadapp.dmdc.osd.mil/personnel/CASUALTY/gwot_reason.pdf. Accessed April 25, 2012.
26. Holcomb JB, Stansbury LG, Champion HR, Wade C, Bellamy RF: Understanding combat casualty care statistics. *J Trauma* 2006; 60(2):397-401.
27. Covey DC: From the frontlines to the home front: The crucial role of military orthopaedic surgeons. *J Bone Joint Surg Am* 2009;91(4): 998-1006.
28. Owens BD, Kragh JF Jr, Wenke JC, Macaitis J, Wade CE, Holcomb JB: Combat wounds in Operation Iraqi Freedom and Operation Enduring Freedom. *J Trauma* 2008;64(2):295-299.
29. Covey DC, Lurate RB, Hatton CT: Field hospital treatment of blast wounds of the musculoskeletal system during the Yugoslav civil war. *J Orthop Trauma* 2000; 14(4):278-286, discussion 277.
30. Jansen JO, Thomas GO, Adams SA, et al: Early management of proximal traumatic lower extremity amputation and pelvic injury caused by improvised explosive devices (IEDs). *Injury* 2012;43(7): 976-979.
31. Beekley AC, Sebesta JA, Blackbourne LH, et al: Prehospital tourniquet use in Operation Iraqi Freedom: Effect on hemorrhage control and outcomes. *J Trauma* 2008;64(2, suppl):S28-S37.
32. Kragh JF Jr, Walters TJ, Baer DG, et al: Survival with emergency tourniquet use to stop bleeding in major limb trauma. *Ann Surg* 2009;249(1):1-7.
33. Covey DC: Blast and fragment injuries of the musculoskeletal system. *J Bone Joint Surg Am* 2002;84(7):1221-1234.
34. Leininger BE, Rasmussen TE, Smith DL, Jenkins DH, Coppola C: Experience with wound VAC and delayed primary closure of contaminated soft tissue injuries in Iraq. *J Trauma* 2006;61(5): 1207-1211.
35. Kaplan FS, Glaser DL, Hebela N, Shore EM: Heterotopic ossification. *J Am Acad Orthop Surg* 2004;12(2):116-125.
36. Potter BK, Burns TC, Lacap AP, Granville RR, Gajewski DA: Heterotopic ossification following traumatic and combat-related amputations: Prevalence, risk factors, and preliminary results of excision. *J Bone Joint Surg Am* 2007;89(3):476-486.
37. Forsberg JA, Pepek JM, Wagner S, et al: Heterotopic ossification in high-energy wartime extremity injuries: Prevalence and risk factors. *J Bone Joint Surg Am* 2009; 91(5):1084-1091.
38. Malone JM, Fleming LL, Roberson J, et al: Immediate, early, and late postsurgical management of upper-limb amputation. *J Rehabil Res Dev* 1984;21(1):33-41.
39. Wartan SW, Hamann W, Wedley JR, McColl I: Phantom pain and sensation among British veteran amputees. *Br J Anaesth* 1997; 78(6):652-659.
40. O'Shaughnessy KD, Dumanian GA, Lipschutz RD, Miller LA, Stubblefield K, Kuiken TA: Targeted reinnervation to improve prosthesis control in transhumeral amputees: A report of three cases. *J Bone Joint Surg Am* 2008;90(2): 393-400.
41. Dharm-Datta S, Etherington J, Mistlin A, Rees J, Clasper J: The outcome of British combat amputees in relation to military service. *Injury* 2011;42(11):1362-1367.
42. Dougherty PJ: Wartime amputations. *Mil Med* 1993;158(12): 755-763.
43. Reiber GE, McFarland LV, Hubbard S, et al: Service members and veterans with major traumatic limb loss from Vietnam War and OIF/OEF conflicts: Survey methods, participants, and summary findings. *J Rehabil Res Dev* 2010; 47(4):275-297.
44. Smith DG, McFarland LV, Sangeorzan BJ, Reiber GE, Czerniecki JM: Postoperative dressing and management strategies for transtibial amputations: A critical review. *J Rehabil Res Dev* 2003; 40(3):213-224.
45. Dougherty PJ: Transtibial amputees from the Vietnam War: Twenty-eight-year follow-up. *J Bone Joint Surg Am* 2001;83(3): 383-389.
46. Smith DG, Horn P, Malchow D, Boone DA, Reiber GE, Hansen ST Jr: Prosthetic history, prosthetic charges, and functional outcome of the isolated, traumatic below-knee amputee. *J Trauma* 1995;38(1):44-47.
47. Dougherty PJ: Long-term follow-up of unilateral transfemoral amputees from the Vietnam

war. *J Trauma* 2003;54(4): 718-723.

48. Gailey R, McFarland LV, Cooper RA, et al: Unilateral lower-limb loss: Prosthetic device use and functional outcomes in servicemembers from Vietnam War and OIF/OEF conflicts. *J Rehabil Res Dev* 2010;47(4):317-331.
49. Yari P, Dijkstra PU, Geertzen JH: Functional outcome of hip disarticulation and hemipelvectomy: A cross-sectional national descriptive study in the Netherlands. *Clin Rehabil* 2008;22(12):1127-1133.
50. Ostlie K, Franklin RJ, Skjeldal OH, Skrondal A, Magnus P: Musculoskeletal pain and overuse syndromes in adult acquired major upper-limb amputees. *Arch Phys Med Rehabil* 2011;92(12): 1967-1973, e1.
51. Flor H: Maladaptive plasticity, memory for pain and phantom limb pain: Review and suggestions for new therapies. *Expert Rev Neurother* 2008;8(5):809-818.
52. Schley MT, Wilms P, Toepfner S, et al: Painful and nonpainful phantom and stump sensations in acute traumatic amputees. *J Trauma* 2008;65(4):858-864.
53. Ebrahimzadeh MH, Fattahi AS: Long-term clinical outcomes of Iranian veterans with unilateral transfemoral amputation. *Disabil Rehabil* 2009;31(22):1873-1877.
54. Ebrahimzadeh MH, Hariri S: Long-term outcomes of unilateral transtibial amputations. *Mil Med* 2009;174(6):593-597.
55. Ostlie K, Franklin RJ, Skjeldal OH, Skrondal A, Magnus P: Assessing physical function in adult acquired major upper-limb amputees by combining the Disabilities of the Arm, Shoulder and Hand (DASH) Outcome Questionnaire and clinical examination. *Arch Phys Med Rehabil* 2011;92(10): 1636-1645.
56. Archer KR, Castillo RC, MacKenzie EJ, Bosse MJ, LEAP Study Group: Perceived need and unmet need for vocational, mental health, and other support services after severe lower-extremity trauma. *Arch Phys Med Rehabil* 2010;91(5):774-780.
57. Copuroglu C, Ozcan M, Yilmaz B, Gorgulu Y, Abay E, Yalniz E: Acute stress disorder and post-traumatic stress disorder following traumatic amputation. *Acta Orthop Belg* 2010;76(1):90-93.

2

Surgical Timing of Treating Injured Extremities: An Evolving Concept of Urgency

Brett D. Crist, MD, FACS
Tania Ferguson, MD
Yvonne M. Murtha, MD
Mark A. Lee, MD

Abstract

The management of some orthopaedic extremity injuries has changed over the past decade because of changing resource availability and the risks of complications. It is helpful to review the current literature regarding orthopaedic extremity emergencies and urgencies. The effects of the techniques of damage control orthopaedic techniques and the concept of the orthopaedic trauma room have also affected the management of these injuries.

The available literature indicates that the remaining true orthopaedic extremity emergencies include compartment syndrome and vascular injuries associated with fractures and dislocations. Orthopaedic urgencies include open fracture management, femoral neck fractures in young patients treated with open reduction and internal fixation, and talus fractures that are open or those with impending skin compromise.

Deciding when the definitive management of orthopaedic extremity injuries will occur has evolved as the concept of damage control orthopaedics has become more commonly accepted. Patient survival rates have improved with current resuscitative protocols. Definitive fixation of extremity injuries should be delayed until the patient's physiologic and extremity soft-tissue status allows for appropriate definitive management while minimizing the risks of complications. In patients with semiurgent orthopaedic injuries, the use of an orthopaedic trauma room has led to more efficient care of patients, fewer complications, and better time management for surgeons who perform on-call service for patients with traumatic orthopaedic injuries.

Instr Course Lect 2013;62:17-28.

After more than a decade of conflicting publications as well as changes in institutional resources, surgeons rightly question the ideal timing of surgical intervention for various extremity injuries. Is this fracture a true emergency? Can it wait until tomorrow morning? Is definitive management best delayed to minimize further trauma to the patient's physiology or soft tissues? How does the availability of protected, daytime operating room time influence these decisions? To address these questions, the evidence regarding the optimal or critical time for surgical intervention in treating various extremity injuries and the influence of a designated orthopaedic trauma room on management strategies were evaluated.

True Emergencies

Compartment Syndrome

Compartment syndrome of the extremities remains a true orthopaedic surgical emergency. Although innovative treatments continue to be developed, little has changed in the diagnosis and management of this condition. After the diagnosis is made, fasciotomy and evaluation of muscle viability is emergent; there are few indications for treatment delay except for a patient in extremis.

Diagnosis

The diagnosis of compartment syndrome remains clinically challenging, and despite technologic developments in pressure detection instruments, physical examination and clinical history remain the mainstays of diagnosis. One of the challenges of diagnosis is physical examination in patients who cannot reliably communicate, such as those who are intubated or those with altered sensorium. In these patients, examination can be unreliable.[1] The so-called classic clinical findings, such as changes on vascular examination or paralysis, occur late and are less helpful in preventing morbidity.

Pain out of proportion with passive stretch of an involved muscle group is one of the earliest and most sensitive clinical signs.[1] Paresthesias are an early sign and likely related to nerve ischemia.[2] Compartment syndromes can develop acutely after injury, after fracture fixation, or in a delayed fashion.[1,3] Although a specific measured value may be controversial, a delta *P* value is supported for diagnosis when invasive monitoring is selected.[4] McQueen and Court-Brown[4] defined the differential pressure between the measured compartment pressure and the systemic diastolic pressure. Their prospective evaluation of tibial fractures showed no compartment syndromes were missed when the delta *P* value was 30 mm Hg or greater.

Treatment

Clinical treatment of compartment syndromes is based primarily on the natural history and management protocols of compartment syndrome of the leg. Treatment of other extremities is by extrapolation from studies of the leg.[5,6] Research has defined thresholds for irreversible injury to nerves and muscle with pressure-related ischemia, and worse outcomes have been reported with delay in diagnosis and treatment.[7] Complete fasciotomies should be performed emergently after the diagnosis of compartment syndrome is determined. In a study of acute compartment syndrome in the leg, complete pressure release was not obtained until the length of the fasciotomy was 16 cm or longer.[8]

Legal Issues

Although there is considerable concern with regard to legal liability, malpractice claims for compartment syndrome are uncommon, with an estimated 0.002 claim per year of practice per surgeon.[9] A recent review evaluated the 20-year history of a single large malpractice insurer.[9] The most prominent risk factor for an indemnity payment was a delay before fasciotomy. In fact, the number of hours from the alleged presentation of the compartment syndrome until fasciotomy was linearly associated with the dollar amount of the indemnity payment. Most plaintiffs were employed, ensured, and white. The average indemnity payment from this insurer was $426,000.

Practice Trends

Compartment syndrome is a true orthopaedic emergency. This chapter's authors proceed with emergency fasciotomies after the diagnosis is made.

Vascular Injuries Associated With Orthopaedic Trauma

Vascular injuries associated with fractures and dislocations are unusual and mostly associated with high-energy trauma. Limb-threatening ischemia requires an organized multiservice approach for limb salvage. One of the most important controversies in management involves the order of repair when combined vascular and osseous injuries and/or dislocations occur. With a pulseless limb, the vascular repair is typically done first, and orthopaedic stabilization follows. This can be a problem when the repair is performed with the fracture and/or dislocation in unreduced position because subsequent reduction, including length restoration and angular correction, can disrupt the vascular repair. Treatment acuity for occult injuries—intimal disruptions—is more controversial. In these settings, the fixation sequence may affect outcome less, and the justification for primary stabilization of the fracture or dislocation is more logical.

Diagnosis

Rapid detection of vascular injury and localization of the lesion is key to successful management. Classic so-called hard signs that require emergency management include pulsatile hemorrhage, expanding hematoma, palpable thrill, audible bruit, and a frankly pulseless limb that persists after closed reduction and/or limb realignment. The ankle-brachial index is an effective noninvasive screening tool for diagnosing vascular injury. Mills et al[10] prospectively demonstrated excellent sensitivity, specificity, and positive predictive value with an ankle-brachial index of less than 0.9 in patients with knee dislocations. Doppler (ultra-

---

Dr. Crist or an immediate family member serves as a board member, owner, officer, or committee member of the Orthopaedic Trauma Association; has received research or institutional support from Medtronic, Novalign, Synthes, and Wound Care Technologies; has stock or stock options held in Amedica Corporation and Orthopaedic Implant Company; and has received nonincome support (such as equipment or services), commercially derived honoraria, or other non–research-related funding (such as paid travel) from Zimmer. Dr. Ferguson or an immediate family member is a member of a speakers' bureau or has made paid presentations on behalf of DePuy and Stryker. Dr. Lee or an immediate family member is a member of a speakers' bureau or has made paid presentations on behalf of Synthes, Zimmer, and the AONA; serves as a paid consultant to or is an employee of Synthes, Zimmer, and Biomet; has received research or institutional support from Synthes and SpineSmith; and has received nonincome support (such as equipment or services), commercially derived honoraria, or other non–research-related funding (such as paid travel) from Synthes Fellowship Support. Neither Dr. Murtha nor any immediate family member has received anything of value from or has stock or stock options held in a commercial company or institution related directly or indirectly to the subject of this chapter.

sound) screening can have excellent sensitivity and specificity but is operator dependent.[11] Multidetector CT angiography may be used and has good sensitivity and specificity.[12]

Treatment

The detection of vascular dissection is more difficult, but delays in repair are associated with high rates of amputation.[13] There is a lack of fracture-specific outcome data to counsel patients with both vascular injuries and fractures. High-energy fractures of the tibial plateau with vascular injuries have been shown to be especially problematic. A single-institution study reported that the presence of a dysvascular limb requiring vascular reconstruction was significantly associated with a deep wound infection.[14] Knee dislocations must be emergently reduced to allow for evaluation of the popliteal artery because there is a high rate of popliteal arterial injury.[15] Poor outcomes have been reported with delayed diagnosis in this setting.

Practice Trends

In the setting of a vascular injury associated with fracture or dislocation, this chapter's authors prefer to have temporary shunting done for arterial injuries that require repair, with definitive vascular repair performed after reduction and stabilization of the fracture or joint, usually with temporary external fixation.

Open Fractures

The treatment of open fractures has evolved over the past decade with the emergence of the orthopaedic trauma room and its ensured daily availability of operating room time for urgent cases. In general, there is a trend toward more delayed treatment of open fractures. However, delayed treatment of open fractures is not well supported in the literature.

The etiology of the 6-hour rule for open fracture débridement remains somewhat elusive. Although it is commonly practiced and taught to surgeons in training, the evidence for this dogma is questionable. Friedrich[16] performed an obscure set of experiments looking at the kinetics of infection using garden mold and dust in a guinea pig surgical wound model. In these rudimentary experiments, simple débridement cleared infection within 6 hours. By screening for bacteria in contaminated wounds, Robson et al[17] determined 10^5 organisms per gram of tissue as the threshold for infection, and it was reached at 5.17 hours after injury. The quality of data supporting a 6-hour threshold for open fracture débridement is quite limited.

The lack of data for early débridement, however, cannot be solely interpreted as support for cavalierly delayed treatment approaches. In fact, the basic science of bacterial colonization suggests that time is an important variable in the establishment of infection. One description of the establishment of infection has suggested that the fundamental first step in bacterial colonization is the process of adhesion or permanent attachment.[18] Many common musculoskeletal pathogens use biofilm formation during colonization to deter host defenses and promote adhesion. Adhesion is based on a time-dependent protein receptor interaction, polymer synthesis, ionic charge, and physical forces. Biofilms participate in cell-cell aggregation and consolidate adhesion. Devitalized bone stripped of periosteum, as with open fractures, presents a collagen protein matrix and acellular crystal surfaces to which bacteria may optimally bind.[19] Several in vitro studies evaluating debris and bacterial removal from biologic tissues have suggested a time-dependent efficacy. Comparing low- and high-pressure pulsatile lavage, Bhandari et al[20] demonstrated the best clearance of *Staphylococcus aureus* in human and canine bone models was within 3 hours of inoculation. Adherence of *S aureus* has also been shown to increase after 6 hours in a rabbit contamination model.[21]

In studies focusing on biomaterial-based infections, several interesting findings were postulated.[22] Within 3 hours of exposure to a surface such as bone, *S aureus* attaches to bone with weak van der Waals forces and hydrophobic interactions. After 3 hours, bone-surface receptor interactions and chemical interactions strengthen the bonds between bacteria and bone. As time continued, the bacteria were able to establish a protective microzone that inhibited clearance (biofilm). Thus, early débridement might prevent adherence and colonization. Extrapolation of this sequence to open fracture-related infection may support early débridement. In addition to the theoretic risks of time-dependent adhesion, there are practical concerns with delaying open fracture débridement. Clinical experience suggests that it is common to discover higher than expected levels of contamination and nonviable tissue in many open fracture wounds, even simple-appearing wounds. This is a problem because any foreign material may promote bacterial colonization.[23] Thus, extensive contamination and tissue injury are possible with benign-appearing soft-tissue wounds. Evaluation of the literature with regard to the timing of surgical débridement is varied, primarily retrospective, and minimally helpful in decision making. There are a minimum of nine retrospective studies that failed to identify increased risk of infection with delayed surgical débridement between 6 and 24 hours.[24] Two small prospective studies showed no increased risk of infection with delayed treatment of up to 24 hours.[25,26] In a

Table 1
Clinical Investigations Supporting Early Surgery for Young Patients With Femoral Neck Fractures

Study (Year)	Study Design	No. of Patients	Summary
Swiontkowski et al[30] (1984)	Retrospective, observational	25	20% had osteonecrosis and none had nonunion; all patients treated within 8 hours of injury.
Gerber et al[36] (1993)	Retrospective, observational	37	11% had osteonecrosis and 18% had nonunion; all treated within 12 hours after injury.
Robinson et al[37] (1995)	Retrospective, observational	32	21% had osteonecrosis and 18% had nonunion; all treated within 12 hours after injury.
Jain et al[33] (2002)	Retrospective, comparative	15 in early fixation group and 23 in late fixation group	No patient had osteonecrosis in early group, and 26% had osteonecrosis in late group. No nonunion in either group. No difference in functional outcomes between groups, leading the authors to suggest early fixation to decrease the radiographic finding of osteonecrosis.

study of 70 patients with open fractures, Merritt[25] took culture samples preoperatively, intraoperatively, and postoperatively, but failed to identify an increased risk of infection with delayed surgical débridement between 6 and 24 hours. A level I study with a variety of open fractures (41 tibiae) and most commonly Gustilo and Anderson type I open fractures (39 of 115) failed to identify an increased risk of infection with a delay of greater than 6 hours.[26] In contrast, three small retrospective series reported an increased risk of infection with surgical delay.[27-29] Overall, the literature does not have high-quality evidence that provides guidance in the timing of treatment of open fractures.

Practice Trends

As bacterial adhesion and colonization appears to be time dependent, this chapter's authors irrigate and débride open fractures urgently—meaning that the patient goes to the operating room when his or her physiologic status and the operating-room resources allow.

Injuries That Might Be Able to Wait Overnight

Femoral neck fractures in young patients and fractures of the talus have been labeled surgical emergencies. The most common justification for emergency care of these patients has been to rapidly reestablish the blood supply to the femoral head and talus and thus decrease the risk of osteonecrosis and nonunion. Controversy exists in the literature regarding the importance of surgical timing in these patients. With the increasing availability of orthopaedic trauma rooms, surgeons can often take these injuries to the operating room as a guaranteed first case of the day after injury. Conflicting evidence and changes in institutional resource allocation have made surgeons question the ideal timing of surgical intervention. Should these injuries be treated as orthopaedic emergencies or are they better treated as relative urgencies?

Should Femoral Neck Fractures in Young Patients Be Treated as Emergencies?

Femoral neck fractures in physiologically young patients are approached differently than those in elderly patients, with the primary goal being preservation of the native femoral head.[30] Complications including nonunion and osteonecrosis are common; the historic rates of osteonecrosis and nonunion have been reported to be as high as 86% and 59%, respectively.[30-34] Anatomic investigations have shown the importance of the intracapsular retinacular branches of the medial femoral circumflex artery on the perfusion of the femoral head. Simulating complete disruption of the femoral neck and these vessels leads to a complete lack of perfusion of the femoral head in cadaver hips.[35]

Timing of management has been debated in the literature. Swiontkowski et al[30] reported low rates of osteonecrosis (20%) and no symptomatic nonunions in 27 patients between ages 15 and 50 years, and attributed this success to the application of an institutional protocol of so-called immediate reduction (within 8 hours of diagnosis) and internal fixation with compression. This pivotal publication labeled these injuries surgical emergencies in young patients. Since the publication of that study, several authors have reported small series supporting an association between time to surgery and the outcomes of nonunion and osteonecrosis[33,36,37] (**Table 1**).

More recent studies have demonstrated no difference in outcomes between cohorts of patients treated emergently or after a delay.[32,38] The time considered as a delay varies (8 hours was used by Swiontkowski et al[30] and 24 hours by Haidukewych et al,[32] for example). However, despite different time intervals used to define a delay, the cohorts identified as having surgery late in these publications had outcomes comparable with the early co-

Table 2
Studies Suggesting No Advantage to Early Surgical Intervention

Study (Year)	Study Design	No. of Patients	Summary
Haidukewych et al[32] (2004)	Retrospective, comparative	73	Patients treated within 24 hours: 23% had osteonecrosis, and 7% had nonunion. Patients treated after 24 hours: 20% had osteonecrosis, and 10% had nonunion.
Upadhyay et al[38] (2004)	Prospective, non-randomized	92	Patients treated within 48 hours: 14% had osteonecrosis, and 18% had nonunion. Patients treated after 48 hours: 19% had osteonecrosis, and 16.7% had nonunion.
Damany et al[42] (2005)	Meta-analysis of seven studies	170	110 patients identified as treated within 12 hours: 13.6% had osteonecrosis, and 11.8% had nonunion. 60 patients identified as treated after 12 hours: 15% had osteonecrosis, and 5% had nonunion.

horts in the studies promoting emergency fixation. Three case series have described cohorts of patients treated after inadvertent delays of 6 days to 2 years, with rates of osteonecrosis and nonunion similar to those in series in which patients were treated emergently (0% to 25%)[39-41] (**Table 2**).

A meta-analysis reviewing 18 retrospective cohort studies of femoral neck fractures in patients between ages 15 and 50 years (547 fractures) found an overall osteonecrosis rate of 22.5%.[42] Seven of those studies described comparative data on 110 patients treated within 12 hours and 60 treated more than 12 hours after fracture. No substantial differences were noted in the rates of either osteonecrosis or nonunion, despite an incidence of nonunion that was more than twice as great in the group treated within 12 hours.

Although the evidence is controversial with regard to the role of surgical timing, other factors have been consistently and more robustly associated with poor outcomes.[30-33,38,43-46] Injury variables, such as initial displacement and posterior comminution, are strongly correlated with the development of osteonecrosis, nonunion, and loss of fixation. The quality of the obtained surgical reduction is strongly correlated with the rate of reported nonunion and is the most consistently predictive variable of poor outcome.

Progression to osteonecrosis, nonunion, and poor functional outcome is multifactorial in these patients. Current best evidence suggests a lack of association between time to reduction (less than 24 hours) and osteonecrosis or nonunion, but is composed of underpowered observational cohorts (levels III and IV) and is far from conclusive.

Practice Trends

This chapter's authors strive for an urgent anatomic reduction. Delaying late or overnight surgery to the first case the next morning is considered if it is expected that operating room conditions will influence the quality of the achieved reduction and if there is guaranteed operating room time available for a first-case start.

Should Talar Neck Fractures Be Treated as Emergencies?

The historically high rates of osteonecrosis (50% among Hawkins type II fractures and 84% among Hawkins type III fractures) associated with talar fractures have been attributed to fracture displacement injuring the fragile retrograde blood supply, preventing vascularization to the talar body.[47,48] Several small observational studies have reported decreased rates of osteonecrosis (< 35% in displaced fractures) with early or immediate surgical stabilization.[49-51] Those authors advocated emergency treatment of talar neck fractures, stating that early reduction promotes revascularization and helps to preserve any remaining blood supply to the posterior aspect of the talus.

Many studies by experts in foot and ankle trauma have subsequently found no correlation between surgical timing and outcomes. Vallier et al[52] reported an overall rate of 36% for osteonecrosis and 5% for nonunion, with no correlation between outcomes and the surgical time interval. Osteonecrosis was associated with Hawkins type fractures (39% of Hawkins type II fractures versus 64% of Hawkins type III fractures), talar neck comminution, and open fractures. Similarly, Lindvall et al[53] evaluated 26 patients, 12 of whom were treated early (within 6 hours) and 14 of whom were treated more than 6 hours after the injury. The rate of osteonecrosis in the open fractures was 85%. No significant difference was seen between the 6 closed fractures fixed within 6 hours and the 13 closed fractures treated more than 6 hours after injury. Collectively, these authors agreed that injury severity and associated soft-tissue injury were strongly associated with patient outcomes and recommended that consideration be given to delayed definitive fixation of the talar neck fracture until the soft tissues were in favorable condition for surgery.

These series were limited by small sample size, study design, and confounding variables. The current best evidence is level IV and inconclusive, but it does not seem to support a relationship between surgical timing and outcomes.

Practice Trends

This chapter's authors urgently débride open talar neck fractures and span the fractures with external fixation (when appropriate) to allow soft-tissue stabilization and wound management. Fracture-dislocations are treated as emergencies when associated with neurovascular compromise. To avoid skin necrosis and wound complications, definitive management is delayed until the soft-tissue swelling has abated.

Damage Control Orthopaedics

History of Damage Control Surgery

The timing of definitive fracture fixation in trauma patients has evolved over the past several decades. As implant options broadened and improved in the 1980s, a more aggressive initial approach to fracture management was undertaken. A subsequent alteration in treatment paradigms, with a shift toward decreasing acute surgical burden in critically injured patients, evolved in the 1990s on the basis of the general surgery concepts of the so-called triad of death—coagulopathy, hypothermia, and hypotension—and the importance of minimization of acute surgical burden in patients with major trauma.[54,55] The goals of damage control surgery were to lessen complications arising from a result of the so-called second hit of increased acute surgical burden. Orthopaedic surgeons began to adopt this concept, and Pape et al[56] added soft-tissue injuries as a fourth consideration in trauma patients with blunt-force injury. Within the orthopaedic trauma field, the staged approach to surgical intervention and a greater respect for the patient's physiologic status have developed, with increased consideration given to the timing and nature of surgical interventions.

Inflammatory and Resuscitation Considerations

Traumatic injury and surgical procedures are known to induce a systemic inflammatory response and a counter-inflammatory response.[57,58] In a prospectively randomized trial, the acute inflammatory marker interleukin (IL)-6 increased more in stable patients with a femoral fracture treated with immediate definitive fixation with an intramedullary nail than in patients undergoing a staged treatment protocol with initial external fixation.[59] The potential for the exacerbation of the trauma inflammatory response by subjecting a patient to longer and more invasive surgery is sustained for several days following the acute traumatic event and is associated with organ dysfunction. Pape et al,[60] in a prospectively randomized group of trauma patients, found those who were converted to intramedullary stabilization of a femoral fracture between days 2 and 4 after the injury had higher postoperative levels of IL-6 compared with those treated with delayed conversion on day 5 or later after the injury. Patients with higher initial IL-6 levels in the day 2 to day 4 conversion group had significantly higher rates of organ dysfunction compared with the delayed conversion group. Although a host of immunomodulators are released during the acute trauma phase and surgical interventions, IL-6 levels can be predictive of clinical outcomes, with higher levels correlated to increased morbidity.[57,61,62] The inflammatory effect of the trauma should be considered along with the inflammatory burden of early and prolonged surgery.

Little controversy exists with regard to treating stable patients with early definitive fixation and treating unstable patients, or those in extremis, with staged management. The question of the best treatment plan arises with respect to the patient with borderline status and how to identify those who fall into that category. Because IL-6 values are not available in most US trauma centers, other methods of determining patients at risk must be used. Pape et al[56] expanded the so-called triad of death to include soft-tissue injuries in blunt trauma patients and provided a reasonable tool to assist in the identification of borderline patients, with reclassification possible as the patient undergoes resuscitation or subsequent deterioration (**Table 3**). Pape et al,[63] using their criteria for stable and borderline status, prospectively randomized patients in these categories who had femoral fractures to initial treatment of intramedullary nailing or external fixation with eventual conversion to intramedullary nailing. Borderline patients managed with provisional external fixation had fewer pulmonary complications. Further analysis also showed longer ventilatory times in stable patients randomized to provisional external fixation rather than definitive fixation. The results underscore the benefits of patient stratification for appropriate initial management. If the patient is stable, early definitive care is appropriate. However, borderline patients seem to benefit from provisional external fixation and delayed definitive management.

Included in the previously mentioned guidelines for patient stratification is the idea of resuscitation, as measured by base deficit and lactate level. The general surgery and orthopaedic trauma literature have reported resus-

Table 3
Assessment of Four Different Clinical Grades and Ranges of Clinical Parameters Determining These Grades

Parameter	Stable (Grade I)	Borderline (Grade II)	Unstable (Grade III)	In Extremis (Grade IV)
Shock				
Blood pressure (mm Hg)	100 or more	80-100	60-90	< 50-60
Blood units (per 2 hours)	0-2	2-8	5-15	> 15
Lactate levels	Normal range	Approximately 2.5	> 2.5	Severe acidosis
Base deficit (mmol/L)	Normal range	No data	No data	> 6-18
ATLS classification	I	II-III	III-IV	IV
Urine output (mL/h)	> 150	50-150	< 100	< 50
Coagulation				
Platelet count (μg/mL)	> 110,000	90,000-110,000	< 70,000-90,000	< 70,000
Factor II and V (%)	90-100	70-80	50-70	< 50
Fibrinogen (g/dL)	> 1	Approximately 1	< 1	DIC
D-dimer	Normal range	Abnormal	Abnormal	DIC
Temperature	> 34°C	33°C-35°C	30°C-32°C	≤ 30°C
Soft-tissue injuries				
Lung function (PaO_2/FiO_2)	> 350	300	200-300	< 200
Chest trauma scores (AIS)	I or II	II or more	II or more	III or more
Thoracic trauma score (TTS)	0	I-II	II-III	IV
Abdominal trauma (Moore)	≤ II	≤ III	III	III or more
Pelvic trauma (AO classification)	A type (AO)	B or C	C	C (crush, rollover abdomen)
Extremities (AIS)	I-II	II-III	III-IV	Crush, rollover extremities
Surgical strategy				
Damage control (DCO) or Definitive surgery (ETC)	ETC	DCO if uncertain ETC if stable	DCO	DCO

(Reproduced with modification from Pape HC, Giannoudis PV, Krettek C, Trentz O: Timing of fixation of major fractures in blunt polytrauma: Role of conventional indicators in clinical decision making. *J Orthop Trauma* 2005;19(8):551-62.)
ATLS = Advanced Trauma and Life Support, AIS = Abbreviated Injury Scale, TTS = thoracic trauma score, DIC = disseminated intravascular coagulation, DCO = damage control orthopaedics, ETC = early total care

citation to be an important predictor of outcome in the trauma patient population, and clinically available parameters such as serum lactate levels and base deficit can be useful.[64-66] O'Toole et al,[67] using resuscitation as a predictor of readiness for surgical intervention, reported low rates of both acute respiratory distress syndrome and death in patients with multiple traumatic injuries treated with intramedullary fixation of femoral shaft fractures after adequate resuscitation (lactate levels trending toward 2.5 mmol/L). Predictably higher rates of mortality were noted in the external fixator group, which had substantially higher lactate levels and less stable cardiopulmonary parameters compared with those in the intramedullary fixation group.

Patients With Head Injuries

Although clinical signs of hypoperfusion and associated laboratory findings are important predictors of patients who may respond well to a limited initial approach, special consideration must also be given to those persons presenting with or at risk for the development of traumatic brain injuries. No prospective randomized trial is available to provide specific criteria indicative of the readiness of a brain-injured patient for definitive surgical intervention. Understanding the diagnosis and management of the head injury can direct the care of these patients and guide clinical decision making. Adequate resuscitation and maintenance of appropriate perfusion of brain tissue is important to avoid further cerebral insult. Cerebral perfusion pressure is quantified by measuring the difference between mean arterial pressure and intracranial pressure. Intracranial pressures of greater than 20 to 25 mm Hg should trigger initiation of therapy to decrease intracranial pressure and thus increase cerebral perfusion pressure.[68] In orthopaedics, the effect that surgical intervention can have on cerebral perfusion pressure should factor into surgical decision making. Anglen et al[69] reported an intraoperative decrease in mean arterial pressure and cerebral perfusion pressure in patients treated with intramedullary femoral fixation. Careful consideration of the specific neurologic condition of a patient, his or her resuscitation status, the expected length of procedures, and the effect of surgery on the cerebral perfusion pressure should be discussed with the neurosurgical team to avoid further cerebral insult.

Practice Trends

Although general surgery trauma colleagues play a critical role in determining when borderline patients are adequately resuscitated for surgery, this chapter's authors take a proactive role with them in determining what definitive and what staged procedures can be done for the patient when he or she is cleared for surgery. In questionable situations, staged management is chosen to avoid major complications.

Damage Control for the Extremity

Two commonly encountered injuries that have been shown to benefit from staged management (damage control orthopaedics), primarily because of the risk of complications secondary to the soft-tissue injuries, are high-energy tibial plateau and pilon fractures. Either injury-related factors (high energy) or patient-related factors (medical comorbidities) place patients at a considerably high risk of complications. Delayed definitive fixation with early temporary joint-spanning external fixation allows improved imaging and evaluation of the fracture and allows the soft-tissue injury to recover before a second surgical procedure.

Tibial plateau fractures vary substantially with regard to fracture pattern and overlying soft-tissue injury, despite the association of more complex fracture patterns with high-energy injuries. In patients with preexisting poor soft tissue due to age or medical comorbidities, such as diabetes mellitus or peripheral vascular disease, a simple low-level fall can create a relatively simple fracture pattern but a substantial soft-tissue injury. High-energy fractures in any patient can create a severe soft-tissue injury and more complex fracture patterns that require multiple surgical approaches to adequately treat the fracture. The use of a temporary knee-spanning external fixator has proven to be safe and effective in decreasing the risk of infection from up to 80% to less than approximately 8%, especially when dual surgical approaches are used.[14,70-73]

The management of tibial pilon fractures has changed notably over the past 10 to 15 years on the basis of a historic complication rate of up to 100% with primary open reduction and internal fixation (ORIF) to less than 10% with staged management.[74-77] Although a recent study retrospectively evaluating early primary ORIF (median time from injury to surgery was 18 hours) showed a deep infection rate of 6% in 95 with AO/OTA (Orthopaedic Trauma Association) type 43C pilon fractures, the condition of the soft-tissue envelope should determine when definitive ORIF is performed to minimize the risk of previously reported major complication rates[78] (**Figure 1**).

Practice Trends

The soft-tissue injury should determine when definitive ORIF is performed for both tibial plateau and pilon fractures. In high-energy injuries or low-energy injuries in patients with a poor preexisting soft-tissue envelope, this chapter's authors use a two-staged approach with delayed definitive ORIF with early joint-spanning external fixation, if indicated. This approach is supported by the literature.

Effect of the Orthopaedic Trauma Room

The orthopaedic trauma room, staffed by experienced orthopaedic support personnel, is a new concept over the past decade that provides dedicated time, separate from the general surgery trauma room, during normal daylight hours. The room is late release, meaning that cases can be scheduled in the room typically up until the same morning without being placed as an add-on. Historically, orthopaedic trauma cases that were not emergencies would be placed on the add-on list to be done at the end of the day when all of the electively scheduled surgeries were completed. This led to inefficient care for patients who were bedridden or had limited mobility secondary to their injury and would have benefited the most from early care. It also led to longer hospital stays and a higher burden on the on-call hospital staff and the associated hospital resources. In addition, it contributed to an orthopaedic trauma surgeon "burning out" and not being able to sustain a full-time acute trauma practice during his or her entire career.

After-hours surgery is associated with a higher rate of complications. Ricci et al[79] prospectively reviewed patients who were treated with intramedullary nailing of femoral and tibial fractures and found a significantly higher rate of unplanned reoperations and deep implant removal in the patients who had a femoral fracture.

Several studies have shown that a dedicated orthopaedic trauma room

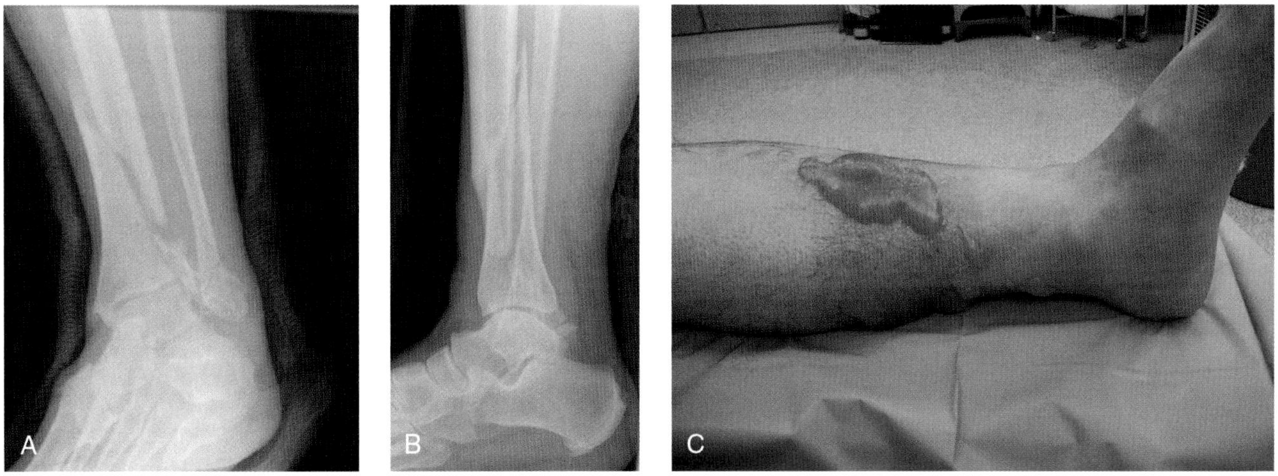

Figure 1 A 64-year-old man fell 4 feet (1.2 m) off a stepladder and sustained an AO/OTA type-43B tibial pilon and distal fibular fracture. **A,** Oblique radiograph made at the time of presentation. **B,** Lateral radiograph made at the time of presentation. **C,** Within 12 hours after the injury, fracture blisters occurred. The patient was treated with initial spanning external fixation and delayed definitive management.

leads to more efficient care with fewer complications. Bhattacharyya et al[80] retrospectively reviewed the efficacy of the orthopaedic trauma room at a level I trauma center. The room was used 88% of the available time, which is above the standard acceptable utilization rate for an operating room. Fewer elective orthopaedic cases were rescheduled, and there was a 72% reduction in the number of hip fractures that were surgically treated after 5 PM. There were also fewer complications and less surgical time for patients treated with femoral nailing before 5 PM. Wixted et al[81] reported that the orthopaedic trauma room led to an improved case flow, with a greater total number of cases being done, fewer after-hours cases, and an increased likelihood of isolated femoral shaft fractures being transferred to the orthopaedic traumatologist. In comparing two level I Canadian trauma centers, one with and one without a dedicated orthopaedic trauma room, Elder et al[82] showed that the availability of the orthopaedic trauma room significantly decreased the time to surgery and morbidity by almost 50% in elderly patients with subcapital femoral neck fractures.

Practice Trends

All of this chapter's authors have the availability of the orthopaedic trauma room and believe it is a critical factor for the efficient care of trauma patients. The trauma operating room also improves career satisfaction and sustainability for orthopaedic traumatologists and those who regularly manage orthopaedic trauma patients.

Summary

Although technical and resource trends have changed over the past few decades, true orthopaedic emergencies related to extremity injuries continue to occur and include compartment syndrome and fractures or dislocations associated with vascular injury. Open fractures, displaced femoral neck fractures in young adults, and open fractures of the talus or those with potential soft-tissue compromise should be managed as soon as the patient's status and medical resources allow. Definitive fixation of extremity injuries should be done when the patient and the soft-tissue status provide the best opportunity to minimize the risk of complications. The orthopaedic trauma operating room has allowed for more efficient care of these potentially critically injured patients and has improved resource utilization, decreased the risk of complications, and improved job satisfaction for orthopaedic surgeons who manage trauma patients.

References

1. McQueen MM, Christie J, Court-Brown CM: Acute compartment syndrome in tibial diaphyseal fractures. *J Bone Joint Surg Br* 1996; 78(1):95-98.
2. Matava MJ, Whitesides TE Jr, Seiler JG III, Hewan-Lowe K, Hutton WC: Determination of the compartment pressure threshold of muscle ischemia in a canine model. *J Trauma* 1994;37(1): 50-58.
3. Olson SA, Glasgow RR: Acute compartment syndrome in lower extremity musculoskeletal trauma. *J Am Acad Orthop Surg* 2005;13 (7):436-444.

4. McQueen MM, Court-Brown CM: Compartment monitoring in tibial fractures: The pressure threshold for decompression. *J Bone Joint Surg Br* 1996;78 (1):99-104.
5. Friedrich JB, Shin AY: Management of forearm compartment syndrome. *Hand Clin* 2007;23 (2):245-254, vii.
6. Ojike NI, Roberts CS, Giannoudis PV: Compartment syndrome of the thigh: A systematic review. *Injury* 2010;41(2): 133-136.
7. Finkelstein JA, Hunter GA, Hu RW: Lower limb compartment syndrome: Course after delayed fasciotomy. *J Trauma* 1996;40 (3):342-344.
8. Cohen MS, Garfin SR, Hargens AR, Mubarak SJ: Acute compartment syndrome: Effect of dermotomy on fascial decompression in the leg. *J Bone Joint Surg Br* 1991; 73(2):287-290.
9. Bhattacharyya T, Vrahas MS: The medical-legal aspects of compartment syndrome. *J Bone Joint Surg Am* 2004;86(4):864-868.
10. Mills WJ, Barei DP, McNair P: The value of the ankle-brachial index for diagnosing arterial injury after knee dislocation: A prospective study. *J Trauma* 2004; 56(6):1261-1265.
11. Bynoe RP, Miles WS, Bell RM, et al: Noninvasive diagnosis of vascular trauma by duplex ultrasonography. *J Vasc Surg* 1991; 14(3):346-352.
12. Rieger M, Mallouhi A, Tauscher T, Lutz M, Jaschke WR: Traumatic arterial injuries of the extremities: Initial evaluation with MDCT angiography. *AJR Am J Roentgenol* 2006;186(3):656-664.
13. Hafez HM, Woolgar J, Robbs JV: Lower extremity arterial injury: Results of 550 cases and review of risk factors associated with limb loss. *J Vasc Surg* 2001;33(6): 1212-1219.
14. Barei DP, Nork SE, Mills WJ, Henley MB, Benirschke SK: Complications associated with internal fixation of high-energy bicondylar tibial plateau fractures utilizing a two-incision technique. *J Orthop Trauma* 2004;18 (10):649-657.
15. Rihn JA, Groff YJ, Harner CD, Cha PS: The acutely dislocated knee: Evaluation and management. *J Am Acad Orthop Surg* 2004;12(5):334-346.
16. Friedrich PL: Die aseptische Versorgung frischer Wundern. *Arch Klin Chir* 1898;57:288-310.
17. Robson MC, Duke WF, Krizek TJ: Rapid bacterial screening in the treatment of civilian wounds. *J Surg Res* 1973;14(5):426-430.
18. Gristina AG, Costerton JW: Bacterial adherence to biomaterials and tissue: The significance of its role in clinical sepsis. *J Bone Joint Surg Am* 1985;67(2):264-273.
19. Gristina AG, Naylor PT, Webb LX: Molecular mechanisms in musculoskeletal sepsis: The race for the surface. *Instr Course Lect* 1990;39:471-482.
20. Bhandari M, Adili A, Lachowski RJ: High pressure pulsatile lavage of contaminated human tibiae: An in vitro study. *J Orthop Trauma* 1998;12(7):479-484.
21. Gracia E, Fernández A, Conchello P, et al: Adherence of Staphylococcus aureus slime-producing strain variants to biomaterials used in orthopaedic surgery. *Int Orthop* 1997;21(1):46-51.
22. Gristina AG, Oga M, Webb LX, Hobgood CD: Adherent bacterial colonization in the pathogenesis of osteomyelitis. *Science* 1985; 228(4702):990-993.
23. Gristina AG, Naylor PT, Myrvik QN: Mechanisms of musculoskeletal sepsis. *Orthop Clin North Am* 1991;22(3):363-371.
24. Werner CM, Pierpont Y, Pollak AN: The urgency of surgical débridement in the management of open fractures. *J Am Acad Orthop Surg* 2008;16(7):369-375.
25. Merritt K: Factors increasing the risk of infection in patients with open fractures. *J Trauma* 1988; 28(6):823-827.
26. Spencer J, Smith A, Woods D: The effect of time delay on infection in open long-bone fractures: A 5-year prospective audit from a district general hospital. *Ann R Coll Surg Engl* 2004;86(2):108-112.
27. Jacob E, Erpelding JM, Murphy KP: A retrospective analysis of open fractures sustained by U.S. military personnel during Operation Just Cause. *Mil Med* 1992; 157(10):552-556.
28. Kindsfater K, Jonassen EA: Osteomyelitis in grade II and III open tibia fractures with late debridement. *J Orthop Trauma* 1995; 9(2):121-127.
29. Kreder HJ, Armstrong P: A review of open tibia fractures in children. *J Pediatr Orthop* 1995;15(4): 482-488.
30. Swiontkowski MF, Winquist RA, Hansen ST Jr: Fractures of the femoral neck in patients between the ages of twelve and forty-nine years. *J Bone Joint Surg Am* 1984; 66(6):837-846.
31. Protzman RR, Burkhalter WE: Femoral-neck fractures in young adults. *J Bone Joint Surg Am* 1976; 58(5):689-695.
32. Haidukewych GJ, Rothwell WS, Jacofsky DJ, Torchia ME, Berry DJ: Operative treatment of femoral neck fractures in patients between the ages of fifteen and fifty years. *J Bone Joint Surg Am* 2004; 86(8):1711-1716.
33. Jain R, Koo M, Kreder HJ, Schemitsch EH, Davey JR, Mahomed NN: Comparison of early and delayed fixation of subcapital hip fractures in patients sixty years of age or less. *J Bone Joint Surg Am* 2002;84(9):1605-1612.

34. Gautier E, Ganz K, Krügel N, Gill T, Ganz R: Anatomy of the medial femoral circumflex artery and its surgical implications. *J Bone Joint Surg Br* 2000;82 (5):679-683.

35. Sevitt S, Thompson RG: The distribution and anastomoses of arteries supplying the head and neck of the femur. *J Bone Joint Surg Br* 1965;47:560-573.

36. Gerber C, Strehle J, Ganz R: The treatment of fractures of the femoral neck. *Clin Orthop Relat Res* 1993;292:77-86.

37. Robinson CM, Court-Brown CM, McQueen MM, Christie J: Hip fractures in adults younger than 50 years of age: Epidemiology and results. *Clin Orthop Relat Res* 1995;312:238-246.

38. Upadhyay A, Jain P, Mishra P, Maini L, Gautum VK, Dhaon BK: Delayed internal fixation of fractures of the neck of the femur in young adults: A prospective, randomised study comparing closed and open reduction. *J Bone Joint Surg Br* 2004;86(7):1035-1040.

39. Butt MF, Dhar SA, Gani NU, et al: Delayed fixation of displaced femoral neck fractures in younger adults. *Injury* 2008;39(2): 238-243.

40. Huang CH: Treatment of neglected femoral neck fractures in young adults. *Clin Orthop Relat Res* 1986;206:117-126.

41. Roshan A, Ram S: Early return to function in young adults with neglected femoral neck fractures. *Clin Orthop Relat Res* 2006;447: 152-157.

42. Damany DS, Parker MJ, Chojnowski A: Complications after intracapsular hip fractures in young adults: A meta-analysis of 18 published studies involving 564 fractures. *Injury* 2005;36 (1):131-141.

43. Liporace F, Gaines R, Collinge C, Haidukewych GJ: Results of internal fixation of Pauwels type-3 vertical femoral neck fractures. *J Bone Joint Surg Am* 2008;90 (8):1654-1659.

44. Tooke SM, Favero KJ: Femoral neck fractures in skeletally mature patients, fifty years old or less. *J Bone Joint Surg Am* 1985;67(8): 1255-1260.

45. Bray TJ: Femoral neck fracture fixation: Clinical decision making. *Clin Orthop Relat Res* 1997; 339:20-31.

46. Scheck M: Intracapsular fractures of the femoral neck: Comminution of the posterior neck cortex as a cause of unstable fixation. *J Bone Joint Surg Am* 1959;41: 1187-1200.

47. Hawkins LG: Fractures of the neck of the talus. *J Bone Joint Surg Am* 1970;52(5):991-1002.

48. Canale ST, Kelly FB Jr: Fractures of the neck of the talus: Long-term evaluation of seventy-one cases. *J Bone Joint Surg Am* 1978; 60(2):143-156.

49. Grob D, Simpson LA, Weber BG, Bray T: Operative treatment of displaced talus fractures. *Clin Orthop Relat Res* 1985;199:88-96.

50. Frawley PA, Hart JA, Young DA: Treatment outcome of major fractures of the talus. *Foot Ankle Int* 1995;16(6):339-345.

51. Elgafy H, Ebraheim NA, Tile M, Stephen D, Kase J: Fractures of the talus: Experience of two level 1 trauma centers. *Foot Ankle Int* 2000;21(12):1023-1029.

52. Vallier HA, Nork SE, Barei DP, Benirschke SK, Sangeorzan BJ: Talar neck fractures: Results and outcomes. *J Bone Joint Surg Am* 2004;86(8):1616-1624.

53. Lindvall E, Haidukewych G, DiPasquale T, Herscovici D Jr, Sanders R: Open reduction and stable fixation of isolated, displaced talar neck and body fractures. *J Bone Joint Surg Am* 2004; 86(10):2229-2234.

54. Rotondo MF, Schwab CW, McGonigal MD, et al: 'Damage control': An approach for improved survival in exsanguinating penetrating abdominal injury. *J Trauma* 1993;35(3):375-383.

55. Burch JM, Ortiz VB, Richardson RJ, Martin RR, Mattox KL, Jordan GL Jr: Abbreviated laparotomy and planned reoperation for critically injured patients. *Ann Surg* 1992;215(5):476-484.

56. Pape HC, Giannoudis PV, Krettek C, Trentz O: Timing of fixation of major fractures in blunt polytrauma: Role of conventional indicators in clinical decision making. *J Orthop Trauma* 2005;19(8):551-562.

57. Nast-Kolb D, Waydhas C, Gippner-Steppert C, et al: Indicators of the posttraumatic inflammatory response correlate with organ failure in patients with multiple injuries. *J Trauma* 1997;42 (3):446-455.

58. Pape HC, Schmidt RE, Rice J, et al : Biochemical changes after trauma and skeletal surgery of the lower extremity: Quantification of the operative burden. *Crit Care Med* 2000;28(10):3441-3448.

59. Pape HC, Grimme K, Van Griensven M, et al: Impact of intramedullary instrumentation versus damage control for femoral fractures on immunoinflammatory parameters: Prospective randomized analysis by the EPOFF Study Group. *J Trauma* 2003; 55(1):7-13.

60. Pape HC, van Griensven M, Rice J, et al: Major secondary surgery in blunt trauma patients and perioperative cytokine liberation: Determination of the clinical relevance of biochemical markers. *J Trauma* 2001;50(6):989-1000.

61. Frink M, van Griensven M, Kobbe P, et al: IL-6 predicts organ dysfunction and mortality in patients with multiple injuries. *Scand J Trauma Resusc Emerg Med* 2009;17:49.

62. Jastrow KM III, Gonzalez EA, McGuire MF, et al: Early cytokine production risk stratifies trauma patients for multiple organ failure. *J Am Coll Surg* 2009; 209(3):320-331.

63. Pape HC, Rixen D, Morley J, et al: Impact of the method of initial stabilization for femoral shaft fractures in patients with multiple injuries at risk for complications (borderline patients). *Ann Surg* 2007;246(3):491-501.

64. Davis JW, Parks SN, Kaups KL, Gladen HE, O'Donnell-Nicol S: Admission base deficit predicts transfusion requirements and risk of complications. *J Trauma* 1996; 41(5):769-774.

65. Crowl AC, Young JS, Kahler DM, Claridge JA, Chrzanowski DS, Pomphrey M: Occult hypoperfusion is associated with increased morbidity in patients undergoing early femur fracture fixation. *J Trauma* 2000;48(2):260-267.

66. Abramson D, Scalea TM, Hitchcock R, Trooskin SZ, Henry SM, Greenspan J: Lactate clearance and survival following injury. *J Trauma* 1993;35(4):584-589.

67. O'Toole RV, O'Brien M, Scalea TM, Habashi N, Pollak AN, Turen CH: Resuscitation before stabilization of femoral fractures limits acute respiratory distress syndrome in patients with multiple traumatic injuries despite low use of damage control orthopedics. *J Trauma* 2009;67(5):1013-1021.

68. Brain Trauma Foundation, American Association of Neurological Surgeons (AANS), Congress of Neurological Surgeons (CNS), AANA/CNS Joint Section on Neurotrauma and Critical Care: *Guidelines for the Management of Severe Traumatic Brain Injury*, ed 3. New York, NY, Brain Trauma Foundation, 2007. https://www.braintrauma.org/pdf/protected/Guidelines_Management_2007w_bookmarks.pdf. Accessed May 2012.

69. Anglen JO, Luber K, Park T: The effect of femoral nailing on cerebral perfusion pressure in head-injured patients. *J Trauma* 2003; 54(6):1166-1170.

70. Anglen JO, Aleto T: Temporary transarticular external fixation of the knee and ankle. *J Orthop Trauma* 1998;12(6):431-434.

71. Egol KA, Tejwani NC, Capla EL, Wolinsky PL, Koval KJ: Staged management of high-energy proximal tibia fractures (OTA types 41): The results of a prospective, standardized protocol. *J Orthop Trauma* 2005;19(7):448-456.

72. Barei DP, Nork SE, Mills WJ, Coles CP, Henley MB, Benirschke SK: Functional outcomes of severe bicondylar tibial plateau fractures treated with dual incisions and medial and lateral plates. *J Bone Joint Surg Am* 2006; 88(8):1713-1721.

73. Young MJ, Barrack RL: Complications of internal fixation of tibial plateau fractures. *Orthop Rev* 1994;23(2):149-154.

74. Wyrsch B, McFerran MA, McAndrew M, et al: Operative treatment of fractures of the tibial plafond: A randomized, prospective study. *J Bone Joint Surg Am* 1996; 78(11):1646-1657.

75. Anglen JO: Early outcome of hybrid external fixation for fracture of the distal tibia. *J Orthop Trauma* 1999;13(2):92-97.

76. Sirkin M, Sanders R, DiPasquale T, Herscovici D Jr: A staged protocol for soft tissue management in the treatment of complex pilon fractures. *J Orthop Trauma* 1999; 13(2):78-84.

77. Patterson MJ, Cole JD: Two-staged delayed open reduction and internal fixation of severe pilon fractures. *J Orthop Trauma* 1999; 13(2):85-91.

78. White TO, Guy P, Cooke CJ, et al: The results of early primary open reduction and internal fixation for treatment of OTA 43.C-type tibial pilon fractures: A cohort study. *J Orthop Trauma* 2010;24(12):757-763.

79. Ricci WM, Gallagher B, Brandt A, Schwappach J, Tucker M, Leighton R: Is after-hours orthopaedic surgery associated with adverse outcomes? A prospective comparative study. *J Bone Joint Surg Am* 2009;91(9):2067-2072.

80. Bhattacharyya T, Vrahas MS, Morrison SM, et al : The value of the dedicated orthopaedic trauma operating room. *J Trauma* 2006; 60(6):1336-1341.

81. Wixted JJ, Reed M, Eskander MS, et al : The effect of an orthopedic trauma room on after-hours surgery at a level one trauma center. *J Orthop Trauma* 2008;22 (4):234-236.

82. Elder GM, Harvey EJ, Vaidya R, Guy P, Meek RN, Aebi M: The effectiveness of orthopaedic trauma theatres in decreasing morbidity and mortality: A study of 701 displaced subcapital hip fractures in two trauma centres. *Injury* 2005;36(9):1060-1066.

3

SYMPOSIUM

Orthopaedic Trauma Mythbusters: Intra-articular Fractures

Robert F. Ostrum, MD

Abstract

Intra-articular fractures of the tibial plateau, pilon, and calcaneus often present a challenge for the treating orthopaedic surgeon. These injuries can have substantial comminution in the joint and the metaphyseal areas and are often accompanied by considerable soft-tissue trauma. In recent years, several questionable beliefs concerning these fractures have emerged and are best considered as myths. These myths include the beliefs that most patients with intra-articular fractures will have poor outcomes even with good surgical treatment, severe intra-articular fractures require a later reconstructive procedure regardless of the treatment, and the surgical treatment of comminuted intra-articular fractures has a high complication rate and may result in infection and limit the available options for limb salvage. A review of the literature regarding the treatment of common intra-articular fractures is helpful in determining if these myths concerning treatment options can be confirmed or disproved.

Instr Course Lect 2013;62:29-33.

Intra-articular fractures are often difficult to treat because of substantial comminution in the articular cartilage and metaphyseal areas. This chapter will examine several questionable beliefs concerning the treatment of intra-articular fractures of the tibial plateau, the pilon, and the calcaneus to determine if these myths can be confirmed or disproved. It examines the literature to determine the validity of three commonly held beliefs: (1) Most patients with intra-articular fractures will have poor outcomes even with good surgical treatment, (2) severe intra-articular fractures will require a later reconstructive procedure regardless of the treatment, and (3) the surgical treatment of comminuted intra-articular fractures has a high complication rate and may result in infection and limit the available options for limb salvage.

Tibial Plateau Fractures

Many tibial plateau fractures, especially those of the lateral plateau, do not progress to severe posttraumatic arthritis and do not require total knee arthroplasty. In part, this is true because 70% of the load of the knee joint passes through the medial tibiofemoral compartment with normal walking.[1] This adductor moment unloads the lateral tibial plateau. From an anatomic viewpoint, the lateral tibial plateau has the thickest cartilage of the proximal tibia (6 mm), which makes slight incongruities less important.[2] The lateral meniscus is large and protects the weight-bearing cartilage from degeneration. Several studies have shown that the degree of articular displacement may not be a good indicator of arthritis development or long-term results.[3-5] The degree of knee instability after a tibial plateau fracture is a better indicator of expected function and the likelihood of the development of arthritis than is the amount of articular displacement. Medial tibial plateau fractures and those having excision of the meniscus have a much poorer prognosis. It has been shown that restoration of mechanical alignment and knee instability of less than 10° with the knee nearly fully extended leads to better functional results.[3-5] Primary osteoarthritis of the knee is much more common than posttraumatic arthritis.[6]

Dr. Ostrum or an immediate family member serves as a paid consultant to or is an employee of Smith & Nephew and has received research or institutional support from AONA and Synthes.

In a current review of open reduction and internal fixation (ORIF) combined with external fixation in treating high-energy tibial plateau fractures, 6.5% of the patients had severe arthritis at 8-year follow-up. This finding indicates that the cartilage of the knee joint is relatively tolerant of both articular injury and displacement.[7]

The incidence of patients with a tibial plateau fracture who ultimately require total knee arthroplasty is low; however, the complication rate is high.[8,9] From 1988 to 1999, surgeons at the Mayo Clinic performed 13,821 total knee arthroplasties, but only 62 (0.0045%) were performed because of a previous tibial plateau fracture.[8] Twenty-six percent of the patients had a postoperative complication, and 21% required another surgical procedure.[8,9]

The literature does not support the belief that an intra-articular tibial plateau fracture will usually progress to arthritis. With appropriate treatment, the rate of severe arthrosis is low, and functional results, even at longer-term follow-up, are good.

Pilon Fractures

Osteoarthritis of the knee is predominantly nontraumatic in origin. Only 9.8% of knee osteoarthritis is related to traumatic injuries; however, almost 80% of all ankle arthritis occurs after a traumatic injury.[10] Consultations for ankle osteoarthritis are less common (4.4%) compared with those for knee osteoarthritis (41.2%).[10] In a review of 270 cases of posttraumatic ankle arthritis, Horisberger et al[11] reported that there was a higher incidence of arthritis in patients with malleolar fractures (53.2%, n = 75) compared with pilon fractures (29.1%, n = 41). The average latency period from the time of fracture to the development of osteoarthritis was 20.9 years, but this latency period was shorter if complications occurred during the healing process. A correlation between the severity of the injury and the latency period to arthritis development was reported in the group with pilon fractures but not in the group with malleolar fractures.[11]

It is reasonable to ask if current techniques of staged fixation, with more consideration given to the soft tissues, decreases the rate of complications and/or subsequent arthritis. A study by Marsh et al[12] showed that at 5 to 12 years after limited joint fixation and the application of an external fixator, radiographic arthrosis was predicted by the severity of the injury and the accuracy of the reduction. However, these variables did not have a significant relationship with ankle function, pain, general health, or return-to-work status. Patient-specific socioeconomic factors had the greatest influence on the assessed outcome measures. Only 5 of 40 patients (12.5%) required ankle fusion, and the symptoms continued to decrease over time.[12]

A study by Harris et al[13] reported that high-energy tibial pilon fractures with comminution and open fractures had a higher complication rate, more secondary procedures, and worse outcomes than less severe fractures at an average follow-up of 2 years. Fewer complications occurred in the patients treated with ORIF compared with the group treated with limited internal fixation and a ring fixator; however, the authors recognized a selection bias because more severe fractures were treated with external fixation. Two small series showed that delayed ORIF after initial temporizing external fixation can lead to fewer soft-tissue complications and infections and possibly better overall results.[14,15] Three treatment techniques were compared for severe Orthopaedic Trauma Association (OTA) type C pilon fractures in three groups with small numbers of patients. One group was treated with immediate one-stage classic ORIF, another with limited internal fixation with longer-term external fixation, and the third group with a two-stage approach with immediate external fixation followed by ORIF when soft-tissue swelling diminished.[14] Twenty-three percent of the patients in the study required later ankle fusion for arthritis; however, none of those patients were in the two-stage treatment group. Range of motion, pain, and limitations of activities were slightly better in the group treated with the two-stage technique, but the difference was not statistically significant. It appears that more advanced soft-tissue techniques may lead to improved results and fewer complications, but the numbers in the literature are small. Although orthopaedic surgeons may believe that staged internal fixation is the better treatment option, the literature indicates that the results of tibial pilon fracture treatment are more likely secondary to the initial degree of articular injury and the ability to achieve an acceptable reduction.[14-18] The rate of ankle fusion is 5% to 30% and appears to be related to the degree and severity of the initial articular damage.[14-18]

Controversy still exists whether the articular injury or the surgical reduction is more important in influencing the final outcome of pilon fracture treatment. In two studies using rank-order analysis, the answer remains unclear.[19,20] With good interobserver reliability, surgeons ranked the severity of the articular injury and the quality of the open reduction. These parameters were correlated with functional ankle scores and radiographs. They found that fractures with the greatest articular injury had the worst reductions, and the best reductions were achieved in the less severely injured ankles. Because the variables of injury severity and articular reduction could

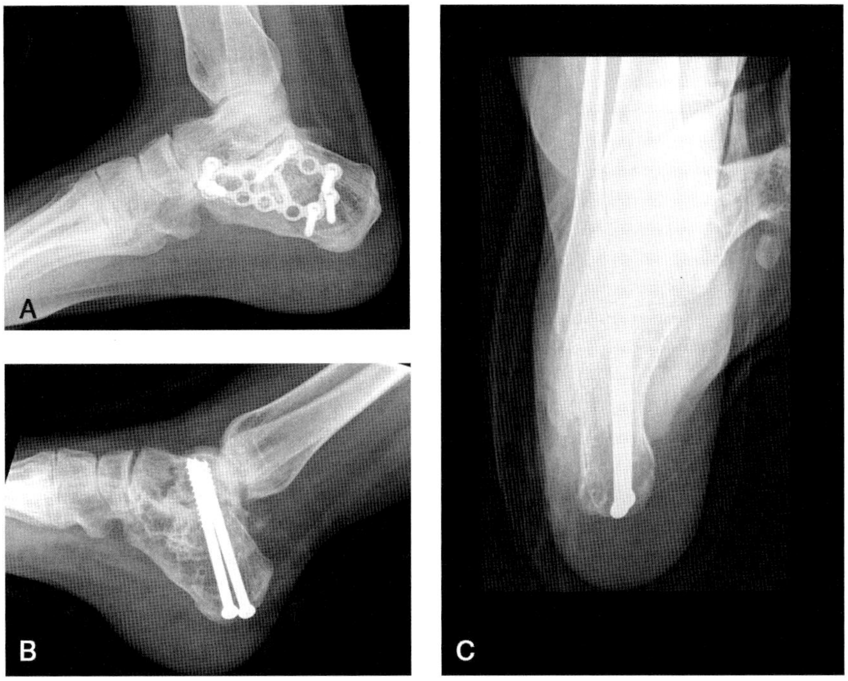

Figure 1 **A,** Radiograph of the foot of a 22-year-old woman with subtalar arthritis 3 years after treatment of a calcaneus fracture with ORIF. Note the overall restoration of the architecture of calcaneus. Lateral (**B**) and axial (**C**) views after subtalar fusion by compression arthrodesis. No additional procedures were needed to prepare the two articular fragments, which were well aligned and congruent.

not be separated, it is unclear which parameter is a better predictor of outcome.[19,20] When further analysis was performed on pilon fractures, neither injury severity nor reduction quality correlated with clinical scores; however, the quality of the reduction was associated with radiographic arthrosis.[20] Whether the severity of the injury or a less than perfect reduction is the causative factor in the development of ankle osteoarthritis remains unanswered because they are intimately linked together. The literature does not support the idea that a better reduction leads to a better clinical result; however, it should be remembered that the rate of fusion for posttraumatic ankle arthritis is only 3% to 9%.[19,20] Because the quality of the reduction correlates with later arthritis, the surgeon should strive for the best possible reduction when treating pilon fractures. With the low incidence of end-stage arthritis requiring arthrodesis, it is prudent to achieve a reasonable open reduction on all pilon fractures; reasonably good clinical results can then be expected.

Calcaneus Fractures

In a large, randomized controlled trial, Buckley et al[21] and Csizy et al[22] reported no substantial differences in Medical Outcomes 36-Item Short Form and visual analog scores when comparing surgically and nonsurgically treated calcaneus fractures. The authors found a statistical difference in the rate of subtalar arthrodesis and reported that ORIF reduced the risk of fusion by 83% when compared with nonsurgical treatment. A recent meta-analysis of calcaneus fracture treatment found that surgical treatment may be superior to nonsurgical care by allowing a faster return to work and fewer restrictions on shoe wear and can potentially be beneficial to women, those with lighter workloads, younger men, and patients with a lower Boehler angle.[23] Patients receiving workers' compensation, those older than 50 years, men, and those in occupations requiring heavy labor may benefit from nonsurgical management.[23]

In a series of 600 calcaneus fractures treated with ORIF by an experienced surgeon, only 6% of these fractures eventually required subtalar fusion[24] (**Figure 1**). A comparison of subtalar fusions in patients treated with ORIF and those treated nonsurgically showed that the surgically treated patients had fewer complications and higher foot and ankle scores than the nonsurgically treated group.[24] The authors concluded that subtalar fusion secondary to arthritis after ORIF yielded better clinical results than arthrodesis after nonsurgical treatment (**Figure 2**).

Patients with nonsurgically treated calcaneus fractures were 1.5 times more likely to have pain than those treated surgically and 6 times more likely to have a fusion.[22,25] Pain and the inability to return to work were much more common after nonsurgical management of calcaneus fractures than after surgical treatment, and the complication rate after subtalar fusion was higher than in those who were initially treated surgically.

Summary

The literature provides the evidence to disprove several myths about intra-articular fractures. Study results show that intra-articular fractures are not best treated by just preserving bone stock. Patients with severe intra-articular fractures do not always require a later reconstructive procedure, regardless of the type of treatment provided. Surgical treatment for commi-

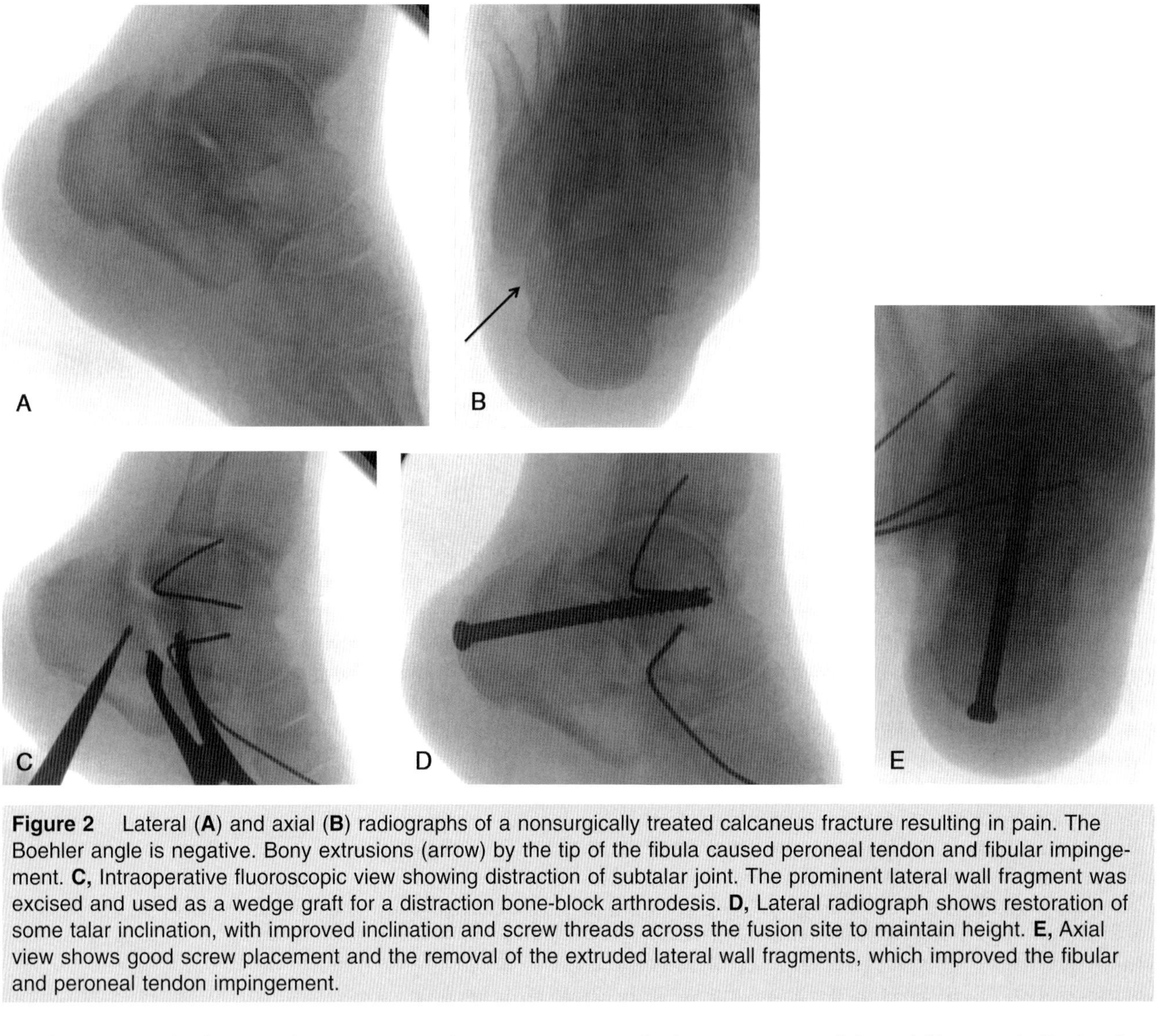

Figure 2 Lateral (**A**) and axial (**B**) radiographs of a nonsurgically treated calcaneus fracture resulting in pain. The Boehler angle is negative. Bony extrusions (arrow) by the tip of the fibula caused peroneal tendon and fibular impingement. **C,** Intraoperative fluoroscopic view showing distraction of subtalar joint. The prominent lateral wall fragment was excised and used as a wedge graft for a distraction bone-block arthrodesis. **D,** Lateral radiograph shows restoration of some talar inclination, with improved inclination and screw threads across the fusion site to maintain height. **E,** Axial view shows good screw placement and the removal of the extruded lateral wall fragments, which improved the fibular and peroneal tendon impingement.

nuted intra-articular fractures does not have high complication or infection rates, and viable salvage plans are still an option; ORIF preceding posttraumatic arthritis may provide better patient outcomes. Patients with tibial plateau fractures have good outcomes with ORIF, and few require later arthroplasty. Pilon fractures with severe comminution may not be able to be reduced perfectly, but it is difficult to establish if the clinical result is determined by the quality of the reduction or the severity of the initial injury. A better reduction may lead to a decrease in later ankle arthritis. Patients with nonsurgically treated calcaneus fractures have more pain, a higher incidence of posttraumatic arthritis, and a higher complication rate after subtalar arthrodesis than those who are initially treated surgically.

References

1. Andriacchi TP: Dynamics of knee malalignment. *Orthop Clin North Am* 1994;25(3):395-403.
2. Huch K, Kuettner KE, Dieppe P: Osteoarthritis in ankle and knee joints. *Semin Arthritis Rheum* 1997;26(4):667-674.
3. Rasmussen PS: Tibial condylar fractures: Impairment of knee joint stability as an indication for surgical treatment. *J Bone Joint Surg Am* 1973;55(7):1331-1350.
4. Honkonen SE: Degenerative arthritis after tibial plateau fractures. *J Orthop Trauma* 1995;9(4):273-277.
5. Lansinger O, Bergman B, Körner L, Andersson GB: Tibial condylar fractures: A twenty-year follow-up. *J Bone Joint Surg Am* 1986;68(1):13-19.
6. Volpin G, Dowd GS, Stein H, Bentley G: Degenerative arthritis after intra-articular fractures of the knee: Long-term results. *J Bone Joint Surg Br* 1990;72(4):634-638.

7. Weigel DP, Marsh JL: High-energy fractures of the tibial plateau: Knee function after longer follow-up. *J Bone Joint Surg Am* 2002;84(9):1541-1551.
8. Weiss NG, Parvizi J, Trousdale RT, Bryce RD, Lewallen DG: Total knee arthroplasty in patients with a prior fracture of the tibial plateau. *J Bone Joint Surg Am* 2003;85(2):218-221.
9. Saleh KJ, Sherman P, Katkin P, et al: Total knee arthroplasty after open reduction and internal fixation of fractures of the tibial plateau: A minimum five-year follow-up study. *J Bone Joint Surg Am* 2001;83(8):1144-1148.
10. Brown TD, Johnston RC, Saltzman CL, Marsh JL, Buckwalter JA: Posttraumatic osteoarthritis: A first estimate of incidence, prevalence, and burden of disease. *J Orthop Trauma* 2006;20(10):739-744.
11. Horisberger M, Valderrabano V, Hintermann B: Posttraumatic ankle osteoarthritis after ankle-related fractures. *J Orthop Trauma* 2009;23(1):60-67.
12. Marsh JL, Weigel DP, Dirschl DR: Tibial plafond fractures: How do these ankles function over time? *J Bone Joint Surg Am* 2003;85(2):287-295.
13. Harris AM, Patterson BM, Sontich JK, Vallier HA: Results and outcomes after operative treatment of high-energy tibial plafond fractures. *Foot Ankle Int* 2006;27(4):256-265.
14. Blauth M, Bastian L, Krettek C, Knop C, Evans S: Surgical options for the treatment of severe tibial pilon fractures: A study of three techniques. *J Orthop Trauma* 2001;15(3):153-160.
15. Sirkin M, Sanders R, DiPasquale T, Herscovici D Jr: A staged protocol for soft tissue management in the treatment of complex pilon fractures. *J Orthop Trauma* 1999;13(2):78-84.
16. Ovadia DN, Beals RK: Fractures of the tibial plafond. *J Bone Joint Surg Am* 1986;68(4):543-551.
17. Teeny SM, Wiss DA: Open reduction and internal fixation of tibial plafond fractures: Variables contributing to poor results and complications. *Clin Orthop Relat Res* 1993;292:108-117.
18. Wyrsch B, McFerran MA, McAndrew M, et al: Operative treatment of fractures of the tibial plafond: A randomized, prospective study. *J Bone Joint Surg Am* 1996;78(11):1646-1657.
19. Marsh JL, Buckwalter J, Gelberman R, et al: Articular fractures: Does an anatomic reduction really change the result? *J Bone Joint Surg Am* 2002;84-A(7):1259-1271.
20. DeCoster TA, Willis MC, Marsh JL, et al: Rank order analysis of tibial plafond fractures: Does injury or reduction predict outcome? *Foot Ankle Int* 1999;20(1):44-49.
21. Buckley R, Tough S, McCormack R, et al: Operative compared with nonoperative treatment of displaced intra-articular calcaneal fractures: A prospective, randomized, controlled multicenter trial. *J Bone Joint Surg Am* 2002;84(10):1733-1744.
22. Csizy M, Buckley R, Tough S, et al: Displaced intra-articular calcaneal fractures: Variables predicting late subtalar fusion. *J Orthop Trauma* 2003;17(2):106-112.
23. Bajammal S, Tornetta P III, Sanders D, Bhandari M: Displaced intra-articular calcaneal fractures. *J Orthop Trauma* 2005;19(5):360-364.
24. Radnay CS, Clare MP, Sanders RW: Subtalar fusion after displaced intra-articular calcaneal fractures: Does initial operative treatment matter? *J Bone Joint Surg Am* 2009;91(3):541-546.
25. Randle JA, Kreder HJ, Stephen D, Williams J, Jaglal S, Hu R: Should calcaneal fractures be treated surgically? A meta-analysis. *Clin Orthop Relat Res* 2000;377:217-227.

4

SYMPOSIUM

Orthopaedic Trauma Mythbusters: Is Limb Salvage the Preferred Method of Treatment for the Mangled Lower Extremity?

Robert A. Probe, MD

Abstract

Orthopaedic education is replete with unsubstantiated recommendations (myths) from predecessors in the field of orthopaedics. Even in the presence of sound evidence, some of these myths can be perpetuated through generations. One such recommendation is that if a mangled lower extremity can be saved, it should be saved. Recent technical and biologic advances allow the salvage of limbs that often required amputation in the past. Today's physicians must decide whether the physical, emotional, and financial costs of limb salvage can be justified by the expected functional outcome. Accumulated evidence suggests that functional outcomes are similar for amputation and limb salvage, whereas those treated with limb salvage have more hospitalizations and longer treatment times.

Instr Course Lect 2013;62:35-40.

In recent decades, orthopaedic advances have made possible the salvage and ultimate reconstruction of limbs that often would have required amputation in the past. Along with the technologic advancements came the recommendation that all limbs that can be saved should be saved. Increasing amounts of clinical outcome data now allow examination of the validity of that recommendation and the clinical decision making that surrounds the treatment of severe limb injuries.

Background

Historically, the value of amputation surgery in the United States was proved by the dramatic improvement in patient survival rates when amputation was used as a definitive treatment for open tibial fractures. During the Civil War, open fractures of the lower extremity had a high mortality rate; that rate was dramatically decreased with the introduction of limb amputation for the most severe wounds.[1] This practice continued through World War II, when most amputations were performed for isolated injuries to bone and muscle rather than for vascular reasons.[2]

During the latter half of the 20th century, advances occurred in antibiotic therapy, internal and external fixation, bone grafting, rotational and free-tissue transfer, and vascular reconstruction. The nascent discipline of orthopaedic traumatology proceeded to use these newfound tools to salvage limbs, with the presumption that a retained extremity would provide better function than a prosthesis. In 1987, this strategy of salvage at all costs was questioned in a retrospective analysis of open tibial shaft fractures by Caudle and Stern.[3] They reported that in Gustilo type IIIB fractures not covered within 7 days and in all type IIIC fractures, the rate of both nonunion and infection was more than 50%, with many patients requiring delayed amputation. The authors concluded that "primary amputation should be seriously considered as a reliable and dependable means of restoring function..." Georgiadis et al[4] retrospectively compared 16 patients with open tibial fractures reconstructed using

Dr. Probe or an immediate family member serves as a board member, owner, officer, or committee member of the Orthopaedic Trauma Association, Scott & White Healthcare, and the Scott & White Memorial Hospital; is a member of a speakers' bureau or has made paid presentations on behalf of Synthes and Stryker; and serves as a paid consultant to or is an employee of Stryker.

free-tissue transfer with a group treated with early amputation. In the limb salvage group, more time was required to full weight bearing, the patients were less willing or able to work, and hospital costs were higher. More of the patients treated with limb salvage considered themselves severely disabled and reported more problems in the performance of occupational and recreational activities than those treated with amputation.

Amputation Versus Limb Salvage: Considerations

Although the Georgiadis et al[4] study suggests that amputation might be a preferable treatment of the mangled lower extremity, the increased energy expenditure of prosthetic walking and the maintenance costs of prosthetic devices present challenges to the amputee.[5] This is particularly true of above-knee amputations because the metabolic cost of walking is 50% greater than in normal individuals.[6]

In the early phases of evaluating patients with mangled lower extremities, treatment decisions are difficult because of the gravity and irreversibility of a decision to amputate. Compounding this dilemma is the fact that the difficulties encountered in attempted reconstruction are speculative, and the long-term outcomes of reconstruction are unknown. Many physicians attempt limb salvage in all situations and choose amputation only when salvage appears futile. This strategy often leads to delayed amputation. The patient ultimately loses his or her limb and also sacrifices both time and resources in the failed attempt at limb salvage. The retention of a compromised extremity also introduces the potential for systemic infection and metabolic complications. Bondurant et al[7] reported that delayed amputation was associated with a substantial increase in the length of the hospital stay (53 days versus 22 days), higher costs ($53,462 versus $28,964), more surgical procedures (6.9 versus 1.6), and a 21% mortality rate from sepsis.

Scoring Systems

In an attempt to avoid delaying a needed amputation, various investigators have created scoring systems to predict the likelihood that a particular patient will require amputation. Developed in the 1990s, these scoring systems include the Mangled Extremity Severity Score;[8] the Limb Salvage Index;[9] the Predictive Salvage Index;[10] the Nerve Injury, Ischemia, Soft-Tissue Injury, Skeletal Injury, Shock, and Age of Patient Score;[11] and the Hannover Fracture Scale-98.[12] Each scoring system was developed by retrospectively reviewing a single institution's management of severely injured limbs. To predict outcomes, these scoring systems variably incorporate the early assessment of anatomic limb injury, perfusion, patient age, the presence of shock, and time to treatment. When these scoring systems were applied prospectively within the multiple centers participating in the Lower Extremity Assessment Project (LEAP) study, the initially reported degrees of accuracy could not be reproduced.[13] Assuming that all predictive tests have error rates, the mandate in selecting the threshold score for amputation would be to select a score that was highly specific and suggest amputation only in patients who were ultimately treated with amputation. This mandate for specificity comes with a requisite compromise in sensitivity to accurately predict all limbs that require amputation.

The practical implication is that these scoring systems can identify some but not all limbs that require amputation. In a prospective analysis by the LEAP study group, the Limb Salvage Index proposed by Russell et al[9] produced the best combination of specificity (97%) and a useful level of sensitivity (51%).[13] The Limb Salvage Index includes seven components: arterial, nerve, bone, skin, muscle, and deep venous injury, along with warm ischemia time (**Table 1**). It is distinguished from the other scoring systems by its more detailed anatomic assessment of the injured limb. This focus on anatomic injury, particularly with regard to sensory deficits, allows better prediction of both the challenges in the reconstructive phase and the ultimate functional return. Although once considered an indication for amputation, a more recent prospective study has demonstrated that most limbs that are insensate at presentation will recover sensation without adverse functional consequences.[14]

Expected Functional Outcome

Although the Limb Salvage Index can provide support for the decision to perform immediate amputation, the expected functional outcome is an important factor in choosing limb salvage or amputation. The understanding of functional outcome was enhanced by a 2002 study of the functional outcomes of 569 patients at risk for limb amputation.[15] In this prospective multicenter trial, the LEAP study group collected and correlated detailed injury data with functional outcome scores using the Sickness Impact Profile (SIP). The 24-month outcomes were poor in the group treated with limb salvage and in those treated with immediate amputation. In both groups, 40% of the patients had a severe disability based on SIP scores, and only 50% had returned to work. When adjusting for injury severity, the SIP impairment scores were identical in both the amputation and the limb salvage groups. At an average follow-up of 7 years after injury, the physical and psychosocial subsections of the SIP scores showed functional deterioration and no discernable differences between the limb salvage and amputation groups.[16]

Complication Rates

The incidence and severity of expected complications is also relevant in the process of choosing amputation or limb salvage. In a study by Harris et al,[17] complications were reported in 34% of the amputation group; however, the complications were typically wound infections or dehiscences that could be readily treated. In contrast, complications in the limb salvage group were more common (89%), severe, and delayed in onset. Most notably, the incidence of osteomyelitis (8.6%) and nonunion (31%) in the limb salvage group led to increased rates of rehospitalization, cost, and disability.[17] Considered in the complication rate were patient factors such as current smoking, which decreased the rate of fracture union by 37%, doubled the infection rate, and increased the risk of osteomyelitis 3.7 times.[18]

Other Variables Affecting Outcomes

Although the choice of definitive treatment did not produce demonstrable differences in outcomes, the presence of a major complication, a low educational level, nonwhite race, poverty, a lack of private health insurance, a poor social support network, low self-efficacy, smoking, and involvement in disability compensation were associated with a poorer outcome. The influence of these variables shows the influence of social determinants on outcomes and suggests that social interventions in addition to medical treatment may improve functional outcomes.[17]

Outcome Findings and Discussion

The findings of the LEAP study were corroborated by subsequent systematic

Table 1
Limb Salvage Index

Points	Components
	Artery Findings
0	Contusion, intimal tear, partial laceration or avulsion (pseudoaneurysm) with no distal thrombosis and palpable pedal pulses; complete occlusion of one of three shank vessels or profunda
1	Occlusion of two or more shank vessels, complete laceration, avulsion or thrombosis of femoral or popliteal vessels without palpable pedal pulses
2	Complete occlusion of femoral, popliteal, or three of three shank vessels with no distal runoff available
	Nerve Findings
0	Contusion or stretch injury; minimal clean laceration of femoral, peroneal, or tibial nerves
1	Partial transection or avulsion of sciatic nerve; complete or partial transection of femoral, peroneal, or tibial nerves
2	Complete transection or avulsion of sciatic nerve; complete transection or avulsion of both peroneal and tibial nerves
	Bone Findings
0	Closed fracture one or two sites; open fracture without comminution or with minimal displacement; closed dislocation without fracture; open joint without foreign body; fibula fracture
1	Closed fracture at three or more sites on same extremity; open fracture with comminution or moderate to large displacement; segmental fracture; fracture-dislocation; open joint with foreign body; bone loss < 3 cm
2	Bone loss > 3 cm; type IIIB or IIIC fracture (open fracture with periosteal stripping, gross contamination, and extensive soft-tissue injury/loss)
	Skin Findings
0	Clean laceration, single or multiple or small avulsion injuries, all with primary repair; first-degree burn
1	Delayed closure due to contamination; large avulsion requiring split-thickness skin graft or flap closure; second- and third-degree burns
	Muscle Findings
0	Laceration or avulsion involving a single compartment or tendon
1	Laceration or avulsion involving two or more compartments; complete laceration or avulsion of two or more tendons
2	Crush injury
	Deep Vein Findings
0	Contusion, partial laceration, or avulsion; complete laceration or avulsion if alternate route of venous return is intact; superficial vein injury
1	Complete laceration, avulsion, or thrombosis with no alternate route of venous return
	Warm Ischemia Time
0	Less than 6 hours
1	6 to 9 hours
2	9 to 12 hours
3	12 to 15 hours
4	More than 15 hours
Total score[a]	**Sum of the scores of the seven components**

[a]An absolute score of 6 or greater after summing the scores of the seven components provides an indication for amputation.

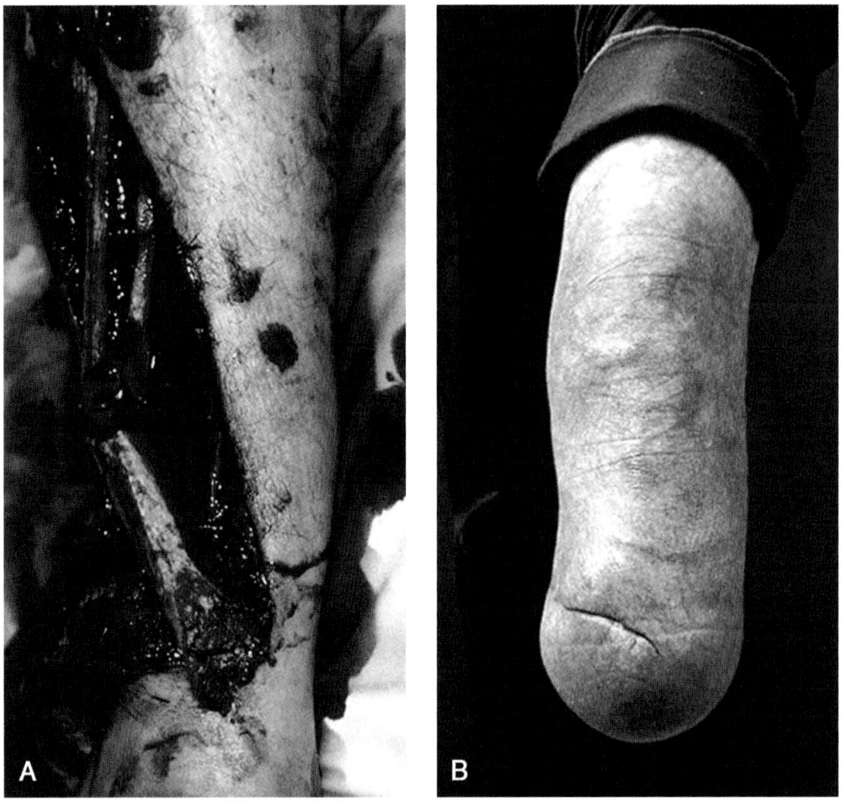

Figure 1 **A,** Clinical photograph shows extensive bone devitalization and wound contamination in the leg of a 66-year-old man injured in a farming accident. **B,** With the expected morbidity associated with reconstruction of this injury, the patient chose immediate amputation. Atypical laterally based flaps were used to preserve the length of the residual limb.

reviews. Busse et al[19] reported on eight observational studies and found no functional difference in patients treated with amputation and those treated with limb salvage. The authors also confirmed the high rates of disability and the dominance of social factors in determining outcomes. In an expanded systematic review of 28 observational studies, Saddawi-Konefka et al[20] reported increased rates of complications in the salvage group, a secondary amputation rate of 7.3%, and a 63.5% rate of return to work (compared with a 73% rate of return to work in those treated with amputation).

There seems to be little correlation between the treatment selected and patient satisfaction. Patient satisfaction is most influenced by the ability to return to work, physical function, residual pain, and walking speed.[21]

With the growing evidence that socioeconomic class, insurance status, and social support opportunities play a role in outcomes, it is appropriate that the resources available to an individual patient be considered in acute treatment decisions. Although the costs of care in the 2 years after injury are relatively comparable for limb salvage and amputation groups ($81,316 versus $91,106, respectively), this comparability does not apply to the lifetime costs. For the limb salvage group, the lifetime costs are estimated at $163,106. Because of the need to repair and replace lower limb prostheses, the average lifetime costs for the amputation group are estimated at $509,275. Even the best amputation will result in functional failure if an appropriate prosthesis cannot be used because of cost considerations.[22]

Pragmatically, there will be a subset of limbs in which the clinical appearance augmented by the Limb Salvage Index will strongly indicate the need for immediate amputation. At the other end of the spectrum, the limited extent of some injuries can predict a satisfactory outcome with limb salvage. In many cases, however, the injury will fall between those extremes, and the ultimate decision will be based on the surgeon's judgment. Given that the long-term functional outcomes are similar, careful consideration of the projected reconstructive path in combination with the patient's psychological profile, education, financial resources, social support system, and expectations and desires are major determinants in the decision-making process. This depth of knowledge about a patient is typically difficult to acquire on the day of injury. In the absence of severe associated injury, there is usually the opportunity to perform débridement and provisional stabilization on the day of injury followed by a thorough discussion with the patient and family regarding the predicted treatment courses and outcomes with limb salvage and amputation.

The Choice for Amputation

When amputation is chosen, the basic tenet of preserving as much limb length as possible while allowing for a quality soft-tissue cover applies. In functional outcome measurements of LEAP study patients, there was no difference in the SIP scores of those treated with above-knee versus below-knee amputations; however, more below-knee amputees could walk at a self-selected speed greater than 4 feet/s.[23] A substantial increase in the disability score and reduction in walking speed was reported in the through-knee amputation group. It

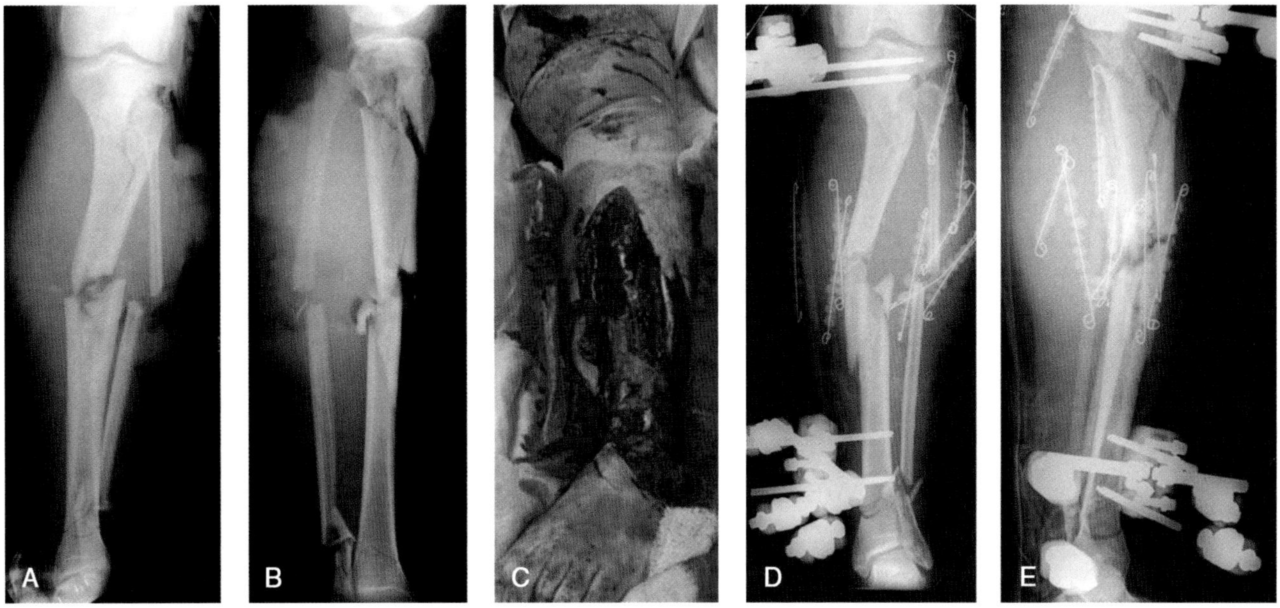

Figure 2 A 22-year-old patient sustained a crush injury resulting from a rollover by heavy machinery. AP (**A**) and lateral (**B**) preoperative radiographs of the tibia and fibula. **C,** Clinical photograph of the injured lower extremity. AP (**D**) and lateral (**E**) radiographs after immediate débridement of contaminated and devitalized tissue, half-pin external fixation, and bead-pouch management.

was theorized that this finding, which was contradictory to findings in the nontrauma literature, was secondary to the limited soft tissues available to cover the femoral condyles in patients with major traumatic injuries.[23] In the setting of trauma, the available reserve of skin often does not allow the use of conventional flaps. With priority given to limb-length preservation, these situations are best managed by using atypical flaps that have not been found to increase complication rates or decrease functional outcomes[23] (**Figure 1**).

The Choice for Limb Salvage

When limb salvage is chosen, the principles of open fracture care dictate initial management. Wounds are often heavily contaminated, with extensive zones of injury in which tissue devitalization often develops over time (**Figure 2**). Often, it is necessary to identify and remove this necrotic tissue with serial irrigation and débridement procedures. Skeletal stabilization is provided during these stages with simple external fixation, dead space is managed with antibiotic-laden cement, and temporary coverage is provided by bead pouches or vacuum-assisted closure devices. In amenable circumstances, external fixation should be converted to intramedullary stabilization after the need for circumferential débridement has passed.[24] Soft-tissue coverage should be done within 7 days of injury, with skeletal defects managed with antibiotic-laden cement spacers and secondary grafting or bone transport. Wounds should be closely monitored for any signs of infection; aggressive treatment is needed when infection is identified.

Summary

The presumption that limb salvage is warranted in all potentially viable traumatized limbs is a myth. A growing body of evidence suggests that functional outcomes are similar for amputation and limb salvage, whereas those treated with limb salvage have more hospitalizations and longer treatment times. It must also be recognized that technologies are advancing for both attempted reconstruction techniques and prosthetic devices. The biologic power of induced membranes, cellular therapies, and infection prevention therapy may someday improve limb salvage outcomes. At the same time, improvements in prosthetic devices, including the increasing use of advanced materials, energy returning designs, microprocessors, and osseointegration, provide optimism for better outcomes for amputees. It is hoped that future generations of patients, whether treated with amputation or limb salvage, will not incur the level of disability that currently exists after severe lower extremity injuries.

References

1. Kuz JE: The ABJS presidential lecture, June 2004: Our orthopaedic heritage. The American Civil War. *Clin Orthop Relat Res* 2004; 429:306-315.

2. Spittler AW, Taylor LW: Causes of amputations performed at Walter Reed General Hospital during 1947 and 1948. *J Bone Joint Surg Am* 1949;31(4):800-804.
3. Caudle RJ, Stern PJ: Severe open fractures of the tibia. *J Bone Joint Surg Am* 1987;69(6):801-807.
4. Georgiadis GM, Behrens FF, Joyce MJ, Earle AS, Simmons AL: Open tibial fractures with severe soft-tissue loss: Limb salvage compared with below-the-knee amputation. *J Bone Joint Surg Am* 1993; 75(10):1431-1441.
5. Waters RL, Perry J, Antonelli D, Hislop H: Energy cost of walking of amputees: The influence of level of amputation. *J Bone Joint Surg Am* 1976;58(1):42-46.
6. Jeans KA, Browne RH, Karol LA: Effect of amputation level on energy expenditure during overground walking by children with an amputation. *J Bone Joint Surg Am* 2011;93(1):49-56.
7. Bondurant FJ, Cotler HB, Buckle R, Miller-Crotchett P, Browner BD: The medical and economic impact of severely injured lower extremities. *J Trauma* 1988;28(8): 1270-1273.
8. Helfet DL, Howey T, Sanders R, Johansen K: Limb salvage versus amputation: Preliminary results of the Mangled Extremity Severity Score. *Clin Orthop Relat Res* 1990; 256:80-86.
9. Russell WL, Sailors DM, Whittle TB, Fisher DF Jr, Burns RP: Limb salvage versus traumatic amputation: A decision based on a seven-part predictive index. *Ann Surg* 1991;213(5):473-481.
10. Howe HR Jr, Poole GV Jr, Hansen KJ, et al: Salvage of lower extremities following combined orthopedic and vascular trauma: A predictive salvage index. *Am Surg* 1987;53(4):205-208.
11. McNamara MG, Heckman JD, Corley FG: Severe open fractures of the lower extremity: A retrospective evaluation of the Mangled Extremity Severity Score (MESS). *J Orthop Trauma* 1994; 8(2):81-87.
12. Tscherne H, Oestern HJ: A new classification of soft-tissue damage in open and closed fractures. *Unfallheilkunde* 1982;85(3):111-115.
13. Bosse MJ, MacKenzie EJ, Kellam JF, et al: A prospective evaluation of the clinical utility of the lower-extremity injury-severity scores. *J Bone Joint Surg Am* 2001; 83(1):3-14.
14. Bosse MJ, McCarthy ML, Jones AL, et al: The insensate foot following severe lower extremity trauma: An indication for amputation? *J Bone Joint Surg Am* 2005;87(12):2601-2608.
15. Bosse MJ, MacKenzie EJ, Kellam JF, et al: An analysis of outcomes of reconstruction or amputation after leg-threatening injuries. *N Engl J Med* 2002;347(24): 1924-1931.
16. MacKenzie EJ, Bosse MJ, Pollak AN, et al: Long-term persistence of disability following severe lower-limb trauma: Results of a seven-year follow-up. *J Bone Joint Surg Am* 2005;87(8):1801-1809.
17. Harris AM, Althausen PL, Kellam J, Bosse MJ, Castillo R; Lower Extremity Assessment Project (LEAP) Study Group: Complications following limb-threatening lower extremity trauma. *J Orthop Trauma* 2009;23(1):1-6.
18. Castillo RC, Bosse MJ, MacKenzie EJ, Patterson BM; LEAP Study Group: Impact of smoking on fracture healing and risk of complications in limb-threatening open tibia fractures. *J Orthop Trauma* 2005;19(3):151-157.
19. Busse JW, Jacobs CL, Swiontkowski MF, Bosse MJ, Bhandari M; Evidence-Based Orthopaedic Trauma Working Group: Complex limb salvage or early amputation for severe lower-limb injury: A meta-analysis of observational studies. *J Orthop Trauma* 2007; 21(1):70-76.
20. Saddawi-Konefka D, Kim HM, Chung KC: A systematic review of outcomes and complications of reconstruction and amputation for type IIIB and IIIC fractures of the tibia. *Plast Reconstr Surg* 2008; 122(6):1796-1805.
21. O'Toole RV, Castillo RC, Pollak AN, MacKenzie EJ, Bosse MJ; LEAP Study Group: Determinants of patient satisfaction after severe lower-extremity injuries. *J Bone Joint Surg Am* 2008; 90(6):1206-1211.
22. MacKenzie EJ, Jones AS, Bosse MJ, et al: Health-care costs associated with amputation or reconstruction of a limb-threatening injury. *J Bone Joint Surg Am* 2007; 89(8):1685-1692.
23. MacKenzie EJ, Bosse MJ, Castillo RC, et al: Functional outcomes following trauma-related lower-extremity amputation. *J Bone Joint Surg Am* 2004;86(8):1636-1645.
24. Webb LX, Bosse MJ, Castillo RC, MacKenzie EJ; LEAP Study Group: Analysis of surgeon-controlled variables in the treatment of limb-threatening type-III open tibial diaphyseal fractures. *J Bone Joint Surg Am* 2007;89(5): 923-928.

5

Locked and Minimally Invasive Plating: A Paradigm Shift? Metadiaphyseal Site-Specific Concerns and Controversies

Stephen A. Kottmeier, MD
Clifford B. Jones, MD, FACS
Paul Tornetta III, MD
Thomas A. Russell, MD

Abstract

Metadiaphyseal fractures of long bones are associated with considerable deforming forces, tenuous soft-tissue envelopes, and, often, severely compromised osseous integrity. Contemporary methods to fix complex metadiaphyseal fractures must achieve a balance between the biomechanical and biologic environments. The advent of precontoured locking plates inserted with evolving minimally invasive techniques may achieve both goals. Enthusiasm for their application demands continued scientific validation. Indications and outcomes must be carefully evaluated, and the benefits and limitations of this combination of implant design and surgical execution must be recognized.

Instr Course Lect 2013;62:41-59.

The advent of locking plate fixation has been described as a paradigm shift. The designation of this term to fixed-angle implant fixation appears valid in several respects. A paradigm shift by definition is not a minor event; it has a considerable effect within the realm of its purpose. In the preparadigm phase, a problem previously deemed difficult or unsolvable is identified. Methods to resolve it are offered, received, and adopted. As the paradigm shift is embraced, its application ascends rapidly and often without validation. As problems are "solved," new problems brought on by the shift become apparent. These new problems often were not previously recognized or deemed relevant. A critical assessment of the shift often ensues, and its acceptance is questioned. The stage is then set for another paradigm shift if conditions are appropriate. Whether locking plate fixation represents a paradigm shift can be viewed from the analysis of individual and collective experiences.

Historical Perspective

Haller offered a theory that bone was deposited from the vascularity around the reparative zone in response to injury.[1] This early understanding of the importance of the vascular network in fracture repair is one of the cornerstones of minimally invasive fracture surgery. Hunter, in support of Haller's theory, offered a four-stage classification of callus repair in fractures (inflammation, soft callus formation, hard callus formation, and remodeling). Goodsir of the University of Edinburgh described osteoblasts as the actual builders of bone. Macewen from the University of Glasgow, an active proponent of Goodsir's theory of osteoblastic formation, relegated the periosteum to insignificance in surgical approaches for fracture repair. Ollier, a surgeon and proponent of Duhamel du Monceau, an 18th century French physician, was convinced that the periosteum, bone marrow, and bone were the sources of osteogenesis. He argued for preservation of the periosteum with surgical approaches.[1]

Dr. Jones or an immediate family member serves as a board member, owner, officer, or committee member of the American Orthopaedic Association Own the Bone, the Mid American Orthopaedic Association Bylaws Committee, the Orthopaedic Trauma Association Outcomes and Classification Committee, and the Michigan Orthopaedic Society President. Dr. Tornetta or an immediate family member serves as a board member, owner, officer, or committee member of the American Orthopaedic Association and the Orthopaeidc Trauma Association; has received royalties from the Smith & Nephew; and serves as a paid consultant to or is an employee of Smith & Newphew. Dr. Russell or an immediate family member has received royalties from Smith & Nephew and Knee Creations; serves as a paid consultant to or is an employee of Innovision; serves as an unpaid consultant to ETEX; and has stock or stock options held in ETEX and Innovision. Neither Dr. Kottmeier nor any immediate family member has received anything of value from or has stock options held in a commercial company or institution related directly or indirectly to the subject of this chapter.

These respective theories are still evident in current surgical practices. Coincidental with the biologic concepts of fracture repair, the concept of open reduction of the fracture to prevent deformity began to be debated.

Danis was the dominant theorist of the 20th century.[2] His work in plating and his discoveries of interfragmentary compression and compression plating resulting in primary bone healing were promulgated and taught by Müller and the AO group. Willenegger, Müller, Allgöwer, and Schneider formed the AO in 1958.[2] Their research and standardization of instrumentation, implants, and educational programs have benefited physicians and patients for more than 50 years. The predominant focus for healing with this philosophy was bone, as was proposed by Macewen and Goodsir.

Difficulties with this primary bone healing theory surfaced in the application of these techniques to open and high-energy fractures, where anatomic reductions were not possible. This problem became a focus for the two other surgical schools of thought in the 20th century: external fixation and intramedullary nailing. These schools focused on callus as the primary method of reparative osteogenesis. Hoffman, although best known for his external fixator designs, contributed to the concept of closed reduction of fractures with the use of external devices through attachment with percutaneous pins. In 1938, he termed this process osteotaxis.[3] In 1939, Küntscher presented his preliminary study of nonreamed intramedullary nailing using the principles of closed reduction and intramedullary fixation. His described technique included the insertion of long nails introduced at a location remote from the fracture site, preserving the vascularity of the fracture periosteal environment. Ilizarov introduced the techniques of osteoreparative osteosynthesis with nonrigid external fixation and temporal sequential distraction; these techniques were diametrically opposed to the philosophy of Danis. The complexity of interactions, which lead to successful reparative osteogenesis, can now be viewed as a synthesis of these researchers' contributions.

Metaphyseal-diaphyseal fracture union is dependent on the effect of the surrounding biomechanical environment and several biologic factors. These consist of the adjacent fracture components; the respective viable periosteum; the void at the fracture site, which acutely and in the inflammatory phase is filled with hematoma and necrotic debris; and the adjacent soft-tissue envelope. These components give rise to a regenerative organ for reparative osteogenesis.

As Goodship and Kenwright[4] and De Bastiani et al[5] have shown, callus is sensitive to mechanical manipulation of the fixation construct during the reparative cycle. The growth and maturation of the cell lines in the torus are controlled by a negative feedback loop that terminates their growth phase after mechanical stability is obtained and the consolidation phase begins. In this model, vascular preservation is mandatory to allow revascularization of the zone of injury and bringing in stem cells and regional cell lines with the capability of metaplasia and cell mitogenesis to form new osteoblasts. This type of model allows for integration of all biologic factors and mechanical behaviors of the fracture repair mechanism. It also explains the benefits of minimally invasive techniques and suggests potential design modification goals for surgical implant constructs. More importantly, it may help surgeons understand the principles behind the various surgical techniques that have proven successful and predict new concepts for invention.

Locked plating with an emphasis on biologic fixation and secondary bone formation has been described as an internal form of external fixation. Interestingly, the first locked plate design, which would be recognized as a contemporary design, was invented by Hey-Groves of Bristol, England.[6] In describing the device mechanism, he stated, "The screw may instead be threaded into the plate, and there fixed by the grip of metal against metal in such a way that it never can become loose from the plate." Reinhold patented a very similar plate design to Hey-Groves in 1931, and it was commercialized by the Collin Company in 1935.[7] Locking plates then reemerged in Europe with the Wolter system (Litos/GmbH, Ahrensburg, Germany) in 1974[8] and the system developed by Zespol in Poland in 1982.[9]

AO designed and repopularized locked plating in the United States with the Less Invasive Stabilization System (LISS; Synthes, Paoli, PA) with its first implantation in 1995.[10] For the AO, this system was a major departure from Danis' theories of fracture repair. The results were impressive and led to a revitalization of plate and screw osteosynthesis, especially in lower extremity fractures.

It is necessary to recognize that all fractures do not require locked plates, but all fractures should be repaired with respect to the viability of the soft-tissue components in the zone of injury. In uncomplicated midshaft fractures of the radius and the ulna (Orthopaedic Trauma Association [OTA]/AO 22A), conventional AO compression plating with 3.5-mm plates and 3.5-mm cortical screws is the standard for care. The advantages of the locking plate systems are demonstrated in osteoporotic bone and metaphyseal–diaphyseal transition fractures that have a high rate of screw pull-out, such as distal femoral

(OTA/AO 33A) and periprosthetic fractures.

The combination of minimally invasive surgery and locking plates is an exciting development in osteosynthesis. Fracture reduction can now be achieved in a closed fashion and can provide an environment that engenders callus or torus formation of reparative bone. Articular components of metadiaphyseal fractures are simultaneously managed with anatomic reduction and interfragmentary compression as advocated by Danis. Contemporary implants and surgical fixation strategies emphasize optimal construct rigidity and strength while permitting early functional mobilization of the extremity.

The development of locking plates and their resultant success has moved orthopaedics away from the theories of primary bone healing for metaphyseal–diaphyseal fractures to view callus-type fracture healing or so-called secondary bone healing as a three-dimensional toroid structure that the surgeon can enhance and manipulate by optimizing the implant-bone construct. This is similar to the application and roles served by intramedullary and nonrigid external fixation devices. Krettek et al[11,12] first reported minimally invasive plate osteosynthesis for supracondylar femoral fractures in 1996. Minimally invasive surgical technique avoids trauma to the noninjured components of the fracture site by preserving the vascularity and substance of bone, the periosteum, and soft-tissue structures. This technique is adapted from the intramedullary and nonrigid external fixation schools of fracture surgery. In a vascular injection study on cadavers, minimally invasive plate osteosynthesis techniques appeared to preserve both endosteal and periosteal blood supply as well as regional nutrient vessels when compared with conventional plating methods.[13]

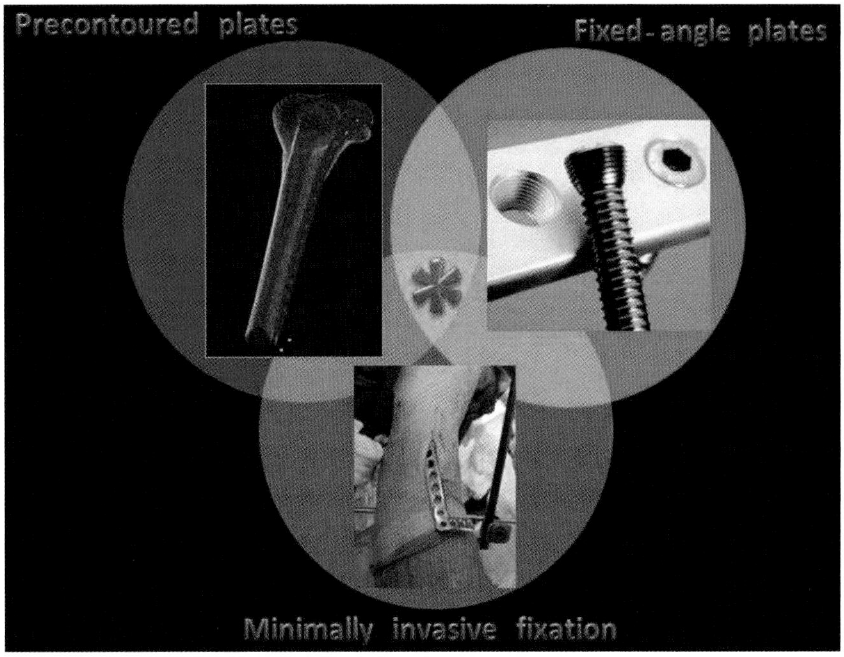

Figure 1 Illustration of the trinity of anatomic precontoured plates with fixed-angle interfaces and minimally invasive fixation. (Courtesy of Zimmer, Warsaw, IN.)

The Metadiaphyseal Trinity

The trinity of anatomic precontoured plates with fixed-angle interfaces using minimally invasive fixation has afforded new avenues in complex metadiaphyseal fracture fixation[3-5] (**Figure 1**). The management of these lesions is often complicated by the presence of a short periarticular segment, a tenuous soft-tissue envelope, regional deforming forces, and impaired bone quality. Contemporary locking plates and surgical methods for their insertion have favorably affected metadiaphyseal fracture fixation in both the upper and the lower extremities; however, there has been an evolving recognition of the limitations and liabilities of these devices and techniques.

Anatomic Precontoured Plate

Plates used for metadiaphyseal fixation before the advent of the anatomic precontoured design were often structurally weak and intolerant of regional biomechanical forces. Implant failure (screw and/or plate breakage) or construct deformity (plate bending) occasionally occurred. Prior to the development of anatomic designs, earlier implants with improper contours were often prone or contributed to malreduction (**Figure 2**). Preoperative designs fashioned on bone models, if incorrectly contoured, tended to induce deformity. Contemporary anatomically precontoured plates do not fit the "average" anatomic site for which they were designed but instead are designed to fit most patients. These designs, however, do not fit all patients.[14]

Fixed-Angle Interface

Fixed-angle plates offer an angular, stable interface that may be beneficial in the presence of impaired bone or regions of increased stress. These plates have been used to counteract varus forces, particularly in the proximal humerus, proximal tibia, and proximal and distal femur. Such devices applied

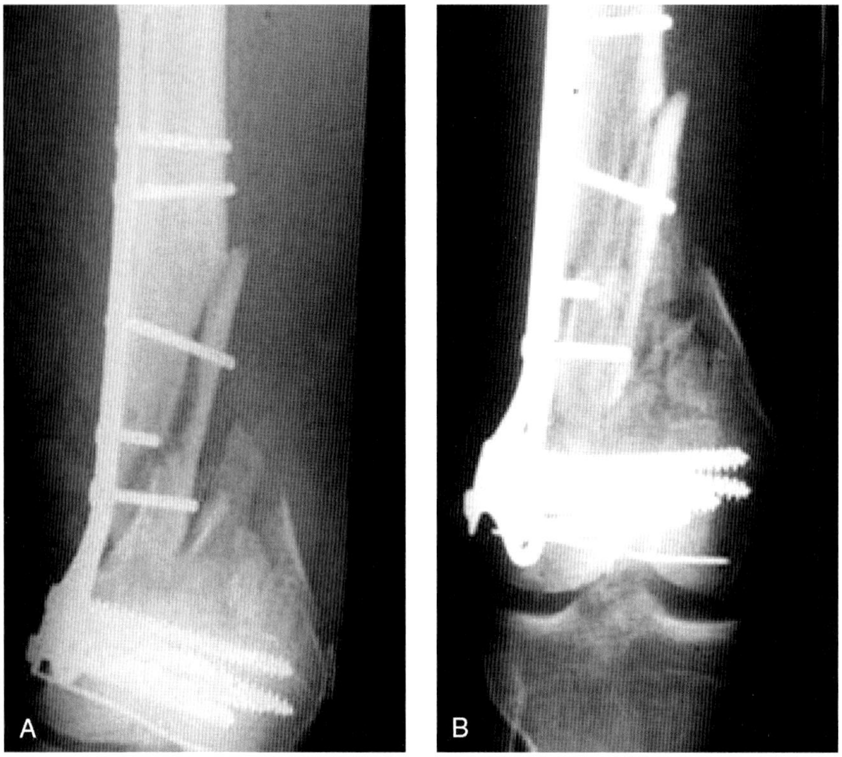

Figure 2 Lateral (**A**) and AP (**B**) radiographs of a lateral condylar buttress plate (circa 1988). Nonanatomically precontoured devices contributed to malreduction (valgus), were structurally weak, and contributed to fracture and implant deformity (varus).

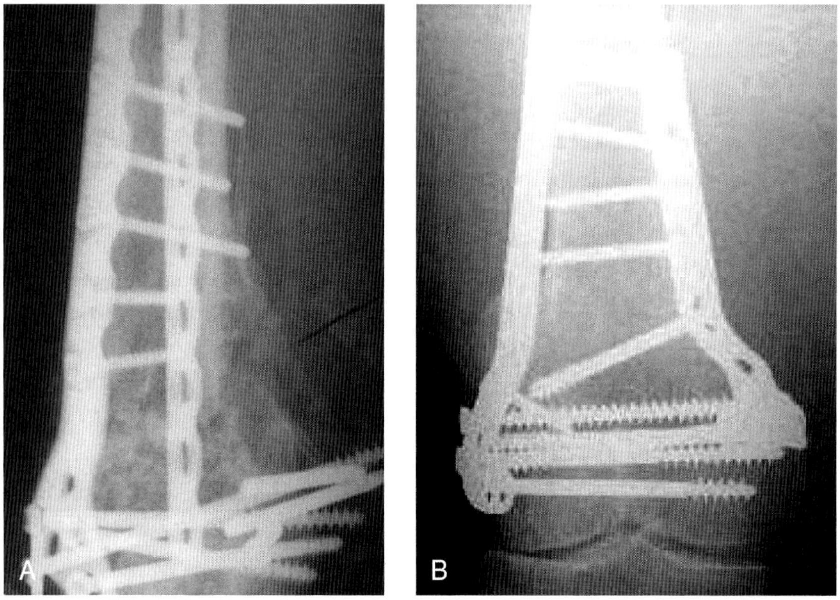

Figure 3 AP radiographs of endosteal substitution (intramedullary adjuvant plating) (**A**) and dual plating (**B**) of the distal femur.

laterally may obviate the need for additional adjuvant medial, endosteal, or dual plate constructs, which can contribute to motion deficits and the increased risk of infection[15-17] (**Figure 3**). If forces exceed the design limitations of these devices or if they are inserted improperly, poor results can be expected.

Minimally Invasive Fixation

Minimally invasive locking plate fixation, when used to manage complex metadiaphyseal fractures, combines implant design and surgical technique. The use of precontoured plates with a fixed-angle interface inserted in submuscular or subcutaneous fashion continues to evolve. The surgical goals include obtaining a satisfactory biomechanical environment while minimizing the risks of injury to soft tissues and osseous viability. Minimally invasive fixation does not mandate the use of locking plates nor does the use of locking plates mandate minimally invasive insertion techniques.

Anatomic reduction of comminuted metadiaphyseal fractures with interfragmentary compression affords absolute stability. Because of soft-tissue stripping, this stability comes at a considerable biologic price. In the presence of substantial metadiaphyseal comminution, indirect reduction techniques may be preferred.[18] Instead of absolute stability via interfragmentary compression, the intercalary fragments are indirectly reduced by traction exerted on the intact osseous soft-tissue attachments (**Figure 4**). Regional fracture biology is accordingly preserved. This results in tolerable instability and satisfactory secondary fracture healing (callus formation).

Although minimally invasive fracture fixation may pose a decreased risk of injury to the soft tissues and osseous blood supply than conventional fracture fixation techniques, it is still an

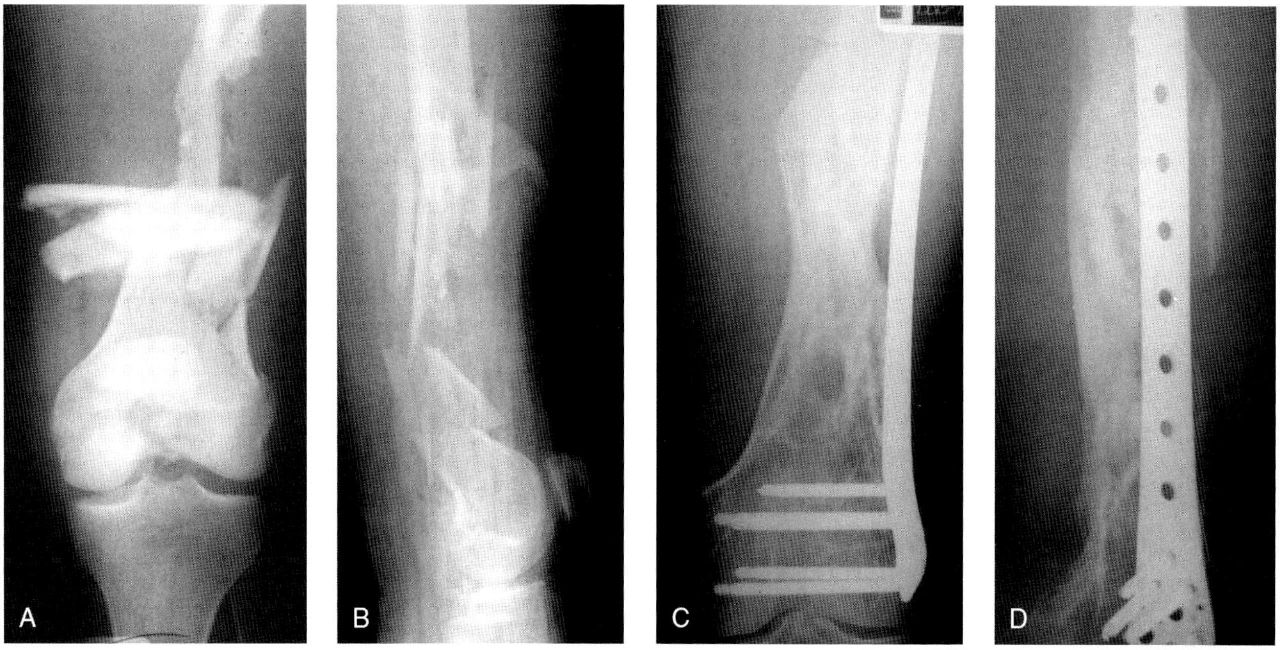

Figure 4 Using indirect reduction, intercalary fragments are reduced by ligamentotaxis with preservation of the osseous soft-tissue attachments and regional fracture biology. AP (**A**) and lateral (**B**) radiographs of a comminuted distal femoral supracondylar fracture. AP (**C**) and lateral (**D**) radiographs of the fracture after insertion of a submuscular LISS plate.

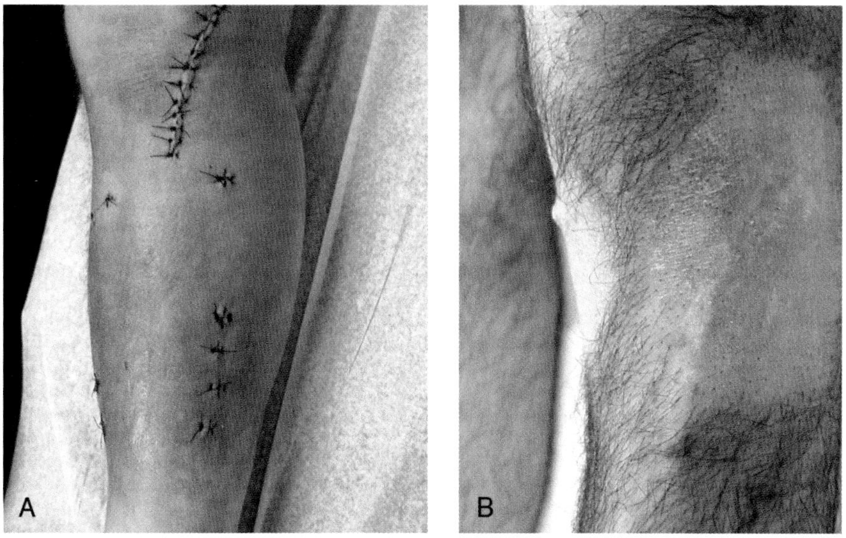

Figure 5 Subcutaneous and submuscular insertion of implants may pose a risk of injury to the soft tissues. Photographs of postoperative swelling (**A**) and implant prominence (**B**) after treatment of a proximal tibial fracture with submuscular locking plate fixation. The anterolateral approach was used, with distal percutaneous screw fixation.

invasive technique. Despite skillful observance to proper technique, the introduction of plates and screws within small subcutaneous and submuscular portals poses a considerable hazard to the cross-sectional anatomy. Iatrogenic injury to regional neurovascular structures has been described.[19-23] Although "overstuffing" limbs with plates when using minimally invasive techniques may not substantially contribute to the development of compartment syndrome, it may complicate wound healing[24,25] (**Figure 5, A**). Implant prominence and patient–implant-size incompatibility warrant consideration when electing minimally invasive fracture fixation (**Figure 5, B**).

Metadiaphyseal Site-Specific Concerns and Controversies

Controversies regarding metadiaphyseal fixation with locking plate technology range from clinical indication to surgical execution to outcome expectations. If the indication is improper or the execution is inadequate, outcome expectations should be low. Reported clinical outcomes suggest that results do not necessarily meet expectations. This section will focus on indications, execution, and

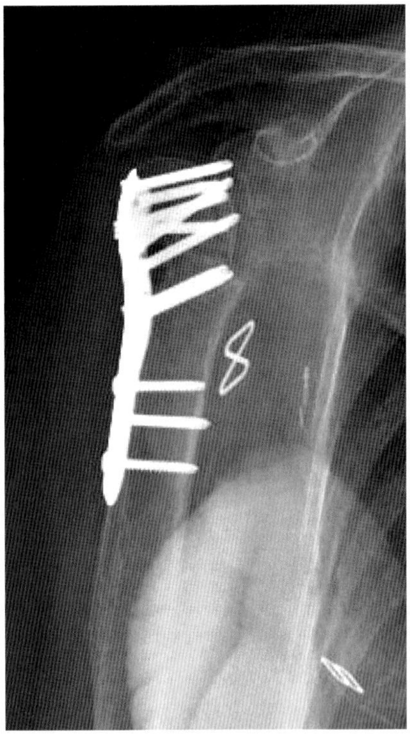

Figure 6 Radiograph showing proximal humeral osteonecrosis after fixation of a proximal humeral fracture. The selected approach and technique of plate insertion may have considerable effect on preservation of the osseous blood supply.

results with metadiaphyseal fracture fixation of the proximal humerus, proximal femur, distal femur, and proximal tibia.

Proximal Humerus

The fixation of proximal humeral fractures requires a balance between required exposure and adequate fixation. Surgical fixation of proximal humeral fractures may contribute to iatrogenically induced osteonecrosis[26,27] (**Figure 6**). Compromise to the viability of both the osseous and soft-tissue elements of the proximal humerus should be minimized. The pursuit of reduction at all costs must be reconsidered and the osseous blood supply preserved. The surgical exposure itself and overzealous dissection during the course of plating have been implicated in contributing to regional vascular impairment.[28] Surgical access strategies include either the familiar deltopectoral approach or a more recently advocated deltoid-splitting approach.[29,30]

The deltopectoral approach requires both considerable soft-tissue dissection and muscular retraction and affords an indirect approach to the osseous site of plate application proximally (the plating zone).[31] Its proximity to the anterior humeral circumflex artery and its terminal ascending branch may further jeopardize the blood supply to the osseous components of the proximal humerus. In this scenario, the surgical approach selected may violate the tenets of minimally invasive skeletal surgery. Another concern is the seemingly required detachment of a portion of the distal deltoid insertion for applying the inferior portion of the plate. This is required to afford a more favorable vector of drilling and screw insertion, owing to the voluminous size of the intact deltoid. Its insertion encompasses 40% of the humeral circumference. This broad attachment explains the need for incomplete detachment and the absence of any reported avulsions. An anatomic study has suggested a required detachment of 50% of the deltoid's insertion during the application of a 4.5-mm plate.[32] Klepps et al[33] described functional compromise to the anterior deltoid with release of as little as 20% of its insertion.

An alternative to the deltopectoral approach is the deltoid-splitting (transdeltoid) approach. The advantages of the deltoid-splitting approach include less required anterior dissection, the avoidance of additional surgical compromise to the osseous blood supply, direct access to the plating zone, and improved fracture plane access to both tuberosities and the surgical neck. Partial detachment of the deltoid insertion is not required because of the more favorable drill and screw trajectory.

The deltoid-splitting approach, as described by Gardner et al,[29,30] is initiated with a 10-cm anterolateral incision (**Figure 7, A**), beneath which is an avascular anterior raphe that is identified as a vertically oriented fat stripe (**Figure 7, B**). The direct plate access site, also referred to as the bare spot, is directly beneath this raphe and encompasses a zone 3 cm in diameter. A cadaver vascular latex polymer injection study suggested this is a hypovascular zone surrounded by anterior and posterior penetrating osseous vessels. Plate application within this region will not disturb these vessels.

The greatest obstacle to performing the deltoid-splitting approach is the risk of injury to the axillary nerve, which traverses the inferiormost portion of the exposure. In contrast to the deltoid-splitting approach, the deltopectoral approach does not carry a similar risk to the axillary nerve. Numerous studies, however, have suggested that there is no substantial detriment to the axillary nerve during dissection and implant insertion with the deltoid-splitting approach.[30,34-36] The anterior branch of the axillary nerve, predictably identified in the inferior portion of the wound, is identified and protected during the course of dissection and plate insertion (**Figure 8, A**). Its mobility is sufficient to allow introduction and fixation of a plate both proximally and distally beneath it (**Figure 8, B**). An inferior window is established for distal plate application and fixation.

Variations of the deltoid-splitting approach to the proximal humerus permit tuberosity fracture fragment reduction from within the fracture surfaces, an attribute not easily offered

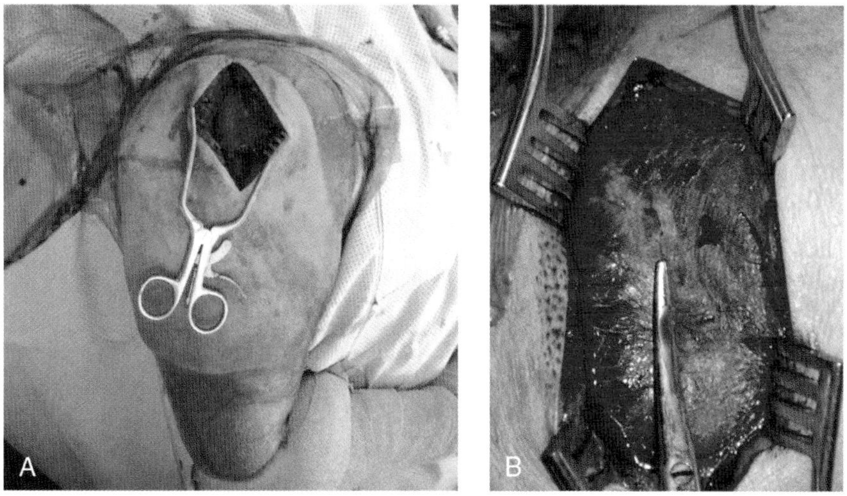

Figure 7 **A,** An anterolateral acromial incision is made with the deltoid-splitting approach to the proximal humerus. **B,** The anterior avascular raphe is identified by a vertically oriented fat stripe.

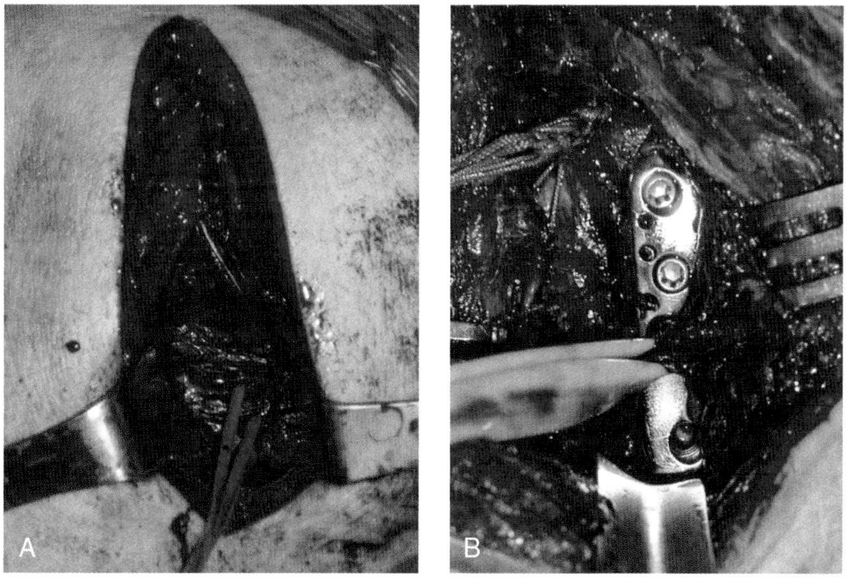

Figure 8 **A,** Using the deltoid-splitting approach, the anterior branch of the axillary nerve is identified in the inferior aspect of the wound. **B,** The axillary nerve is sufficiently mobile to allow plate insertion and afford upper and lower windows for proximal and distal screw insertion.

with the deltopectoral approach.[34] This invites the opportunity for more indirect reduction techniques, including external jig-facilitated fixation with the inclusion of distal percutaneous portals. A dual approach technique has been described in which both the deltopectoral and deltoid-splitting approaches are used.[37] This technique offers both the advantages of deltopectoral and deltoid-splitting access, as well as the risks and limitations of both approaches.

The mechanical performance of proximal humeral locking plates in clinical studies has been variable. Locking screws within laterally applied plates may not reliably prevent reduction loss when managing proximal humeral fractures.[38-41] Several studies have expressed concerns regarding loss of fixation, varus malunion, and the negative effect of varus alignment on both loss of fixation and resultant nonunion (**Figure 9, A**). It has been suggested that fixation adequacy may be in part proportional to the adequacy of reduction. Important factors in fixation failure include initial varus reduction and the absence of medial column support. The presence of medial column comminution may contribute to varus malreduction, and both conditions may contribute to fixation failure and resultant malunion or nonunion. Methods of manipulating the mechanical environment have been described to improve the adequacy of fixation. The surgical objective should be the re-creation of a medial buttress. A method to resolve a deficient medial column includes the introduction of inferomedial oblique locking screws within the fixation construct[26,42] (**Figure 9, B**). Endosteal substitution with an intramedullary allograft may also serve to counteract varus deforming forces[43,44] (**Figure 9, C**). A similar construct may be used to address refractory proximal humeral nonunions[45] (**Figure 10**). Conflicting data exist regarding the mechanical benefits of augmentation with calcium phosphate bone cement agents.[42,46]

Proximal Femur

Controversy exists regarding the indications for proximal femoral locking plate fixation. The challenges of managing subtrochanteric variants include displacement of the proximal fragment caused by the deforming forces of flexion, abduction, and external rotation. Unique regional anatomic, biomechanical, and biologic concerns also exist.

Indirect reduction techniques have been described to address comminuted

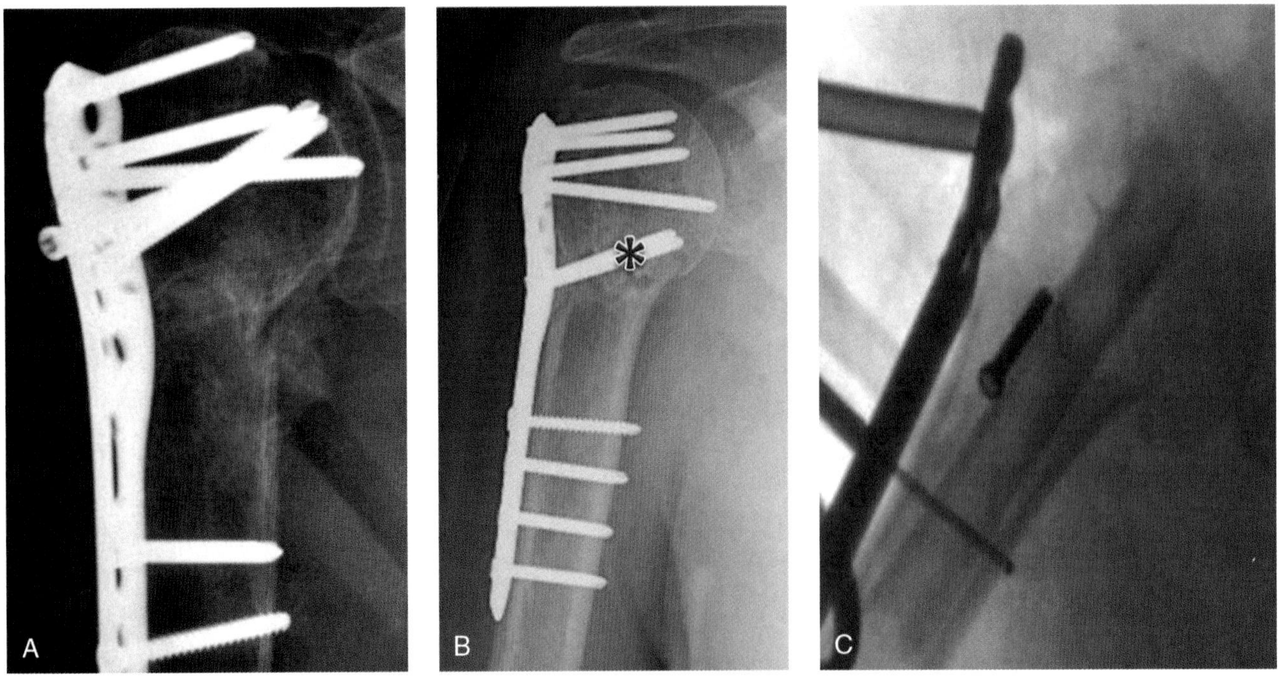

Figure 9 Radiographs of the proximal humerus. **A,** Varus reduction and the absence of medial reduction and support may contribute to malunion and nonunion. **B,** Inferomedial oblique locking screws (asterisk) enhance the stability of the construct. **C,** Intramedullary fibular allograft (endosteal implant) may offer medial columnar support. The graft is preferentially positioned medially at its proximal limit by screws within the plate or a blocking screw (shown here).

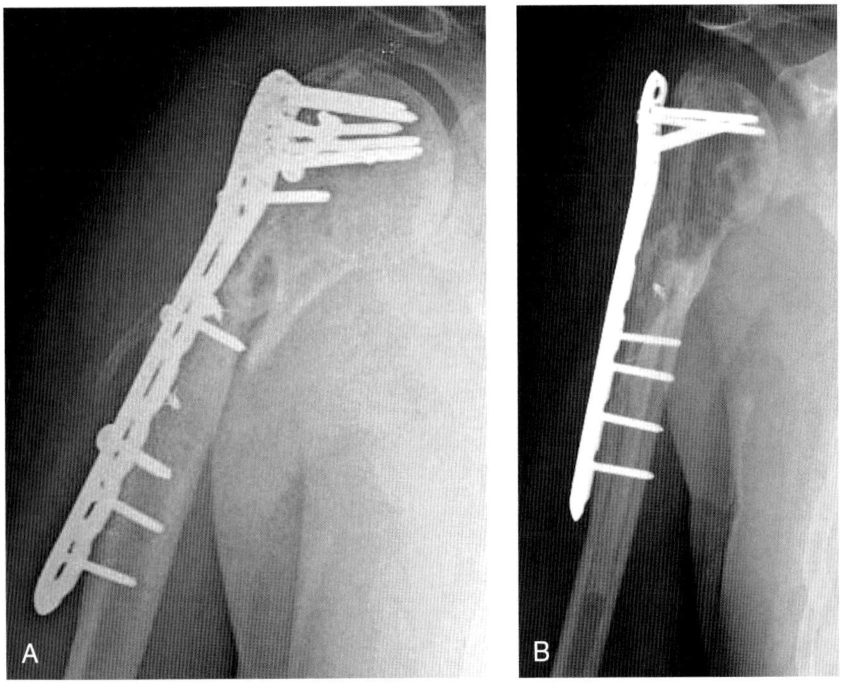

Figure 10 **A,** Radiograph of a comminuted metadiaphyseal proximal humeral fracture managed with a locking plate that resulted in aseptic nonunion and construct failure. **B,** Successful revision fixation was achieved with a locking plate and adjuvant intramedullary fibular allograft and cancellous autograft.

variants. Avoiding medial dissection and osseous devitalization serve to promote medial callous formation and consolidation. Conventional implants (dynamic condylar screw and blade plate) in combination with conventional open methods of indirect reduction have achieved satisfactory results[47-49] (**Figure 11**). These earlier efforts emphasized preserving regional biology and providing stability and weight-bearing restriction. Low infection and implant failure rates were described in combination with high rates of union. In the absence of medial surgical dissection, more predictable rates of consolidation were described when compared with direct techniques of reduction. Malreduction parameters of length and rotation, however, were described and remain a concern with more current techniques advocating minimally invasive surgery with contemporary implants.

The use of conventional implants with minimally invasive submuscular techniques of fixation to manage comminuted fractures of the proximal femur have been described.[50-52] Preserving biology and providing stability with protected loading were emphasized. No instances of nonunion or low nonunion rates were described, and implant failure was either minimal or nonexistent. Similar to open methods of indirect reduction, concern was directed toward outcomes showing nonanatomic reduction, which was primarily limited to length and rotational concerns, and, to a lesser degree, coronal plane malalignment.

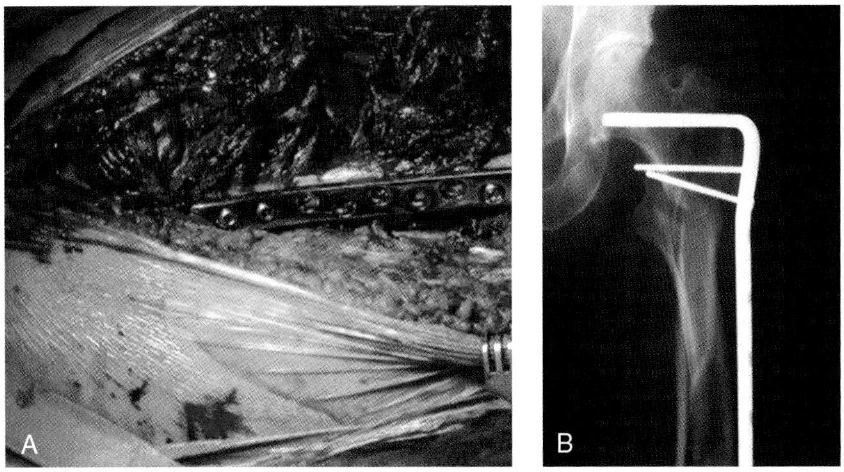

Figure 11 **A,** Open technique of indirect reduction of the proximal femur. Soft-tissue stripping is minimized, and osseous soft-tissue attachments are preserved. Screw fixation is performed proximal and distal to sites of interfragmentary comminution. **B,** Radiograph of blade plate fixation of a comminuted proximal femoral fracture using indirect reduction.

The role of contemporary proximal femoral locking devices remains undetermined. Indications include complex proximal femoral fracture patterns, including those with trochanteric extension, and reverse obliquity patterns. Perhaps the best use of these devices is to treat lesions when intramedullary implant applications cannot be considered, such as in patients with indwelling intramedullary hardware or small intramedullary dimensions.

Few studies have been done on proximal femoral locking plate fixation. Kregor et al[53] described 20 patients with complex subtrochanteric femoral fractures treated with locked plating. Submuscular techniques of insertion were described, and a union rate of 95% was reported. The authors reported no surgical infections and a single case of implant failure (plate breakage).

Proximal femoral locking plate fixation may be uniquely indicated for lesions with a deficient proximal segment or a preexisting deformity that is not suitable for intramedullary stabilization.[54,55] An additional attribute of laterally applied plate fixation in contrast to intramedullary nail fixation may include abductor preservation. Depending on the method of insertion, an intramedullary device may contribute to malreduction, whereas a laterally applied plate can facilitate alignment.

As with plating techniques in general and particularly metadiaphyseal fracture fixation of the proximal femur, the role of the plate must be defined before its selection and insertion. Bridge-plating techniques for simple fracture patterns can induce high strain and may result in nonunion and subsequent implant failure. Of particular concern are perceived simple fracture patterns with medial cortical compromise (**Figure 12**). Constructs incorporating relative stability with long working lengths and proper screw balance may preferentially induce secondary healing and result in satisfactory union. Several case studies have recently described the mechanical failure of proximal locking plates within the proximal femur.[56,57] Individual variables, such as appropriate indications, proper technique, and potential design flaws of the implant, must be assessed to determine the reasons for undesirable outcomes. If indirect reduction techniques are pursued, medial dissection must be minimized because this represents a region of both impaired vascular supply and substantial biomechanical stress (**Figure 13**). If the blood supply is surgically violated and construct adequacy or medial reduction are not achieved, this combination of poor blood supply and heightened stress can result in implant failure.

The use of proximal femoral locking plates to manage lesions proximal to the subtrochanteric region has been described. Catastrophic mechanical failure has been reported for both unstable intertrochanteric and femoral neck fractures.[58,59] Construct stiffness and increased implant mechanical burden have been implicated.

Distal Femur

Lateral plate fixation of the distal femur in contrast to other metadiaphyseal sites affords a robust and often intact soft-tissue envelope. From the perspective of the surgical approach, articular access and reconstitution are more easily achieved and are aided by multiplanar fluoroscopic imaging. Based on these attributes, contemporary techniques of minimally invasive

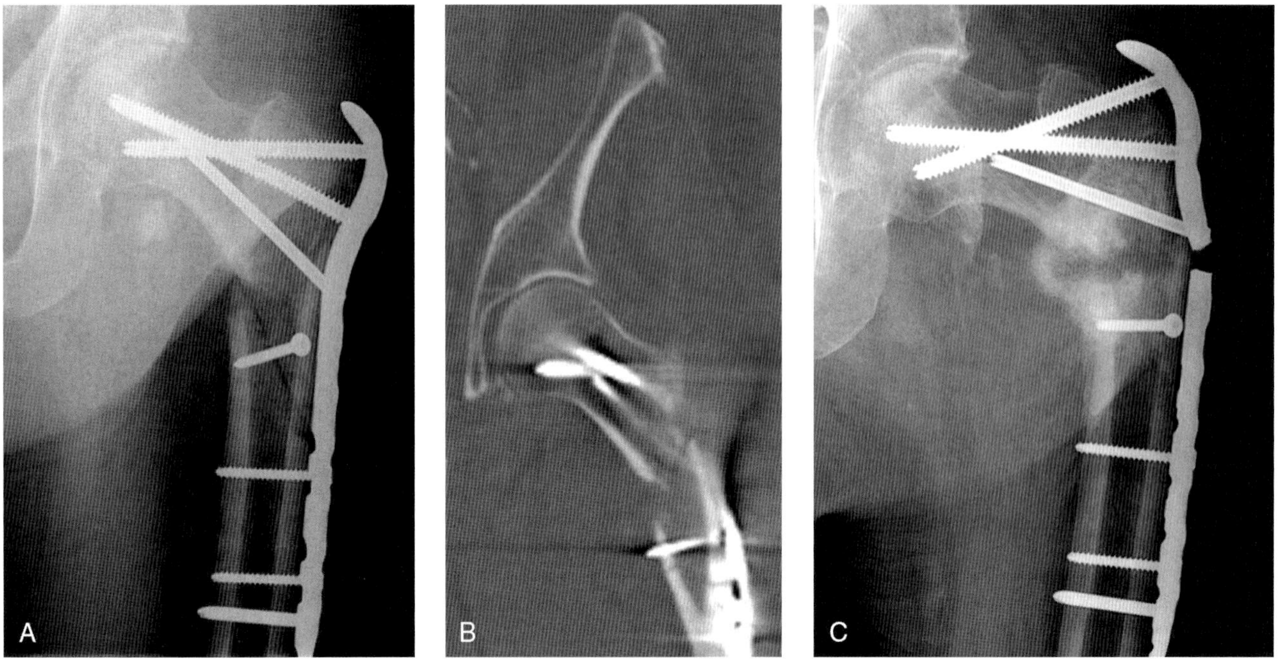

Figure 12 **A,** Radiograph of proximal femoral locking plate fixation of a minimally comminuted subtrochanteric fracture. Interfragmentary reduction and lag screw fixation required additional surgical dissection without establishing medial cortical continuity. **B,** Postoperative CT scan shows deficient medial cortical reconstitution. **C,** High regional biomechanical forces and surgical osseous devitalization contributed to nonunion and implant failure.

fracture fixation are appropriate for lateral plate fixation of the distal femur.

Open techniques of indirect reduction with the inclusion of conventional implants have achieved high union rates and low infection rates. Similarly, the introduction of submuscular (minimally invasive) techniques of indirect reduction and contemporary locking plate fixation have offered similar results.[60,61] Contemporary techniques (biologically benign) and contemporary implants (locking plate devices) appear to offer satisfactory biomechanical and biologic environments for positive outcomes. If reduction is achieved and maintained and the construct is sufficiently stable, union can be expected.

The limits of indirect reduction and the adequacies of implant capability still need to be defined. Limitations to indirect techniques of reduction on patient selection are difficult to recognize and establish. Open and higher energy fractures may lack sufficient biologic healing potential.

Union may be difficult to characterize from both clinical and conventional radiographic perspectives. Several studies have focused on methods to measure and maximize adequate callous formation.[60-62] One study reported enhanced callus formation with titanium rather than stainless-steel implants; this was particularly evident with open fractures.[62] Another study suggested that locking plate fixation of distal femoral fractures may result in inconsistent and asymmetric callus formation.[63,64]

In the management of distal femoral fractures, the optimal plate material, the length of the plate construct, and the location of the plate (medial versus lateral) have not been convincingly established. Multiple factors may contribute to implant failure in nonunited or incompletely united fractures with distal femoral locking plate constructs.[65,66] Implant design and composition; patient compliance; implantation techniques; and the use or absence of allograft, autograft, and osteoblastic grafts and fixation supplements should be considered when evaluating implant failure. Catastrophic failure of fixation may be subtle and delayed[67] (**Figure 14**). Implant failure may occur late in the treatment process, and the patient may not have clinical suggestions of impending implant failure. As with revision fixation of the proximal humerus, a unique concern associated with failed locking plate constructs is the presence of coronally oriented split fractures[68] (**Figure 15, A** through **C**). These fractures are caused by the multiple fixed-angle anchorage points of the locking plate and result in additional compromise to osseous integrity; this further complicates revision fixation (**Figure 15, D**).

The effect of the construct design in terms of plate length and screw and plate balance remains a subject of ongoing clinical and biomechanical study. Implant composition and de-

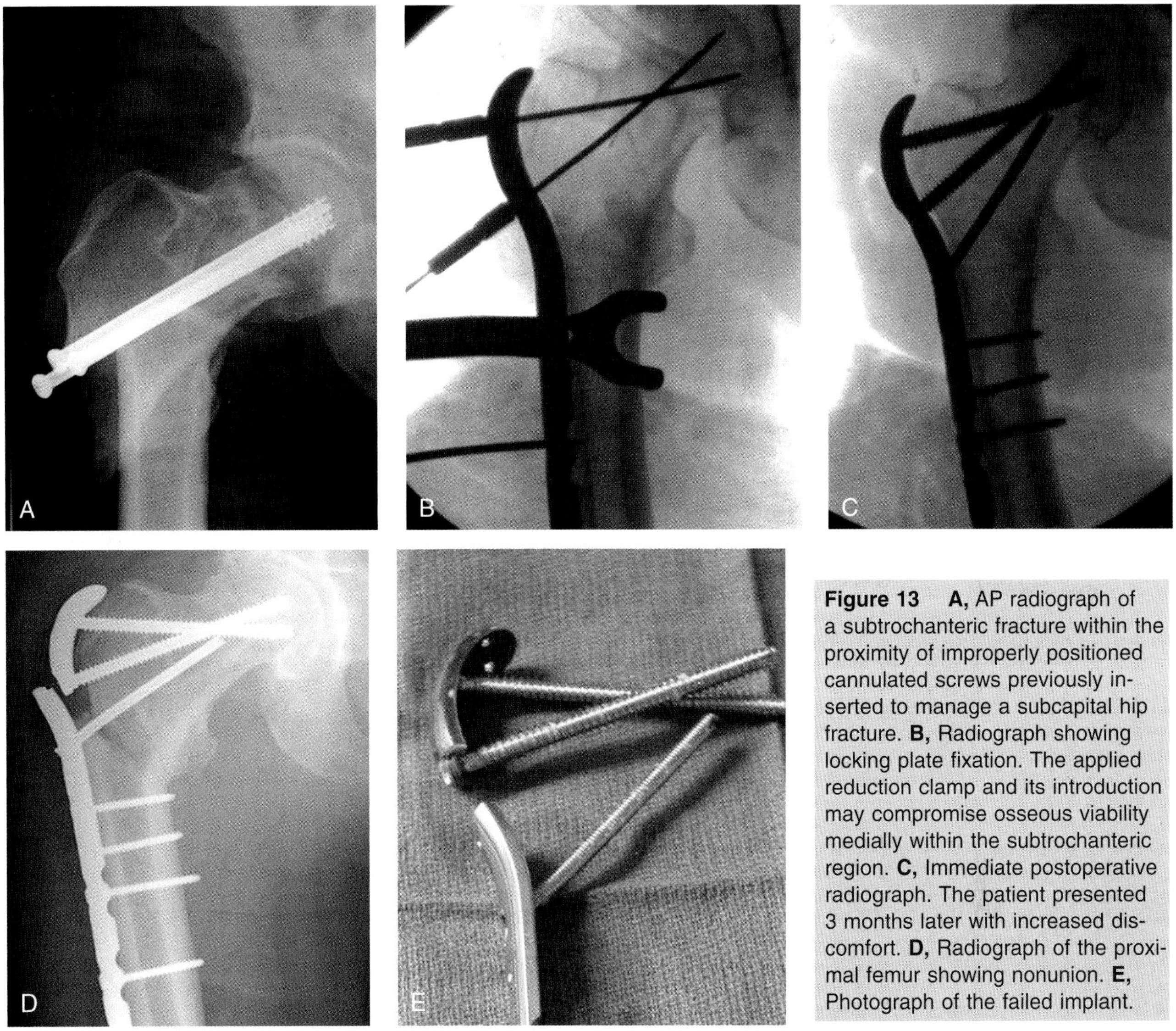

Figure 13 **A,** AP radiograph of a subtrochanteric fracture within the proximity of improperly positioned cannulated screws previously inserted to manage a subcapital hip fracture. **B,** Radiograph showing locking plate fixation. The applied reduction clamp and its introduction may compromise osseous viability medially within the subtrochanteric region. **C,** Immediate postoperative radiograph. The patient presented 3 months later with increased discomfort. **D,** Radiograph of the proximal femur showing nonunion. **E,** Photograph of the failed implant.

sign may affect the adequacy of union. As with other sites of metadiaphyseal locking plate fracture fixation, additional covariables include patient selection, fixation techniques, and the use of adjuvant bone-stimulating agents.

Proximal Tibia

Locking plate application to the proximal tibia poses intricate and unique fixation challenges, including the complexities of articular access and reconstitution and the risks of surgically induced soft-tissue compromise. The priorities of reestablishing limb axis, articular congruity, and joint function cannot come at a biologic price that may compromise osteoarticular viability and union. Laterally applied fixed-angle plate constructs appear particularly attractive in the proximal tibia because of the often tenuous soft-tissue envelope. These devices are intended to resist varus collapse and are compatible with minimally invasive insertion techniques. The introduction of locking screws within a nonreduced subchondral joint surface will not restore articular congruity and will result in sustained malreduction.

Results of proximal tibial locking plate fixation have been promising, but additional scientific validation is needed. Clinical success with the LISS has been reported for locked plating of proximal tibial fractures.[69-74] Excellent results with high union rates, high functional scores, the preservation of motion, and low complication rates were reported in early studies. Many of the lesions within these cohorts were low-energy injuries, and some had no articular involvement. Subsequent to these studies, several single-center and multicenter studies that included data on fracture patterns caused by higher-energy mechanisms reported higher rates of intraoperative malalignment,

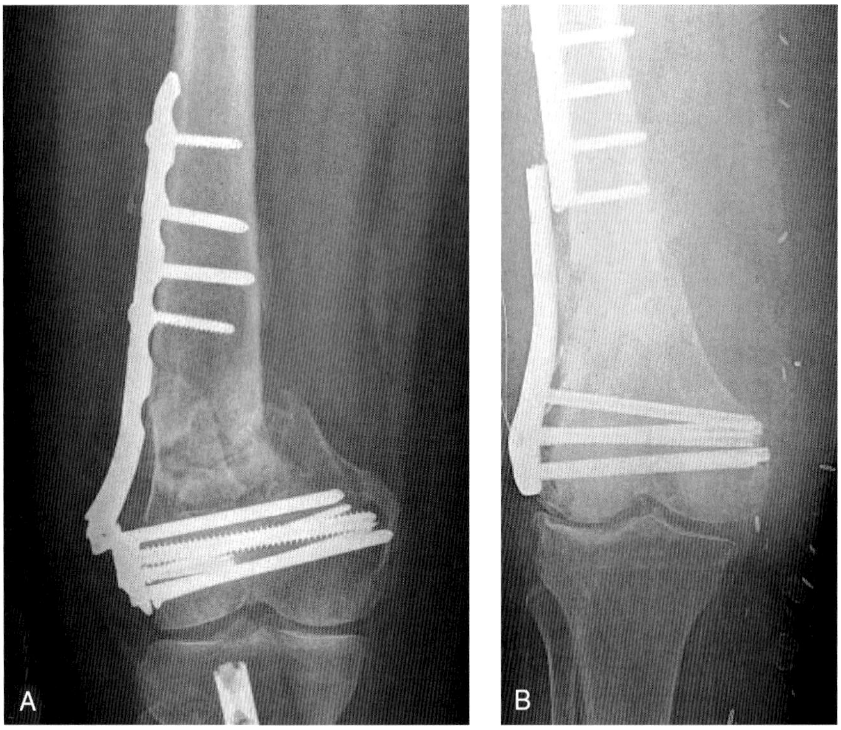

Figure 14 Radiographs showing failure of distal femoral stainless steel (**A**) and titanium (**B**) locking plates. Patients with failed implants may present late with only mild antecedent symptoms of discomfort. The screw balance and the proximity of the screws to the fracture site may influence fracture site strain, which can contribute to nonunion and implant failure.

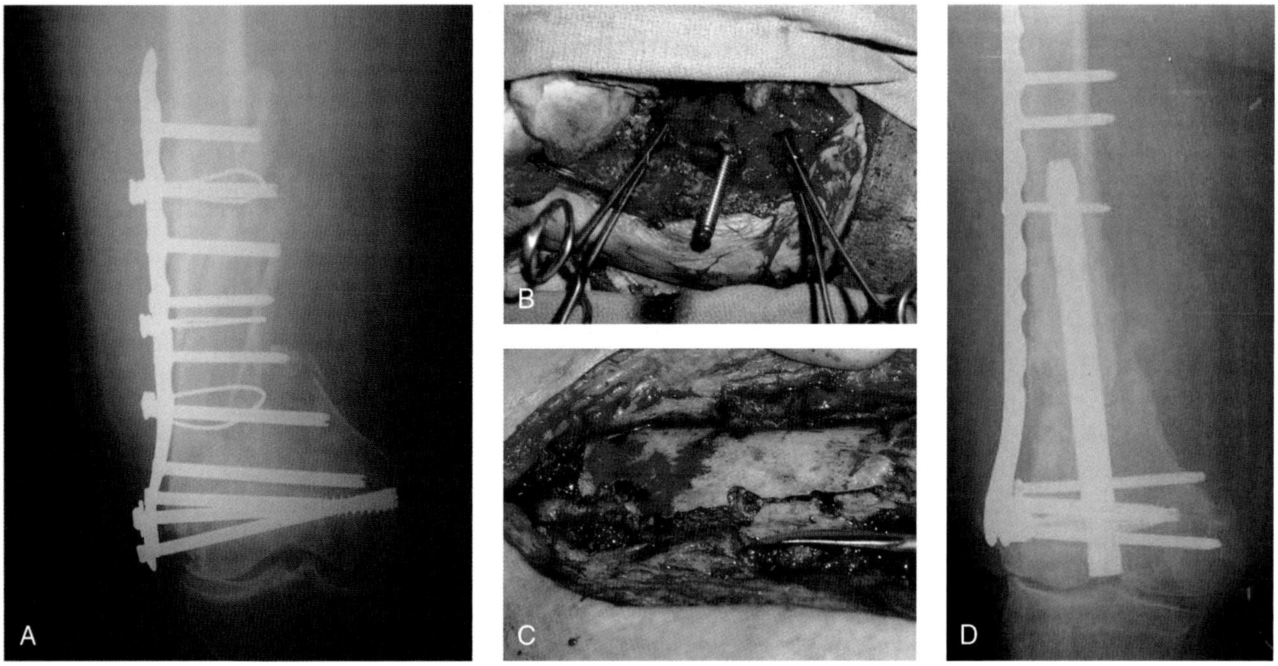

Figure 15 **A,** Radiograph of a locking plate used to treat a comminuted, closed, low-energy, distal femoral supracondylar fracture. The tenets of indirect reduction were violated with inclusion of cerclage wires and the proximity of the screws to the fracture site. **B** and **C,** The fixed anchorage points of the locking plate further compromised the osseous integrity and complicated revision fixation (**D**).

postoperative loss of alignment, and deep infection rates.[75,76] More recent reports have raised concern for potential varus collapse, particularly with fracture patterns associated with posteromedial fragments that may have been inadequately managed and fixed with single, laterally applied, fixed-angle plates.

There is growing concern over dependence on the anglular, stable screw-plate interface to manage varus forces on a sustained and sufficient basis. The amount of stability required and the cost to the regional anatomy of maintaining that stability are undetermined. Biomechanical laboratory studies have tried to establish the limitations of these fixation devices for managing fractures of the proximal tibia.[77-80] The inherent weaknesses of these studies do not allow for comparisons because the studies include nonphysiologic loading of varying fracture patterns with varying instability and the use of implants of different designs. Additionally, extrapolating clinically meaningful information from study designs using synthetic bone may be misleading.

Clinically, the potential inadequacies of using lateral locking plates to address the medial component of transcondylar and bicondylar fractures must be considered. Watson et al[81] described the importance of ascertaining the integrity of the medial osseous column of the proximal tibia in addition to its reduction parameters. The authors suggested that a lateral locking plate will suffice without subsequent varus collapse only if certain criteria, including medial condylar reduction, medial cortical opposition, and an adequate medial fracture capture size, are present or established (**Figure 16**). Laterally applied devices were best suited for fractures with established inherent medial cortical stability. This would primarily include patterns without medial comminution and satisfactory medial reduction. In contrast, inherent cortical instability was defined as the presence of medial comminution, the absence of medial reduction, or both. Such fracture patterns may prove problematic with the use of laterally based fixed-angle devices alone. A protocol was offered emphasizing caution when using laterally based locking plates in the presence of medial condylar apical comminution. Further study will determine whether these investigators identified or forecasted a problem. In the absence of medial reduction or in the presence of medial comminution, adjunctive medial plating should be considered. This method has been described incorporating minimally invasive techniques.[82]

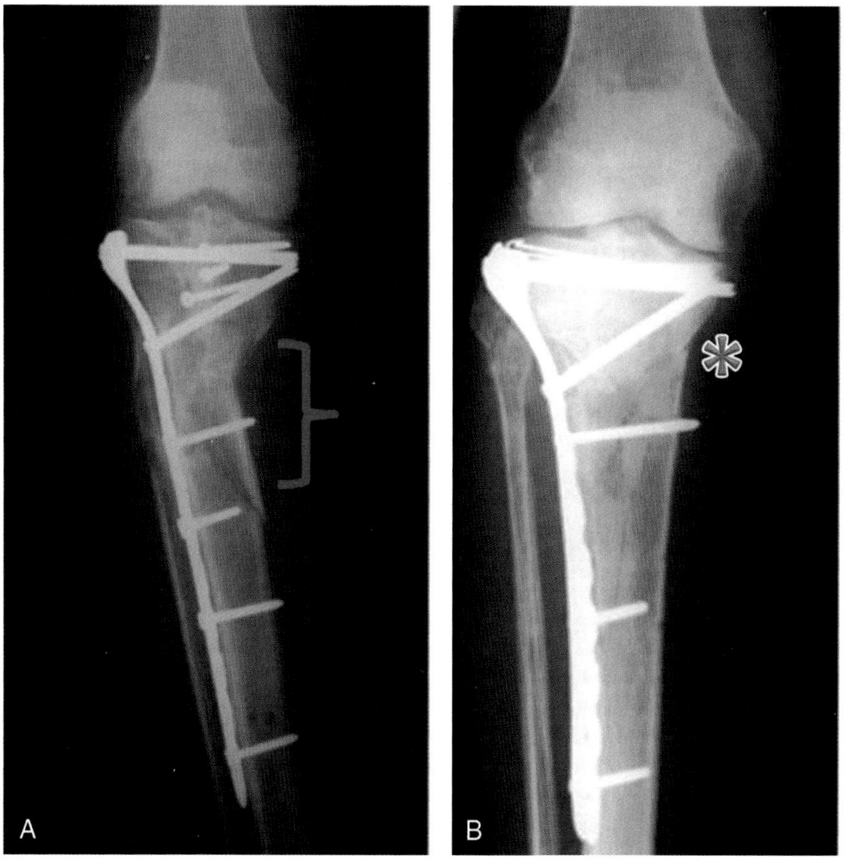

Figure 16 Laterally based locking plates may yield to varus forces, which can result in a loss of alignment. This is particularly concerning in the presence of medial comminution (bracketed area; **A**) or in the presence of inadequate medial reduction (**B**; asterisk).

The clear contribution of posteromedial fragments to postoperative malalignment has been described.[82] To treat bicondylar fractures with a laterally based fixed-angle device, the fracture morphology from coronal and sagittal perspectives must be characterized, and the unique attributes or limitations of the selected implant and its ability to capture multiplanar fracture components must be appreciated. Inadequate capture of the medial condyle in coronally oriented fractures can precipitate varus collapse. Coronally oriented posteromedial fragments may often be underrecognized and undertreated (**Figure 17**).

In two studies of multiplanar articular fractures, specific attention was directed toward coronally oriented posteromedial fragments.[83,84] The frequency of these fragments ranged from 60% to 70% for OTA type C fracture patterns. Because these posteromedial lesions encompassed as much as 20% to 25% of the entire joint surface, they had a considerable effect on the adequacy of reduction and the stability of fracture fixation. Inadequate capture

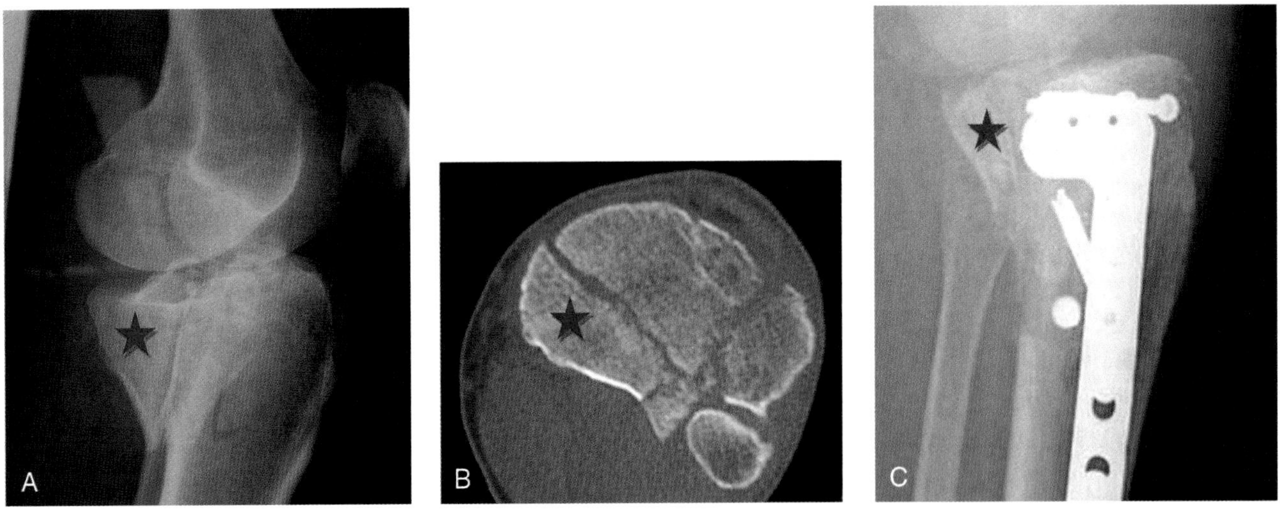

Figure 17 Coronally oriented posteromedial fragments are often underrecognized. Radiograph (**A**) and CT scan (**B**) show the position of the fragments (stars). **C,** Laterally based locking plates may provide inadequate fixation to the fragments (star).(Panel C adapted with permission from Higgins TF, Kemper D, Klatt J: Incidence and morphology of th posteromedial fragment in condylar tibial plateau fracture. *J Orthop Trauma* 2009;23:45-51.)

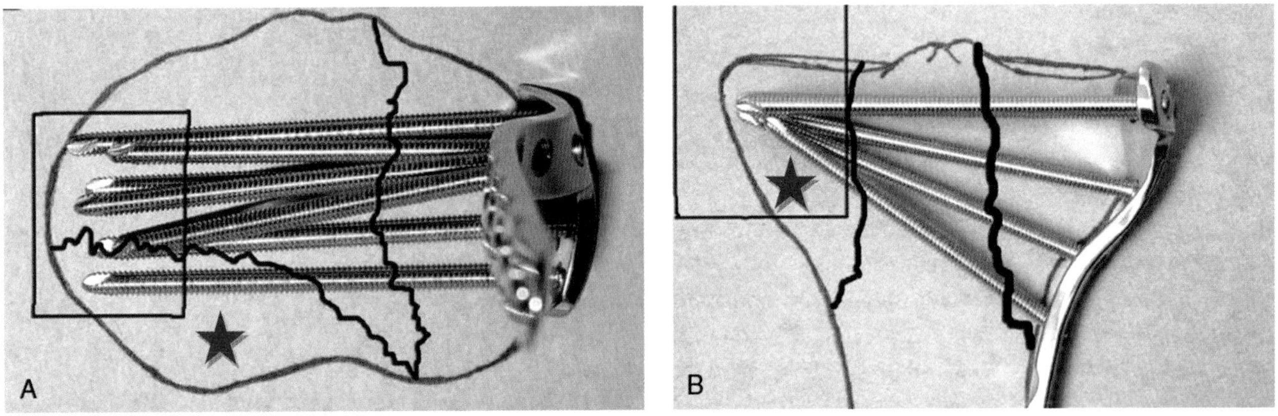

Figure 18 **A** and **B,** Laterally based fixed-angle implants have a fixed-screw pattern based on the design of the individual manufacturer. The location of the fragments is shown by the stars.

of these fragments and a resultant inferior fixation construct may contribute to posterior subluxation of the femur, resulting in both knee instability and arthrosis.

Laterally based fixed-angle implants have a fixed screw pattern and unique "capture area" medially based on the individual manufacturer's design (**Figure 18**). In some instances, the predetermined screw trajectory is inadequate when managing posteromedial fragments. The location and design of the plate may have a substantial influence on the adequate capture of fragments medially and posteromedially. The biomechanical reliability of these laterally based devices for managing fracture patterns with posteromedial components has been studied clinically and biomechanically.[85] Of increasing concern is the unreliable and inconsistent fixation of posteromedial fragments with laterally based, fixed-angle locking plates. Dual plating techniques using two incisions (lateral and posteromedial) may afford the best outcomes (**Figure 19**). Concerning rates of infection with dual plating have been reported despite attempts to respect the soft-tissue envelope and without violation of the anteromedial skin bridge.[86]

Discussion

The optimization of minimally invasive surgery combined with locking plates is an exciting development in osteosynthesis. Metadiaphyseal comminution can be addressed in a closed fashion (indirect reduction), which engenders an environment promoting

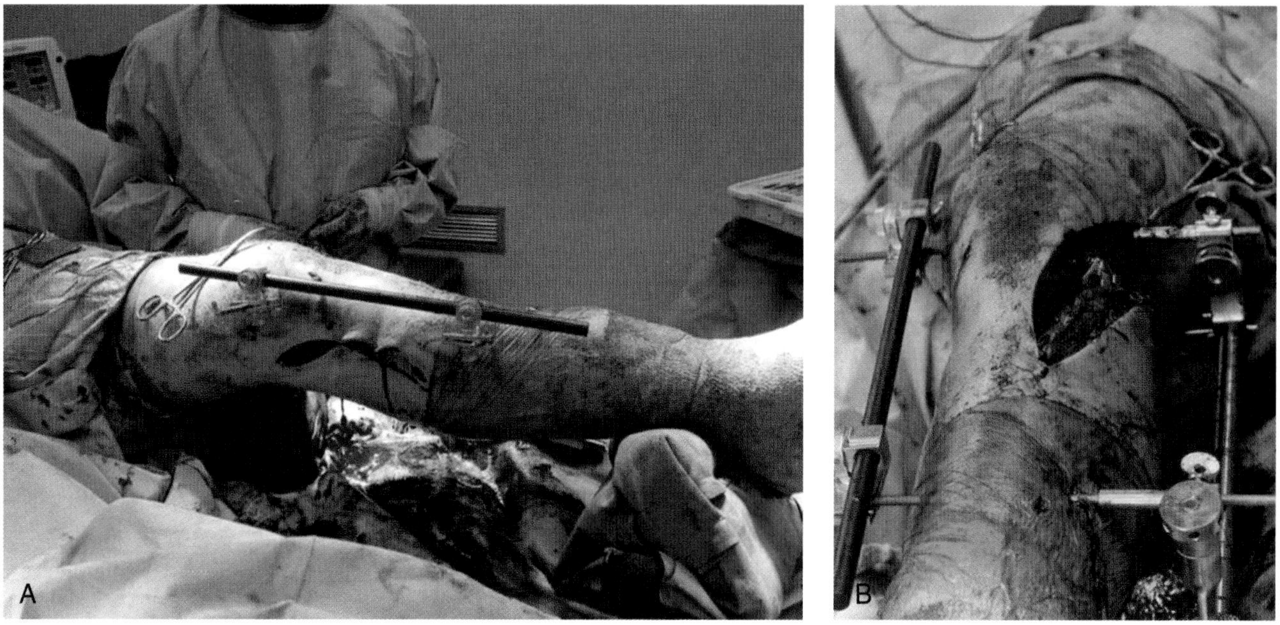

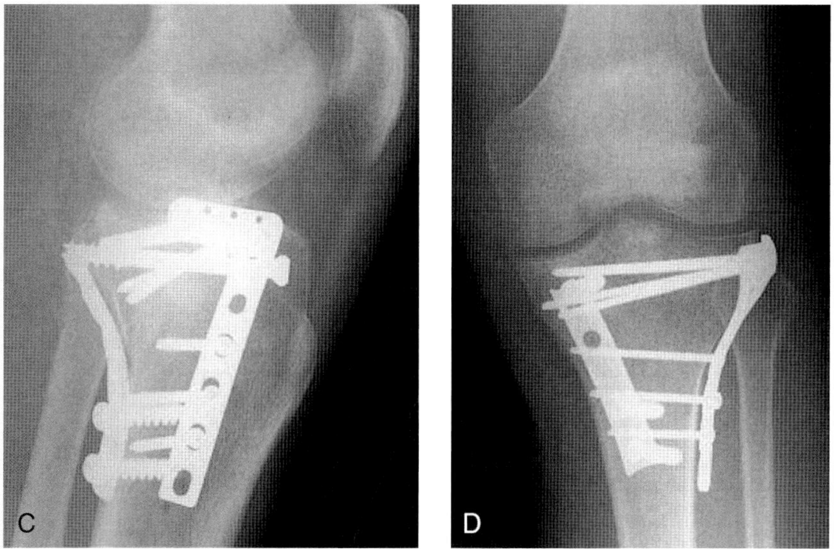

Figure 19 Bicondylar tibial plateau fractures with posteromedial coronally oriented fragments may be preferentially managed with a dual-plate and a dual-incision technique. Photographs of dual-incision fixation of a proximal tibial (left knee) fracture show the medial wound (**A**) and the anterolateral wound (**B**). Postoperative AP (**C**) and lateral (**D**) radiographs.

callus or torus formation of healing bone. Osteoarticular components are simultaneously managed with anatomic reduction and interfragmentary compression. Implants must be engineered to accommodate metadiaphyseal and articular priorities and bone reparative processes. Implant rigidity and strength must permit early functional mobilization of the extremity while encouraging osseous union. For metadiaphyseal fractures, the use of anatomic precontoured plates with fixed-angle interfaces and minimally invasive fixation has resulted in a mix of favorable and unfavorable outcomes.

Methods of minimally invasive fracture fixation continue to evolve and strike a balance between biomechanical demands and biologic price.[87] The surgeon must continue to respect the goals of restoration of limb alignment, length, rotation, and articular reconstitution. In a 2004 editorial, Sanders[88] suggested that minimal incision surgery may be taken too far. He suggests that "a 2-inch incision is an obvious improvement over a 10-inch incision. If one needs a 3-inch incision, however, struggling instead of extending the wound 1 inch may be a true example of triumph of technique over reason." The pursuit of a small incision should not take priority over the risk of fracture malreduction.

Minimally invasive techniques are not noninvasive. Numerous studies describe substantial hazards to cross-sectional anatomy when attempts are made to introduce plates via small subcutaneous and submuscular portals with sharp instruments. Krettek[89] observed that current minimally invasive techniques may appear maximally invasive to future generations. He further suggested that the term minimally invasive is imperfect because by definition it precludes the development of even less invasive techniques. The future of less invasive fracture surgery may shift to more surgeries (staged) and multiple strategically positioned incisions rather than fewer and smaller surgical access sites.

Recent clinical studies emphasizing minimally invasive fixation with locking plate devices, although often elegant, may have design flaws. Such studies often include heterogeneous groups, inadequate or varying lengths of follow-up, imperfect radiographic reduction assessment, differing functional scores, and no control group. Many studies often include different implants with different designs. Some laboratory studies also have design flaws, including nonphysiologic loading and mechanisms of load application. Cadaver and synthetic bone comparisons are complicated by the inclusion of varying fractures, varying instability, and constructs of dissimilar metals. Accordingly, the data retrieved from such studies result in conflicting information.

Summary

It is apparent from clinical and biomechanical studies of locking plates and minimally invasive surgical techniques that acceptance of this new paradigm is based on faith more than scientific validity. Personal surgical preferences should be replaced by scientific validation. This is not to imply that individual preferences should not arise from personal experience. Surgeons must question if undesired outcomes are caused by improper indications, poor implant designs, or improper surgical techniques. Orthopaedic surgeons must learn from individual and collective experiences. New technologies breed new problems. This in turn may set the stage for yet another paradigm shift.

References

1. Marzona L, Pavolini B: Play and players in bone fracture healing match. *Clin Cases Miner Bone Metab* 2009;6(2):159-162.
2. Müller ME, Allgöwer M, Schneider R, Willenegger H: *Manual of Internal Fixation: Techniques Recommended by the AO-ASIF Group*, ed 3. Berlin, Germany, Springer-Verlag, 1991.
3. Hoffmann R: Closed osteosynthesis. *Acta Chir Scand* 1942;86: 235-266.
4. Goodship AE, Kenwright J: The influence of induced micromovement upon the healing of experimental tibial fractures. *J Bone Joint Surg Br* 1985;67(4): 650-655.
5. De Bastiani G, Aldegheri R, Renzi Brivio L: The treatment of fractures with a dynamic axial fixator. *J Bone Joint Surg Br* 1984;66(4): 538-545.
6. Hey-Groves E: *On Modern Methods of Treating Fractures*. Bristol, United Kingdom, John Wright and Sons, 1916.
7. Uniderectional locking screw technology. Litos website. http://www.litos.com/locking_screw_technology.html. Accessed October 13, 2012.
8. Lin KC. Innovative locking plate system. US patent 5,085,660. February 4, 1992.
9. Ramotowski W, Granowski R: Zespol: An original method of stable osteosynthesis. *Clin Orthop Relat Res* 1991;272:67-75.
10. Frigg R: Development of the locking compression plate. *Injury* 2003;34(suppl 2):B6-B10.
11. Krettek C, Schandelmaier P, Tscherne H: Distal femoral fractures: Transarticular reconstruction, percutaneous plate osteosynthesis and retrograde nailing. *Unfallchirurg* 1996;99(1):2-10.
12. Krettek C, Müller M, Miclau T: Evolution of minimally invasive plate osteosynthesis (MIPO) in the femur. *Injury* 2001; 32(suppl 3):SC14-SC23.
13. Farouk O, Krettek C, Miclau T, Schandelmaier P, Guy P, Tscherne H: Minimally invasive plate osteosynthesis: Does percutaneous plating disrupt femoral blood supply less than the traditional technique? *J Orthop Trauma* 1999;13(6):401-406.
14. Goyal KS, Skalak AS, Marcus RE, Vallier HA, Cooperman DR: Analysis of anatomic periarticular tibial plate fit on normal adults. *Clin Orthop Relat Res* 2007;461: 245-257.
15. Matelic TM, Monroe MT, Mast JW: The use of endosteal substitution in the treatment of recalcitrant nonunions of the femur: Report of seven cases. *J Orthop Trauma* 1996;10(1):1-6.
16. Prayson MJ, Datta DK, Marshall MP: Mechanical comparison of endosteal substitution and lateral plate fixation in supracondylar fractures of the femur. *J Orthop Trauma* 2001;15(2):96-100.
17. Sanders R, Swiontkowski M, Rosen H, Helfet D: Double-plating of comminuted, unstable fractures of the distal part of the femur. *J Bone Joint Surg Am* 1991; 73(3):341-346.
18. Leunig M, Hertel R, Siebenrock KA, Ballmer FT, Mast JW, Ganz R: The evolution of indirect reduction techniques for the treatment of fractures. *Clin Orthop Relat Res* 2000;375:7-14.
19. Demey K, Haeck L, Sioen W: False aneurysm of the superficial femoral artery following minimally invasive plate osteosynthesis

of a femoral shaft fracture. *Acta Orthop Belg* 2008;74(5):700-703.

20. Wolinsky P, Lee M: The distal approach for anterolateral plate fixation of the tibia: An anatomic study. *J Orthop Trauma* 2008; 22(6):404-407.
21. Mirza A, Moriarty AM, Probe RA, Ellis TJ: Percutaneous plating of the distal tibia and fibula: Risk of injury to the saphenous and superficial peroneal nerves. *J Orthop Trauma* 2010;24(8): 495-498.
22. van Hensbroek PB, Ponsen KJ, Reekers JA, Goslings JC: Endovascular treatment of anterior tibial artery pseudoaneurysm following locking compression plating of the tibia. *J Orthop Trauma* 2007;21(4):279-282.
23. Deangelis JP, Deangelis NA, Anderson R: Anatomy of the superficial peroneal nerve in relation to fixation of tibia fractures with the less invasive stabilization system. *J Orthop Trauma* 2004;18(8): 536-539.
24. Cole PA, Zlowodzki M, Kregor PJ: Compartment pressures after submuscular fixation of proximal tibia fractures. *Injury* 2003; 34(suppl 1):A43-A46.
25. Wilson FB, Sargent MC, Dickson KF, et al: Abstract: Soft tissue complications in the treatment of complex fractures of the proximal tibia with use of the Less Invasive Stabilization System. 2003 Annual Meeting of the Orthopaedic Trauma Association. Paper No. 17. October 10, 2003. http://www.hwbf.org/ota/am/ota03/otapa/OTA03317.htm. Accessed August 27, 2012.
26. Gerber C, Werner CM, Vienne P: Internal fixation of complex fractures of the proximal humerus. *J Bone Joint Surg Br* 2004;86(6): 848-855.
27. Gerber C, Hersche O, Berberat C: The clinical relevance of posttraumatic avascular necrosis of the humeral head. *J Shoulder Elbow Surg* 1998;7(6):586-590.
28. Hepp P, Theopold J, Voigt C, Engel T, Josten C, Lill H: The surgical approach for locking plate osteosynthesis of displaced proximal humeral fractures influences the functional outcome. *J Shoulder Elbow Surg* 2008;17(1):21-28.
29. Gardner MJ, Griffith MH, Dines JS, Briggs SM, Weiland AJ, Lorich DG: The extended anterolateral acromial approach allows minimally invasive access to the proximal humerus. *Clin Orthop Relat Res* 2005;434:123-129.
30. Gardner MJ, Boraiah S, Helfet DL, Lorich DG: The anterolateral acromial approach for fractures of the proximal humerus. *J Orthop Trauma* 2008;22(2):132-137.
31. Gardner MJ, Voos JE, Wanich T, Helfet DL, Lorich DG: Vascular implications of minimally invasive plating of proximal humerus fractures. *J Orthop Trauma* 2006; 20(9):602-607.
32. Morgan SJ, Furry K, Parekh AA, Agudelo JF, Smith WR: The deltoid muscle: An anatomic description of the deltoid insertion to the proximal humerus. *J Orthop Trauma* 2006;20(1):19-21.
33. Klepps S, Auerbach J, Calhon O, Lin J, Cleeman E, Flatow E: A cadaveric study on the anatomy of the deltoid insertion and its relationship to the deltopectoral approach to the proximal humerus. *J Shoulder Elbow Surg* 2004;13(3): 322-327.
34. Robinson CM, Page RS: Severely impacted valgus proximal humeral fractures: Results of operative treatment. *J Bone Joint Surg Am* 2003;85(9):1647-1655.
35. Laflamme GY, Rouleau DM, Berry GK, Beaumont PH, Reindl R, Harvey EJ: Percutaneous humeral plating of fractures of the proximal humerus: Results of a prospective multicenter clinical trial. *J Orthop Trauma* 2008; 22(3):153-158.
36. Saran N, Bergeron SG, Benoit B, Reindl R, Harvey EJ, Berry GK: Risk of axillary nerve injury during percutaneous proximal humerus locking plate insertion using an external aiming guide. *Injury* 2010;41(10):1037-1040.
37. Gallo RA, Zeiders GJ, Altman GT: Two-incision technique for treatment of complex proximal humerus fractures. *J Orthop Trauma* 2005;19(10):734-740.
38. Fankhauser F, Boldin C, Schippinger G, Haunschmid C, Szyszkowitz R: A new locking plate for unstable fractures of the proximal humerus. *Clin Orthop Relat Res* 2005;430:176-181.
39. Björkenheim JM, Pajarinen J, Savolainen V: Internal fixation of proximal humeral fractures with a locking compression plate: A retrospective evaluation of 72 patients followed for a minimum of 1 year. *Acta Orthop Scand* 2004; 75(6):741-745.
40. Owsley KC, Gorczyca JT: Fracture displacement and screw cutout after open reduction and locked plate fixation of proximal humeral fractures. *J Bone Joint Surg Am* 2008;90(2):233-240.
41. Agudelo J, Schürmann M, Stahel P, et al: Analysis of efficacy and failure in proximal humerus fractures treated with locking plates. *J Orthop Trauma* 2007;21(10): 676-681.
42. Gardner MJ, Weil Y, Barker JU, Kelly BT, Helfet DL, Lorich DG: The importance of medial support in locked plating of proximal humerus fractures. *J Orthop Trauma* 2007;21(3):185-191.
43. Gardner MJ, Boraiah S, Helfet DL, Lorich DG: Indirect medial reduction and strut support of proximal humerus fractures using an endosteal implant. *J Orthop Trauma* 2008;22(3):195-200.

44. Hettrich CM, Neviaser A, Beamer BS, Paul O, Helfet DL, Lorich DG: Locked plating of the proximal humerus using an endosteal implant. *J Orthop Trauma* 2012; 26(4):212-215.
45. Badman BL, Mighell M, Kalandiak SP, Prasarn M: Proximal humeral nonunions treated with fixed-angle locked plating and an intramedullary strut allograft. *J Orthop Trauma* 2009;23(3): 173-179.
46. Egol KA, Sugi M, Ong C, Davidovitch RI, Zuckerman JD: Abstract: Fracture-site augmentation with calcium phosphate cement prevents screw penetration following open reduction and internal fixation (ORIF) of proximal humerus. 2010 Annual Meeting of the Orthopaedic Trauma Association. Paper No. 28. October 14, 2010. http://www.hwbf.org/ota/am/ota10/otapa/OTA100128.htm. Accessed August 27, 2012.
47. Siebenrock KA, Müller U, Ganz R: Indirect reduction with a condylar blade plate for osteosynthesis of subtrochanteric femoral fractures. *Injury* 1998;29(suppl 3): C7-C15.
48. Vaidya SV, Dholakia DB, Chatterjee A: The use of a dynamic condylar screw and biological reduction techniques for subtrochanteric femur fracture. *Injury* 2003;34(2):123-128.
49. Kinast C, Bolhofner BR, Mast JW, Ganz R: Subtrochanteric fractures of the femur: Results of treatment with the 95 degrees condylar blade-plate. *Clin Orthop Relat Res* 1989;238:122-130.
50. Krettek C, Schandelmaier P, Miclau T, Tscherne H: Minimally invasive percutaneous plate osteosynthesis (MIPPO) using the DCS in proximal and distal femoral fractures. *Injury* 1997; 28(suppl 1):A20-A30.
51. Celebi L, Can M, Muratli HH, Yagmurlu MF, Yuksel HY, Bicimolu A: Indirect reduction and biological internal fixation of comminuted subtrochanteric fractures of the femur. *Injury* 2006; 37(8):740-750.
52. Lee PC, Hsieh PH, Yu SW, Shiao CW, Kao HK, Wu CC: Biologic plating versus intramedullary nailing for comminuted subtrochanteric fractures in young adults: A prospective, randomized study of 66 cases. *J Trauma* 2007;63(6): 1283-1291.
53. Kregor PJ, Corr BR, Zlowodzki MP: Abstract: Submuscular proximal femoral locked plating for subtrochanteric femur fractures. *73rd Annual Meeting Proceedings*. Rosemont, IL, American Academy of Orthopaedic Surgeons, 2006, p 778.
54. Schmidt AH: Locked plating for subtrochanteric fractures: The next big thing. *Tech Orthop* 2008; 23(2):106-112.
55. Zhou F, Zhang ZS, Yang H, et al: Less invasive stabilization system (LISS) versus proximal femoral nail anti-rotation (PFNA) in treating proximal femoral fractures: A prospective randomized study. *J Orthop Trauma* 2012;26(3): 155-162.
56. Floyd JC, O'Toole RV, Stall A, et al: Biomechanical comparison of proximal locking plates and blade plates for the treatment of comminuted subtrochanteric femoral fractures. *J Orthop Trauma* 2009;23(9):628-633.
57. Glassner PJ, Tejwani NC: Failure of proximal femoral locking compression plate: A case series. *J Orthop Trauma* 2011;25(2):76-83.
58. Streubel PN, Moustoukas MJ, Obremskey WT: Mechanical failure after locking plate fixation of unstable intertrochanteric femur fractures. [published online ahead of print April 28, 2012.] *J Orthop Trauma*. PMID: 22549030.
59. Berkes MB, Little MT, Lazaro LE, Cymerman RM, Helfet DL, Lorich DG: Catastrophic failure after open reduction internal fixation of femoral neck fractures with a novel locking plate implant. [published online ahead of print March 16, 2012.] *J Orthop Trauma* PMID 22430524.
60. Kregor PJ, Stannard JA, Zlowodzki M, Cole PA: Treatment of distal femur fractures using the less invasive stabilization system: Surgical experience and early clinical results in 103 fractures. *J Orthop Trauma* 2004; 18(8):509-520.
61. Weight M, Collinge C: Early results of the less invasive stabilization system for mechanically unstable fractures of the distal femur (AO/OTA types A2, A3, C2, and C3). *J Orthop Trauma* 2004; 18(8):503-508.
62. Gains RJ, Sanders R, Sagi HC, Haidukewych GJ: Abstract: Titanium versus stainless steel locked plates for distal femur fractures: Is there any difference? 2008 Annual Meeting of the Orthopaedic Trauma Association. Paper No. 55. October 18, 2008. http://www.hwbf.org/ota/am/ota08/otapa/OTA080655.htm. Accessed August 27, 2012.
63. Lujan TJ, Henderson CE, Madey SM, Fitzpatrick DC, Marsh JL, Bottlang M: Locked plating of distal femur fractures leads to inconsistent and asymmetric callus formation. *J Orthop Trauma* 2010;24(3):156-162.
64. Henderson CE, Kuhl LL, Fitzpatrick DC, Marsh JL: Locking plates for distal femur fractures: Is there a problem with fracture healing? *J Orthop Trauma* 2011; 25(suppl 1):S8-S14.
65. Button G, Wolinsky P, Hak D: Failure of less invasive stabilization system plates in the distal femur: A report of four cases. *J Orthop Trauma* 2004;18(8): 565-570.
66. Vallier HA, Hennessey TA, Sontich JK, Patterson BM: Failure of LCP condylar plate fixation in the

distal part of the femur: A report of six cases. *J Bone Joint Surg Am* 2006;88(4):846-853.

67. Vallier HA, Immler W: Comparison of the 95-degree angled blade plate and the locking condylar plate for the treatment of distal femoral fractures. *J Orthop Trauma* 2012;26(6):327-332.
68. Hall JA, Phieffer LS, McKee MD: Humeral shaft split fracture around proximal humeral locking plates: A report of two cases. *J Orthop Trauma* 2006;20(10): 710-714.
69. Egol KA, Su E, Tejwani NC, Sims SH, Kummer FJ, Koval KJ: Treatment of complex tibial plateau fractures using the less invasive stabilization system plate: Clinical experience and a laboratory comparison with double plating. *J Trauma* 2004;57(2):340-346.
70. Stannard JP, Wilson TC, Volgas DA, Alonso JE: Fracture stabilization of proximal tibial fractures with the proximal tibial LISS: Early experience in Birmingham, Alabama (USA). *Injury* 2003; 34(suppl 1):A36-A42.
71. Stannard JP, Wilson TC, Volgas DA, Alonso JE: The less invasive stabilization system in the treatment of complex fractures of the tibial plateau: Short-term results. *J Orthop Trauma* 2004;18(8): 552-558.
72. Schütz M, Kääb MJ, Haas N: Stabilization of proximal tibial fractures with the LIS-System: Early clinical experience in Berlin. *Injury* 2003;34(suppl 1):A30-A35.
73. Ricci WM, Rudzki JR, Borrelli J Jr: Treatment of complex proximal tibia fractures with the less invasive skeletal stabilization system. *J Orthop Trauma* 2004; 18(8):521-527.
74. Cole PA, Zlowodzki M, Kregor PJ: Treatment of proximal tibia fractures using the less invasive stabilization system: Surgical experience and early clinical results in 77 fractures. *J Orthop Trauma* 2004;18(8):528-535.
75. Gosling T, Schandelmaier P, Muller M, Hankemeier S, Wagner M, Krettek C: Single lateral locked screw plating of bicondylar tibial plateau fractures. *Clin Orthop Relat Res* 2005;439:207-214.
76. Phisitkul P, McKinley TO, Nepola JV, Marsh JL: Complications of locking plate fixation in complex proximal tibia injuries. *J Orthop Trauma* 2007;21(2): 83-91.
77. Peindl RD, Zura RD, Vincent A, Coley ER, Bosse MJ, Sims SH: Unstable proximal extraarticular tibia fractures: A biomechanical evaluation of four methods of fixation. *J Orthop Trauma* 2004; 18(8):540-545.
78. Horwitz DS, Bachus KN, Craig MA, Peters CL: A biomechanical analysis of internal fixation of complex tibial plateau fractures. *J Orthop Trauma* 1999;13(8): 545-549.
79. Ratcliff JR, Werner FW, Green JK, Harley BJ: Medial buttress versus lateral locked plating in a cadaver medial tibial plateau fracture model. *J Orthop Trauma* 2007;21(7):444-448.
80. Mueller KL, Karunakar MA, Frankenburg EP, Scott DS: Bicondylar tibial plateau fractures: A biomechanical study. *Clin Orthop Relat Res* 2003;412:189-195.
81. Watson TJ, Phillips M, Karges D, Jackman J: Abstract: Lateral locking plates for the treatment of bicondylar tibial plateau fractures: A treatment protocol, indications, and results. 2007 Annual Meeting of the Orthopaedic Trauma Association. Paper No. 24. October 19, 2007. http://www.hwbf.org/ota/am/ota07/otapa/OTA070424.htm. Accessed August 27, 2012.
82. Krettek C, Gerich T, Miclau T: A minimally invasive medial approach for proximal tibial fractures. *Injury* 2001;32(suppl 1): SA4-SA13.
83. Higgins TF, Kemper D, Klatt J: Incidence and morphology of the posteromedial fragment in bicondylar tibial plateau fractures. *J Orthop Trauma* 2009;23(1):45-51.
84. Barei DP, O'Mara TJ, Taitsman LA, Dunbar RP, Nork SE: Frequency and fracture morphology of the posteromedial fragment in bicondylar tibial plateau fracture patterns. *J Orthop Trauma* 2008; 22(3):176-182.
85. Yoo BJ, Beingessner DM, Barei DP: Stabilization of the posteromedial fragment in bicondylar tibial plateau fractures: A mechanical comparison of locking and nonlocking single and dual plating methods. *J Trauma* 2010; 69(1):148-155.
86. Barei DP, Nork SE, Mills WJ, Henley MB, Benirschke SK: Complications associated with internal fixation of high-energy bicondylar tibial plateau fractures utilizing a two-incision technique. *J Orthop Trauma* 2004;18(10): 649-657.
87. Perren SM: Evolution of the internal fixation of long bone fractures: The scientific basis of biological internal fixation. Choosing a new balance between stability and biology. *J Bone Joint Surg Br* 2002; 84(8):1093-1110.
88. Sanders R: When evolution begets revolution. *J Orthop Trauma* 2004;18(8):481-482.
89. Krettek C: Foreword: Concepts of minimally invasive plate osteosynthesis. *Injury* 1997;28(suppl 1): A1-A2.

6

Extra-articular Proximal Tibial Fractures: Nail or Plate?

John C. Kurylo, MD
Paul Tornetta III, MD

Abstract

The surgical goals for treating proximal tibial fractures are to restore articular congruity, the mechanical axis, and knee motion while avoiding soft-tissue complications. The fracture pattern should be correctly identified and understood. For fractures with minimal intra-articular extension, fracture fixation with an intramedullary nail can decrease the risk of infection because it uses a small incision that is not placed directly over the injured soft tissue, and it provides better axial load sharing than a plate. Using the semiextended technique, choosing the correct starting portal, incorporating blocking screws or stability screws into the fixation construct, and using mini-open reduction and internal fixation of the fracture will help achieve the goals of fracture fixation with an intramedullary nail.

All proximal tibial fractures can be treated successfully with a plate or multiple plates. When a plate is used, the surgical approach and technique should minimize soft-tissue damage and account for future surgical procedures that may be needed. Fractures with intra-articular involvement and/or comminution of the medial metaphyseal region are appropriately treated with dual plating. Extra-articular fractures without major medial comminution may be treated with a locked lateral plate. Final union rates for patients treated with either intramedullary nail or plate fixation are reported at 96% and 97%, respectively. A prospective, randomized, multicenter study is currently in progress to further clarify and advance the treatment of proximal tibial fractures.

Instr Course Lect 2013;62:61-77.

Proximal tibial fractures are challenging to treat because of the frequency of substantial soft-tissue injury, the strong deforming forces involved, and the need for accurate alignment. This chapter will focus primarily on extra-articular proximal tibial fractures and those with minimally displaced intra-articular extension that can be treated with intramedullary (IM) nailing or plate fixation.

Proximal tibial fractures make up 5% to 11% of all tibial injuries and typically are caused by a high-energy mechanism.[1] Because of the location of these fractures in the highly vascular and muscular area of the lower extremity, there is a higher incidence of arterial injury, muscle damage, and compartment syndrome than in diaphyseal fractures.[2,3] Burgess et al[4] reported that the most proximal tibial fractures result from pedestrians being struck by automobiles; the extent of the soft-tissue injury is often grossly underestimated.

The AO/Orthopaedic Trauma Association (OTA) system is the most widely used system for classifying proximal tibial fractures. Type A fractures are extra-articular, type B fractures are partially articular, and type C fractures are articular with a metaphyseal component. Both IM nails and plates are appropriate for treating type A and simple intra-articular type C1 fracture patterns[5] (**Figure 1**).

Regardless of the fixation method chosen, traditional fracture care principles should be followed. Open fractures are treated with urgent irrigation and débridement of the devitalized tis-

Dr. Tornetta or an immediate family member serves as a board member, owner, officer, or committee member of the American Orthopaedic Association and the Orthopaedic Trauma Association; has received royalties from Smith & Nephew; and serves as a paid consultant to or is an employee of Smith & Nephew. Neither Dr. Kurylo nor any immediate family member has received anything of value from or owns stock in a commercial company or institution related directly or indirectly to the subject of this chapter.

sue. Temporary external fixation may be used, particularly if initial definitive soft-tissue coverage cannot be obtained or if the surgeon chooses to perform the definitive reduction and fixation under more ideal conditions. These fractures should be closely monitored because of the substantial risk for compartment syndrome.

Imaging

The surgical goals for treating proximal tibial fractures are to restore articular congruity, the mechanical axis, and knee motion while avoiding soft-tissue complications. To accomplish these goals, correct identification of the fracture pattern is necessary. AP and lateral radiographs may not provide adequate information on fracture comminution, displacement, planes, and, especially, intra-articular displacement. A caudad plateau view, with the x-ray beam directed 10° caudal on the AP orientation, will provide a better understanding of the articular extension. Oblique internal and external rotation views may provide additional information about the fracture. CT will provide the best information about intra-articular extension, if present. This is particularly helpful in determining if a fracture extends into the area of portal placement for nailing (**Figure 2**). This chapter's authors typically obtain a CT scan if an intra-articular fracture is seen on radiographic studies.

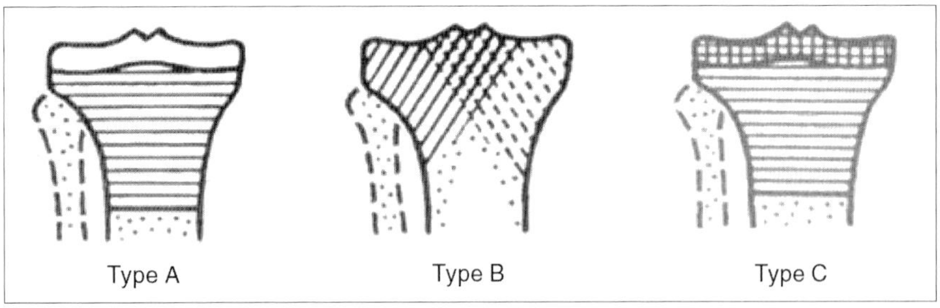

Figure 1 Illustration of the AO classification system of proximal tibial fractures. Type A fractures are extra-articular, type B fractures are partially articular, and type C fractures are articular with a metaphyseal component. (Reproduced from Hiesterman TG, Shafiq BX, Cole PA: Intramedullary nailing of extra-articular proximal tibia fractures. *J Am Acad Orthop Surg* 2011;19(10): 690-700.)

Closed Treatment

Although closed treatment of proximal tibial fractures is beyond the scope of this chapter, it is an option that should be considered. Sarmiento et al[6] championed the nonsurgical management

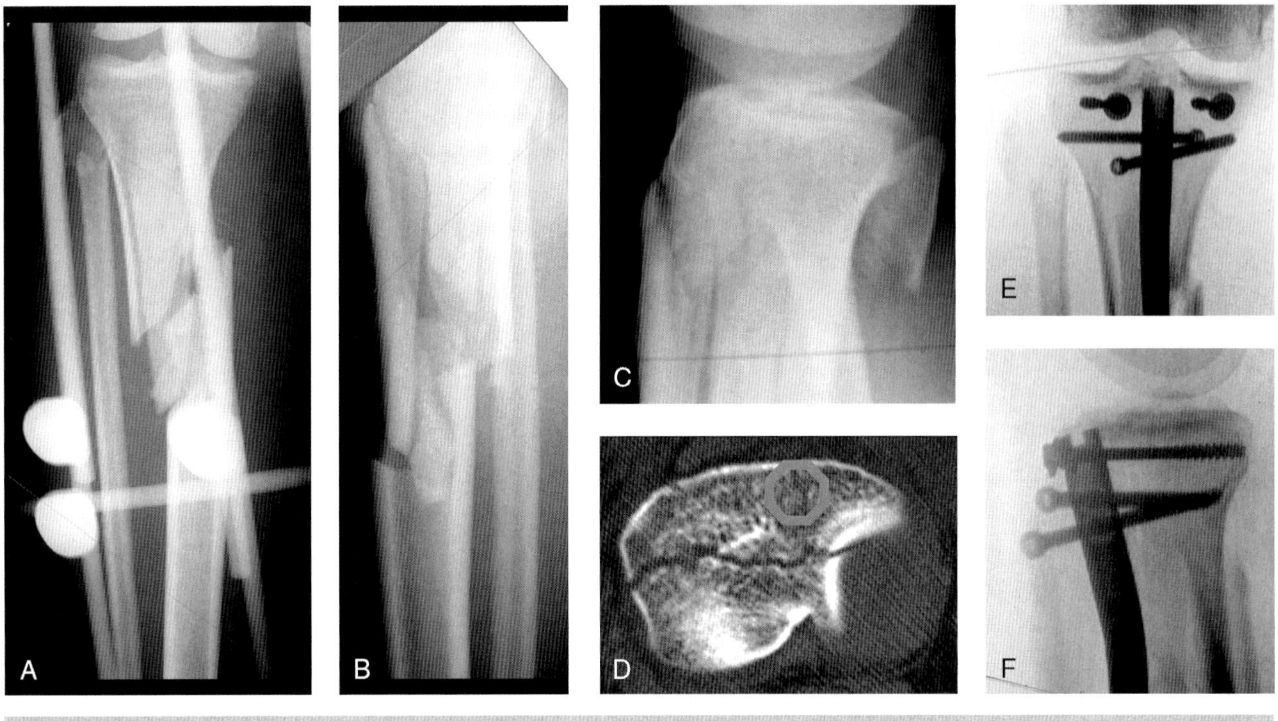

Figure 2 AP tibia (**A**), lateral tibia (**B**), and lateral knee (**C**) radiographs and CT scan (**D**) of a proximal tibial fracture showing fracture extension into the nail portal (circle). Postoperative AP (**E**) and lateral (**F**) radiographs show joint reduction with two anterior-to-posterior screws after IM nailing.

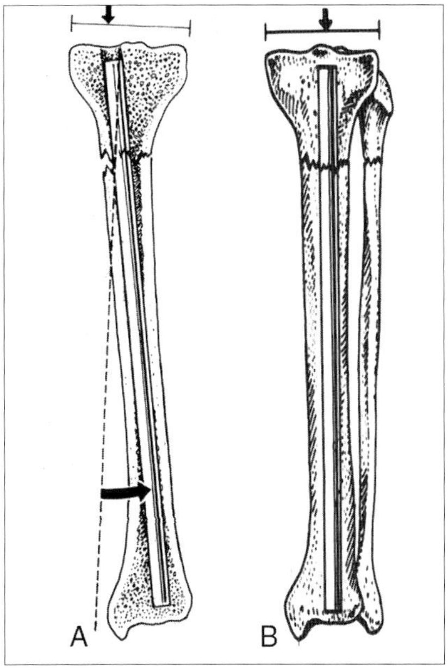

Figure 3 **A,** A medial starting portal for nail placement will create a valgus deformity at the fracture site. The short arrow represents a starting portal that is too medial. The dashed line represents the nail trajectory if the nail were to follow the original trajectory. However, with a starting portal that is too medial, the fracture gaps medially, a valgus deformity results, and the nail's final position is different than originally planned (large curved arrow). **B,** A more lateral starting portal aids in proper angulation. The short arrow represents the correct starting portal. The nail is introduced and follows the correct trajectory without causing a varus or a valgus deformity. (Reproduced from Tornetta P III: Technical considerations in the surgical management of tibial fractures. *Instr Course Lect* 1997;46:271-280.)

Table 1
Tips for Treating Proximal Tibial Fractures With IM Nailing

Use the semiextended technique. The knee is flexed from 20° to 30°. A medial parapatellar approach with lateral subluxation of the patella is used to establish the starting portal. Special cannulas are used to protect the articular surface of the patella and trochlea.
Locate the safe zone for nail entry. On the AP view, it is located just medial to the lateral tibial spine. On the lateral view, it is located just at or behind the anterior articular surface.
Use blocking screws before nail placement to address malalignment.
Stability screws can be placed after the nail is inserted to provide additional support for the nail.
Proximal locking in the nail should use at least two multiplanar interlocking screws. Locking the screws to the nail is helpful.

of proximal tibial fractures. The authors reported on 68 patients with nonarticular proximal tibial fractures who were treated with a long leg cast. In patients with proximal tibial and fibular fractures, 84% had acceptable outcomes (less than 5° of angulation in any plane) at union. Based on these results, nonsurgical treatment can be considered for patients with good alignment in the initial cast or those who present without fracture displacement.

Treatment With an IM Nail

In early reports, proximal tibial fracture treatment with IM nailing was associated with high rates of malalignment and loss of proximal fragment fixation. In 1995, Lang et al[1] reported that 84% of their patients treated with IM nailing had sagittal malunion, and 25% had loss of reduction. Freedman and Johnson[7] reported that 58% of proximal tibial fractures treated with IM nailing resulted in malalignment, and 83% of these fractures were segmental or comminuted. It is important to note that unlocked transverse screws were used in these early series; these screws provided only uniaxial stability and may have contributed to the loss of reduction.

Malreductions are mainly caused by errant portal placement. The most common error is a starting portal that is too medial. When nailing a proximal tibial fracture, the nail tends to lie against the lateral portion of the proximal tibia. If the portal is medial, this will result in a valgus deformity (**Figure 3**). A more lateral starting portal will prevent a valgus deformity. Flexion and posterior translation at the fracture site is the second most common deformity. Early IM nail designs exacerbated the posterior translational deformity of the proximal tibial fracture when the proximal bend of the tibial nail was distal to the fracture site.[8]

The relative contraindications for using IM nailing for proximal tibial fractures include a narrow IM canal, inability to pass a nail because of an existing canal deformity, or the presence of a tibial base plate in a total knee arthroplasty or knee fusion. IM nailing for tibial fractures in pediatric patients should be approached with caution. Court-Brown et al[9] reported on 52 adolescent patients between the ages of 13 and 16 years who had a tibial fracture treated with IM nailing. Partial growth arrest of the proximal tibial physis did not develop in any of the patients.

Many techniques have been shown to be helpful with complex proximal tibial nailing (**Table 1**). In general, IM nailing is an attractive method for treating proximal tibial fractures. It may decrease the risk of infection because it uses a small incision that is not placed directly over the injured soft tissue, and it provides better axial load sharing than a plate. To achieve adequate reduction with IM nailing, it is necessary to understand the characteristics of the fracture and the deforming mechanical forces acting on the proximal tibia.[7] The patella tendon,

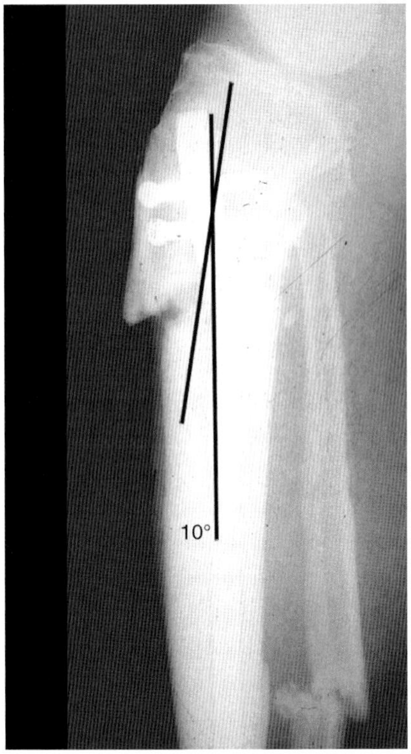

Figure 4 Radiograph showing a 10° extension deformity at the proximal tibial fracture site caused by hyperflexion nailing of the fracture. (Reproduced from Tornetta P III: Technical considerations in the surgical management of tibial fractures. *Instr Course Lect* 1997;46:271-280.)

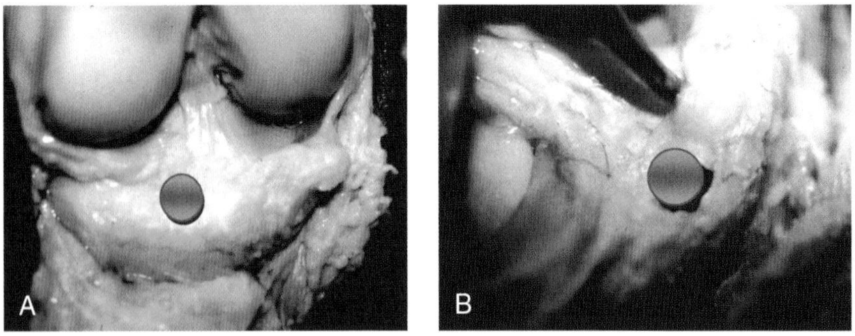

Figure 5 AP (**A**) and lateral (**B**) views of the tibia showing the safe zone (red circle) for IM nailing of a proximal tibial fracture as described by Tornetta et al.[18]

which is attached on the anterior tibial tubercle, will pull the proximal fragment into extension; this is a common problem seen with traditional hyperflexion nailing techniques (**Figure 4**). The strong muscular attachments on the lateral aspect of the proximal tibia restrict lateral gapping and may favor a valgus deformity. With large forces acting at the fracture gap, these forces must be reduced either directly or indirectly through the nailing approach and before fixation to prevent deformity.

Portal Placement

As with all nailing procedures, the starting portal is paramount to achieving a good outcome. Various IM nailing methods and techniques have been reported for treating proximal tibial fractures.[10-17] Each method uses the same overall approach: correct starting portal, fracture reduction through direct or indirect means, and guidance of the nail down the tibial canal without creating a deformity.

Technically, the correct starting portal for nailing proximal fractures is intra-articular and as in line with the center of the canal distally as possible without causing intra-articular damage. This positioning makes nail passage easier and tends to prevent the creation of a deformity. As described by Tornetta et al,[18] the safe zone for the starting portal for IM nailing of proximal tibial fractures is located 3 mm lateral to the center of the tibial tubercle, 9 ± 5 mm lateral to the midline of the tibial plateau, and 23 ± 9 mm in width (**Figure 5**). This zone allows nail placement without damaging the meniscal or articular cartilage of the knee. On an AP view of the knee, the average position of the safe zone is just medial to the lateral tibial spine.[19] On the lateral view, the position is at the joint line (**Figure 6**). The proximal tibia is triangular in shape and has a large metaphyseal area. Because of the geometry of the proximal tibia, the fit is not tight at the metaphyseal bone-nail interface. The medullary center of the tibia is just lateral to the midline[13] (**Figure 7**). A more lateral starting portal is important because it helps prevent a valgus deformity and provides a greater propensity for the nail to be colinear with the tibial axis.

Nailing in Relative Extension

In the semiextended approach to IM nailing, the leg is positioned in approximately 20° to 30° of flexion with a small bolster under the thigh.[14] A midline skin incision approximately 5 cm long is made from just above the upper pole of the patella. The deep incision is made medial to the patella and extends slightly into the vastus proximally and down as low as the upper portion of the patella tendon distally. This allows for lateral subluxation of the patella during the procedure. The tibial portal, which is located on the superior surface of the tibia, is made accessible using the trochlear groove as a conduit. A straight awl may be used to start the portal (**Figure 8**).

It is essential that the direction of the awl or the starting guidewire and reamer be checked with fluoroscopy as they are driven into the tibia. They must be directed as anteriorly as possible in the proximal tibia. In a recent study, none of the 192 patients treated with this method had greater than 5° of apex anterior angulation.[20] This ap-

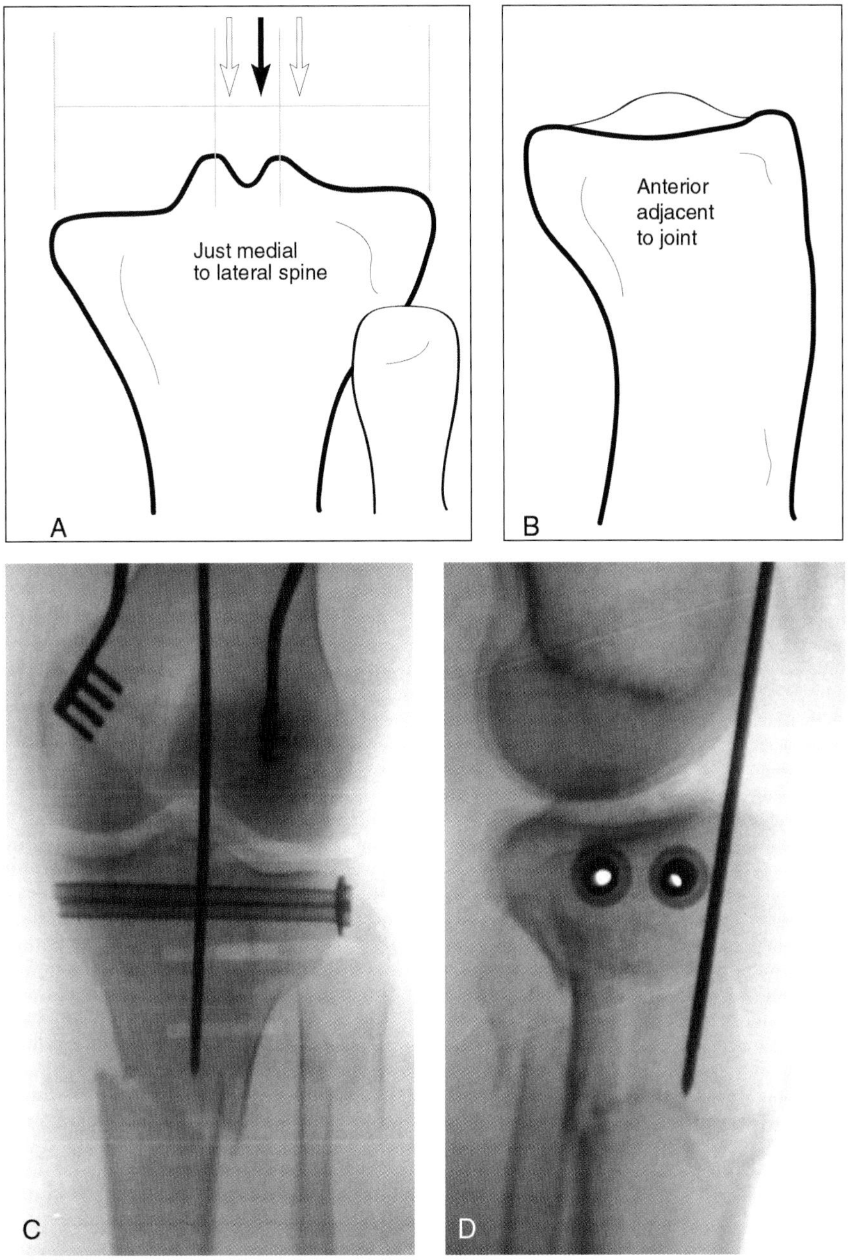

Figure 6 Illustrations of the correct nail starting point for IM nailing from AP (**A**) and lateral (**B**) views. Radiographs show the location of the correct starting portal for IM nailing. **C,** AP radiograph of the guidewire placed just medial to the lateral tibial spine. **D,** Lateral radiograph of the guidewire placed just anterior to the joint line.

proach has the potential for decreased postoperative anterior knee pain because the infrapatellar branch of the saphenous nerve and patellar tendon are avoided.[21]

A common criticism of the semiextended technique is the potential for patella or trochlear groove injury during nailing. Since the original technique was described, special instrumentation has been developed to protect the fragile articular surface of the patella and the trochlear groove during instrumentation and nailing of the tibial canal. The current technique uses only a 3-cm incision and cannulas to protect the trochlea and undersurface of the patella. A recent study reported that knee pain is the same in patients treated with a semiextended approach as those treated with standard hyperflexion nailing, despite a higher percentage of fractures with intra-articular extension.[20]

Other methods for nailing proximal tibial fractures have recently been reported. These methods describe nailing in a fully or a partially extended position. The suprapatellar portal, a 2-cm vertical incision in the quadriceps mechanism directly superior to the patella, is used for nailing in full extension.[13] Although this technique is appealing, the starting portal in the tibia is more distal and anterior than the ideal starting portal, which is not accessible until the knee is flexed 30°.[13,22]

Proximal Fixation

To increase the stability of a proximal tibial fracture treated with IM nailing, multiplanar proximal locking is offered by various nailing systems and increases the stability of fixation.[23,24] At least two proximal interlocking screws in different planes are recommended for proximal tibial fractures; three or more screws offer greater stability.[23,24] The development of angular, stable interlocking screws placed through an IM nail decreases fragmentary motion and increases the stiffness of the construct.[25] In most systems, some method is used to lock at least the most proximal screw to the nail using an end cap. Different nailing systems offer proximal locking screw locations closer to or further from the most proximal portion of the nail.

Blocking Screws

Blocking screws essentially tighten the canal and force the nail to take a par-

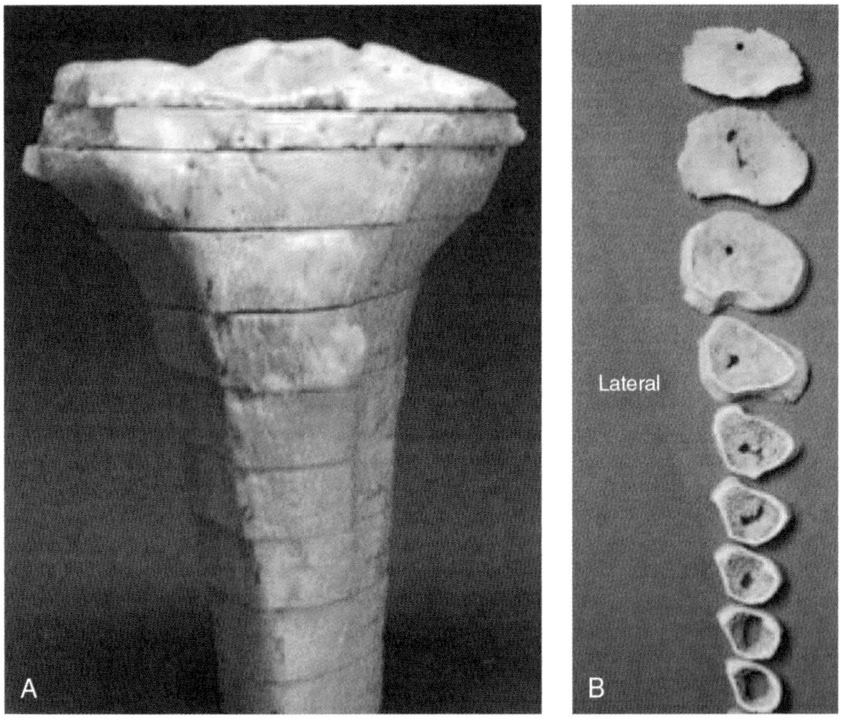

Figure 7 **A,** Photograph of the proximal tibia. Sectioning demonstrates the wide metaphyseal region that narrows distally to a well-defined cortical tube. **B,** Enface view of the tibial sections arranged in order from proximal to distal shows the more lateral trajectory a nail will take within the medullary canal of the tibia. (Reproduced with permission from Buehler KC, Green J, Woll TS, Duwelius PJ: A technique for intramedullary nailing of proximal third tibia fractures. *J Orthop Trauma* 1997;11:218-223.)

ticular path to avoid malalignment in the sagittal and coronal planes. The screws are placed before nail insertion and reaming. Krettek et al[15] and Cole[26] described their techniques for blocking screw placement to address malreduction. To prevent apex anterior angulation, a coronal blocking screw can be placed in the posterior half of the proximal fragment (**Figure 9**). Valgus malalignment can be related to a medial entry point and a laterally directed nailing insertion angle in the proximal fragment. To correct this, a blocking screw can be placed on the lateral side of the proximal fracture. If the portal is too medial, then it must be widened, even when using a lateral blocking screw. Both coronal and sagittal blocking screws can be used simultaneously to reduce multidirectional forces. Krettek et al[15] reported a mean loss of reduction between placement of the initial blocking screw and follow-up as 0.5° in the frontal plane and 0.4° in the sagittal plane. No complications were related to the use of blocking screws. When blocking screws are used appropriately, reproducible results can be expected for acceptable alignment, and the biomechanical stability of the bone-implant construct is increased 25%.[12,27] If blocking screws are placed after IM nailing to add stability to the construct, they are called stability screws rather than blocking screws.[12]

Mini-Open Reduction and Internal Fixation

The treatment of a proximal tibial fracture with an IM nail can be aided by using percutaneous clamps or small plates, which can be placed to obtain and maintain the reduction before nail or lag screw placement. Percutaneous reduction clamps do not increase the rate of infection.[28] If clamp fixation is not sufficient, unicortical plating is an option.[29,30] A small, four- or six-hole plate is placed over the fracture or fracture fragment and is held in place with at least two unicortical screws. The plate can be placed percutaneously or via a mini-open approach. If possible, the plate should lie anteriorly to avoid the canal. Potential complications from this method include an additional incision and dissection. However, the plate may provide excellent stability for fracture reduction, and the unicortical screws can be replaced by bicortical screws after IM nailing to improve overall stability[17] (**Figure 10**). This technique is not needed for all proximal tibial fractures, but it offers another method of providing stability. This is particularly helpful in open injuries in which further soft-tissue dissection is not necessary and can be detrimental.

Outcomes

Most complications seen with IM nailing of proximal tibial fractures involve malreduction (greater than 5° in any plane). The advent of the semiextended technique; angular, stable interlocking screws; and improved implant designs have resulted in average malreduction rates between 0% and 8.2%.[20,31] Nork et al[17] evaluated 456 patients with a tibial shaft fracture; 37 had a tibial fracture in the proximal quarter that was treated with IM nailing. Postoperative angulation was less than 5° in any plane for 34 of the 37 fractures (92%). Two infections were reported in the 37 patients treated with IM nailing, with both infections involving open fractures. The authors concluded that satisfactory ra-

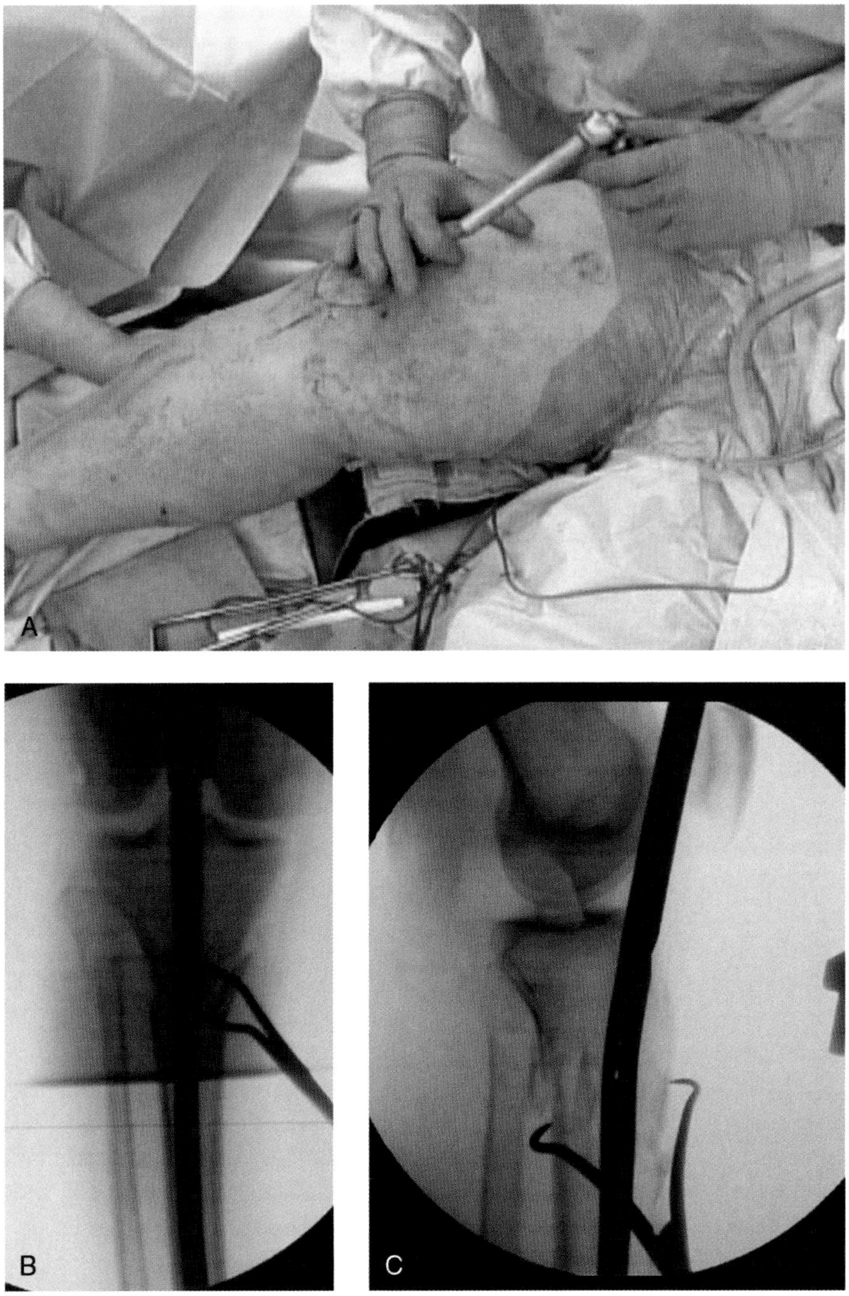

Figure 8 **A,** Intraoperative photograph showing protective cannula placement for semiextended nailing via a small surgical incision. AP (**B**) and lateral (**C**) fluoroscopic images showing the correct starting portal with the semiextended technique. On the lateral view, the knee is flexed 20° to allow proper access to the correct nail entry site.

diographic alignment and union rates can be achieved; however, it is necessary to obtain the reduction before inserting the nail.

In studies of patients with anterior knee pain, 78% had sensory deficits in the distribution area of the infrapatellar nerve.[32-34] Even after nail removal, pain persisted in 7 of 12 patients (58%). The authors concluded that the incidence of iatrogenic damage to the infrapatellar nerve after tibial nailing is high and lasting. In one study, 67% of the patients treated with transtendinous nailing reported anterior knee pain at the final evaluation, whereas 71% of the patients treated with paratendinous nailing reported anterior knee pain.[34] Katsoulis et al[21] reported a 56% incidence of anterior knee pain. Tornetta et al[20] compared postoperative pain in patients treated with IM nailing in extension and in hyperflexion. Of the 192 patients studied, the same number of patients in each nailing group experienced knee pain (**Table 2**). None of these patients had greater than 5° of angulation in any plane.

Treatment With a Plate

Proximal tibial fractures can be successfully treated with one or multiple plates. Plates may be locked, unlocked, placed in an open fashion with clear reduction of the fracture, or placed using minimally invasive techniques and fluoroscopy. Regardless of the type of plate used or the surgical technique, the goal is to accurately restore alignment and achieve stable fracture fixation with minimal soft-tissue damage.

Anatomy of the Fracture

Most proximal tibial fractures are caused by a direct blow to the tibia. For extra-articular fractures (type A), the length of the plate used and the orientation of the fixation will depend on the amount of comminution at the fracture site and whether the fracture is purely metaphyseal or has diaphyseal extension. The two most common extra-articular patterns are oblique in nature, going from anteroinferior to posterosuperior or inferomedial to superolateral. For the simple articular (type C1) fracture pattern, intra-articular involvement is minimal, although all of the proximal tibial condyle is fractured from the remaining tibia. Bicondylar fractures with greater

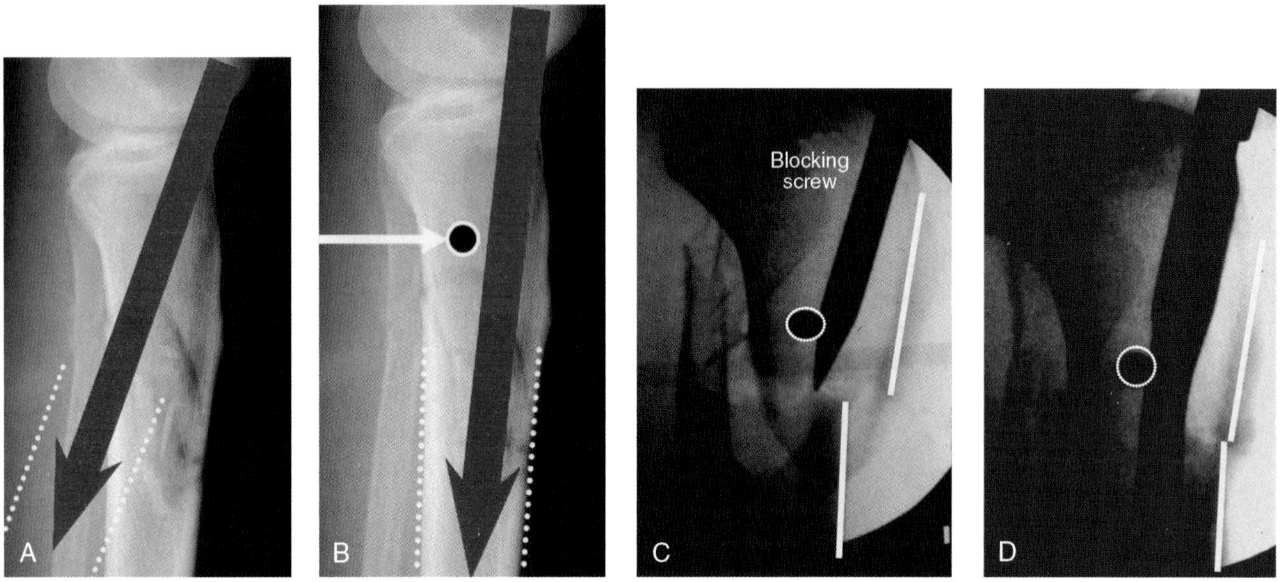

Figure 9 **A,** Lateral radiograph of a proximal tibial fracture. The red arrow shows the trajectory of the posterior nail. The dotted yellow lines show where the shaft will end if the nail trajectory is not changed. **B,** With the placement of a blocking screw (black circle) the nail trajectory changes, and the fracture is aligned (dotted yellow lines). **C,** Lateral radiograph of a posteriorly placed blocking screw in the proximal fragment. Note the fracture gap (yellow lines). **D,** After placement of the IM nail, the fracture has been reduced (yellow lines).

displacement at the level of the joint (C2 and C3 fractures), as well as fracture-dislocations, are beyond the scope of this chapter but are typically best treated with plating or fine wire external fixation (**Figure 11**).

The fracture anatomy and stability required to maintain fracture alignment will dictate the type of plate used and the location of the plate(s). A laterally based plate is frequently used for extra-articular fractures and lateral condyle fractures. Dual plating with a lateral plate combined with a medial or a posteromedial plate is more appropriate for proximal tibial fractures with greater intra-articular involvement and/or comminution of the medial metaphyseal region. The morphologic features of the medial condyle play a critical role in deciding on the type of plate(s). Laterally based, thick, locking plates are well suited for stabilizing the proximal tibia if the medial fracture is a basic transverse pattern or believed to be axially stable. The axial stability of the medial side will take pressure off the lateral plate. The greater the metaphyseal comminution is medially, the more one may lean toward using a medial plate to help support the medial side. In such cases, a thinner locked or unlocked plate laterally will diminish soft-tissue concerns and provide adequate lateral stability unless the fracture has a long diaphyseal extension. In contrast, if the medial fracture is not complete, as in the typical fracture-dislocation pattern with a coronal plane fracture, a posteromedial plate is obligatory (**Figure 12**). This type of medial injury is observed in almost one third of bicondylar plateau fractures.[35]

Surgical Approaches

The approach used for fracture fixation is equally as important as stabilizing the fracture itself. A lateral proximal tibial fracture can be approached with a vertical incision or an incision shaped like a lazy S or a hockey stick to allow appropriate treatment using a buttress plating technique (**Figure 13**). These approaches can be extended distally to treat diaphyseal extension if a percutaneous reduction cannot be achieved. A direct posterior medial approach between the gastrocnemius and semimembranous muscles will allow access to the posterior aspect of the tibial plateau and posterior metaphyseal area[36] (**Figure 14**). With this approach, placement of a buttress plate on the posterior medial cortex will allow treatment of the fracture, with fragment-specific reduction through placement of a plate at the apex of the fracture. With any surgical approach chosen, the need for future surgical incisions over the knee, such as for a total knee arthroplasty, should be considered. Vertical incisions are generally preferred for complex intra-articular fractures (**Figure 15**). For extra-articular fractures, the joint does not have to be opened, and the incision should be large enough only to elevate the anterior compartment sufficiently to fit the head of the plate.

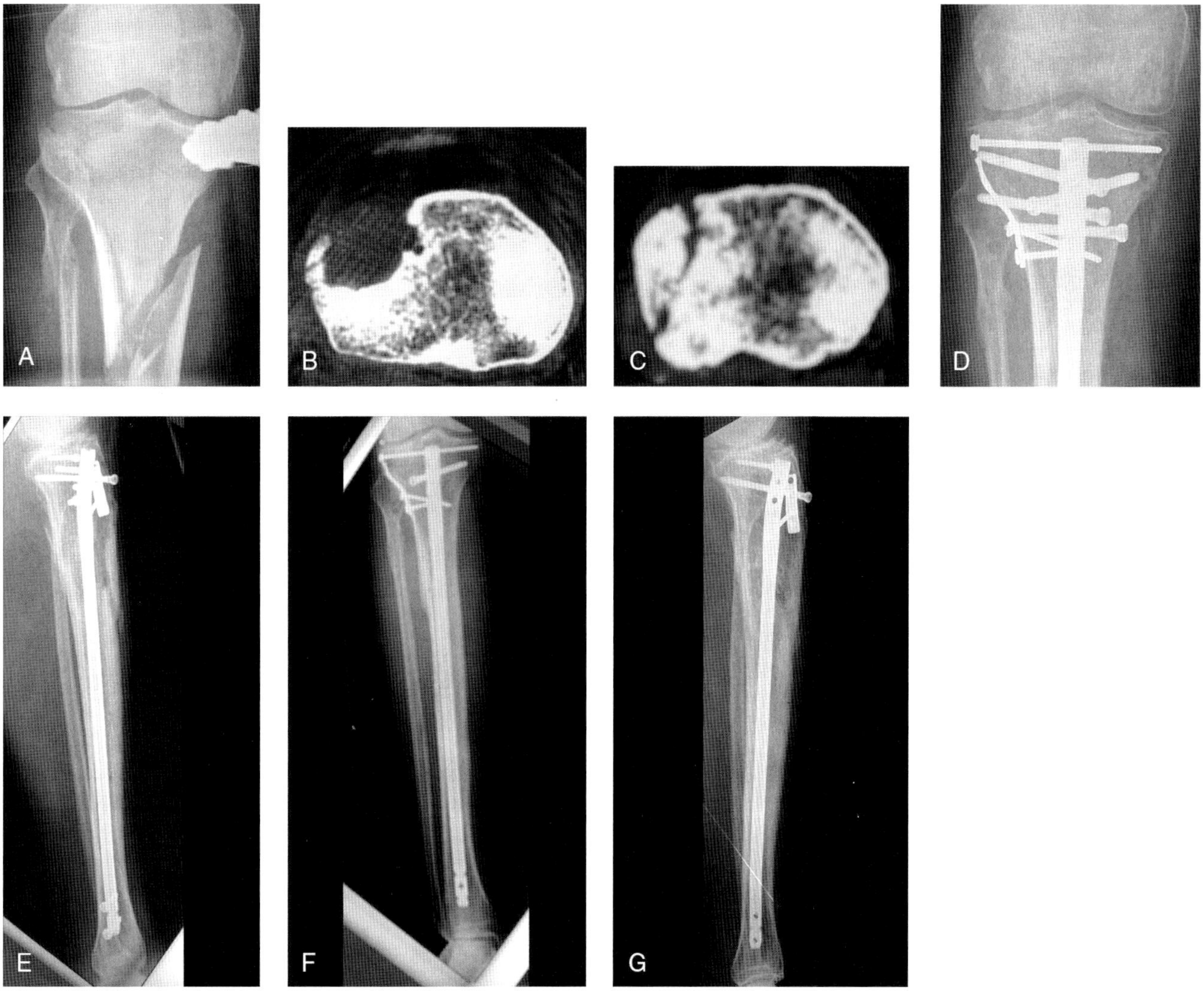

Figure 10 Preoperative AP radiograph (**A**) and CT scans (**B** and **C**) of an interarticular proximal tibial fracture with diaphyseal extension. Immediate postoperative AP (**D**) and lateral (**E**) radiographs after treatment with IM nailing and mini-open reduction and internal fixation. AP (**F**) and lateral (**G**) radiographs taken at the 5-year follow-up examination.

Locking Plates

Locked plating offers improved fixation of fractures prone to collapse on the opposite side of the plate, as seen on the medial side of proximal tibial fractures. The locked screws placed in the proximal fragment from the lateral side provide support to the medial side to aid in preventing varus collapse. In a retrospective review of 54 patients treated with locked plating for periarticular fractures of the knee, 94% of the fractures united, and no varus collapse or screw fixation failure occurred.[37]

Table 2
Postoperative Knee Pain: Intramedullary Nailing (Semiextended Technique) Versus Standard Nailing (Hyperflexion)

Pain (0 = none, 3 = severe)	Extension Nailing	Standard Nailing
0	79%	78%
1	19%	10%
2	2%	8%
3	0%	4%

To improve fracture fixation, specific techniques and tips are helpful (**Table 3**). This chapter's authors recommend that metaphyseal fixation for locked plates should use as many large diameter screws (for example, 5.7 mm) as the system allows. Using a larger screw diameter and a large number of

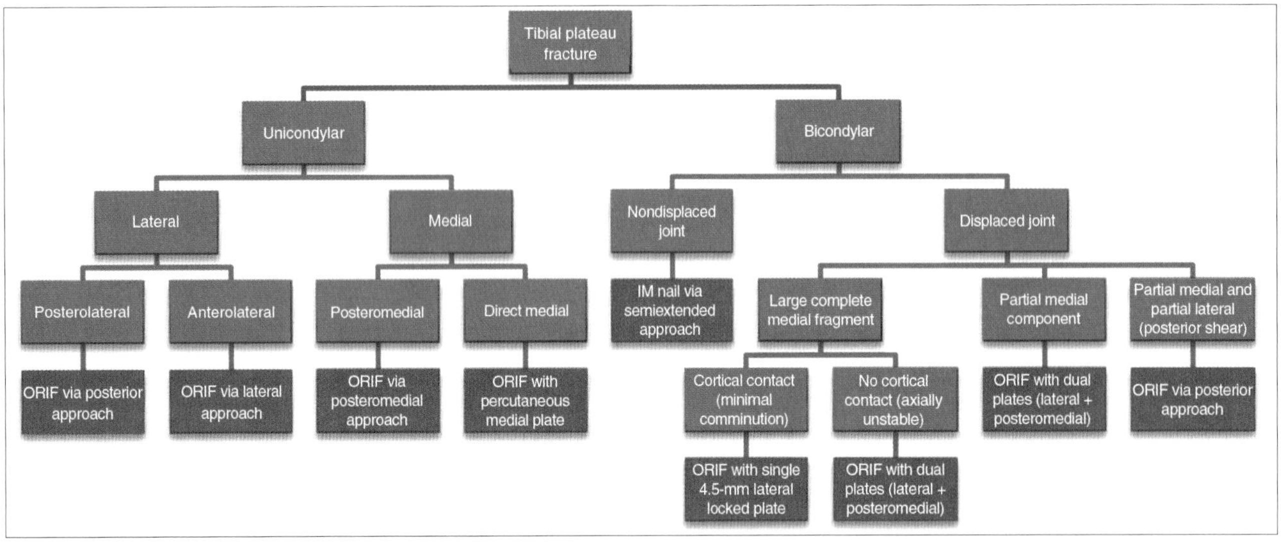

Figure 11 This chapter's authors treatment algorithm for the fixation of proximal tibial fractures. ORIF = open reduction and internal fixation.

screws in the metaphysis provides a larger area of metaphyseal bone support. When adding locking screws to a plate construct in the diaphysis, bicortical screws will increase the construct's rigidity.[38] The mechanical strength of the plate-fracture construct with unicortical diaphyseal locking screws is inferior to bicortical fixation, especially in torsion.[37,39,40] However, it is unclear how many fixation points are needed in the diaphysis. Although stable fixation is needed, a construct that is too stiff can diminish callus formation. The working length must be optimized for each fracture. If an anatomic reduction is achieved, a stiff construct may be beneficial. In contrast, if a bridge plate technique is used, leaving several holes open near the fracture may benefit healing. The surgeon must determine the goals of fixation and choose a construct that meets those criteria.

After metaphyseal reduction has been obtained, provisional fixation and a formal radiographic check of the alignment should be done. Extramedullary guides can be used to confirm alignment from the knee to the ankle in proximal tibial fractures. An alignment board, a radiopaque board with a single vertical line down the tibial shaft and multiple horizontal lines at 90° angles to the single vertical line, can be placed on top of the leg to assess the plateau-to-shaft alignment and the plateau-to-ankle alignment (**Figure 16**). Using the board, starting at the level of the knee joint down to the ankle, locking plate fixation can be performed with confidence that the alignment of the knee to the ankle is correct. Although no studies have been performed comparing final alignment with and without the use of an alignment board, additional intraoperative tools to verify alignment may provide the surgeon with more information to aid in fracture reduction and alignment. If such a board is not available, this chapter's authors suggest provisional fixation of the plate and obtaining full-length AP and lateral tibial radiographs to confirm alignment.

After alignment is confirmed, an unlocked screw or large clamp typically is used to compress the proximal portion of the plate to the metaphyseal region, creating friction before the fixation is locked. In younger patients with good bone quality, the diaphyseal portion of the fracture can be fixed with all unlocked screws. In revision cases or in patients with osteoporotic bone, a hybrid technique is used. Nonlocking screws are placed within the locking plate to reduce the fracture/bone to the plate. The nonlocking screws can then be replaced by locking screws. The hybrid system offers the benefits of using nonlocking screws for fracture compression and locking screws for fracture stability. The expense of locked constructs is substantially higher than for nonlocked constructs, with most of the cost attributed to the price of the locked screws.[41,42]

A limitation of locking plates is that reduction must be maintained before placing any locked screws. Capturing smaller fractures or portions of the articular surface, especially the posterior medial proximal tibial fracture fragment, is not predictable with laterally placed locking plate systems.[41,43-45]

Nonlocking Plates

Nonlocking plates rely on friction generated by the compression force between the head of the screw and plate for fracture fixation. These types of

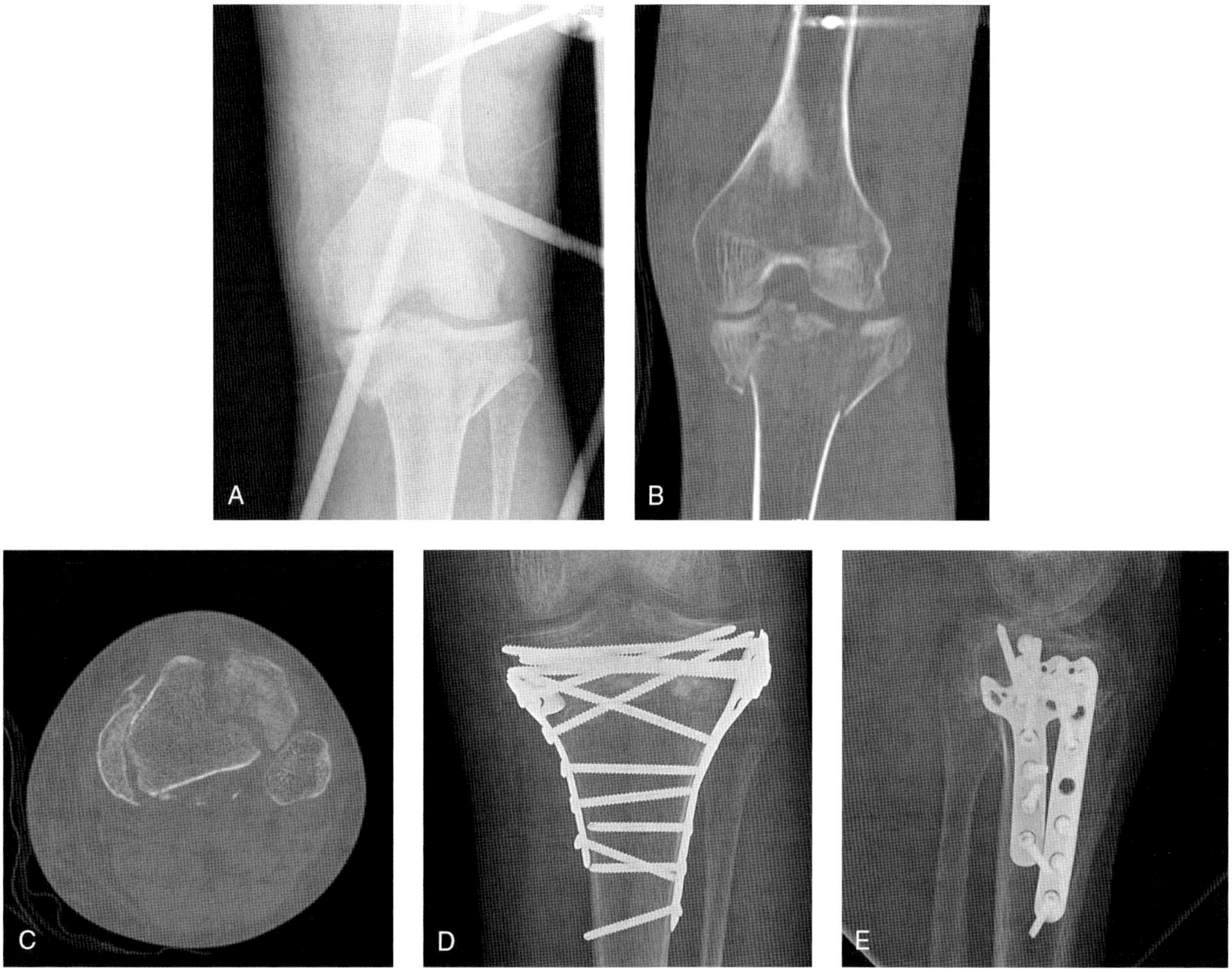

Figure 12 Example of bicondylar tibial plateau fracture treated with dual plating. AP radiograph (**A**) and CT scans (**B** and **C**) of a bicondylar tibial plateau fracture treated initially with a spanning external fixator. AP (**D**) and lateral (**E**) postoperative radiographs after the fracture was treated with condylar plate fixation

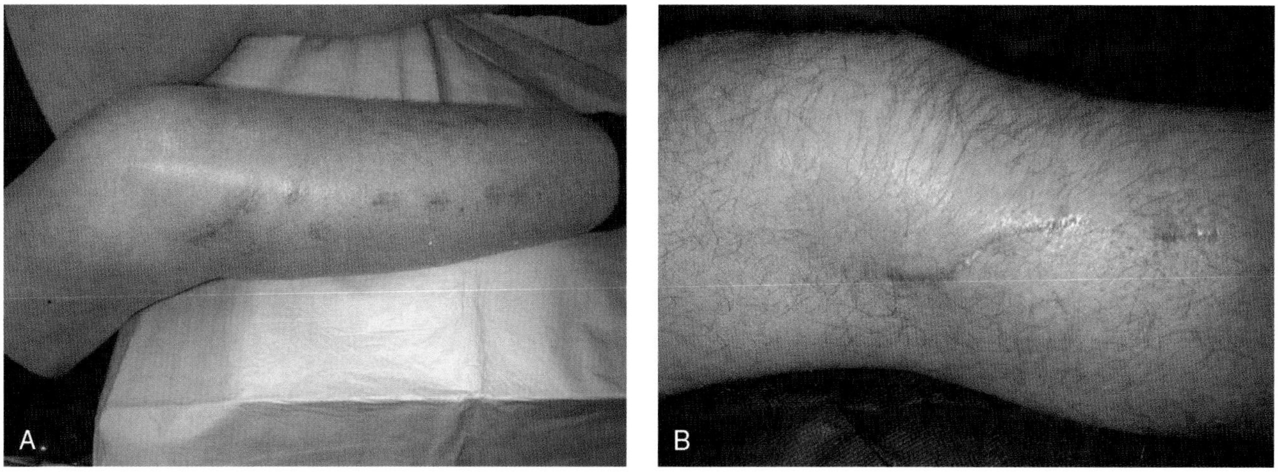

Figure 13 Clinical photographs of the leg after healing of a proximal tibial fracture treated with a mini-open approach (**A**) and the lazy S approach (**B**).

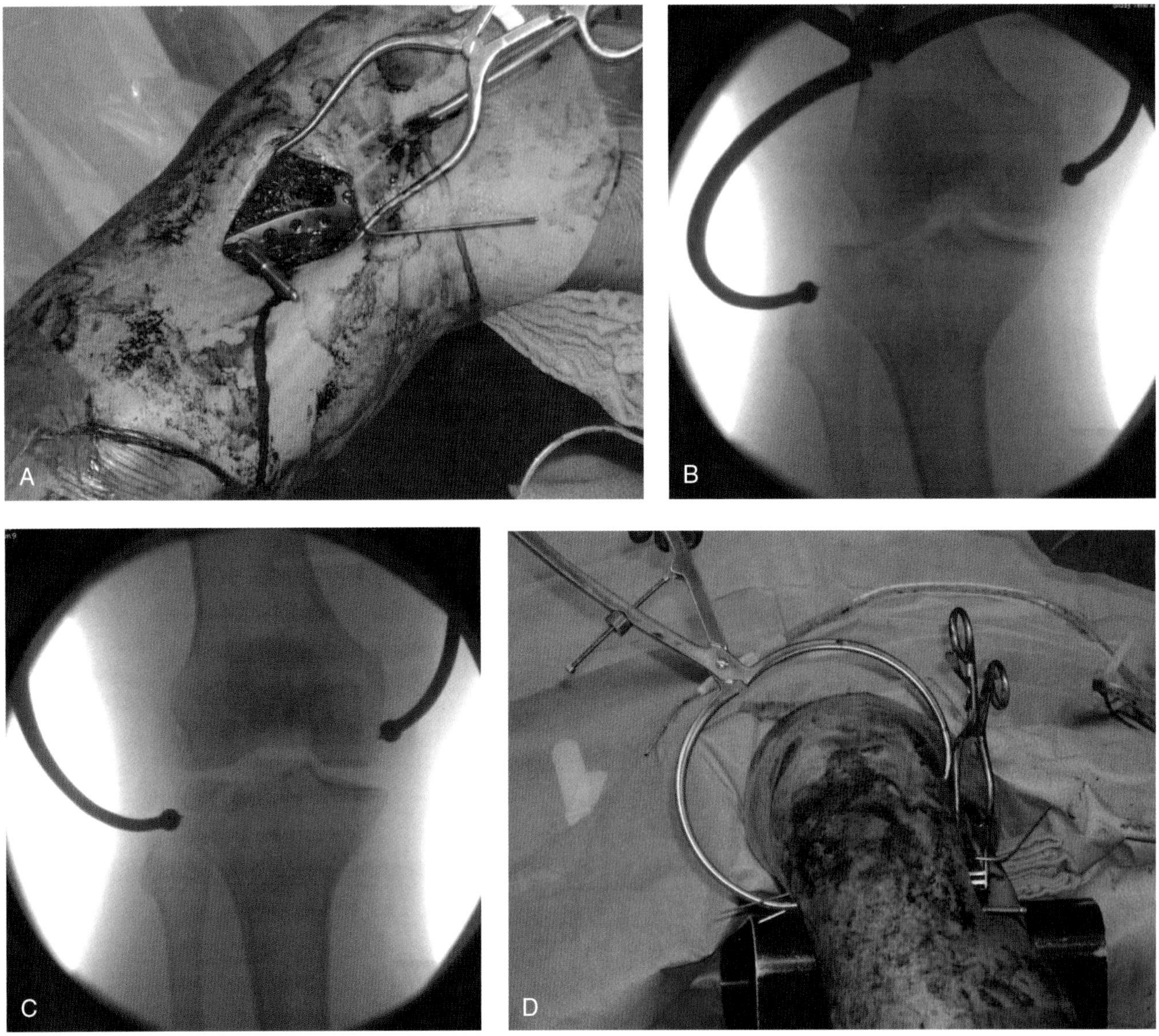

Figure 14 **A,** Intraoperative photograph of the location of the posterior medial plate on completion of the posterior proximal approach to the medial fracture. Wire and a provisional fixation pin are used to temporarily hold the plate in place. Intraoperative fluoroscopic images of the location of the clamp before (**B**) and after (**C**) reduction. **D,** AP view of the periarticular reduction clamp.

constructs fail because of the loss of force at the screw-plate interface and have limited ability to provide axial stability (the bone fracture fragment and screw move as a single unit and become displaced). Because of their design, fracture fixation using only nonlocking plates has limited use in extra-articular proximal tibial fractures. For unstable proximal tibial fractures, both medial and lateral column plates should be used because a single lateral plate will lead to varus collapse. In rare instances of a very stable medial extension, a single unlocked lateral plate will suffice.

Nonlocking fixation can be augmented with external fixation. The addition of an external fixator can help prevent fracture malalignment and provide time for soft-tissue healing. A low malunion rate and a 5% deep infection rate have been reported in treating medial and lateral proximal tibial fractures with a medial external fixator and a 4.5-mm, contoured, dynamic compression plate placed laterally.[46,47]

Percutaneous Plating

The fracture pattern, the need for stability, the condition of the soft-tissue sleeve, and the judgment of the treat-

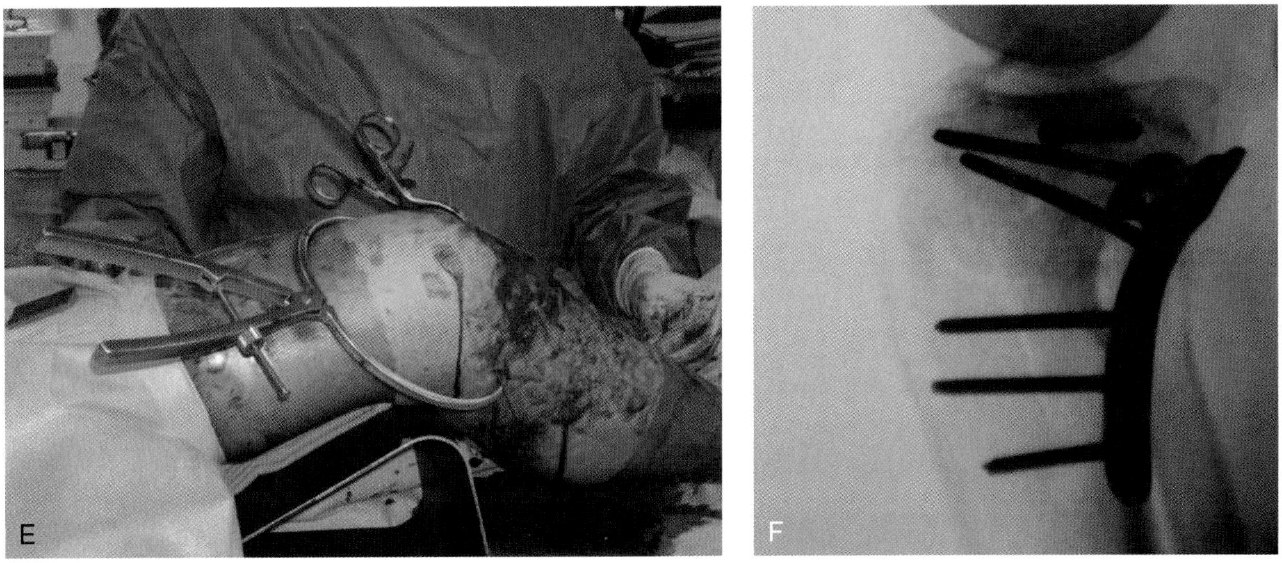

Figure 14 (continued) **E,** Lateral view of the periarticular reduction clamp. **F,** Lateral radiograph showing the final location of the plate on the posterior medial aspect of the tibia.

ing surgeon regarding his or her ability to reduce the fracture percutaneously should be considered when choosing percutaneous fixation versus an open approach.[48] Percutaneous placement and locked fixation are not synonymous. Any plate may be placed with minimally invasive techniques. The decision to open the fracture is based on the ability to reduce it closed or with percutaneous clamps, external distractors, and plating as well as the desired type of fixation (anatomic with compression versus bridge plating).

The Less Invasive Stabilization System (LISS; Synthes, Paoli, PA) was the first implant used in percutaneous treatment of proximal tibial fractures. It is a precontoured lateral implant placed in a submuscular manner. The reported advantages of the LISS system, and percutaneous plating in general, are a smaller incision and less muscle dissection.[49,50]

Studies of percutaneous plating have reported that malalignment occurs in 10% of patients, submuscular fixation of the tibia does not cause a substantial rise in leg compartment pressures, and the incidence of compartment syndrome is not increased.[50,51] Ricci et al[52] confirmed that percutaneous plating can be used to successfully treat complex proximal tibial fractures without the need for additional medial stabilization. However, because the plate is placed without direct surgical visualization of its entire length, the superficial peroneal nerve is at substantial risk for injury during lateral percutaneous screw placement.[53] When the plate is in the region of the neurovascular structures, a small 1- to 2-cm incision should be made, and the anterior compartment should be retracted posteriorly to expose the plate for safe screw placement.

Complications

Infection, malunion, nonunion, and painful hardware necessitating removal are possible complications of plating. Postoperative infection rates range from 1.6% with lateral fixation only to 8.4% with dual plating.[54] The infection rate for percutaneous plating ranges from 0% to 6%.[51,53-57] Even with open visualization and reduction of a proximal tibial fracture, malreduction can occur. The rate of initial loss of fracture reduction using percutaneous plating ranges from 0% to 4%.[51,53-57] Phisitkul et al[58] reported on 37 proximal tibial fractures treated with plate fixation. Complications included eight deep wound infections (22%), eight fracture malalignments (22%), and three fractures with loss of reduction (8%). Fractures treated initially with an external fixator followed by plating had a 5% deep wound infection rate and 4% nonunion rate.[56] Cole et al[49] reported a 5% incidence of hardware removal after plate fixation.

Outcomes

Lindvall et al[59] reported on 29 patients with proximal tibial fractures treated with IM nailing and 42 treated with plating. There was no statistical difference in the final union rate after any additional procedures, with 96% union in the IM nailing group and 97% in the plate group. Apex anterior malreduction was the most preventable form of malreduction in both

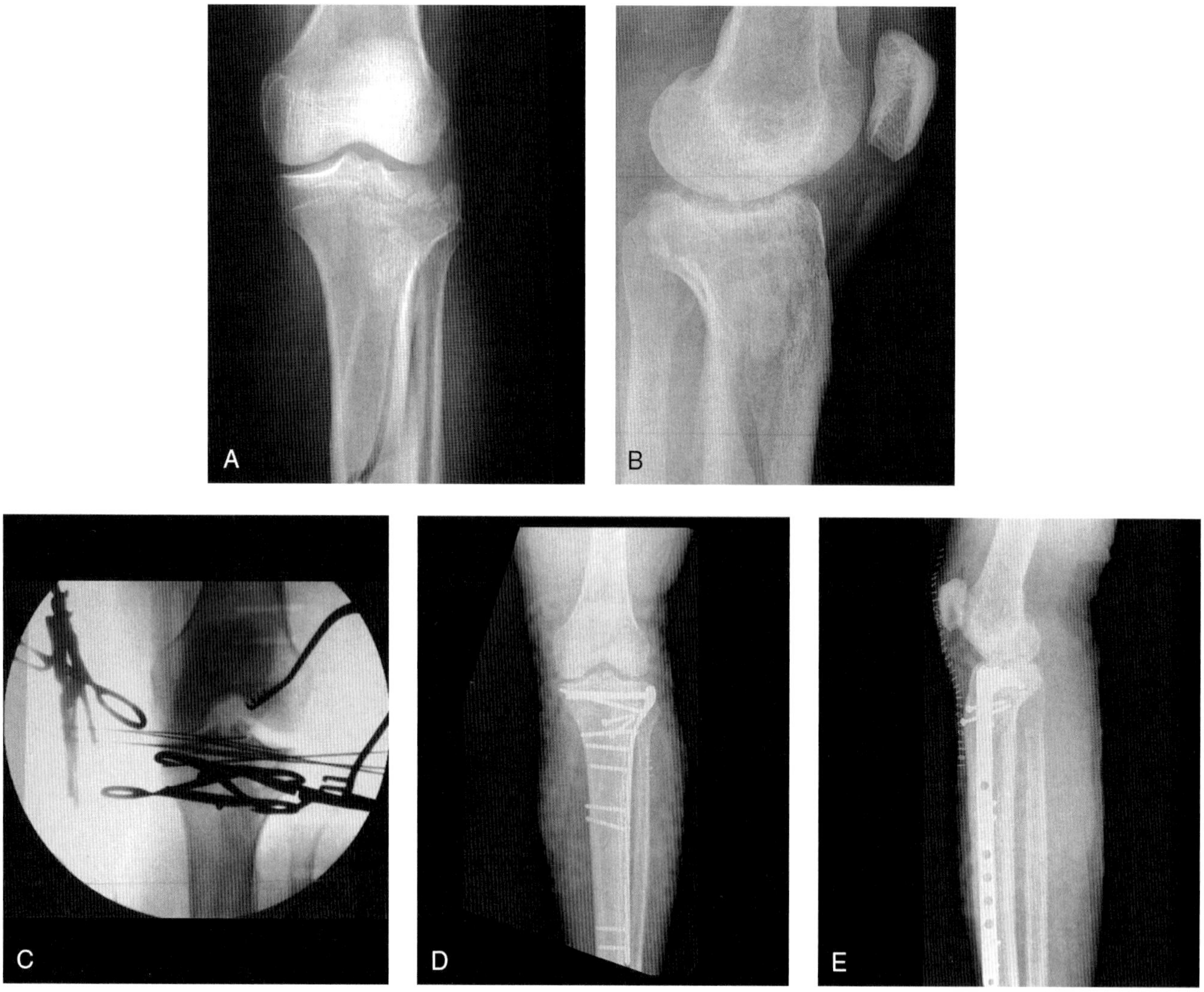

Figure 15 AP (**A**) and lateral (**B**) radiographs of a proximal tibial intra-articular fracture with diaphyseal extension. **C,** Intraoperative fluoroscopic view of the temporary reduction of the proximal fracture using wires and clamps. The fracture was approached via a single middle incision. Postoperative AP (**D**) and lateral (**E**) radiographs. Note the staple line going down the midline of the knee and the limited extent of the incision that stops just distal to the proximal portion of the plate. The distal end of the plate is placed with elevation of the anterior compartment.

groups (36% in the IM nailing group and 15% in the plate group). The rate of implant removal was three times greater in the plating group, and additional surgical techniques were used during reduction in the IM nailing group. The interval change from immediate postoperative radiographs to healed radiographs was substantially different between the groups.

Treatment choice also influences the time to weight bearing. Studies of IM nailing reported commencement of full weight bearing 0 to 16 weeks after surgery. For fractures treated with plating, full weight bearing began 6 to 13 weeks after surgery.[15,49,60]

Future Directions

A prospective multicenter study is currently in progress to evaluate plating or nailing of proximal tibial fractures. The Intramedullary Nails Versus Plate Fixation Re-Evaluation study (IMPRESS) is a randomized controlled trial in which patients with a fracture of the proximal metaphysis of the tibia will be surgically managed with one of two strategies. The first strategy involves fracture fixation with a reamed, interlocking IM nail. The second strategy involves open reduction and internal fixation of the fracture with a locking periarticular plate. The hypothesis of the study is that there will be no difference in the two groups with respect to primary and secondary outcome measures. It is hoped that the results from this study

Table 3
Tips for Treating Proximal Tibial Fractures With a Plate

The surgical approach and technique should minimize soft-tissue damage and account for future surgical procedures that may be needed, such as a total knee arthroplasty.
Fractures with intra-articular involvement and/or comminution of the medial metaphyseal region are appropriately treated with dual plating (a lateral plate combined with a medial or posteromedial plate). Extra-articular fractures without major medial comminution may be treated with a locked lateral plate.
The reduction can be aided with a distractor or an external fixator to gain length.
An alignment guide or a full-length lower extremity radiograph should be used to confirm intraoperative alignment before full definitive fixation.
The number and size of locking screws should be maximized for metaphyseal fixation.
If diaphyseal fixation is required, a long plate is recommended to provide appropriate stability.
Distal diaphyseal fixation of a lateral plate should be done by mobilizing the anterior compartment posteriorly to place screws under direct vision.

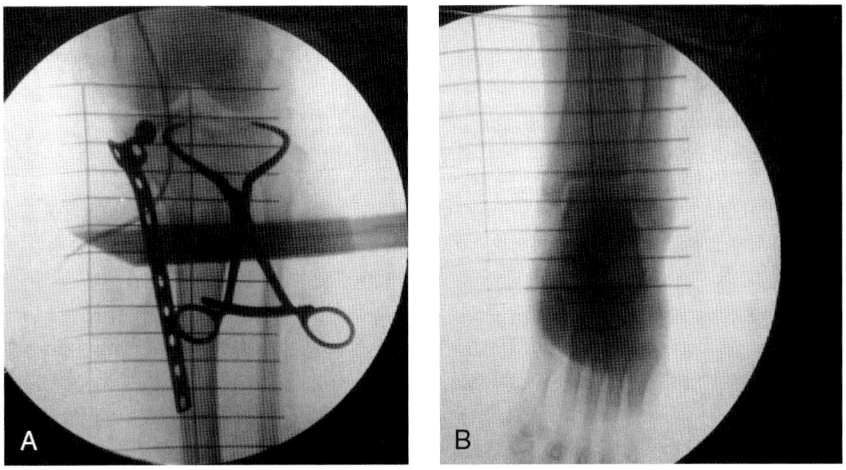

Figure 16 **A,** Intraoperative radiograph of the proximal tibia just before placement of the plate. The horizontal lines are from the alignment board placed behind the lower extremity. **B,** The alignment board aids in visualizing the axis of the tibia and the joint line at the knee and ankle to help prevent malalignment.

will further clarify and advance the treatment of proximal tibial fractures.

Summary

Plates provide excellent fixation of intra-articular extension fractures and are most useful when the soft-tissue environment is amenable to dissection in the area of the proximal tibia. IM nailing provides added stability through diaphyseal extension, but it requires special techniques and an understanding of the nail's relationship to medullary canal mechanics. Direct incisions in the area of the proximal tibia are avoided, and the soft-tissue sleeve is respected. Hybrid constructs of both minimal plating and IM nailing are viable options. The optimal method of treating a proximal tibial fracture is the method that best balances soft-tissue management and fracture reduction and alignment.

References

1. Lang GJ, Cohen BE, Bosse MJ, Kellam JF: Proximal third tibial shaft fractures: Should they be nailed? *Clin Orthop Relat Res* 1995;315:64-74.
2. Halpern AA, Nagel DA: Anterior compartment pressures in patients with tibial fractures. *J Trauma* 1980;20(9):786-790.
3. Borrelli J Jr, Prickett W, Song E, Becker D, Ricci W: Extraosseous blood supply of the tibia and the effects of different plating techniques: A human cadaveric study. *J Orthop Trauma* 2002;16(10): 691-695.
4. Burgess AR, Poka A, Brumback RJ, Flagle CL, Loeb PE, Ebraheim NA: Pedestrian tibial injuries. *J Trauma* 1987;27(6):596-601.
5. AO Foundation: Müller AO classification of fractures: Long bones. Switzerland, AO Foundation website. http://www.aofoundation.org/ Documents/ mueller_ao_class.pdf. Accessed August 6, 2012.
6. Sarmiento A, Kinman PB, Latta LL, Eng P: Fractures of the proximal tibia and tibial condyles: A clinical and laboratory comparative study. *Clin Orthop Relat Res* 1979;145:136-145.
7. Freedman EL, Johnson EE: Radiographic analysis of tibial fracture malalignment following intramedullary nailing. *Clin Orthop Relat Res* 1995;315:25-33.
8. Henley MB, Meier M, Tencer AF: Influences of some design parameters on the biomechanics of the unreamed tibial intramedullary nail. *J Orthop Trauma* 1993;7(4): 311-319.
9. Court-Brown CM, Byrnes T, McLaughlin G: Intramedullary nailing of tibial diaphyseal fractures in adolescents with open physes. *Injury* 2003;34(10): 781-785.
10. Benirschke SK: Proximal one-third tibial fracture solutions. *Orthop Trans* 1995;18:1055-1056.
11. Vidyadhara S, Sharath KR: Prospective study of the clinico-

radiological outcome of interlocked nailing in proximal third tibial shaft fractures. *Injury* 2006;37(6):536-542.

12. Ricci WM, O'Boyle M, Borrelli J, Bellabarba C, Sanders R: Fractures of the proximal third of the tibial shaft treated with intramedullary nails and blocking screws. *J Orthop Trauma* 2001;15(4):264-270.
13. Buehler KC, Green J, Woll TS, Duwelius PJ: A technique for intramedullary nailing of proximal third tibia fractures. *J Orthop Trauma* 1997;11(3):218-223.
14. Tornetta P III, Collins E: Semiextended position of intramedullary nailing of the proximal tibia. *Clin Orthop Relat Res* 1996;328:185-189.
15. Krettek C, Stephan C, Schandelmaier P, Richter M, Pape HC, Miclau T: The use of Poller screws as blocking screws in stabilising tibial fractures treated with small diameter intramedullary nails. *J Bone Joint Surg Br* 1999;81(6):963-968.
16. Wysocki RW, Kapotas JS, Virkus WW: Intramedullary nailing of proximal and distal one-third tibial shaft fractures with intraoperative two-pin external fixation. *J Trauma* 2009;66(4):1135-1139.
17. Nork SE, Barei DP, Schildhauer TA, et al: Intramedullary nailing of proximal quarter tibial fractures. *J Orthop Trauma* 2006;20(8):523-528.
18. Tornetta P III, Riina J, Geller J, Purban W: Intraarticular anatomic risks of tibial nailing. *J Orthop Trauma* 1999;13(4):247-251.
19. McConnell T, Tornetta P III, Tilzey J, Casey D: Tibial portal placement: The radiographic correlate of the anatomic safe zone. *J Orthop Trauma* 2001;15(3):207-209.
20. Tornetta P III, Steen B, Ryan S: Tibial metaphyseal fractures: Nailing in extension. Orthopaedic Trauma Association 2008 Annual Meeting. Scientific Program Papers: Session 2: Tibia/Polytrauma. http://www.hwbf.org/ota/am/ota08/otapa/OTA080207.htm. Accessed August 6, 2012.
21. Katsoulis E, Court-Brown C, Giannoudis PV: Incidence and aetiology of anterior knee pain after intramedullary nailing of the femur and tibia. *J Bone Joint Surg Br* 2006;88(5):576-580.
22. Eastman J, Tseng S, Lo E, Li CS, Yoo B, Lee M: Retropatellar technique for intramedullary nailing of proximal tibia fractures: A cadaveric assessment. *J Orthop Trauma* 2010;24(11):672-676.
23. Hansen M, Blum J, Mehler D, Hessmann MH, Rommens PM: Double or triple interlocking when nailing proximal tibial fractures? A biomechanical investigation. *Arch Orthop Trauma Surg* 2009;129(12):1715-1719.
24. Sayana MK, Davis BJ, Kapoor B, Rahmatalla A, Maffulli N: Fracture strain and stability with additional locking screws in intramedullary nailing: A biomechanical study. *J Trauma* 2006;60(5):1053-1057.
25. Horn J, Linke B, Höntzsch D, Gueorguiev B, Schwieger K: Angle stable interlocking screws improve construct stability of intramedullary nailing of distal tibia fractures: A biomechanical study. *Injury* 2009;40(7):767-771.
26. Cole D: Intramedullary fixation of proximal tibia fractures. *Tech Orthop* 1998;13(1).
27. Krettek C, Miclau T, Schandelmaier P, Stephan C, Möhlmann U, Tscherne H: The mechanical effect of blocking screws ("Poller screws") in stabilizing tibia fractures with short proximal or distal fragments after insertion of small-diameter intramedullary nails. *J Orthop Trauma* 1999;13(8):550-553.
28. Tang P, Gates C, Hawes J, Vogt M, Prayson MJ: Does open reduction increase the chance of infection during intramedullary nailing of closed tibial shaft fractures? *J Orthop Trauma* 2006;20(5):317-322.
29. Matthews DE, McGuire R, Freeland AE: Anterior unicortical buttress plating in conjunction with an unreamed interlocking intramedullary nail for treatment of very proximal tibial diaphyseal fractures. *Orthopedics* 1997;20(7):647-648.
30. Kim KC, Lee JK, Hwang DS, Yang JY, Kim YM: Provisional unicortical plating with reamed intramedullary nailing in segmental tibial fractures involving the high proximal metaphysis. *Orthopedics* 2007;30(3):189-192.
31. Hiesterman TG, Shafiq BX, Cole PA: Intramedullary nailing of extra-articular proximal tibia fractures. *J Am Acad Orthop Surg* 2011;19(11):690-700.
32. Leliveld MS, Verhofstad MH: Injury to the infrapatellar branch of the saphenous nerve: A possible cause for anterior knee pain after tibial nailing? *Injury* 2012;43(6):779-783.
33. Keating JF, Orfaly R, O'Brien PJ: Knee pain after tibial nailing. *J Orthop Trauma* 1997;11(1):10-13.
34. Toivanen JA, Väistö O, Kannus P, Latvala K, Honkonen SE, Järvinen MJ: Anterior knee pain after intramedullary nailing of fractures of the tibial shaft: A prospective, randomized study comparing two different nail-insertion techniques. *J Bone Joint Surg Am* 2002;84(4):580-585.
35. Barei DP, O'Mara TJ, Taitsman LA, Dunbar RP, Nork SE: Frequency and fracture morphology of the posteromedial fragment in bicondylar tibial plateau fracture patterns. *J Orthop Trauma* 2008;22(3):176-182.

36. Medvecky MJ, Noyes FR: Surgical approaches to the posteromedial and posterolateral aspects of the knee. *J Am Acad Orthop Surg* 2005;13(2):121-128.

37. Haidukewych G, Sems SA, Huebner D, Horwitz D, Levy B: Results of polyaxial locked-plate fixation of periarticular fractures of the knee. *J Bone Joint Surg Am* 2007;89(3):614-620.

38. Dougherty PJ, Kim DG, Meisterling S, Wybo C, Yeni Y: Biomechanical comparison of bicortical versus unicortical screw placement of proximal tibia locking plates: A cadaveric model. *J Orthop Trauma* 2008;22(6):399-403.

39. Kregor PJ, Stannard J, Zlowodzki M, Cole PA, Alonso J: Distal femoral fracture fixation utilizing the Less Invasive Stabilization System (L.I.S.S.): The technique and early results. *Injury* 2001;32(suppl 3): SC32-SC47.

40. Egol KA, Kubiak EN, Fulkerson E, Kummer FJ, Koval KJ: Biomechanics of locked plates and screws. *J Orthop Trauma* 2004; 18(8):488-493.

41. Haidukewych GJ: Innovations in locking plate technology. *J Am Acad Orthop Surg* 2004;12(4): 205-212.

42. Gardner MJ, Helfet DL, Lorich DG: Has locked plating completely replaced conventional plating? *Am J Orthop (Belle Mead NJ)* 2004;33(9):439-446.

43. Althausen PL, Lee MA, Finkemeier CG, Meehan JP, Rodrigo JJ: Operative stabilization of supracondylar femur fractures above total knee arthroplasty: A comparison of four treatment methods. *J Arthroplasty* 2003;18(7): 834-839.

44. Fulkerson E, Koval K, Preston CF, Iesaka K, Kummer FJ, Egol KA: Fixation of periprosthetic femoral shaft fractures associated with cemented femoral stems: A biomechanical comparison of locked plating and conventional cable plates. *J Orthop Trauma* 2006;20(2):89-93.

45. Raab GE, Davis CM III: Early healing with locked condylar plating of periprosthetic fractures around the knee. *J Arthroplasty* 2005;20(8):984-989.

46. Bolhofner BR: Indirect reduction and compositie fixation of extraarticular proximal tibia fractures. *Clin Orthop Relat Res* 1995;315: 75-83.

47. Gerber A, Ganz R: Combined internal and external osteosynthesis: A biological approach to the treatment of complex fractures of the proximal tibia. *Injury* 1998; 29(suppl):C22-C28.

48. Lowe JA, Tejwani N, Yoo BJ, Wolinsky PR: Surgical techniques for complex proximal tibial fractures. *Instr Course Lect* 2012;61:39-51.

49. Cole PA, Zlowodzki M, Kregor PJ: Treatment of proximal tibia fractures using the less invasive stabilization system: Surgical experience and early clinical results in 77 fractures. *J Orthop Trauma* 2004;18(8):528-535.

50. Cole PA, Zlowodzki M, Kregor PJ: Compartment pressures after submuscular fixation of proximal tibia fractures. *Injury* 2003; 34(suppl 1):A43-A46.

51. Boldin C, Fankhauser F, Hofer HP, Szyszkowitz R: Three-year results of proximal tibia fractures treated with the LISS. *Clin Orthop Relat Res* 2006;445:222-229.

52. Ricci WM, Rudzki JR, Borrelli J Jr: Treatment of complex proximal tibia fractures with the less invasive skeletal stabilization system. *J Orthop Trauma* 2004; 18(8):521-527.

53. Deangelis JP, Deangelis NA, Anderson R: Anatomy of the superficial peroneal nerve in relation to fixation of tibia fractures with the less invasive stabilization system. *J Orthop Trauma* 2004;18(8): 536-539.

54. Higgins TF, Klatt J, Bachus KN: Biomechanical analysis of bicondylar tibial plateau fixation: How does lateral locking plate fixation compare to dual plate fixation? *J Orthop Trauma* 2007;21(5): 301-306.

55. Stannard JP, Wilson TC, Volgas DA, Alonso JE: Fracture stabilization of proximal tibial fractures with the proximal tibial LISS: Early experience in Birmingham, Alabama (USA). *Injury* 2003; 34(suppl 1):A36-A42.

56. Egol KA, Tejwani NC, Capla EL, Wolinsky PL, Koval KJ: Staged management of high-energy proximal tibia fractures (OTA types 41): The results of a prospective, standardized protocol. *J Orthop Trauma* 2005;19(7):448-456.

57. Schütz M, Kääb MJ, Haas N: Stabilization of proximal tibial fractures with the LIS-System: Early clinical experience in Berlin. *Injury* 2003;34(suppl 1): A30-A35.

58. Phisitkul P, McKinley TO, Nepola JV, Marsh JL: Complications of locking plate fixation in complex proximal tibia injuries. *J Orthop Trauma* 2007;21(2): 83-91.

59. Lindvall E, Sanders R, Dipasquale T, Herscovici D, Haidukewych G, Sagi C: Intramedullary nailing versus percutaneous locked plating of extra-articular proximal tibial fractures: Comparison of 56 cases. *J Orthop Trauma* 2009; 23(7):485-492.

60. Gustilo RB, Simpson L, Nixon R, Ruiz A, Indeck W: Analysis of 511 open fractures. *Clin Orthop Relat Res* 1969;66:148-154.

7

Fractures and Dislocations of the Midfoot: Lisfranc and Chopart Injuries

Stephen K. Benirschke, MD
Eric G. Meinberg, MD
Sarah A. Anderson, MD
Clifford B. Jones, MD, FACS
Peter A. Cole, MD

Abstract

The midfoot is a complex association of five bones and many articulations between the forefoot metatarsals and the talus and calcaneus, which make up the hindfoot. These anatomic relationships are connected and restrained by an even more complex network of ligaments, capsules, and fascia, which must function as a unit to provide normal and painless locomotion. The common eponyms of Lisfranc and Chopart refer to the distal and proximal joint relationships of the midfoot, respectively. Midfoot injuries range from single ligament strains to complicated fracture-dislocations involving multiple bones and joints. To provide best outcomes for patients, it is important to understand the anatomy and the mechanical function of the midfoot; to review the epidemiology, mechanism, and classification of injuries encountered in an orthopaedic clinical practice; and to review the principles, indications, and surgical techniques for managing midfoot fractures and dislocations.

Instr Course Lect 2013;62:79-91.

Definitions and Epidemiology

The Chopart joint, also known as the midtarsal or transverse tarsal joint, consists of the calcaneocuboid and talonavicular joints. These two joints lie in a plane perpendicular to the longitudinal arch of the foot and act as a single unit with respect to the hindfoot. The Lisfranc joint consists of the tarsometatarsal joint complex, which includes the medial, middle, and lateral cuneiforms; the cuboid; and the articulations with the five metatarsal bases. The navicular cuneiform articulations and the articulation between the navicular and cuboid bones do not specifically have their own eponym. The Lisfranc joint forms the osseous and ligamentous foundation of the longitudinal and transverse arches (**Figure 1**).

Midfoot fractures, including those involving the Chopart and Lisfranc joints, can be very easy to miss because of their rarity, the lack of obvious radiographic findings in up to 33% of such injuries, and the lack of familiarity with such fractures by many treating physicians.[1] Chopart joint injuries are extremely rare.[2] Injuries to the Lisfranc joint complex are uncommon, accounting for only 0.2% of fractures, or 1 in 55,000 people each year.[3] Approximately one third are caused by low-energy trauma, such as sports injuries.[4,5] Adding to the confusion, injuries to the Lisfranc or Chopart joint

Dr. Benirschke or an immediate family member serves as an unpaid consultant to Synthes and Zimmer. Dr. Meinberg or an immediate family member serves as a board member, owner, officer, or committee member of the Northern California Chapter, Western Orthopaedic Association; is a member of a speakers' bureau or has made paid presentations on behalf of Synthes; and serves as a paid consultant to or is an employee of Amgen, Medtronic, and Synthes. Dr. Jones or an immediate family member serves as a board member, owner, officer, or committee member of the AOA Own the Bone Board, the Mid-American Orthopaedic Association Bylaws Committee, the OTA Outcomes and Classification Committee, and is the Michigan Orthopaedic Society President. Dr. Cole or an immediate family member serves as a paid consultant to or is an employee of Synthes and has received research or institutional support from Synthes, DePuy, Zimmer, Acumed, Smith & Nephew, and Stryker. Neither Dr. Anderson nor any immediate family member has received anything of value from or owns stock in a commercial company or institution related directly or indirectly to the subject of this chapter.

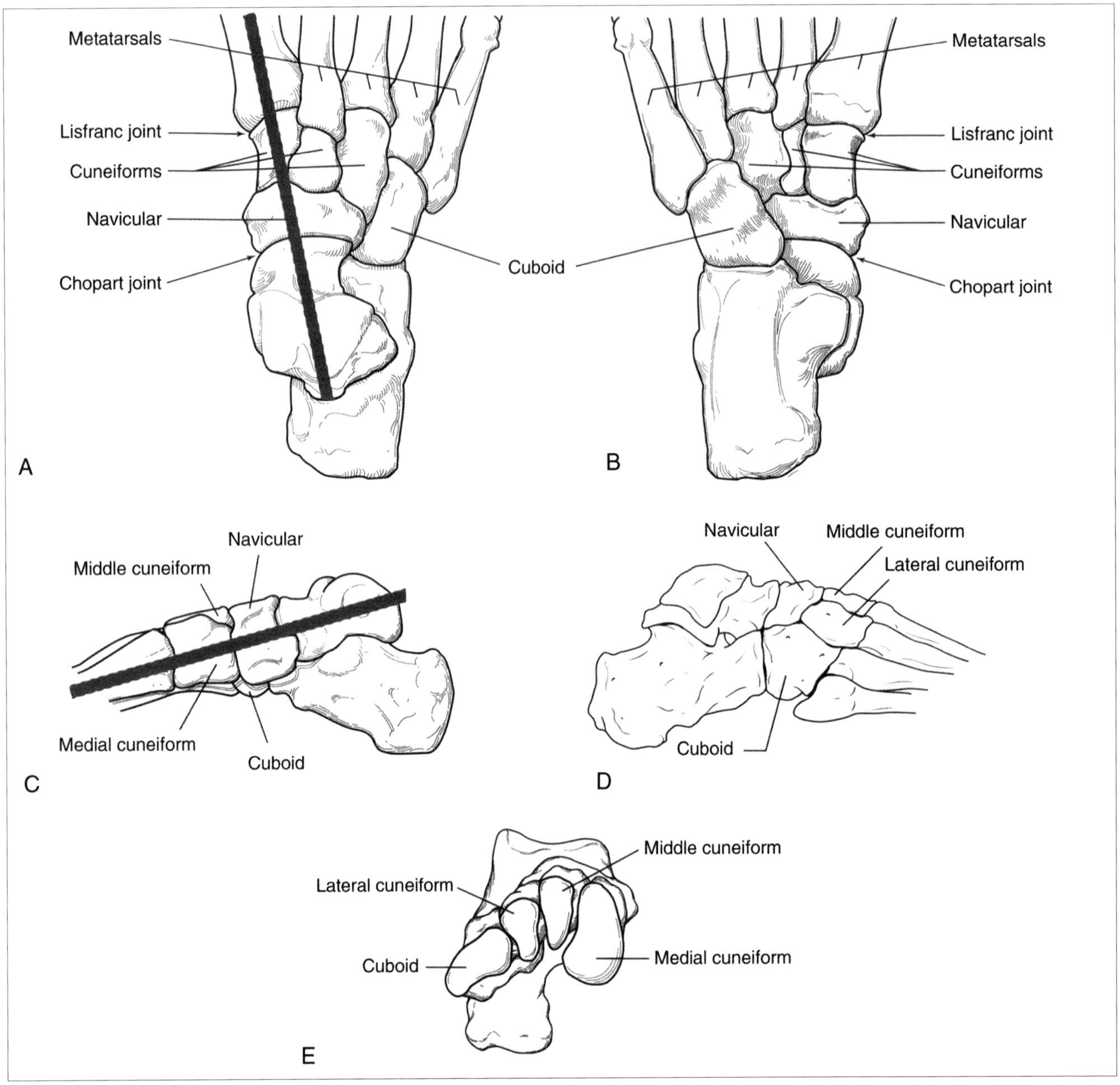

Figure 1 Illustrations of the osseous anatomy of the midfoot showing superior view (**A**), inferior view (**B**), medial view (**C**), lateral view (**D**), and coronal view (**E**). Note the modification of images with the red lines (**A** and **C**), which show normal alignment of the midfoot, with the talus, navicular, medial cuneiform, and first metatarsal. (Adapted with permission from Reid JJ, Early JS: Osseous anatomy of the midfoot, in Bucholz RW, Heckman JD, Court-Brown CM, Tornetta P, eds: *Rockwood and Green's Fractures in Adults*, ed 7. Philadelphia, PA, Lippincott Williams and Wilkins, 2010, p 2111.)

frequently occur in combination with other midfoot injuries.

Osseous and Soft-Tissue Anatomy

The Chopart joint is composed of the condyloid talonavicular joint and the saddle-shaped calcaneocuboid joint. These two joints invert and evert with the subtalar joint. The talonavicular joint is stabilized in part by the acetabulum pedis, a deep socket that contains the head of the talus. It is composed of the concave proximal surface of the navicular, the anterior and middle facets of the calcaneus, the spring ligament, and the bifurcate Y-shaped ligament (**Figure 2**). The calcaneocuboid joint is concave vertically and convex transversely, forming the articulation between the anterior process of

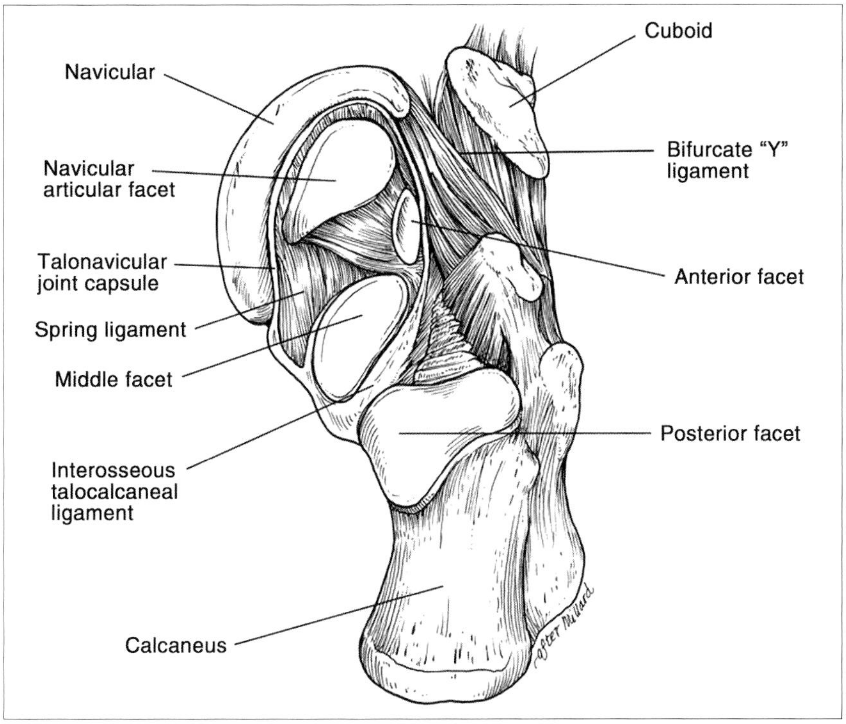

Figure 2 Illustration showing the anatomy of the acetabulum pedis. (Reproduced from Kou JX, Fortin PT: Commonly missed peritalar injuries. *J Am Acad Orthop Surg* 2009;17:775-786.)

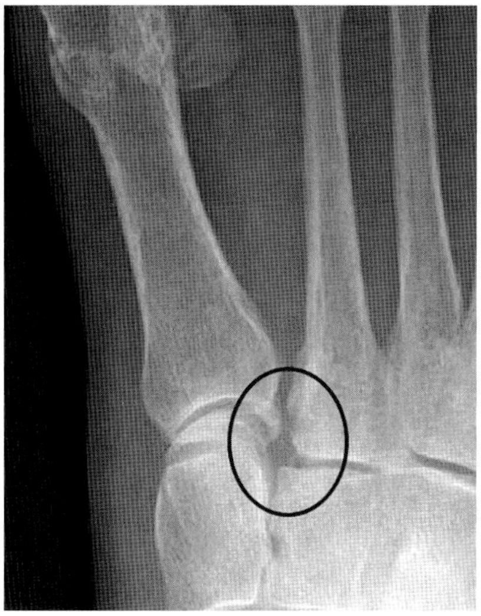

Figure 3 Non–weight-bearing AP radiograph of the foot showing a diastasis of greater than 2 mm (circle) between the medial border of the second metatarsal base and the lateral border of the medial cuneiform. Note the avulsion fragment in this interspace.

the calcaneus and the cuboid. This highly congruent joint "locks in" during step-off.

The Lisfranc joint is a combination of the tarsometatarsal, anterior intertarsal, and proximal intermetatarsal joints and is critical to the longitudinal and transverse arches of the foot. Transverse stability is provided by the trapezoidal Roman arch architecture of the complex. Longitudinal stability is provided primarily by the second metatarsal base, which acts as a keystone to the joint complex. The first three metatarsals each articulate with a cuneiform, whereas the fourth and fifth metatarsals each articulate with a separate facet of the cuboid (**Figure 1**). The stability of these joints is dependent on ligamentous support.

The joint capsules of the Lisfranc complex are divided into three compartments: medial (first tarsometatarsal joint), central (second and third tarsometatarsal joints), and lateral (fourth and fifth tarsometatarsal joints). Ligaments are best grouped as dorsal, interosseous, and plantar. Dorsal ligaments follow a transverse, oblique, and longitudinal orientation. The interosseous ligaments are the strongest of the Lisfranc complex and are important in the stability of the joint. Interosseous ligaments join the second through fifth metatarsals together, but there are none between the first and second metatarsal. Rather, the Lisfranc ligament joins the second metatarsal to the medial cuneiform, securing the medial column to the intermediate and lateral columns. The Lisfranc ligament is the largest and strongest interosseous ligament and is responsible for the avulsion fragment off the plantar second metatarsal base commonly seen in fracture-dislocations (**Figure 3**). Plantar ligaments are substantially stronger than their corresponding dorsal counterparts, helping to maintain the Roman arch architecture of the midfoot.

The dorsalis pedis artery crosses the Lisfranc joint and courses between the first and second metatarsal bases to the plantar surface to form the plantar arch. It may be avulsed or thrombosed in a fracture-dislocation, resulting in hematoma or compartment syndrome. The deep peroneal nerve follows the dorsalis pedis artery and provides innervation to the first dorsal web space.

Although many tendons cross the Chopart and Lisfranc joints, the tibialis anterior and peroneus longus are the most important. The tibialis anterior inserts onto the dorsum of the first metatarsal base and the medial cuneiform, providing dynamic stability to the first tarsometatarsal joint. In ipsilateral dislocations, the tibialis anterior tendon may become entrapped between the middle and medial cuneiforms, blocking reduction. The peroneus longus inserts onto the plantar-

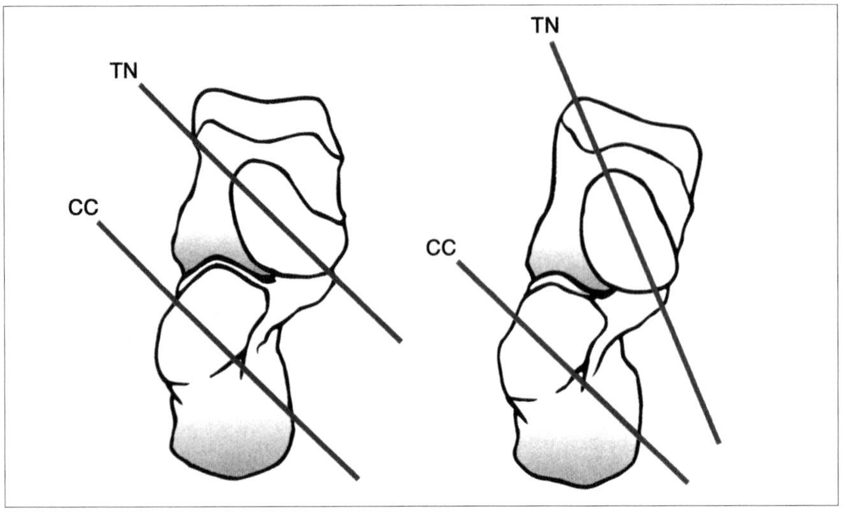

Figure 4 Function of the transverse tarsal joint. When the foot is in an everted position as shown in the left image, the lines bisecting the two joints are parallel. In the right image, the foot is shown in an inverted position, and the two joints are not parallel. This highlights the complexity of the subtalar joint and the multiplanar motion of the hindfoot. TN = talonavicular joint, CC = calcaneocuboid joint. (Adapted with permission from Mann RA, Haskell A: Biomechanics of the foot and ankle, in Coughlin MJ, Mann RA, Saltzman CL, eds: *Surgery of the Foot and Ankle*, ed 8. Philadelphia, PA, Mosby, 2007, p 21.)

lateral surface of the first metatarsal, dynamically supporting the transverse and longitudinal arches of the foot.

Video 7.1: Midfoot Anatomy. Eric G. Meinberg, MD (6 min)

Biomechanics of the Midfoot

Normal anatomy and biomechanics of the midfoot are best understood with use of the column theories. The Chopart joint is the flexible medial column, involving the talus and navicular, and the lateral column, which includes the calcaneus and the cuboid. The rest of the medial column is rigid and made up of the cuneiforms and the first, second, and third metatarsals, whereas the rest of the lateral column is flexible and is made up of the fourth and fifth metatarsals. In the midfoot, the middle and medial cuneiform, second and third metatarsals, and their associated rays are the intermediate or the middle column. Approximately 3.5 mm of dorsal-plantar motion occurs in the medial column. Rigidity is provided by the intermediate column, whereas the mobile lateral column provides shock absorption.

The Chopart joint allows the hindfoot to pivot while the forefoot remains stationary. This joint complex, together with the subtalar joint, functions as a unit to invert and evert the foot.[6] When the heel is everted, the calcaneocuboid and talonavicular joints are parallel, allowing for motion across the Chopart joint. When the heel is inverted, the two joints are not parallel and "lock," becoming immobile to stabilize the midfoot during the push-off phase of gait (**Figure 4**). Furthermore, a windlass mechanism is provided by the plantar aponeurosis, which locks the midfoot and stiffens the longitudinal arch. During push-off, dorsiflexion of the first metatarsophalangeal joint tightens the aponeurosis and plantar fascia, elevating the arch and inverting the calcaneus.

Mechanism of Injury

Most midtarsal joint and tarsometatarsal joint injuries occur through an axial load or twisting force applied to the plantar-flexed foot.[7,8] Fracture-dislocations most frequently occur at the first and second metatarsal bases, with secondary medial or lateral dislocation depending on the direction of the force. Forceful abduction often leads to fracture-dislocation of the second metatarsal base, with an associated cuboid crush fracture referred to as a nutcracker injury.

Although less common, a crush injury or direct blow from a falling object onto the dorsum of the midfoot may lead to injury.[7-9] These injuries can be devastating, with associated severe soft-tissue injury, neurovascular injury and/or compromise, and the potential development of compartment syndrome of the foot.[10]

If the tarsometatarsal joint is disrupted on the radiograph but the clinical history is unremarkable, the clinician must consider Charcot neuroarthropathy. Although Charcot neuroarthropathy affects a small percentage of diabetic neuropathic patients,[11,12] the midfoot is the most common location. It can be the presenting finding of diabetes in some patients. In this setting, the appropriate diagnosis and treatment can be limb saving and lifesaving.

Classification of Injury

Main and Jowett,[2] in 1975, suggested a classification system based on the mechanism of midfoot injury; however, the classification system described by Quénu and Küss[13] in 1909, which was later modified in 1982 by Hardcastle et al,[9] noting three primary patterns of injury—divergent, isolated,

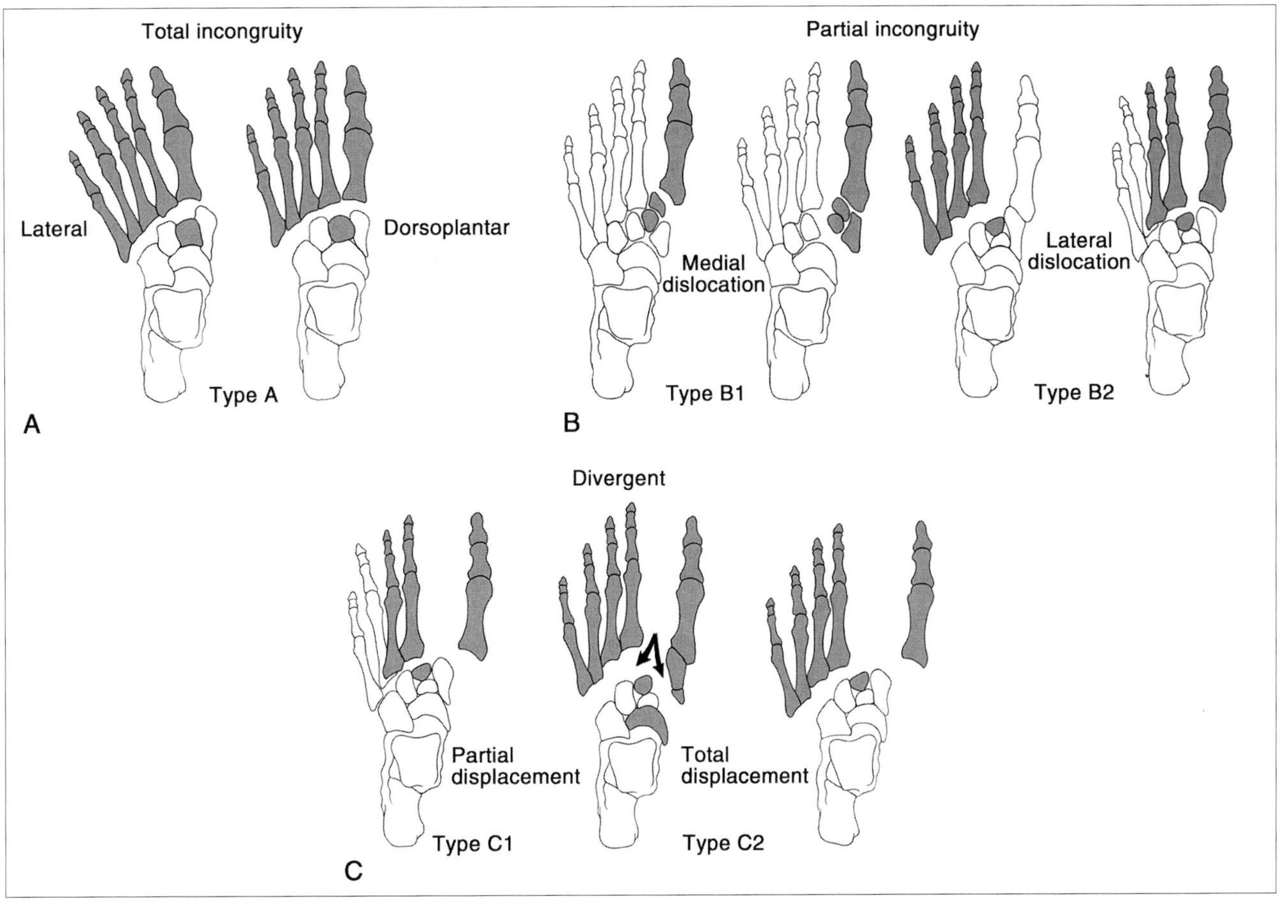

Figure 5 **A** through **C,** Myerson classification of tarsometatarsal injury. The arrows in part C are showing divergence. (Reproduced with permission from Myerson MS, Fisher RT, Burgess AR, Kenzora JE: Fracture-dislocations of the tarsometatarsal joints: End results correlated with pathology and treatment. *Foot Ankle* 1986;6:225-242.)

and homolateral—has maintained greater acceptance. This classification system provides a helpful framework because it implies that energy enters and exits the midfoot at different locations, a principle that is fundamental to diagnostic and treatment options. Those authors divided the injuries into three patterns: type A, indicating total incongruity; type B, partial incongruity; and type C, divergent. In 1986, Myerson et al[7] further divided types B and C into type B1, indicating partial incongruity with medial displacement; type B2, partial incongruity with lateral displacement; type C1, a divergent pattern with partial displacement; and type C2, total displacement. They described these injuries as involving not only the tarsometatarsal joints but also the intercuneiform and naviculocuneiform joints (**Figure 5**).

Diagnosis of Midfoot Injury

A high clinical suspicion for midfoot injury is indicated when a patient has pain and swelling of the foot with plantar ecchymosis on presentation.[14] Up to 20% of injuries are initially missed.[15] Standard imaging includes AP, lateral, and oblique radiographs of the foot, made parallel to the tarsometatarsal joints. Displacement of more than 2 mm between the medial cuneiform and the second metatarsal base indicates instability (**Figure 3**). The pathognomic finding of tarsometatarsal injury, the fleck sign, may also be seen on radiographs. This is a fleck of bone between the first and second metatarsal bases and represents an avulsion fracture of the Lisfranc ligament.[7] A CT scan may be used to better visualize fracture patterns, but as CT scans are static and made without weight bearing, they are not generally helpful in determining stability. Fleck signs or avulsion fractures can be subtle yet represent instability.

If non–weight-bearing radiographs have normal findings, then weight-bearing radiographs should be made. Standing AP radiographs of both feet on one cassette are particularly helpful to look for subtle side-to-side differences. In addition to looking for subluxation of joints and fractures, align-

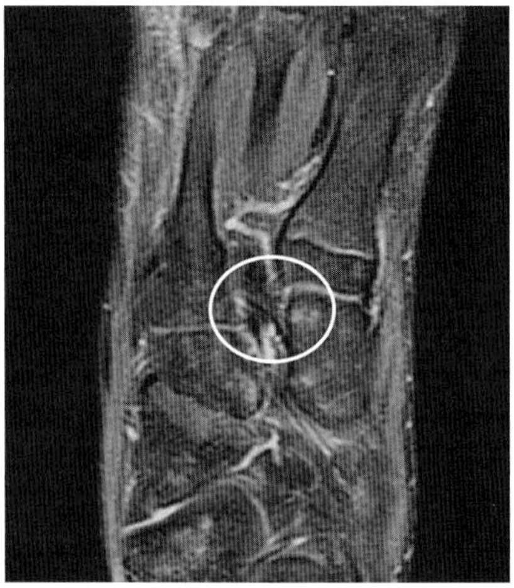

Figure 6 Coronal T2-weighted MRI scan showing an intact plantar Lisfranc ligament in an adolescent with midfoot pain.

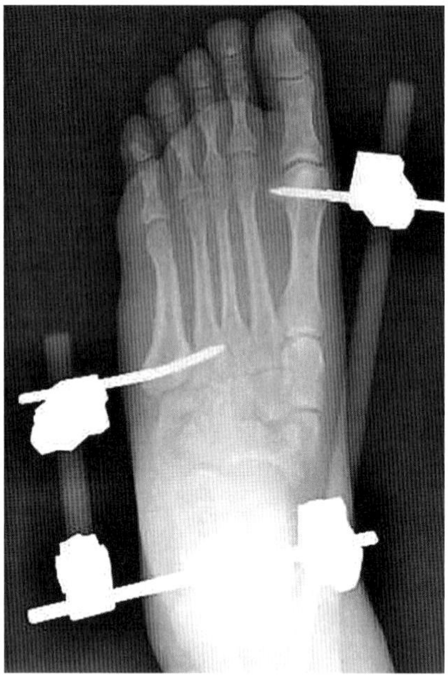

Figure 7 AP radiograph of a foot with a bicolumnar frame. The medial and lateral frames are anchored by the Schanz pin through the calcaneal tuberosity.

ment of the foot must be assessed radiographically because the talus-navicular-medial cuneiform-first metatarsal should be lined up on both a lateral and AP radiograph of the foot (**Figure 1, A** and **C**). Patients may be unable to fully bear weight, leading to an inconclusive study. In this situation, a manual stress examination with the patient under anesthesia is recommended to rule out instability.[4,16,17] Although the patient is under anesthesia, two stresses are applied. First, the foot is abducted and pronated. Second, the medial and middle columns are compressed together. Either of these provocative maneuvers may create displacement through the tarsometatarsal joints. It is also helpful to attempt to flex the midfoot through the Lisfranc joint on a lateral dynamic image to assess for subluxation or gapping of the dorsal joints.

If the diagnosis is still unclear, MRI can evaluate the midfoot soft tissues (**Figure 6**). Recently, Raikin et al[18] correlated MRI findings with stress examinations. They showed a high correlation between rupture of the plantar Lisfranc ligament and instability. They also described a clinical algorithm to help determine which patients need to undergo stress examinations, which are generally reserved for patients with intact plantar Lisfranc ligament but a positive fleck sign. An MRI is a static image that cannot detect instability.

Indications for Treatment

Nonsurgical treatment is reserved for nondisplaced and stable injuries only. A short leg cast is applied, and no weight bearing is allowed for 4 to 6 weeks. As symptoms resolve, the patient can begin weight bearing in a boot or custom-molded orthosis.[19,20] Joint displacement through the tarsometatarsal joint complex with or without a stress examination is an indication for surgical intervention.

Preoperative Planning and/or Initial Treatment

Initially, the acute Lisfranc and Chopart injury is reduced to relieve pressure on the surrounding soft tissues to ensure skin viability. When the reduction is stable, the patient can be managed with a splint until definitive treatment is done, usually within 2 weeks. Unfortunately, most high-energy Lisfranc injury reductions are not stable. In these cases, the reduction is stabilized by placing an external fixator and, if necessary, one or two Kirschner wires are added. Unstable interim reductions may lead to soft-tissue damage, which can compromise foot viability, sometimes with full-thickness skin necrosis. Malaligned midfoot fractures are difficult or impossible to reduce anatomically after soft-tissue swelling has resolved and too much time has elapsed. Satisfactory interim provisional reduction promotes resolution of swelling more quickly.

Unicolumnar frames stabilize a shortened lateral column, which is caused by displacement of the fourth and fifth metatarsal-cuboid complex or a crushed cuboid. Bicolumnar frames are used when both the lateral and medial columns are injured or shortened, such as in injuries caused by an axial load through the midfoot, where the cuboid, navicular, and/or cuneiforms are crushed (**Figure 7**). Details of the techniques used to place external fixators and the care required before definitive treatment have been described previously.[21] Patients with Lisfranc injuries should be assessed for gastrocnemius tightness, which is associated with a relative equinus condition at the ankle.[22] If patients have gastrocnemius tightness, a gastrocnemius recession should be performed in the same surgical setting in advance of the definitive treatment of the Lisfranc injury itself.[21] Definitive open reduction and internal fixation (ORIF) is done when soft-tissue swelling is sufficiently decreased.

Technique for Definitive Treatment

There are essential and nonessential joints of the midfoot. Essential joints are those essential to midfoot function because of the motion required at those joints. Nonessential joints have minimal to no motion. Every attempt must be made to reconstruct and preserve essential joints. Nonessential joints may be fused, and permanent implants may be placed across these joints. The essential joints of the midfoot include the talonavicular and the calcaneocuboid, as well as the articulations between the cuboid and the fourth and fifth metatarsals. The nonessential joints include all of the other midfoot joints: the first, second, and third metatarsocuneiform joints; the intercuneiform joints; and the naviculocuneiform joint.

Internal fixation is guided by two basic strategies. First, stability of the medial column must be obtained even at the cost of restriction of tarsometatarsal motion by fixing the first, second, and third metatarsals to the adjacent cuneiforms. Second, motion of the lateral column (between the fourth and fifth metatarsal and the cuboid) and of the talonavicular joint must be maintained.

In general, reduction of the Lisfranc injury follows a pattern of proximal to distal and of medial to lateral. Reductions are performed and maintained with provisional fixation with Kirschner wires, if needed. The medial frame is removed before the medial column is reduced, and if maintenance of length is a problem, then provisional Kirschner wires can be placed before the external fixator is removed.

Navicular fractures are reduced first, followed by the cuneiform fractures. Cuboid fractures are reduced after definitive fixation of the medial column tarsometatarsal disruptions. The tarsometatarsal disruptions are reduced as needed through skin incisions and muscle dissections detailed in **Table 1**.[21] It is important to be familiar with these common intervals, but often variations are necessary to incorporate fracture combinations or lacerations in the foot. The foot may be accessed from medial, lateral, and dorsal, but it is never approached via the plantar surface despite the plantar comminution often seen in CT scans at the bases of the metatarsal cuneiform joints. The lateral frame may be left in place as long as 8 weeks after definitive fixation if the fixation of the cuboid or calcaneal anterior process is complex, to protect the fixation of a comminuted lateral column during the phase of earlier mobilization, stretching, and massage.

Table 1
Skin Incisions and Muscular Dissections Needed to Access the Tarsometatarsal Joints[a]

Skin Incision	Access Lateral to Specified Muscle	Access Medial to Specified Muscle	Allows Visualization of Specified Metatarsal Base
A	NA	EHL	Medial MT1
	EHL	EHB	Lateral MT1
			Medial MT2
	EHB	EDB2 and EDL2	Lateral MT2
	EDB2	EDB3	Medial MT3
B	EDB3	EDB4	Lateral MT3
			Medial MT4
C	EDB4	PB and PT	Medial MT4
			Lateral MT4
			Medial MT5
			Lateral MT5

[a]Note that not all incisions are needed in every patient. EHL = extensor hallucis longus; EHB = extensor hallucis brevis; EDLx = extensor digitorum longus, where x refers to the muscular head attached to pedal ray x; EDBx = extensor digitorum brevis, where x refers to the muscular head attached to pedal ray x; MTx = metatarsal of pedal ray x; PB = peroneus brevis; PT = peroneus tertius; and NA = not applicable. (Adapted with permission from Benirschke SK, Kramer PA: High energy acute Lisfranc fractures and dislocations. *Tech Foot Ankle Surg* 2010;9(3):82-91.)

Step 1: Provisional Fixation of the Medial Column

The first metatarsal is manipulated to reduce its proximal joint surface onto the articulation of the medial cuneiform. The soft tissues are retracted medially to allow visualization and assessment of the reduction of the medial border of the medial cuneiform to the first metatarsal. Any gap or translational displacement must be eliminated for a perfect reduction. Provisional fixation is done with Kirschner wires until definitive fixation is complete. At the first, second, and third tarsometatarsal reductions, one Kirschner wire provides stability, and the second wire is a guide for the definitive fixation (**Figure 8, A** through **C**).

Through incision A, the second metatarsal base is keyed into its position as the keystone of the arch (**Table 1**). The lateral side is viewed via a capsulotomy of the second metatarsal-intermediate cuneiform joint. It is important to ensure that both the medial and lateral sides are reduced. Provisional fixation is done with a Kirschner wire placed just lateral to the medial

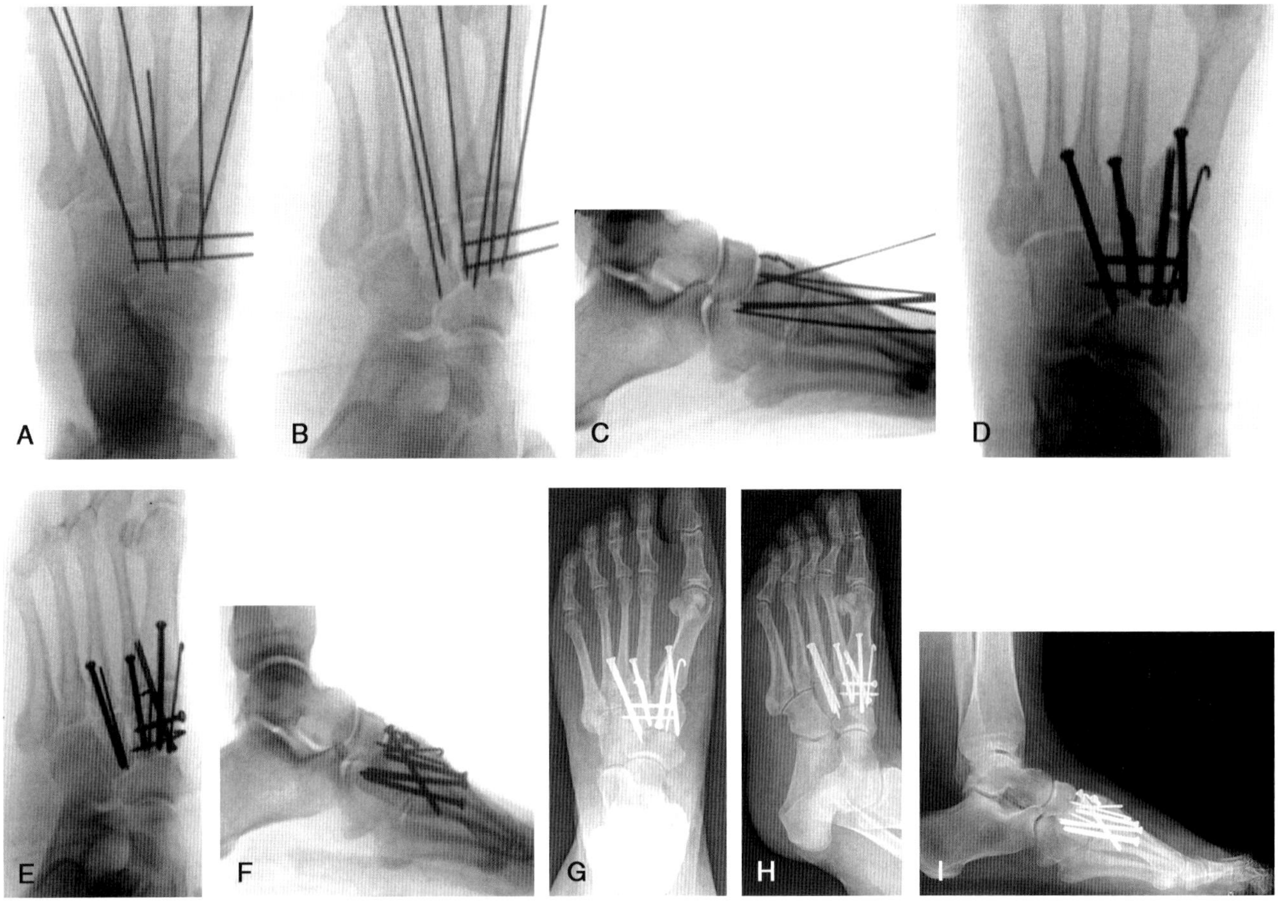

Figure 8 A patient with a midfoot fracture. Intraoperative AP (**A**), oblique (**B**), and lateral (**C**) radiographs made after provisional fixation of the medial column. The crisp joint margins of the third metatarsal and lateral cuneiform indicate that the joint is articulated correctly. AP (**D**), oblique (**E**), and lateral radiographs (**F**) made after definitive fixation. Note the crisscross pattern of screw placement across the joint of the first metatarsal and medial cuneiform, and the Kirschner wires remaining after definitive fixation are bent over flush to the surface of the metatarsals, which allows them to be low profile and permanent. AP (**G**), oblique (**H**), and lateral (**I**) radiographs, made 3 months postoperatively, show anatomically reduced columns and facets with fixation across the nonessential joints of the midfoot. Note the lateral insertion sites at each of the first, second, and third metatarsal necks, which are less prominent and irritating.

edge and central to the second metatarsal. Incision B is used to access the base of the third metatarsal and lateral cuneiform (**Table 1**).

Step 2: Definitive Fixation of the Lateral Column

The lateral column is managed after the medial column has been temporarily fixed. The bases of the fourth and fifth metatarsals are often dorsally displaced, which is seen radiographically as a diffuse separation rather than a crisp joint surface. Reduction by manipulation is recognized when there is a congruent joint line on the oblique radiograph at the medial edge of the cuboid. Direct visualization of the lateral reduction is possible through incision C (**Table 1**). A Kirschner wire is placed from the fourth metatarsal base through the joint surfaces to the medial corner of cuboid. From the lateral surface of the fifth metatarsal, another wire is placed in the fifth metatarsal through the center of the joint to the medial corner of the cuboid.

This chapter's authors prefer to clip all wires under the skin to mitigate skin problems, which are common because of swelling.

Step 3: Definitive Fixation of the Medial Column

Definitive fixation of the navicular and cuneiforms can be done with joint-spanning implants, which provide maximal stability. The first tarsometatarsal joint is definitively fixed with two screws (**Figure 8, D** through **F**). A screw is inserted from the lateral side of the first metatarsal, in a proximal and plantar direction, into the medial cuneiform. This screw placement creates no prominence of the screw head, which, if placed dorsally, can irritate the extensor hallucis longus. Another screw is placed from the medial cuneiform to the plantar prominence of the first metatarsal base. The central Kirschner wire is replaced with a 3.5-mm screw or Lisfranc 4.0-mm screw to definitively fix the second and third metatarsals. The 3.5-mm and 4.0-mm screws with 2.7-mm heads are less irritating to the extensor tendons. Donati-Allgöwer sutures are used to close the skin incision because this technique has been shown to preserve blood supply to the skin edges.[23]

DVD **Video 7.2:** Case Presentation: Complex Chopart and Lisfranc injury. Peter A. Cole, MD (8 min)

Postoperative Management

The foot is placed in a well-padded dressing and is maintained in a plantigrade position and splinted with well-molded plaster held on with an elastic bandage, which allows volumetric changes of the ankle caused by swelling. If a lateral column frame was used, the patient continues to be managed with antibiotics (trimethoprim and sulfamethoxazole or ciprofloxacin) for 6 to 8 weeks, until the frame is removed. Quadriceps-locking exercises, designed to straighten the knee to stretch the gastrocnemius, are begun immediately. Care is taken to prevent an ankle equinus contracture.

Sutures are removed 2 weeks after surgery. If a gastrocnemius recession was performed, the foot is placed in a short-leg fiberglass cast with the ankle in neutral position unless there is an external fixator frame on the foot, in which case it is splinted. Passive range of motion of the metatarsophalangeal joints and active range of motion of the hip and knee are started. Six weeks postoperatively, the cast is removed and the patient wears a boot. Between 6 and 10 weeks after surgery, patients with lateral frames have the frames removed as well as the pins that were placed across the fourth and fifth metatarsal-cuboid joint. Active ankle and subtalar joint motion is begun, and weight bearing on the heel with the boot on is allowed as tolerated.

The patient walks with a flatfoot gait in a boot with compressive stockings. Orthotics can be used at this juncture. Three months postoperatively, the patient begins to roll over the forefoot with the boot on (**Figure 8, G** through **I**), and at this time normal shoe wear is initiated. At 6 to 9 months, a fitted semicustom insert is made for shoe use if the patient is symptomatic or if needed because of the severity of the initial injury. Exercises that strengthen and stretch the gastrocnemius to keep the motion provided by the gastrocnemius recession should be emphasized to the patient. Advanced balance and proprioceptive training for lower extremity function is begun at this time. At 1 year postoperatively, the patient returns for a final follow-up evaluation.

Complications

Complications related to midfoot injuries are common. Complications can be grouped into nonsurgical and surgical categories. The nonsurgical complications are a missed injury or deformity, such as planovalgus,[24] and posttraumatic arthritis. Skin or wound-healing problems are related to surgical timing (too early), surgical technique (undermining wound edges or creating flaps), and wound spacing between intervals. Dorsal neural structures, such as the deep peroneal (first web space), superficial peroneal, and sural nerves, may be injured with the surgical approach or with aggressive retraction. Attention to detail and knowledge of the neighboring anatomy are paramount. Allowing unstable injuries to shorten without maintenance of length, followed by surgical lengthening and stabilization, or missed compartment syndrome may create regional pain syndrome and can be avoided with temporary external fixation.[25] Injury to the anterior tibialis artery is the most common vascular injury. Because of the subcutaneous position of the implants, prominent screw heads or plates can be extremely bothersome to surrounding neural structures or with shoe wear. Failed fixation from inadequate stability or fixation can result in loss of fixation, broken implants, and midfoot collapse.[26] In addition, continued foot pain, whether or not it is surgically treated, can be associated with posttraumatic contracture of the heel cord.[27-29]

Outcomes

In a retrospective evaluation of 48 tarsometatarsal injuries at an average follow-up of 4.5 years, the average functional outcome scores were 77 points on the American Orthopaedic Foot and Ankle Society (AOFAS) scoring system and 19 points on the Musculoskeletal Function Assessment scoring system.[30] Twenty-five percent of the patients had posttraumatic arthritis, and 12.5% of the patients required revision salvage arthrodesis. Rigid anatomic fixation produced the best results. The purely ligamentous injuries performed the worst, with 40% having symptomatic posttraumatic arthritis compared with only 18% of the combined ligamentous and osseous injuries. In an analysis of 25 patients who had midfoot injuries treated with ORIF, injuries to one column of the foot resulted in patients preferentially bearing weight on the noninjured column or loading the longer column.[31] The amount and severity of arthritis did not influence gait. Comminution with loss of column length shifted the foot axis in the sagittal or coronal plane, affecting the gait pattern and subsequent symptoms. Bicolumnar injuries have worse clinical and functional outcomes compared with medial or lateral column injuries. Obesity was also a predictor of inferior results.[32]

The Debate of Fusion Versus ORIF

The foot has functional columns and joints.[22] The medial column, where the navicular is the keystone, requires rigidity for stability, whereas the lateral column, where the cuboid is the keystone, requires flexibility for mobility. This principle was discussed earlier with use of the terms essential joints (those that require motion) and nonessential joints (those that have minimal motion to begin with). Therefore, the role of the columns and joints are important to potential treatment options, such as temporary Kirschner wire fixation, ORIF, or arthrodesis.

In a prospective randomized trial of primary arthrodesis compared with ORIF of the medial three rays (first, second, and third tarsometatarsals), 20 patients were treated with ORIF and 21 had a primary arthrodesis.[33] Anatomic reductions were performed in 18 of 20 patients who had ORIF and in 20 of 21 patients who had primary arthrodesis. After a mean 4.5-year follow-up period, reoperations were done in 5 of 20 patients who had ORIF secondary to posttraumatic arthritis, whereas none of the patients who had primary arthrodesis required secondary surgery. The average AOFAS score was 68.6 points for the ORIF group and 88 points for the group that had primary arthrodesis. The average postoperative activity level was 65% of the preinjury level for the ORIF group and 92% for the primary arthrodesis group. Better short- and medium-term function was noted with primary arthrodesis compared with ORIF.

In another analysis of ORIF compared with primary arthrodesis, 22 patients were randomized to ORIF and 17 to primary arthrodesis.[34] Patients were followed for a minimum of 2 years. Anatomic reductions were performed in 21 of 22 patients who had ORIF and in 16 of 17 who had primary arthrodesis. The reoperation rate was 78.6% after ORIF because of posttraumatic arthritis and implant removal compared with a rate of 16.7% after primary arthrodesis because of prominent bothersome implants. The Medical Outcomes Study 36-Item Short Form and Short Musculoskeletal Function Assessment scores were not significantly different at each time interval, but a trend for improved function after primary arthrodesis compared with ORIF was noted. The primary arthrodesis group had better short- and medium-term function.

In a review of 185 consecutive patients with Lisfranc injuries,[35] the overall infection rate was 4.3%. Pain was present in 30% of the patients. The number of tarsometatarsal injuries did not correlate to outcome. Increased reoperation rates were seen in patients with polytrauma, application of initial spanning external fixation, and associated ipsilateral cuboid and navicular injuries correlating with higher-energy mechanisms and injury patterns. Injuries treated with ORIF and those occurring in males were associated with worse mobility outcome subscores. The removal of prominent implants compared with implant retention positively affected bother outcome subscores but not any other functional measurements.[36] Pain and polytrauma were the greatest predictors of more dysfunction and worse bother subscores. Compared with normative data,[37] tarsometatarsal injuries have more long-term mobility but no other functional outcome impairment. Return-to-work status was excellent, with 91% returning to work and 42% standing throughout the day.[35] Of the patients who were unable to return to work, all had polytrauma and other injuries that precluded working. If surgical treatment of tarsometatarsal injuries was performed well, resulting in a stable, well-aligned foot and no prominent implants, the foot functioned well in the long term.

Cuboid and Navicular Fractures

The optimal management and outcome of cuboid fractures continues to be controversial. Historically, the cuboid was presumed to be protected between the calcaneus and the fourth and fifth metatarsal base; therefore, surgical intervention was not necessary.[38,39] Displaced fractures with subluxation or dislocation were potentially treated with surgical fixation to decrease convalescence time and improve functional results.[39] With marginal impaction, articular reconstruction with bone grafting and ORIF could restore articular congruity.[40,41] In the event of cuboid fractures, the cuboid must be restored anatomically to properly gain lateral column length and foot alignment (**Figure 9**). Arthrodesis of the cuboid articulations produced less satisfactory results.[40]

In a comparison of surgical and nonsurgical treatment of 90 cuboid fractures, surgical intervention was performed on subluxated or displaced fractures.[42] No difference was noted between groups with regard to complications, but the surgically treated group had a higher rate of secondary surgery because of implant irritation. Associated navicular fractures correlated with changes to normal shoe wear and independently contributed

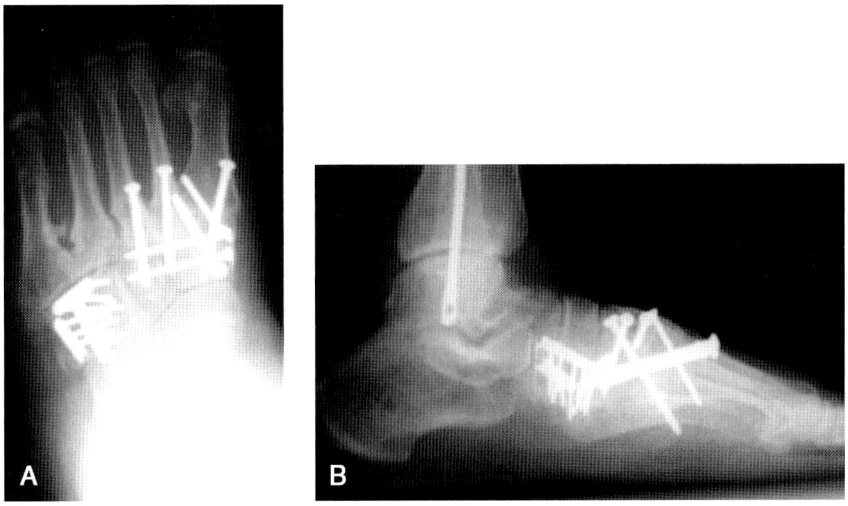

Figure 9 AP (**A**) and lateral radiographs (**B**) of a 67-year-old man, made 10 years after ORIF of a cuboid fracture with allograft and rigid anatomic fixation of the medial column (first, second, and third tarsometatarsals). At the time of the latest follow-up examination, the patient functioned without pain, had no restrictions on activities of daily living, and used standard shoes.

to secondary osteoarthritis. The AO/Orthopaedic Trauma Association (OTA) fracture classification was not predictive of outcome.[43] Reduction quality was associated with increased rates of posttraumatic osteoarthritis.

Navicular injuries consisting of a fracture or subluxation can be occult and result in a painful and problematic foot.[44] Despite poor subjective results, patients are able to perform many routine activities without disabling pain.[45] Most fractures had associated lateral column injuries requiring stabilization of both the medial and lateral columns.[46] Anatomic reduction is better achieved with ORIF, and correction of the length and shape of the longitudinal arch of both the lateral and medial columns improves patient outcomes.[47]

In a large series of 90 navicular fractures treated with or without surgery, patients with worse injury patterns (such as those with three or more associated foot injuries) had worse outcomes.[48] Patients with associated cuboid fracture patterns had increased rates of posttraumatic arthritis, pain, and need for custom shoe wear. Associated talar and tibial pilon injuries independently predicted the inability to return to work. Bone grafting of fractures was associated with improved quality of fracture reduction. Reduction quality was inversely related to pain, posttraumatic arthritis, and activity level. Obese patients had higher rates of pain and posttraumatic arthritis and poorer maintenance of reduction quality. As with cuboid fractures, the AO/OTA fracture classification[43] did not predict outcomes.

Navicular fractures are debilitating injuries that require restoration of medial column length and articular surface congruity. Reduction quality influences the development of posttraumatic arthritis in the long term. Pain, posttraumatic arthritis, and inability to wear normal shoes are related to inferior results. Current classification systems do not adequately predict outcome.

Summary

The midfoot is a complex anatomic association of many bones and articulations, restrained by an even more complex network of ligaments, capsules, and fascia, which must work in concert to provide normal and painless locomotion. The common eponyms of Lisfranc and Chopart refer to the distal and proximal joint relationships of the midfoot, respectively. An understanding of the essential joints in the midfoot, which require motion to be restored, and nonessential joints in the midfoot, which can be fused with impunity, guide the surgical tactic used to address these fractures. Careful diagnostic work-up with three high-quality radiographs of the foot (weight-bearing radiographs when possible) and CT are used to detect associated injuries and fractures, and MRI is used to assess the Lisfranc ligament. Careful consideration should be given to the timing of surgery, as well as to the use of temporizing external fixation for the medial and/or lateral columns when these are shortened and severely fractured. After an appropriate waiting period, surgery is carefully planned to address each disrupted column with its corresponding tarsometatarsal and intertarsal joints. Treatment and rehabilitation should emphasize prevention of heel-cord contracture, which can amplify poor outcomes. Outcomes for these injuries should be measured, but good results have been associated even with grave injuries when anatomic reductions of all bones can be achieved with restoration of proper alignment. Such results are more likely to be achieved by the expert surgeon who has spent substantial time on the learning curve, given the rarity of the injury and the technical tricks necessary to accomplish successful results.

References

1. Wei CJ, Tsai WC, Tiu CM, Wu HT, Chiou HJ, Chang CY: Systematic analysis of missed extremity fractures in emergency radiol-

ogy. *Acta Radiol* 2006;47(7): 710-717.

2. Main BJ, Jowett RL: Injuries of the midtarsal joint. *J Bone Joint Surg Br* 1975;57(1):89-97.
3. Mantas JP, Burks RT: Lisfranc injuries in the athlete. *Clin Sports Med* 1994;13(4):719-730.
4. Curtis MJ, Myerson M, Szura B: Tarsometatarsal joint injuries in the athlete. *Am J Sports Med* 1993;21(4):497-502.
5. Vuori JP, Aro HT: Lisfranc joint injuries: Trauma mechanisms and associated injuries. *J Trauma* 1993;35(1):40-45.
6. Elftman H: The transverse tarsal joint and its control. *Clin Orthop* 1960;16:41-46.
7. Myerson MS, Fisher RT, Burgess AR, Kenzora JE: Fracture dislocations of the tarsometatarsal joints: End results correlated with pathology and treatment. *Foot Ankle* 1986;6(5):225-242.
8. Wiley JJ: The mechanism of tarso-metatarsal joint injuries. *J Bone Joint Surg Br* 1971;53(3): 474-482.
9. Hardcastle PH, Reschauer R, Kutscha-Lissberg E, Schoffmann W: Injuries to the tarsometatarsal joint: Incidence, classification and treatment. *J Bone Joint Surg Br* 1982;64(3):349-356.
10. Myerson MS, McGarvey WC, Henderson MR, Hakim J: Morbidity after crush injuries to the foot. *J Orthop Trauma* 1994;8(4): 343-349.
11. Pinzur MS: Current concepts review: Charcot arthropathy of the foot and ankle. *Foot Ankle Int* 2007;28(8):952-959.
12. van der Ven A, Chapman CB, Bowker JH: Charcot neuroarthropathy of the foot and ankle. *J Am Acad Orthop Surg* 2009; 17(9):562-571.
13. Quénu E, Küss G: Study on the dislocations of the metatarsal bones (tarsometatarsal dislocations) and diastasis between the 1st and 2nd metatarsal. *Rev Chir* 1909;39:281-336, 720-791, 1093-1134.
14. Ross G, Cronin R, Hauzenblas J, Juliano P: Plantar ecchymosis sign: A clinical aid to diagnosis of occult Lisfranc tarsometatarsal injuries. *J Orthop Trauma* 1996; 10(2):119-122.
15. Trevino SG, Kodros S: Controversies in tarsometatarsal injuries. *Orthop Clin North Am* 1995; 26(2):229-238.
16. Arntz CT, Veith RG, Hansen ST Jr: Fractures and fracture-dislocations of the tarsometatarsal joint. *J Bone Joint Surg Am* 1988; 70(2):173-181.
17. Coss HS, Manos RE, Buoncristiani A, Mills WJ: Abduction stress and AP weightbearing radiography of purely ligamentous injury in the tarsometatarsal joint. *Foot Ankle Int* 1998;19(8): 537-541.
18. Raikin SM, Elias I, Dheer S, Besser MP, Morrison WB, Zoga AC: Prediction of midfoot instability in the subtle Lisfranc injury: Comparison of magnetic resonance imaging with intraoperative findings. *J Bone Joint Surg Am* 2009;91(4):892-899.
19. Myerson MS, Cerrato RA: Current management of tarsometatarsal injuries in the athlete. *J Bone Joint Surg Am* 2008;90(11):2522-2533.
20. Nunley JA, Vertullo CJ: Classification, investigation, and management of midfoot sprains: Lisfranc injuries in the athlete. *Am J Sports Med* 2002;30(6):871-878.
21. Benirschke SK, Kramer PA: High energy acute Lisfranc fractures and dislocations. *Tech Foot Ankle Surg* 2010;9(3):82-91.
22. Hansen ST: *Functional Reconstruction of the Foot and Ankle.* Philadelphia, PA, Lippincott Williams & Wilkins, 2000.
23. Sagi HC, Papp S, Dipasquale T: The effect of suture pattern and tension on cutaneous blood flow as assessed by laser Doppler flowmetry in a pig model. *J Orthop Trauma* 2008;22(3):171-175.
24. Bohay DR, Johnson KD, Manoli A II: The traumatic bunion. *Foot Ankle Int* 1996;17(7):383-387.
25. Manoli A II: Compartment syndromes of the foot: Current concepts. *Foot Ankle* 1990;10(6): 340-344.
26. Habbu R, Holthusen SM, Anderson JG, Bohay DR: Operative correction of arch collapse with forefoot deformity: A retrospective analysis of outcomes. *Foot Ankle Int* 2011;32(8):764-773.
27. DiGiovanni CW, Kuo R, Tejwani N, et al: Isolated gastrocnemius tightness. *J Bone Joint Surg Am* 2002;84-A(6):962-970.
28. Pinney SJ, Hansen ST Jr, Sangeorzan BJ: The effect on ankle dorsiflexion of gastrocnemius recession. *Foot Ankle Int* 2002; 23(1):26-29.
29. Maskill JD, Bohay DR, Anderson JG: Gastrocnemius recession to treat isolated foot pain. *Foot Ankle Int* 2010;31(1):19-23.
30. Kuo RS, Tejwani NC, Digiovanni CW, et al: Outcome after open reduction and internal fixation of Lisfranc joint injuries. *J Bone Joint Surg Am* 2000;82(11):1609-1618.
31. Mittlmeier T, Krowiorsch R, Brosinger S, Hudde M: Gait function after fracture-dislocation of the midtarsal and/or tarsometatarsal joints. *Clin Biomech (Bristol, Avon)* 1997;12(3):S16-S17.
32. Coulibaly MO, Jones CB, Sietsema DL, Ringler JR, Endres TJ: Functional outcomes of operatively treated midfoot fractures. Mid-America Orthopaedic Association 2010 Annual Meeting. http://www.maoa.org/downloads/maoa2010abstracts.pdf. Accessed July 19, 2012.

33. Ly TV, Coetzee JC: Treatment of primarily ligamentous Lisfranc joint injuries: Primary arthrodesis compared with open reduction and internal fixation. A prospective, randomized study. *J Bone Joint Surg Am* 2006;88(3): 514-520.

34. Henning JA, Jones CB, Sietsema DL, Bohay DR, Anderson JG: Open reduction internal fixation versus primary arthrodesis for Lisfranc injuries: A prospective randomized study. *Foot Ankle Int* 2009;30(10):913-922.

35. Henning J, Jones CB, Sietsema DL: Abstract: Review of 185 consecutive Lisfranc injuries treated with open reduction and internal fixation or primary arthrodesis. *75th Annual Meeting Proceedings*. Rosemont, IL, American Academy of Orthopaedic Surgeons, 2008, pp 720-721.

36. Henning JA, Jones CB, Sietsema DL, et al: Abstract: Lisfranc injuries: Is hardware removal necessary following ORIF? Mid-American Orthopaedic Association 2008 Annual Meeting. http://www.maoa.org/downloads/maoa2008abstracts.pdf. Accessed July 19, 2012.

37. Hunsaker FG, Cioffi DA, Amadio PC, Wright JG, Caughlin B: The American Academy of Orthopaedic Surgeons outcomes instruments: Normative values from the general population. *J Bone Joint Surg Am* 2002;84(2):208-215.

38. McKeever FM: Fractures of tarsal and metatarsal bones. *Surg Gynecol Obstet* 1950;90(6):735-745.

39. Hermel MB, Gershon-Cohen J: The nutcracker fracture of the cuboid by indirect violence. *Radiology* 1953;60(6):850-854.

40. Sangeorzan BJ, Swiontkowski MF: Displaced fractures of the cuboid. *J Bone Joint Surg Br* 1990; 72(3):376-378.

41. Weber M, Locher S: Reconstruction of the cuboid in compression fractures: Short to midterm results in 12 patients. *Foot Ankle Int* 2002;23(11):1008-1013.

42. Coulibaly MO, Jones CB, Sietsema DL, Ringler JR, Endres TJ: Results of 90 consecutive cuboid fractures. Mid-America Orthopaedic Association 2009 Annual Meeting. http://www.maoa.org/downloads/maoa2009abstracts.pdf. Accessed July 19, 2012.

43. Marsh JL, Slongo TF, Agel J, et al: Fracture and dislocation classification compendium, 2007: Orthopaedic Trauma Association classification, database and outcomes committee. *J Orthop Trauma* 2007;21(10, suppl): S1-S133.

44. Eichenholtz SN, Levine DB: Fractures of the tarsal navicular bone. *Clin Orthop Relat Res* 1964;34: 142-157.

45. Sangeorzan BJ, Benirschke SK, Mosca V, Mayo KA, Hansen ST Jr: Displaced intra-articular fractures of the tarsal navicular. *J Bone Joint Surg Am* 1989;71(10):1504-1510.

46. Dhillon MS, Nagi ON: Total dislocations of the navicular: Are they ever isolated injuries? *J Bone Joint Surg Br* 1999;81(5): 881-885.

47. Richter M, Wippermann B, Krettek C, Schratt HE, Hufner T, Therman H: Fractures and fracture dislocations of the midfoot: Occurrence, causes and long-term results. *Foot Ankle Int* 2001;22(5): 392-398.

48. Coulibaly MO, Jones CB, Sietsema DL, Ringler JR, Endres TJ: Paper No. 475. Results of 90 consecutive navicular fractures. *AAOS 2010 Annual Meeting Proceedings*. CD-ROM. Rosemont, IL, American Academy of Orthopaedic Surgeons, 2010, p 495.

Video References

7.1: Meinberg EG: Video. *Midfoot Anatomy* San Francisco, CA, 2012

7.2: Cole PA: Video. *Case Presentation:-Complex Chopart and Lisfranc Injury* Saint Paul, MN, 2012.

SECTION

2

Shoulder

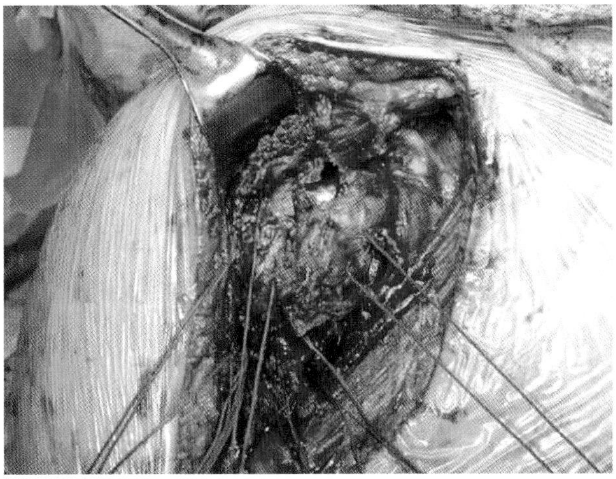

DVD 8 Revision Open Capsular Shift for Atraumatic and Multidirectional Instability of the Shoulder

9 General Surgical Principles of Open Rotator Cuff Repair in the Management of Failed Arthroscopic Cuff Repairs

DVD 10 Prevention of Complications in Shoulder Arthroplasty: Understanding Options and Critical Steps

11 Complications in Total Shoulder Arthroplasty

DVD 12 Proximal Humeral Fractures: Internal Fixation

13 Proximal Humeral Fractures: Prosthetic Replacement

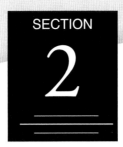

8

Revision Open Capsular Shift for Atraumatic and Multidirectional Instability of the Shoulder

Aaron J. Bois, MD, FRCSC
Michael A. Wirth, MD

Abstract

Shoulder stability is critical for proper functioning of the upper extremity and is dependent on the interplay between static and dynamic stabilizers of the glenohumeral joint. Surgical management of patients with atraumatic and multidirectional instability is effective if the capsular redundancy is properly reconstructed to restore glenohumeral joint biomechanics. Residual capsular laxity is a common cause of recurrent glenohumeral joint dislocation in patients who had previous stabilization procedures; surgical results become less predictable in patients who had multiple revision procedures. It is important to detect capsular laxity at the time of the index surgery and use reliable surgical techniques to obtain optimal results.

Instr Course Lect 2013;62:95-103.

Diagnosing Multidirectional Instability

The glenohumeral joint is one of the most frequently dislocated joints in humans.[1] Shoulder instability is best understood as a spectrum of disease; traumatic unidirectional instability exists at one end of the spectrum, whereas atraumatic and multidirectional instability lies at the other extreme.[2] Although capsular laxity is necessary to allow a wide range of glenohumeral motion, patients with multidirectional instability have pathologically increased capsular volume, which results in instability of the glenohumeral joint in more than one direction, primarily inferiorly.[3-5] In contrast, patients with traumatic unidirectional instability are less likely to have abnormal capsular volumes and more commonly have pathologic lesions involving the capsulolabral complex.[6,7]

Multidirectional instability was first described by Neer and Foster[3] in 1980 and is categorized into several clinical subtypes. Some patients may present with an inherited disorder of collagen, such as Ehlers-Danlos syndrome, and exhibit generalized ligamentous laxity. Other patients may have acquired instability following repetitive microtrauma, as seen in those who participate in baseball, swimming, or gymnastics.[2] A small subset of patients may be able to dislocate their shoulders on command using techniques of asymmetric muscle pull or because of the development of improper muscle-firing patterns.[2] These patients may have an accompanying psychiatric disorder or secondary gain issues that must be recognized and considered before recommending surgery because of their deleterious effects on surgical outcomes. Patients with capsular insufficiency may present with pain as their only symptom, a condition known as the unstable painful shoulder.[8]

Diagnosing multidirectional instability can be challenging because of the wide spectrum of clinical presentations. Patients with classic multidirectional instability have symptomatic glenohumeral instability in more than one direction; however, there may be

Dr. Wirth or an immediate family member serves as a board member, owner, officer, or committee member of the American Shoulder and Elbow Surgeons; has received royalties from DePuy; is a member of a speakers' bureau or has made paid presentations on behalf of DePuy and Tornier; serves as a paid consultant to or is an employee of DePuy and Tornier; and owns stock or stock options in Tornier. Neither Dr. Bois nor any immediate family member has received anything of value from or owns stock in a commercial company or institution related directly or indirectly to the subject of this chapter.

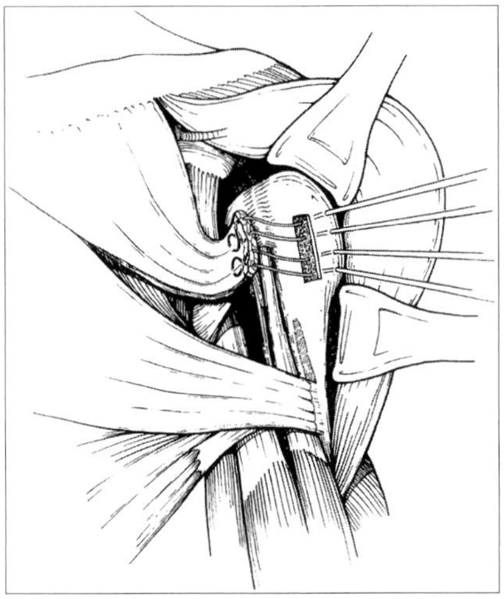

Figure 1 Surgical technique for pectoralis major transfer for irreparable rupture of the subscapularis tendon. Stay sutures, which had been placed in the superior half of the pectoralis major tendon, are passed into a bone trough made lateral to the bicipital groove and out through cortical drill holes. (Reproduced with permission from Wirth MA, Rockwood CA Jr: Operative treatment of irreparable rupture of the subscapularis. *J Bone Joint Surg Am* 1997;79:722-731.)

elements of both asymptomatic laxity and symptomatic instability in the same shoulder, and accurate differentiation between these two entities is crucial for surgical decision making.[2] On physical examination, subtle differences between laxity and symptomatic instability can be delineated by specific maneuvers to detect anterior, posterior, and inferior capsular insufficiencies.[3,9-11] The integrity of the inferior capsule and rotator interval should be assessed with the sulcus test.[3] With the affected arm in adduction and neutral rotation, the examiner grasps the distal aspect of the humerus just above the epicondyles and applies downward traction to the limb. In patients with inferior laxity, a sulcus is visible between the lateral acromial edge and the humeral head. Patients with inferior instability exhibit apprehension when the sulcus test is performed. To assess the rotator cuff interval, the maneuver is repeated with the arm in 30° of external rotation; if the sulcus decreases, the rotator interval is intact. Such a distinction is important because of the role of the rotator cuff interval in both posterior and inferior instability patterns.[12] Although the diagnosis of multidirectional instability is dependent on a thorough history and physical examination, magnetic resonance arthrography is a useful adjunct to assess capsular redundancy and other soft-tissue and/or osseous causes of shoulder pain and dysfunction. This is especially important if revision surgery is needed.[13]

Nonsurgical Treatment of Multidirectional Instability

Standard initial treatment of multidirectional instability is a rehabilitation program focused on rotator cuff strengthening, scapular stabilization, and proprioception exercises, in addition to activity modification.[11] Nonsurgical treatment was reported to be effective in 80% of patients compliant with an exercise program;[14] however, a recent long-term study of nonsurgical treatment indicated that only 47% of patients had a satisfactory result on the basis of shoulder stability and Rowe scores, and only 64% had good to excellent results with regard to pain.[15] In 2010, Nyiri et al[16] reported that kinematic parameters and activity patterns of muscles around the glenohumeral joint can be normalized after surgery and physical therapy but not with physical therapy alone. Whether these kinematic parameters and muscle activity patterns correlate clinically to better overall patient satisfaction and shoulder stability has yet to be determined. Regardless of the results of the latter two studies, the initial standard of care for patients with multidirectional instability is nonsurgical rehabilitation; when such measures are unsuccessful, surgical options can be considered.

Revision Surgery After Failed Stabilization Surgery

Traditionally, an open inferior capsular shift procedure is performed to address the capsular laxity that is present in multidirectional instability;[3] however, advances in arthroscopic techniques have revealed results comparable to those reported for open capsular shift[17-20] and primary Bankart repairs.[21,22] With revision surgery, arthroscopic techniques are appropriate in properly selected patients to treat residual capsular laxity or perform repeat Bankart repairs.[23-25] Furthermore, arthroscopic examination should be considered before open reconstruction to allow the surgeon to identify and arthroscopically address other associated pathology found in patients with recurrent instability, including superior labral and rotator cuff tears.[26,27]

Despite the advances in arthroscopic techniques, there is still a role for the open capsular shift procedure; the choice of surgical treatment is predominantly based on surgeon experience and individual patient pathology.[28-30] Generally, open treatment is indicated for patients with specific soft-tissue pathology, including humeral avulsion of the glenohumeral ligaments, midsubstance capsular rupture, capsular deficiency, and subscapularis deficiency[31-35] (**Figure 1**). The latter two abnormalities are more common with revision surgery or after previous thermal capsulorrhaphy.[29,35,36] In addition to soft-tissue pathology, osseous deficiency of the glenoid and/or humeral head or abnormal glenoid version (**Figure 2**) must be addressed with open reconstructive procedures to restore normal shoulder mechanics.[37,38] Although uncommon in atraumatic

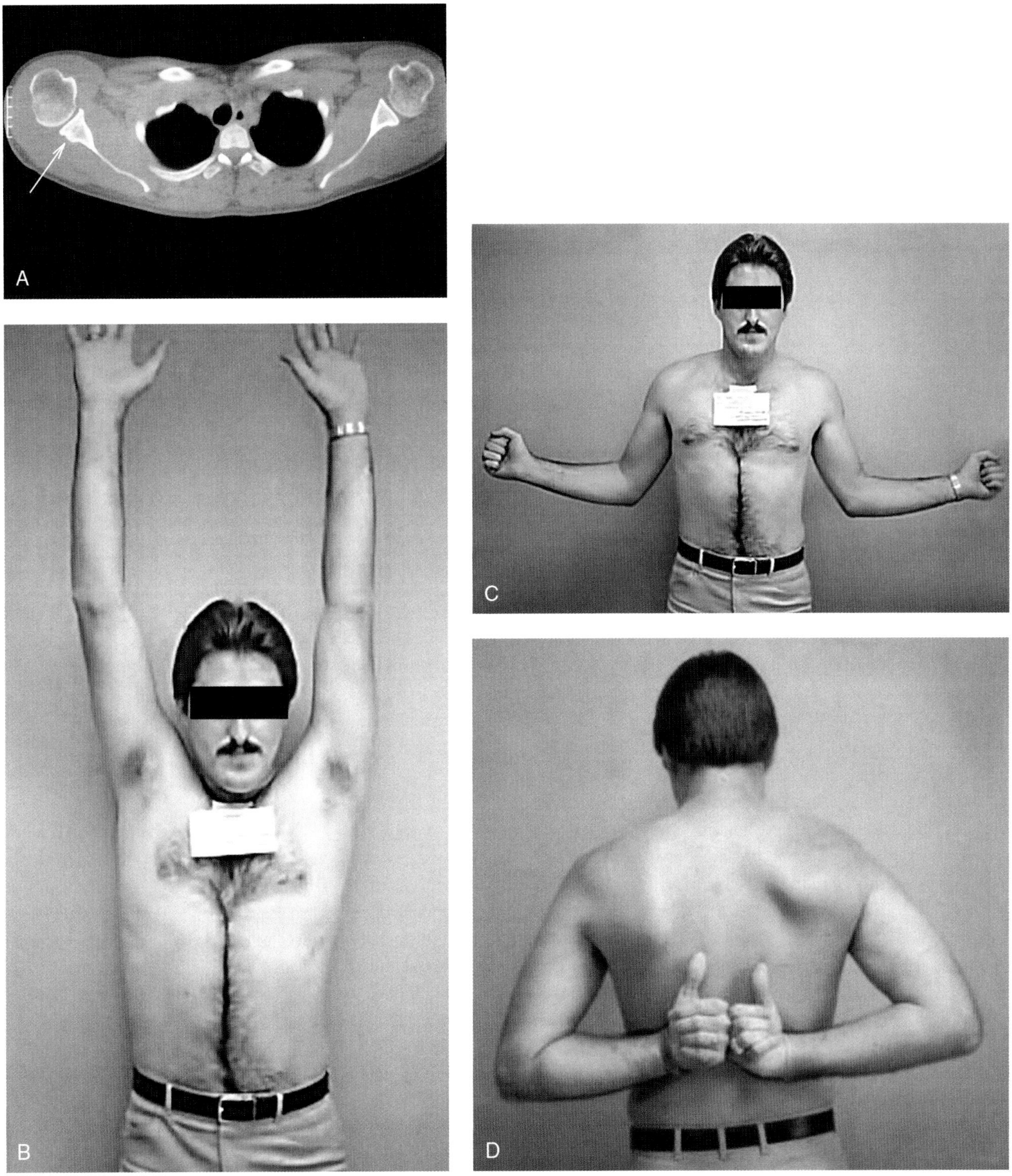

Figure 2 **A,** Postoperative axial CT scan showing symmetric glenoid version and incorporation of the tricortical bone graft (arrow) after a posterior opening wedge osteotomy of the glenoid for glenoid retroversion of approximately 50°. **B** through **D,** Clinical photographs showing full and symmetric motion. (Panel A adapted with permission from Wirth MA, Seltzer DG, Rockwood CA Jr: Recurrent posterior glenohumeral dislocation associated with increased retroversion of the glenoid: A case report. *Clin Orthop Relat Re*s 1994;308:98-101. Panels B, C, and D adapted with permission from Matsen FA III, Lippitt SB, Bertlesen A, Rockwood CA Jr, Wirth MA: Glenohumeral instability, in Rockwood CA Jr, Matsen FA III, Wirth MA, Lippitt SB, eds: *The Shoulder,* ed 4. Philadelphia, PA, WB Saunders, 2009, pp 617-770.)

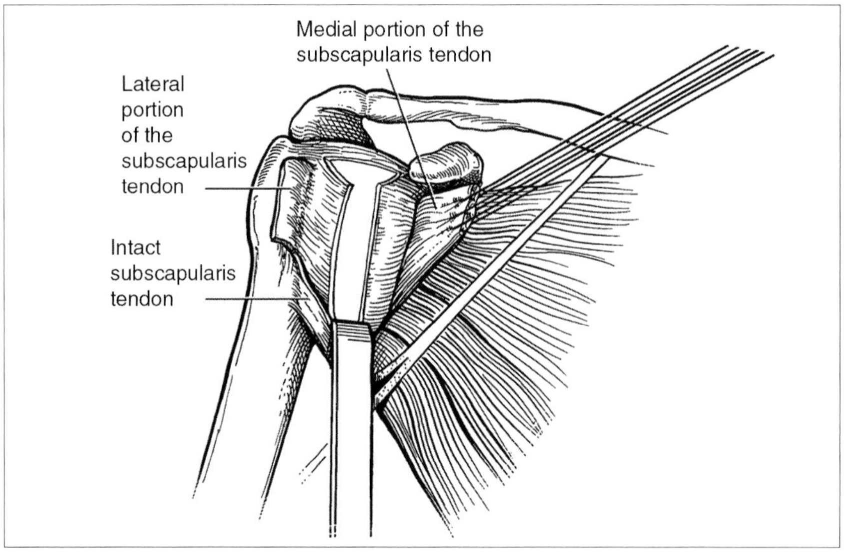

Figure 3 Illustration showing the vertical division of the anterior capsule, midway between its attachments on the glenoid rim and humeral head. (Reproduced with permission from Wirth MA, Groh GI, Rockwood CA Jr: Capsulorrhaphy through an anterior approach for the treatment of atraumatic posterior glenohumeral instability with multidirectional laxity of the shoulder. *J Bone Joint Surg Am* 1998;80:1570-1578.)

instability or multidirectional instability, bone augmentation procedures are performed when bone loss exceeds approximately 25% to 30% of the posterosuperior humeral head (measured as a percentage of either the diameter of the humeral head or the articular arc)[39-42] or anterior glenoid margin (anteroposterior diameter of the inferior aspect of the glenoid).[43-46] Both humeral and glenoid bone loss can be quantified preoperatively, with advanced imaging such as CT, or intraoperatively, with direct measurements or arthroscopic techniques.

Surgical Technique: Open Capsular Shift

Surgical efforts for shoulder instability are directed toward the specific pathoanatomy. In general, all pathologic lesions involving the static and dynamic shoulder stabilizers must be identified and, when indicated, corrected simultaneously to restore shoulder mechanics. The primary goal of surgical management in patients with multidirectional instability typically involves shifting or imbricating the redundant inferior capsule to reduce excessive glenohumeral volume and restore joint stability.[3] These procedures should be combined with open Bankart repairs when indicated.

Open capsular shift procedures were originally performed with a laterally based capsular incision, through which the inferior capsule is shifted superiorly to reduce capsular volume and restore tension to the glenohumeral ligaments.[3] Modifications to the original open capsular shift procedure involve variations in the location of the capsulotomy and include medially based[47] and midline-based[48] techniques. The concept of a selective capsular shift was introduced to refine the final step of a standard open capsulolabral repair, in which the capsuloligamentous complex is tensioned with the arm in a position of approximately 30° of abduction and external rotation to selectively tension the capsule in a functional position.[49,50]

The surgical technique for the midline capsular imbrication procedure is performed through an axillary incision in the deltopectoral interval.[48] The axillary nerve is identified along the anteroinferior border of the subscapularis muscle and is protected. With the arm in external rotation, the borders of the subscapularis tendon are identified and the superior two thirds of the tendon is incised vertically 2 cm from its insertion on the lesser tuberosity. The tendon is incised down to but not into the capsule. Mayo scissors are used to reflect the medial part of the subscapularis tendon off the capsule.

Video 8.1: Tendon Incision. Aaron J. Bois, MD; Michael A. Wirth, MD (2 min)

Video 8.2: Reflecting the Medial Part of the Subscapularis Tendon Off the Capsule. Aaron J. Bois, MD; Michael A. Wirth, MD (1 min)

The capsule is then divided vertically, midway between its attachments on the humeral neck and the glenoid rim (**Figure 3**). The incision begins at the inferior border of the rotator interval and extends inferiorly beyond the 6-o'clock position. The more laxity in the posterior aspect of the capsule, the more the capsular incision should be extended posteriorly (**Figure 4**). Stay sutures are placed sequentially along the free edge of the medial capsular leaflet; these sutures allow traction on the medial capsular leaflet, which makes it possible to divide the most posteroinferior portion of the inferior glenohumeral ligament complex. This degree of capsular incision allows subsequent anterior advancement of the

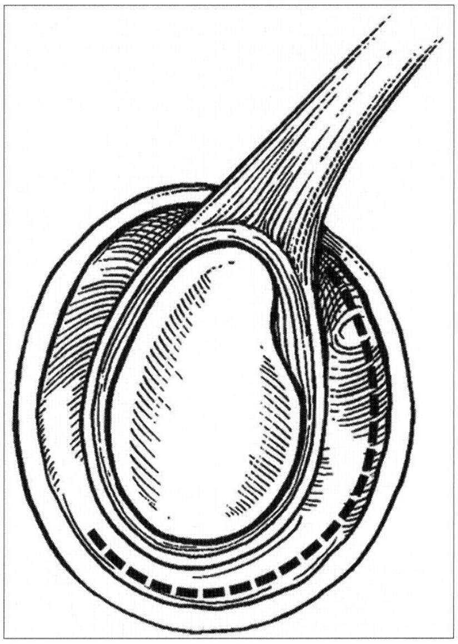

Figure 4 Illustration showing a medial (en face) view of the glenoid fossa with attached glenohumeral joint capsule. The capsular incision (broken line) begins at the rotator interval superiorly and extends to the posteroinferior aspect of the capsule. (Reproduced with permission from Wirth MA, Groh GI, Rockwood CA Jr: Capsulorrhaphy through an anterior approach for the treatment of atraumatic posterior glenohumeral instability with multidirectional laxity of the shoulder. *J Bone Joint Surg Am* 1998;80:1570-1578.)

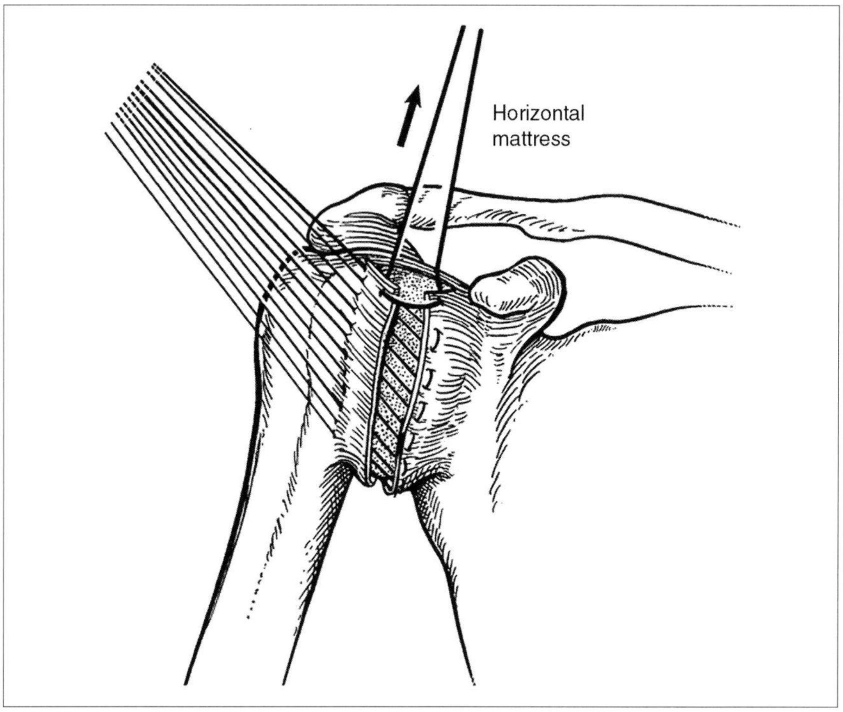

Figure 5 Illustration showing the placement of sutures along the medial capsular leaflet to allow traction (arrow) and permit division of the most posteroinferior capsular complex. These sutures are then passed through the lateral capsule as part of the first imbrication step. (Reproduced with permission from Wirth MA, Groh GI, Rockwood CA Jr: Capsulorrhaphy through an anterior approach for the treatment of atraumatic posterior glenohumeral instability with multidirectional laxity of the shoulder. *J Bone Joint Surg Am* 1998;80: 1570-1578.)

posterior portion of the inferior glenohumeral ligament complex.

After the capsulotomy is completed, the capsular tissue within the rotator interval is closed with a horizontal mattress suture (**Figure 5**). This is followed by two capsular imbrication phases; during each phase, the arm is held in 25° of external rotation, 20° of abduction, and 0° of forward elevation. The first imbrication step shifts the medial aspect of the inferior glenohumeral ligament complex anteriorly and laterally, and the remaining portion of the medial aspect of the capsule is shifted laterally and superiorly under the lateral capsular leaflet. This step should eliminate any posterior capsular laxity. Next, the lateral aspect of the capsule is shifted superomedially and is sutured to the anterior surface of the medial aspect of the capsule (**Figure 6**). If less than 30° of passive external rotation is present at the conclusion of the procedure, there has been excessive tightening of the anterior structures and the procedure may push the humeral head out posteriorly.[51]

Video 8.3: Eliminate Posterior Capsule Laxity. Aaron J. Bois, MD; Michael A. Wirth, MD (2 min)

Postoperatively, the patient wears a shoulder immobilizer for comfort. During this time, the patient is encouraged to use the involved extremity for activities of daily living and is instructed to exercise the hand, wrist, and elbow but is cautioned to avoid adduction, forward elevation, and internal rotation maneuvers. Pendulum exercises are initiated at 14 days after surgery; however, the stretching phase of the rehabilitation program is not started until 6 weeks after surgery. Muscle strengthening is initiated only after the patient has regained active elevation to within 20° to 30° of that of the normal side and rotation is about 50% to 60% of that of the normal side. The strengthening program is performed three or four times daily and emphasizes conditioning of the deltoid and rotator cuff muscles, as well as the muscles that stabilize the scapula.

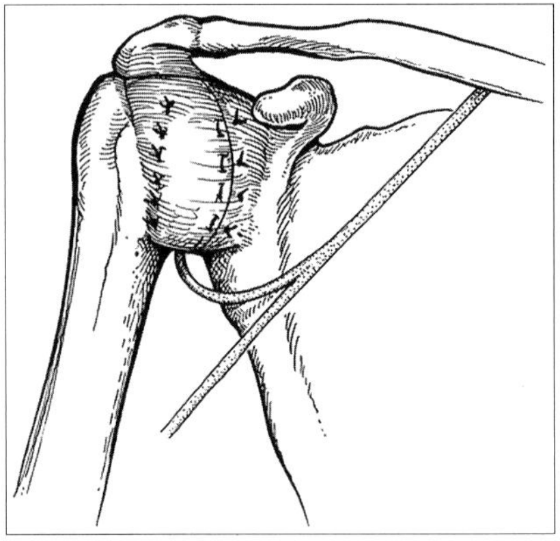

Figure 6 Illustration showing double-breasting of the lateral aspect of the capsule. (Reproduced with permission from Wirth MA, Groh GI, Rockwood CA Jr: Capsulorrhaphy through an anterior approach for the treatment of atraumatic posterior glenohumeral instability with multidirectional laxity of the shoulder. *J Bone Joint Surg Am* 1998;80:1570-1578.)

Risk Factors for Failed Stabilization Procedures

The most common complication of any stabilization procedure, whether open or arthroscopic, is recurrent glenohumeral joint instability. In patients with multidirectional instability, surgical intervention is aimed at treating the specific type of capsular laxity present.[2,3,11] When the capsulolabral complex is not appropriately managed, higher failure rates have been reported.[45,52-55]

Rowe et al[52] reviewed the intraoperative findings in 32 patients treated with revision surgery for recurrent anterior instability. In that series, capsular laxity was found in 80% of the 32 shoulders with unsuccessful index surgery. In 1991, Young and Rockwood[53] reported a good or excellent outcome in only 50% of patients with revision anterior shoulder reconstruction after an unsuccessful Bristow procedure. At the time of revision surgery, 32 shoulders (80%) had excessive capsular laxity, and 8 (20%) had an untreated Perthes-Bankart lesion. In 2006, Boileau et al[45] attempted to identify risk factors for recurrent instability after an arthroscopic stabilization procedure and found that the presence of (1) a stretched inferior glenohumeral ligament, (2) anterior hyperlaxity, or (3) a glenoid compression fracture involving more than 25% of the glenoid surface led to a 75% recurrence rate. Balg and Boileau[56] later incorporated shoulder hyperlaxity as one of six risk factors listed as part of a 10-point "preoperative instability severity index score." This preoperative checklist serves to identify patients at risk for the development of recurrent instability after an arthroscopic Bankart procedure.

Failure to surgically address critical bone loss of the glenoid or humeral head has also been correlated with higher recurrence rates after isolated repairs of the capsulolabral complex in patients with recurrent instability.[37,45,52,54] In a review of 29 shoulders treated with revision stabilization surgery, Rowe et al[52] reported that a Hill-Sachs defect was found in 23 patients and a glenoid rim defect in 22 patients. In addition to the capsular laxity in these patients, glenohumeral bone loss may have affected the results of the index instability procedure. In a series of 194 patients treated with a primary soft-tissue repair, Burkhart and De Beer[37] reported 21 recurrent dislocations and subluxations; 14 of those shoulders had substantial bone defects, including 3 engaging Hill-Sachs lesions and 11 inverted-pear glenoid lesions, for a combined recurrence rate of 67%. Boileau et al[45] similarly reported higher rates of postoperative recurrent instability in patients with considerable glenohumeral bone loss.

Results of Open Capsular Shift

The results after a primary capsular shift procedure addressing multidirectional instability are encouraging. This chapter's authors believe that Neer and Foster[3] were the first to describe the surgical technique and early results of an open inferior capsular shift in 36 patients (40 shoulders) with involuntary multidirectional instability. Only one patient in that series experienced recurrent instability within the first year of follow-up. In 1992, Cooper and Brems[57] reported the results of an inferior capsular shift procedure using an anterior approach in 38 patients (43 shoulders) with multidirectional instability. Overall, 89% of the patients were satisfied, with no recurrent instability after a minimum follow-up of 2 years. More recently, Pollock et al[58] reported on 46 patients (49 shoulders) with multidirectional instability treated with an inferior capsular shift procedure (mean follow-up, 61 months). Good or excellent results were found in 94% of the shoulders, and 96% of the shoulders remained stable; however, the results were less favorable in athletes because only 69% of this cohort returned to their prior level of participation.

Less reliable results can be expected after revision stabilization surgery in patients with preexisting arthritis, glenohumeral bone loss, residual capsular laxity, a history of two or more unsuccessful surgical procedures for glenohumeral joint instability, or those older than 30 years.[59-64]

Zabinski et al[59] evaluated the results of revision shoulder stabilization surgery in 20 patients (21 shoulders) with multidirectional instability. At the time of the revision, the primary lesion in all patients was capsular laxity; 15 patients required a capsular shift procedure. At a mean follow-up of 61.5 months, only nine shoulders had good or excellent results despite multiple reoperations, with four requiring glenohumeral arthrodesis. Levine et al[60] reported the results of revision anterior stabilization surgery in 50 patients. At the time of revision surgery, all patients required an anteroinferior capsular shift for residual capsular laxity. After an average of 4.7 years of follow-up, the results in 11 shoulders (22%) were considered unsatisfactory. Factors associated with poor results included an atraumatic cause of failure, voluntary dislocations, unaddressed capsular laxity, and multiple prior stabilization procedures. Four of 9 shoulders (44%) that had been treated with more than one prior stabilization attempt had recurrent instability after the revision procedure compared with only 7 of 41 shoulders (17%) that had one prior stabilization procedure. Other investigators reported similar results for patients with multidirectional instability who had multiple unsuccessful stabilization procedures, with less predictable results in terms of postoperative pain relief.[62] In severe cases of multidirectional instability refractory to conservative management, a glenohumeral arthrodesis can be considered in this subgroup of young patients.

Summary

In general, good surgical outcomes can be achieved in patients with glenohumeral joint instability if the soft-tissue and osseous pathology identified during the primary stabilization surgery is appropriately addressed. Capsular abnormalities in atraumatic and multidirectional instability typically represent a combination of asymptomatic laxity and symptomatic instability. Open capsular shift procedures offer a reliable and effective surgical solution in appropriately selected patients with capsular redundancy; however, less favorable results should be expected after revision surgery in patients with multidirectional instability. Future work should be directed at improving the ability to diagnose and anatomically repair capsular redundancy at the time of the index surgery to prevent the long-term adverse outcomes after revision surgery.

References

1. Zacchilli MA, Owens BD: Epidemiology of shoulder dislocations presenting to emergency departments in the United States. *J Bone Joint Surg Am* 2010;92(3): 542-549.
2. Lo IK, Bishop JY, Miniaci A, Flatow EL: Multidirectional instability: Surgical decision making. *Instr Course Lect* 2004;53:565-572.
3. Neer CS II, Foster CR: Inferior capsular shift for involuntary inferior and multidirectional instability of the shoulder: A preliminary report. *J Bone Joint Surg Am* 1980;62(6):897-908.
4. Mallon WJ, Speer KP: Multidirectional instability: Current concepts. *J Shoulder Elbow Surg* 1995; 4(1 pt 1):54-64.
5. Dewing CB, McCormick F, Bell SJ, et al: An analysis of capsular area in patients with anterior, posterior, and multidirectional shoulder instability. *Am J Sports Med* 2008;36(3):515-522.
6. Bankart AS: The pathology and treatment of recurrent dislocation of the shoulder-joint. *Br J Surg* 1938;26:23-29.
7. Stefko JM, Tibone JE, Cawley PW, ElAttrache NE, McMahon PJ: Strain of the anterior band of the inferior glenohumeral ligament during capsule failure. *J Shoulder Elbow Surg* 1997;6(5): 473-479.
8. Boileau P, Zumstein M, Balg F, Penington S, Bicknell RT: The unstable painful shoulder (UPS) as a cause of pain from unrecognized anteroinferior instability in the young athlete. *J Shoulder Elbow Surg* 2011;20(1):98-106.
9. Gagey OJ, Gagey N: The hyperabduction test. *J Bone Joint Surg Br* 2001;83(1):69-74.
10. Matsen FA III, Chebli C, Lippitt S; American Academy of Orthopaedic Surgeons: Principles for the evaluation and management of shoulder instability. *J Bone Joint Surg Am* 2006;88(3):648-659.
11. Bell JE: Arthroscopic management of multidirectional instability. *Orthop Clin North Am* 2010; 41(3):357-365.
12. Harryman DT II, Sidles JA, Harris SL, Matsen FA III: The role of the rotator interval capsule in passive motion and stability of the shoulder. *J Bone Joint Surg Am* 1992;74(1):53-66.
13. Mohana-Borges AV, Chung CB, Resnick D: MR imaging and MR arthrography of the postoperative shoulder: Spectrum of normal and abnormal findings. *Radiographics* 2004;24(1):69-85.
14. Burkhead WZ Jr, Rockwood CA Jr: Treatment of instability of the shoulder with an exercise program. *J Bone Joint Surg Am* 1992; 74(6):890-896.
15. Misamore GW, Sallay PI, Didelot W: A longitudinal study of patients with multidirectional instability of the shoulder with seven- to ten-year follow-up. *J Shoulder Elbow Surg* 2005;14(5):466-470.
16. Nyiri P, Illyés A, Kiss R, Kiss J: Intermediate biomechanical analysis of the effect of physiotherapy only compared with capsular shift and physiotherapy in multidirectional shoulder instability. *J Shoulder Elbow Surg* 2010;19(6): 802-813.
17. Duncan R, Savoie FH III: Arthroscopic inferior capsular shift for multidirectional instability of the shoulder: A preliminary report. *Arthroscopy* 1993;9(1):24-27.
18. Treacy SH, Savoie FH III, Field LD: Arthroscopic treatment of

multidirectional instability. *J Shoulder Elbow Surg* 1999;8(4): 345-350.

19. Gartsman GM, Roddey TS, Hammerman SM: Arthroscopic treatment of multidirectional glenohumeral instability: 2- to 5-year follow-up. *Arthroscopy* 2001; 17(3):236-243.
20. Sekiya JK, Willobee JA, Miller MD, Hickman AJ, Willobee A: Arthroscopic multi-pleated capsular plication compared with open inferior capsular shift for reduction of shoulder volume in a cadaveric model. *Arthroscopy* 2007; 23(11):1145-1151.
21. Fabbriciani C, Milano G, Demontis A, Fadda S, Ziranu F, Mulas PD: Arthroscopic versus open treatment of Bankart lesion of the shoulder: A prospective randomized study. *Arthroscopy* 2004; 20(5):456-462.
22. Petrera M, Patella V, Patella S, Theodoropoulos J: A meta-analysis of open versus arthroscopic Bankart repair using suture anchors. *Knee Surg Sports Traumatol Arthrosc* 2010;18(12): 1742-1747.
23. Kim SH, Ha KI, Kim YM: Arthroscopic revision Bankart repair: A prospective outcome study. *Arthroscopy* 2002;18(5):469-482.
24. Patel RV, Apostle K, Leith JM, Regan WD: Revision arthroscopic capsulolabral reconstruction for recurrent instability of the shoulder. *J Bone Joint Surg Br* 2008; 90(11):1462-1467.
25. Boileau P, Richou J, Lisai A, Chuinard C, Bicknell RT: The role of arthroscopy in revision of failed open anterior stabilization of the shoulder. *Arthroscopy* 2009; 25(10):1075-1084.
26. Yiannakopoulos CK, Mataragas E, Antonogiannakis E: A comparison of the spectrum of intra-articular lesions in acute and chronic anterior shoulder instability. *Arthroscopy* 2007;23(9):985-990.
27. Arrigoni P, Huberty D, Brady PC, Weber IC, Burkhart SS: The value of arthroscopy before an open modified Latarjet reconstruction. *Arthroscopy* 2008;24(5): 514-519.
28. Cole BJ, L'Insalata J, Irrgang J, Warner JJ: Comparison of arthroscopic and open anterior shoulder stabilization: A two to six-year follow-up study. *J Bone Joint Surg Am* 2000;82(8):1108-1114.
29. Millett PJ, Clavert P, Warner JJ: Open operative treatment for anterior shoulder instability: When and why? *J Bone Joint Surg Am* 2005;87(2):419-432.
30. Boselli KJ, Cody EA, Bigliani LU: Open capsular shift: There still is a role! *Orthop Clin North Am* 2010;41(3):427-436.
31. Wolf EM, Cheng JC, Dickson K: Humeral avulsion of glenohumeral ligaments as a cause of anterior shoulder instability. *Arthroscopy* 1995;11(5):600-607.
32. Iannotti JP, Antoniou J, Williams GR, Ramsey ML: Iliotibial band reconstruction for treatment of glenohumeral instability associated with irreparable capsular deficiency. *J Shoulder Elbow Surg* 2002;11(6):618-623.
33. Warner JJ, Venegas AA, Lehtinen JT, Macy JJ: Management of capsular deficiency of the shoulder: A report of three cases. *J Bone Joint Surg Am* 2002;84(9):1668-1671.
34. Alcid JG, Powell SE, Tibone JE: Revision anterior capsular shoulder stabilization using hamstring tendon autograft and tibialis tendon allograft reinforcement: Minimum two-year follow-up. *J Shoulder Elbow Surg* 2007;16(3): 268-272.
35. Wirth MA, Rockwood CA Jr: Operative treatment of irreparable rupture of the subscapularis. *J Bone Joint Surg Am* 1997;79(5): 722-731.
36. Wong KL, Williams GR: Complications of thermal capsulorrhaphy of the shoulder. *J Bone Joint Surg Am* 2001;83(suppl 2, pt 2): 151-155.
37. Burkhart SS, De Beer JF: Traumatic glenohumeral bone defects and their relationship to failure of arthroscopic Bankart repairs: Significance of the inverted-pear glenoid and the humeral engaging Hill-Sachs lesion. *Arthroscopy* 2000;16(7):677-694.
38. Wirth MA, Seltzer DG, Rockwood CA Jr: Recurrent posterior glenohumeral dislocation associated with increased retroversion of the glenoid: A case report. *Clin Orthop Relat Res* 1994;308: 98-101.
39. Miniaci A, Gish MW: Management of anterior glenohumeral instability associated with large Hill-Sachs defects. *Tech Shoulder Elbow Surg* 2004;5:170-175.
40. Cho SH, Cho NS, Rhee YG: Preoperative analysis of the Hill-Sachs lesion in anterior shoulder instability: How to predict engagement of the lesion. *Am J Sports Med* 2011;39(11):2389-2395.
41. Sekiya JK, Wickwire AC, Stehle JH, Debski RE: Hill-Sachs defects and repair using osteoarticular allograft transplantation: Biomechanical analysis using a joint compression model. *Am J Sports Med* 2009;37(12):2459-2466.
42. Kaar SG, Fening SD, Jones MH, Colbrunn RW, Miniaci A: Effect of humeral head defect size on glenohumeral stability: A cadaveric study of simulated Hill-Sachs defects. *Am J Sports Med* 2010; 38(3):594-599.
43. Bigliani LU, Newton PM, Steinmann SP, Connor PM, Mcllveen SJ: Glenoid rim lesions associated with recurrent anterior dislocation of the shoulder. *Am J Sports Med* 1998;26(1):41-45.
44. Lo IK, Parten PM, Burkhart SS: The inverted pear glenoid: An indicator of significant glenoid

bone loss. *Arthroscopy* 2004;20(2): 169-174.

45. Boileau P, Villalba M, Héry JY, Balg F, Ahrens P, Neyton L: Risk factors for recurrence of shoulder instability after arthroscopic Bankart repair. *J Bone Joint Surg Am* 2006;88(8):1755-1763.
46. Yamamoto N, Itoi E, Abe H, et al: Effect of an anterior glenoid defect on anterior shoulder stability: A cadaveric study. *Am J Sports Med* 2009;37(5):949-954.
47. Jobe FW, Giangarra CE, Kvitne RS, Glousman RE: Anterior capsulolabral reconstruction of the shoulder in athletes in overhand sports. *Am J Sports Med* 1991; 19(5):428-434.
48. Wirth MA, Groh GI, Rockwood CA Jr: Capsulorrhaphy through an anterior approach for the treatment of atraumatic posterior glenohumeral instability with multidirectional laxity of the shoulder. *J Bone Joint Surg Am* 1998; 80(11):1570-1578.
49. Warner JJ, Johnson D, Miller M, Caborn DN: Technique for selecting capsular tightness in repair of anterior-inferior shoulder instability. *J Shoulder Elbow Surg* 1995; 4(5):352-364.
50. Gerber C, Werner CM, Macy JC, Jacob HA, Nyffeler RW: Effect of selective capsulorrhaphy on the passive range of motion of the glenohumeral joint. *J Bone Joint Surg Am* 2003;85(1):48-55.
51. Lusardi DA, Wirth MA, Wurtz D, Rockwood CA Jr: Loss of external rotation following anterior capsulorrhaphy of the shoulder. *J Bone Joint Surg Am* 1993;75(8): 1185-1192.
52. Rowe CR, Zarins B, Ciullo JV: Recurrent anterior dislocation of the shoulder after surgical repair: Apparent causes of failure and treatment. *J Bone Joint Surg Am* 1984;66(2):159-168.
53. Young DC, Rockwood CA Jr: Complications of a failed Bristow procedure and their management. *J Bone Joint Surg Am* 1991;73(7): 969-981.
54. Tauber M, Resch H, Forstner R, Raffl M, Schauer J: Reasons for failure after surgical repair of anterior shoulder instability. *J Shoulder Elbow Surg* 2004;13(3):279-285.
55. Araghi A, Prasarn M, St Clair S, Zuckerman JD: Revision anterior shoulder repair for recurrent anterior glenohumeral instability. *Bull Hosp Jt Dis* 2005;62(3-4): 102-104.
56. Balg F, Boileau P: The instability severity index score: A simple preoperative score to select patients for arthroscopic or open shoulder stabilisation. *J Bone Joint Surg Br* 2007;89(11):1470-1477.
57. Cooper RA, Brems JJ: The inferior capsular-shift procedure for multidirectional instability of the shoulder. *J Bone Joint Surg Am* 1992;74(10):1516-1521.
58. Pollock RG, Owens JM, Flatow EL, Bigliani LU: Operative results of the inferior capsular shift procedure for multidirectional instability of the shoulder. *J Bone Joint Surg Am* 2000;82(7):919-928.
59. Zabinski SJ, Callaway GH, Cohen S, Warren RF: Revision shoulder stabilization: 2- to 10-year results. *J Shoulder Elbow Surg* 1999;8(1):58-65.
60. Levine WN, Arroyo JS, Pollock RG, Flatow EL, Bigliani LU: Open revision stabilization surgery for recurrent anterior glenohumeral instability. *Am J Sports Med* 2000;28(2):156-160.
61. Millett PJ, Clavert P, Warner JJ: Arthroscopic management of anterior, posterior, and multidirectional shoulder instability: Pearls and pitfalls. *Arthroscopy* 2003; 19(suppl 1):86-93.
62. Krishnan SG, Hawkins RJ, Horan MP, Dean M, Kim YK: A soft tissue attempt to stabilize the multiply operated glenohumeral joint with multidirectional instability. *Clin Orthop Relat Res* 2004;429: 256-261.
63. Marquardt B, Garmann S, Schulte T, Witt KA, Steinbeck J, Pötzl W: Outcome after failed traumatic anterior shoulder instability repair with and without surgical revision. *J Shoulder Elbow Surg* 2007;16(6):742-747.
64. Cheung EV, Sperling JW, Hattrup SJ, Cofield RH: Long-term outcome of anterior stabilization of the shoulder. *J Shoulder Elbow Surg* 2008;17(2):265-270.

Video References

8.1: Bois AJ, Wirth MA: Video. *Tendon Incision.* San Antonio, TX, 2012.
8.2: Bois AJ, Wirth MA: Video. *Reflecting the Medial Part of the Subscapularis Tendon Off the Capsule.* San Antonio, TX, 2012.
8.3: Bois AJ, Wirth MA: Video. *Eliminate Posterior Capsule Laxity.* San Antonio, TX, 2012.

9

General Surgical Principles of Open Rotator Cuff Repair in the Management of Failed Arthroscopic Cuff Repairs

Wayne Z. Burkhead Jr, MD
Todd C. Moen, MD
Glen H. Rudolph, MD

Abstract

Open management of failed rotator cuff repair is currently rare because of the advancements in arthroscopic techniques in rotator cuff surgery. Minimally invasive arthroscopic treatment of rotator cuff injuries has eclipsed the traditional open approach at most institutions around the world. Many residents complete their training in orthopaedic surgery without exposure to traditional open rotator cuff repair. When open repair is chosen, an understanding of the necessary preoperative evaluation, surgical techniques, and postoperative care regimens will provide patients with the best possible outcomes.

Instr Course Lect 2013;62:105-114.

Shoulder surgery has undergone a paradigm shift in the past 10 to 20 years. The introduction, development, and refinement of arthroscopic instrumentation and surgical techniques have prompted many surgeons to abandon traditional open surgical procedures in favor of arthroscopic repairs. This shift is readily apparent in rotator cuff surgery. The minimally invasive, deltoid-sparing approach of arthroscopic rotator cuff repair has led to a substantial increase in the popularity of this procedure. Based on the experience of one of this chapter's authors (TCM) and his classmates, it is possible for a resident to complete his or her orthopaedic training without performing a traditional open rotator cuff repair.

Open surgery remains an important tool for treating rotator cuff disease. Open cuff repair requires a deltoid takedown; however, the morbidity of this maneuver, when performed carefully, is likely overstated. Because tendon healing after rotator cuff surgery can lag months behind deltoid healing, the rate of success is more often limited by tendon healing, making the takedown of the deltoid a less important factor in measuring the success of the procedure.

The clinical results are largely equivalent among arthroscopic, mini-open, and open rotator cuff repairs; therefore, it can be argued that primary open rotator cuff repair remains a reasonable surgical option. Open surgery is especially important in revision scenarios. In any failed surgery, an alternative approach to the failed approach is an attractive option. Open rotator cuff repair in revision surgery is well suited to treat complications of arthroscopic cuff repair such as a failed repair, stiff shoulder, inadequate distal clavicle excision, recurrent impingement, biceps issues, and anchor-related chondrolysis. This chapter reviews the evolution and general surgical principles of open rotator cuff revision surgery as applied to failed arthroscopic rotator cuff repairs for massive rotator cuff tears.

Dr. Burkhead or an immediate family member serves as a board member, owner, officer, or committee member of the American Shoulder and Elbow Surgeons and the International Board of Shoulder and Elbow Surgery; has received royalties from Tornier; is a member of a speakers' bureau or has made paid presentations on behalf of Tornier; serves as a paid consultant to or is an employee of Tornier, Wright Medical Technology, and Stryker; has received research or institutional support from Wright Medical Technology; and has stock or stock options in Tornier. Neither of the following authors nor any immediate family member has received anything of value from or has stock or stock options in a commercial company or institution related directly or indirectly to the subject of this chapter: Dr. Moen and Dr. Rudolph.

Preoperative Evaluation

The first step in the successful treatment of a failed rotator cuff repair is establishing a correct diagnosis. It is imperative to identify the etiology of the patient's symptoms. Favorable clinical results can be achieved after rotator cuff repair despite a failure of the tear to heal.[1-3] It should not be assumed that the source of residual pain is from the tendon tear itself. Infection, adhesive capsulitis, residual acromioclavicular (AC) osteoarthritis, biceps tendinopathy or instability, and suprascapular neuropathy are among the multiple etiologies of pain or dysfunction after rotator cuff surgery.

The initial workup consists of a careful history and physical examination, along with plain radiography, MRI, or CT arthrography. The workup also includes aspiration, with cultures held for 14 days; serology, including a complete blood count, erythrocyte sedimentation rate, and C-reactive protein level; and nerve conduction velocity studies of the axillary and suprascapular nerves and an electromyogram of their innervated muscles. After obtaining the necessary studies, sequential selective injections with a low dose of lidocaine can help to localize the source of the patient's symptoms. After the major pain generators are identified, if the patient is healthy and nonarthritic and the coracoacromial arch is intact or reconstructible, revision surgery to repair the cuff can be performed. This removal of all major pain generators has been termed the RAMPAGE procedure.

Technique

The RAMPAGE procedure is performed under general endotracheal anesthesia. Preoperative antibiotics are not given because tissue will be obtained for intraoperative biopsy and cultures. After the patient is anesthetized, an examination is performed. The patient is then placed in the modified beach chair position and is prepped and draped. After establishing an anterior portal, standard diagnostic arthroscopy is performed, and tissue is obtained for frozen section biopsies and cultures. Prophylactic antibiotics are given after the cultures are obtained. At the time of arthroscopy, the quality and mobility of the rotator cuff is assessed with a tissue grasper. The tendon is assessed arthroscopically to determine if it is appropriate to proceed with open repair or perform only a simple arthroscopic débridement. When indicated, biceps tenotomy and/or selective primarily inferior capsular releases can be performed. Because the coracohumeral ligament is an extra-articular structure, it is released from the coracoid during the open portion of the procedure without violating the capsule. The rotator cuff remains intact in contrast to an interval slide procedure in which the natural connection and interdigitation of the collagen fibers of the rotator cuff are divided.

Skin Incision

After initial arthroscopy, the open portion of the procedure is performed. The shoulder is reprepped with 2% povidone iodine. The skin incisions are marked and infiltrated with 0.25% bupivacaine hydrochloride with epinephrine. The skin incisions are placed in the relaxed skin tension lines to minimize scarring. The internervous plane is respected to avoid neuroma formation (**Figure 1**). In female patients, a 5-cm incision is made into these lines just medial to the lateral border of the acromion. In male patients, an oblique incision measuring approximately 6 cm is made from the AC joint to the lateral border of the acromion. After the initial skin incision, generous subcutaneous flaps are raised to allow optimal exposure of the deltoid, trapezius, deltotrapezial fascia, acromion, clavicle, and AC joint.

Deltotrapezial Approach

The deltotrapezial approach is the product of both good and bad experiences of multiple surgeons. Prior to the Neer technique of limited acromioplasty, which respects the lateral deltoid, many poorly designed procedures for the shoulder detached the lateral deltoid and/or acromion and resulted in poor outcomes.[4,5] Some open approaches, with or without acromioplasty, risk injury to the acromial attachment of the deltoid. This chapter's senior author (WZB) has tried to combine the best features of the Kessell approach learned in 1982 at the Royal National Orthopaedic Hospital in London, the Rockwood approach learned in 1983 at the University of Texas Health Science Center in San Antonio, and the Rowe approach, which creates robust flaps of tissue and minimizes the risk of failed deltoid repair[6,7] (**Figure 2**).

The deltotrapezial incision starts medial to the AC joint and proceeds anterolaterally toward the anterolateral corner of the acromion and into the raphe between the anterior and the middle heads of the deltoid. By orienting this fascial incision 20° anterior to the spine of the scapula, the incision is made parallel with the plane of maximum forward elevation of the arm (**Figure 3**). At closure, this creates a tensionless side-to-side repair parallel to the plane of maximum elevation of the arm.[8] The thickest part of the deltotrapezial fascia is within 1 cm of the AC joint. Electrocautery is used for the initial incision down to bone. Slow, controlled pressure with the bevel of a No. 15 blade turned toward the bone is applied to harvest the thickest fascial flaps possible. This technique incorporates Sharpey fibers and strengthens the flaps (**Figure 4**).

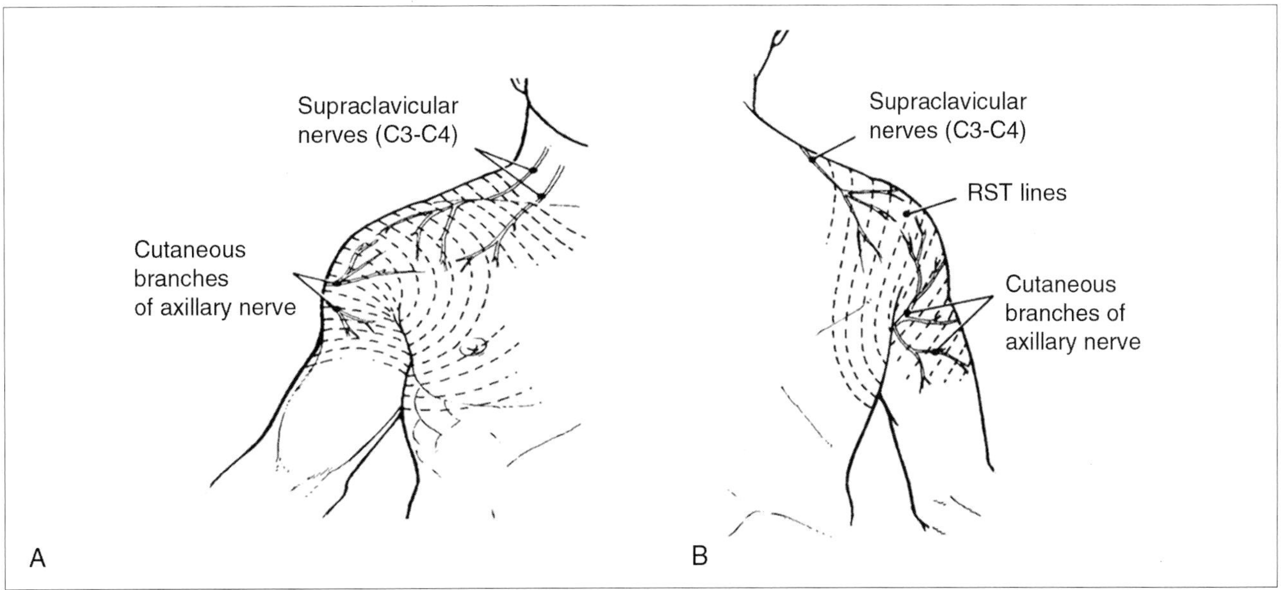

Figure 1 Illustrations of the anterior (**A**) and posterior (**B**) shoulder showing nerves and relaxed skin tension (RST) lines. Placing an incision on the relaxed skin tension lines in the internervous plane will minimize scarring and neuroma formation.

Incorporating this tissue in all flaps for rotator cuff repair and extending the incision into the thick raphe between the anterior and middle thirds of the deltoid will ensure, to the extent possible, the creation of flaps capable of holding sutures for optimal repair of the deltoid takedown. This fascial incision, which exploits the interval between the anterior and middle heads of the deltoid, is the key to exposing all portions of the rotator cuff. As described by Codman,[9] extension down this interval anteriorly and distally from the acromion allows the treating surgeon or his or her assistant to rotate the arm so that nearly all parts of the rotator cuff are accessible. Extension via splitting the trapezius allows better mobilization of the supraspinatus and suprascapular nerve release if indicated.

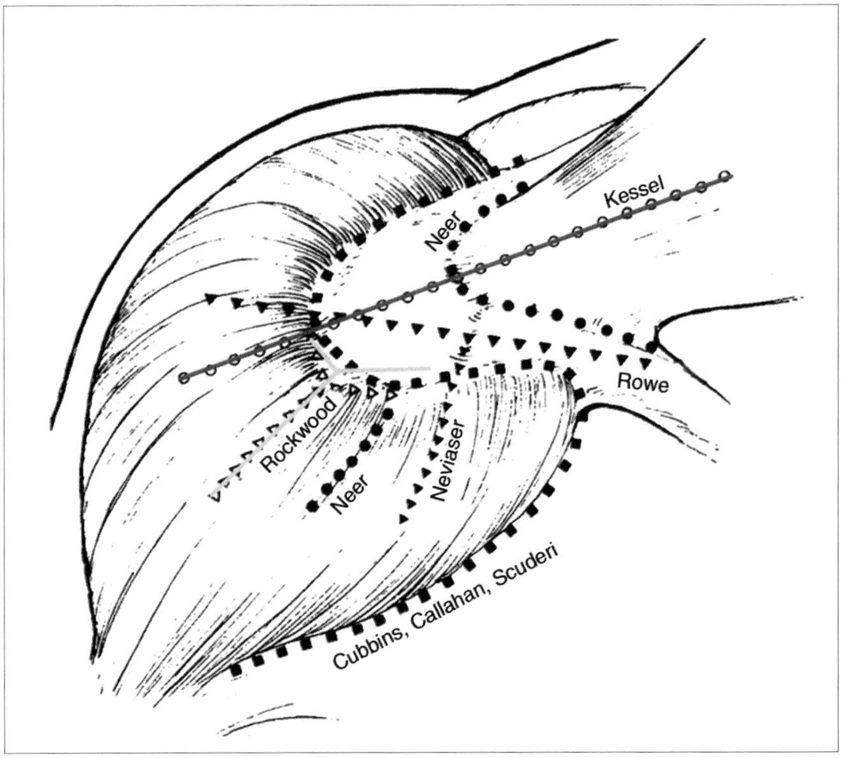

Figure 2 Illustration showing various deltotrapezial fascial incisions for open cuff repair. The senior author's approach combines elements of the Rockwood technique (use of the raphe) for visualization, the Rowe technique (increased thickness of tissue at the AC joint) for secure repair fixation, and the Kessel technique (extension into the trapezius) for an extensile approach into the supraspinatus fossae for suprascapular nerve release if indicated.

Exploration of the Residual AC Joint

Persistent pain after arthroscopic rotator cuff repair can be the result of an incompletely resected or completely

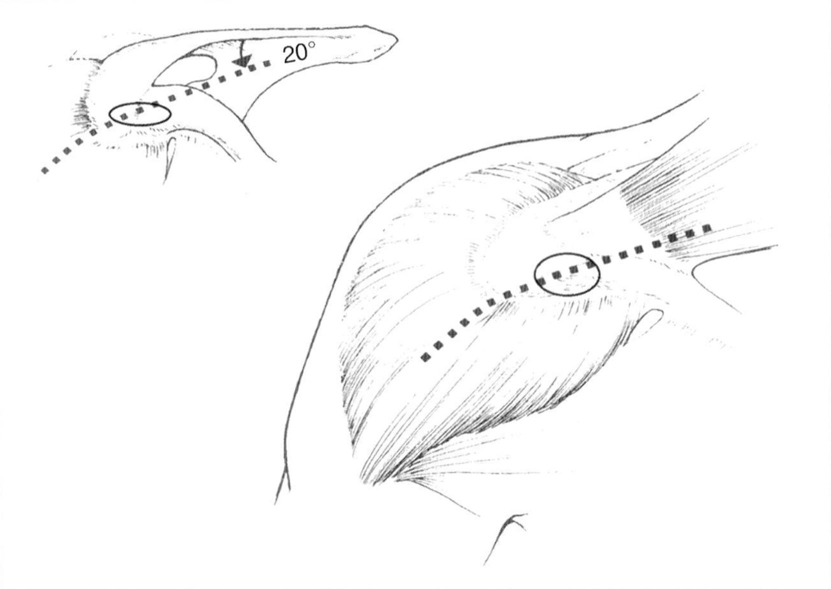

Figure 3 The deltotrapezial fascial incision (dashed line) is made 20° anterior to the spine of the scapula using the senior author's approach.

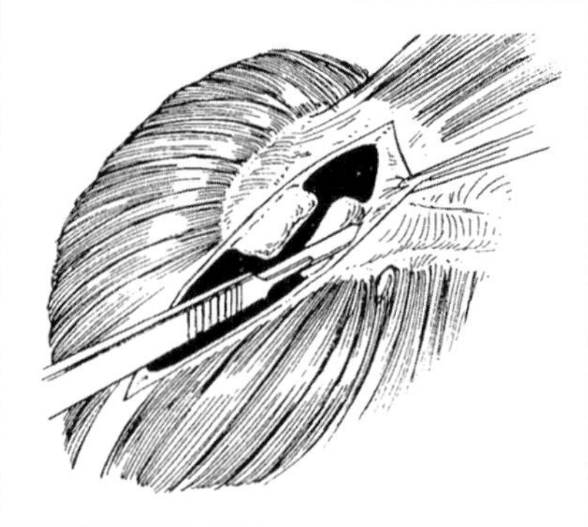

Figure 4 Care should be exercised to elevate the flaps and incorporate the Sharpey fibers using a blade rather than a cautery.

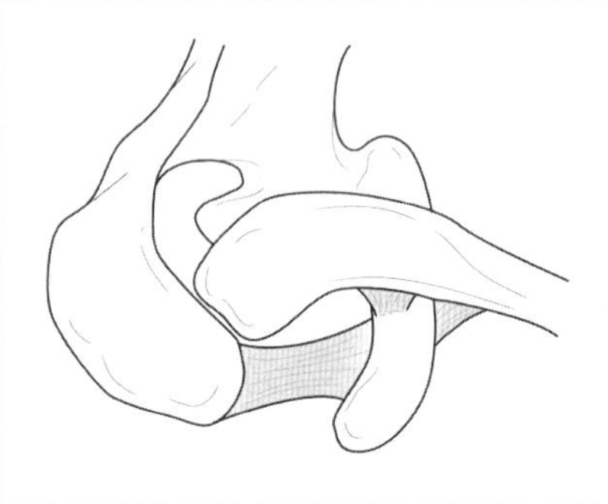

Figure 5 The coracoacromial ligament can be seen coursing under the surface of the acromion for more than 1 cm in many patients. It should be harvested in its entirety and repaired back to the acromion. Care should be taken not to shorten the acromion in massive rotator cuff tears.

unresected distal clavicle and clavicular facet of the acromion. These residual structures, if present, are routinely resected at the time of revision rotator cuff repair. Although the literature suggests that a 5-mm clavicle resection is satisfactory when applied arthroscopically, recent data suggest that open distal claviculectomy yields superior results (F. Gohike, MD, Edinburgh, Scotland, unpublished data, 2010). Excision of the distal clavicle and the clavicular facet eliminates pain emanating from the AC joint, removes tension on the underlying musculotendinous portion of the rotator cuff from bulbous inferior osteophytes, and improves exposure and suture passage through larger medially retracted tears. This chapter's senior author has found that persistent pain is common after inferior osteophyte removal.

Residual Acromion and Coracoacromial Ligament

Care is taken not to shorten the acromion. Inferior spurs are removed after the coracoacromial ligament is harvested by peeling it from the undersurface (**Figure 5**). The ligament is tagged and repaired at the end of the procedure. If the rotator cuff adheres to the undersurface of the acromion, it is peeled off with a No. 15 blade.

A thorough subacromial and subcoracoid bursectomy is then performed. The notion that the bursa somehow participates in healing has been dismissed.[10] Postoperative adhesions and scarring, especially at the posterior portal site and subcoracoid recess, may be extensive and require sharp dissection. The subacromial bursa contains a rich network of sympathetic nerves. It is quite common that, despite a surgical report stating that a bursectomy was performed, both the floor and the roof of the subacromial bursa are still present and are often thickened and fibrotic or inflamed.

Next, control of the rotator cuff is gained, and it is mobilized for repair. The leading edges of the rotator cuff are tagged with No. 2 nonabsorbable suture, and the cuff is sequentially mobilized with various releases— both extra-articular and intra-articular releases. Structures creating a static deforming force are addressed in order. First, the coracohumeral ligament (**Figure 6**) and then the capsulolabral attachments (**Figure 7**) are released. A Darrach retractor can be passed all the way into the supraspinatus and infraspinatus fossae to free the muscle bellies of both tendons if necessary (**Figure 8**). These releases allow the tendon to be more anatomically restored to the rotator cuff footprint and

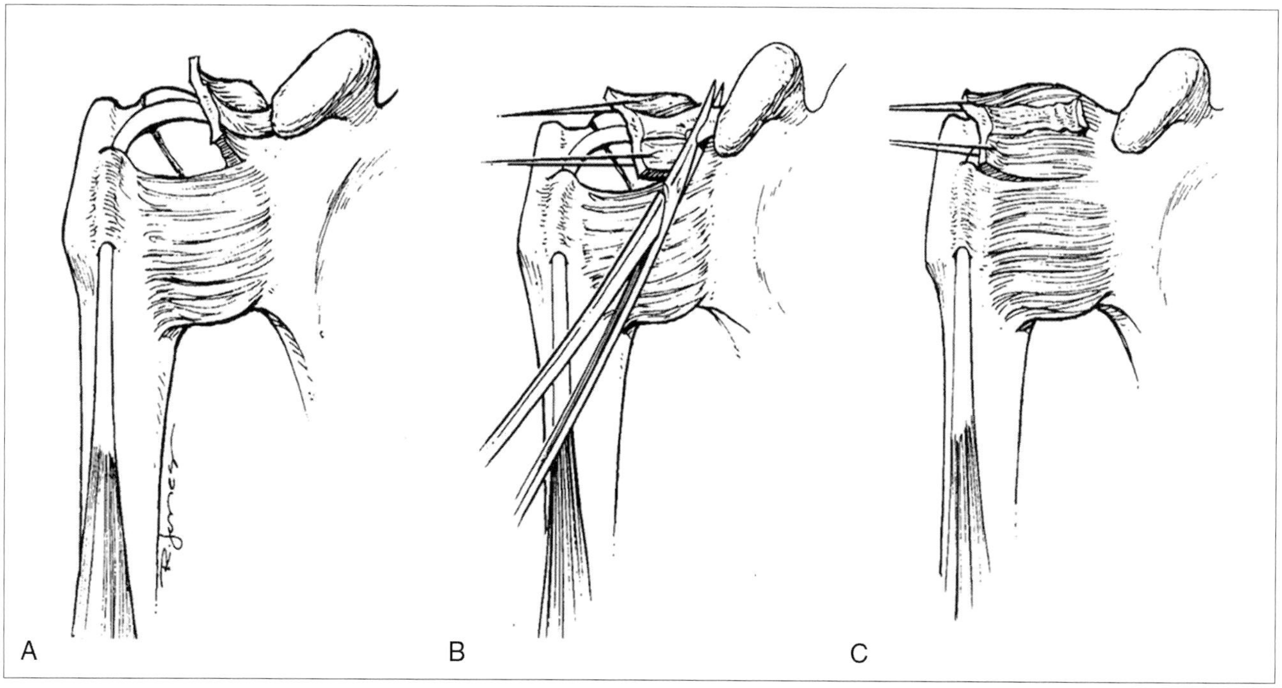

Figure 6 The coracohumeral ligament is excised on its bursal surface, preserving the capsular layer beneath. **A,** A rotator cuff tear, with a tight and contracted coracohumeral ligament tethering the tear medially. **B,** The coracohumeral ligament if sharply released. **C,** The excursion of the rotator cuff tear is improved after the release.

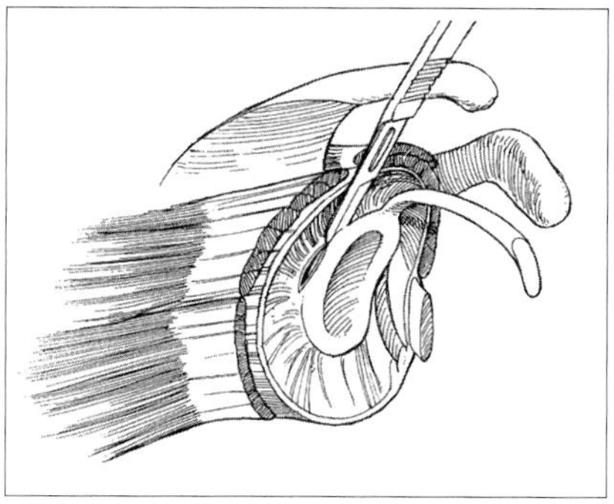

Figure 7 Care should be taken to stay within 1 cm of the labrum at the posterosuperior corner to avoid injury to the branch of the suprascapular nerve to the infraspinatus.

diminish tension on the repair construct.

After the cuff has been sufficiently mobilized, it is critical to understand the configuration and characteristics of the tear to determine the optimal repair construct. The tear pattern dictates the repair construct, be it a side-to-side, margin convergence repair or an end-to-end, massive avulsion-type repair. The key principle in identifying the tear pattern is determining the amount of exposure of the rotator cuff footprint. A boutonniere-type deformity will expose a relatively small amount of the sulcus and the tuberosity, whereas a massive avulsion will expose the entire sulcus and, occasionally, both tuberosities (**Figure 9**). L-shaped and reverse L-shaped tears are reduced in opposite directions and should be immobilized in opposite directions.

In patients with massive avulsions, it is wise to widen the sulcus by encroaching onto the articular surface for 5 mm to decrease tension on the repair and broaden the surface area of exposed bone. Abduction of the arm intraoperatively and postoperatively will take tension off the repair. With margin convergence, the sulcus may need to be widened in a chevron shape to create end-to-end fixation for each leaf of the boutonniere. This chapter's senior author prefers using metal anchors in the humerus. Because the rotator cuff will not heal to a hole in the bone, the smallest diameter anchor should be used; poly-L-lactic anchors should be avoided.

From 1991 until 2007, this chapter's senior author used a combination of a medial anchor with lateral transosseous suture passage, with the same suture as the transosseous anchor double-knot technique. In essence, this technique is both a dual-row and a suture-bridging technique (**Figure 10**). The initial study performed with first-generation anchors and No. 2 polyester suture showed a marked improvement in pullout strength when compared with anchor only or transosseous only repairs (**Figure 11**). When the study was repeated 10 years later with screw-in anchors and high tensile strength No. 2 suture, the pullout strength nearly doubled

(**Figure 12**). More recently, the senior author has preferred metal anchors that are vented for the medial row and an anchor-based lateral row using a press-in anchor that achieves excellent fixation in bone (**Figure 13, A** and **B**). Over the past 8 years, an allograft dermal matrix has been used in revisions as augmentation on the superior aspect of the repair to improve the biology, promote healing, and prevent suture cutout in tears larger than 5 cm (**Figure 13, C** and **D**). The grafts are soaked in platelet-rich plasma to improve incorporation and apply growth factors.

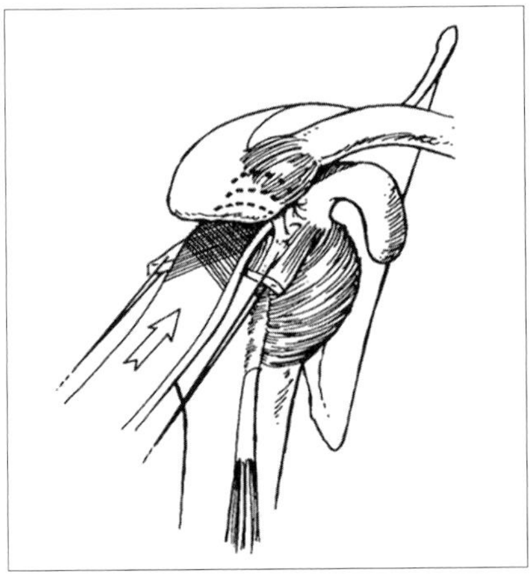

Figure 8 A Darrach retractor has been the tool of choice among shoulder surgeons for decades and helps define the bursal plane and eliminate adhesions. Here the Darrach retractor is being passed superior to the supraspinatus and infraspinatus muscles to release bursal adhesions. The arrow shows the direction in which the retractor is moving.

Recent literature has shown that double-row repairs are superior to single-row repairs in vitro, although clinical results have not mirrored these findings. Multiple biomechanical studies have shown the superior strength of double-row rotator cuff repairs to single-row repairs.[11-18] Double-row repairs have been shown to provide a more anatomic restoration of the rotator cuff footprint compared with single-row repairs.[19] More recently, transosseous equivalent double-row repair with suture anchors was found to be biomechanically superior to pure transosseous repair regardless of the suture configuration (MJ Salata, MD, et al, San Francisco, CA, unpublished data presented at the American Shoulder and Elbow Surgeons Open Meeting, 2012). Despite the laboratory results, some recently published data regarding the clinical outcomes associated with dual-row versus single-row constructs have shown equivalent outcomes with the techniques.[20-24] Other studies of double-row repair, however, have shown improved healing rates, lower retear rates, and improved strength, especially in patients with larger tears. These findings seem to confirm the biomechanical advantages of the double-row repair.[25-27] For massive tears, this chapter's authors recommend a dual-row, suture-bridging configuration.

Closure

Closure of the deltoid is accomplished with No. 1 and 2 antibiotic-impregnated, polyglactin 910 suture.

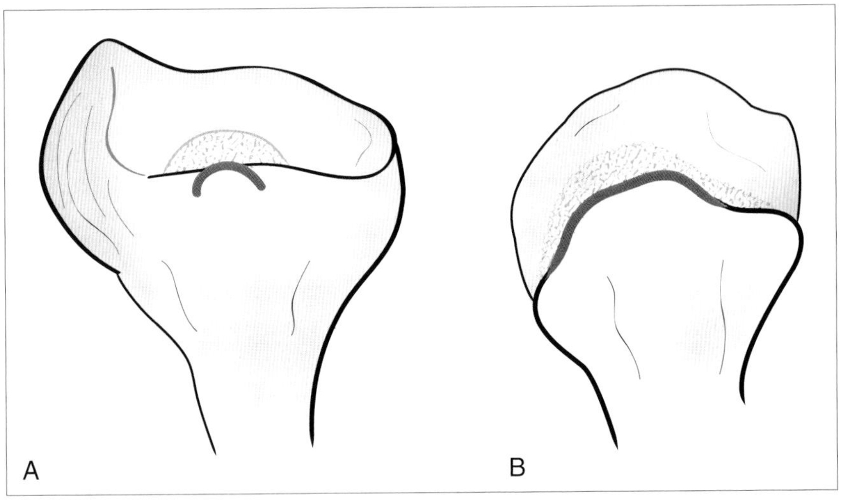

Figure 9 **A,** A boutonniere-type deformity has a relatively small amount of exposed sulcus and tuberosity. It is reduced with downward traction and a side-to-side repair. **B,** A massive avulsion will expose the entire sulcus and occasionally both tuberosities. These avulsions are reduced by abducting the arm. Side-to-side repairs of massive avulsion-type deformities shorten the rotator cuff and make it impossible to reach even the sulcus with the converged tendon.

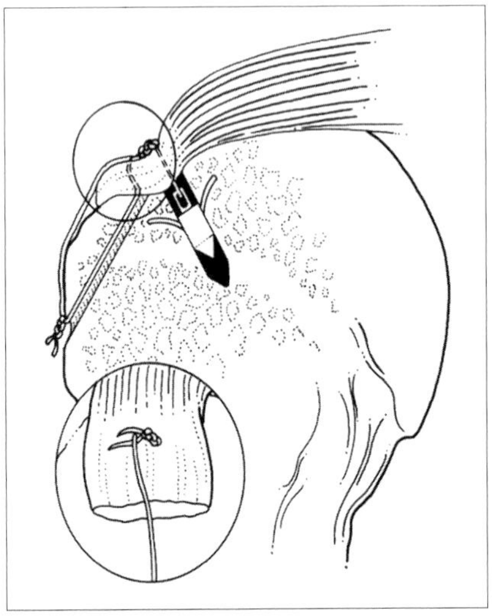

Figure 10 Illustration of the original transosseous anchor double-knot technique (circa 1991), with a first-generation anchor and a second grasping stitch (insert) through the tendon before transosseous suture passage.

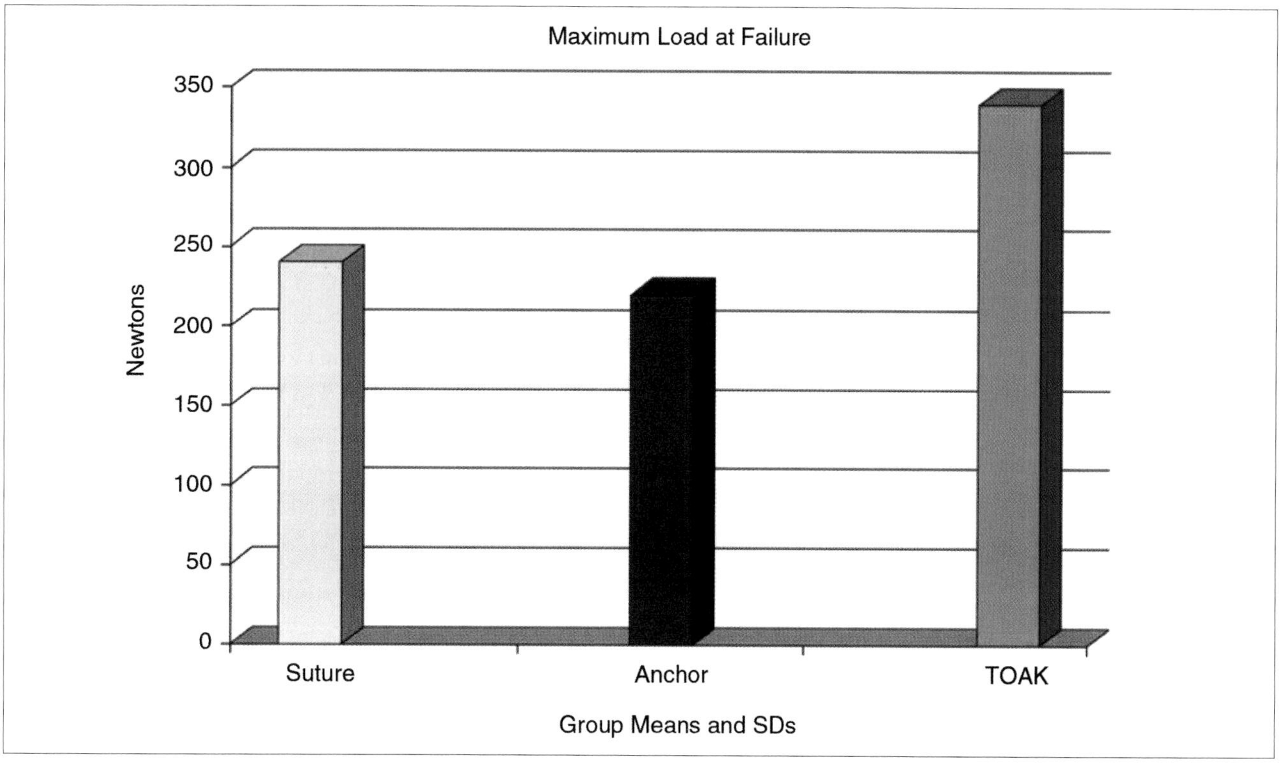

Figure 11 Bar graph comparing maximum load to failure of rotator cuff repairs with suture only, anchors only, and the transosseous anchor double-knot (TOAK) technique.

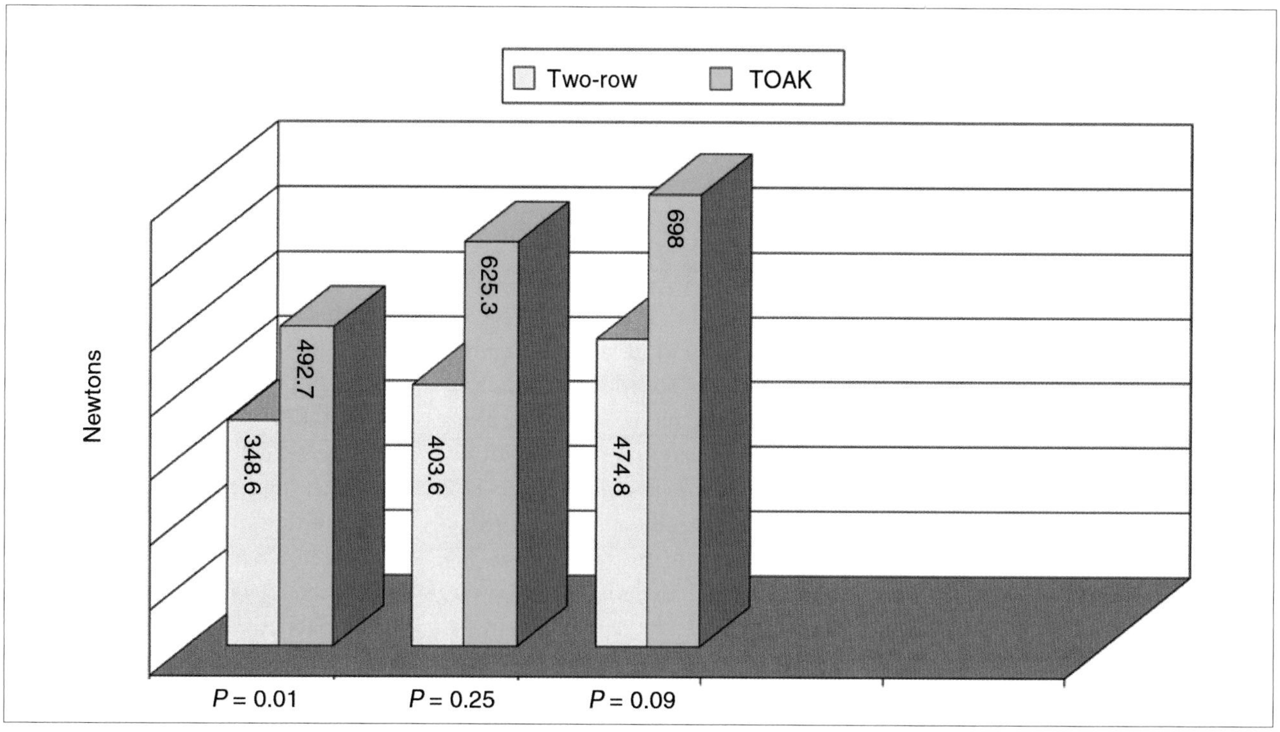

Figure 12 Bar graph comparing the pullout strength of the two-row technique and the transosseous anchor double-knot (TOAK) technique of rotator cuff repair.

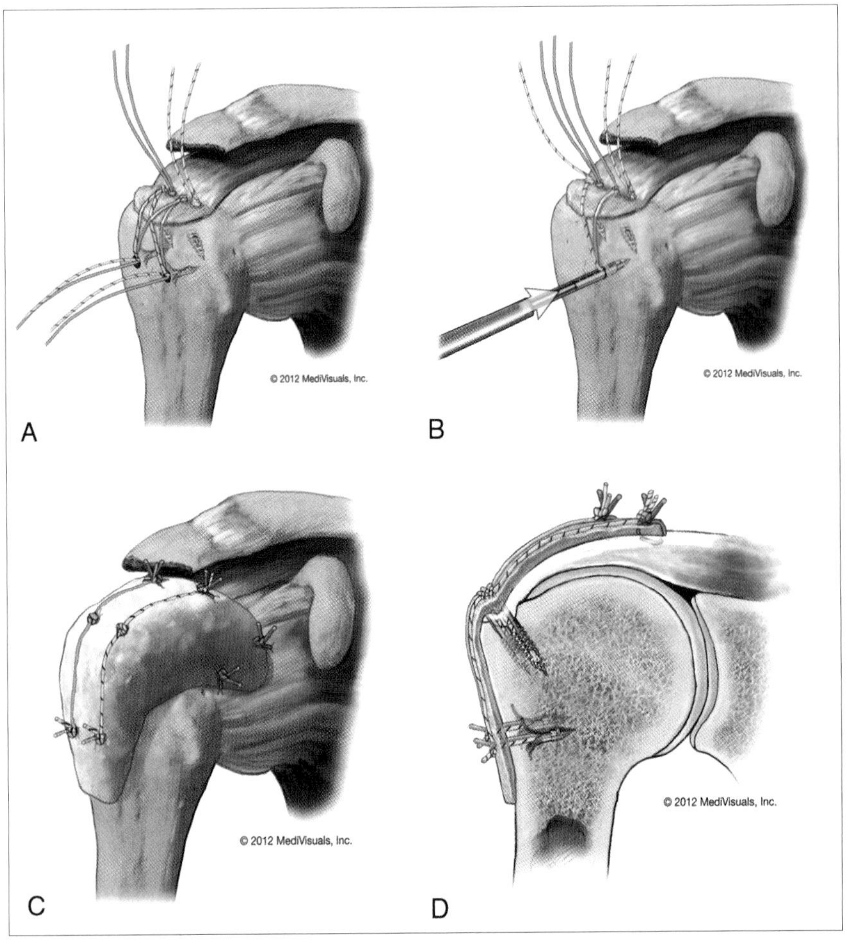

Figure 13 **A,** In a more recent version of the transosseous anchor double-knot technique, the medial row involves a horizontal mattress suture from a vented screw in the anchor. **B,** The lateral row is a push-in–type anchor with nitinol flanges that deploy and become rigid at body temperature. **C,** The lateral anchors are strong enough to secure an allograft dermal matrix graft with the sutures still attached. **D,** Coronal view of the lateral anchors. (Courtesy of MediVisuals, Dallas, TX.)

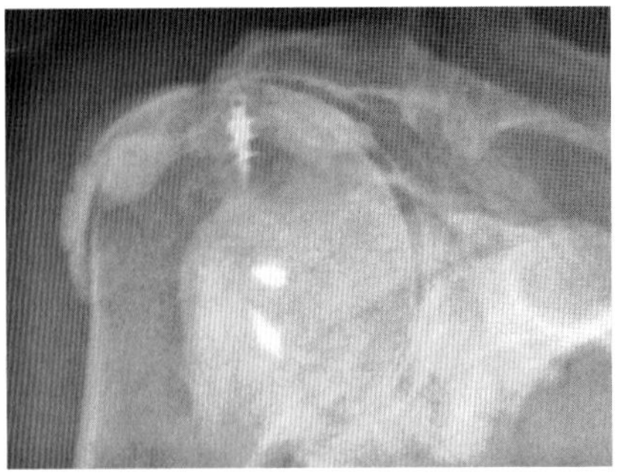

Figure 14 A 57-year-old patient presented with pain and pseudoparalysis 10 weeks after an arthroscopic rotator cuff repair. A scout radiograph for magnetic resonance arthrography shows an obliterated acromiohumeral distance medially, prominent anchor placement, and an unresected AC joint.

The thick deltotrapezial flaps hold sutures well. Usually one of the sutures is placed through the anterior acromion. A subcuticular closure results in a cosmetically acceptable scar.

Postoperative Immobilization and Rehabilitation

Patients with massive avulsion pattern tears are placed in an abduction pillow. For the first 3 weeks, only elbow, wrist, and finger range of motion are allowed. Any passive motion at the shoulder potentially pumps joint fluid with its associated metalloproteinases and collagenases into and through the repair site. At 3 weeks, passive elevation above the pillow is allowed along with passive external rotation. In patients with a margin-convergence–type repair, a small pillow sling is used to keep the arm in neutral rotation. The sling is worn loosely to avoid upward pressure against the repair. At 3 weeks, pendulum exercises are started. Active-assisted exercise is begun with a pulley at 6 weeks, along with internal rotation up the back. Active range of motion begins at 6 to 8 weeks and strengthening at 12 to 14 weeks. This chapter's senior author prefers a home rehabilitation program for at least the first 8 to 10 weeks. Residual stiffness usually resolves over the next 3 to 6 months. Postoperative stiffness, such as adhesive capsulitis, after successful rotator cuff repair is a time-dependent and, often, self-limiting condition. Preoperative counseling should inform the patient of the expectation of a prolonged, gradual recovery. This chapter's authors believe that a common cause for rotator cuff failure after arthroscopic repair may be overly aggressive rehabilitation, such as manipulation under anesthesia at 3 months postoperatively.

Case Example

A 57-year-old man who worked as a firefighter injured his right shoulder during lifting at work 2 years before his expected retirement. He presented for treatment with shoulder pain and pseudoparalysis 10 weeks after arthroscopic rotator cuff repair. Scout radiographs showed medial and prominent hardware and untreated severe AC arthritis (**Figure 14**). Magnetic resonance arthrography confirmed failure of the repair, a high-riding humerus,

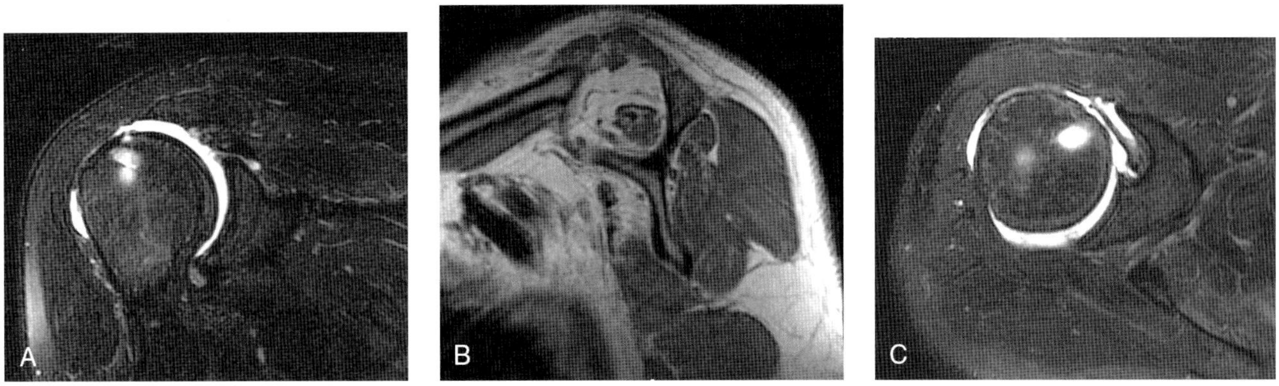

Figure 15 MRI scans of the shoulder of the patient described in Figure 14. **A,** Coronal T2-weighted MRI scan showing retraction of the cuff tendon to the glenoid rim. **B,** T1-weighted sagittal MRI scan shows atrophy of the supraspinatus and fatty infiltration of the subscapularis. **C,** Axial MRI scan confirms subscapularis involvement.

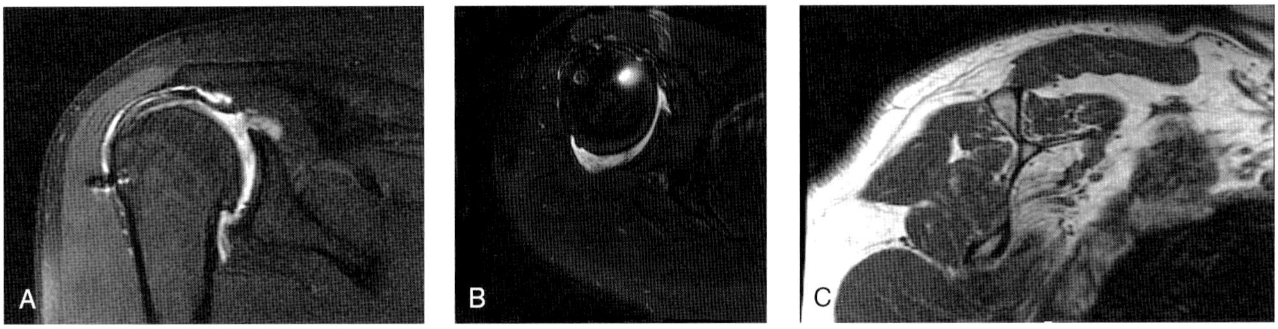

Figure 16 MRI scans of the patient described in Figure 14 taken at 3-year follow-up. **A,** Coronal MRI scan confirms tendon healing across the humeral head. **B,** Axial MRI scan shows the healed subscapularis with improved coracohumeral distance. **C,** Sagittal T1-weighted MRI scan shows improvement in muscle trophicity. The patient reported that his shoulder felt nearly normal.

atrophy of the supraspinatus, and marked fatty infiltration of the subscapularis (**Figure 15**). The patient was treated according to the principles described in this chapter along with dermal matrix augmentation. At 7 months, he returned to active duty as a firefighter. At 3-year follow-up, he had retired, lived in the country, and did ranch work without pain. His strength score on supraspinatus and infraspinatus testing was more than 4 on a 5-point scale. MRI showed improved acromiohumeral distance, graft and tendon healing, and improvement in muscle trophicity (**Figure 16**). Fatty infiltration of the subscapularis was unchanged, although the patient had a negative belly-press test.

Summary

To achieve a successful outcome, open treatment is sometimes needed after a failed rotator cuff repair. With the continuing advances in arthroscopic treatment of the rotator cuff, open treatment of rotator cuff injuries is becoming a lost art. Patients with a previously failed rotator cuff repair should be carefully evaluated. After the decision is made to surgically treat the patient through an open approach, the principles and techniques of the deltotrapezial approach described in this chapter, along with postoperative care and rehabilitation, can achieve a positive outcome for the patient.

References

1. Jost B, Pfirrmann CW, Gerber C, Switzerland Z: Clinical outcome after structural failure of rotator cuff repairs. *J Bone Joint Surg Am* 2000;82(3):304-314.
2. Jost B, Zumstein M, Pfirrmann CW, Gerber C: Long-term outcome after structural failure of rotator cuff repairs. *J Bone Joint Surg Am* 2006;88(3):472-479.
3. Zumstein MA, Jost B, Hempel J, Hodler J, Gerber C: The clinical and structural long-term results of open repair of massive tears of the rotator cuff. *J Bone Joint Surg Am* 2008;90(11):2423-2431.
4. Hammond G: Complete acromionectomy in the treatment

of chronic tendinitis of the shoulder: A follow-up of ninety operations on eighty-seven patients. *J Bone Joint Surg Am* 1971;53(1): 173-180.

5. Neer CS II, Marberry TA: On the disadvantages of radical acromionectomy. *J Bone Joint Surg Am* 1981;63(3):416-419.
6. Watson M: Major ruptures of the rotator cuff: The results of surgical repair in 89 patients. *J Bone Joint Surg Br* 1985;67(4):618-624.
7. Rockwood CA Jr, Williams GR Jr, Burkhead WZ Jr: Débridement of degerative, irreparable lesions of the rotator cuff. *J Bone Joint Surg Am* 1995;77(6): 857-866.
8. An KN, Browne AO, Korinek S, Tanaka S, Morrey BF: Three-dimensional kinematics of glenohumeral elevation. *J Orthop Res* 1991;9(1):143-149.
9. Codman EA: *The Shoulder*. Boston, MA, Thomas Todd, 1934.
10. Uhthoff HK, Trudel G, Himori K: Relevance of pathology and basic research to the surgeon treating rotator cuff disease. *J Orthop Sci* 2003;8(3):449-456.
11. Baums MH, Spahn G, Buchhorn GH, Schultz W, Hofmann L, Klinger HM: Biomechanical and magnetic resonance imaging evaluation of a single- and double-row rotator cuff repair in an in vivo sheep model. *Arthroscopy* 2012; 28(6):769-777.
12. Kim DH, Elattrache NS, Tibone JE, et al: Biomechanical comparison of a single-row versus double-row suture anchor technique for rotator cuff repair. *Am J Sports Med* 2006;34(3):407-414.
13. Lorbach O, Kieb M, Raber F, Busch LC, Kohn D, Pape D: Comparable biomechanical results for a modified single-row rotator cuff reconstruction using triple-loaded suture anchors versus a suture-bridging double-row repair. *Arthroscopy* 2012;28(2):178-187.
14. Lorbach O, Bachelier F, Vees J, Kohn D, Pape D: Cyclic loading of rotator cuff reconstructions: Single-row repair with modified suture configurations versus double-row repair. *Am J Sports Med* 2008;36(8):1504-1510.
15. Ma CB, Comerford L, Wilson J, Puttlitz CM: Biomechanical evaluation of arthroscopic rotator cuff repairs: Double-row compared with single-row fixation. *J Bone Joint Surg Am* 2006;88(2): 403-410.
16. Milano G, Grasso A, Zarelli D, Deriu L, Cillo M, Fabbriciani C: Comparison between single-row and double-row rotator cuff repair: A biomechanical study. *Knee Surg Sports Traumatol Arthrosc* 2008;16(1):75-80.
17. Smith CD, Alexander S, Hill AM, et al: A biomechanical comparison of single and double-row fixation in arthroscopic rotator cuff repair. *J Bone Joint Surg Am* 2006; 88(11):2425-2431.
18. Wall LB, Keener JD, Brophy RH: Double-row vs single-row rotator cuff repair: A review of the biomechanical evidence. *J Shoulder Elbow Surg* 2009;18(6):933-941.
19. Nelson CO, Sileo MJ, Grossman MG, Serra-Hsu F: Single-row modified Mason-Allen versus double-row arthroscopic rotator cuff repair: A biomechanical and surface area comparison. *Arthroscopy* 2008;24(8):941-948.
20. Aydin N, Kocaoglu B, Guven O: Single-row versus double-row arthroscopic rotator cuff repair in small- to medium-sized tears. *J Shoulder Elbow Surg* 2010;19(5): 722-725.
21. Koh KH, Kang KC, Lim TK, Shon MS, Yoo JC: Prospective randomized clinical trial of single- versus double-row suture anchor repair in 2- to 4-cm rotator cuff tears: Clinical and magnetic resonance imaging results. *Arthroscopy* 2011;27(4):453-462.
22. Pauly S, Gerhardt C, Chen J, Scheibel M: Single versus double-row repair of the rotator cuff: Does double-row repair with improved anatomical and biomechanical characteristics lead to better clinical outcome? *Knee Surg Sports Traumatol Arthrosc* 2010; 18(12):1718-1729.
23. Reardon DJ, Maffulli N: Clinical evidence shows no difference between single- and double-row repair for rotator cuff tears. *Arthroscopy* 2007;23(6):670-673.
24. Saridakis P, Jones G: Outcomes of single-row and double-row arthroscopic rotator cuff repair: A systematic review. *J Bone Joint Surg Am* 2010;92(3):732-742.
25. DeHaan AM, Axelrad TW, Kaye E, Silvestri L, Puskas B, Foster TE: Does double-row rotator cuff repair improve functional outcome of patients compared with single-row technique? A systematic review. *Am J Sports Med* 2012; 40(5):1176-1185.
26. Mihata T, Watanabe C, Fukunishi K, et al: Functional and structural outcomes of single-row versus double-row versus combined double-row and suture-bridge repair for rotator cuff tears. *Am J Sports Med* 2011;39(10):2091-2098.
27. Ma HL, Chiang ER, Wu HT, et al: Clinical outcome and imaging of arthroscopic single-row and double-row rotator cuff repair: A prospective randomized trial. *Arthroscopy* 2012;28(1):16-24.

10

Prevention of Complications in Shoulder Arthroplasty: Understanding Options and Critical Steps

Curtis A. Bush, MD
Richard J. Hawkins, MD

Abstract

Total shoulder arthroplasty provides reliable pain relief of osteoarthritic shoulder pain. The keys to success with shoulder arthroplasty are adhering to appropriate indications, understanding the surgical implications of various pathologies, and applying good surgical technique. Many complications of total shoulder arthroplasty may be avoided with good preoperative preparation. Some key surgical steps that may help avoid the more common complications include proper patient positioning, adequate soft-tissue releases for rebalancing, identification of the axillary nerve, correction of glenoid version, the adjustment of humeral component size and version as needed for stability, and meticulous subscapularis repair. Additional precautions can include postoperative immobilization to protect soft-tissue repairs followed by structured rehabilitation.

Instr Course Lect 2013;62:115-133.

The principal goals of shoulder arthroplasty are to resurface the joint to provide pain relief, balance the soft tissues to provide stability, and restore motion to improve function. Total shoulder arthroplasty (TSA) provides reliable pain relief of osteoarthritic shoulder pain. The keys to successful TSA are adhering to appropriate indications, understanding the surgical indications of various pathologies, and applying good surgical technique. A recent study reported that the overall complication and revision rates in TSA have declined.[1] Most of the complications occurred within 90 days of surgery; early complications tended to be of a technical nature, and many were likely avoidable. Understanding the options and critical steps in TSA may help avoid the most common complications associated with the procedure.

Preoperative Assessment

A thorough evaluation of active and passive range of motion and functional limitations is a key component in preoperative planning. Limited external rotation is a common finding in patients with advanced osteoarthritis (OA) because of contractures of anterior soft tissues. Depending on the extent of such limitations, the surgical approach may vary. Assessment of the condition and function of the rotator cuff is essential and should begin with a good patient history and physical examination. Although the incidence of concomitant OA and rotator cuff tears is very low (especially in young patients), occult rotator cuff or subscapularis tears may lead to early failure of TSA.[2-8] A thorough neurologic examination is also important, especially in patients with traumatic injuries. Any concerns regarding neurologic deficits may warrant electromyographic evaluation.

Radiographic studies include true AP, outlet, and axillary views. Preoperative radiographs may be useful for templating component sizes in preparation for surgery. Thorough evaluation of glenohumeral morphology is an important step, with emphasis on

Dr. Hawkins or an immediate family member has received royalties from Ossur; serves as a paid consultant to or is an employee of DJ Orthopaedics; and has received research or institutional support from DJ Orthopaedics, Breg, Smith & Nephew, OrthoRehab, Ferring Pharmaceuticals, Tornier, and Ossur. Neither Dr. Bush nor any immediate family member has received anything of value from or owns stock in a commercial company or institution related directly or indirectly to the subject of this chapter.

Table 1
Summary of Literature Reporting Proximal Humerus Fractures Treated With Reverse Total Shoulder Arthroplasty

Study	No. of Patients	Mean Age (Years)	Mean Follow-up (Months)	Mean Active Forward Flexion
Boileau et al[12]	5	72	40	122°
Cazeneuve and Cristofari[13]	36	75	78	NA
Bufquin et al[14]	41	78	22	97°
Gallinet et al[15]	16	74	12	98°
Klein et al[16]	20	75	33	122°
Lenarz et al[17]	30	76	23	138°

NA = not available.

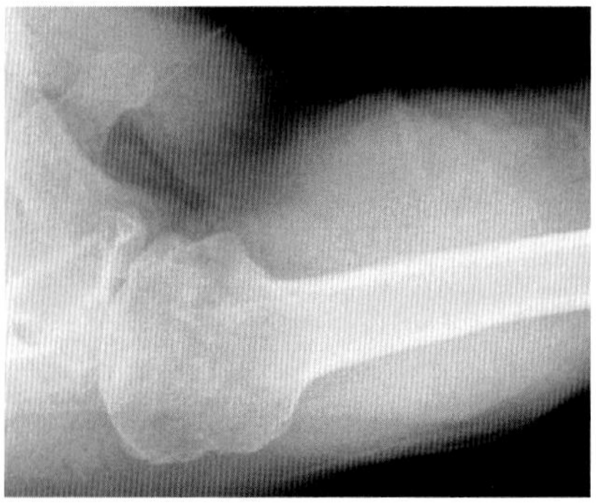

Figure 1 The axillary radiographic view is helpful for evaluating posterior glenoid wear and subluxation.

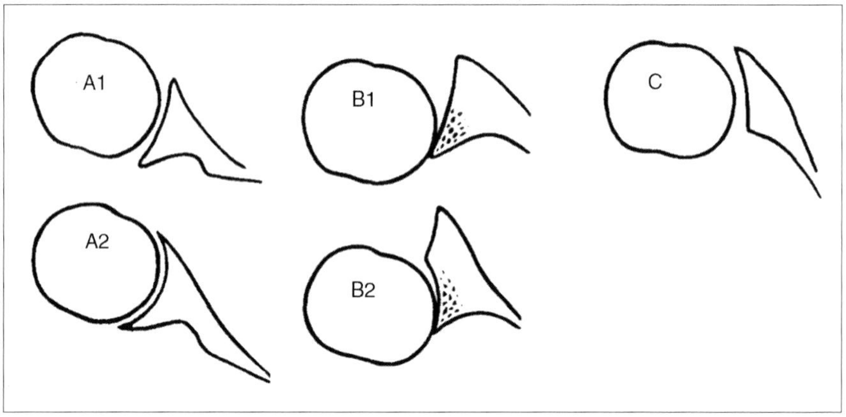

Figure 2 Illustration of the Walch classification system for glenoid morphology. Type A erosions are well centered. Type A1, minor erosion; type A2, deeper, central erosion. In type B erosions the head is subluxated posteriorly. Type B1, posterior wear; Type B2, severe biconcave wear; type C, glenoid retroversion of more than 25° (dysplastic in origin).

determining whether the articulation is concentric and posterior glenoid bone wear is evident. The axillary view is most useful in making these assessments (**Figure 1**). This chapter's authors emphasize the use of the Walch classification system, which is helpful in guiding surgical decision making[9] (**Figure 2**). Determining the Walsh grade may dictate which implants and surgical techniques are used at the time of surgery.

Standard or three-dimensional CT can be helpful for assessing glenoid version and quantifying bone loss in complex reconstructions (**Figure 3**). Scalise et al[10] reported that three-dimensional CT imaging can affect the interpretation of glenoid morphology, judgment regarding the fit of the prosthetic glenoid implant, and selection of the surgical technique related to glenoid preparation. Some surgeons routinely use CT.

MRI is helpful when the integrity of the rotator cuff is questionable. Al-

Table 1 (Continued)
Summary of Literature Reporting Proximal Humerus Fractures Treated With Reverse Total Shoulder Arthroplasty

Mean Active External Rotation	Mean Pain Score	Complications	Mean Outcome Scores
9°	VAS, 1.7	1 intraoperative glenoid fracture, scapular notching and heterotopic ossification noted for the entire group, but not specifically for the fracture sequelae group	Constant-Murley, 61
NA	Constant-Murley, 12	11% dislocation rate, 3% infections with *Acinetobacter*, 19 scapular notchings, 1 aseptic loosening of base plate	Constant-Murley, 55
8° (neutral) 30° (abducted)	Constant-Murley, 12.5	1 glenoid fracture, 5 neurologic complications, 1 acromial stress fracture, 3 reflex sympathetic dystrophy, 1 dislocation, deltoid dehiscence, 14 tuberosity nonunions, 5 tuberosity malunions, 5 scapular notchings, heterotopic ossification in 36 shoulders	Constant-Murley, 44; DASH, 44
9°	Constant-Murley, 13	1 deep infection, 1 superficial infection, 1 reflex sympathetic dystrophy	Constant-Murley, 53
25°	NA	Recurrent dislocation in 1 patient, 2 infections	Constant-Murley, 68; ASES, 68
27°	VAS, 1.0 ASES, 0.6	1 patient with complex regional pain syndrome, deep venous thrombosis, and tuberosity resorption; 1 patient with tuberosity malunion; 1 patient with grade 1 scapular notching	ASES, 78

NA = not available, VAS = Visual Analog Scale, ASES = American Shoulder and Elbow Sugeons, DASH = Disabilities of the Arm, Shoulder and Hand.

though the incidence of concomitant rotator cuff tears in primary OA is low, it is common in patients with rheumatoid arthritis (RA); therefore, MRI may be especially helpful in these patients. Attention should be paid to the integrity and quality of the supraspinatus, infraspinatus, and subscapularis muscles and tendons. Because outcomes of TSA are negatively affected by subscapularis insufficiency, preoperative evaluation of this tissue may be important.

Common Indications for TSA

The most common pathologies treated with TSA are OA, RA, posttraumatic arthritis, osteonecrosis, and capsulorrhaphy arthropathy. Understanding the underlying diagnosis is important in achieving a good outcome in shoulder arthroplasty. Choosing the right candidate for TSA requires the correct diagnosis and respect for the functional demands and goals of the patient.

TSA is indicated in most patients with OA if nonsurgical treatment is unsuccessful, although hemiarthroplasty can be considered in younger patients with a concentric glenohumeral joint and little glenoid erosion. TSA is indicated in patients with RA if the rotator cuff is intact. Posttraumatic arthritis and osteonecrosis with glenoid involvement are less common indications for TSA.

Common Indications for Hemiarthroplasty

Patients with acute four-part, three-part, or head-split fractures may be candidates for hemiarthroplasty. In recent years, reverse total shoulder arthroplasty (RTSA) has been popularized as a treatment for three- and four-part fractures in patients older than 65 years. Although there is controversy on this topic, several studies support the use of RTSA in patients older than 70 years with lower functional demands, those with severe tuberosity and metaphyseal comminution and a high likelihood of tuberosity nonunion or malunion, patients with severe osteoporosis or comorbidities that limit tuberosity healing, and those with irreparable rotator cuff tears.[11-17] (**Table 1**).

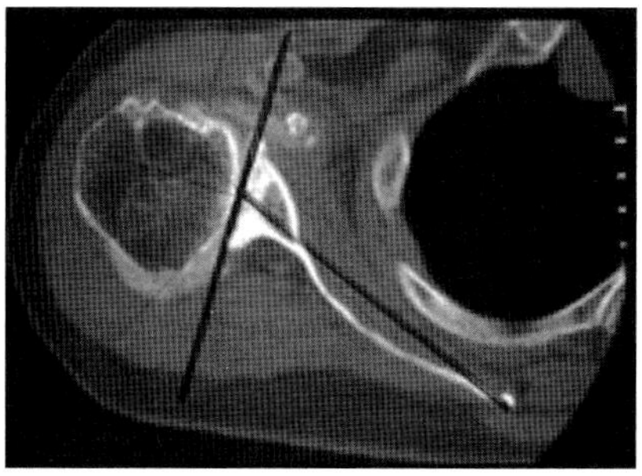

Figure 3 CT may be helpful for evaluating glenoid morphology, particularly when determining version and bone stock within the glenoid vault. Two lines are drawn, one in the scapular plane and the other along the face of the glenoid to subtend an angle that determines the glenoid version. In this figure, the glenoid has approximately 22° of retroversion.

Stage 3 or 4 (head collapse) osteonecrosis without glenoid involvement is also an acceptable indication

Table 2
Studies Comparing Outcomes of Hemiarthroplasty and Total Shoulder Arthroplasty for Osteoarthritis

Authors	No. of Patients	Mean Age (Years)	Follow-up	Revisions	Results
Radnay et al[20] (systematic review)	1,952 (23 studies)	66	43.4 months	TSA: 6.5% 1.7% polyethylene glenoids revised HHR: 10.2% revised to TSA	TSA: Improved: pain relief ($P < 0.0001$) forward elevation ($P < 0.0001$) gains in forward elevation ($P < 0.0001$), gain in external rotation ($P < 0.0001$) patient satisfaction ($P < 0.0001$)
Bryant et al[21] (systematic review; 4 RCTs)	112 HHR = 50 TSA = 62	68	Minimum 2 years	HHR: 10 (20%) revised to TSA	TSA: Improved UCLA function score ($P < 0.0001$) Improved pain relief ($P < 0.0001$) Forward elevation ($P < 0.008$)
Edwards et al[22]	790 HHR = 89 TSA = 601	HHR: 66 TSA: 67	43.3 months	68 TSA: 25 glenoid revisions HHR: 7 revised because of pain related to glenoid wear	HHR: 86% good/excellent results TSA: 94% good/excellent results
Gartsman et al[23]	47 HHR = 22 TSA = 25	65	35 months	HHR: 3 revised to TSA	TSA: superior pain relief and internal rotation; equivocal satisfaction and function Five of 6 poor outcomes from hemiarthroplasty group, 3 converted to TSA and subsequently satisfied

HHR = humeral head replacement, TSA = total shoulder arthroplasty, UCLA = University of California Los Angeles.

for hemiarthroplasty.[18] In a small subset of patients with cuff tear arthropathy (CTA), standard hemiarthroplasty or CTA hemiarthroplasty may be indicated. CTA in a patient with poor shoulder motion and function is best treated with RTSA; however, in a patient older that 65 years with good motion, a centered humeral head, and low functional demands, cuff tear hemiarthroplasty may be an acceptable treatment.[19] Patients with RA with rotator cuff insufficiency and inadequate glenoid bone stock may be better treated with CTA hemiarthroplasty rather than RTSA.

Hemiarthroplasty Versus TSA in Patients With OA

Several studies have shown that TSA with glenoid resurfacing results in less pain, a better fulcrum for active motion, and better strength than hemiarthroplasty[20-23] (**Table 2**). The American Academy of Orthopaedic Surgeon's clinical practice guideline recommends shoulder arthroplasty instead of hemiarthroplasty for the treatment of glenohumeral arthritis. The strength of the recommendation is moderate.[24]

OA in Young, Active Patients

OA in a young patient or a patient who works as a manual laborer presents a challenge to shoulder surgeons based on predicted activity levels and associated concerns about prosthesis durability. Management of these patients is controversial. Surgical options include hemiarthroplasty or TSA. Shoulder fusion was once the standard treatment method but is now rarely performed. Arthroscopic capsular release is a surgical option in early stages of OA with a stiff shoulder. The literature on this topic is limited and is beyond the scope of this chapter.

In response (perhaps) to increased patient expectations, the indications for shoulder arthroplasty have been expanded to include younger, more active patients. Hemiarthroplasty has led to good results in patients with concentric glenoid wear, but it is important to limit the use of hemiarthroplasty to patients with a concentric glenohumeral joint.[25] When used in young patients, hemiarthroplasty frequently requires revision surgery to treat persistent glenoid erosion and pain. The results of converting hemiarthroplasty to TSA are not as good as

Table 3
Studies Comparing Hemiarthroplasty and Total Shoulder Arthroplasty in Patients Older Than 55 Years

Study	No. of Patients	Follow-up	TSA Survivorship	Hemiarthroplasty Survivorship	Outcomes
Bartelt et al[31]	66	7 years	5 years: 100% 10 years: 92%	5 years: 85% 10 years: 72%	Hemiarthroplasty: 60% unsatisfactory results TSA: better pain relief, active elevation, patient satisfaction; 48% unsatisfactory results
Sperling et al[29]	114	Minimum 15 years	5 years: 97% 10 years: 97% 20 years: 84%	5 years: 91% 10 years 82% 20 years 75%	Hemiarthroplasty: Unsatisfactory results increased from 47% to 60% after 5 years TSA: unsatisfactory results remained little changed after 5 years (49% to 50%)

TSA = total shoulder arthroplasty.

those of primary TSA.[26,27] Even though TSA has historically been contraindicated in young patients because of concerns about accelerated glenoid wear, loosening, and subsequent failure, several studies of patients younger than 50 years have shown equivalent or sometimes better implant survival rates than those achieved with hemiarthroplasty.[28-30] Outcomes of the two procedures in patients 55 years or younger are summarized in **Table 3**.[29,31] Sperling et al[29] reported that, after a minimum 15-year follow-up, 60% of young patients treated with hemiarthroplasty and 48% treated with TSA had unsatisfactory results based on a modified Neer rating system. Although neither procedure achieved encouraging results in young patients, TSA appears to be the better treatment.

Radnay et al[20] compared the revision rate in TSA related to glenoid loosening with the rate of hemiarthroplasty revision for glenoid wear and found the rates to be 1.7% and 8.1%, respectively. Carroll et al[26] and Sperling and Cofield[27] demonstrated poorer outcomes when converting a hemiarthroplasty to TSA compared with primary TSA. In contrast, revision TSA for glenoid implant-related problems seems to improve function, patient satisfaction, and pain.[32] Glenoid component loosening or wear can be treated with component removal (arthroscopic or open) or open reimplantation. The results of excision and reimplantation are both favorable, but reimplantation seems to be better.[32-35] The decision to either remove or reimplant a glenoid component is primarily dictated by the amount of glenoid bone stock.

Dissatisfaction with both hemiarthroplasty and TSA, given their respective disadvantages in younger patients, has led to the development of glenoid biologic resurfacing arthroplasty.[36-38] This technique typically involves the implantation of a porous-coated, cementless, humeral head replacement along with biologic resurfacing of the glenoid.[36-39] Thus far, the published results have been mixed, if not poor. Surface replacement is another alternative for the treatment of OA. This technique has gained popularity despite limited data supporting its use.[40]

Common Pathologies: Surgical Implications and Outcomes

Rheumatoid Arthritis

Multiple studies have reported a relatively high rate of long-term complications in patients with RA.[41-47] The complications include component-related problems (radiographic lucency around the glenoid component and loosening of glenoid and humeral components), rotator cuff failure with proximal humeral migration, increased susceptibility to infection, an increased rate of periprosthetic humeral fracture, and delayed healing.[41-52] Despite these reports of complications, published midterm and long-term revision rates in patients with RA are less than 5%.[41,53] Interestingly, this rate is lower than published revision rates for patients without RA.[54-57]

The most important technical considerations in treating patients with RA are central glenoid erosion (in contrast to the posterior wear patterns in OA) and rotator cuff disease. Excessive medial wear may preclude glenoid component implantation and be an indication for either bone grafting or hemiarthroplasty rather than TSA or RTSA.[58,59] Patients with RA are more likely to have concomitant rotator cuff deficiency and arthritis. In such cases, anatomic TSA is contraindicated, and RTSA may be more suitable. TSA has proven success in patients with RA with an intact rotator cuff, and it has been shown to be more successful than hemiarthroplasty.[60] There are no direct comparisons to date between TSA and RTSA in patients with RA.

Cuff Tear Arthropathy

In patients with end-stage arthropathy, which can be characterized by anterior-superior escape of the humeral head, RTSA is the preferred procedure to maximize function and relieve pain. However, the role of CTA hemiarthroplasty in patients who have CTA but good motion is controversial. In a series of 60 shoulders with CTA managed with CTA hemiarthroplasty, motion, pain, and American Shoulder and Elbow Surgeon scores improved.[19] Based on published results, hemiarthroplasty with a CTA head may be considered in a young patient if the humeral head is contained by the coracoacromial arch. In a patient with a nonconcentric humeral head and anterosuperior instability, hemiarthroplasty is unlikely to restore motion and function; RTSA should be considered.[40]

Osteonecrosis

Symptomatic osteonecrosis is usually treated with TSA or hemiarthroplasty, depending on the extent of glenoid involvement. Multiple outcome studies[42,61-67] on osteonecrosis-related arthroplasty have reported excellent results, which are often superior to results in patients with other diagnoses, such as OA.

Posttraumatic Arthritis

The surgical management of posttraumatic arthritis is challenging, in part because of proximal humeral bone loss, malunion, nonunion, rotator cuff tendon and muscle loss, soft-tissue contractures and scarring, obliteration of tissue planes, heterotopic ossification, nerve injury, regional pain syndrome, failed prior surgeries, and a greater risk of complications. Management options include humeral head replacement, TSA, or glenohumeral arthrodesis. The results of hemiarthroplasty in this population are less satisfactory than when used to treat acute fractures or primary OA.[68-78] TSA for posttraumatic arthritis provides reliable pain relief but less reliable improvement in range of motion or function.[79] If rotator cuff insufficiency exists either in the form of an irreparable tear or tuberosity resorption, RTSA is the preferred treatment. The most common complication of the surgical treatment of posttraumatic arthritis is stiffness.[79] Instability, another common complication, was reported in 19% of the patients in one study.[72] Successful TSA requires extensive release of adhesions and the mobilization of soft-tissue planes. Aggressive postoperative rehabilitation is important in preventing the re-formation of adhesions. Nerves in the posttraumatic setting may be obscured or tethered by scar tissue, which increases the risk of nerve injury from retraction or dissection.

Dislocation Arthropathy/ Capsulorrhaphy Arthropathy

The development of OA is a recognized complication of shoulder instability surgery.[80-84] Arthroplasty in patients who had prior instability surgery may be challenging because of the young age of many patients and the presence of soft-tissue contractures and bone deficiencies.[85] Capsulorrhaphy arthropathy can result in internal rotation contracture and eccentric wear posteriorly.[86] Sperling et al[85] reported that hemiarthroplasty for capsulorrhaphy arthropathy in a relatively young population provides pain relief and improved motion but is associated with high rates of revision surgery and unsatisfactory results caused by instability and glenoid arthritis. Matsoukis et al,[87] in a multicenter series, showed no difference in outcomes of arthroplasty in patients previously treated surgically versus nonsurgically for shoulder instability. At an average follow-up of 16 years, Bigliani et al[88] reported good results with hemiarthroplasty and TSA to treat arthritis after instability surgery. Pain was relieved in 94% of patients, results were satisfactory in 77% of patients, and elevation improved an average of 37° and external rotation an average of 53°. Bauer et al[89] reported that 3 of 33 patients (10%) treated with TSA after instability surgery had subscapularis rupture, whereas such ruptures occur in approximately 3% of patients with primary OA treated with TSA (MA Frankel, MD, et al, Orlando, FL, unpublished data presented at the American Shoulder and Elbow Surgeons Third Biennial Meeting, 2002).

Shoulder arthroplasty for locked posterior dislocations is challenging because substantial alterations in the bony and soft-tissue anatomy can make balancing difficult. Inadequate anterior soft-tissue length and flexibility and posterior soft-tissue laxity after surgery may result in recurrent posterior instability. Instability usually manifests early in the postoperative period.[90] Arthroplasty in this subset of patients is associated with satisfactory pain relief and improvement in motion if anatomic distortions are corrected. Surgical techniques include lengthening the anterior capsule and/or the subscapularis, releasing the anterior-inferior capsule, decreasing humeral retroversion, inserting a glenoid component (TSA, if there is substantial glenoid wear), selecting a larger humeral head size for added stability, and tightening the posterior capsule.[90]

Surgical Techniques

Positioning

Successful patient positioning requires that the entire shoulder be placed at the edge of the operating table so that the arm can clear the table and be extended to expose the shaft. The head and neck should be securely stabilized (**Figure 4**).

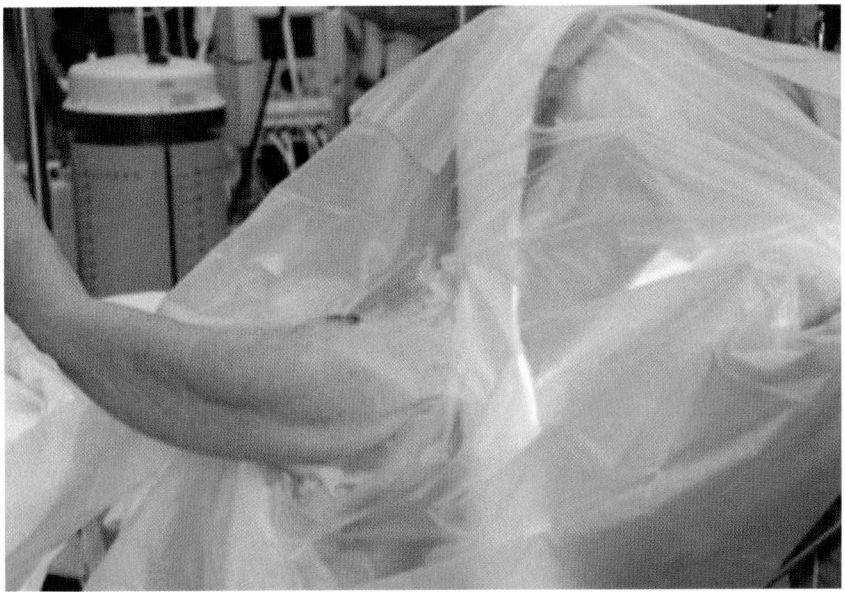

Figure 4 Effective patient positioning requires that the entire shoulder be placed at the edge of the operating table so that the arm can clear the table and be extended to expose the shaft. The head and neck should be securely stabilized.

Preparation

After prepping and draping the patient in the usual sterile fashion, an adhesive microbial drape can be applied for barrier protection. Sterile hoods help prevent shedding and protect the surgeon from debris. A first-generation cephalosporin, with the dosage based on the patient's weight, is given 30 minutes before the incision is made. The cephalosporin will not cover anaerobes, methicillin-resistant *Staphylococcus aureus*, or *Staphylococcus epidermidis*. *Propionibacterium* is a slow growing, aerotolerant, anaerobic, gram-positive rod that is part of normal skin flora and particularly thrives on the fatty acids in the sebaceous glands and sebum in hair follicles. This organism is susceptible to peroxide, chlorhexidine, tetracycline (a resistant strain is common), and clindamycin. Because of the incidence of *Propionibacterium* infections, both chlorhexidine antiseptic and clindamycin antibiotic may be beneficial; however, there is no clear evidence available to justify their use. Another simple measure of decreasing infection risk may include decreasing traffic in the operating room.[91]

Incision

An extended deltopectoral approach directed in line with the coracoid toward the deltoid insertion is the most commonly used approach. The cephalic vein is usually identified and should be preserved, especially in patients with any preexisting venous compromise. However, ligation of the vein does not seem to have major consequences. If the cephalic vein is taken medially, injury from retractors will be minimized. When using the routine deltopectoral approach, the vein may be taken laterally to preserve the deltoid branches. Releasing the upper border of the pectoralis major insertion may help gain exposure. Careful, gentle palpation of the axillary nerve helps the surgeon maintain awareness of its proximity throughout the procedure. Gentle tugging on the lateral deltoid will create some tension in the nerve and may help identify its location. The axillary nerve courses anterior to the subscapularis, then under and around the inferior capsule (on average 3.2 mm inferior to the inferior capsule).[92-94]

Humeral Exposure

For less experienced surgeons, glenoid exposure is often the most challenging aspect of the procedure, but it is the humeral exposure and preparation that allows for good glenoid exposure. The subscapularis is released first. The three most common methods of releasing the subscapularis are tenotomy, tendon peel, and the lesser tuberosity osteotomy (**Figure 5**). Meticulous attention should be given to this step because subscapularis deficiency after shoulder arthroplasty often requires revision surgery and has a negative effect on long-term outcomes.[95]

Subscapularis

In a biomechanical study, Van Thiel et al[96] reported no difference in the initial strength of subscapularis fixation between three different types of fixation: tendon-to-bone, combined tendon-tendon/bone, and lesser tuberosity osteotomy. Giuseffi et al[97] reported more displacement through cyclical loading in osteotomy specimens compared with tenotomy specimens in a biomechanical study. In contrast, Ponce et al[98] showed that osteotomy repairs were stronger than transosseous sutures and tendon-to-tendon repairs and could also lead to good clinical results. Scalise et al[99] reviewed the clinical results of subscapularis tenotomy compared with lesser tuberosity osteotomy for TSA. This retrospective

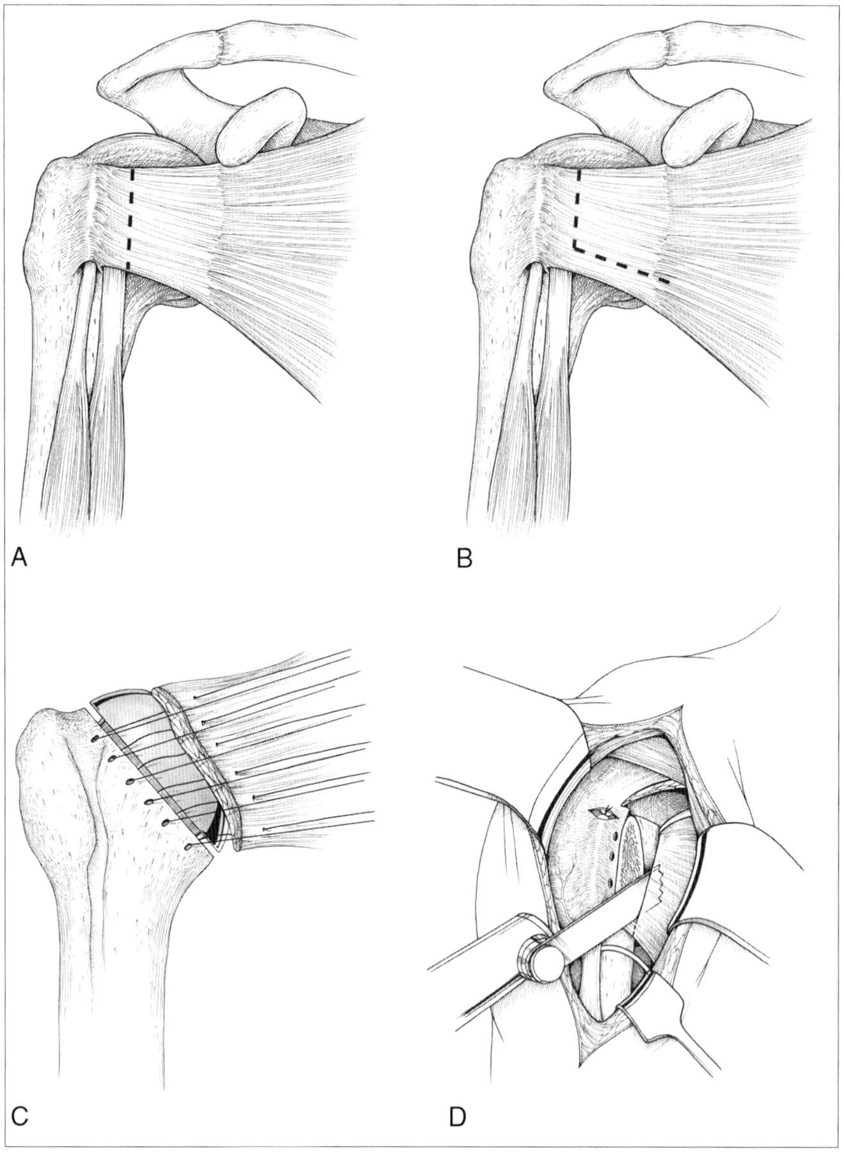

Figure 5 **A,** Illustration of complete subscapularis tenotomy. **B,** Subscapularis tenotomy with the inferior one third of the tendon preserved. **C,** Subscapularis peel with bone tunnels shown for repair. **D,** Lesser tuberosity osteotomy.

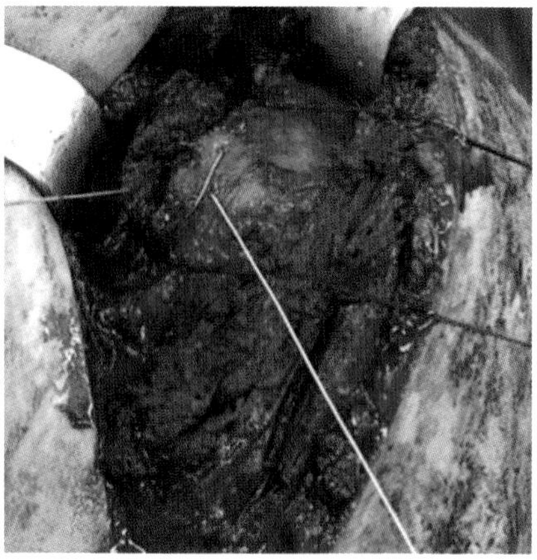

Figure 6 Intraoperative photograph of the suture repair technique that this chapter's senior author (RJH) uses to repair the subscapularis tendon. Note the dark tag sutures in the subscapularis being used to hold the tendon to its footprint and maintain tension as knots are tied. The white sutures are passed according to the Mason-Allen technique and used to repair the tendon.

review, which had a limited number of patients (34), demonstrated a higher rate of subscapularis tears and lower clinical outcome scores in the patients treated with tenotomy. Similarly, Jandhyala et al[100] compared the two techniques in a small series and reported that patients treated with osteotomy had better functional outcomes based on graded belly-press tests.

The perceived advantages of tuberosity osteotomy are potential bone-to-bone healing and its safety and effectiveness in patients with a prior subscapularis-splitting stabilization procedure. Disadvantages of the tuberosity osteotomy are the time requirements, technical difficulty, obstruction of the surgical field by the bone fragment, and difficulties achieving good fixation. There are a variety of osteotomy repair techniques. Heckman et al[101] compared the backpack and the dual-row techniques. The dual-row technique appeared biomechanically stronger, with less displacement and greater ultimate tensile strength.

There is no consensus on the optimal technique for treating the subscapularis; the choice depends on the preference of the treating surgeon. Subscapularis tenotomy and repair using the Mason-Allen suture technique is the preferred technique of this chapter's senior author (RJH) (**Figure 6**).

Subscapularis rupture is a worrisome complication and the most common cause of anterior instability after TSA.[102,103] The rates of subscapularis weakness diagnosed by the belly-press test after TSA have been reported to be as high as 67%, and the rates of subscapularis deficiency, diagnosed by ultrasound, as high as 30% to 46%.[104-106] However, current studies show that ultrasound and physical examination findings do not correlate well in the diagnosis of subscapularis failure. Risk factors associated with

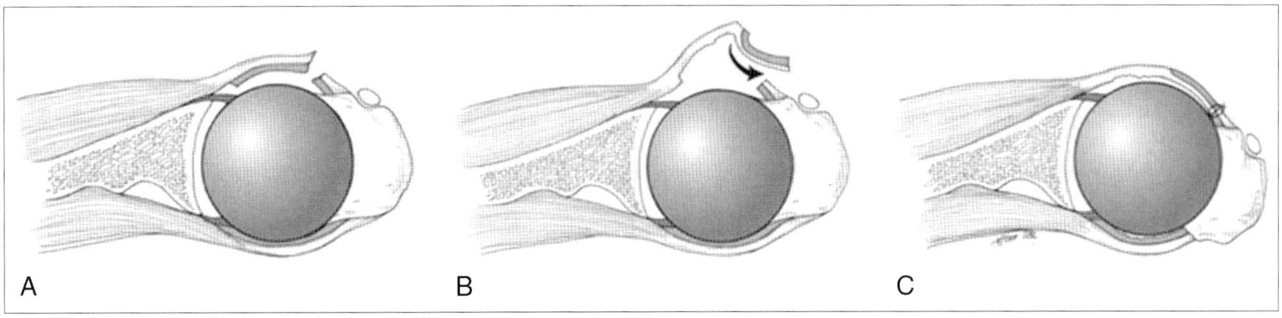

Figure 7 Illustration of Z-plasty lengthening of the subscapularis. **A,** Subscapularis tenotomy extending through the anterior glenohumeral joint capsule. **B,** Parts of the subscapularis tendon and the glenohumeral joint capsule have been dissected, leaving the lateral edge intact (Z-plasty technique). **C,** Soft-tissue repair.

subscapularis rupture include previous surgical insults and lengthening procedures.[95] Surgical treatment is usually required for subscapularis ruptures that cause symptoms or instability. Revision repair or reconstruction seems to be more successful when performed early.[107] The first step in a salvage situation usually involves a pectoralis transfer. Augmentation may be necessary; hamstring autograft or allograft and Achilles allograft are common graft choices. If supraspinatus and/or infraspinatus tears accompany a subscapularis tear, conversion to RTSA may be the best option.

Subscapularis Release

After release of the subscapularis from its insertion, either by tenotomy, peel, or osteotomy, further releases are necessary. The purpose of further releases is to gain length and excursion to maximize external rotation. Subscapularis releases may provide only 1 to 1.5 cm of additional length.[108,109] On average, 1 cm of additional length translates to approximately 20° of increased external rotation.[110,111]

A complete 360° release of the muscle-tendon unit entails anterior interval release to the base of the coracoid, inferior border release (known as the inferior slide), Bankart release, and a subcoracoid release. These releases alone may not provide enough length when there is substantial internal rotation contracture. The need for more extensive releases may be predicted preoperatively with the physical examination (external rotation ≤ -20°). Coronal Z-plasty is one type of lengthening procedure that may be useful in such situations (**Figure** 7). The disadvantage to the Z-plasty is that it weakens the anterior soft-tissue construct while relying on an often tenuous end-to-end repair. To avoid an end-to-end repair, Nicholson et al[112] described a technique that effectively lengthens the capsulotendinous complex while creating perhaps a more reliable overlapping slide-type repair (**Figure 8**). Using this technique, external rotation increased from -2° preoperatively to 46° postoperatively.

Capsule

The safest approach to the capsule is to perform all releases around the humerus and glenoid subperiosteally. A capsulectomy may be necessary to obtain adequate external rotation. The disadvantage of capsulectomy is that it weakens the anterior repair. If external rotation is dramatically limited (≤ -20° external rotation), a lengthening procedure can be considered.

Exposure

Proper exposure is of paramount importance in shoulder arthroplasty and requires the proper retractors, including glenoid neck and humeral retractors (**Figure 9**). Surgeons vary as to which retractors they use and where the retractors are placed. Anterior glenoid retractors are usually placed along the anterior neck of the glenoid, and posterior glenoid retractors, Fukuda retractors, or Hohmann retractors are usually placed along the posterior glenoid neck.

Humeral Head Cut

The first step in making the proper humeral head cut is to identify and remove the osteophyte shelf surrounding the native head. Some surgeons choose to do this step after the humeral head osteotomy. Osteophyte removal allows accurate determination of the native humeral head size and version. Failure to remove osteophytes may lead to oversizing of the humeral head implant. Some surgeons use guides (**Figure 10**) designed to orient the humeral cut, whereas others base the cut off the anatomic neck. Regardless of the surgeon's preference, the cut should be made at the anatomic neck, and care should be taken to avoid cutting the rotator cuff. Normally, the humeral implant should be retroverted 30°; however, when substantial posterior glenoid wear is present, as in a Walch type B2 glenoid, the humeral cut is made with less retroversion to avoid

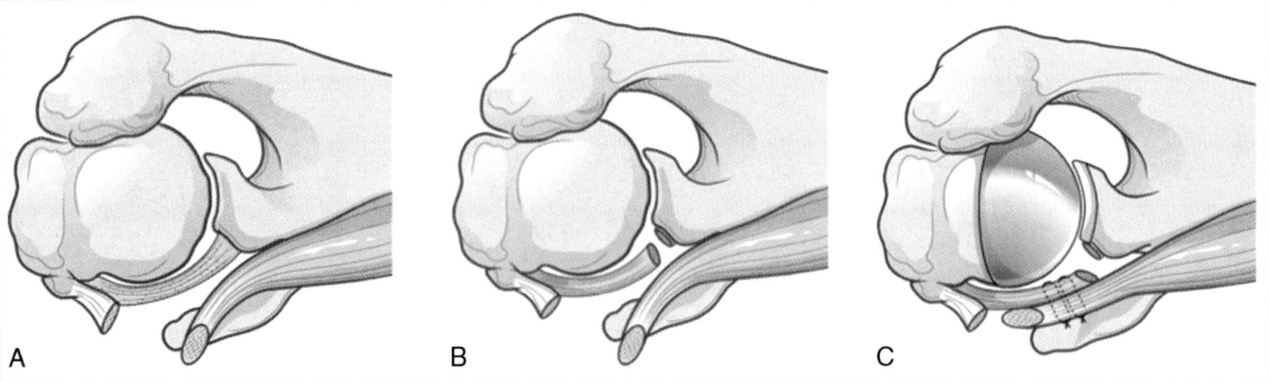

Figure 8 The subscapularis lengthening technique as described by Nicholson et al.[112] Note the use of an overlapping slide-type repair as opposed to end-to-end repair. **A,** Superior view. The subscapularis tendon is incised approximately 5 to 8 mm medial to the lesser tuberosity. The tendon is elevated off the underlying intact capsule and reflected medially. The muscle-tendon unit is elevated off the glenoid rim to provide access to the capsule medially. **B,** The capsule (blue) is incised off the glenoid as far medially as possible. The capsule is released from the glenoid to form a rectangular-shaped, laterally based flap. This flap is composed of the subscapularis tendon insertion and the anterior capsule. **C,** After shoulder arthroplasty, the shoulder is rotated to 30° of external rotation. The subscapularis tendon (anterior flap) is repaired with vertical mattress sutures to the underlying capsule (posterior flap) under light tension. There is excellent surface area available for repair and healing. This demonstrates the sliding overlap of the flaps to gain length and is not an end-to-end repair.

posterior instability or eccentric loading of the glenohumeral articulation.

Glenoid Preparation

Glenoid exposure can be the most difficult step in TSA. Adequate capsular release from the humerus and the humeral osteotomy are the first steps in obtaining good exposure. Next, the labrum is removed; this allows full appreciation of the glenoid borders and determination of the presence of any osteophytes. If glenoid osteophytes are present, they should be removed to appreciate the true glenoid borders and avoid oversizing or eccentric placement of the prosthesis. Posterior capsular releases may be detrimental in patients with advanced OA because of the risk of creating posterior instability. Long-standing internal rotation contractures and posterior wear predispose the shoulder to posterior instability; release of the capsule may place the shoulder at further risk. The glenoid prosthetic component is normally placed in the center of the glenoid. To accurately place a centering hole, crosshairs are drawn on the glenoid face, with a centered vertical line and an intersecting, centered horizontal line.

Normal glenoid version ranges from 2° anteversion to 9° retroversion, but changes in version occur in pathologic conditions such as OA.[113-116] Several studies have reported increased retroversion in OA by as much as 9° to 13°.[114,117] Shapiro et al[118] showed that uncorrected glenoid retroversion leads to eccentric loading and increases the likelihood of implant wear and loosening. To correct excessive retroversion, the high side of the glenoid can be taken down with eccentric reaming. The reaming process can continue to the level of punctate subchondral bone but no further. Although eccentric reaming is a useful technique, there are limits to how much version can be corrected. In a cadaver analysis, Gillespie et al[119] showed that 10° of anterior correction leads to substantial decreases in glenoid width (normal range, approximately 23 mm in the cephalad portion to 29 mm in the caudad portion).[120] Fifteen degrees of anterior correction resulted in an inability to seat the glenoid in 50% of specimens because of inadequate bone stock, and 20° of anterior correction resulted in an inability to seat the glenoid in 75% of specimens. The authors recommended limiting anterior correction to 10°. If more correction is necessary, bone grafting or augmentation should be considered (**Figure 11**). Bone graft can be easily taken from the resected humeral head.

Glenoid Implant

The three general variations in glenoid implant designs are cemented versus uncemented, pegged versus keeled, and flat versus a curved backside contour. Several studies show that pegged implants have improved seating, fixation, and radiographic appearance compared with keeled implants.[121-123] Seating, stability, and radiolucency scores appear to be better in curved-back as opposed to flatback implants.[124,125] It is theorized that gle-

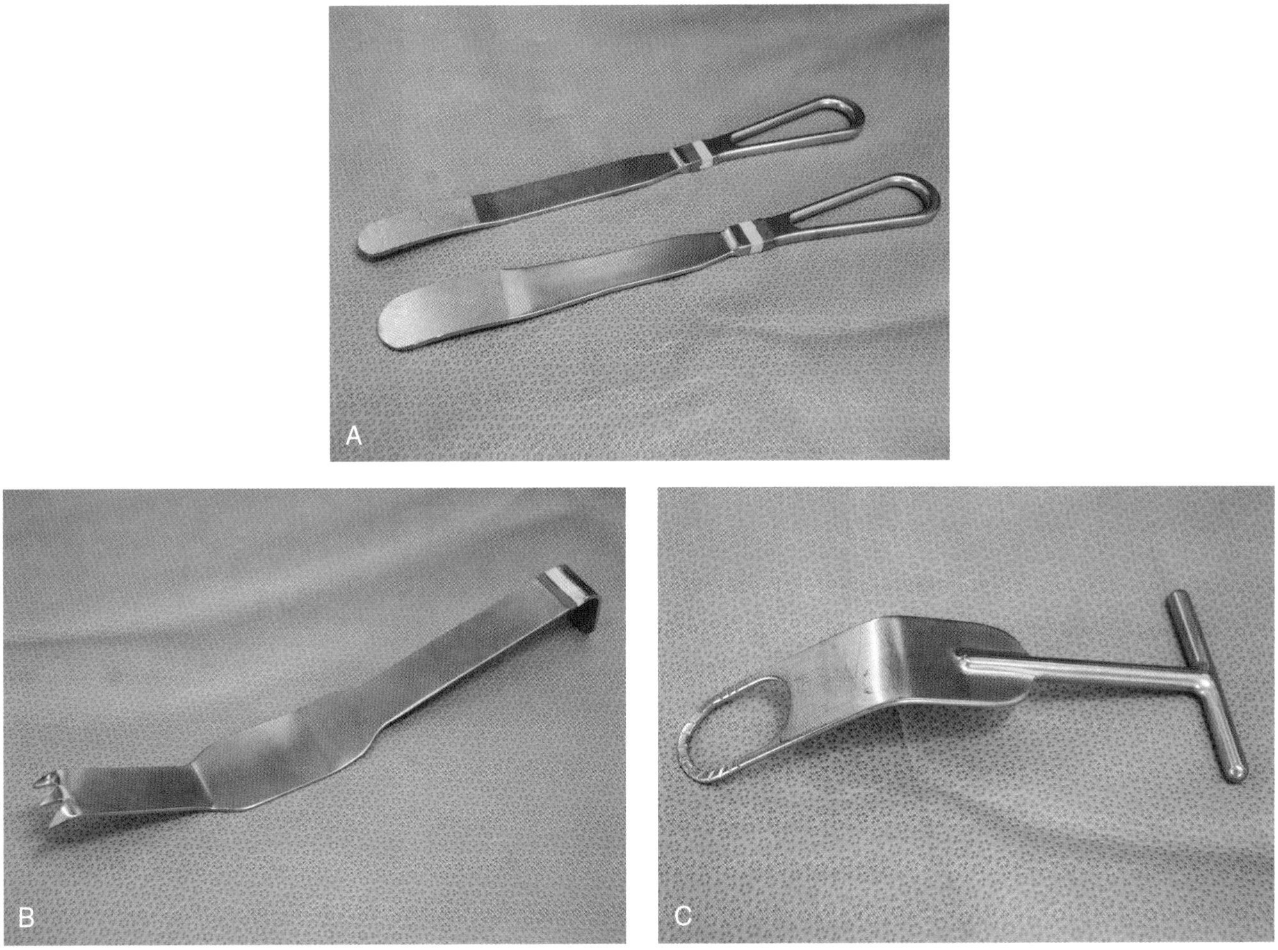

Figure 9 **A,** Darrach-type retractors. **B,** Anterior glenoid neck retractor. **C,** Fukuda-type retractor.

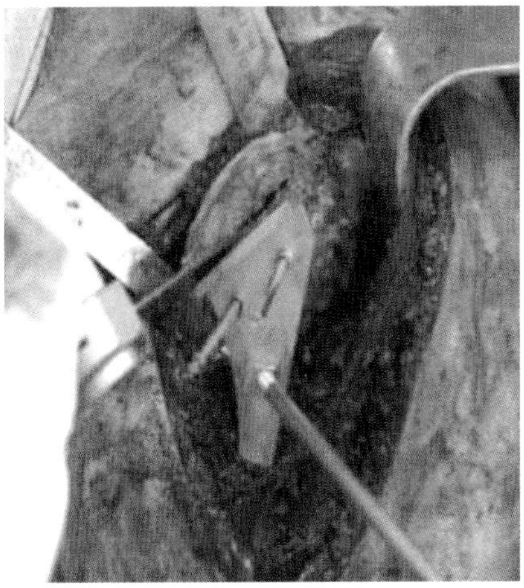

Figure 10 Intraoperative view showing a humeral cutting guide.

noid implants with a curved backside preserve more bone during implantation and are exposed to less shear stresses. The designs with a curved back convert shear stresses to compressive stresses; this accounts for their improved stability. Iannotti et al[126] used finite element analysis to show that glenoid implants with curved backs are more resistant to failure from malpositioning than flatback designs.

Controversy also exists regarding cemented versus uncemented (metal-backed) implant designs. The gold standard is the cemented, all-polyethylene implant; however, the rate of periprosthetic radiolucent line formation is a concern.[127,128] Early results of uncemented, metal-backed glenoid components is also concerning. More recent results involving more current, uncemented, metal-backed implant designs using softer metal have been more favorable.[129,130]

Cementing Techniques

Despite variability in cementing techniques, some fundamental principles apply. Creating a uniform cement mantle is of foremost importance. Based on finite element analysis, the ideal thickness must be at least 1.0 mm.[131] Nyffeler et al[132] assessed the effect of cement mantle thickness, implant surface finish (smooth versus rough), and peg design (cylindrical versus notched versus threaded pegs). Threaded pegs had a substantially higher pullout strength compared with notched pegs, and notched pegs had

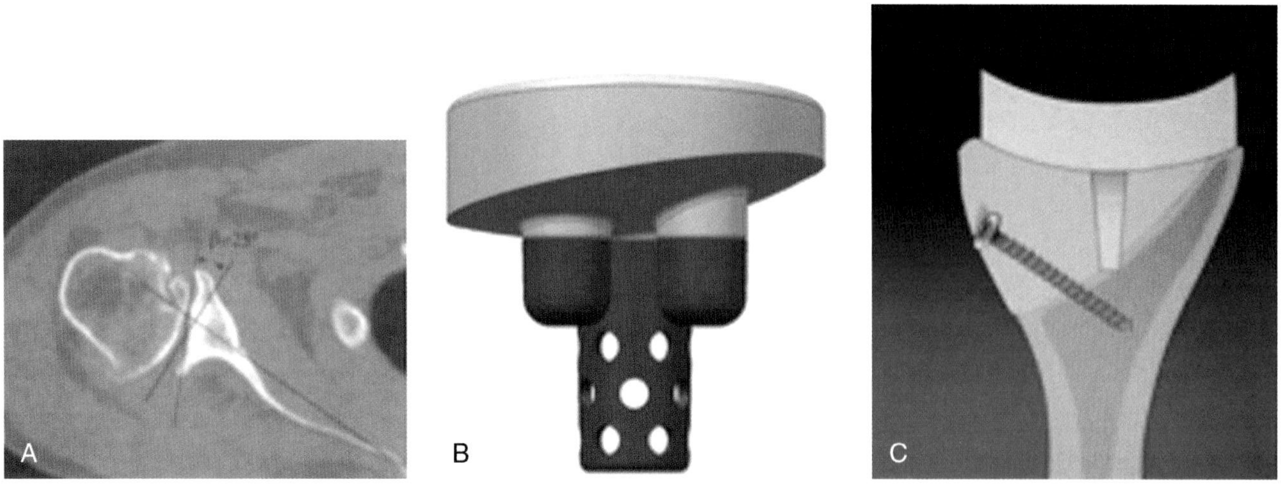

Figure 11 **A,** CT scan showing Walch type B2 glenoid morphology. **B,** Augmented glenoid component. **C,** Bone graft technique used in cases of severe posterior bone loss.

higher pullout strength than cylindrical pegs. Increasing the cement mantle thickness increased resistance to pullout for all peg types. A rougher surface resulted in higher pullout strength for the notched and cylindrical pegs. Anglin et al[125] reported improved resistance to loosening with rough-back glenoid components compared with components with smooth backs. Although the cement mantle thickness is important to glenoid component stability, excess cement causes thermal-induced bone necrosis, and this may contribute to glenoid loosening.[133] By using cement pressurization techniques, Boileau et al[127] and Klepps et al[134] reported a substantial reduction in radiolucencies. Nyffeler et al[135] reported better fixation and better cement mantle formation around pegs when a syringe instead of finger pressure was used to apply cement into peg holes. The authors also found better fixation when cement was applied to the backside of the glenoid component in combination with the peg holes rather than only filling the peg holes.

Radial Mismatch

Without some degree of radial mismatch between the glenoid and the humeral components, the glenohumeral articulation becomes constrained and is subject to loosening. Karduna et al[136] found that a mismatch of 4 mm best simulated the normal glenohumeral kinematics, and Walch et al[137] reported that 6 to 7 mm radial mismatch maximizes clinical results while minimizing the incidence of radiolucent lines around the glenoid. Commercial designs generally account for an appropriate amount of radial mismatch in their sizing options.

Glenoid Malpositioning

A glenoid placed in a central position has the lowest potential for mechanical failure. Placement of the glenoid in a superiorly or an inferiorly inclined position has the highest probability of failure. A retroverted glenoid position has a higher likelihood of loosening compared with an anteverted position.[138] Retroversion causes posterior displacement of contact points during rotational motion, which leads to increased micromotion and stress at the bone-cement interface.[118,139] Yian et el[140] correlated glenoid retroversion with clinical outcomes in 47 shoulders and reported that increased retroversion correlated with significantly lower Constant scores. Glenoid retroversion of more than 10° is probably unacceptable.[139] If the version cannot be improved beyond 10° retroversion, then it is probably better not to implant a glenoid component or to use an augmented component.

Humeral Component Preparation

Currently, more than 90% of implanted humeral components are press-fit components. The key to success with this type of device is metaphyseal security, although line-to-line broaching may also be considered. Cement should be reserved for poor fitting implants or thin and/or delicate cortices. For added stability and a better immediate fit, autograft bone taken from the humeral head can be used to fill metaphyseal bone defects and/or for compaction bone grafting.

The humeral head component should match the footprint of the metaphyseal humeral cut. Severe shoulder OA may require a large head with increased offset to confer stability to the construct. Modular systems make adjustments easier. The disadvantage of increasing the head size is that subscapularis closure is more difficult.

After the trial components are in place, assessing version and sizing is somewhat subjective. By convention, a good fit is indicated by a humeral head that can be manually translated posteriorly by 50% and easily reduces when released. The same test can be done for inferior translation. It is also important to internally rotate the arm to the abdomen to make sure no posterior subluxation occurs. Internal rotation also can be tested with the arm in abduction; 40° of internal rotation can be considered acceptable, although there is no absolute established number. To test external rotation, the subscapularis is reduced to its footprint, and the arm is then externally rotated to determine the point at which the eventual repair site may come under tension. Assessing humeral head height is usually easy because the greater tuberosity is intact; the implant should be at the same height or slightly above it. Alternatively, the pectoralis major tendon can be used to determine the correct humeral head height. Murachovsky et al[141] reported that the humeral head averages 5.6 ± 0.5 cm from the upper border of the pectoralis tendon.

As described previously, alterations in the posterior capsule resulting from long-standing OA can be problematic. As a preventive measure, posterior capsular release should be avoided because it can exacerbate preexisting capsular insufficiency and increase the risk of posterior subluxation or instability (**Figure 12**). Posterior instability that persists even after appropriate adjustments in sizing and version may make it necessary for the surgeon to redress the posterior capsule. In rare instances, posterior capsular plication may be used to correct persistent posterior instability.

One of the final steps in TSA is to reevaluate the safe range of external rotation after the subscapularis has been repaired, specifically noting the point at which the repair is under tension. The postoperative range of motion should be restricted to no more than 10° to 20° minus the maximum external rotation allowable in the operating room (until the subscapularis repair heals). In patients at high risk for posterior instability, further protective measures may be necessary, including postoperative bracing in external rotation and/or delaying physical therapy.

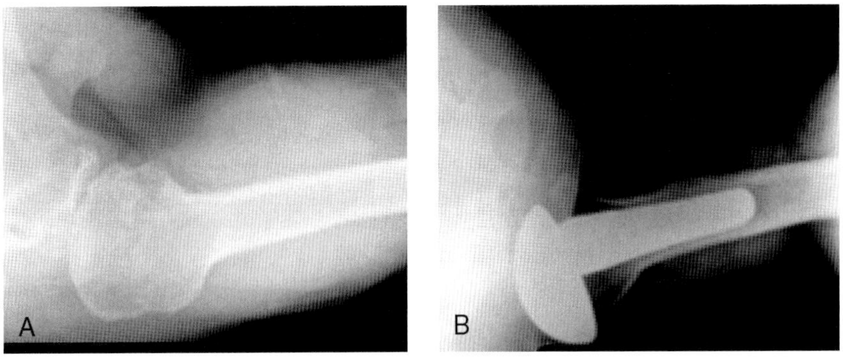

Figure 12 **A,** Preoperative radiograph of Walch type B2 glenoid morphology with posterior subluxation. This radiograph shows posterior capsular attenuation, which is a risk factor for posterior subluxation. **B,** Radiograph showing subsequent posterior instability following TSA, possibly caused by excess humeral retroversion, glenoid retroversion, or posterior capsular release.

DVD **Video 10.1:** Total Shoulder Arthroplasty: Steps to Get It Right. Richard J. Hawkins, MD (12 min)

Key Steps in Treatment

Figure 13 shows the steps that may help address many of the challenges associated with difficult cases of shoulder OA, such as Walch type B2 glenoid morphology. An overzealous approach to these steps could cause anterior instability. In the future, RTSA may be used for patients with Walch type B2 glenoid morphology.

Postoperative Rehabilitation

The postoperative rehabilitation protocol in patients treated with TSA may influence final function and motion. Most protocols adhere to a progression from gentle, passive mobilization to active motion and finally to strengthening. The primary concern during the early postoperative period is protecting the subscapularis. If the subscapularis repair is reliable, early mobilization within a safe range is acceptable. When there are concerns about the strength of the repair or when passive external rotation in the operating room is 20° or less, postoperative protection of the repair with immobilization or conservative limits on external rotation should be considered. Successful rehabilitation has been reported in heavily supervised programs and in home-based programs involving minimal supervision by a therapist.[142-147] Mulieri et al[148] reported better forward flexion, abduction, and physical component scores on the Medical Outcomes Study 36-Item Short Form in patients using a home therapy program compared with those participating in supervised therapy. Even with minimal external rotation obtained at the completion of surgery, eventual external rotation is

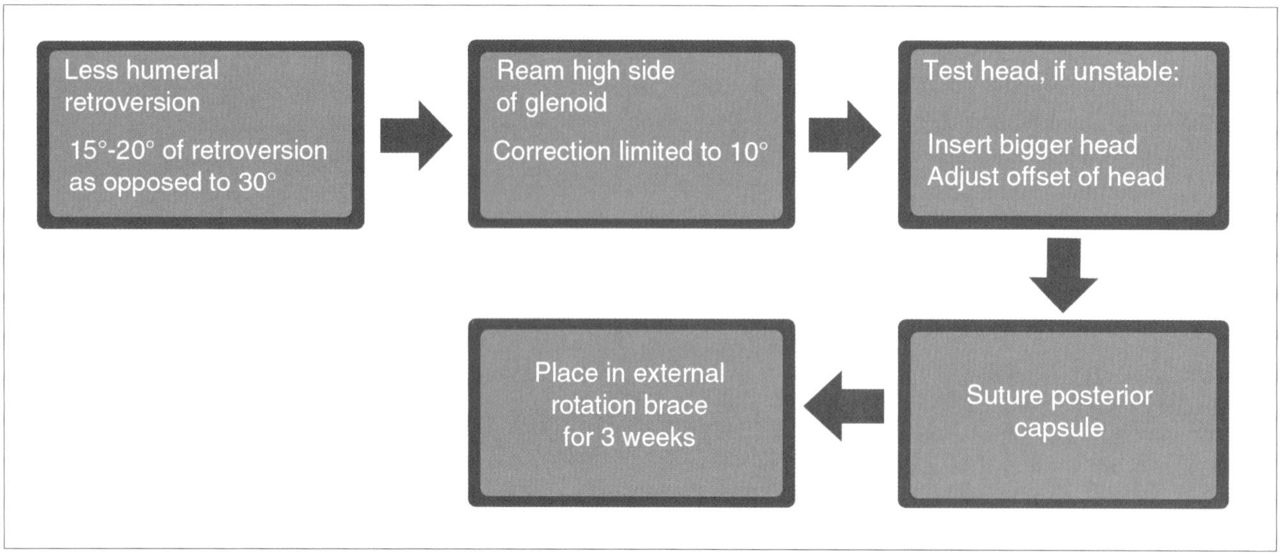

Figure 13 Key surgical steps in treating severe shoulder OA.

usually satisfactory with time and stretching.

Summary

Many complications of TSA can be avoided by the appropriate choice of indications, understanding the pathology, and preoperative preparation. The key surgical steps that may help avoid complications include proper positioning of the patient, adequate soft-tissue release for exposure and rebalancing, identifying the axillary nerve, correcting glenoid version, adjusting humeral component size and version as needed for stability, and meticulous subscapularis repair. Postoperatively, precautions may be necessary to protect soft-tissue repairs before progressing with physical therapy.

References

1. Chin PY, Sperling JW, Cofield RH, Schleck C: Complications of total shoulder arthroplasty: Are they fewer or different? *J Shoulder Elbow Surg* 2006;15(1):19-22.
2. Neer CS II: Replacement arthroplasty for glenohumeral osteoarthritis. *J Bone Joint Surg Am* 1974;56(1):1-13.
3. Boyd AD Jr, Thornhill TS: Surgical treatment of osteoarthritis of the shoulder. *Rheum Dis Clin North Am* 1988;14(3):591-611.
4. Cofield RH: Total shoulder arthroplasty with the Neer prosthesis. *J Bone Joint Surg Am* 1984;66(6):899-906.
5. Fenlin JM Jr, Ramsey ML, Allardyce TJ, Frieman BG: Modular total shoulder replacement: Design rationale, indications, and results. *Clin Orthop Relat Res* 1994;307:37-46.
6. Godeneche A, Boulahia A, Noel E, Boileau P, Walch G: Total shoulder arthroplasty in chronic inflammatory and degenerative disease. *Rev Rhum Engl Ed* 1999;66(11):560-570.
7. Hawkins RJ, Bell RH, Jallay B: Total shoulder arthroplasty. *Clin Orthop Relat Res* 1989;242:188-194.
8. Kempf JF, Walch G, Lacaze F: Results of shoulder arthroplasty in primary gleno-humeral osteoarthritis, in Walch G, Boileau P, eds: *Shoulder Arthroplasty*. New York, NY, Springer, 1999, pp 203-210.
9. Walch G, Badet R, Boulahia A, Khoury A: Morphologic study of the glenoid in primary glenohumeral osteoarthritis. *J Arthroplasty* 1999;14:756-760.
10. Scalise JJ, Codsi MJ, Bryan J, Brems JJ, Iannotti JP: The influence of three-dimensional computed tomography images of the shoulder in preoperative planning for total shoulder arthroplasty. *J Bone Joint Surg Am* 2008;90(11):2438-2445.
11. Voos JE, Dines JS, Dines DM: Arthroplasty for fractures of the proximal part of the humerus. *J Bone Joint Surg Am* 2010;92(6):1560-1567.
12. Boileau P, Tinsi L, Walch G, Kishnan SG: Tuberosity osteosynthesis and hemiarthroplasty for four-part fractures of the proximal humerus. *Tech Shoulder Elbow Surg* 2000;1:96-109.
13. Cazeneuve JF, Cristofari D: The reverse shoulder prosthesis in the treatment of fractures of the proximal humerus in the elderly. *J Bone Joint Surg Br* 2010;92:535-539.
14. Bufquin T, Hersan A, Hubert L, Massin P: Reverse shoulder arthroplasty for the treatment of

three- and four-part fractures of the proximal humerus in the elderly. *J Bone Joint Surg Br* 2007; 89:516-520.

15. Gallinet D, Clappaz P, Garbuio P, Tropet Y, Obert L: Three or four parts complex humerus fractures: Hemiarthroplasty versus reverse prosthesis. A comparative study of 40 cases. *Orthop Traumatol Surg Res* 2009;95(1):48-55.
16. Klein M, Juschka M, Hinkenjann B, Scherger B, Ostermann P: Treatment of comminuted fractures of the proximal humerus in elderly patients with the Delta III reverse shoulder prosthesis. *J Orthop Trauma* 2008;22:698-704.
17. Lenarz C, Shishani Y, McCrum C, Nowinski RJ, Edwards TB, Goebezie R: Is reverse shoulder arthroplasty appropriate for the treatment of fractures in the older patient? *Clin Orthop Relat Res* 2011;469:3324-3331.
18. Smith RG, Sperling JW, Cofield RH, Hattrup SJ, Schleck CD: Shoulder hemiarthroplasty for steroid-associated osteonecrosis. *J Shoulder Elbow Surg* 2008;17(5): 685-688.
19. Visotsky JL, Basamania C, Seebauer L, Rockwood CA, Jensen KL: Cuff tear arthropathy: Pathogenesis, classification, and algorithm for treatment. *J Bone Joint Surg Am* 2004;86(suppl 2):35-40.
20. Radnay CS, Setter KJ, Chambers L, Levine WN, Bigliani LU, Ahmad CS: Total shoulder replacement compared with humeral head replacement for the treatment of primary glenohumeral osteoarthritis: A systematic review. *J Shoulder Elbow Surg* 2007;16(4): 396-402.
21. Bryant D, Litchfield R, Sandow M, Gartsman GM, Guyatt G, Kirkley A: A comparison of pain, strength, range of motion, and functional outcomes after hemiarthroplasty and total shoulder arthroplasty in patients with osteoarthritis of the shoulder: A systematic review and meta-analysis. *J Bone Joint Surg Am* 2005;87(9):1947-1956.
22. Edwards TB, Kadakia NR, Boulahia A, et al: A comparison of hemiarthroplasty and total shoulder arthroplasty in the treatment of primary glenohumeral osteoarthritis: Results of a multicenter study. *J Shoulder Elbow Surg* 2003;12(3):207-213.
23. Gartsman GM, Roddey TS, Hammerman SM: Shoulder arthroplasty with or without resurfacing of the glenoid in patients who have osteoarthritis. *J Bone Joint Surg Am* 2000;82(1):26-34.
24. American Academy of Orthopaedic Surgeons: *Clinical Practice Guideline on the Treatment of Glenohumeral Joint Osteoarthritis.* Rosemont, IL, American Academy of Orthopaedic Surgeons. December 2009. http://www.aaos.org/research/guidelines/gloguideline.pdf.
25. Levine WN, Djurasovic M, Glasson JM, Pollock RG, Flatow EL, Bigliani LU: Hemiarthroplasty for glenohumeral osteoarthritis: Results correlated to degree of glenoid wear. *J Shoulder Elbow Surg* 1997;6(5):449-454.
26. Carroll RM, Izquierdo R, Vazquez M, Blaine TA, Levine WN, Bigliani LU: Conversion of painful hemiarthroplasty to total shoulder arthroplasty: Long-term results. *J Shoulder Elbow Surg* 2004;13(6): 599-603.
27. Sperling JW, Cofield RH: Revision total shoulder arthroplasty for the treatment of glenoid arthrosis. *J Bone Joint Surg Am* 1998;80(6):860-867.
28. Burroughs PL, Gearen PF, Petty WR, Wright TW: Shoulder arthroplasty in the young patient. *J Arthroplasty* 2003;18(6): 792-798.
29. Sperling JW, Cofield RH, Rowland CM: Minimum fifteen-year follow-up of Neer hemiarthroplasty and total shoulder arthroplasty in patients aged fifty years or younger. *J Shoulder Elbow Surg* 2004;13(6):604-613.
30. Sperling JW, Cofield RH, Rowland CM: Neer hemiarthroplasty and Neer total shoulder arthroplasty in patients fifty years old or less: Long-term results. *J Bone Joint Surg Am* 1998;80(4): 464-473.
31. Bartelt R, Sperling JW, Schleck CD, Cofield RH: Shoulder arthroplasty in patients aged fifty-five years or younger with osteoarthritis. *J Shoulder Elbow Surg* 2011;20(1):123-130.
32. Deutsch A, Abboud JA, Kelly J, et al: Clinical results of revision shoulder arthroplasty for glenoid component loosening. *J Shoulder Elbow Surg* 2007;16(6):706-716.
33. Phipatanakul WP, Norris TR: Treatment of glenoid loosening and bone loss due to osteolysis with glenoid bone grafting. *J Shoulder Elbow Surg* 2006;15(1): 84-87.
34. Cheung EV, Sperling JW, Cofield RH: Revision shoulder arthroplasty for glenoid component loosening. *J Shoulder Elbow Surg* 2008;17(3):371-375.
35. Antuna SA, Sperling JW, Cofield RH, Rowland CM: Glenoid revision surgery after total shoulder arthroplasty. *J Shoulder Elbow Surg* 2001;10(3):217-224.
36. Burkhead WZ Jr, Hutton KS: Biologic resurfacing of the glenoid with hemiarthroplasty of the shoulder. *J Shoulder Elbow Surg* 1995;4(4):263-270.
37. Ball CM, Galatz LM, Yamaguchi K: Meniscal allograft interposition arthroplasty for the arthritic shoulder: Description of a new surgical technique. *Tech Shoulder Elbow Surg* 2001;2:247-254.
38. Themistocleous GS, Zalavras CG, Zachos VC, Itamura JM: Biologic resurfacing of the glenoid using a meniscal allograft. *Tech Hand Up Extrem Surg* 2006;10(3):145-149.

39. Krishnan SG, Nowinski RJ, Harrison D, Burkhead WZ: Humeral hemiarthroplasty with biologic resurfacing of the glenoid for glenohumeral arthritis: Two to fifteen-year outcomes. *J Bone Joint Surg Am* 2007;89(4):727-734.
40. Wiater JM, Fabing MH: Shoulder arthroplasty: Prosthetic options and indications. *J Am Acad Orthop Surg* 2009;17(7):415-425.
41. Betts HM, Abu-Rajab R, Nunn T, Brooksbank AJ: Total shoulder replacement in rheumatoid disease: A 16- to 23-year follow-up. *J Bone Joint Surg Br* 2009;91(9): 1197-1200.
42. Boyd AD Jr, Aliabadi P, Thornhill TS: Postoperative proximal migration in total shoulder arthroplasty: Incidence and significance. *J Arthroplasty* 1991;6(1):31-37.
43. Sneppen O, Fruensgaard S, Johannsen HV, Olsen BS, Sojbjerg JO, Andersen NH: Total shoulder replacement in rheumatoid arthritis: Proximal migration and loosening. *J Shoulder Elbow Surg* 1996;5(1):47-52.
44. Wirth MA, Rockwood CA Jr: Complications of total shoulder-replacement arthroplasty. *J Bone Joint Surg Am* 1996;78(4): 603-616.
45. Boyd AD Jr, Thornhill TS, Barnes CL: Fractures adjacent to humeral prostheses. *J Bone Joint Surg Am* 1992;74(10):1498-1504.
46. Steinmann SP, Cheung EV: Treatment of periprosthetic humerus fractures associated with shoulder arthroplasty. *J Am Acad Orthop Surg* 2008;16(4):199-207.
47. Wright TW, Cofield RH: Humeral fractures after shoulder arthroplasty. *J Bone Joint Surg Am* 1995;77(9):1340-1346.
48. Hambright D, Henderson RA, Cook C, Worrell T, Moorman CT, Bolognesi MP: A comparison of perioperative outcomes in patients with and without rheumatoid arthritis after receiving a total shoulder replacement arthroplasty. *J Shoulder Elbow Surg* 2011;20(1): 77-85.
49. Goronzy JJ, Weyand CM: Developments in the scientific understanding of rheumatoid arthritis. *Arthritis Res Ther* 2009; 11(5):249.
50. Gravallese EM: Bone destruction in arthritis. *Ann Rheum Dis* 2002; 61(suppl 2):ii84-ii86.
51. Lichtman EA: Candida infection of a prosthetic shoulder joint. *Skeletal Radiol* 1983;10(3): 176-177.
52. Wirth MA, Rockwood CA Jr: Complications of shoulder arthroplasty. *Clin Orthop Relat Res* 1994; 307:47-69.
53. Hedtmann A, Werner A: Shoulder arthroplasty in rheumatoid arthritis. *Orthopade* 2007;36(11):1050-1061.
54. Brenner BC, Ferlic DC, Clayton ML, Dennis DA: Survivorship of unconstrained total shoulder arthroplasty. *J Bone Joint Surg Am* 1989;71(9):1289-1296.
55. Neer CS II, Kirby RM: Revision of humeral head and total shoulder arthroplasties. *Clin Orthop Relat Res* 1982;170:189-195.
56. van de Sande MA, Brand R, Rozing PM: Indications, complications, and results of shoulder arthroplasty. *Scand J Rheumatol* 2006;35(6):426-434.
57. Wirth MA, Seltzer DG, Senes HR, Pannone A, Lee J, Rockwood CA: A analysis of failed humeral head and total shoulder arthroplasty. *J Shoulder Elbow Surg* 1995;4:S13.
58. Collins DN, Harryman DT II, Wirth MA: Shoulder arthroplasty for the treatment of inflammatory arthritis. *J Bone Joint Surg Am* 2004;86(11):2489-2496.
59. Kelly IG, Foster RS, Fisher WD: Neer total shoulder replacement in rheumatoid arthritis. *J Bone Joint Surg Br* 1987;69(5): 723-726.
60. Sperling JW, Cofield RH, Schleck CD, Harmsen WS: Total shoulder arthroplasty versus hemiarthroplasty for rheumatoid arthritis of the shoulder: Results of 303 consecutive cases. *J Shoulder Elbow Surg* 2007;16(6):683-690.
61. Amstutz HC, Thomas BJ, Kabo JM, Jinnah RH, Dorey FJ: The Dana total shoulder arthroplasty. *J Bone Joint Surg Am* 1988;70(8): 1174-1182.
62. Bade HA II, Wrren RF, Ranawat CS, et al: Long-term results of Neer total shoulder replacement, in Bateman JE, Welch RP, eds: *Surgery of the Shoulder*. St. Louis, MO, Mosby, 1984, pp 294-302.
63. Boyd AD Jr, Thomas WH, Scott RD, Sledge CB, Thornhill TS: Total shoulder arthroplasty versus hemiarthroplasty: Indications for glenoid resurfacing. *J Arthroplasty* 1990;5(4):329-336.
64. Dines DM, Warren RF, Altchek DW, Moechel B: Post traumatic changes of proximal humerus: Malunion, nonunion, and osteonecrosis. Treatment with modular hemiarthroplasty or total shoulder arthroplasty. *J Shoulder Elbow Surg* 1993;2:11-21.
65. Kay SP, Amstutz HC: Shoulder hemiarthroplasty at UCLA. *Clin Orthop Relat Res* 1988;228:42-48.
66. Neer CS II: Articular replacement for the humeral head. *J Bone Joint Surg Am* 1955;37(2):215-228.
67. Warren RF, Ranawat CS, Inglis AE: Total shoulder replacement, indications and results of the Neer nonconstrained prosthesis, in Inglis AE, ed: *American Academy of Orthopaedic Surgeons: Symposium on Total Joint Replacement of the Upper Extremity*. St. Louis, MO, Mosby, 1982, pp 56-67.
68. Beredjiklian PK, Iannotti JP, Norris TR, Williams GR: Operative treatment of malunion of a frac-

ture of the proximal aspect of the humerus. *J Bone Joint Surg Am* 1998;80(10):1484-1497.

69. Bosch U, Fremerey RW, Skutek M, Lobenhoffer P, Tscherne H: Primary or secondary measure for 3- and 4-fragment fractures of the proximal humerus in the elderly? *Unfallchirurg* 1996;99(9): 656-664.
70. Bosch U, Skutek M, Fremerey RW, Tscherne H: Outcome after primary and secondary hemiarthroplasty in elderly patients with fractures of the proximal humerus. *J Shoulder Elbow Surg* 1998;7(5):479-484.
71. Cofield RH, Briggs BT: Glenohumeral arthrodesis: Operative and long-term functional results. *J Bone Joint Surg Am* 1979;61(5): 668-677.
72. Frich LH, Søjbjerg JO, Sneppen O: Shoulder arthroplasty in complex acute and chronic proximal humeral fractures. *Orthopedics* 1991;14(9):949-954.
73. Habermeyer P, Schweiberer L: Corrective interventions subsequent to humeral head fractures. *Orthopade* 1992;21(2):148-157.
74. Huten D, Duparc J: Prosthetic arthroplasty in recent and old complex injuries of the shoulder. *Rev Chir Orthop Reparatrice Appar Mot* 1986;72(8):517-529.
75. Muldoon MP, Cofield RH: Complications of humeral head replacement for proximal humeral fractures. *Instr Course Lect* 1997; 46:15-24.
76. Norris TR, Green A, McGuigan FX: Late prosthetic shoulder arthroplasty for displaced proximal humerus fractures. *J Shoulder Elbow Surg* 1995;4(4):271-280.
77. Neer CS II: Glenohumeral arthroplasty, in *Shoulder Reconstruction.* Philadelphia, PA, WB Saunders, 1990, pp 143-271.
78. Neer CS II, Watson KC, Stanton FJ: Recent experience in total shoulder replacement. *J Bone Joint Surg Am* 1982;64(3):319-337.
79. Wiater JM, Flatow EL: Posttraumatic arthritis. *Orthop Clin North Am* 2000;31(1):63-76.
80. Hawkins RJ, Angelo RL: Glenohumeral osteoarthrosis: A late complication of the Putti-Platt repair. *J Bone Joint Surg Am* 1990; 72(8):1193-1197.
81. Lombardo SJ, Kerlan RK, Jobe FW, Carter VS, Blazina ME, Shields CL Jr: The modified Bristow procedure for recurrent dislocation of the shoulder. *J Bone Joint Surg Am* 1976;58(2): 256-261.
82. Samilson RL, Prieto V: Dislocation arthropathy of the shoulder. *J Bone Joint Surg Am* 1983;65(4): 456-460.
83. Young DC, Rockwood CA Jr: Complications of a failed Bristow procedure and their management. *J Bone Joint Surg Am* 1991;73(7): 969-981.
84. Zuckerman JD, Matsen FA III: Complications about the glenohumeral joint related to the use of screws and staples. *J Bone Joint Surg Am* 1984;66(2):175-180.
85. Sperling JW, Antuna SA, Sanchez-Sotelo J, Schleck C, Cofield RH: Shoulder arthroplasty for arthritis after instability surgery. *J Bone Joint Surg Am* 2002; 84(10):1775-1781.
86. Miller LS, Donahue JR, Good RP, Staerk AJ: The Magnuson-Stack procedure for treatment of recurrent glenohumeral dislocations. *Am J Sports Med* 1984; 12(2):133-137.
87. Matsoukis J, Tabib W, Guiffault P, et al: Shoulder arthroplasty in patients with a prior anterior shoulder dislocation: Results of a multicenter study. *J Bone Joint Surg Am* 2003;85(8):1417-1424.
88. Bigliani LU, Weinstein DM, Glasgow MT, Pollock RG, Flatow EL: Glenohumeral arthroplasty for arthritis after instability surgery. *J Shoulder Elbow Surg* 1995; 4(2):87-94.
89. Bauer GS, Freehill MQ, Masters C, et al: Poster: Glenohumeral arthroplasty for arthritis after instability surgery. *2002 Annual Meeting Proceedings*, Rosemont, IL, American Academy of Orthopaedic Surgeons, 2002, p 511.
90. Sperling JW, Pring M, Antuna SA, Cofield RH: Shoulder arthroplasty for locked posterior dislocation of the shoulder. *J Shoulder Elbow Surg* 2004;13(5):522-527.
91. Dalstrom DJ, Venkatarayappa I, Manternach AL, Palcic MS, Heyse BA, Prayson MJ: Time-dependent contamination of opened sterile operating-room trays. *J Bone Joint Surg Am* 2008;90(5):1022-1025.
92. Bryan WJ, Schauder K, Tullos HS: The axillary nerve and its relationship to common sports medicine shoulder procedures. *Am J Sports Med* 1986;14(2):113-116.
93. Loomer R, Graham B: Anatomy of the axillary nerve and its relation to inferior capsular shift. *Clin Orthop Relat Res* 1989;243: 100-105.
94. Boardman ND III, Cofield RH: Neurologic complications of shoulder surgery. *Clin Orthop Relat Res* 1999;368:44-53.
95. Miller BS, Joseph TA, Noonan TJ, Horan MP, Hawkins RJ: Rupture of the subscapularis tendon after shoulder arthroplasty: Diagnosis, treatment, and outcome. *J Shoulder Elbow Surg* 2005;14(5):492-496.
96. Van Thiel GS, Wang VM, Wang FC, et al: Biomechanical similarities among subscapularis repairs after shoulder arthroplasty. *J Shoulder Elbow Surg* 2010;19(5): 657-663.
97. Giuseffi SA, Wongtriratanachai P, Omae H, et al: Biomechanical comparison of lesser tuberosity osteotomy versus subscapularis tenotomy in total shoulder arthroplasty. *J Shoulder Elbow Surg* 2012;21(8):1087-1095.

98. Ponce BA, Ahluwalia RS, Mazzocca AD, Gobezie RG, Warner JJ, Millett PJ: Biomechanical and clinical evaluation of a novel lesser tuberosity repair technique in total shoulder arthroplasty. *J Bone Joint Surg Am* 2005;87(suppl 2):1-8.
99. Scalise JJ, Ciccone J, Iannotti JP: Clinical, radiographic, and ultrasonographic comparison of subscapularis tenotomy and lesser tuberosity osteotomy for total shoulder arthroplasty. *J Bone Joint Surg Am* 2010;92(7):1627-1634.
100. Jandhyala S, Unnithan A, Hughes S, Hong T: Subscapularis tenotomy versus lesser tuberosity osteotomy during total shoulder replacement: A comparison of patient outcomes. *J Shoulder Elbow Surg* 2011;20(7):1102-1107.
101. Heckman DS, Hoover SA, Weinhold PS, Spang JT, Creighton RA: Repair of lesser tuberosity osteotomy for shoulder arthroplasty: Biomechanical evaluation of the backpack and dual row techniques. *J Shoulder Elbow Surg* 2011;20(3):491-496.
102. Gerber A, Ghalambor N, Warner JJ: Instability of shoulder arthroplasty: Balancing mobility and stability. *Orthop Clin North Am* 2001;32(4):661-670, ix.
103. Moeckel BH, Altchek DW, Warren RF, Wickiewicz TL, Dines DM: Instability of the shoulder after arthroplasty. *J Bone Joint Surg Am* 1993;75(4):492-497.
104. Miller SL, Hazrati Y, Klepps S, Chiang A, Flatow EL: Loss of subscapularis function after total shoulder replacement: A seldom recognized problem. *J Shoulder Elbow Surg* 2003;12(1):29-34.
105. Armstrong A, Lashgari C, Teefey S, Menendez J, Yamaguchi K, Galatz LM: Ultrasound evaluation and clinical correlation of subscapularis repair after total shoulder arthroplasty. *J Shoulder Elbow Surg* 2006;15(5):541-548.
106. Jackson JD, Cil A, Smith J, Steinmann SP: Integrity and function of the subscapularis after total shoulder arthroplasty. *J Shoulder Elbow Surg* 2010;19(7):1085-1090.
107. Gerber C, Krushell RJ: Isolated rupture of the tendon of the subscapularis muscle: Clinical features in 16 cases. *J Bone Joint Surg Br* 1991;73(3):389-394.
108. Boileau P, Kontakis GM, Trossarello P, Coste JS: Release of the subscapularis tendon and muscle: A limited gain in length. *Orthopedics* 2007;30(8):657-661.
109. Cleeman E, Brunelli M, Gothelf T, Hayes P, Flatow EL: Releases of subscapularis contracture: An anatomic and clinical study. *J Shoulder Elbow Surg* 2003;12(3):231-236.
110. Matsen FA, Leppitt SB, Sidles JA, Harryman DT: *Practical Evaluation of Management of the Shoulder*. Philadelphia, PA, WB Saunders, 1994.
111. Rockwood CA Jr: The technique of total shoulder arthroplasty. *Instr Course Lect* 1990;39:437-447.
112. Nicholson GP, Twigg S, Blatz B, Sturonas-Brown B, Wilson J: Subscapular lengthening in shoulder arthroplasty. *J Shoulder Elbow Surg* 2010;19(3):427-433.
113. Churchill RS, Brems JJ, Kotschi H: Glenoid size, inclination, and version: An anatomic study. *J Shoulder Elbow Surg* 2001;10(4):327-332.
114. Friedman RJ, Hawthorne KB, Genez BM: The use of computerized tomography in the measurement of glenoid version. *J Bone Joint Surg Am* 1992;74(7):1032-1037.
115. Nyffeler RW, Jost B, Pfirrmann CW, Gerber C: Measurement of glenoid version: Conventional radiographs versus computed tomography scans. *J Shoulder Elbow Surg* 2003;12(5):493-496.
116. Randelli M, Gambrioli PL: Glenohumeral osteometry by computed tomography in normal and unstable shoulders. *Clin Orthop Relat Res* 1986;208:151-156.
117. Scalise JJ, Codsi MJ, Bryan J, Iannotti JP: The three-dimensional glenoid vault model can estimate normal glenoid version in osteoarthritis. *J Shoulder Elbow Surg* 2008;17(3):487-491.
118. Shapiro TA, McGarry MH, Gupta R, Lee YS, Lee TQ: Biomechanical effects of glenoid retroversion in total shoulder arthroplasty. *J Shoulder Elbow Surg* 2007;16(3, suppl):S90-S95.
119. Gillespie R, Lyons R, Lazarus M: Eccentric reaming in total shoulder arthroplasty: A cadaveric study. *Orthopedics* 2009;32(1):21.
120. Iannotti JP, Gabriel JP, Schneck SL, Evans BG, Misra S: The normal glenohumeral relationships: An anatomical study of one hundred and forty shoulders. *J Bone Joint Surg Am* 1992;74(4):491-500.
121. Lazarus MD, Jensen KL, Southworth C, Matsen FA III : The radiographic evaluation of keeled and pegged glenoid component insertion. *J Bone Joint Surg Am* 2002;84(7):1174-1182.
122. Gartsman GM, Elkousy HA, Warnock KM, Edwards TB, O'Connor DP: Radiographic comparison of pegged and keeled glenoid components. *J Shoulder Elbow Surg* 2005;14(3):252-257.
123. Nuttall D, Haines JF, Trail II: A study of the micromovement of pegged and keeled glenoid components compared using radiostereometric analysis. *J Shoulder Elbow Surg* 2007;16(3, suppl):S65-S70.
124. Szabo I, Buscayret F, Edwards TB, Nemoz C, Boileau P, Walch G: Radiographic comparison of flat-back and convex-back glenoid components in total shoulder ar

throplasty. *J Shoulder Elbow Surg* 2005;14(6):636-642.

125. Anglin C, Wyss UP, Pichora DR: Mechanical testing of shoulder prostheses and recommendations for glenoid design. *J Shoulder Elbow Surg* 2000;9(4):323-331.

126. Iannotti JP, Spencer EE, Winter U, Deffenbaugh D, Williams G: Prosthetic positioning in total shoulder arthroplasty. *J Shoulder Elbow Surg* 2005;14(1, suppl S): 111S-121S.

127. Boileau P, Avidor C, Krishnan SG, Walch G, Kempf JF, Molé D: Cemented polyethylene versus uncemented metal-backed glenoid components in total shoulder arthroplasty: A prospective, double-blind, randomized study. *J Shoulder Elbow Surg* 2002;11(4): 351-359.

128. Fox TJ, Cil A, Sperling JW, Sanchez-Sotelo J, Schleck CD, Cofield RH: Survival of the glenoid component in shoulder arthroplasty. *J Shoulder Elbow Surg* 2009;18(6):859-863.

129. Clement ND, Mathur K, Colling R, Stirrat AN: The metal-backed glenoid component in rheumatoid disease: Eight- to fourteen-year follow-up. *J Shoulder Elbow Surg* 2010;19(5):749-756.

130. Castagna A, Randelli M, Garofalo R, Maradei L, Giardella A, Borroni M: Mid-term results of a metal-backed glenoid component in total shoulder replacement. *J Bone Joint Surg Br* 2010;92(10): 1410-1415.

131. Terrier A, Büchler P, Farron A: Bone-cement interface of the glenoid component: Stress analysis for varying cement thickness. *Clin Biomech (Bristol, Avon)* 2005; 20(7):710-717.

132. Nyffeler RW, Anglin C, Sheikh R, Gerber C: Influence of peg design and cement mantle thickness on pull-out strength of glenoid component pegs. *J Bone Joint Surg Br* 2003;85(5):748-752.

133. Churchill RS, Boorman RS, Fehringer EV, Matsen FA III: Glenoid cementing may generate sufficient heat to endanger the surrounding bone. *Clin Orthop Relat Res* 2004;419:76-79.

134. Klepps S, Chiang AS, Miller S, Jiang CY, Hazrati Y, Flatow EL: Incidence of early radiolucent glenoid lines in patients having total shoulder replacements. *Clin Orthop Relat Res* 2005;435: 118-125.

135. Nyffeler RW, Meyer D, Sheikh R, Koller BJ, Gerber C: The effect of cementing technique on structural fixation of pegged glenoid components in total shoulder arthroplasty. *J Shoulder Elbow Surg* 2006;15(1):106-111.

136. Karduna AR, Williams GR, Williams JL, Iannotti JP: Glenohumeral joint translations before and after total shoulder arthroplasty: A study in cadavera. *J Bone Joint Surg Am* 1997;79(8):1166-1174.

137. Walch G, Edwards TB, Boulahia A, Boileau P, Mole D, Adeleine P: The influence of glenohumeral prosthetic mismatch on glenoid radiolucent lines: Results of a multicenter study. *J Bone Joint Surg Am* 2002;84-A(12):2186-2191.

138. Hopkins AR, Hansen UN, Amis AA, Emery R: The effects of glenoid component alignment variations on cement mantle stresses in total shoulder arthroplasty. *J Shoulder Elbow Surg* 2004;13(6): 668-675.

139. Farron A, Terrier A, Büchler P: Risks of loosening of a prosthetic glenoid implanted in retroversion. *J Shoulder Elbow Surg* 2006;15(4): 521-526.

140. Yian EH, Werner CM, Nyffeler RW, et al: Radiographic and computed tomography analysis of cemented pegged polyethylene glenoid components in total shoulder replacement. *J Bone Joint Surg Am* 2005;87(9):1928-1936.

141. Murachovsky J, Ikemoto RY, Nascimento LG, Fujiki EN, Milani C, Warner JJ: Pectoralis major tendon reference: A new method for accurate restoration of humeral length with hemiarthroplasty for fracture. *J Shoulder Elbow Surg* 2006;15(6):675-678.

142. Boardman ND III, Cofield RH, Bengtson KA, Little R, Jones MC, Rowland CM: Rehabilitation after total shoulder arthroplasty. *J Arthroplasty* 2001;16(4):483-486.

143. Brems JJ: Rehabilitation following total shoulder arthroplasty. *Clin Orthop Relat Res* 1994;307:70-85.

144. Brown DD, Friedman RJ: Postoperative rehabilitation following total shoulder arthroplasty. *Orthop Clin North Am* 1998;29(3):535-547.

145. Hughes M, Neer CS II: Glenohumeral joint replacement and postoperative rehabilitation. *Phys Ther* 1975;55(8):850-858.

146. Jackins S: Postoperative shoulder rehabilitation. *Phys Med Rehabil Clin N Am* 2004;15(3):vi, 643-682.

147. Wilcox RB, Arslanian LE, Millett P: Rehabilitation following total shoulder arthroplasty. *J Orthop Sports Phys Ther* 2005;35(12): 821-836.

148. Mulieri PJ, Holcomb JO, Dunning P, et al: Is a formal physical therapy program necessary after total shoulder arthroplasty for osteoarthritis? *J Shoulder Elbow Surg* 2010;19(4):570-579.

Video Reference

10.1: Hawkins RJ: Video. Excerpt. *Total Shoulder Arthroplasty: Steps to Get It Right.* Greenville, SC, 2012.

11

Complications in Total Shoulder Arthroplasty

John W. Sperling, MD, MBA
Richard J. Hawkins, MD
Gilles Walch, MD
Andrew P. Mahoney, MD
Joseph D. Zuckerman, MD

Abstract

A wider spectrum of complications associated with shoulder arthroplasty is expected because of the substantial increase in the prevalence of this procedure over the past decade. It is helpful to review the management and methods needed to prevent the most common complications associated with shoulder arthroplasty.

Instr Course Lect 2013;62:135-141.

Over the past decade, there has been a substantial increase in the prevalence of shoulder arthroplasty.[1] As a result, a wider spectrum of complications associated with shoulder arthroplasty is expected. This chapter will discuss the management and methods of preventing the most common complications associated with shoulder arthroplasty.

Periprosthetic Fractures

The reported prevalence of periprosthetic fractures associated with shoulder arthroplasty is between 1.6% and 2.3%.[2] Potential etiologies include osteopenia, cortical thinning from osteolysis, excess reaming of the humeral cortex, and eccentric placement of the humeral component.

Initially, AP and axillary radiographs are necessary. It is important that the radiographs include the entire humerus to determine the exact length of the fracture and clearly evaluate for evidence of component loosening. CT may be useful in evaluating for component loosening, particularly for the glenoid.

The most widely used classification system was described by Wright and Cofield.[3] This system is based on the location of the fracture in relation to the tip of the prosthesis. Type A fractures occur at the tip of the prosthesis and extend proximally. Type B fractures occur at the tip of the prosthesis without extension. Type C fractures occur at the prosthetic tip and have distal extension.

The literature indicates that classification of the fracture helps to predict the outcome of treatment. Boyd et al[4] reported on the outcome of seven periprosthetic fractures, six of which did not heal with nonsurgical treatment. All of the fractures were type B and were centered at the tip of the prosthesis. Type B fractures have a high rate of nonunion with nonsurgical treatment.[2] Campbell et al[5] reported on five fractures that healed with nonsurgical treatment, with four fractures distal to the tip of the humeral stem (type C). These type C fractures have a high rate of healing with nonsurgical treatment.[5]

Kumar et al[2] reported on the outcome of 16 periprosthetic humeral fractures, all followed until union

Dr. Sperling or an immediate family member has received royalties from Biomet and DJ Orthopaedics; serves as a paid consultant to or is an employee of Tornier; and has stock or stock options in Emerge Medical and Tornier. Dr. Hawkins or an immediate family member has received royalties from Ossur; serves as a paid consultant to or is an employee of DJ Orthopaedics; and has received research or institutional support from DJ Orthopaedics, Breg, Smith & Nephew, OrthoRehab, Ferring Pharmaceuticals, Tornier, and Ossur. Dr. Walch or an immediate family member has received royalties from Tornier and has received nonincome support (such as equipment or services), commercially derived honoraria, or other non–research-related funding (such as paid travel) from Tornier. Dr. Zuckerman or an immediate family member has received royalties from Exactech and has stock or stock options in Neostem and Joint Innovation Technology. Neither Dr. Mahoney nor any immediate family member has received anything of value from or has stock or stock options in a commercial company or institution related directly or indirectly to the subject of this chapter.

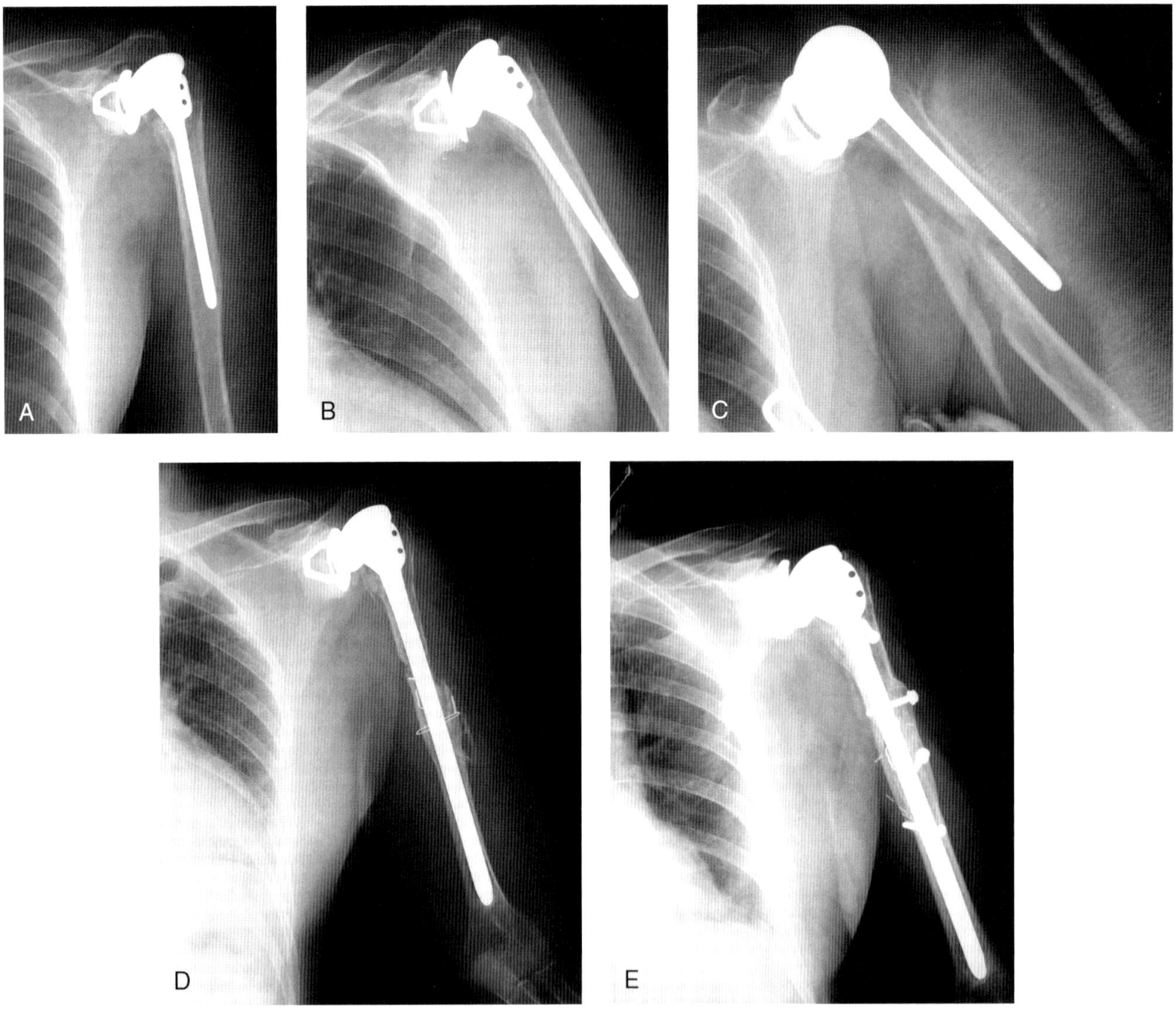

Figure 1 Radiographs of the shoulder of a patient who had a shift in the humeral component position with a subsequent fracture that was noted over a 2-year period. **A**, AP radiograph made immediately after total shoulder arthroplasty. **B**, Progressive eccentric shift of the humeral component was seen. **C**, A periprosthetic fracture subsequently developed. **D**, Treatment of the fracture with a long-stemmed component and cerclage wire failed. **E**, Successful treatment was achieved with a free fibular graft. (Reproduced with permission from Kumar S, Sperling JW, Haidukewych GH, Cofield RH: Periprosthetic humeral fractures after shoulder arthroplasty. *J Bone Joint Surg Am* 2004;86(4):680-689.)

(**Figure 1**). The mean interval from arthroplasty to fracture was 49 months. None of the patients had an ipsilateral total elbow arthroplasty. The most common mechanism of injury was a fall onto the upper extremity. Six fractures healed with nonsurgical treatment at a mean of 180 days (range, 49 to 332 days). Five fractures were treated surgically after failing to heal with nonsurgical management. Five fractures were treated with immediate surgery. Excluding one patient who required multiple surgical procedures (including a free vascularized fibular graft to heal), the mean time to healing was 230 days. At the most recent follow-up at a mean of 5.5 years, the average shoulder abduction was 107°, and the average external rotation was 43°.

Kumar et al[2] recommended various treatments depending on the fracture type and the fixation status of the humeral component.

Type C (Loose Humeral Component)

When the humeral component is loose, placing a long-stemmed component with bone graft at the fracture site is considered.

Type C (Well-Fixed Humeral Component)

When the humeral component is well fixed, the fracture is treated as a closed humeral shaft fracture. A trial of nonsurgical treatment using an orthosis is recommended if an acceptable closed reduction can be obtained.

Type B (Loose Humeral Component)

When the humeral component is loose, the prosthesis should be revised to a long-stemmed humeral component with allograft at the fracture site. The additional use of a strut allograft or a plate and screws can be considered to improve fracture fixation.

Type B (Well-Fixed Humeral Component)

A trial of nonsurgical treatment should be considered initially. However, Kumar et al[2] found that four of five type B fractures treated nonsurgically failed to heal and eventually required surgery. If surgery is performed, a plate and screws or allograft strut fixation distally and cerclage fixation proximally, with or without autogenous bone graft, should be considered because this approach is often an attractive alternative to revising a well-fixed prosthesis.

Type A (Loose Humeral Component)

In a type A fracture with a loose humeral component, revision arthroplasty using a long stem with allograft is necessary, and a strut allograft or plate and screws to improve fixation should be considered.

Type A (Well-Fixed Humeral Component)

The management of a type A fracture with a well-fixed humeral component is debated. However, if there is substantial overlap of the fracture and the humeral stem, the humeral component has an increased likelihood of being loose, and revision arthroplasty is necessary.

Infection After Shoulder Arthroplasty

Infection is a rare but devastating complication after shoulder arthroplasty. The prevalence has been reported to range between 0% and 4%.[6,7] Because there is minimal information to guide decision making, the rationale behind evaluation and treatment is derived in large part from the reported experience in managing infection at the site of total knee arthroplasty and total hip arthroplasty.

A humeral component that has become loose is considered to be associated with infection until proven otherwise. First, the time course of the pain and whether the patient had a recent procedure, such as dental work, that may have caused bacterial seeding of the joint should be determined. Did the patient have wound-healing problems or prolonged antibiotic use at the time of the initial shoulder arthroplasty? The prior surgical reports should be reviewed to determine the indication for the original procedure. All prior radiographs should be reviewed.

Diagnosing an infection can be challenging. Most patients do not present with overt signs of infection. Topolski et al[8] evaluated the outcome of 75 patients with positive cultures at the time of revision shoulder arthroplasty without overt signs of infection. The white blood cell count was normal in 67 of 72 patients (93%), polymorphonuclear cell or neutrophil distribution was normal in 64 of 70 patients (91%), the erythrocyte sedimentation rate was normal in 36 of 42 patients (86%), and the C-reactive protein level was normal in 12 of 16 patients (75%). For these patients, the intraoperative histologic studies were negative for acute inflammation in 67 of 73 patients (92%). *Propionibacterium acnes* is the most common organism responsible for infection after shoulder arthroplasty.[7] However, as shown by Topolski et al,[8] the first culture to become positive required an average of 5.1 days, so reviewing culture data after shoulder aspiration is necessary for at least 1 week.

Coste et al[6] reported on eight shoulders that had débridement for infection. Each of two arthroscopic débridements failed, and four of six open débridements failed. Sperling et al[7] reported that three of six open débridements failed. Ince et al[9] reported on nine patients with a one-stage reimplantation without any recurrent infection. Strickland et al[10] reported on the outcome of two-stage reimplantation in 19 patients. At the time of the most recent follow-up of these patients, the mean shoulder elevation was 89°, and the mean external rotation was 48°. There were a substantial number of complications, including the need for secondary surgical procedures in five patients and chronic antibiotic treatment of infection suppression in six patients.

Classification and Treatment of Periprosthetic Infection

Type I: Positive Cultures at Time of Revision Surgery

Organism-specific antibiotic treatment is instituted with close clinical observation. There are no good data to determine the optimal length of antibiotic treatment.

Type II: Acute Infection Within 30 Days After Surgery

Surgical débridement with prosthetic retention is used, although there are minimal data available on the outcomes of this approach.

Type III: Acute Hematogenous Infection More Than 30 Days After Surgery

Surgical débridement with retention of the implants or two-stage treatment with the use of an antibiotic spacer impregnated with gentamicin and vancomycin between explantation and reimplantation is recommended.

Type IV: Chronic Infection

Surgical débridement with implant removal, temporary placement of an antibiotic spacer impregnated with gentamicin and vancomycin, and reimplantation approximately 8 weeks later are recommended.

Instability After Shoulder Arthroplasty

Different patterns of shoulder instability occur after arthroplasty. Superior instability is usually associated with a deficient rotator cuff and/or coracoacromial arch. Although superior instability is characterized by a loss of contact between the glenoid and the proximal part of the humerus, this pattern of instability is a separate topic. The focus of this section is anterior and posterior instability after shoulder arthroplasty. The causes, characteristics, and treatment of prosthetic instability are different after nonconstrained anatomic arthroplasty or semiconstrained reverse arthroplasty and are discussed separately.

Anterior Instability With an Anatomic Prosthesis

The reported frequency of anterior instability after total shoulder arthroplasty with an anatomic prosthesis has ranged from 0.9% to 1.8%.[11,12] The two main causes are soft-tissue abnormality (subscapularis rupture or insufficiency) or component malposition (humeral and/or glenoid anteversion). Some patients may have both.

Treatment results are generally discouraging when an anatomic prosthesis is revised to another anatomic prosthesis. Sanchez-Sotelo et al[13] reported that after subscapularis repair, component revision, and humeral head exchange were performed in 19 shoulders, stability was obtained in only 5 shoulders. Ahrens et al[11] repaired the subscapularis, transferred the pectoralis major tendon, and reoriented the humeral and glenoid components in 35 shoulders. Recurrent instability occurred in more than 50% of the shoulders. However, all three shoulders treated with revision to a reverse shoulder arthroplasty were stable. Moeckel et al[14] described repair of the subscapularis in seven patients with anterior instability. Three of the patients continued to have instability and were treated with subsequent reconstruction with an Achilles tendon allograft with successful results.

Posterior Instability With an Anatomic Prosthesis

The rate of posterior instability after arthroplasty with an anatomic prosthesis has been reported to range from 1% to 1.3%.[11,12] The two primary causes are soft-tissue abnormality (excess posterior capsular laxity) or component malposition (humeral and/or glenoid retroversion). Patients with preoperative posterior static instability with an associated biconcave glenoid have a predisposition to posterior instability after arthroplasty with an anatomic prosthesis.

A variety of strategies are available to restore stability in shoulders with posterior instability. It is critical to address all potential causes of instability, including restoration of normal retroversion of the components, posterior capsular tightening, and potential immobilization in neutral rotation. Sanchez-Sotelo et al[13] reported that the outcome after the treatment of 14 patients with posterior instability was categorized as good for 9 patients and as a failure for 5. After revision surgery in 29 patients, Ahrens et al[11] reported 15 good results and 14 failures. All four patients who had revision to a reverse arthroplasty had a stable shoulder.

Instability After Arthroplasty With a Reverse Semiconstrained Prosthesis

Instability after a reverse arthroplasty is more frequent in revision arthroplasty and primary arthroplasty for posttraumatic arthritis. The causes are soft-tissue abnormalities (inadequate deltoid tension), component malpositioning, or both. The key to avoiding instability after reverse arthroplasty is to restore the humeral length. The surgical approach may influence the rate of instability. A superior approach has been noted to have a lower prevalence of instability compared with a deltopectoral approach.[15] There is increasing interest in repairing the subscapularis and then protecting this repair by limiting shoulder motion for 4 to 6 weeks.

It is necessary to carefully assess the humeral length in a patient with unstable reverse arthroplasty components. It may be helpful to obtain a CT scan to evaluate the position of the glenosphere to ensure proper version. In the acute setting, a closed reduction can be attempted. If open reduction is done, it is essential to have the appropriate instrumentation available to place a thicker humeral bearing surface, to increase the diameter and/or thickness of the glenosphere, or to place a retentive insert.

Rotator Cuff Tearing After Shoulder Arthroplasty

There are a variety of presentations of rotator cuff tearing after shoulder arthroplasty.[12,16] Rupture of the subscapularis is the most frequent and may present with anterior subluxation of the humeral head on the axillary radiograph.[12] The rate of postoperative rupture of the subscapularis is likely underestimated.[12] There may be a traumatic or an atraumatic onset. Often, the tear is asymptomatic, with a loss of strength discovered at clinical examination, including excessive external rotation with the elbow at the side or a positive belly-press test.

The rate of rotator cuff tearing after shoulder arthroplasty has been reported to range from 1.3% to 7.8%.[12,17-20] Rupture of the posterosuperior aspect of the cuff (the supraspinatus and/or the infraspinatus and/or the teres minor) may occur and typically presents with upward migration of the humeral head with a decreased acromiohumeral distance on AP radiographs.

There are several important factors to consider to avoid this complication. Because subscapularis fatty infiltration may be associated with a high risk for nonhealing and secondary insufficiency, knowing that it exists before surgery may reduce the risk. This may be determined by physical examination and possible imaging studies, including MRI. The key technical steps at the time of surgery include intraoperative mobilization of the superior tendon with release of subcoracoid adhesions, release of the middle and inferior glenohumeral ligaments, and sparing the innervation of the subscapularis. It is important to avoid overstuffing the joint. A secure repair of the subscapularis is critical, along with postoperative protection of the subscapularis repair. The postoperative safe range of motion for physical therapy is determined at the time of surgery.

Treatment of the postoperative subscapularis tear is challenging. Miller et al[21] reported on early repeat repair with gentle mobilization in patients with symptomatic rupture. For patients with a chronic rupture, augmentation of the repair with a pectoralis major tendon transfer should be considered.

Deprey[19] described attempted tendon repair with placement of a smaller prosthetic humeral head, as well as possible pectoralis major transfer. In that report of 22 shoulders, the functional gain was minimal.

In patients with a traumatic acute subscapularis rupture with good-quality tendon and muscle, an immediate revision to repair the tendon is likely the best treatment. In patients with a chronic tear with fatty infiltration, nonsurgical treatment is preferred if there are minimal symptoms because repair with or without pectoralis major transfer does not provide good results.[22] For the patients with symptoms, a reverse arthroplasty may be considered.

Postoperative Rupture of the Posterosuperior Aspect of the Rotator Cuff

The frequency of postoperative rupture of the posterosuperior aspect of the rotator cuff has been reported to be variable but is usually associated with rheumatoid arthritis.[23-26] It may occur secondary to trauma or degeneration without trauma but increases with time from surgery. Young et al[20] reported on the outcome of 518 total shoulder arthroplasties for primary osteoarthritis with a mean follow-up of 8.7 years. The survivorship free of secondary cuff failure was 100% at 5 years, 84% at 10 years, and 43% at 15 years after surgery.

There are several potential predisposing factors,[20,27] including preoperative fatty infiltration of the rotator cuff muscles as detected on MRI ($P < 0.05$), superior tilt of the glenoid component on immediate postoperative radiographs ($P < 0.01$), and a longer duration of follow-up ($P < 0.001$).

Weakness in shoulder forward elevation and external rotation is the common symptom. Patients with a postoperative tear have a worse clinical outcome with respect to the Constant score, subjective results, and shoulder motion.[20] Results using radiographic criteria are also worse. However, Young et al[20] reported that the revision rate was not substantially different between patients with and those without secondary rotator cuff failure.

Patients with minimal symptoms can be treated without surgery because attempts at repair have not been successful. In the series by Hattrup et al,[24] repair was successful in only 4 of 18 shoulders. For the patient with symptoms, the use of revision to reverse arthroplasty, with or without latissimus dorsi transfer, appears to be the best treatment.

Glenoid Component Loosening

Glenoid components remain a primary concern in shoulder arthroplasty. The presence of radiolucent lines around the glenoid component may not be clinically important. Miller and Bigliani[28] reported that radiolucent lines were common, but there was no direct correlation to the level of clinical symptoms. Brems[29] reported on the association between radiolucent lines and revision procedures with an analysis of 20 reported series of total shoulder arthroplasties. At a mean follow-up of 5 years, radiolucent lines were seen around 39% of all total shoulder replacements. For all of the shoulders with periprosthetic lucency, the rate of revision surgery was 8%. This chapter's authors have found that radiolucent lines may be reflective of the surgical technique, glenoid bone quality, and changes that may result from stress shielding or disuse osteoporosis. Careful preparation of the glenoid bone and the use of a minimal amount of cement may reduce the prevalence of glenoid loosening. Loosening of the glenoid component is associated with rotator cuff deficiency. Franklin et al[30] reported on seven patients with glenoid component loosening associated with rotator cuff insufficiency.

The evaluation of glenoid loosening requires proper radiographs, preferably made with fluoroscopically positioned views. If it is difficult to determine whether the glenoid component is loose, CT is useful.

The prevention of loosening is critical. The surgeon must have a clear understanding of the glenoid anatomy, including the specific wear pattern. Careful review of preoperative radiographs is essential. CT will aid in planning if the wear pattern is not determined with radiographs. Key technical steps to prevent loosening include preserving as much native glenoid bone stock as possible during preparation and removal of only that amount of bone essential to place the implant, including minimal reaming. Additional preparation includes pulsatile saline solution lavage, careful drying of the glenoid bone, mixing the bone cement to diminish porosity, and pressurizing the bone cement.

Overall, a substantial number of loose glenoid components do not require revision surgery. If a patient becomes symptomatic, it is imperative to rule out other problems as a reason for the symptoms, including rotator cuff insufficiency or low-grade infection. Each of these complications may occur alone or together with loosening of the glenoid.

This chapter's authors believe that the largest series on revision for glenoid component loosening was reported by Cheung et al.[31] Those authors reviewed the results after revision for glenoid loosening in 68 shoulders in 66 patients. In the study, 33 shoulders were treated with the placement of a new glenoid component, and component removal and bone grafting without glenoid reimplantation were done in 35 shoulders. The authors reported substantial overall improvement with regard to pain in both groups. Twenty-four of 33 patients (73%) who received a new glenoid component were satisfied compared with 19 of 35 patients (54%) who had only bone grafting. Nine shoulders with a new glenoid component and three with bone grafting had an excellent or satisfactory result ($P = 0.0432$). Interestingly, 20 shoulders had positive cultures, with *P acnes* detected most frequently.

References

1. Kim SH, Wise BL, Zhang Y, Szabo RM: Increasing incidence of shoulder arthroplasty in the United States. *J Bone Joint Surg Am* 2011;93(24):2249-2254.
2. Kumar S, Sperling JW, Haidukewych GH, Cofield RH: Periprosthetic humeral fractures after shoulder arthroplasty. *J Bone Joint Surg Am* 2004;86(4):680-689.
3. Wright TW, Cofield RH: Humeral fractures after shoulder arthroplasty. *J Bone Joint Surg Am* 1995;77(9):1340-1346.
4. Boyd AD Jr, Thornhill TS, Barnes CL: Fractures adjacent to humeral prostheses. *J Bone Joint Surg Am* 1992;74(10):1498-1504.
5. Campbell JT, Moore RS, Iannotti JP, Norris TR, Williams GR: Periprosthetic humeral fractures: Mechanisms of fracture and treatment options. *J Shoulder Elbow Surg* 1998;7(4):406-413.
6. Coste JS, Reig S, Trojani C, Berg M, Walch G, Boileau P: The management of infection in arthroplasty of the shoulder. *J Bone Joint Surg Br* 2004;86(1):65-69.
7. Sperling JW, Kozak TK, Hanssen AD, Cofield RH: Infection after shoulder arthroplasty. *Clin Orthop Relat Res* 2001;382:206-216.
8. Topolski MS, Chin PY, Sperling JW, Cofield RH: Revision shoulder arthroplasty with positive intraoperative cultures: The value of preoperative studies and intraoperative histology. *J Shoulder Elbow Surg* 2006;15(4):402-406.
9. Ince A, Seemann K, Frommelt L, Katzer A, Loehr JF: One-stage exchange shoulder arthroplasty for peri-prosthetic infection. *J Bone Joint Surg Br* 2005;87(6): 814-818.
10. Strickland JP, Sperling JW, Cofield RH: The results of two-stage re-implantation for infected shoulder replacement. *J Bone Joint Surg Br* 2008;90(4):460-465.
11. Ahrens P, Boileau P, Walch G: Anterior and posterior instability after unconstrained shoulder arthroplasty, in Walch G, Boileau P, Molé D, eds: *2000 Shoulder Prostheses: Two to Ten Year Follow-Up*. Montpellier, France, Sauramps Medical, 2001, pp 359-393.
12. Bohsali KI, Wirth MA, Rockwood CA Jr: Complications of total shoulder arthroplasty. *J Bone Joint Surg Am* 2006;88(10):2279-2292.
13. Sanchez-Sotelo J, Sperling JW, Rowland CM, Cofield RH: Instability after shoulder arthroplasty: Results of surgical treatment. *J Bone Joint Surg Am* 2003;85(4): 622-631.
14. Moeckel BH, Altchek DW, Warren RF, Wickiewicz TL, Dines DM: Instability of the shoulder after arthroplasty. *J Bone Joint Surg Am* 1993;75(4):492-497.
15. Walch G, Wall B, Mottier F: A multicenter study of 457 cases, in Walch G, Boileau P, Mole D, Favard L, Lévigne C, Sirveaux F, eds: *Reverse Shoulder Arthroplasty: Clinical Results, Complications, Revision*. Montpellier, France,

Sauramps Médical, 2006, pp 335-342.

16. Wirth MA, Rockwood CA Jr: Complications of total shoulder-replacement arthroplasty. *J Bone Joint Surg Am* 1996;78(4): 603-616.
17. Chin PY, Sperling JW, Cofield RH, Schleck C: Complications of total shoulder arthroplasty: Are they fewer or different? *J Shoulder Elbow Surg* 2006;15(1):19-22.
18. Cofield RH, Edgerton BC: Total shoulder arthroplasty: Complications and revision surgery. *Instr Course Lect* 1990;39:449-462.
19. Deprey F: Problèmes de coiffe après prothèse d'épaule, in Walch G, Boileau P, Molé D, eds: *2000 Shoulder Prostheses: Two to Ten Year Follow-Up*. Montpellier, France, Sauramps Medical, 2001, pp 393-399.
20. Young AA, Walch G, Pape G, Gohlke F, Favard L: Secondary rotator cuff dysfunction following total shoulder arthroplasty for primary glenohumeral osteoarthritis: Results of a multicenter study with more than five years of follow-up. *J Bone Joint Surg Am* 2012;94(8):685-693.
21. Miller BS, Joseph TA, Noonan TJ, Horan MP, Hawkins RJ: Rupture of the subscapularis tendon after shoulder arthroplasty: Diagnosis, treatment, and outcome. *J Shoulder Elbow Surg* 2005;14(5):492-496.
22. Elhassan B, Ozbaydar M, Massimini D, Diller D, Higgins L, Warner JJ: Transfer of pectoralis major for the treatment of irreparable tears of subscapularis: Does it work? *J Bone Joint Surg Br* 2008;90(8):1059-1065.
23. Betts HM, Abu-Rajab R, Nunn T, Brooksbank AJ: Total shoulder replacement in rheumatoid disease: A 16- to 23-year follow-up. *J Bone Joint Surg Br* 2009;91(9): 1197-1200.
24. Hattrup SJ, Cofield RH, Cha SS: Rotator cuff repair after shoulder replacement. *J Shoulder Elbow Surg* 2006;15(1):78-83.
25. Sneppen O, Fruensgaard S, Johannsen HV, Olsen BS, Sojbjerg JO, Andersen NH: Total shoulder replacement in rheumatoid arthritis: Proximal migration and loosening. *J Shoulder Elbow Surg* 1996;5(1):47-52.
26. Stewart MP, Kelly IG: Total shoulder replacement in rheumatoid disease: 7- to 13-year follow-up of 37 joints. *J Bone Joint Surg Br* 1997;79(1):68-72.
27. Edwards TB, Boulahia A, Kempf JF, Boileau P, Nemoz C, Walch G: The influence of rotator cuff disease on the results of shoulder arthroplasty for primary osteoarthritis: Results of a multicenter study. *J Bone Joint Surg Am* 2002; 84(12):2240-2248.
28. Miller SR, Bigliani LU: *Complications of Shoulder Surgery*. Baltimore, MD, Williams & Wilkins, 1993, pp 59-72.
29. Brems J: The glenoid component in total shoulder arthroplasty. *J Shoulder Elbow Surg* 1993;2(1): 47-54.
30. Franklin JL, Barrett WP, Jackins SE, Matsen FA III: Glenoid loosening in total shoulder arthroplasty: Association with rotator cuff deficiency. *J Arthroplasty* 1988;3(1):39-46.
31. Cheung EV, Sperling JW, Cofield RH: Revision shoulder arthroplasty for glenoid component loosening. *J Shoulder Elbow Surg* 2008;17(3):371-375.

12

Proximal Humeral Fractures: Internal Fixation

Daniel Aaron, MD
Joshua Shatsky, MD
Juan Carlos S. Paredes, MD
Chunyan Jiang, MD, PhD
Bradford O. Parsons, MD
Evan L. Flatow, MD

Abstract

Fractures of the proximal humerus are common injuries that are increasing in incidence as the population ages. These fractures are often treated nonsurgically; however, surgery is indicated if displacement, concurrent dislocation, or unacceptable alignment is present. Knowledge of the anatomic and physiologic characteristics of the proximal humerus and shoulder joint and familiarity with the available fixation elements will help surgeons make informed and patient-specific decisions regarding treatment. Reduction and internal fixation of proximal humeral fractures has expanding indications in comparison with arthroplasty, in part because of improvements in fixation technology and a better understanding of anatomy and physiology. The outcomes of proximal humeral fractures managed with percutaneous pinning, open reduction and locked-plate fixation, and intramedullary fixation are being actively investigated.

Instr Course Lect 2013;62:143-154.

Fractures of the proximal part of the humerus represent 4% to 5% of all fractures.[1,2] Older individuals are more likely to sustain these injuries, with 71% of proximal humeral fractures occurring in patients older than 60 years.[3,4] As the population ages, such data suggest a potential increase in the total number of proximal humeral fractures. Some authors have estimated a threefold increase in the next 30 years.[5] Neer[6] reported that most proximal humeral fractures are minimally displaced or nondisplaced, allowing nonsurgical treatment to yield high rates of union and functional restoration; however, a recent multicenter study noted that 64% were displaced.[7] Management strategies for displaced fractures have recently evolved because of advances in technology and improved understanding of pathophysiology. Unless contraindications exist, surgery, with the use of various forms of internal fixation, is the recommended general strategy for managing displaced proximal humeral fractures. Internal fixation includes pins, screws, tension-band wires, plate and screw constructs, heavy sutures, and intramedullary devices. Arthroplasty, which has also undergone dramatic advances in recent years, is an additional option. Each technique has particular indications, and each has its own set of potential complications. Familiarity with all of these techniques is essential for the practitioner caring for fractures of the proximal part of the humerus.

Dr. Parsons or an immediate family member is a member of a speakers' bureau or has made paid presentations on behalf of Zimmer and Arthrex; serves as a paid consultant to or is an employee of Zimmer and Arthrex; and has received research or institutional support from Wyeth. Dr. Flatow or an immediate family member serves as a board member, owner, officer, or committee member of the American Shoulder and Elbow Surgeons and the Arthroscopy Association of North America; has received royalties from Innomed and Zimmer; is a member of a speakers' bureau or has made paid presentations on behalf of Zimmer; serves as an unpaid consultant to Zimmer; and has received research or institutional support from Wyeth. None of the following authors nor any immediate family member has received anything of value from or has stock or stock options in a commercial company or institution related directly or indirectly to the subject of this chapter: Dr. Aaron, Dr. Shatsky, Dr. Paredes, and Dr. Jiang.

Anatomy

To understand the pathophysiology of fractures of the proximal part of the humerus, knowledge of the osseous, muscular, and vascular anatomy is imperative. The commonly used classification schemes rely on this anatomy, as do the deforming forces that must be overcome by reduction maneuvers and fixation. Prognostic information is a direct correlate of the specific sites of anatomic disruption. The proximal part of the humerus initially had a primary ossification center and two secondary ossification centers (greater and lesser tuberosities) that fuse, but as Codman first recognized, fractures tend to occur along these physeal lines, even with skeletal maturity.[6]

The supraspinatus, infraspinatus, and teres minor muscles attach to the greater tuberosity and exert abduction and external rotation forces. The subscapularis tendon attaches to the lesser tuberosity and exerts a medial and internal rotation vector. The deltoid, pectoralis major, and latissimus dorsi muscles all insert distal to the tuberosities. The pectoralis major muscle is a strong deforming force, and it is important to recognize this during reduction maneuvers and when fracture fixation is selected and placed.[8]

The vascular anatomy of the proximal part of the humerus is complex and has implications for the risk of the development of osteonecrosis of the humeral head after a fracture. The principal vascular supply to the humeral head is via the anterolateral branch of the anterior humeral circumflex artery, which arises from the axillary artery.[9,10] The anterior circumflex system courses at the inferior border of the subscapularis tendon near its insertion to the lesser tuberosity and then underneath the biceps tendon to penetrate bone at the superomedial border of the greater tuberosity.[9,11,12] A relatively minor segment of the posteromedial aspect of the humeral head is directly supplied by the posterior circumflex artery.[9] There is a rich network of other arteries, including the profunda brachii and thoracoacromial, subscapular, and suprascapular arteries,[10] that can sustain the humeral head even in the event of injury to both circumflex systems or axillary artery disruption.[13,14] An injury in which both tuberosities are fractured with a concomitant metaphyseal fracture places the patient at high risk for osteonecrosis of the humeral head.[15] The treating surgeon must be aware of this risk to make educated decisions about fixation or arthroplasty, the importance of anatomic reductions, and to appropriately counsel the patient.

Classification

The most widely used classification scheme for proximal humeral fractures is the Neer classification system.[6,16,17] In this system, the humeral articular surface, greater tuberosity, lesser tuberosity, and humeral shaft are considered the parts of the proximal aspect of the humerus. A part is considered to be displaced if it is angulated 45° or more or displaced 1 cm or more. Recently, a valgus-impacted subset of four-part fractures was added.[18] This is an important addition because valgus-impacted fractures retain an intact medial calcar hinge, which makes them relatively stable biomechanically and likely to have a preserved blood supply to the humeral head. Therefore, percutaneous fixation is a viable option and the prognosis is good.[8] Head-splitting fractures and large (40%) humeral impression fractures compose a separate category, for which arthroplasty is considered.

The AO classification system is based on the vascular supply to the humeral head.[19] It consists of three main types: extra-articular unifocal, extra-articular bifocal, and intra-articular. Each type contains three subtypes based on the severity of the injury as indicated by displacement, comminution, or glenohumeral joint dislocation. This scheme is more complex than the Neer classification system, but there is no evidence that it is more reliable.[17,20]

Evaluation

Evaluation of the patient with a fracture of the proximal part of the humerus begins with a history and a physical examination. Relevant medical comorbidities must be identified. A social history should be obtained to assess the patient's level of activity and demand on the shoulder, as well as his or her expectations after treatment. The physical examination should begin with an assessment of the skin condition and the neurovascular status. Motor function of the deltoid muscle should include voluntary isometric contraction of all three heads. Palpation of the distal pulses and careful inspection for signs of arterial injury should be performed acutely. Any question about vascular compromise should prompt Doppler examination and, if necessary, angiography.

Imaging assessment begins with a standard series of radiographs, including AP, true AP, axillary lateral, and scapular-Y radiographs of the proximal humeral fracture. AP radiographs, with the arm in internal and external rotation, may better characterize tuberosity fractures or occult fractures of the surgical neck. CT can provide additional information for both classification and preoperative planning, particularly with a fracture of the lesser tuberosity.[21,22] CT is also helpful in fractures with articular surface involvement and for the enumeration of fracture fragments (**Figure 1**). The number of fragments in the setting of severe

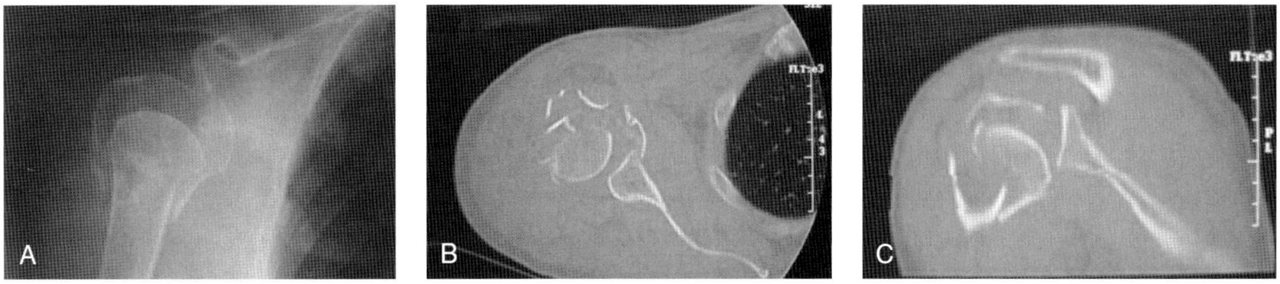

Figure 1 AP radiograph (**A**), axial CT scan (**B**), and coronal CT scan (**C**) of a comminuted head-splitting fracture.

comminution is underestimated by standard radiography in more than 60% of cases.[23]

MRI is not part of the routine evaluation of proximal humeral fractures. Although traumatic rotator cuff tearing at the time of a proximal humeral fracture is rare, some authors have recommended consideration of MRI.[24] Rutten et al[25] recently described an ultrasonographic sign that reliably detected occult proximal humeral fractures. The so-called double-line sign was present in 93% of the patients with occult fractures.

Surgical Indications

Many proximal humeral fractures with minimal displacement are amenable to nonsurgical treatment. Displaced two-, three-, and four-part fractures are indications for surgical management to optimize anatomic healing and improve functional outcome. Displacement of the tuberosities above the humeral head, as in three- or four-part fractures or in varus two-part fractures, often yields a poor functional outcome, even if healing occurs nonsurgically. Surgery is aimed at restoring the proximal humeral anatomy, including the neck-shaft angle, version, and tuberosity-to-head and tuberosity-to-tuberosity relationships. Bone-preserving options include percutaneous techniques, intramedullary nailing, and locked plating.

Percutaneous Fixation

Indications

Percutaneous fixation with pins is a minimally invasive strategy with a theoretically lower rate of osteonecrosis than that with open fixation. However, it offers less stability than other forms of fixation and is technically demanding. It is advocated for unstable two-part surgical neck fractures but also has a role in more complex three-part and valgus-impacted four-part fractures[8] (**Figure 2**). This form of fixation is generally reserved for patients with good bone quality; minimal comminution, particularly involving the tuberosity; and an intact medial calcar. It is also essential that patients are compliant with postoperative follow-up and immobilization requirements.[8]

Technique

A detailed description of the percutaneous pinning technique has been previously published.[26] Pearls of management are discussed in this chapter. Percutaneous techniques should be performed within 5 to 7 days of injury to avoid difficulties associated with early callous and scarring.

Proper setup and timing of surgery is critical to the outcome. The patient is placed in a supine or modified beach-chair position on a radiolucent table, with the shoulder and arm off the edge of the table. Good AP and axillary radiographs must be ensured before skin preparation. After the C-arm fluoroscopic image intensifier is properly positioned, sterile preparation and draping of the shoulder is performed.

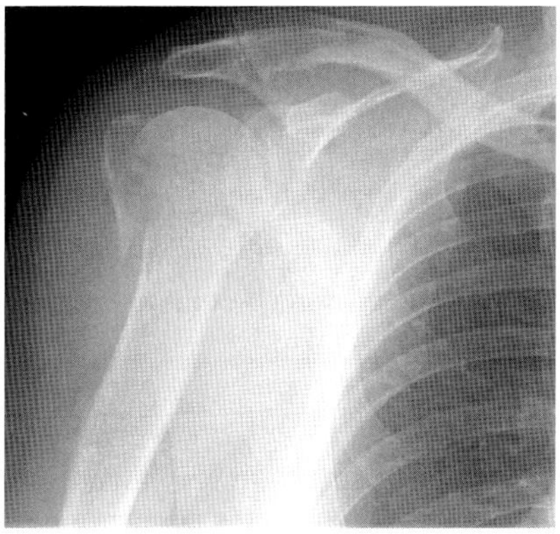

Figure 2 AP radiograph of a valgus-impacted four-part fracture.

Careful pin placement is essential to avoid neurovascular injury. Lateral pins should be distal to the anterior branch of the axillary nerve but proximal to the deltoid insertion to avoid the radial nerve.[27] The musculocutaneous nerve, cephalic vein, and biceps tendon are at risk from the placement of the anterior pins.

Reduction of the humeral shaft under the humeral head is done by applying longitudinal traction with a posterolateral force to the arm. If this does not reduce the fracture, a 2.5-mm terminally threaded pin inserted through the greater tuberosity into the humeral head can be used as a so-called joystick. Another reduction technique is to use a small so-called reduction

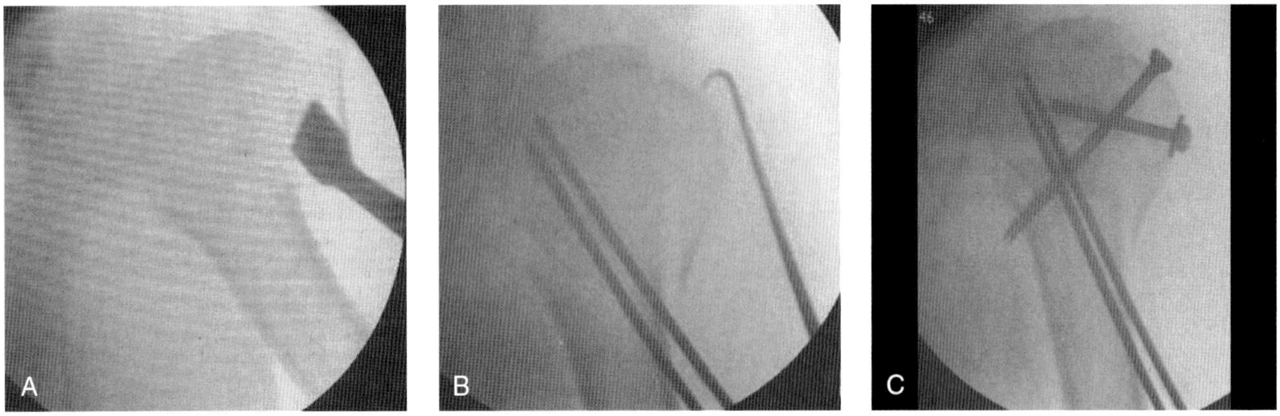

Figure 3 Use of an elevator (**A**) and a hook (**B**) in fracture reduction during percutaneous pinning. **C**, Final construct after percutaneous pinning.

portal to manipulate the fragments with instruments such as elevators, tamps, or hooks[28] (**Figure 3, A** and **B**).

After adequate reduction is achieved, a 2.5-mm terminally threaded pin is driven from the lateral metaphysis into the humeral head. As the pin nears the articular surface of the humeral head, driving it in by hand with the use of a T-handled chuck rather than a power driver provides better tactile feedback and minimizes the risk of penetrating the articular cartilage. Insertion should also be done under image guidance to further minimize the risk of pin penetration. If penetration occurs, the pin must be removed and a completely new track created—if the pin is simply partially withdrawn, it may migrate and penetrate over time. When inserting the pin, the surgeon must recognize that the humeral head is retroverted 20° to 40°. Two or three antegrade pins in a parallel configuration are usually adequate for fixation of the humeral head to the shaft, although a retrograde pin from the greater tuberosity to the humeral shaft is sometimes used to augment stability.[29,30] Fixation of the tuberosities in displaced three- and four-part fractures is achieved with 3.5- or 4.0-mm cannulated screws placed antegrade from the tuberosity either bicortically into the calcar (for the greater tuberosity) or unicortically into the head (for the lesser tuberosity). Pins and screws are buried underneath the skin (**Figure 3, C**). The arm is immobilized for 3 to 4 weeks, and the pins are removed after 4 to 6 weeks.

Prognosis and Outcomes

Functional outcome is correlated with the adequacy of reduction and the residual deformity. Union rates are high, and good results should be expected with two- and three-part fractures.[28,31,32] If acceptable alignment cannot be obtained at the time of surgery, open reduction is recommended.

Complications

Malunion

Malunion rates have been reported to be as high as 28%.[31] Patients with osteoporotic bone and those who have fracture comminution have the highest risk. Varus angulation of the humeral head with posterosuperior displacement of the greater tuberosity is the most common deformity.[8]

Pin Migration and/or Loosening

Despite the use of terminally threaded pins, the migration of pins occurs in up to one third of patients.[28,31] Migration into the chest and other vital structures has been described.[8] Weekly evaluation and radiographs are performed to monitor fracture reduction and pin alignment. Pins that become loose or migrate should be removed before 4 weeks.

Pin Tract Infection

Superficial infections are treated with local wound care, antibiotics, and pin removal. Ensuring that the pins remain below the skin lessens the chance of infection. It is important to be aware of deeper infections, including osteomyelitis.

Osteonecrosis

Osteonecrosis of the humeral head is most likely related to the magnitude of the injury, with four-part fractures associated with a prevalence of osteonecrosis in up to 28% of patients.[28,31,33] Kralinger et al[34] reported a substantially lower rate of osteonecrosis after percutaneous pinning compared with open reduction and internal fixation.

Harrison et al[26] reported on a series of 27 patients treated with percutaneous pin fixation, with follow-up at a minimum of 3 years after surgery. Osteonecrosis was reported in 26% of the patients at an average follow-up of 50 months (range, 11 to 101 months), including 5 of 10 patients (50%) who had four-part fractures, 2 of 12 patients (17%) who had three-part fractures, and none of the patients who had two-part fractures. The mean American Shoulder and Elbow Surgeons (ASES) score was 65 for patients with osteonecrosis and 84 for patients without osteonecrosis.

Neurovascular Injury

Despite cadaver studies demonstrating potential neurovascular injury with percutaneous fixation, clinical rates are low.[27,35,36] A good knowledge of anatomy and normal variants is essential to prevent complications.

Intramedullary Nailing

Indications

Intramedullary nails are accepted as an effective method to treat two-part surgical neck fractures, although their use in more complex proximal humeral fractures has varied.[37-39] Small incisions, closed reduction, and excellent nail-bone purchase in osteoporotic bone are advantages.

Gradl et al[40] treated displaced proximal humeral fractures with an antegrade nail (Targon PH; Aesculap, Tuttlingen, Germany) and had better functional results in patients with two- and three-part fractures than in those with four-part fractures. The published results have varied.[41-45] The intramedullary nail may be rigid and locked or flexible and unlocked. Locked intramedullary nails are axially and rotationally stable, whereas flexible intramedullary nails are not. Shoulder impairment and iatrogenic fractures are risks with locked intramedullary nails.[46-48] The advantages of flexible intramedullary nails are relatively little blood loss, no soft-tissue stripping at the fracture site, minimal muscular trauma, and a low risk of radial nerve injury. The disadvantages of flexible intramedullary nails, particularly among patients with osteoporotic bone, are restricted early motion and delayed physiotherapy because of the relatively low construct stability.[49]

Technique

Rigid Intramedullary Nail

The patient is placed supine in the beach-chair position, and the image intensifier device is positioned to ensure that AP and axillary radiographs of the affected shoulder can be obtained intraoperatively.

A 4-cm longitudinal incision is made anterolateral to the acromion. The deltoid is split from the anterolateral corner of the acromion distally for 4 cm. The humeral head fragment is exposed, and the head fragment is reduced with either a 2.5-mm Kirschner wire or a Steinmann pin under fluoroscopic guidance. For displaced four-part fractures, 1.25-mm Kirschner wires can be used for temporary fragment reduction. A 1-cm incision is made in the supraspinatus tendon in line with its fibers. An awl or a guide pin is used to enter the medullary canal. For the straight 150-mm Targon PH nail (Aesculap), the recommended entry point is approximately 8 mm medial to the cartilage-bone transitional zone at the sulcus, between the humeral head and the greater tuberosity.[50] For the 6° angled Stryker T2 Proximal Humerus nail (Stryker, Kiel, Germany), the recommended entry point is 10 mm posterior to the anterior edge of the supraspinatus and at the junction of the greater tuberosity and the articular cartilage.[50] The entry point for the proximal humeral nail (Synthes, West Chester, Pennsylvania) is just lateral to the articular margin in the sulcus between the greater tuberosity and the articular margin.[38] The entry point of the intramedullary nail is important; however, cortical apposition may be lost after inserting the nail because of the specific humeral pathology and anatomic characteristics.[50] The medullary canal is reamed. The nail is inserted manually with its targeting device. The depth of nail insertion may vary according to the manufacturer and design. Precise orientation of the targeting device is necessary to avoid injury to the long head of the biceps and neurovascular structures.[51] Fixation screws are inserted. This chapter's authors recommend placement of all of the proximal screws, particularly if the tuberosities are fractured. The rotator cuff tendon and deltoid are repaired, and active-assisted to active shoulder motion is begun on the third postoperative day.

Flexible Intramedullary Nails

Retrograde flexible intramedullary nailing uses more than one 2-mm-diameter, curved, flexible nail to achieve multiple-point intramedullary fixation. The fracture pattern and the diameter of the medullary canal dictate the number of nails that are inserted. Usually, three, four, or five nails are necessary to obtain sufficient stability. After closed reduction has been achieved, the nails are advanced from distal to proximal from an entry point 3 cm proximal to the olecranon tip under fluoroscopic guidance to the medial half of the humeral head, diverging in the subchondral region.[37]

Pendulum movements of the shoulder are started on the first postoperative day, with mobilization of the elbow joint. Passive movement exercises may be initiated the third week, and active exercises may be started from the fourth week onward.

Prognosis and Outcomes

When appropriate patients are chosen, careful placement of the nail entry point and effective postoperative rehabilitation lead to a successful result.[38,40,50]

Rigid Intramedullary Nail

Several recent cohort studies have reported 100% union rates, low complication rates, and favorable subjective outcomes with rigid intramedullary nailing.[38,52,53] Three recent comparisons of rigid intramedullary nailing and locked plate fixation did not reveal a substantial difference in objective or subjective outcomes.[54-56] One study showed a trend of more complications and lower relative Constant scores with nail fixation, but this did not reach significance.[55] Another showed a higher rate of complications but better outcome scores with locked plate fixation at 1 year; however, no difference was detected between the locked plate group and the nail fixation group at 3 years.[56]

Matziolis et al[37] found no significant difference in absolute Constant scores between Zifko nailing and fixed-angle plating for two-part fractures. The score for the subitem "activity of daily life" was significantly higher in the plate group than in the Zifko group.

Complications

Nonunion

In a systematic review by Lanting et al[39] (66 articles with results on 2,653 fractures), nonunion was as high as 4% in two- and three-part fractures.

Nail Migration

Verbruggen and Stapert[48] reported rates of flexible nail migration as high as 29% and rates of fracture distraction of up to 41%.

Malunion

Malunion is one of the commonly reported complications, and the rate of postoperative varus deformity of the humeral neck has been reported to be as high as 7.7% to 37%.[39,54,57]

Nerve Injury

The locking screws that are used with the nails may pose an injury risk to the axillary nerve.[51] Closed reduction and implant insertion place the radial nerve at risk. Blunt dissection and the use of protection sleeves during drilling and screw insertion can prevent this injury.

Rotator Cuff Injury

Insertion of the nail through the rotator cuff tendon causes different degrees of injury to the supraspinatus tendon that can lead to shoulder pain.[38,46,52] Care should be taken in the dissection of the supraspinatus tendon and in its meticulous repair.

Open Reduction and Locked Plate Fixation

Background

Prior to the advent of locked plating, hemiarthroplasty had been advocated for most three- and four-part fractures. Anatomic proximal humeral locking plates represent an advance in construct stability and have a lower rate of implant failure compared with unlocked plating.[58,59] However, the complication rate remains substantial. Continued innovation in technology (such as polyaxial systems and suture eyelets) and technique (such as structural allograft and rotator cuff sutures) are aimed at improving current outcomes.

The importance of medial cortical support has been shown with the locking construct; the screw buttressing the inferomedial portion of the proximal segment aids in medial column support.[60] Restoration of medial calcar and medial support plays an important role in maintaining reduction.[61] This screw functions as a so-called kickstand and is beneficial in maintaining the stability and ultimate reduction of the construct. Additionally, anatomic or slightly impacted reductions aid in construct stability.[61]

Other constructs have attempted to use pegs as alternatives to screws to prevent articular perforation. Schumer et al[62] found no significant difference in joint perforation between the two constructs. Newer locking constructs offer polyaxial locking mechanisms. In a comparison of monoaxial and polyaxial constructs, the polyaxial system had equal biomechanical performance with the advantage of more head fixation.[63]

In a comparison of a locked plate and locked nail, plates were found to be stronger in torsion, equivalent in axial stiffness,[64] and superior in varus bending.[65] In comparison with proximal humeral blade plates, locking plates provided better torsional fatigue resistance and stiffness.[66]

Proximal humeral fracture fixation fails because of bending and rotational moments.[60-67] Because locking plates are biomechanically more stable than the tested constructs under these circumstances, the added stability may reduce the fracture failure rate.

Indications

Most displaced two-, three-, or four-part fractures of the proximal part of the humerus can be treated with locked plates. Fracture-dislocations and head-splitting fractures in patients older than 40 years are relative contraindications to plate fixation. Both are higher-energy injuries associated with the risk of osteonecrosis of the humeral head; however, in younger patients in whom joint-preserving strategies are most appropriate, head-splitting and high-energy fractures may be fixed with a locked plate (**Figure 4**). Few other contraindications exist, except prohibitive medical comorbidities, pediatric fractures, or patterns of injury amenable to less invasive techniques.[68,69]

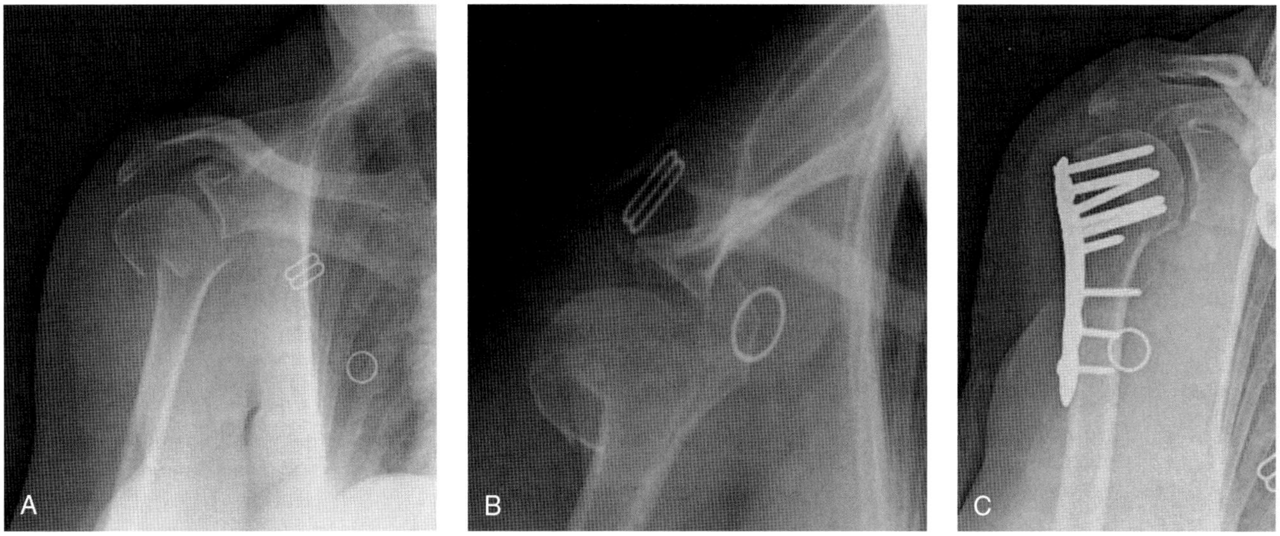

Figure 4 AP radiographs of a comminuted proximal humeral fracture with a head split made preoperatively (**A** and **B**) and immediately after open reduction and locked-plate fixation (**C**).

Proximal Humeral Exposures

Multiple exposures for the proximal part of the humerus, including the classic deltopectoral, anterolateral deltoid-splitting, and two-incision approaches, have been described.[9,70-73] Each has advantages and disadvantages. The anterolateral and two-incision approaches were developed with the primary purposes of improving visualization, minimizing soft-tissue dissection, and allowing more direct plate application, which may permit improved preservation of the blood supply. However, these approaches may place the axillary nerve at risk.[72-77] Conversely, the classic deltopectoral approach is the only truly internervous approach and is the most widely used exposure. Controversy exists as to what approach to use for locking plate fixation.[9,71-74] This chapter's authors use the deltopectoral approach because of its extensile nature and long track record of safety.

Deltopectoral Approach

The deltopectoral approach uses the internervous plane between the deltoid (axillary nerve) and the pectoralis major (medial and lateral pectoral nerves).[70] The patient can be positioned in the beach-chair position or supine, depending on the available equipment and the surgeon preference. The skin incision is approximately 10 to 15 cm long, beginning at the coracoid and angled distally to the deltoid tuberosity.

The cephalic vein is identified in the deltopectoral interval and is usually mobilized laterally to protect the many deltoid branches;[78] however, it may be taken medially as well. The clavipectoral fascia is opened, and the conjoint tendon is retracted medially. Deltoid or pectoralis major detachment is not needed, and no more than one fifth of each should be released.[79]

Continuity of the axillary nerve can be tested with the so-called tug test at the inferior border of the subscapularis and beneath the deltoid.[80] The distance from the coracoid to the point of entrance of the main musculocutaneous nerve trunk into the coracobrachialis averages 5.6 cm (range, 3 to 8 cm).[81]

The rotator cuff interval may be incised at the level of penetration of the biceps tendon to mobilize the tuberosities and to allow visualization and palpation of the articular surfaces. The long head of the biceps tendon is uncovered in its groove and is followed proximally to its insertion on the superior aspect of the glenoid. The tendon may be tenotomized and tenodesed to the pectoralis major, removing a source of postoperative pain.[82] It is important to avoid excessive dissection and cauterization in the bicipital groove to preserve the ascending branch of the anterior humeral circumflex artery.

Reduction

Control of the rotator cuff is the most important step to reduce and control the multiple fracture fragments. Nonabsorbable sutures are placed in the subscapularis to control the lesser tuberosity and in the supraspinatus and infraspinatus to control the greater tuberosity and humeral head. Elevators, if necessary, are placed in the fracture planes to disimpact the fragments and correct varus or valgus positioning of the head. The tuberosities are reduced to their anatomic position with respect to the head and the metaphysis and shaft. Tuberosity reduction is a key predictor of functional outcome.[83,84] If there is insufficient metaphyseal bone, the surgeon may place a fibular strut allograft within the intramedullary canal and impact the head onto it to provide control and structural support.[85]

Fixation

Locking plates have a low profile, a hole for a kickstand screw to buttress the medial calcar, divergent proximal locking screws, and eyelets to allow passage of rotator cuff sutures through the plate.[68] The plate should be placed lateral to the bicipital groove, 1.5 to 2 cm distal to the greater tuberosity (2 to 3 cm from the superior aspect of the head). If the plate is placed too high, there is a risk of impingement. If it is placed too low, head fixation can be compromised. Proximal screws should remain short of the subchondral bone to reduce the risk of perforation with humeral head collapse. Rotator cuff sutures are then tied to the plate to neutralize the displacing force of the cuff muscles and offload the proximal screws. Screw penetration into the joint is a risk, and rotator cuff sutures add additional stability and are believed to stabilize the fracture enough to allow early motion and decrease fixation failure.[86-88] After completion of fixation, fluoroscopy should be used, and the humeral articular surface should be palpated to ensure that no screws violate the joint.

DVD **Video 12.1:** Proximal Humeral Fractures: Open Reduction and Internal Fixation With a Plate. Bradford O. Parsons, MD (20 min)

Rehabilitation

Postoperative rehabilitation is a balance between early motion and not disrupting the fixation.[89] Initially, the arm is placed in a sling. Active range of motion of elbow, wrist, and hand, as well as pendulum exercises may begin on the first postoperative day. Gentle passive range of motion of the shoulder is started as soon as the patient is comfortable. Active shoulder motion should begin at 4 to 6 weeks, and strengthening exercises should not be started until 12 weeks.

Results and Complications

The results of locked plate fixation are evolving, but the overall complication rate remains high.[86,90-94] The most common complications are screw joint perforation (13.7% to 23%) and osteonecrosis (3.1% to 16.4%). The rate of revision surgery has been reported to range from 13% to 26.7%. However, in a study comparing the functional outcomes of patients with three- and four-part proximal humeral fractures treated with locked plating or with a hemiarthroplasty, the University of California at Los Angeles shoulder score, the Constant score, patient satisfaction, and motion were superior in the locked-plate group.[95]

Strategies to augment locked plate fixation and minimize complications are being developed. Improved results and decreased complications were detailed in a series by Ricchetti et al[69] in which the authors supplemented plate-and-screw fixation with suturing of the rotator cuff tendons to the plate. Hettrich et al[96] used endosteal fibular strut allografts or medial semitubular plates and reported only one substantial loss of reduction and no implant failures or screw cutout. Egol et al[97] used calcium phosphate cement to prevent settling and screw cutout, and less humeral settling was seen.

Locked plating has been a major advance in the treatment of displaced proximal humeral fractures and has allowed many more fractures to be successfully treated with a joint-preserving method instead of arthroplasty. Complications remain substantial, but the techniques and technology of proximal humeral locked plating are areas of active research.

Summary

Percutaneous, intramedullary, and locked-plate fixation can be reliable fixation strategies for proximal humeral fractures with the correct indications and careful patient selection, which are based on an understanding of the anatomy and biomechanics of the injury. Each method has advantages and disadvantages that the surgeon must consider and individualize for a particular patient. Regardless of the technique selected, meticulous surgical technique and anatomic reduction are essential. Careful postoperative rehabilitation is essential. Each method also has specific complications, which may be mitigated as techniques and technology continue to evolve.

References

1. Buhr AJ, Cooke AM: Fracture patterns. *Lancet* 1959;1(7072): 531-536.
2. Court-Brown CM, Garg A, McQueen MM: The epidemiology of proximal humeral fractures. *Acta Orthop Scand* 2001;72(4): 365-371.
3. Lind T, Krøner K, Jensen J: The epidemiology of fractures of the proximal humerus. *Arch Orthop Trauma Surg* 1989;108(5): 285-287.
4. Horak J, Nilsson BE: Epidemiology of fracture of the upper end of the humerus. *Clin Orthop Relat Res* 1975;112:250-253.
5. Kannus P, Palvanen M, Niemi S, Parkkari J, Järvinen M, Vuori I: Increasing number and incidence of osteoporotic fractures of the

proximal humerus in elderly people. *BMJ* 1996;313(7064):1051-1052.

6. Neer CS II: Displaced proximal humeral fractures: I. Classification and evaluation. *J Bone Joint Surg Am* 1970;52(6):1077-1089.
7. Tamai K, Ishige N, Kuroda S, et al: Four-segment classification of proximal humeral fractures revisited: A multicenter study on 509 cases. *J Shoulder Elbow Surg* 2009;18(6):845-850.
8. Magovern B, Ramsey ML: Percutaneous fixation of proximal humerus fractures. *Orthop Clin North Am* 2008;39(4):405-416, v.
9. Gerber C, Schneeberger AG, Vinh TS: The arterial vascularization of the humeral head: An anatomical study. *J Bone Joint Surg Am* 1990; 72(10):1486-1494.
10. Laing PG: The arterial supply of the adult humerus. *J Bone Joint Surg Am* 1956;38(5):1105-1116.
11. Brooks CH, Revell WJ, Heatley FW: Vascularity of the humeral head after proximal humeral fractures: An anatomical cadaver study. *J Bone Joint Surg Br* 1993; 75(1):132-136.
12. Netter FH: *The CIBA Collection of Medical Illustrations.* Summit, NJ, CIBA-Geigy, 1987, vol 8, pp 20-74.
13. Fitzgerald JF, Keates J: False aneurysm as a late complication of anterior dislocation of the shoulder. *Ann Surg* 1975;181(6): 785-786.
14. Gerber C, Lambert SM, Hoogewoud HM: Absence of avascular necrosis of the humeral head after post-traumatic rupture of the anterior and posterior humeral circumflex arteries: A case report. *J Bone Joint Surg Am* 1996;78(8): 1256-1259.
15. Neer CS II: Displaced proximal humeral fractures: II. Treatment of three-part and four-part displacement. *J Bone Joint Surg Am* 1970;52(6):1090-1103.
16. Sidor ML, Zuckerman JD, Lyon T, Koval K, Cuomo F, Schoenberg N: The Neer classification system for proximal humeral fractures: An assessment of interobserver reliability and intraobserver reproducibility. *J Bone Joint Surg Am* 1993;75(12):1745-1750.
17. Siebenrock KA, Gerber C: The reproducibility of classification of fractures of the proximal end of the humerus. *J Bone Joint Surg Am* 1993;75(12):1751-1755.
18. Neer CS II: Four-segment classification of proximal humeral fractures: Purpose and reliable use. *J Shoulder Elbow Surg* 2002;11(4): 389-400.
19. Müeller ME: The principle of classification, in Müeller ME, Allgöwer M, Schneider R, Willenegger H, eds: *Manual of Internal Fixation: Techniques Recommended by the AO-ASIF Group*, ed 2. New York, NY, Springer-Verlag, 1995, pp 118-125.
20. Sjödén GO, Movin T, Güntner P, et al: Poor reproducibility of classification of proximal humeral fractures: Additional CT of minor value. *Acta Orthop Scand* 1997; 68(3):239-242.
21. Edelson G, Kelly I, Vigder F, Reis ND: A three-dimensional classification for fractures of the proximal humerus. *J Bone Joint Surg Br* 2004;86(3):413-425.
22. Mora Guix JM, Gonzalez AS, Brugalla JV, Carril EC, Baños FG: Proposed protocol for reading images of humeral head fractures. *Clin Orthop Relat Res* 2006;448: 225-233.
23. Haapamaki VV, Kiuru MJ, Koskinen SK: Multidetector CT in shoulder fractures. *Emerg Radiol* 2004;11(2):89-94.
24. Gallo RA, Altman DT, Altman GT: Assessment of rotator cuff tendons after proximal humerus fractures: Is preoperative imaging necessary? *J Trauma* 2009;66(3): 951-953.
25. Rutten MJ, Jager GJ, de Waal Malefijt MC, Blickman JG: Double line sign: A helpful sonographic sign to detect occultfractures of the proximal humerus. *Eur Radiol* 2007;17(3):762-767.
26. Harrison AK, Gruson KI, Zmistowski B, et al: Intermediate outcomes following percutaneous fixation of proximal humeral fractures. *J Bone Joint Surg Am* 2012; 94(13):1223-1228.
27. Liu KY, Chen TH, Shyu JF, Wang ST, Liu JY, Chou PH: Anatomic study of the axillary nerve in a Chinese cadaveric population: Correlation of the course of the nerve with proximal humeral fixation with intramedullary nail or external skeletal fixation. *Arch Orthop Trauma Surg* 2011; 131(5):669-674.
28. Keener JD, Parsons BO, Flatow EL, Rogers K, Williams GR, Galatz LM: Outcomes after percutaneous reduction and fixation of proximal humeral fractures. *J Shoulder Elbow Surg* 2007;16(3): 330-338.
29. Jiang C, Zhu Y, Wang M, Rong G: Biomechanical comparison of different pin configurations during percutaneous pinning for the treatment of proximal humeral fractures. *J Shoulder Elbow Surg* 2007;16(2):235-239.
30. Durigan A Jr, Barbieri CH, Mazzer N, Shimano AC: Two-part surgical neck fractures of the humerus: Mechanical analysis of the fixation with four Shanz-type threaded pins in four different assemblies. *J Shoulder Elbow Surg* 2005;14(1):96-102.
31. Calvo E, de Miguel I, de la Cruz JJ, López-Martín N: Percutaneous fixation of displaced proximal humeral fractures: Indications based on the correlation between clinical and radiographic results.

J Shoulder Elbow Surg 2007;16(6): 774-781.

32. Jaberg H, Warner JJ, Jakob RP: Percutaneous stabilization of unstable fractures of the humerus. *J Bone Joint Surg Am* 1992;74(4): 508-515.
33. Hertel R, Hempfing A, Stiehler M, Leunig M: Predictors of humeral head ischemia after intracapsular fracture of the proximal humerus. *J Shoulder Elbow Surg* 2004;13(4):427-433.
34. Kralinger F, Irenberger A, Lechner C, Wambacher M, Golser K, Sperner G: Comparison of open versus percutaneous treatment for humeral head fracture. *Unfallchirurg* 2006;109(5):406-410.
35. Kamineni S, Ankem H, Sanghavi S: Anatomical considerations for percutaneous proximal humeral fracture fixation. *Injury* 2004; 35(11):1133-1136.
36. Rowles DJ, McGrory JE: Percutaneous pinning of the proximal part of the humerus: An anatomic study. *J Bone Joint Surg Am* 2001; 83(11):1695-1699.
37. Matziolis D, Kaeaeb M, Zandi SS, Perka C, Greiner S: Surgical treatment of two-part fractures of the proximal humerus: Comparison of fixed-angle plate osteosynthesis and Zifko nails. *Injury* 2010; 41(10):1041-1046.
38. Zhu Y, Lu Y, Wang M, Jiang C: Treatment of proximal humeral fracture with a proximal humeral nail. *J Shoulder Elbow Surg* 2010; 19(2):297-302.
39. Lanting B, MacDermid J, Drosdowech D, Faber KJ: Proximal humeral fractures: A systematic review of treatment modalities. *J Shoulder Elbow Surg* 2008;17(1): 42-54.
40. Gradl G, Dietze A, Arndt D, et al: Angular and sliding stable antegrade nailing (Targon PH) for the treatment of proximal humeral fractures. *Arch Orthop Trauma Surg* 2007;127(10):937-944.
41. Koike Y, Komatsuda T, Sato K: Internal fixation of proximal humeral fractures with a Polarus humeral nail. *J Orthop Traumatol* 2008;9(3):135-139.
42. Lin J: Effectiveness of locked nailing for displaced three-part proximal humeral fractures. *J Trauma* 2006;61(2):363-374.
43. Park JY, An JW, Oh JH: Open intramedullary nailing with tension band and locking sutures for proximal humeral fracture: Hot air balloon technique. *J Shoulder Elbow Surg* 2006;15(5):594-601.
44. Agel J, Jones CB, Sanzone AG, Camuso M, Henley MB: Treatment of proximal humeral fractures with Polarus nail fixation. *J Shoulder Elbow Surg* 2004;13(2): 191-195.
45. Bernard J, Charalambides C, Aderinto J, Mok D: Early failure of intramedullary nailing for proximal humeral fractures. *Injury* 2000;31(10):789-792.
46. Lin J, Inoue N, Valdevit A, Hang YS, Hou SM, Chao EY: Biomechanical comparison of antegrade and retrograde nailing of humeral shaft fracture. *Clin Orthop Relat Res* 1998;351:203-213.
47. Chao TC, Chou WY, Chung JC, Hsu CJ: Humeral shaft fractures treated by dynamic compression plates, Ender nails and interlocking nails. *Int Orthop* 2005;29(2): 88-91.
48. Verbruggen JP, Stapert JW: Humeral fractures in the elderly: Treatment with a reamed intramedullary locking nail. *Injury* 2007;38(8):945-953.
49. Durbin RA, Gottesman MJ, Saunders KC: Hackethal stacked nailing of humeral shaft fractures: Experience with 30 patients. *Clin Orthop Relat Res* 1983;179: 168-174.
50. Noda M, Saegusa Y, Maeda T: Does the location of the entry point affect the reduction of proximal humeral fractures? A cadaveric study. *Injury* 2011; 42(suppl 4):S35-S38.
51. Nijs S, Sermon A, Broos P: Intramedullary fixation of proximal humerus fractures: Do locking bolts endanger the axillary nerve or the ascending branch of the anterior circumflex artery? A cadaveric study. *Patient Saf Surg* 2008;2(1):33.
52. Hatzidakis AM, Shevlin MJ, Fenton DL, Curran-Everett D, Nowinski RJ, Fehringer EV: Angular-stable locked intramedullary nailing of two-part surgical neck fractures of the proximal part of the humerus: A multicenter retrospective observational study. *J Bone Joint Surg Am* 2011; 93(23):2172-2179.
53. Georgousis M, Kontogeorgakos V, Kourkouvelas S, Badras S, Georgaklis V, Badras L: Internal fixation of proximal humerus fractures with the Polarus intramedullary nail. *Acta Orthop Belg* 2010; 76(4):462-467.
54. Gradl G, Dietze A, Kääb M, Hopfenmüller W, Mittlmeier T: Is locking nailing of humeral head fractures superior to locking plate fixation? *Clin Orthop Relat Res* 2009;467(11):2986-2993.
55. Krivohlávek M, Lukás R, Taller S, Srám J: Use of angle-stable implants for proximal humeral fractures: Prospective study. *Acta Chir Orthop Traumatol Cech* 2008; 75(3):212-220.
56. Zhu Y, Lu Y, Shen J, Zhang J, Jiang C: Locking intramedullary nails and locking plates in the treatment of two-part proximal humeral surgical neck fractures: A prospective randomized trial with a minimum of three years of follow-up. *J Bone Joint Surg Am* 2011;93(2):159-168.
57. van den Broek CM, van den Besselaar M, Coenen JM, Vegt PA: Displaced proximal humeral fractures: Intramedullary nailing versus conservative treatment.

Arch Orthop Trauma Surg 2007; 127(6):459-463.

58. Seide K, Triebe J, Faschingbauer M, et al: Locked vs. unlocked plate osteosynthesis of the proximal humerus: A biomechanical study. *Clin Biomech (Bristol, Avon)* 2007;22(2):176-182.
59. Strauss EJ, Schwarzkopf R, Kummer F, Egol KA: The current status of locked plating: The good, the bad, and the ugly. *J Orthop Trauma* 2008;22(7):479-486.
60. Lescheid J, Zdero R, Shah S, Kuzyk PR, Schemitsch EH: The biomechanics of locked plating for repairing proximal humerus fractures with or without medial cortical support. *J Trauma* 2010; 69(5):1235-1242.
61. Gardner MJ, Weil Y, Barker JU, Kelly BT, Helfet DL, Lorich DG: The importance of medial support in locked plating of proximal humerus fractures. *J Orthop Trauma* 2007;21(3):185-191.
62. Schumer RA, Muckley KL, Markert RJ, et al: Biomechanical comparison of a proximal humeral locking plate using two methods of head fixation. *J Shoulder Elbow Surg* 2010;19(4):495-501.
63. Zettl R, Müller T, Topp T, et al: Monoaxial versus polyaxial locking systems: A biomechanical analysis of different locking systems for the fixation of proximal humeral fractures. *Int Orthop* 2011;35(8):1245-1250.
64. Foruria AM, Carrascal MT, Revilla C, Munuera L, Sanchez-Sotelo J: Proximal humerus fracture rotational stability after fixation using a locking plate or a fixed-angle locked nail: The role of implant stiffness. *Clin Biomech (Bristol, Avon)* 2010;25(4): 307-311.
65. Edwards SL, Wilson NA, Zhang LQ, Flores S, Merk BR: Two-part surgical neck fractures of the proximal part of the humerus: A biomechanical evaluation of two fixation techniques. *J Bone Joint Surg Am* 2006;88(10):2258-2264.
66. Weinstein DM, Bratton DR, Ciccone WJ II, Elias JJ: Locking plates improve torsional resistance in the stabilization of three-part proximal humeral fractures. *J Shoulder Elbow Surg* 2006;15(2): 239-243.
67. Wheeler DL, Colville MR: Biomechanical comparison of intramedullary and percutaneous pin fixation for proximal humeral fracture fixation. *J Orthop Trauma* 1997;11(5):363-367.
68. Badman BL, Mighell M: Fixed-angle locked plating of two-, three-, and four-part proximal humerus fractures. *J Am Acad Orthop Surg* 2008;16(5):294-302.
69. Ricchetti ET, Warrender WJ, Abboud JA: Use of locking plates in the treatment of proximal humerus fractures. *J Shoulder Elbow Surg* 2010;19(2):66-75.
70. Hoppenfeld S, deBoer P, eds: *Surgical Exposures in Orthopaedics: The Anatomic Approach*, ed 2. Philadelphia, PA, Lippincott Williams & Wilkins, 1994.
71. Gardner MJ, Griffith MH, Dines JS, Briggs SM, Weiland AJ, Lorich DG: The extended anterolateral acromial approach allows minimally invasive access to the proximal humerus. *Clin Orthop Relat Res* 2005;434:123-129.
72. Gardner MJ, Boraiah S, Helfet DL, Lorich DG: The anterolateral acromial approach for fractures of the proximal humerus. *J Orthop Trauma* 2008;22(2):132-137.
73. Gallo RA, Zeiders GJ, Altman GT: Two-incision technique for treatment of complex proximal humerus fractures. *J Orthop Trauma* 2005;19(10):734-740.
74. Wu CH, Ma CH, Yeh JJ, Yen CY, Yu SW, Tu YK: Locked plating for proximal humeral fractures: Differences between the deltopectoral and deltoid-splitting approaches. *J Trauma* 2011;71(5): 1364-1370.
75. Gardner MJ, Voos JE, Wanich T, Helfet DL, Lorich DG: Vascular implications of minimally invasive plating of proximal humerus fractures. *J Orthop Trauma* 2006; 20(9):602-607.
76. Neviaser AS, Hettrich CM, Dines JS, Lorich DG: Rate of avascular necrosis following proximal humerus fractures treated with a lateral locking plate and endosteal implant. *Arch Orthop Trauma Surg* 2011;131(12):1617-1622.
77. Cetik O, Uslu M, Acar HI, Comert A, Tekdemir I, Cift H: Is there a safe area for the axillary nerve in the deltoid muscle? A cadaveric study. *J Bone Joint Surg Am* 2006;88(11):2395-2399.
78. Radkowski CA, Richards RS, Pietrobon R, Moorman CT III: An anatomic study of the cephalic vein in the deltopectoral shoulder approach. *Clin Orthop Relat Res* 2006;442:139-142.
79. Klepps S, Auerbach J, Calhon O, Lin J, Cleeman E, Flatow E: A cadaveric study on the anatomy of the deltoid insertion and its relationship to the deltopectoral approach to the proximal humerus. *J Shoulder Elbow Surg* 2004;13(3): 322-327.
80. Flatow EL, Bigliani LU: Tips of the trade: Locating and protecting the axillary nerve in shoulder surgery. The tug test. *Orthop Rev* 1992;21(4):503-505.
81. Flatow EL, Bigliani LU, April EW: An anatomic study of the musculocutaneous nerve and its relationship to the coracoid process. *Clin Orthop Relat Res* 1989; 244:166-171.
82. Tosounidis T, Hadjileontis C, Georgiadis M, Kafanas A, Kontakis G: The tendon of the long head of the biceps in complex proximal humerus fractures: A histological perspective. *Injury* 2010;41(3):273-278.

83. Gerber C, Hersche O, Berberat C: The clinical relevance of posttraumatic avascular necrosis of the humeral head. *J Shoulder Elbow Surg* 1998;7(6):586-590.

84. Hintermann B, Trouillier HH, Schäfer D: Rigid internal fixation of fractures of the proximal humerus in older patients. *J Bone Joint Surg Br* 2000;82(8):1107-1112.

85. Gardner MJ, Boraiah S, Helfet DL, Lorich DG: Indirect medial reduction and strut support of proximal humerus fractures using an endosteal implant. *J Orthop Trauma* 2008;22(3):195-200.

86. Brunner F, Sommer C, Bahrs C, et al: Open reduction and internal fixation of proximal humerus fractures using a proximal humeral locked plate: A prospective multicenter analysis. *J Orthop Trauma* 2009;23(3):163-172.

87. Egol KA, Ong CC, Walsh M, Jazrawi LM, Tejwani NC, Zuckerman JD: Early complications in proximal humerus fractures (OTA Types 11) treated with locked plates. *J Orthop Trauma* 2008;22(3):159-164.

88. Vallier HA: Treatment of proximal humerus fractures. *J Orthop Trauma* 2007;21(7):469-476.

89. Hawkins RJ, Kiefer GN: Internal fixation techniques for proximal humeral fractures. *Clin Orthop Relat Res* 1987;223:77-85.

90. Südkamp N, Bayer J, Hepp P, et al: Open reduction and internal fixation of proximal humeral fractures with use of the locking proximal humerus plate: Results of a prospective, multicenter, observational study. *J Bone Joint Surg Am* 2009;91(6):1320-1328.

91. Owsley KC, Gorczyca JT: Fracture displacement and screw cutout after open reduction and locked plate fixation of proximal humeral fractures. *J Bone Joint Surg Am* 2008;90(2):233-240.

92. Yang H, Li Z, Zhou F, Wang D, Zhong B: A prospective clinical study of proximal humerus fractures treated with a locking proximal humerus plate. *J Orthop Trauma* 2011;25(1):11-17.

93. Clavert P, Adam P, Bevort A, Bonnomet F, Kempf JF: Pitfalls and complications with locking plate for proximal humerus fracture. *J Shoulder Elbow Surg* 2010;19(4):489-494.

94. Röderer G, Erhardt J, Kuster M, et al: Second generation locked plating of proximal humerus fractures: A prospective multicentre observational study. *Int Orthop* 2011;35(3):425-432.

95. Wild JR, DeMers A, French R, et al: Functional outcomes for surgically treated 3- and 4-part proximal humerus fractures. *Orthopedics* 2011;34(10):e629-e633.

96. Hettrich CM, Neviaser A, Beamer BS, Paul O, Helfet DL, Lorich DG: Locked plating of the proximal humerus using an endosteal implant. *J Orthop Trauma* 2012;26(4):212-215.

97. Egol KA, Sugi MT, Ong CC, Montero N, Davidovitch R, Zuckerman JD: Fracture site augmentation with calcium phosphate cement reduces screw penetration after open reduction-internal fixation of proximal humeral fractures. *J Shoulder Elbow Surg* 2012;21(6):741-748.

Video Reference

12.1: Parsons BO: Video. Exerpt. *Open Reduction and Internal Fixation With a Plate for Proximal Humeral Fracture.* Rosemont, IL, American Academy of Orthopaedic Surgeons, 2012.

13

Proximal Humeral Fractures: Prosthetic Replacement

Daniel Aaron, MD
Bradford O. Parsons, MD
Francois Sirveaux, MD, PhD
Evan L. Flatow, MD

Abstract

Shoulder arthroplasty has emerged as a reliable treatment for displaced or comminuted fractures of the proximal humerus. The outcomes of humeral head replacement have improved as technology and techniques have evolved. Reverse shoulder arthroplasty has yielded promising results in early investigations. With either type of instrumentation, meticulous surgical technique is critical to achieving a good outcome. Prosthesis height and version and the stable fixation of anatomically reduced tuberosities are essential variables. Shoulder arthroplasty for fracture treatment remains a technically challenging procedure that demands knowledge of shoulder anatomy and implant options.

Instr Course Lect 2013;62:155-162.

Since being described by Neer,[1] shoulder arthroplasty has developed into an effective and commonly performed treatment for certain fractures of the proximal humerus. Humeral head replacement (or hemiarthroplasty) has been the standard of care; however, as reverse shoulder arthroplasty (RSA) has emerged as a treatment for rotator cuff–deficient arthritis, many surgeons have begun to explore its potential in fracture management. This chapter presents a review of indications, techniques of implantation, and current outcomes data for hemiarthroplasty and RSA for proximal humeral fractures.

Hemiarthroplasty

Indications

Advances in percutaneous, intramedullary, and locked-plate fixation technology and techniques have narrowed the indications for shoulder hemiarthroplasty for fracture of the proximal humerus in favor of joint-preserving strategies. Currently, the two principal indications for hemiarthroplasty are classic four-part fracture-dislocations and intra-articular or head-splitting fractures[2] (**Figure 1**). It is important to distinguish classic four-part fractures from valgus-impacted four-part fractures. Although both types of fractures meet the Neer criteria of displacement or angulation, the valgus-impacted fracture maintains a medial calcar hinge. In this situation, the vascular supply to the humeral head is usually preserved, so fixation is a viable option. The preserved medial mechanical support resists varus malalignment, making percutaneous fixation, as opposed to more rigid constructs, adequate in many cases. In contrast, the classic four-part fracture-dislocation, with the head segment in the axilla, maintains neither perfusion nor mechanical stability. Fixation of such four-part fractures or dislocations is prone to failure, progressive varus malalignment, and nonunion and/or osteonecrosis. Thus, all of these sequelae are associated with poor outcomes.

Dr. Parsons or an immediate family member is a member of a speakers' bureau or has made paid presentations on behalf of Zimmer and Arthrex; serves as a paid consultant to or is an employee of Zimmer and Arthrex; and has received research or institutional support from Wyeth. Dr. Sirveaux or an immediate family member has received royalties from Tornier and is a member of a speakers' bureau or has made paid presentations on behalf of DePuy and Sanofi-Aventis. Dr. Flatow or an immediate family member has received royalties from Innomed and Zimmer; is a member of a speakers' bureau or has made paid presentations on behalf of Zimmer; and serves as an unpaid consultant to Zimmer. Neither Dr. Aaron nor any immediate family member has received anything of value from or owns stock or stock options in a commercial company or institution related directly or indirectly to the subject of this chapter.

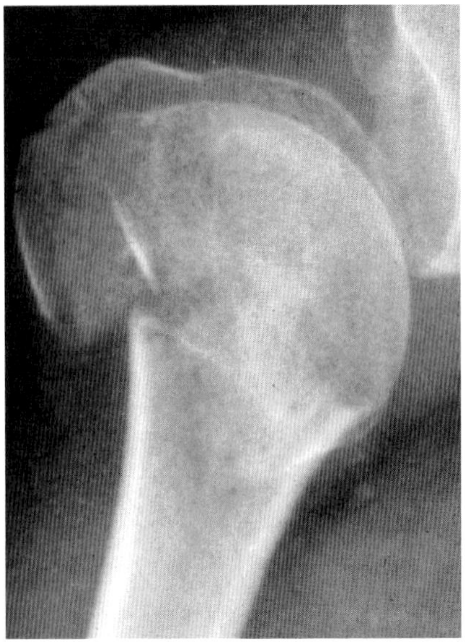

Figure 1 AP radiograph of a head-splitting fracture.

Although head-splitting fractures are difficult to fix, perfect reduction is desirable. The cancellous bone is often crushed (as in a tibial plateau fracture), and there is a substantial risk of posttraumatic arthritis even with anatomic reduction; therefore, replacement of the humeral head is often the selected treatment. Other indications for hemiarthroplasty include three-part fractures in patients with poor bone quality.[2] These patients include the elderly population and patients with comorbid conditions, such as osteoporosis, which can increase the risk of fixation failure. Chronic fracture situations, such as malunion or nonunion, may sometimes be best treated with hemiarthroplasty.

Surgical Technique

Hemiarthroplasty for fracture treatment can be one of the most challenging procedures in shoulder surgery. It is a technically demanding procedure that requires familiarity with bony, musculotendinous, neurologic, and vascular anatomy and allows only a small margin of error for good outcomes. The surgeon should also be familiar with the large variety of available component choices.

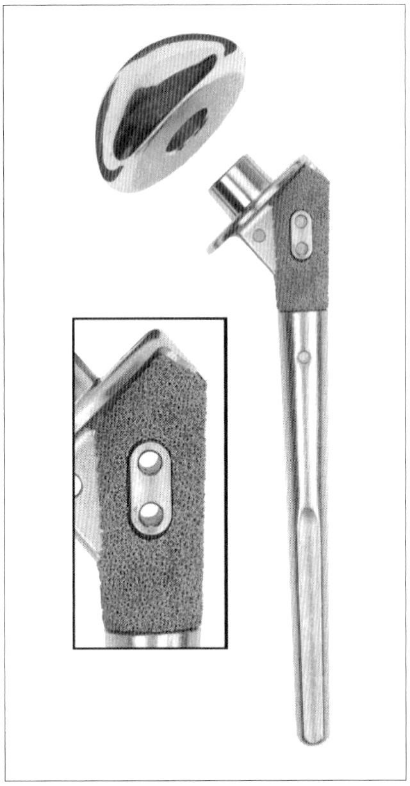

Figure 2 Illustration of a humeral implant with proximal porous tantalum to encourage bone ingrowth and tuberosity healing. (Courtesy of Zimmer, Warsaw, IN.)

Implant Choices

Some humeral implants are specifically designed for proximal humeral fractures. Many have specific features to encourage healing of the tuberosities, which is a strong determinant of postoperative function. Such features include a smaller metaphyseal body to allow room for tuberosity placement, slots in the metaphyseal body for placement of bone graft from the humeral head or other sources, and eyelets in the prosthesis for passing sutures that have been passed through the rotator cuff tendons attached to the tuberosities.[3] Some fracture systems have specific jigs, trial components, and other instrumentation to facilitate provisional placement before final reconstruction. Krishnan et al[4] reported improved tuberosity healing, range of motion, and American Shoulder and Elbow Surgeons (ASES) scores when using a fracture-specific stem compared with a conventional stem.

Newer implant developments include hydroxyapatite coatings and ingrowth metals, such as porous tantalum (**Figure 2**), which may improve tuberosity healing rates.[3] Systems are also available with adaptors for standard convex humeral head components or concave reverse components if the construct requires future revision to an RSA. The wide array of options allows the surgeon to customize the implant for a specific patient, but it demands knowledge of the available choices.

Restoration of Normal Anatomy

Despite advances in implant technology, surgical technique remains a critical factor in achieving a good outcome. The restoration of normal proximal humeral anatomy involves the correct placement of the humeral implant and anatomic reduction of the tuberosities. Proper prosthesis placement includes using the correct prosthesis height and version with respect to the epicondylar axis. Placing the humeral stem at the correct height and version and reducing the tuberosities anatomically without undue soft-tissue stripping or tension on the repair will maximize the chance for a successful outcome.

Boileau et al[5] showed that the height of the humeral stem directly affects tuberosity osteosynthesis, which is the most important factor affecting the functional outcome. Several methods of judging the prosthesis height do not rely on computer navigation. The first method involves direct measurement of the distance from the elbow to the shoulder with a ruler or a jig and comparison with the contralateral side (**Figure 3**). This method relies on preoperative measurements of the contralateral side to obtain symmetry. Another method, called the jigsaw method, involves assembling the various fracture fragments and assessing the fit of the native head on the calcar (**Figure 4**). That relationship can be re-created with the prosthesis. The jigsaw method may not be appropriate in fractures with severe comminution and may not achieve a level of precision within millimeters; however, it is usually sufficient to prevent large, clinically meaningful errors in the prosthesis height.

The ease of tuberosity reduction with respect to the head also can be used to confirm the appropriate height of the humeral stem. Another technique uses tension in the long head of the biceps tendon as a guide.[6] However, this method can be inaccurate, and it is sometimes impossible to use if there is a concomitant biceps rupture or if a biceps tenotomy or a tenodesis has previously been performed. A more recently developed method relies on the consistent relationship between the insertion of the pectoralis major tendon and the top of the humeral head, which was shown to be 5.6 cm ± 5 mm.[6] There may be variability in this relationship in individuals at the extremes of the limb-length spectrum, but it is reliable in most patients. Radiographic findings can also provide information about the height of the prosthesis. The Shenton line of the medial cortex of the proximal humerus should be restored. Krishnan et al[7] described a radiographic Gothic arch and provided calculations for obtaining it based on contralateral radiographs. The authors reported that re-creating the Gothic arch facilitated anatomic tuberosity reduction.

Prosthesis version is also an important factor in restoring normal anatomy. Although normal retroversion can vary, Boileau et al[5] suggested that it is better to set retroversion at the lower end of the range (approximately 20°), with the arm placed in internal rotation in a sling, to avoid undue tension on the greater tuberosity repair. To judge version intraoperatively, some authors advocate placing the arm in neutral rotation and positioning the humeral implant so that the head is pointed directly at the glenoid.[7] Hempfing et al[8] showed that the mean distance from the distal biceps groove to the equatorial plane of the humeral head is 8.0 mm ± 1.4 mm. The distal biceps groove is a reliable bony landmark. Other systems have jigs that base the version relative to the forearm. Inaccurate version has been associated with tuberosity malreduction and poor outcomes.[5]

Managing the Tuberosities

Intraoperative tuberosity management is of paramount importance because anatomic reduction and healing of the tuberosities are principal determinants of shoulder function after hemiarthro-

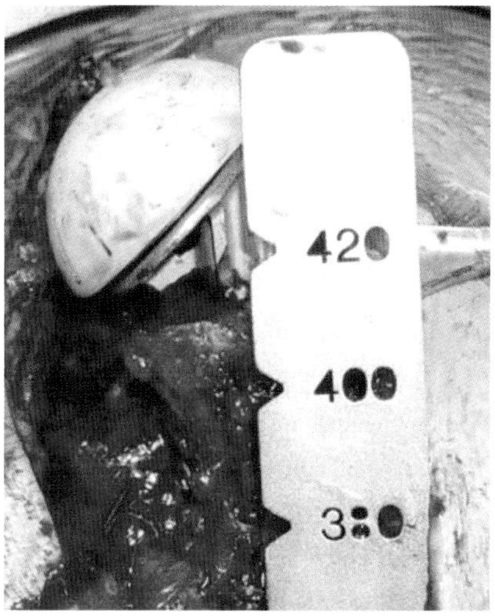

Figure 3 Intraoperative photograph of the direct measurement of prosthesis height using a radiopaque ruler.

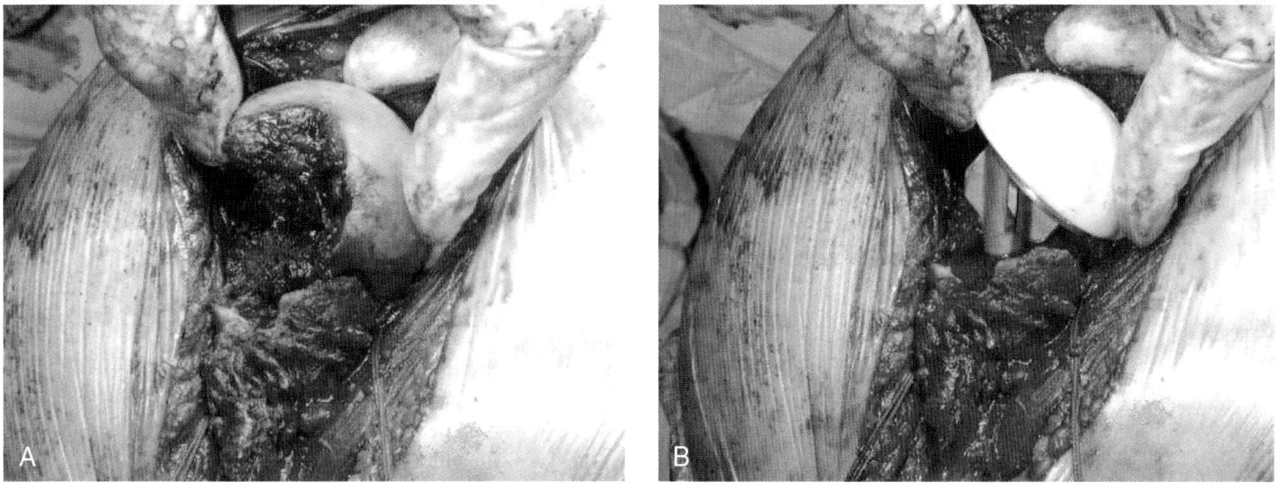

Figure 4 Intraoperative photographs of the jigsaw method of reassembling fracture fragments (**A**) to allow assessment of the head-calcar relationship with the prosthesis (**B**).

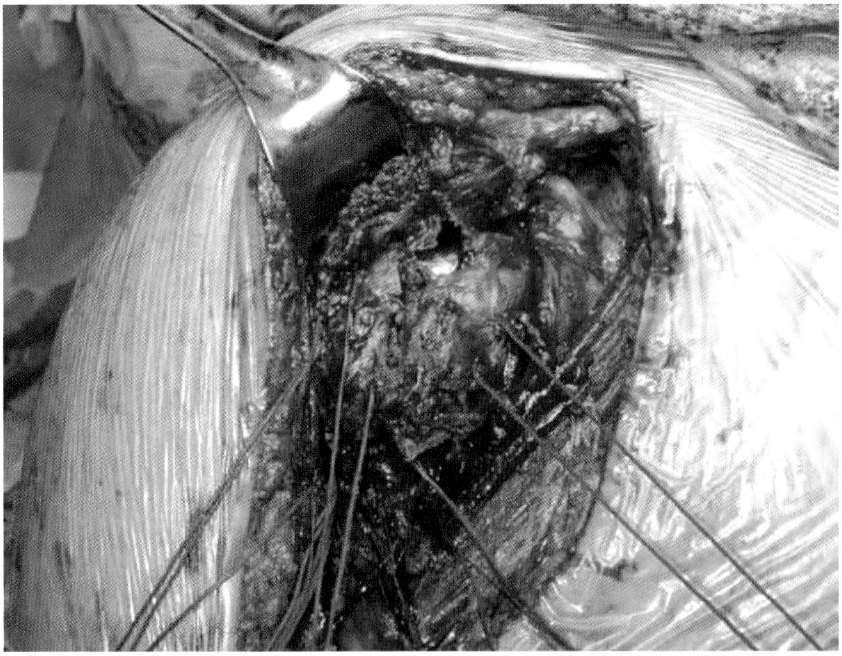

Figure 5 The tuberosity suture repair includes cerclage stitches.

plasty for fracture. The goals of tuberosity management are obtaining a tension-free anatomic reduction and strong fixation. Even when these goals are achieved, there is a substantial incidence of tuberosity displacement or osteolysis. Boileau et al[5] reported a 27% rate of tuberosity malreduction and a 23% overall rate of migration after initial malreduction and initial anatomic reduction. Greater tuberosity malpositioning is defined as placement greater than 1 cm below or 5 mm above the humeral head apex in the vertical plane or if the greater tuberosity is not visible on a postoperative neutral rotation AP radiograph in the horizontal plane. Boileau et al[5] reported that risk factors for tuberosity osteosynthesis failure included being a woman older than 75 years, poor initial prosthesis height or version, and poor initial positioning of the greater tuberosity. Tuberosity malpositioning correlated with superior migration of the prosthesis; shoulder stiffness, weakness, and pain; and low patient satisfaction.[5] Frankle et al[9] demonstrated an eightfold increase in the torque needed to produce 50° of external rotation if the greater tuberosity was malpositioned.

These studies highlight the importance of anatomic tuberosity reduction.[5,9] Other studies have focused on fixation methods to maintain the initial anatomic reduction. Frankle et al[10] showed that a cerclage suture incorporating both the tuberosities and the prosthesis is a critical adjunct to any fixation method (**Figure 5**). Maximal displacement, interfragmentary motion, and strain decreased with the use of a cerclage suture. The use of cables in addition to sutures also has been advocated.[11] Vertical control should also be obtained with sutures from the shaft to each tuberosity. Care must be taken to prevent overreduction of the fragments.

Bone graft from the resected head is often inserted into the space between the tuberosities and the prosthesis. If bone cement is used, it should be placed distally in the shaft, not proximally under the tuberosities.

Rehabilitation

This chapter's authors advocate a judicious pace for rehabilitation, with range of motion and strengthening exercises after hemiarthroplasty for proximal humeral fractures to protect the tuberosity repairs and provide the best opportunity for anatomic healing. This regimen consists of using a sling for the first 6 weeks; only pendulum exercises are allowed. In patients with good bone quality and excellent tuberosity reduction and fixation, passive elevation to 120° in the scapular plane and passive external rotation to 20° may also be incorporated in the early stages of rehabilitation. Formal stretching exercises or active motion is not started for 6 weeks, and strengthening does not begin until 12 weeks after surgery.

Results

The results of hemiarthroplasty are variable. In 57 patients treated with hemiarthroplasty for proximal humeral fractures, Antuña et al[12] reported mean active forward elevation of 100° and external rotation of 30° at a minimum 5-year follow-up. Sixteen percent of the patients had moderate to severe pain, and more than 50% were dissatisfied with the results of the procedure. The greater tuberosities were well positioned in 46 of 57 shoulders (81%). Similar results were reported by Goldman et al[13] who treated 22 patients (26 shoulders) with three- and four-part proximal humeral fractures. The authors reported forward elevation of 107° and external rotation of 31°. No pain or slight pain was reported by 73% of the patients. In a study of 71 patients (80 shoulders) treated with hemiarthroplasty, Mighell et al[14] reported mean forward elevation of 128° and external rotation of 43°. Ninety-three percent of the patients had no pain and were satisfied with their results. The tuberosities were well positioned in 64 of 80 shoulders. Tuberosity malunion was the most common complication. In a retrospective review of 130 patients treated with the Gothic arch reconstruction technique, Krishnan et al[7] reported that the forward elevation averaged 129°, and anatomic tuberosity healing was reported in 114 of 130 patients (88%). The authors also reported better results with a fracture-specific stem. Improvement in active forward elevation, active external rotation, ASES scores, and tuberosity healing were reported.[4]

In a study of 16 shoulders (15 patients) treated using a tantalum ingrowth stem and cerclage-style tuberosity fixation, Kaback et al[15] reported 93.75% tuberosity healing and average forward elevation of 115.9°, external rotation of 55°, internal rotation to L1, and an ASES score of 79.7 (**Figure 6**).

Overall, hemiarthroplasty for the treatment of proximal humeral fractures has achieved reliable pain relief for most patients; however, improvements in range of motion have been less reliable. Prosthesis height, version, and, above all, anatomic tuberosity healing are the main determinants of postoperative function.

Reverse Shoulder Arthroplasty

Arthroplasty has been increasingly indicated for treating fractures of the proximal humerus.[15-18] Because advancing age and medical comorbidities correlate with poor hemiarthroplasty results and tuberosity migration remains the main cause of failure, reverse shoulder arthroplasty was introduced in Europe as an alternative treatment of acute proximal humeral fractures for selected indications.[5,19-29] In a fashion similar to its function in rotator cuff–deficient arthritic shoulders and regardless of the status of the tuberosities, RSA may restore active anterior elevation in the fracture setting.

Influence of Tuberosity Integrity on Functional Outcomes

Initially, RSA for fracture treatment was considered a salvage procedure, and fixation of the tuberosities was not recommended. However, as is the case in rotator cuff tear arthropathy, active external rotation cannot be regained if the infraspinatus and teres minor are not functional, leading to the so-called hornblower sign.[29] Recent studies of RSA for fracture treatment reported that the recovery of active external rotation was better when the tuberosities were fixed and anatomic healing occurred.[26,27] This finding is consistent with results showing markedly decreased active external rotation in the presence of teres minor atrophy.[30]

Wall et al[31] reported that patients treated with RSA had greater improvement in internal rotation if the subscapularis was repaired, suggesting that the status of the lesser tuberosity may have implications for postoperative function after RSA for fracture treatment. To assess the effect of tuberosity integrity on function, a series of patients with four-part fractures treated with RSA and tuberosity fixation was evaluated (F Sirveaux, MD, and D Molé, MD, unpublished data, Nancy, France). The supraspinatus was removed in all cases. Postoperatively, the arm was immobilized in a simple sling. The rates of greater and lesser tuberosity healing were 85% and 98%, respectively. One hundred percent tuberosity healing was achieved using a fracture-dedicated stem compared with 78% healing with the standard stem ($P < 0.05$). The rate of tuberosity healing was better than the rate reported after hemiarthroplasty in a similar population.[32] Anatomic greater tuberosity healing significantly improved

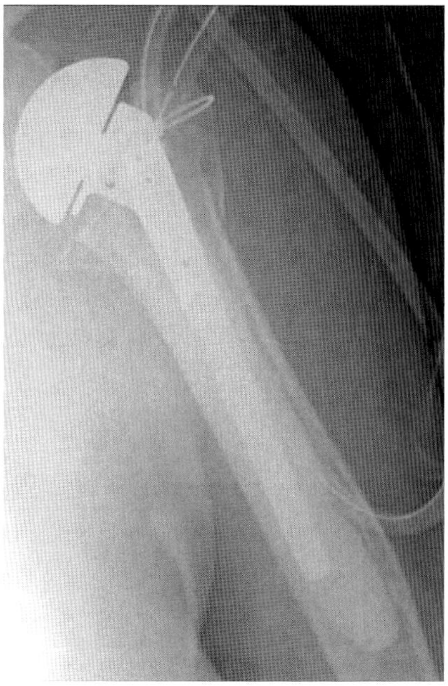

Figure 6 AP radiograph of a porous tantalum hemiarthroplasty with a well-positioned greater tuberosity that is fixed with a cable and sutures.

active external rotation (−4° versus 10°, $P < 0.05$), active elevation (88° versus 124°, $P < 0.05$), and the Constant score (41 versus 57 points, $P < 0.05$).

Analysis of the role of lesser tuberosity fixation on outcomes was not possible because of the high rate of lesser tuberosity healing. In light of previous studies showing that repairing the subscapularis improves active internal rotation and lowers the risk of instability,[33-35] this chapter's authors believe that the lesser tuberosity should be fixed in patients with shoulder fractures.

There may be less tension on the rotator cuff after RSA compared with hemiarthroplasty because of resection of the supraspinatus and medialization of the proximal humerus. This may decrease forces leading to proximal migration of the tuberosities. Biomechanically, RSA applies force directly on the glenosphere during elevation and can decrease torque on the rotator

Table 1
Clinical Results in Hemiarthroplasty and RSA Groups in the Clinique de Traumatologie et d'Orthopédie Study

	Hemiarthroplasty Group	RSA Group
Active anterior elevation	109°	122°
Active external rotation	26°	18°
Pain relief[a]	10	12
Constant score	63 points	57 points

[a]Derived from the Constant score (scale 0-15).

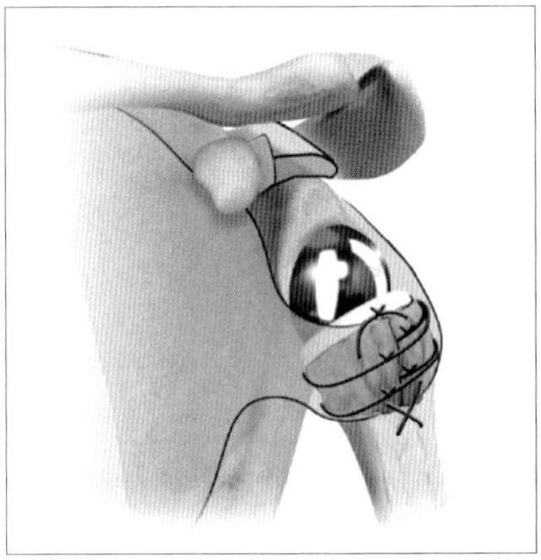

Figure 7 Illustration of the tuberosity suture technique with RSA.

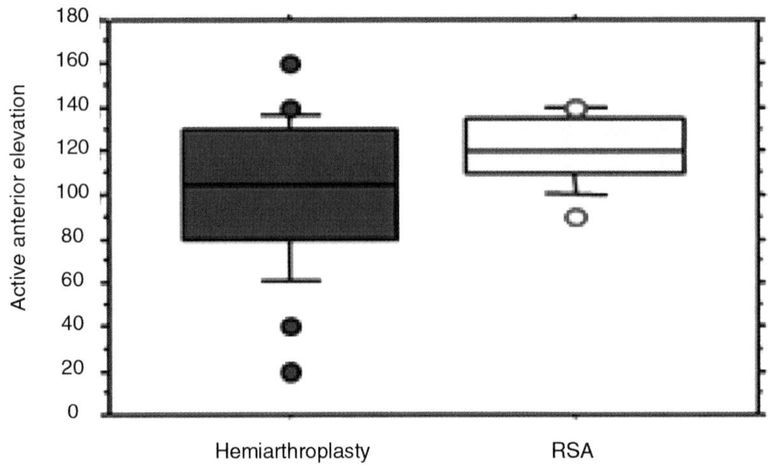

Figure 8 Graph comparing anterior elevation after hemiarthroplasty and RSA.

cuff and tuberosities. Although tuberosity fixation may be protected in RSA, this chapter's authors advocate the rigorous repair technique described by Boileau et al[5] for hemiarthroplasty (**Figure 7**).

Results of RSA Versus Hemiarthroplasty

At the Clinique de Traumatologie et d'Orthopédie in Nancy, France, patients older than 70 years with proximal humeral fractures warranting prosthetic replacement were enrolled in a prospective randomized study (F Sirveaux, MD, and D Molé, MD, unpublished data presented at the 22nd Annual Meeting of the American Shoulder and Elbow Surgeons, Palm Beach, FL, 2005). One group was treated with hemiarthroplasty and the other with RSA. Pain relief was substantially better in the group treated with RSA. No other important differences in the clinical results between the two groups were found (**Table 1**). In the hemiarthroplasty group, a large distribution in active anterior elevation was noted, whereas the results were more predictable in the RSA group (**Figure 8**).

Complications of RSA

The overall complication rate of RSA for fracture is 13% to 28%,[26,27,29] which is similar to the rate for RSA for rotator cuff tear arthropathy.[36] Zumstein et al[36] reported an overall rate of infection of 3.8% for RSA. In patients with fractures, the risk is similar and can be related to hematoma, subacromial dead space, and the compromised general health status of the typically elderly patient population. The risk of acromial fractures exists with RSA and rotator cuff tear arthropathy.[37]

In the unpublished study at the Clinique de Traumatologie et d'Orthopédie mentioned previously, four complications were reported: one acromial fracture (treated conservatively); one traumatic humeral shaft fracture (treated with open reduction and internal fixation with a plate); one infection (treated with removal of the prosthesis at 48 months after surgery); and one early glenoid component loosening, which was associated with an unrecognized preoperative glenoid fracture that likely compromised fixation of the baseplate (never revised). No dislocations or neurologic complications occurred.

Summary

Both hemiarthroplasty and RSA can be effective treatments for proximal humeral fractures; however, improvements in functional outcomes are needed. As technology and techniques continue to develop, particularly with respect to prosthesis height and version and tuberosity management, outcomes will likely improve. At the present time, hemiarthroplasty or RSA is reserved for classic four-part fractures, head-splitting fractures, selected three-part fractures, and patients with poor bone quality. The treating surgeon should be familiar with the indications, the choices of instrumentation, and implantation techniques and should discuss reasonable functional expectations with patients.

RSA for fracture may allow more predictably good functional improvement compared with hemiarthroplasty, especially for elderly patients with poor bone quality. Regardless of the arthroplasty technique chosen, stable fixation of the tuberosities is imperative to maximize functional results and decrease the risk of instability.

References

1. Neer CS II: Prosthetic replacement of the humeral head: Indications and operative technique. *Surg Clin North Am* 1963;43: 1581-1597.
2. Naranja RJ Jr, Iannotti JP: Displaced three- and four-part proximal humerus fractures: Evaluation and management. *J Am Acad Orthop Surg* 2000;8(6):373-382.
3. Cadet ER, Ahmad CS: Hemiarthroplasty for three- and four-part proximal humerus fractures. *J Am Acad Orthop Surg* 2012;20(1): 17-27.
4. Krishnan SG, Reineck JR, Bennion PD, Feher L, Burkhead WZ Jr: Shoulder arthroplasty for fracture: Does a fracture-specific stem make a difference? *Clin Orthop Relat Res* 2011;469(12):3317-3323.
5. Boileau P, Krishnan SG, Tinsi L, Walch G, Coste JS, Molé D: Tuberosity malposition and migration: Reasons for poor outcomes after hemiarthroplasty for displaced fractures of the proximal humerus. *J Shoulder Elbow Surg* 2002;11(5):401-412.
6. Murachovsky J, Ikemoto RY, Nascimento LG, Fujiki EN, Milani C, Warner JJ: Pectoralis major tendon reference (PMT): A new method for accurate restoration of humeral length with hemiarthroplasty for fracture. *J Shoulder Elbow Surg* 2006;15(6):675-678.
7. Krishnan SG, Bennion PW, Reineck JR, Burkhead WZ: Hemiarthroplasty for proximal humeral fracture: Restoration of the Gothic arch. *Orthop Clin North Am* 2008;39(4):441-450.
8. Hempfing A, Leunig M, Ballmer FT, Hertel R: Surgical landmarks to determine humeral head retrotorsion for hemiarthroplasty in fractures. *J Shoulder Elbow Surg* 2001;10(5):460-463.
9. Frankle MA, Greenwald DP, Markee BA, Ondrovic LE, Lee WE III: Biomechanical effects of malposition of tuberosity fragments on the humeral prosthetic reconstruction for four-part proximal humerus fractures. *J Shoulder Elbow Surg* 2001;10(4):321-326.
10. Frankle MA, Ondrovic LE, Markee BA, Harris ML, Lee WE III: Stability of tuberosity reattachment in proximal humeral hemiarthroplasty. *J Shoulder Elbow Surg* 2002;11(5):413-420.
11. Dietz SO, Broos P, Nijs S: Suture fixation versus cable cerclage of the tuberosities in shoulder arthroplasty: Clinical and radiologic results. *Arch Orthop Trauma Surg* 2012;132(6):793-800.
12. Antuña SA, Sperling JW, Cofield RH: Shoulder hemiarthroplasty for acute fractures of the proximal humerus: A minimum five-year follow-up. *J Shoulder Elbow Surg* 2008;17(2):202-209.
13. Goldman RT, Koval KJ, Cuomo F, Gallagher MA, Zuckerman JD: Functional outcome after humeral head replacement for acute three- and four-part proximal humeral fractures. *J Shoulder Elbow Surg* 1995;4(2):81-86.
14. Mighell MA, Kolm GP, Collinge CA, Frankle MA: Outcomes of hemiarthroplasty for fractures of the proximal humerus. *J Shoulder Elbow Surg* 2003;12(6):569-577.
15. Kaback LA, Aaron D, Neviaser AS, et al: Abstract: Functional and radiographic outcomes using a porous tantalum implant in the treatment of three- and four-part proximal humerus fractures. *American Shoulder and Elbow Surgeons Program Book, Closed Meeting White Sulphur Springs, WV.* Rosemont, IL, American Shoulder and Elbow Surgeons, 2011, pp 60-61.
16. Palvanen M, Kannus P, Niemi S, Parkkari J: Update in the epidemiology of proximal humeral fractures. *Clin Orthop Relat Res* 2006; 442:87-92.
17. Robinson CM, Akhtar A, Mitchell M, Beavis C: Complex posterior fracture-dislocation of the shoulder: Epidemiology, injury patterns, and results of operative treatment. *J Bone Joint Surg Am* 2007;89(7):1454-1466.
18. Robinson CM, Page RS, Hill RM, Sanders DL, Court-Brown CM, Wakefield AE: Primary hemiarthroplasty for treatment of proximal humeral fractures. *J Bone Joint Surg Am* 2003;85(7):1215-1223.
19. Kabir K, Burger C, Fischer P, et al: Health status as an important outcome factor after hemiarthroplasty. *J Shoulder Elbow Surg* 2009;18(1):75-82.

20. Nijs S, Broos P: Outcome of shoulder hemiarthroplasty in acute proximal humeral fractures: A frustrating meta-analysis experience. *Acta Orthop Belg* 2009; 75(4):445-451.
21. Plausinis D, Kwon YW, Zuckerman JD: Complications of humeral head replacement for proximal humeral fractures. *Instr Course Lect* 2005;54:371-380.
22. Kralinger F, Schwaiger R, Wambacher M, et al: Outcome after primary hemiarthroplasty for fracture of the head of the humerus: A retrospective multicentre study of 167 patients. *J Bone Joint Surg Br* 2004;86(2):217-219.
23. Prakash U, McGurty DW, Dent JA: Hemiarthroplasty for severe fractures of the proximal humerus. *J Shoulder Elbow Surg* 2002;11(5):428-430.
24. Agorastides I, Sinopidis C, El Meligy M, Yin Q, Brownson P, Frostick SP: Early versus late mobilization after hemiarthroplasty for proximal humeral fractures. *J Shoulder Elbow Surg* 2007;16(3): S33-S38.
25. Sirveaux F, Navez G, Roche O, Mole D: Reverse prosthesis for proximal humerus fracture, technique and results. *Tech Shoulder Elbow Surg* 2008;9(1):15-22.
26. Cazeneuve JF, Cristofari DJ: Grammont reversed prosthesis for acute complex fracture of the proximal humerus in an elderly population with 5 to 12 years follow-up. *Rev Chir Orthop Reparatrice Appar Mot* 2006; 92(6):543-548.
27. Bufquin T, Hersan A, Hubert L, Massin P: Reverse shoulder arthroplasty for the treatment of three- and four-part fractures of the proximal humerus in the elderly: A prospective review of 43 cases with a short-term follow-up. *J Bone Joint Surg Br* 2007; 89(4):516-520.
28. Klein M, Juschka M, Hinkenjann B, Scherger B, Ostermann PA: Treatment of comminuted fractures of the proximal humerus in elderly patients with the Delta III reverse shoulder prosthesis. *J Orthop Trauma* 2008;22(10): 698-704.
29. Gallinet D, Clappaz P, Garbuio P, Tropet Y, Obert L: Three or four parts complex proximal humerus fractures: Hemiarthroplasty versus reverse prosthesis. A comparative study of 40 cases. *Orthop Traumatol Surg Res* 2009;95(1): 48-55.
30. Simovitch RW, Helmy N, Zumstein MA, Gerber C: Impact of fatty infiltration of the teres minor muscle on the outcome of reverse shoulder arthroplasty. *J Bone Joint Surg Am* 2007;89(5):934-939.
31. Wall B, Nové-Josserand L, O'Connor DP, Edwards TB, Walch G: Reverse total shoulder arthroplasty: A review of results according to etiology. *J Bone Joint Surg Am* 2007;89(7):1476-1485.
32. Dietrich M, Meier C, Zeller D, Grueninger P, Berbig R, Platz A: Primary hemiarthroplasty for proximal humeral fractures in the elderly: Long term functional outcome and social implications. *Eur J Trauma Emerg Surg* 2009;5: 512-519.
33. Gallo RA, Gamradt SC, Mattern CJ, et al: Instability after reverse total shoulder replacement. *J Shoulder Elbow Surg* 2011;20(4): 584-590.
34. Edwards TB, Williams MD, Labriola JE, Elkousy HA, Gartsman GM, O'Connor DP: Subscapularis insufficiency and the risk of shoulder dislocation after reverse shoulder arthroplasty. *J Shoulder Elbow Surg* 2009;18(6):892-896.
35. Trappey GJ IV, O'Connor DP, Edwards TB: What are the instability and infection rates after reverse shoulder arthroplasty? *Clin Orthop Relat Res* 2011;469(9): 2505-2511.
36. Zumstein MA, Pinedo M, Old J, Boileau P: Problems, complications, reoperations, and revisions in reverse total shoulder arthroplasty: A systematic review. *J Shoulder Elbow Surg* 2011;20(1): 146-157.
37. Walch G, Mottier F, Wall B, Boileau P, Molé D, Favard L: Acromial insufficiency in reverse shoulder arthroplasties. *J Shoulder Elbow Surg* 2009;18(3):495-502.

SECTION

3

Hand and Wrist

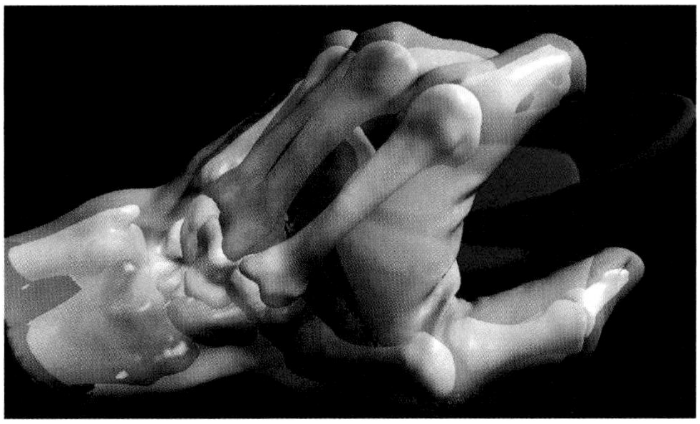

DVD

Symposium

14 The Thumb Carpometacarpal Joint: Anatomy, Hormones, and Biomechanics

15 What Every Resident Should Know About Wrist Fractures: Case-Based Learning

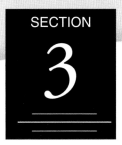

14

SYMPOSIUM

The Thumb Carpometacarpal Joint: Anatomy, Hormones, and Biomechanics

Amy L. Ladd, MD
Arnold-Peter C. Weiss, MD
Joseph J. Crisco, PhD
Elisabet Hagert, MD, PhD
Jennifer Moriatis Wolf, MD
Steven Z. Glickel, MD
Jeffrey Yao, MD

Abstract

Although there are many surgical options to treat thumb carpometacarpal (CMC) arthritis, a precise etiology for this common disorder remains obscure. To better understand the physiology of the thumb CMC joint and treat pathology, it is helpful to examine the biomechanics, hormonal influences, and available surgical treatment options, along with the evolutionary roots of the thumb; its form and function, its functional demands; and the role of supporting ligaments based on their location, stability, and ultrastructure. It is important to appreciate the micromotion of a saddle joint and the role that sex, age, and reproductive hormones play in influencing laxity and joint disease. Minimally invasive surgery is now challenging prevailing treatment principles of ligament reconstruction and plays a role in thumb CMC joint procedures.

Instr Course Lect 2013;62:165-179.

A Marvelous Piece of Machinery

Stability and mobility represent the functional paradox of the thumb carpometacarpal (CMC) joint. The thumb requires a breadth of motion to perform tasks that are uniquely human, from forceful grasp to fine pinch. The joint morphology of the metacarpal on the trapezium affords this functional spectrum. Although in circumduction it behaves like a ball and socket, providing close lateral pinch to the index finger or wide prehension of large objects within the palm, its configuration is more complex. The

Dr. Ladd or an immediate family member serves as a board member, owner, officer, or committee member of the Ruth Jackson Orthopaedic Society; has received royalties from Extremity Medical and Orthohelix; has received research or institutional support from the National Institutes of Health (NIAMS and NICHD) and OREF; and owns stock or stock options in Articulinx, Extremity Medical, Illuminoss Medical, and OsteoSpring Medical. Dr. Weiss or an immediate family member serves as a board member, owner, officer, or committee member of the American Society for Surgery of the Hand; has received royalties from DePuy, Extremity Medical, and Medartis; serves as a paid consultant to or is an employee of Illuminoss Medical; and owns stock or stock options in Articulinx, Illuminoss Medical, and OsteoSpring Medical. Dr. Crisco or an immediate family member serves as a board member, owner, officer, or committee member of the American Society of Biomechanics; has received royalties from Extremity Medical; serves as a paid consultant to or is an employee of Extremity Medical and Illuminoss Medical; and has received research or institutional support from Extremity Medical. Dr. Hagert or an immediate family member serves as an unpaid consultant to Osteomed. Dr. Wolf or an immediate family member serves as a board member, owner, officer, or committee member of the American Association for Hand Surgery, the American Society for Surgery of the Hand, and the American Academy of Orthopaedic Surgeons. Dr. Glickel or an immediate family member serves as a board member, owner, officer, or committee member of the American Society for Surgery of the Hand, the American Orthopaedic Association, and the Dupuytren Foundation. Dr. Yao or an immediate family member serves as a board member, owner, officer, or committee member of the American Society for Surgery of the Hand and the Arthroscopy Association of North America; has received royalties from Arthrex; is a member of a speakers' bureau or has made paid presentations on behalf of Arthrex; and serves as a paid consultant to or is an employee of Smith & Nephew, Arthrex, and Axogen.

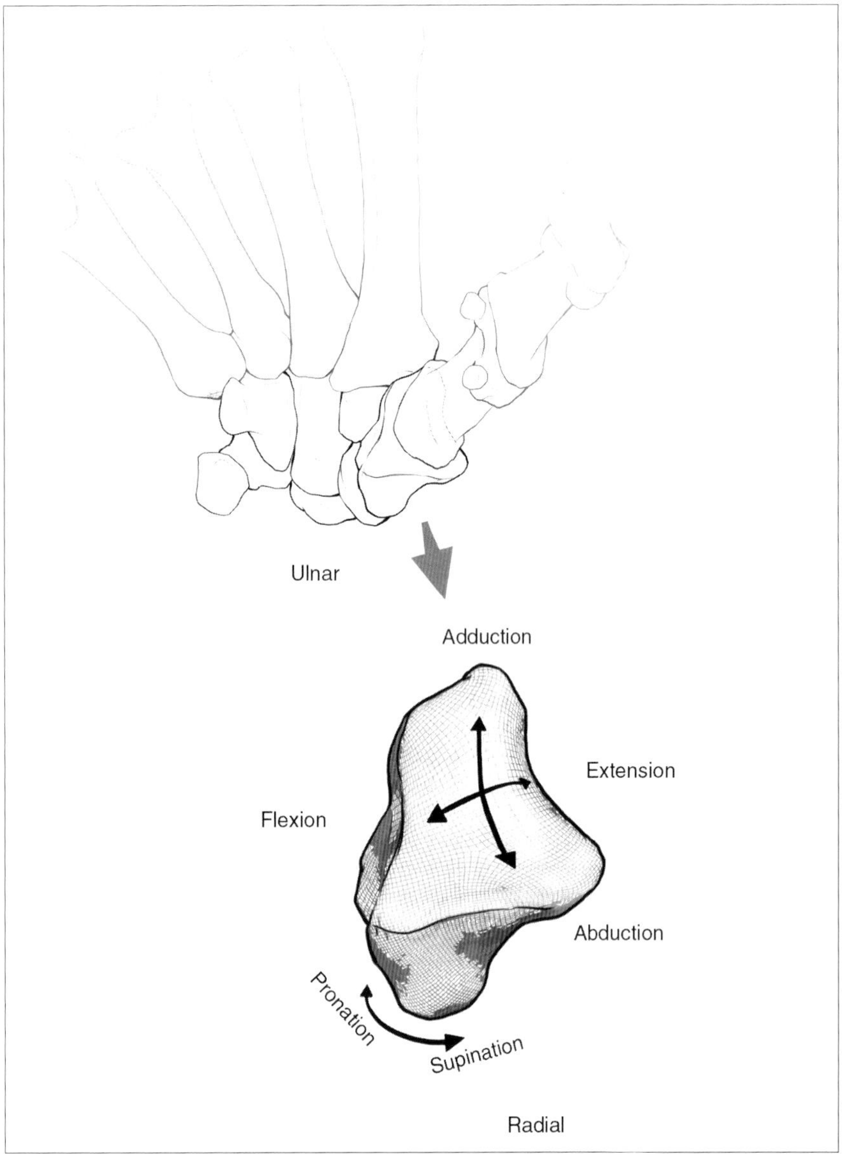

Figure 1 Topography of the distal trapezial joint surface, redrawn from a CT surface rendering of a normal right hand. The CMC-I motion arcs of the metacarpal on the trapezium are flexion-extension and abduction-adduction. Pronation-supination represents composite rotation and translation of this joint based on morphology and muscular activity. The thumb position in relation to the fingers represents a completion of the carpal arch, which places the CMC-I oblique to the adjacent fingers. The arcs of motion thus are out of phase with the fingers, depending on the thumb's position in space. (Courtesy of Sarah Hegmann, Stanford University, Stanford, CA.)

concavo-convex saddle design, described as "articulation by reciprocal reception" in Gray's seminal anatomy textbook,[1] imparts arcs of motion in flexion-extension and abduction-adduction. Pronation-supination represents composite rotation and translation of this joint based on morphology and muscular activity in planes out of phase with the fingers. The metacarpal base is concave dorsovolarly and convex radioulnarly. Conversely, the trapezial concave arc is radioulnar, and the convex arc is dorsovolar. The trapezial and metacarpal articular surfaces have disparate radii of curvature that are congruous only at the extremes of motion[2-5] (**Figure 1**). The concavity of each articular surface is shallow, so the skeleton affords little intrinsic stability. The ligaments and muscles play varying roles in stability, laxity, and proprioception of this complex joint.[6-10]

The evolutionary demands for prehension and manipulative activity accompanied the ability of hominid species to stand upright, freeing the torso and upper limbs. These demands and capabilities coevolved with a larger brain and neurologic complexity.[11,12] Bipedalism and club wielding in *Homo sapiens* are closely associated; other primates and their ancestors use the comparatively hypoplastic thumb as a post, given its shorter, stiffer configuration and absence of intrinsic muscular development.[13,14]

Biomechanical studies have shown that forces increase exponentially from the tip of the thumb to the CMC joint with grasp and forceful pinch. The joint reactive force at the base of the thumb is 12 times greater than that generated at the tip of the thumb with lateral pinch, and compressive forces of as much as 120 kg may occur at the trapeziometacarpal joint with forceful grasp.[8] Cadaver biomechanical studies have suggested that most of the force in pinch is transmitted proximally and dorsoradially.[8] The precise position of the metacarpal on the trapezium during these activities in live subjects can be visualized with various imaging techniques (**Figures 2** and **3**), although correlating the force generated in these positions has yet to be quantified. The functional importance of the thumb is underscored by its effect on disability; loss of thumb function imparts a 40% to 50% rate of impair-

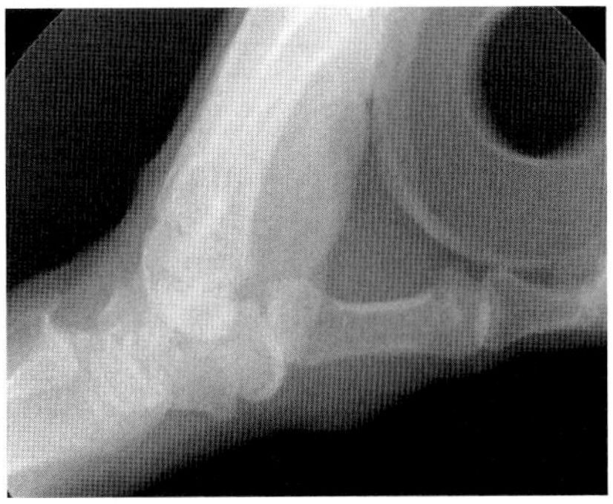

Figure 2 A cine radiograph of the hand during functional, loaded grasp. The position of the metacarpal on the trapezium demonstrates apparent abduction; however, the two-dimensional nature and image overlap prevent precise location and relationship of the two surfaces. (Courtesy of Amy L. Ladd, MD and Stanford University, Stanford, CA.)

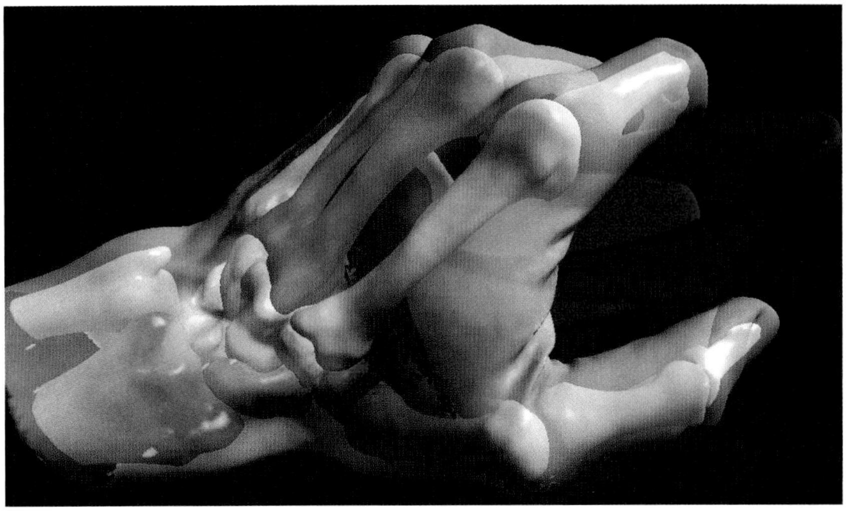

Figure 3 Surface three-dimensional rendering from CT (depicted here as a two-dimensional image) permits quantifying the position of the trapezium and the metacarpal relative to each other in functional grasp. The shading and coloring are added for clarity. (Courtesy of Amy L. Ladd, MD and Stanford University, Stanford, CA.)

ment to the upper extremity because of its central role in nearly all grasping and handling maneuvers.[3]

Video 14.1: Animation of Grasp, Jar Opening, and Pinch. Amy L. Ladd, MD (30 sec)

CMC joint osteoarthritis is traditionally viewed as a disease endemic in postmenopausal women.[4,15,16] Demographic radiographic studies show a 6:1 female-to-male incidence of arthrosis of the trapeziometacarpal joint, although this difference decreases with age, with the incidence in women and men at age 75 years of 40% and 25%, respectively.[17,18] The surgical literature and the institutional experience of one of this chapter's authors (AL) indicates that the average age of patients at the time of surgery for CMC osteoarthritis is 60 years, and the incidence of men undergoing surgery is higher than the radiographic incidence.[4,18-22] One of this chapter's authors (AL) reported on her consecutive surgical experience in 2010 to 2011 with articular wear in 39 trapezia in 37 patients (average age, 62 years). The incidence of female and male specimens in this study was 69% and 31%, respectively.[23] The roles of sex, ethnicity, age, and hand use likely contribute to both the incidence of arthritis and the decision for surgical treatment. Future improvements in surgical treatment will rely on a better understanding of the pathomechanics of the disease.

Thumb CMC Kinematics and Osteoarthritis Progression

Despite the prevalence of thumb CMC joint osteoarthritis, there is little definitive understanding of how altered joint biomechanics relate to the natural history of the disease. Basic science and clinical studies have correlated increases in general joint laxity with the development of CMC osteoarthritis.[24] Radial subluxation of the metacarpal on the trapezium has been noted with functional activities.[25]

In an attempt to further define the kinematic factors that influence the development of thumb osteoarthritis, a state-of-the-art, markerless bone registration (MBR) technique was used for three-dimensional in vivo kinematic analysis in normal individuals and in an ongoing study evaluating patients with early CMC osteoarthritis. Data on thumb CMC kinematics were obtained over several years.[26] Key pinch, progressing from unloaded to loaded, in 12 asymptomatic men (age, 38.7 ± 11.7 years) and 12 women (age, 43.2 ± 15.8 years) was evaluated. These normal individuals demonstrated metacarpal volar translation, internal rotation, and flexion on the distal trapezial surface in key pinch (**Figure 4**). In object grasp, progressing from unloaded to loaded, the metacarpal bone undergoes ulnar translation, flexion, and abduction relative to the distal trapezial surface (**Figure 5**). There appears to be a definite functional coupling of flexion-extension and abduction-adduction (statistical significance, $P < 0.001$) from the neutral position on performing each task (**Figure 6**). Extension of the thumb metacarpal relative to the trapezium couples with adduction, and flexion

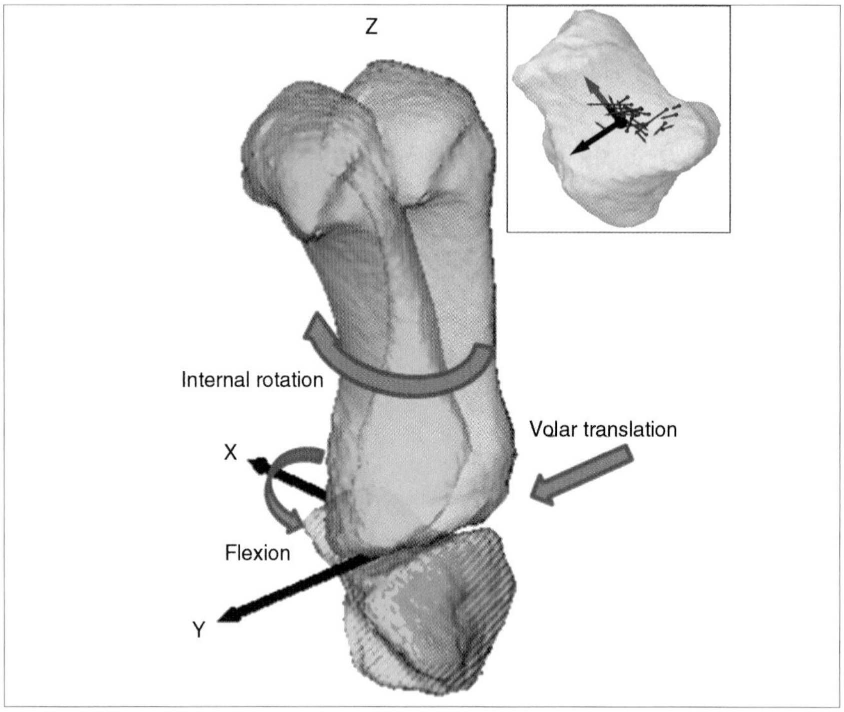

Figure 4 Illustration of MBR kinematic analysis of loaded key pinch. The thumb metacarpal undergoes volar translation, internal rotation, and flexion relative to the trapezium. (Courtesy of Arnold-Peter C. Weiss, MD, Providence, RI.)

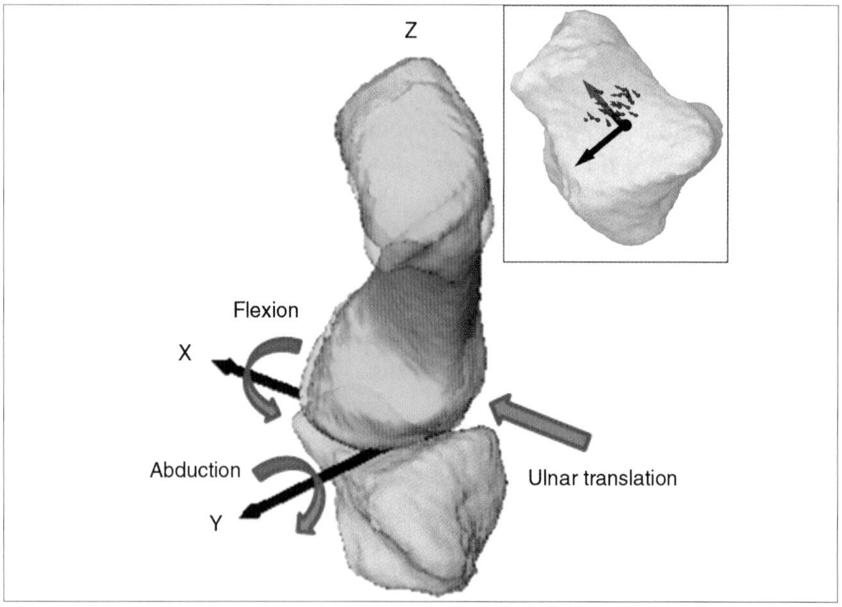

Figure 5 Illustration of MBR kinematic analysis of loaded object grasp. The thumb metacarpal undergoes ulnar translation, flexion, and abduction relative to the trapezium.(Courtesy of Arnold-Peter C. Weiss, MD, Providence, RI.)

couples with abduction. These studies provide a solid framework to further analyze the kinematics of patients with early thumb osteoarthritis and determine whether changes in motion over time (abnormal motion or laxity) can predict osteoarthritis progression in symptomatic patients with little evidence of radiographic disease.

CMC Ligament Anatomy: New Evidence to Change Old Ideas

Although the first accounts of basal thumb ligament anatomy date back to the mid 18th century, an accurate description and reproducible measurements of thumb CMC ligament anatomy remain elusive.[27] As few as 3 and as many as 16 ligaments have been identified. Volar, dorsal, and ulnar ligaments have been named as primary stabilizers of the CMC joint.[7,14,28-30]

Ligaments play an important role in the static stability and the dynamic neuromuscular control of a joint. Studies of knee, shoulder, ankle, and wrist joints have established the concept of proprioception, in which nerve endings within the joint capsule and the ligaments contribute afferent information to the spinal cord for efferent control of periarticular muscles.[31-35] The Hilton law states that "any nerve innervating a joint will also innervate the muscles moving that joint."[36] The thumb CMC joint receives innervation from the dorsal sensory radial nerve and the volar thenar median nerve branches, but the innervation of the ligaments has not been delineated.[37-39]

To better understand thumb CMC stability and function, a study of CMC ligament morphometry, histology, and neuroanatomy (to investigate the anatomy and proprioceptive role of the CMC ligaments) was performed.[9,10,39] Some of the main findings include those associated with the

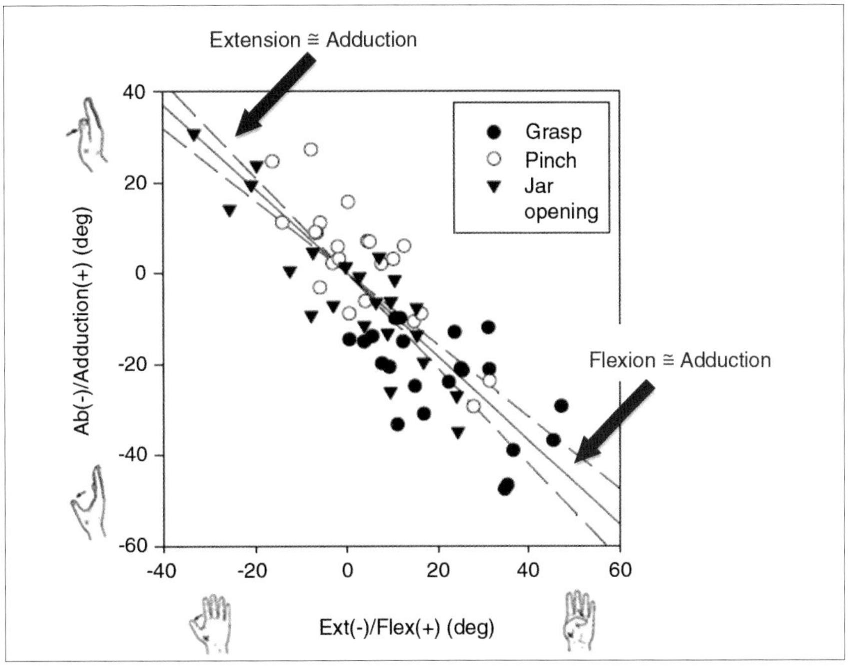

Figure 6 A specific CMC functional coupling occurs in multiple tasks. Coupling occurs with extension/adduction and flexion/abduction. Ab = abduction, deg = degrees, ext = extension, flex = flexion. (Courtesy of Arnold-Peter C. Weiss, MD, Providence, RI.)

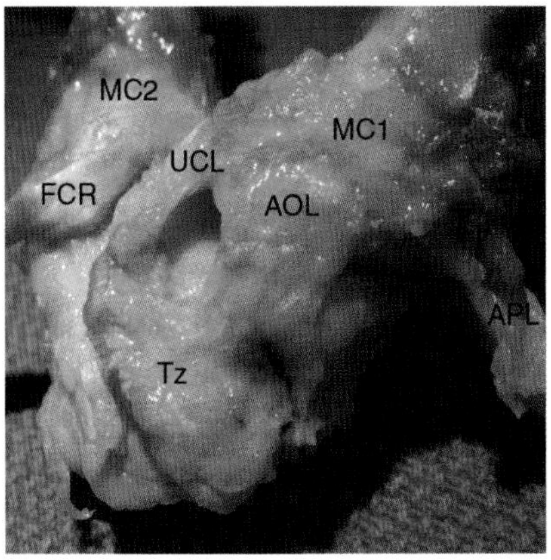

Figure 7 The volar thumb CMC ligaments from a right hand, showing the attenuated volar anterior oblique ligament (AOL) and ulnar collateral ligament (UCL), which course from the trapezial ridge (Tz) onto the volar base of metacarpal 1 (MC1). Also seen are the abductor pollicis longus (APL) and the flexor carpi radialis (FCR) tendons, as well as the base of metacarpal 2 (MC2).(Courtesy of Arnold-Peter C. Weiss, MD, Providence, RI.)

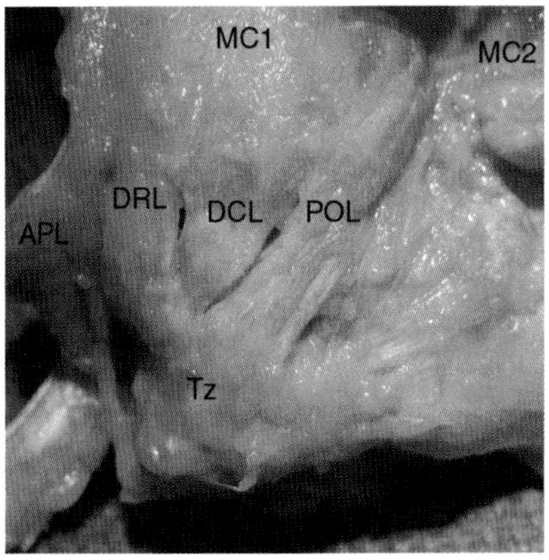

Figure 8 The dorsal thumb CMC ligaments from a right hand showing the dorsal deltoid ligament complex consisting of the dorsal radial ligament (DRL), dorsal central ligament (DCL), and posterior oblique ligament (POL), all emanating from the dorsal tubercle of the trapezium (Tz). Also seen are the dorsal bases of metacarpal 1 and 2 (MC1, MC2) and the abductor pollicis longus (APL). (Courtesy of Amy L. Ladd, MD and Stanford University, Palo Alto, CA.)

volar anterior oblique ligament, the dorsal deltoid ligament, and CMC ligament innervation.

Volar Anterior Oblique Ligament

The volar anterior oblique ligament is consistently described but variably situated in anatomic studies of the CMC joint (**Figure 7**). Pieron[40] described it as a curtain-like structure covering the volar joint surface, which was later affirmed by other studies.[7,10] Bettinger et al[7] and Pellegrini[19] described a deep, intra-articular ligament (the so-called beak ligament), but this finding was not confirmed in a study of low-arthritic cadaver specimens.[10] Morphometric data revealed that the volar anterior oblique ligament is a thin, capsular structure with a mean thickness of 0.71 mm (SD = 11) and variable width.[10] Histomorphometric analysis, including hematoxylin-eosin and 4',6'-diamidino-2-phenylindole (DAPI) staining to determine morphology and cellularity, also support the notion that the volar anterior oblique ligament is primarily a capsular structure consisting of disorganized connective tissue.

Dorsal Deltoid Ligament

In contrast to the volar anterior oblique ligament, the dorsal deltoid ligament in the cadaver study by Ladd et al[10] consisted of three stout ligaments, all emanating from the dorsal tubercle of the triquetrum and inserting fan shaped onto the dorsal base of the first metacarpal (**Figure 8**). These ligaments were consistently found in the same location, had a mean thickness of 1.85 mm (SD = 0.14), and showed histologic findings consistent with a stout ligament with grouped collagen bundles.[10] Macroscopic findings were consistent with articles purporting that the dorsal ligaments are the primary stabilizers of the thumb

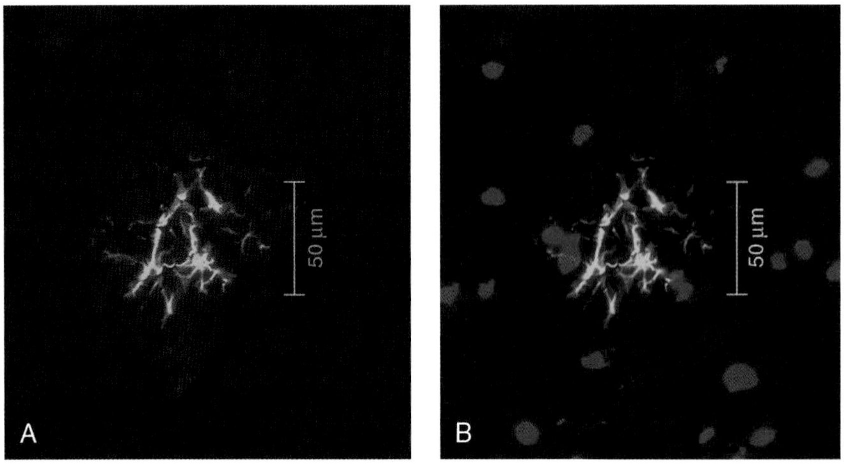

Figure 9 **A,** Ruffini ending from a dorsal radial ligament, as seen in an immunofluorescent protein gene product 9.5 stain. **B,** The Ruffini ending is superimposed on the collagen fibers in the DAPI stain, which highlights the nuclei of fibrocytes. (Courtesy of Amy L. Ladd, MD and Standford University, Stanford, CA.)

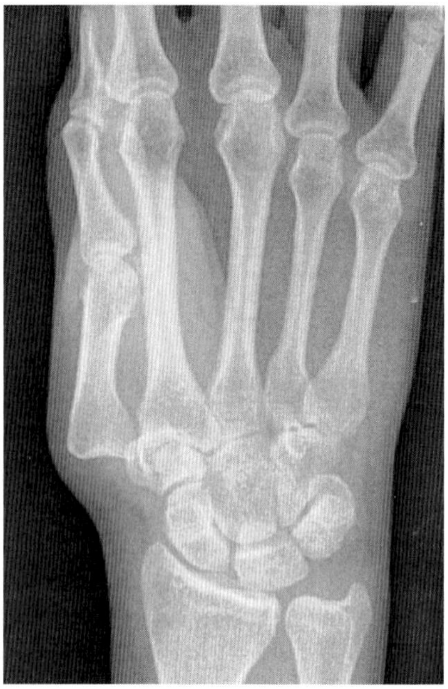

Figure 10 Radiograph showing trapeziometacarpal joint dislocation in a patient with intrinsic ligament laxity after a minor fall. (Courtesy of Jennifer M. Wolf, MD, Farmington, CT.)

CMC joint,[7,30] and a recent study comparing the arthroscopic and macroscopic appearance of the thumb CMC ligaments.[41]

CMC Ligament Innervation

A new, triple-stain immunofluorescent technique was used to investigate the innervation patterns of the three dorsal and two volar thumb CMC ligaments[9] (**Figure 9**). Sensory nerve endings, so-called mechanoreceptors, were identified and classified according to Freeman and Wyke.[42] Ordinal grading of the nerve endings showed that the dorsal deltoid ligament complex was consistently innervated with mechanoreceptors and free nerve endings, with a predominance of nerve endings located close to the insertion into bone and, significantly ($P < 0.05$) more often, closer to the mobile metacarpal insertion than the stable triquetral insertion.[39] The most common mechanoreceptor type was the Ruffini ending, which is known for its ability to monitor joint position and kinesthesia.

Influence of Laxity and Hormones on Basilar Thumb Arthritis

The prevalence in women of both symptomatic and radiographic CMC osteoarthritis has led to speculation that reproductive hormones or joint laxity are responsible for this disparity between the sexes.[17,42] Sodha et al[17] reviewed the radiographs of 615 patients with distal radius fractures. The authors reported a 6:1 female-to-male ratio of radiographic trapeziometacarpal arthritis and found the disorder increases in prevalence with advancing age in both sexes.

Joint Laxity

Joint hypermobility is defined as greater than normal motion at multiple joints. Patients with this condition are often characterized as double jointed because of the hyperextensibility of various joints.[43] In patients with joint laxity, studies have shown a higher correlation with anterior cruciate ligament (ACL) tears, shoulder instability, and ankle sprains.[44,45] Joint laxity is also associated with a higher rate of knee arthritis, implying that greater joint mobility leads to abnormal biomechanical stresses on the joint.[46]

Studies in subjects with extremes of joint laxity, as well as normative populations, have suggested that joint laxity affects the thumb CMC joint. Gamble et al[47] reported thumb CMC joint subluxation and dislocation in more than 75% of a cohort of 24 young patients with Ehlers-Danlos syndrome, with radiographic evidence of CMC arthritis in 16% (**Figure 10**). Jónsson et al[24] noted a higher prevalence of CMC osteoarthritis in Icelandic patients with joint laxity compared with those without hypermobility. Another study showed a significant correlation between the radiographic stress ratio at the trapeziometacarpal joint and the Beighton score of generalized joint laxity.[48,49]

Hormonal Influences

The sex differences in multiple musculoskeletal diseases have led to theories that differences in reproductive hormones may account for these disparities. More women than men sustain ACL tears playing soccer and basketball.[50] Women also have shown less anterior shoulder stiffness and greater shoulder hypermobility than men.[45] In studies of the effect of hormones in these joints, it has been shown that ACL tears occur most frequently during the ovulatory phase in menstruating women.[51] Focusing on the hand joints, Cooley et al[52] reported a higher rate of overall hand osteoarthritis in women who had an earlier onset of menarche and later menopause, implying greater exposure to reproductive hormones.

There is some evidence that reproductive hormones affect various joints. Estrogen and relaxin receptors have been described in the ACL in both women and men.[53] Kapila et al[54] reported that estrogen and relaxin caused dose-dependent matrix degradation of temporomandibular fibrocartilage explants, an effect attenuated by the addition of progesterone.

Relaxin, a hormone produced by the corpus luteum during pregnancy, loosens the pelvic ligaments in preparation for childbirth.[55] It has been proposed as a specific hormone target in the development of trapeziometacarpal arthritis because of attenuation of the supporting joint ligaments. Relaxin is a member of the insulin superfamily that is produced both in pregnant and nonpregnant women and in men.[56,57] Its mechanism of action is mediated through upregulation of matrix metalloproteases and suppression of tissue inhibitors of metalloproteases within the extracellular matrix.[58]

In a prospective study, Dragoo et al[59] demonstrated that serum relaxin levels were higher in female collegiate athletes who sustained ACL tears compared with noninjured athletes. In the basilar thumb joint, Lubahn et al[60] performed an immunohistochemical evaluation of surgically sampled anterior oblique ligaments and showed the presence of relaxin receptors, indicating that relaxin may affect the trapeziometacarpal joint. Fifty anterior oblique ligaments were sampled, RNA was extracted, and reverse-transcriptase polymerase chain reaction analyses were performed (JM Wolf, MD, unpublished data, 2011). A significant correlation was shown between serum relaxin and the presence of relaxin receptors and matrix metalloproteases-1 in the anterior oblique ligament ($P = 0.02$ and 0.05, respectively).

The relaxin knockout mouse model shows progressive fibrosis with interstitial collagen deposition in the lungs, kidney, and heart.[61] These findings suggest that relaxin is a naturally occurring inhibitor of collagen deposition. The effect of relaxin on the supporting ligaments of the CMC joint may involve attenuation of the ligaments or inhibition of repair, potentially during the peak of a woman's reproductive potential.

Reconstructing the Joint: Restoring the Anatomy

Because the skeletal architecture of the trapeziometacarpal joint affords little intrinsic bony stability, the ligaments are critically important for resisting the natural tendency to subluxate with pinch and grasp maneuvers (**Figure 11**). There is no consensus about which ligament or ligaments are most important in preventing the metacarpal from shifting with load. Biddulph[62] focused on the intermetacarpal ligament and Eaton and Littler[63] emphasized the volar or anterior oblique ligament. They pointed out that in a Bennett fracture, the stable fragment is the volar fragment of the metacarpal that is attached to the anterior oblique ligament. By cutting cadaver ligaments, Strauch et al[64] reported that the primary restraint to dorsal subluxation of the trapeziometacarpal joint is the dorsoradial ligament; however, the anterior oblique ligament had to subperiosteally strip off the volar cortex of the metacarpal to dislocate the joint. Arguably, stability of the basal joint is provided by the additive and synergistic effect of each ligament.

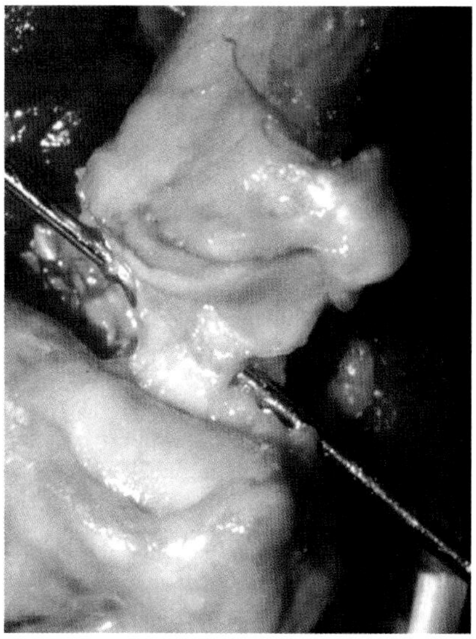

Figure 11 View of a left thumb: The CMC joint is a biconcavo-convex saddle in which the longitudinal axes of the trapezial and metacarpal articular surfaces are perpendicular to each other. The (primarily) concave surface of the metacarpal and the convex surface of the trapezium are sufficiently shallow, so little skeletal intrinsic stability is observed. (Courtesy of Steven Z. Glickel, MD, New York, NY.)

A series of studies has provided compelling evidence to support the hypothesis that the degeneration of the anterior oblique ligament is the precursor of basal joint degenerative disease.[3,19,65] Based on cadaver studies, the volar part of the trapezial articular surface is considered the primary contact area during flexion adduction and, particularly, with key pinch. Degeneration and subsequent detachment of the anterior oblique ligament potentially creates magnified shear forces volarly and dorsal translation of the contact area, predisposing the patient to progressive degeneration of the joint. One study indicted that severely degenerated joints had a nonfunctional anterior oblique ligament.[65]

In 1949, Gervis[66] reported good initial results in a series of 18 trapezium excisions for basal joint osteoarthritis. In 1960, Murley[67] reviewed 39 trapeziectomies and reported that surgery usually relieved pain, but there was a high incidence of loss of strength and decreased range of motion in abduction. Because of the loss of grip strength, he believed that the procedure was most appropriate for less active patients and was not suitable for "men doing heavy work." In a study by Weilby,[68] 17 patients were treated with excision of the trapezium. He reported that five patients had symptoms of weakness, painful spasms, and difficulty holding objects, which were attributed to joint instability. In general, patients regained 75% of their motion, but strength was materially reduced.

Persistent weakness after simple trapeziectomies was likely an impetus for the development of methods to stabilize and resurface or eliminate the trapeziometacarpal joint to provide a more physiologic reconstruction by attempting to restore normal anatomy. Froimson[69] cited the problem of metacarpal subsidence and weakness after trapeziectomy and recommended interposition of a tendon spacer between the metacarpal and the scaphoid. Other investigators pursued the approach of stabilizing the metacarpal with a ligament reconstruction that would tether the metacarpal base (usually to the adjacent index metacarpal). The rationale was to prevent subluxation, prevent metacarpal subsidence in the absence of all or part of the trapezium, and fix the relationship of the thumb metacarpal to the index metacarpal by suspension.

Eaton and Littler[63] and Eaton et al[70] reported that idiopathic hypermobility of the basal joint caused pain, particularly in young women, and also predisposed the joint to progressive degeneration. They developed a method of volar ligament reconstruction using half of the distally based flexor carpi radialis (FCR) tendon, which is passed through a volar-to-dorsal hole in the base of the thumb metacarpal.[63] The tendon is tensioned and sutured to the adjacent periosteum. It is then passed deep to the abductor pollicis longus (APL) tendon, to which it is sutured, and again volarly where it previously passed under the intact part of the FCR tendon and back dorsally where it is again sutured. It was theorized that the reconstruction restored the function of the lax volar ligament and reinforced the thin radial capsule. This reconstruction supported the joint in two planes, rendering it more stable than uniplanar reconstruction. In the initial study reported in 1973, volar ligament reconstruction was used to treat patients with all four stages of basal joint disease.[63] Eaton and Littler[63] reported good or excellent results in 16 of 18 patients and 2 fair results, which occurred in patients with stage IV basal joint disease. In 38 patients who were followed for approximately 7 years, 32 (84%) had good or excellent results, and 6 (16%) had fair results.[70] After segregating the results of 19 patients with stage I or II disease, for whom the procedure is most appropriate, 95% good or excellent results were reported. A 14.7-year average follow-up study of 19 patients treated with volar ligament reconstruction showed no pain in 7, mild pain with strenuous use in 13, and pain with activities of daily living in 4.[71] This reconstructive procedure achieves good but not ideal results, which may in part be related to the fact that seven patients advanced one stage of disease and two patients advanced two disease stages. Volar ligament reconstruction also was used to stabilize the metacarpal after partial trapeziectomy and tendon interposition in patients with stage II or III basal joint disease.[63,70,71]

Burton and Pelligrini[72] popularized the procedure that has become known as ligament reconstruction tendon interposition (LRTI), extending the volar ligament reconstruction to combine it with partial and complete trapeziectomies (**Figures 12** through **14**). The concept is similar to that of volar ligament reconstruction except that the tendon is routed obliquely through the base of the thumb metacarpal and exits dorsally approximately 1 cm distal to the articular surface and perpendicular to the plane of the thumbnail. The remaining tissue is folded and interposed into the space created by the trapezial excision. The reconstruction is stabilized with Kirschner wire fixation. Initially, half of the FCR tendon was used for reconstruction and, more recently, the entire tendon has been used, thus providing more tissue for interposition. A 2-year postoperative review of 25 thumbs treated with LRTI for basal joint laxity showed that the thumb metacarpal subsided proximally 11% of the arthroplasty space, and subluxation was limited to 7%.[71] Ninety-two percent of the patients had pain relief and were satisfied with the procedure. In a 9-year follow-up study of 24 of the patients, Tomaino et al[73] reported little change in metacarpal subsidence (13%) and subluxation (11%) and continued satisfaction and pain relief (95%). Strength increased and grip improved 93%, key pinch improved 34%, and tip pinch im-

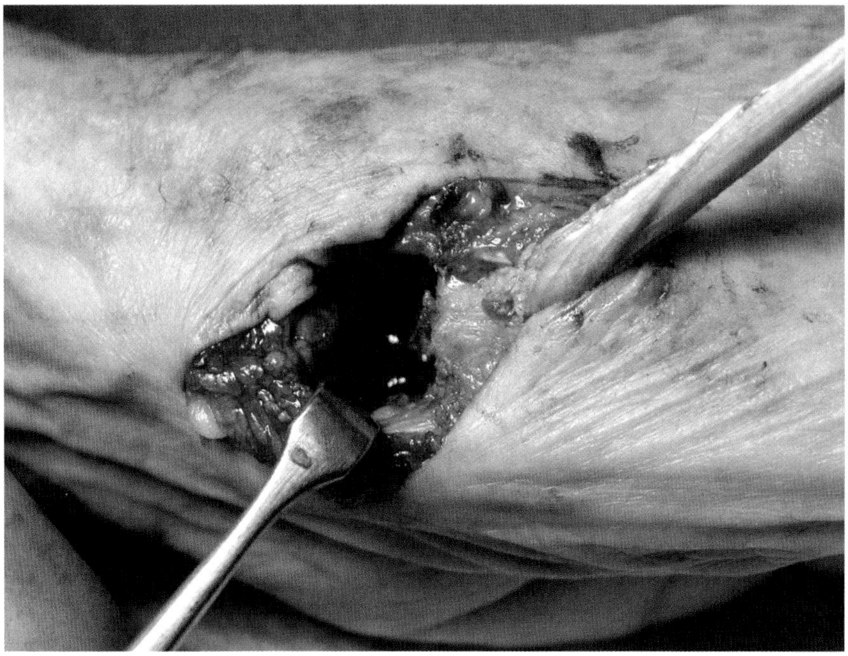

Figure 12 The volar ligament reconstruction (left thumb) reconstructs the lax or incompetent volar anterior oblique ligament complex, with the routing of the tendon dorsally to volarly and back dorsally, thus reinforcing the dorsal ligament complex. Intraoperative photograph of the FCR tendon pulled in maximal tension to restore an abducted thumb position, prior to weaving and securing it in the trapezial void in this set position. (Courtesy of Steven Z. Glickel, MD, New York, NY.)

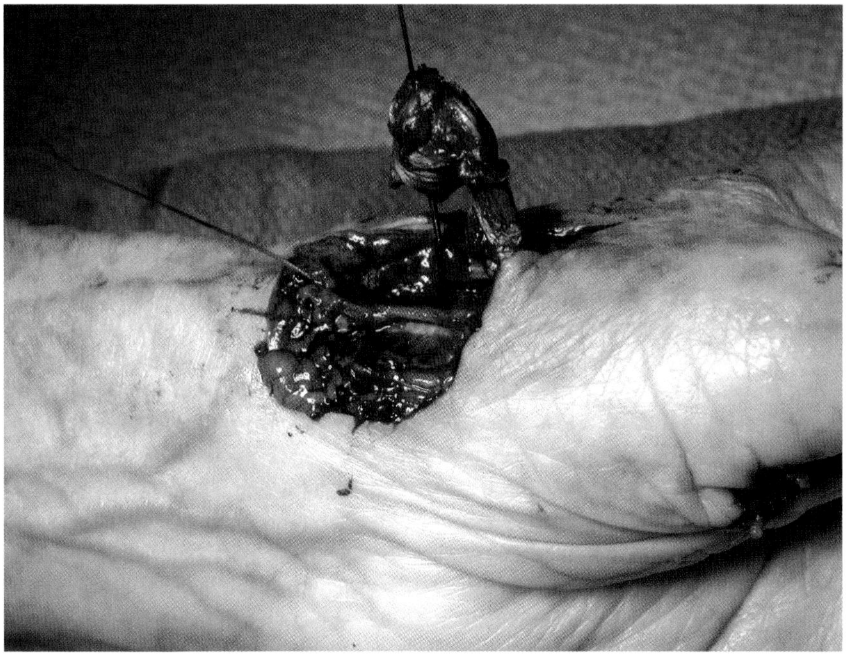

Figure 13 At the completion of the LRTI procedure, the correct tension is set on the FCR tendon that is sutured to the adjacent periosteum. (Courtesy of Steven Z. Glickel, MD, New York, NY.)

proved 65%. LRTI is arguably the most commonly used procedure to treat arthritis of the basal joint. The technique of LRTI includes interposition of the tendon not used for the reconstruction into the space created by the trapezial excision.

Several alternative procedures to LRTI use different rerouting pathways for the FCR tendon (with or without bone tunnels) or use different tendons to tether the thumb to the index metacarpal. The suspensionplasty uses part of the APL tendon to stabilize the thumb metacarpal. The procedure was originated by Thompson[74] as a means of salvaging failed arthroplasties with Silastic implants after trapeziectomy for basal joint osteoarthritis. Because the procedure was effective, the indications were extended to include the primary treatment of stage II to IV basal joint disease. The technique uses part of the APL tendon divided just distal to the musculotendinous junction, mobilizing it from proximal to distal, and leaving it attached to the dorsal base of the thumb metacarpal. An oblique hole is made in the thumb metacarpal base, similar to the hole used for LRTI. The hole starts dorsally approximately 1 cm distal to the articular surface and exits proximally just volar to the center of the base of the metacarpal. A second hole is made dorsally to volarly 1 cm distal to the base of the index metacarpal. Using wire, suture, or a tendon passer, the slip of the APL is passed through the base of the thumb metacarpal and then volarly to dorsally in the index metacarpal. After appropriate tension is set, the APL is fixed dorsally by weaving it into the adjacent extensor carpi radialis longus tendon. Thompson[74] described the technique but did not report results. Soejima et al[75] reported on 18 patients (21 thumbs) treated with suspensionplasty and followed for an average of 33 months. No pain was re-

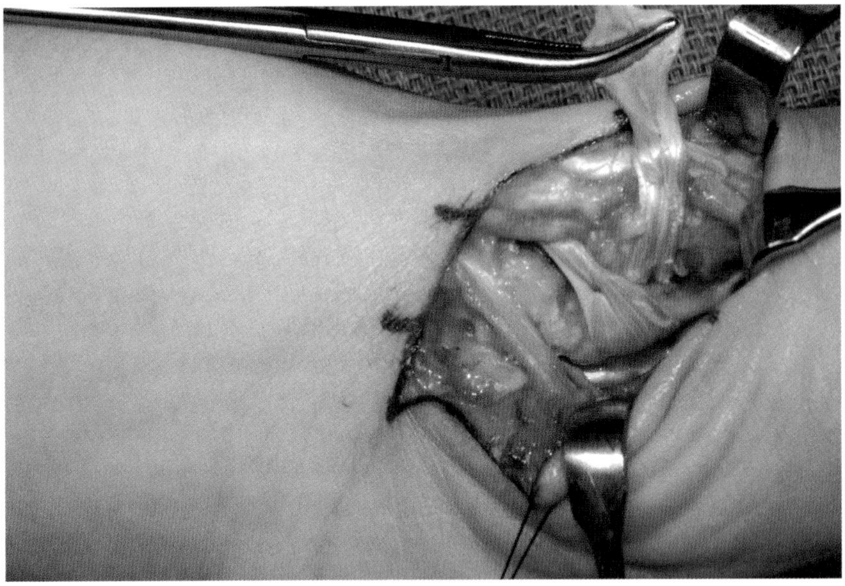

Figure 14 The remainder of the FCR tendon is rolled or folded and interposed in the space created by excision of the trapezium. (Courtesy of Steven Z. Glickel, MD, New York, NY.)

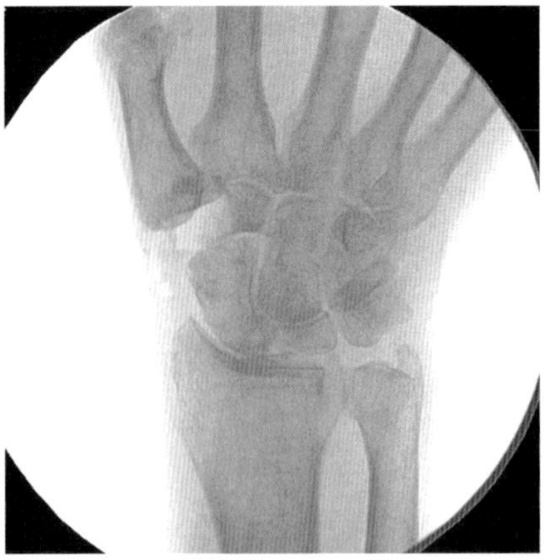

Figure 15 Radiograph of the thumb after a simple trapeziectomy. (Courtesy of Jeffrey Yao, MD, Palo Alto, CA.)

ported in 13 thumbs, 5 had mild pain with strenuous use, and 3 had mild pain with light use. Metacarpal subsidence was 15% of the arthroplasty space. Radial and palmar abduction were both 56°. These results are comparable to those of LRTI, as reported by Burton and Pellegrini.[72]

Comparing Treatment Options

When nonsurgical measures fail to definitively treat a patient's pain from disabling arthritis of the thumb CMC joint, many treatment options exist. Gervis[66] was the first to champion simple excision of the trapezium to remove the bone-on-bone pain generator created by the thumb metacarpal articulating with the trapezium without the benefit of an interposed layer of articular cartilage (**Figure 15**). Subsequent procedures have emphasized height retention and reconstruction of ligament support, with the LRTI procedures, APL suspensionplasty, allograft and other interposition procedures, implant arthroplasty, unloading osteotomy, and arthrodesis.[76,77]

Ligament reconstruction is believed to be important based on the theory that attenuation and incompetence of the anterior oblique ligament is the fundamental cause of thumb CMC joint degeneration. LRTI and APL suspensionplasty techniques are usually performed to reinforce or reconstruct important ligaments; however, simple trapeziectomy with hematoma distraction without ligament reconstruction has recently regained popularity because of the results of medium-term and long-term follow-up studies by Kuhns and Meals[78] and Gray and Meals.[79] Their results challenge the need for more elaborate and time-consuming procedures for reconstructing the anterior oblique ligament.

Outcome studies support the benefits of both reconstructive procedures and excisional arthroplasty. Because comparable pain relief and improvements in range of motion and strength have been reported, it is unclear if any one surgical option is superior to the others.[76,77] In 2005, Wajon et al[76] evaluated 384 patients from seven studies treated with five different techniques. The authors found no significant differences among the techniques in regard to postoperative pain levels, physical function, patient global assessment, range of motion, and strength. However, they reported 16% fewer complications in the patients treated with trapeziectomy alone. In a follow-up study in 2009, Wajon et al[77] reported on 477 patients from nine studies treated with seven different techniques. The authors again found no differences in outcome variables, except fewer complications were again found in the cohort treated with trapeziectomy alone. In a comparison of three techniques (LRTI, costochondral allograft interposition, and trapeziectomy alone), Gray and Meals[79] found no differences in pinch and grip strength and subjective patient-reported outcome using Disability of the Arm, Shoulder and Hand scores. However, surgical time was substantially increased for LRTI procedures when compared with costochondral allograft interposition and trapeziectomy.[22] The conclusions of these three recent studies suggest that any of the described surgical techniques for man-

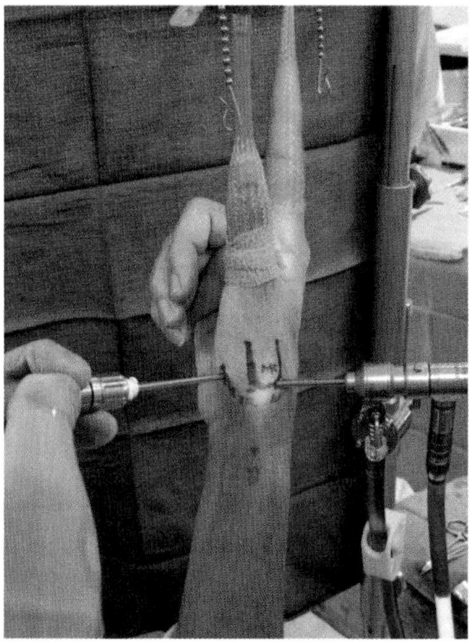

Figure 16 Clinical photograph of thumb CMC joint arthroscopy. (Courtesy of Jeffrey Yao, MD, Palo Alto, CA.)

aging arthritis of the thumb CMC will adequately treat symptoms with comparable subjective and objective outcomes. In contrast, secondary outcomes measures, including overall procedural costs (including surgical time), complications, shorter recovery times, and time off work, influence the treatment choices. A recent publication with long-term follow-up further supports the "less is more" concept over reconstruction of the anatomy.[80]

More recently, arthroscopic management of thumb CMC arthritis has gained popularity. First described by Berger[81] and Menon,[82] arthroscopy is an accepted method for treating the thumb CMC joint (**Figure 16**). Either hemitrapeziectomy or complete trapeziectomy can be performed arthroscopically, with or without interposition of material within the newly created space (**Figure 17**). The benefits of arthroscopy include smaller incisions, less dissection, and, theoretically, faster healing of the CMC joint capsule. Minimal capsular violation with the arthroscopic technique sup-

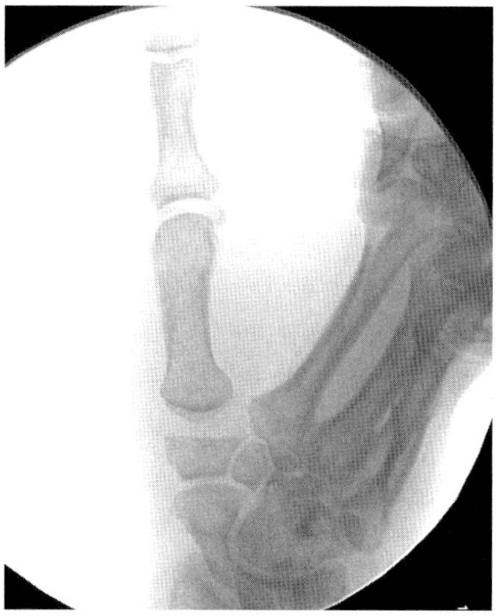

Figure 17 Radiograph of the CMC joint following arthroscopic hemitrapeziectomy. (Courtesy of Jeffrey Yao, MD, Palo Alto, CA.)

ports the concept of less painful and more rapid recovery for patients. Short- and medium-term results are similar to those seen with open techniques.[81-87]

With rising medical costs and the emphasis on cost containment, improving short-term quality of life parameters, and expediting a patient's return to work, secondary outcomes measures have an undoubtable influence on the selection of surgical options. The literature supports a spectrum of surgical procedures for treating thumb CMC arthritis. Because the well-accepted reconstructive procedures are linked to longer recovery periods and higher costs and complication rates, less extensive and invasive procedures may be preferred by many surgeons. Currently, however, the literature is not sufficiently robust to compare the spectrum of anatomic reconstructive procedures focused on ligament reconstruction with minimally invasive procedures that emphasize arthroscopy and excisional arthroplasty.

The ideal surgical procedure expands beyond trapeziectomy. Trapeziectomy, the root treatment in current CMC arthritis surgery, predictably achieves pain relief. The ideal surgical procedure will achieve versatile mobility, with strength and precise docking in the myriad of positions required for fine and gross motor function. This versatility is not currently achieved with any single popular surgical technique. Surgical options that combine a basic science approach and clinical relevance that address strength, mobility, stability, and proprioception, either through emulation (soft-tissue reconstruction), or re-creation (implant arthroplasty), will constitute the ideal surgical procedure.

Summary

The CMC joint, with its complex demands of both stability and mobility, is prone to arthritis for a variety of reasons: evolutionary pressure for a less constrained joint, intricate kinematics and compressive loads with functional activity, and hormonal influences related to sex and age. The joint is primarily stabilized by stout dorsal ligaments that are richly innervated with mechanoreceptors and nerve endings. The volar aspect of the joint has a thin capsular tissue, intimately connected to the thenar muscles, which provide volar muscular stability of the joint. The dynamic proprioceptive function of the joint is the subject of continuing investigations.

Surgical procedures that provide CMC joint pain relief are universal, but the precise combination of treatments to restore stability and strength is yet to be determined. Reconstructive ligament stabilizing procedures are currently being challenged by simpler, less invasive techniques. Improved characterization of the CMC joint as it relates to anatomy, function, and genetic influences will expand and clarify future treatments for CMC arthritis.

Acknowledgments

The section titled "Thumb CMC Kinematics and Osteoarthritis Progression" was funded by the American Foundation for Surgery of the Hand and National Institutes of Health AR059185. The section titled "CMC Ligament Anatomy: New Evidence to Change Old Ideas" was funded by the Williams Charitable Trust and the Orthopaedic Research Education Foundation/Ruth Jackson Orthopaedic Society/DePuy Career Development Award.

References

1. Lewis WH (ed): *Gray's Anatomy of the Human Body*, ed 20. Philadelphia, PA, Lea & Febiger, 1918.
2. Haines RW: The mechanism of rotation at the first carpometacarpal joint. *J Anat* 1944; 78(pt 1-2):44-46.
3. Pellegrini VD Jr: Osteoarthritis and injury at the base of the human thumb: Survival of the fittest? *Clin Orthop Relat Res* 2005; 438:266-276.
4. Haara MM, Heliövaara M, Kröger H, et al: Osteoarthritis in the carpometacarpal joint of the thumb: Prevalence and associations with disability and mortality. *J Bone Joint Surg Am* 2004;86(7): 1452-1457.
5. Matullo KS, Ilyas A, Thoder JJ: CMC arthroplasty of the thumb: A review. *Hand (N Y)* 2007;2(4): 232-239.
6. Berger RA: The anatomy of the ligaments of the wrist and distal radioulnar joints. *Clin Orthop Relat Res* 2001;383:32-40.
7. Bettinger PC, Linscheid RL, Berger RA, Cooney WP III, An KN: An anatomic study of the stabilizing ligaments of the trapezium and trapeziometacarpal joint. *J Hand Surg Am* 1999; 24(4):786-798.
8. Cooney WP III, Lucca MJ, Chao EY, Linscheid RL: The kinesiology of the thumb trapeziometacarpal joint. *J Bone Joint Surg Am* 1981;63(9):1371-1381.
9. Lee J, Ladd A, Hagert E: Immunofluorescent triple-staining technique to identify sensory nerve endings in human thumb ligaments. [published online ahead of print August 10, 2011] *Cells Tissues Organs*. PMID: 21832813.
10. Ladd AL, Lee J, Hagert E: Macroscopic and microscopic analysis of the thumb carpometacarpal ligaments: A cadaveric study of ligament anatomy and history. *J Bone Joint Surg Am* 2012;94(16):1468-1477.
11. Marzke MW, Wullstein KL, Viegas SF: Evolution of the power ("squeeze") grip and its morphological correlates in hominids. *Am J Phys Anthropol* 1992;89(3):283-298.
12. Ladd AL: Upper-limb evolution and development: Skeletons in the closet. Congenital anomalies and evolution's template. *J Bone Joint Surg Am* 2009;91(suppl 4):19-25.
13. Schultz AH: *The Life of Primates*. London, England, Weidenfeld and Nicolson, 1969.
14. Napier JR: The form and function of the carpo-metacarpal joint of the thumb. *J Anat* 1955;89(3): 362-369.
15. Dahaghin S, Bierma-Zeinstra SM, Ginai AZ, Pols HA, Hazes JM, Koes BW: Prevalence and pattern of radiographic hand osteoarthritis and association with pain and disability (the Rotterdam study). *Ann Rheum Dis* 2005;64(5): 682-687.
16. Wilder FV, Barrett JP, Farina EJ: Joint-specific prevalence of osteoarthritis of the hand. *Osteoarthritis Cartilage* 2006;14(9):953-957.
17. Sodha S, Ring D, Zurakowski D, Jupiter JB: Prevalence of osteoarthrosis of the trapeziometacarpal joint. *J Bone Joint Surg Am* 2005; 87(12):2614-2618.
18. Van Heest AE, Kallemeier P: Thumb carpal metacarpal arthritis. *J Am Acad Orthop Surg* 2008; 16(3):140-151.
19. Pellegrini VD Jr : Osteoarthritis of the trapeziometacarpal joint: The pathophysiology of articular cartilage degeneration. I: Anatomy and pathology of the aging joint. *J Hand Surg Am* 1991;16(6): 967-974.
20. Wolf JM: The influence of ligamentous laxity and gender: Implications for hand surgeons. *J Hand Surg Am* 2009;34(1):161-163.
21. Armstrong AL, Hunter JB, Davis TR: The prevalence of degenerative arthritis of the base of the thumb in post-menopausal women. *J Hand Surg Br* 1994; 19(3):340-341.
22. Park MJ, Lichtman G, Christian JB, et al: Surgical treatment of thumb carpometacarpal joint arthritis: A single institution experience from 1995-2005. *Hand (NY)* 2008;3(4):304-310.
23. Van Nortwick SV, Lee J, Cheng R, Ladd AL: Paper No. 404. Divergent patterns of trapezial articular degeneration in thumb carpometacarpal (CMC-I) arthritis. *AAOS 2012 Annual Meeting Proceedings*. CD-ROM. Rosemont, IL, American Academy of Orthopaedic Surgeons, 2012, pp 792-793.
24. Jónsson H, Valtýsdóttir ST, Kjartansson O, Brekkan A: Hypermobility associated with osteoarthritis of the thumb base: A clinical and radiological subset of hand osteoarthritis. *Ann Rheum Dis* 1996; 55(8):540-543.
25. Imaeda T, An KN, Cooney WP III: Functional anatomy and biomechanics of the thumb. *Hand Clin* 1992;8(1):9-15.
26. Crisco JJ, Coburn JC, Moore DC, Akelman E, Weiss AP, Wolfe SW:

In vivo radiocarpal kinematics and the dart thrower's motion. *J Bone Joint Surg Am* 2005;87(12):2729-2740.

27. Weitbrecht J: *Syndesmology or a Description of the Ligaments of the Human Body Arranged in Accordance With Anatomical Dissections and Illustrated With Figures Drawn From Fresh Subjects, 1742.* Philadelphia, PA, WB Saunders, 1969.
28. Ateshian GA, Ark JW, Rosenwasser MP, Pawluk RJ, Soslowsky LJ, Mow VC: Contact areas in the thumb carpometacarpal joint. *J Orthop Res* 1995;13(3):450-458.
29. Bojsen-Moller F: Osteoligamentous guidance of the movements of the human thumb. *Am J Anat* 1976;147(1):71-80.
30. Van Brenk B, Richards RR, Mackay MB, Boynton EL: A biomechanical assessment of ligaments preventing dorsoradial subluxation of the trapeziometacarpal joint. *J Hand Surg Am* 1998; 23(4):607-611.
31. Johansson H: Role of knee ligaments in proprioception and regulation of muscle stiffness. *J Electromyogr Kinesiol* 1991;1(3): 158-179.
32. Diederichsen LP, Nørregaard J, Krogsgaard M, Fischer-Rasmussen T, Dyhre-Poulsen P: Reflexes in the shoulder muscles elicited from the human coracoacromial ligament. *J Orthop Res* 2004;22(5): 976-983.
33. Michelson JD, Hutchins C: Mechanoreceptors in human ankle ligaments. *J Bone Joint Surg Br* 1995;77(2):219-224.
34. Hagert E, Persson JK, Werner M, Ljung BO: Evidence of wrist proprioceptive reflexes elicited after stimulation of the scapholunate interosseous ligament. *J Hand Surg Am* 2009;34(4):642-651.
35. Sjölander P, Johansson H, Djupsjöbacka M: Spinal and supraspinal effects of activity in ligament afferents. *J Electromyogr Kinesiol* 2002;12(3):167-176.
36. Hilton J: *On Rest and Pain: A Course of Lectures on the Influence of Mechanical and Physiological Rest in the Treatment of Accidents and Surgical Diseases, and the Diagnostic Value of Pain* (1863). Charleston, South Carolina, Nabu Press, 2010.
37. Lorea DP, Berthe JV, De Mey A, Coessens BC, Rooze M, Foucher G: The nerve supply of the trapeziometacarpal joint. *J Hand Surg Br* 2002;27(3):232-237.
38. Poupon M, Duteille F, Cassagnau E, Leborgne J, Pannier M: Fifteen dissections. *Rev Chir Orthop Reparatrice Appar Mot* 2004; 90(4):346-352.
39. Hagert E, Lee J, Ladd AL: Innervation patterns of thumb trapeziometacarpal joint ligaments. *J Hand Surg Am,* in press.
40. Pieron AP: The mechanism of the first carpometacarpal (CMC) joint: An anatomical and mechanical analysis. *Acta Orthop Scand Suppl* 1973;148(suppl):1-104.
41. Zhang A, van Nortwick S, Hagert E, Yao J, Ladd AL: A comparative study of arthroscopic and gross anatomy. *J Wrist Surg,* in press.
42. Freeman MA, Wyke B: The innervation of the knee joint: An anatomical and histological study in the cat. *J Anat* 1967;101(pt 3): 505-532.
43. Bird HA: Joint hypermobility. *Musculoskeletal Care* 2007;5(1): 4-19.
44. Myer GD, Ford KR, Paterno MV, Nick TG, Hewett TE: The effects of generalized joint laxity on risk of anterior cruciate ligament injury in young female athletes. *Am J Sports Med* 2008;36(6):1073-1080.
45. Borsa PA, Sauers EL, Herling DE: Patterns of glenohumeral joint laxity and stiffness in healthy men and women. *Med Sci Sports Exerc* 2000;32(10):1685-1690.
46. Sharma L, Lou C, Felson DT, et al: Laxity in healthy and osteoarthritic knees. *Arthritis Rheum* 1999;42(5):861-870.
47. Gamble JG, Mochizuki C, Rinsky LA: Trapeziometacarpal abnormalities in Ehlers-Danlos syndrome. *J Hand Surg Am* 1989; 14(1):89-94.
48. Beighton P, Solomon L, Soskolne CL: Articular mobility in an African population. *Ann Rheum Dis* 1973;32(5):413-418.
49. Wolf JM, Schreier S, Tomsick S, Williams A, Petersen B: Radiographic laxity of the trapeziometacarpal joint is correlated with generalized joint hypermobility. *J Hand Surg Am* 2011;36(7): 1165-1169.
50. Prodromos CC, Han Y, Rogowski J, Joyce B, Shi K: A meta-analysis of the incidence of anterior cruciate ligament tears as a function of gender, sport, and a knee injury-reduction regimen. *Arthroscopy* 2007;23(12):1320-1325, e6.
51. Zazulak BT, Paterno M, Myer GD, Romani WA, Hewett TE: The effects of the menstrual cycle on anterior knee laxity: A systematic review. *Sports Med* 2006; 36(10):847-862.
52. Cooley HM, Stankovich J, Jones G: The association between hormonal and reproductive factors and hand osteoarthritis. *Maturitas* 2003;45(4):257-265.
53. Faryniarz DA, Bhargava M, Lajam C, Attia ET, Hannafin JA: Quantitation of estrogen receptors and relaxin binding in human anterior cruciate ligament fibroblasts. *In Vitro Cell Dev Biol Anim* 2006; 42(7):176-181.
54. Kapila S, Wang W, Uston K: Matrix metalloproteinase induction by relaxin causes cartilage matrix degradation in target synovial joints. *Ann N Y Acad Sci* 2009; 1160:322-328.

55. Weiss G: Relaxin. *Annu Rev Physiol* 1984;46:43-52.
56. Weiss G: Relaxin in the male. *Biol Reprod* 1989;40(2):197-200.
57. Tregear GW, Bathgate RA, Hossain MA, et al: Structure and activity in the relaxin family of peptides. *Ann N Y Acad Sci* 2009; 1160:5-10.
58. Samuel CS, Lekgabe ED, Mookerjee I: The effects of relaxin on extracellular matrix remodeling in health and fibrotic disease. *Adv Exp Med Biol* 2007;612:88-103.
59. Dragoo JL, Castillo TN, Braun HJ, Ridley BA, Kennedy AC, Golish SR: Prospective correlation between serum relaxin concentration and anterior cruciate ligament tears among elite collegiate female athletes. *Am J Sports Med* 2011;39(10):2175-2180.
60. Lubahn J, Ivance D, Konieczko E, Cooney T: Immunohistochemical detection of relaxin binding to the volar oblique ligament. *J Hand Surg Am* 2006;31(1):80-84.
61. Samuel CS, Zhao C, Bathgate RA, et al: Relaxin deficiency in mice is associated with an age-related progression of pulmonary fibrosis. *FASEB J* 2003;17(1): 121-123.
62. Biddulph SL: The extensor sling procedure for an unstable carpometacarpal joint. *J Hand Surg Am* 1985;10(5):641-645.
63. Eaton RG, Littler JW: Ligament reconstruction for the painful thumb carpometacarpal joint. *J Bone Joint Surg Am* 1973;55(8): 1655-1666.
64. Strauch RJ, Rosenwasser MP, Behrman MJ: A biomechanical assessment of ligaments preventing dorsoradial subluxation of the trapeziometacarpal joint. *J Hand Surg Am* 1999;24(1):198-199.
65. Doerschuk SH, Hicks DG, Chinchilli VM, Pellegrini VD Jr: Histopathology of the palmar beak ligament in trapeziometacarpal osteoarthritis. *J Hand Surg Am* 1999;24(3):496-504.
66. Gervis WH: Excision of the trapezium for osteoarthritis of the trapezio-metacarpal joint. *J Bone Joint Surg Br* 1949;31B(4): 537-539.
67. Murley AH: Excision of the trapezium in osteoarthritis of the first carpo-metacarpal joint. *J Bone Joint Surg Br* 1960;42:502-507.
68. Weilby A: Surgical treatment of osteoarthritis of the carpometacarpal joint of the thumb: Indications for arthrodesis, excision of the trapezium, and alloplasty. *Scand J Plast Reconstr Surg* 1971;5(2):136-141.
69. Froimson AI: Tendon arthroplasty of the trapeziometacarpal joint. *Clin Orthop Relat Res* 1970;70: 191-199.
70. Eaton RG, Lane LB, Littler JW, Keyser JJ: Ligament reconstruction for the painful thumb carpometacarpal joint: A long-term assessment. *J Hand Surg Am* 1984;9(5):692-699.
71. Freedman DM, Eaton RG, Glickel SZ: Long-term results of volar ligament reconstruction for symptomatic basal joint laxity. *J Hand Surg Am* 2000;25(2): 297-304.
72. Burton RI, Pellegrini VD Jr: Surgical management of basal joint arthritis of the thumb: Part II. Ligament reconstruction with tendon interposition arthroplasty. *J Hand Surg Am* 1986;11(3): 324-332.
73. Tomaino MM, Pellegrini VD Jr, Burton RI: Arthroplasty of the basal joint of the thumb: Long-term follow-up after ligament reconstruction with tendon interposition. *J Bone Joint Surg Am* 1995;77(3):346-355.
74. Thompson JS: Complications and salvage of trapeziometacarpal arthroplasties. *Instr Course Lect* 1989;38:3-13.
75. Soejima O, Hanamuura T, Kikuta T, Iida H, Naito M: Suspensionplasty with the abductor pollicus longus tendon for osteoarthritis in the carpometacarpal joint of the thumb. *J Hand Surg Am* 2006; 31(3):425-428.
76. Wajon A, Ada L, Edmunds I: Surgery for thumb (trapeziometacarpal joint) osteoarthritis. *Cochrane Database Syst Rev* 2005;19(4): CD004631.
77. Wajon A, Carr E, Edmunds I, Ada L: Surgery for thumb (trapeziometacarpal joint) osteoarthritis. *Cochrane Database Syst Rev* 2009;4:CD004631.
78. Kuhns CA, Meals RA: Hematoma and distraction arthroplasty for basal thumb osteoarthritis. *Tech Hand Up Extrem Surg* 2004; 8(1):2-6.
79. Gray KV, Meals RA: Hematoma and distraction arthroplasty for thumb basal joint osteoarthritis: Minimum 6.5-year follow-up evaluation. *J Hand Surg Am* 2007; 32(1):23-29.
80. Gangopadhyay S, McKenna H, Burke FD, Davis TR: Five- to 18-year follow-up for treatment of trapeziometacarpal osteoarthritis: A prospective comparison of excision, tendon interposition, and ligament reconstruction and tendon interposition. *J Hand Surg Am* 2012;37(3):411-417.
81. Berger RA: A technique for arthroscopic evaluation of the first carpometacarpal joint. *J Hand Surg Am* 1997;22(6):1077-1080.
82. Menon J: Arthroscopic management of trapeziometacarpal joint arthritis of the thumb. *Arthroscopy* 1996;12(5):581-587.
83. Badia A: Arthroscopic indications and technique for artelon interposition arthroplasty of the thumb trapeziometacarpal joint. *Tech Hand Up Extrem Surg* 2008; 12(4):236-241.
84. Hofmeister EP, Leak RS, Culp RW, Osterman AL: Arthroscopic

hemitrapeziectomy for first carpometacarpal arthritis: Results at 7-year follow-up. *Hand (N Y)* 2009;4(1):24-28.

85. Earp BE, Leung AC, Blazar PE, Simmons BP: Arthroscopic hemitrapeziectomy with tendon interposition for arthritis at the first carpometacarpal joint. *Tech Hand Up Extrem Surg* 2008;12(1): 38-42.

86. Edwards SG, Ramsey PN: Prospective outcomes of stage III thumb carpometacarpal arthritis treated with arthroscopic hemitrapeziectomy and thermal capsular modification without interposition. *J Hand Surg Am* 2010;35(4): 566-571.

87. Culp RW, Rekant MS: The role of arthroscopy in evaluating and treating trapeziometacarpal disease. *Hand Clin* 2001;17(2):315-319, x-xi.

Video Reference

14.1: Ladd AL: Video. *Animation of Grasp, Jar Opening, and Pinch.* Palo Alto, CA, 2012.

15

What Every Resident Should Know About Wrist Fractures: Case-Based Learning

Kevin Lutsky, MD
Steven Z. Glickel, MD
Andrew Weiland, MD
Martin I. Boyer, MD, FRCSC

Abstract

The treatment of patients with distal radius fractures can be challenging and requires a thorough understanding of the condition. Many treatment options are available. The choice of treatment is based on patient factors, such as age and activity level, along with the characteristics of the fracture. It is helpful to use a case-based format to review the anatomy, the radiographic evaluation, and the initial and definitive treatment options for patients with distal radius fractures.

Instr Course Lect 2013;62:181-197.

Distal radius fractures are common injuries that account for approximately one sixth of the fractures seen in emergency departments.[1] In older patients, these fractures can occur from low-energy trauma, such as a fall from a standing height. In younger patients, distal radius fractures are often caused by high-energy injuries, such as motor vehicle crashes, falls from a substantial height, or sporting activities. The nature of the injury and age, activity level, and occupation of the patient has important implications in both the initial evaluation and the definitive management of patients with these injuries. A thorough understanding of the anatomy, evaluation, and management options is important in treating patients with distal radius fractures.

Case Study 1

A 42-year-old, right-hand–dominant woman presented for treatment after a fall onto her outstretched right hand. The patient sustained an isolated injury to the wrist. Her skin and neurovascular status were intact, and there was mild visible deformity. The patient's radiographs are shown in **Figure 1**.

Clinical Evaluation

A complete description of the traumatic event, along with pertinent medical (such as sickle cell disease), surgical, social, and family histories and information on medications and allergies, should be obtained. Patients with a distal radius fracture should have the entire ipsilateral upper extremity assessed (as tolerated) for deformity, point tenderness, swelling, and instability. A neurologic examination is done to evaluate motor function of the median (abductor pollicis brevis) and the ulnar (first dorsal interosseous) nerves, as well as a sensory examination of the median (thumb pulp), the palmar cutaneous median (proximal thenar eminence), the ulnar (pulp of fifth finger), the dorsal cutaneous ulnar (dorsal aspect of fifth metacarpal), and the radial (skin over first dorsal interosseous muscle) nerves. Circumferential inspection of the skin is performed to evaluate for

Dr. Lutsky or an immediate family member serves as a board member, owner, officer, or committee member of the American Society for Surgery of the Hand. Dr. Glickel or an immediate family member serves as a board member, owner, officer, or committee member of the American Society for Surgery of the Hand and the American Orthopaedic Association. Dr. Weiland or an immediate family member serves as a board member, owner, officer, or committee member of IBRA; has received royalties from Wright Medical Technology, Inc.; and serves as a paid consultant to or is an employee of Acumed, LLC. Dr. Boyer or an immediate family member serves as a board member, owner, officer, or committee member of the American Society for Surgery of the Hand; has received royalties from OrthoHelix; and owns stock or stock options in MiMedX and OrthoHelix.

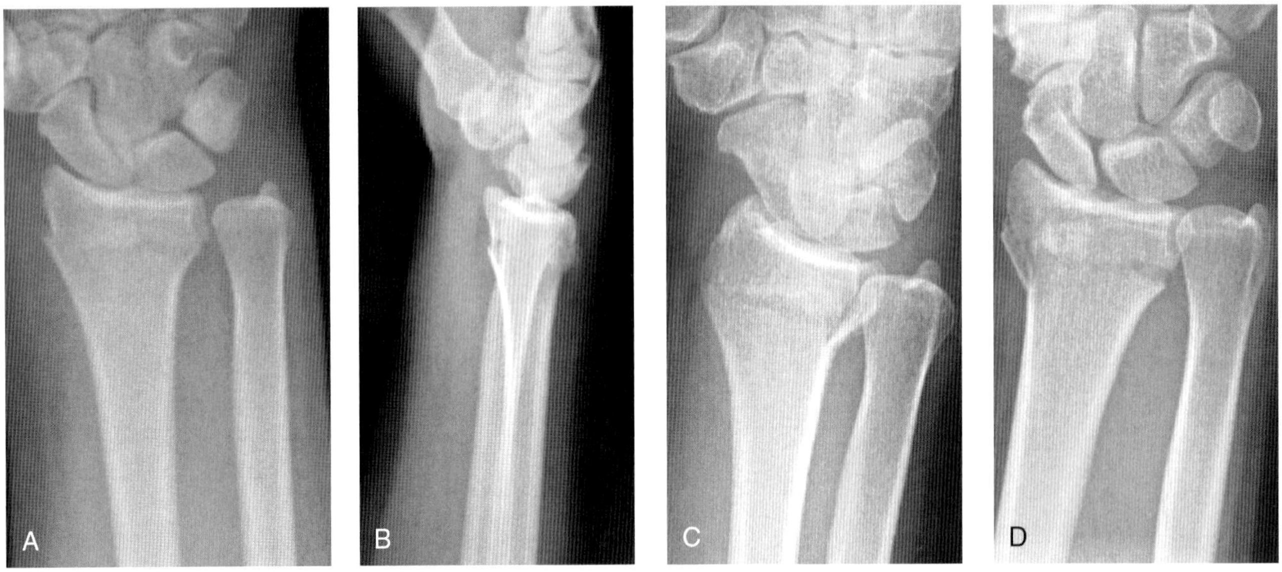

Figure 1 Prereduction PA (**A**), lateral (**B**), and oblique (**C** and **D**) radiographic views of the wrist of a 42-year-old right-hand–dominant woman after a fall onto her outstretched right hand.

open wounds. Wounds are dressed sterilely, and the forearm is immobilized in a splint before radiographic examination.

Radiographic Evaluation

Standard radiographic evaluation includes PA, lateral, and oblique views of the wrist and PA and lateral views of the forearm. Anatomic tilt views can assist in evaluating the articular surface of the distal radius in patients with an intra-articular fracture.[2] These views are obtained by positioning the wrist so the x-ray beam is parallel to the articular surface. The degree of articular displacement, however, can be underestimated on radiographs.[3,4] CT can be useful in assessing the joint surface in these patients.[5] Radiographs should be evaluated for injuries of the distal radius and concomitant bony or ligamentous injuries to the elbow, forearm, or carpus.

On the PA view, the radial styloid, distal radial articular surface, distal radial ulnar joint (DRUJ), distal ulna, and Gilula arcs[6] are seen. Articular displacement, radial inclination, ulnar variance, and radial height are measured, and subluxation of the DRUJ is assessed. Small degrees of rotation can alter the appearance of the wrist on the PA view, and appropriate positioning can be verified by the radial position of the extensor carpi ulnaris groove relative to the midaxis of the ulnar styloid.[7]

Radial inclination (**Figure 2, A**) is defined as the angle between a line perpendicular to the shaft of the radius and a line connecting the tip of the radial styloid to the ulnar margin of the distal radius. This line is best referenced to the center of the dorsal and volar ulnar corners of the radius, a location known as the central reference point.[8] Normal radial inclination measures 23°. Radial height is the difference in length between the tip of the radial styloid and the central reference point; it averages 11 mm (**Figure 2, B**). Ulnar variance is measured as the difference in length between the distal aspect of the ulna and the central reference point; it averages –0.6 mm, which indicates that the ulna is typically 0.6 mm shorter than the radius (**Figure 2, C**). Fractures of the base of the ulnar styloid, widening of the DRUJ, or more than 5 mm shortening of the distal radius may suggest DRUJ disruption visible on a PA radiographic view.[9]

The lateral view is used to measure the volar tilt of the distal radius (**Figure 2, D**). Small degrees of rotation can alter the interpretation with this view. On an appropriately positioned lateral radiographic view, the volar aspect of the pisiform can be seen midway between the volar margins of the scaphoid and capitate.[10] Volar tilt is defined as the angle between a line parallel to the shaft of the radius and a line that connects the apex of the volar and dorsal lips of the distal radius. Normal volar tilt averages 11°. The distal ulna should be reduced relative to the radius on the lateral view, and the radius, the lunate, and the capitate should appear collinear.

Additional imaging studies such as CT scanning can be helpful, particularly in intra-articular fractures. CT can be more accurate in assessing intra-articular extension, gapping or step-off, comminution or metaphyseal defects, and extension into the DRUJ, and can influence management decisions or the choice of surgical

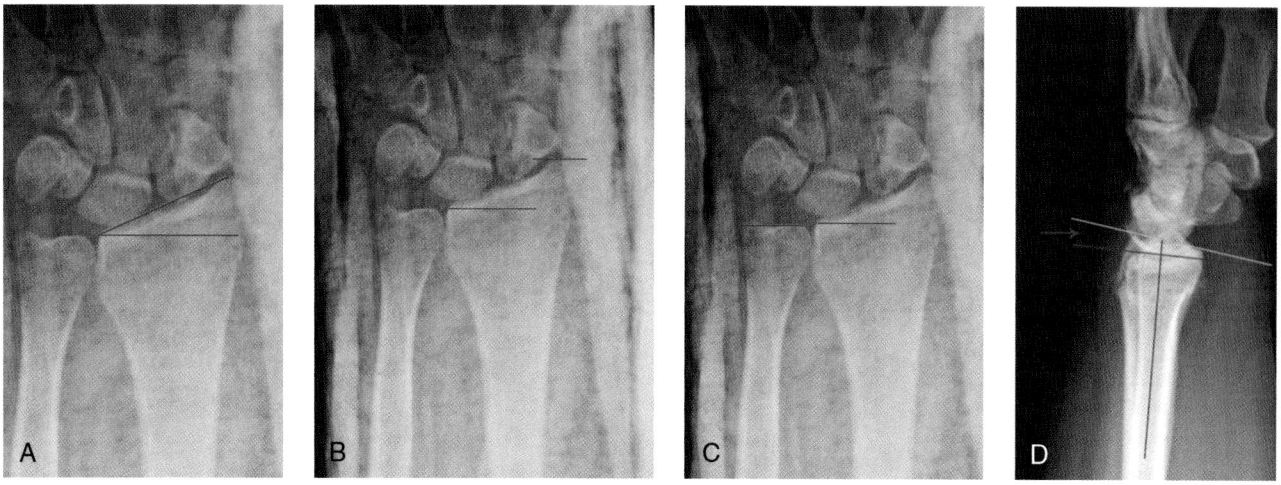

Figure 2 Radiographs showing the radial inclination angle (**A**), radial height (**B**), ulnar variance (**C**), and volar tilt angle (**D**; arrow). See the text for a description of how these measurements are determined.

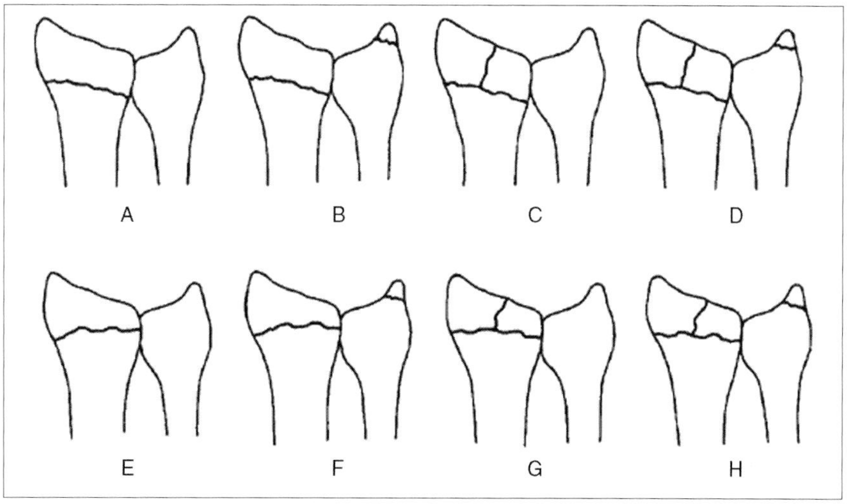

Figure 3 The Frykman classification system for distal radius fractures. **A,** Type I, extra-articular radial fracture. **B,** Type II, extra-articular radial plus ulnar fracture. **C,** Type III, intra-articular radial fracture (radiocarpal joint). **D,** Type IV, intra-articular radial (radiocarpal joint) plus ulnar fracture. **E,** Type V, intra-articular DRUJ fracture. **F,** Type VI, intra-articular DRUJ plus ulnar fracture. **G,** Type VII, intra-articular radial plus DRUJ fracture. **H,** Type VIII, intra-articular radial plus DRUJ plus ulnar fracture.

approach.[4,11-14] Sagittal plane CT can be useful in evaluating the presence of a volar lunate facet rim fracture. If present, volar subluxation of the carpus is possible if this fragment, which is attached to the radioscapholunate ligament and volar capsule, is not identified and fixed.

Classification

There is no universally accepted system for classifying distal radius fractures, and interobserver reliability is low among the systems commonly used.[15] The Frykman[16] classification (**Figure 3**) describes the intra-articular or extra-articular nature and location of the fracture line and the presence or absence of a distal ulnar fracture. The Jupiter and Fernandez[17] classification (**Figure 4**) describes the mechanism of injury and includes bending, shearing, compression, avulsion, and combined categories. This chapter's authors use the Jupiter and Fernandez classification system most frequently in initially evaluating the fracture because it helps determine whether surgery is necessary and which surgical techniques might be the most efficacious. The Melone[18] classification (**Figure 5**) is appropriate for intra-articular fractures and describes the location, the orientation, and the displacement of the fracture fragments. This classification is useful to plan fixation for a comminuted lunate facet after CT evaluation of the fracture. The AO comprehensive classification (**Figure 6**) is a valuable tool for research and documentation and, currently, is probably the most commonly used clinical system.[19]

Relevant Anatomy

An appreciation of the normal anatomy of the distal radius is essential to understand the potential effect of fractures on the normal function and biomechanics of the distal radius. The

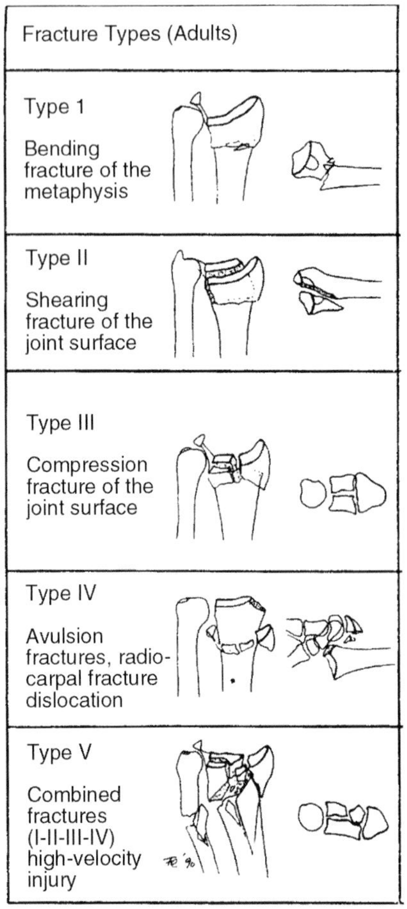

Fracture Types (Adults)
Type 1
Bending fracture of the metaphysis
Type II
Shearing fracture of the joint surface
Type III
Compression fracture of the joint surface
Type IV
Avulsion fractures, radio-carpal fracture dislocation
Type V
Combined fractures (I-II-III-IV) high-velocity injury

Figure 4 The Jupiter and Fernandez classification system for distal radius fractures describes the mechanism of injury.

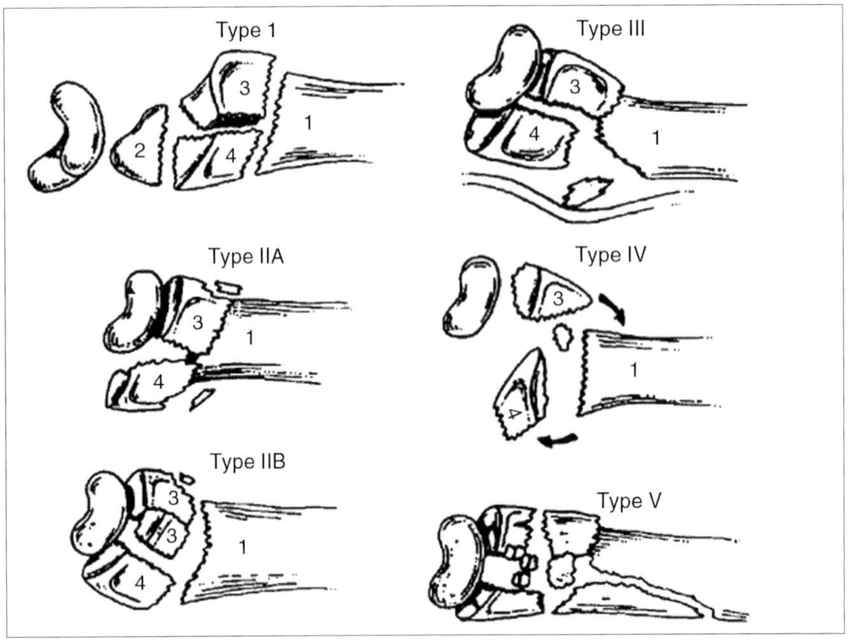

Figure 5 The Melone classification of distal radius fractures describes the location, the orientation, and the displacement of the fracture fragments. Fractures are classified based on the amount of displacement, the degree of volar metaphyseal comminution, and extension into the diaphysis. 1 = Radial shaft. 2 = Radial styloid. 3 = Volar ulnar fragment. 4 = Dorsal ulnar fragment.

anatomy of the distal radius and its surrounding tendons and neurovascular structures has important implications for fracture fixation.

The distal forearm has been described as a three-column construct.[20] The radial column includes the radial styloid and the scaphoid facet; the intermediate column includes the ulnar aspect of the distal radius, with the lunate facet and the sigmoid notch; and the ulnar column includes the distal ulna, triangular fibrocartilage complex, and ulnar aspect of the DRUJ. Werner et al[21] showed that in the ulnar neutral wrist, 80% of the load is transmitted through the distal radius and 20% through the distal ulna. Changes in the relative lengths of the radius and ulna can dramatically alter this relationship. Increasing the ulnar length by 2.5 mm increases force transmission to more than 40%, whereas shortening the ulna by 2.5 mm decreases the load to less than 5%.

The distal radius is concave on its volar surface, where the thick cortical bone is covered by the pronator quadratus muscle. Just proximal to the insertion of the wrist capsule and volar extrinsic ligaments is a transverse ridge or watershed line, which runs roughly perpendicular to the long axis of the radius.[22] Distal to the watershed line, the flexor pollicis longus and digital flexor tendons run more closely over the volar lip of the distal radius, where there is less soft-tissue protection. Plates placed distal to the watershed line may impinge on the flexor pollicis longus and deep digital flexor tendons, causing tendinitis, tenosynovitis, or rupture.[23,24]

Dorsally, the thin, well-vascularized cortical bone is closely invested by the extensor tendons and their sheaths. The dorsal surgical approach and plate fixation require elevation of the extensor tendons; dorsal plate fixation has been associated with potential extensor tendon transfixion, irritation, and rupture.[25,26] The tendons must be protected during percutaneous Kirschner wire (K-wire) placement to avoid injury.[27]

The median nerve travels distally in the forearm between the flexor digitorum superficialis and the flexor digitorum profundus. The nerve emerges distally from beneath the flexor digitorum superficialis and lay deeply in the interval between the palmaris longus and the flexor carpi radialis (FCR) before entering the carpal tunnel. The nerve becomes superficial from beneath the tendon of the ring finger flexor digitorum superficialis tendon. The ulnar nerve runs distally along the

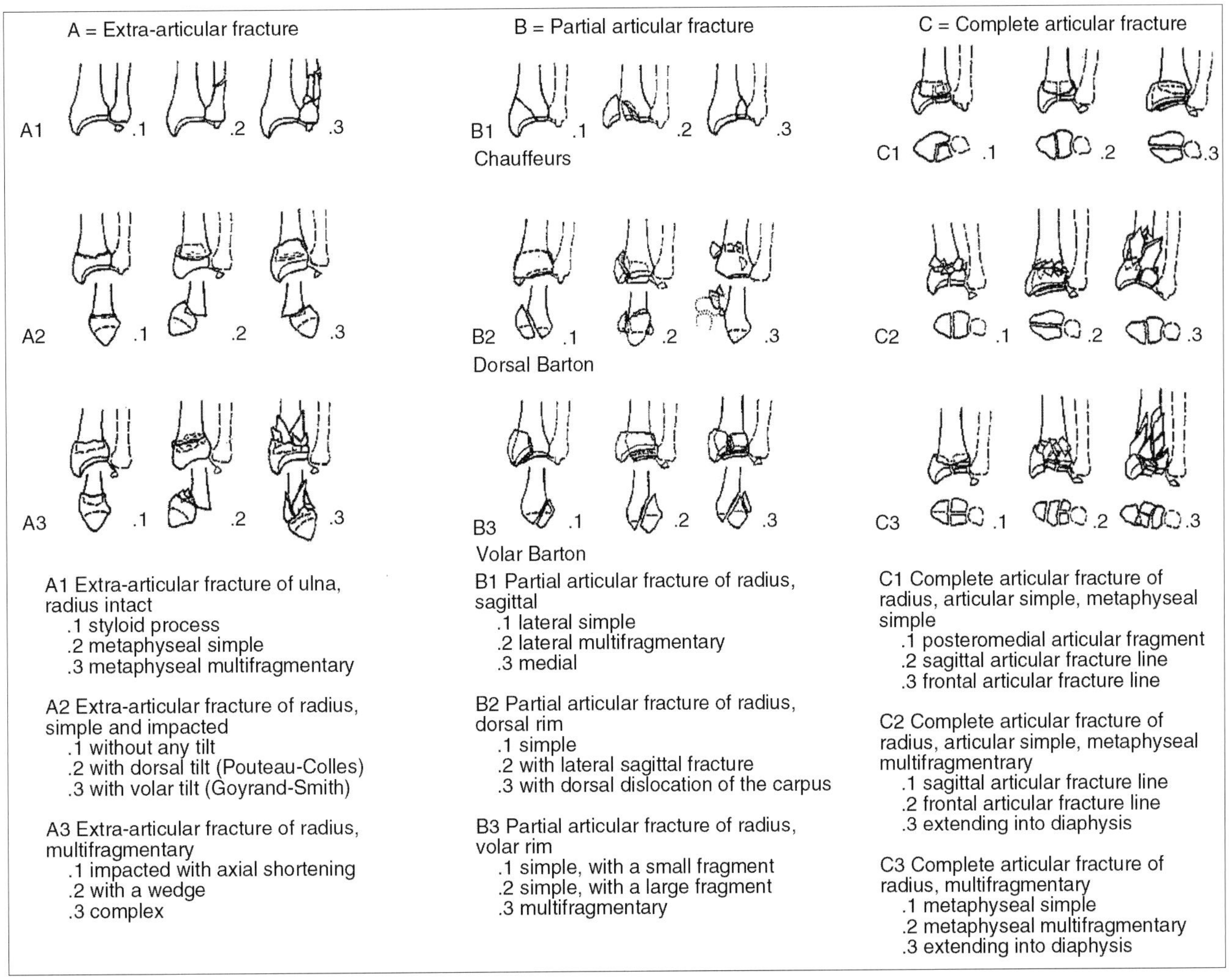
A = Extra-articular fracture
B = Partial articular fracture
C = Complete articular fracture
A1 .1 .2 .3
B1 .1 .2 .3
Chauffeurs
C1 .1 .2 .3
A2 .1 .2 .3
B2 .1 .2 .3
Dorsal Barton
C2 .1 .2 .3
A3 .1 .2 .3
B3 .1 .2 .3
Volar Barton
C3 .1 .2 .3
A1 Extra-articular fracture of ulna, radius intact
.1 styloid process
.2 metaphyseal simple
.3 metaphyseal multifragmentary
A2 Extra-articular fracture of radius, simple and impacted
.1 without any tilt
.2 with dorsal tilt (Pouteau-Colles)
.3 with volar tilt (Goyrand-Smith)
A3 Extra-articular fracture of radius, multifragmentary
.1 impacted with axial shortening
.2 with a wedge
.3 complex
B1 Partial articular fracture of radius, sagittal
.1 lateral simple
.2 lateral multifragmentary
.3 medial
B2 Partial articular fracture of radius, dorsal rim
.1 simple
.2 with lateral sagittal fracture
.3 with dorsal dislocation of the carpus
B3 Partial articular fracture of radius, volar rim
.1 simple, with a small fragment
.2 simple, with a large fragment
.3 multifragmentary
C1 Complete articular fracture of radius, articular simple, metaphyseal simple
.1 posteromedial articular fragment
.2 sagittal articular fracture line
.3 frontal articular fracture line
C2 Complete articular fracture of radius, articular simple, metaphyseal multifragmentrary
.1 sagittal articular fracture line
.2 frontal articular fracture line
.3 extending into diaphysis
C3 Complete articular fracture of radius, multifragmentary
.1 metaphyseal simple
.2 metaphyseal multifragmentary
.3 extending into diaphysis

Figure 6 The AO classification system of distal radius fractures is a comprehensive system.

volar surface of the flexor digitorum profundus, and it distally runs deep and radial to the flexor carpi ulnaris tendon before entering the Guyon canal. The median and ulnar nerves are not typically exposed during routine fixation of distal radius fractures; however, exposure and/or protection may be necessary in the presence of nerve compression that requires release or if an ulnar-sided approach is needed for fracture fixation. The location of the median and ulnar nerves must be appreciated to avoid iatrogenic injury.

An awareness of the position of the relevant cutaneous nerves is useful in surgical planning. The palmar cutaneous branch of the median nerve arises approximately 5 cm proximal to the wrist crease from the radial aspect of the median nerve and becomes superficial approximately halfway to the wrist crease. The nerve travels immediately adjacent to the FCR tendon (**Figure 7**) on its ulnar side (or rarely within or radial to the FCR sheath)[28] and provides sensation to the thenar eminence. Injury to this nerve can result in a painful neuroma when an incision is placed to the ulnar side of the FCR, with injudicious dissection or with excessive retraction.

The superficial radial nerve emerges on the dorsoradial forearm from beneath the brachioradialis 7 to 9 cm proximal to the tip of the radial styloid. It then divides into its terminal branches approximately 5 cm proximal to the styloid.[29] Half pins used for external fixation, percutaneous K-wires, and dorsal surgical approaches place this nerve at risk.

The dorsal ulnar sensory nerve emerges from beneath the flexor carpi ulnaris 5 cm proximal to the pisiform and travels subcutaneously to supply sensation to the dorsoulnar hand. Just distal to the ulnar head, the nerve is in the midaxial line, where it is at risk during exposure and fixation of ulnar head or styloid fractures.

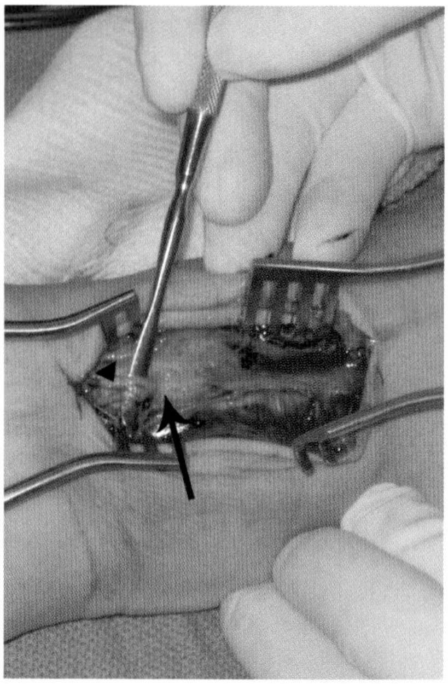

Figure 7 Intraoperative photograph of the volar aspect of the FCR sheath after incision and retraction of the FCR radially. The palmar cutaneous nerve can be seen piercing the ulnar aspect of the FCR sheath (arrow). An anomalous branch can be seen crossing further radially into the FCR sheath (arrowhead).

Treatment

Treatment decisions focus on whether the initial alignment is acceptable or satisfactory after reduction and immobilization. Extra-articular malalignment can lead to incongruency of the DRUJ, subluxation of the ulnar head, or impingement of the lunate and triquetrum with the head of the ulna. Progressive dorsal tilt shifts the load distribution dorsally at the radial articular surface and increases the load on the ulna.[30] It can contribute to DRUJ incongruency, result in adaptive midcarpal instability, and potentially limit motion.[31,32] Combined deformities, particularly dorsal angulation plus translation or dorsal angulation plus shortening, may result in limitations of motion.[33] Articular displacement of greater than 1 to 2 mm increases contact pressures and can lead to progressive arthrosis.[34,35]

Articular malalignment may result in poor radiographic outcomes. Despite the unsatisfactory radiographic appearance, many studies have documented that functional outcomes do not necessarily correlate with radiographic appearance; many patients with healed, malaligned fractures have good functional outcomes despite the radiographic deformity.[34,36-45] This is particularly true in older, more sedentary patients. Nonsurgical treatment in the presence of deformity may be less appropriate for younger or more active patients because residual articular displacement of 1 to 2 mm can lead to radiographic progression of arthrosis.[34,35,46] Because the presence of arthritis on follow-up radiographs does not necessarily correlate with functional outcomes, treatment must be individualized. The American Academy of Orthopaedic Surgeons clinical practice guidelines suggest that acceptable alignment includes postreduction radial shortening of less than 3 mm, dorsal tilt less 10°, or intra-articular displacement less than 2 mm.[47]

After an appropriate radiographic evaluation and a physical examination, most patients with a displaced fracture are initially managed with closed reduction. This treatment decreases soft-tissue swelling, improves provisional alignment, and can obviate the need for surgical reduction and fixation if a satisfactory position can be obtained and maintained.

Closed reduction can be performed in the office or the emergency department by using a hematoma block and/or intravenous sedation. Adequate analgesia is necessary to ensure muscle relaxation. The fracture fragments are initially disimpacted with gentle longitudinal traction. The deformity is accentuated (that is, the wrist is extended for dorsally displaced fractures) and then is reversed. Final reduction is obtained through a palmarly directed force and translation of the carpus and distal fragment. The fracture is then locked in place with the wrist in a position of slight flexion, ulnar deviation, and pronation. Excessive wrist flexion (greater than 15° to 20°) or the Cotton-Loder position of hyperflexion and ulnar deviation should be avoided because those positions greatly increase pressure in the carpal tunnel and can lead to median nerve dysfunction.[48] If fracture instability is such that these extreme positions are required to obtain or maintain a reduction, surgical fixation is indicated.

In nonsurgically treated patients, closed reduction is performed if necessary, and the wrist is generally initially immobilized in a splint. The initial splinting can include the elbow, although evidence suggests there is no difference between long and short arm splints in maintaining reduction. Short arm splints are less functionally limiting and may be of particular benefit to older patients or those who live alone.[49] Serial radiographs are obtained weekly for the first 3 to 4 weeks to ensure stability;[50] the splint is changed to a cast after the first 2 weeks if stable alignment has been maintained. Cast immobilization is continued until 6 weeks postinjury or until evidence of fracture healing is present. For two- and three-part fractures that redisplace after an initially acceptable reduction, repeat reduction and percutaneous K-wire fixation can be considered.[51]

Older patients with low-energy injuries require special consideration. Fragility fractures are those that occur from a low-energy traumatic event, such as a fall from a standing height.[52] The orthopaedic surgeon may be the first physician to see patients with these injures. Patients with fragility fractures of the distal radius have a high incidence of abnormal bone mineral density. A history of a fragility fracture is a strong predictor of future fragility fractures, including hip fractures, and patients with fragility fractures should be evaluated or treated for osteoporosis. The treating orthopaedic surgeon should initiate a bone mineral density evaluation or ensure appropriate follow-up for these patients.[53]

A postreduction neurovascular examination is critical because neurologic symptoms are common after a distal radius fracture. A median nerve contusion causes symptoms that begin at the time of fracture, may improve after reduction, and typically resolve over a period of days to weeks. Surgical intervention may be warranted if symptoms persist. Acute carpal tunnel syndrome is caused by increased pressure and a localized compartment syndrome within the carpal tunnel.[54,55] Median nerve dysfunction is progressive, and urgent surgical decompression is necessary if reduction does not relieve signs and symptoms.

Patients with acute neurologic symptoms associated with a distal radius fracture should be treated with closed reduction, application of a splint, and elevation of the extremity. Serial examinations are performed. If symptoms are progressive or unremitting, urgent decompression and fracture stabilization is performed. Decompression for acute carpal tunnel syndrome associated with a distal radius fracture requires an extensile exposure of the median nerve and release of the transverse carpal ligament and distal volar forearm fascia. The approach for fracture fixation is performed through a separate volar-radial incision, which should be placed well toward the radial side to avoid a narrow skin bridge. Using a single incision for both fixation and carpal tunnel release is not recommended.[56]

A 500 mg per day dose of vitamin C for 50 days after injury should be considered in the management of a patient with a distal radius fracture. Vitamin C administration has been suggested in several studies to decrease the rate of complex regional pain syndrome.[57-59] Although its efficacy may still be unproven, it constitutes a simple intervention with few downside risks. At present, few surgeons who treat these injuries use vitamin C in their postoperative treatment regimens.

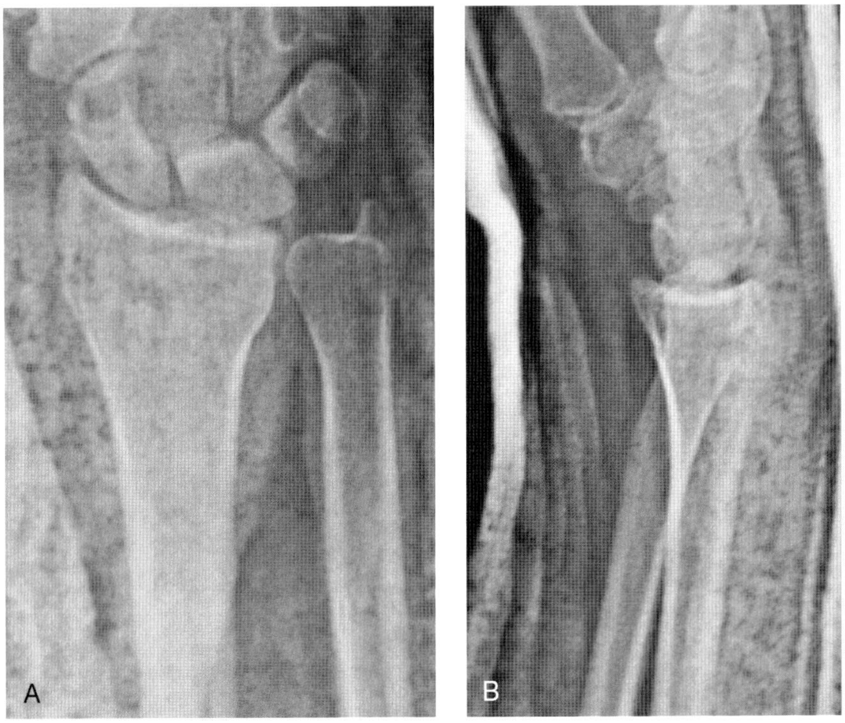

Figure 8 Postreduction PA (**A**) and lateral (**B**) radiographs of the wrist of the patient in Figure 1 showing restoration of anatomic alignment.

Outcome

This patient was treated with closed reduction and the application of a short-arm plaster cast (**Figure 8**). Weekly radiography performed for 3 weeks revealed stable alignment. The fracture healed uneventfully in a cast.

Case Study 2

A 43-year-old right-hand–dominant woman presented with an isolated injury to the right wrist after a fall while biking. Prereduction and postreduction radiographs and CT scans are shown in **Figure 9**.

Several absolute indications for the surgical treatment of distal radius fractures are an open fracture, a fracture with associated neurovascular injury, and a fracture with an associated compartment syndrome. Relative indications for surgical treatment include a polytraumatized patient, the presence of bilateral fractures, or a patient whose functional status would preclude cast immobilization. Beyond these indications there is little consensus regarding the use of surgical treatment of distal radius fractures.

Lafontaine et al[60] described five features that are suggestive of instability (and eventual displacement of the fracture fragment in the absence of surgical fixation): patient age older than 60 years, initial dorsal angulation greater than 20°, dorsal cortical comminution greater than 50%, a distal ulna fracture, and intra-articular fracture exten-

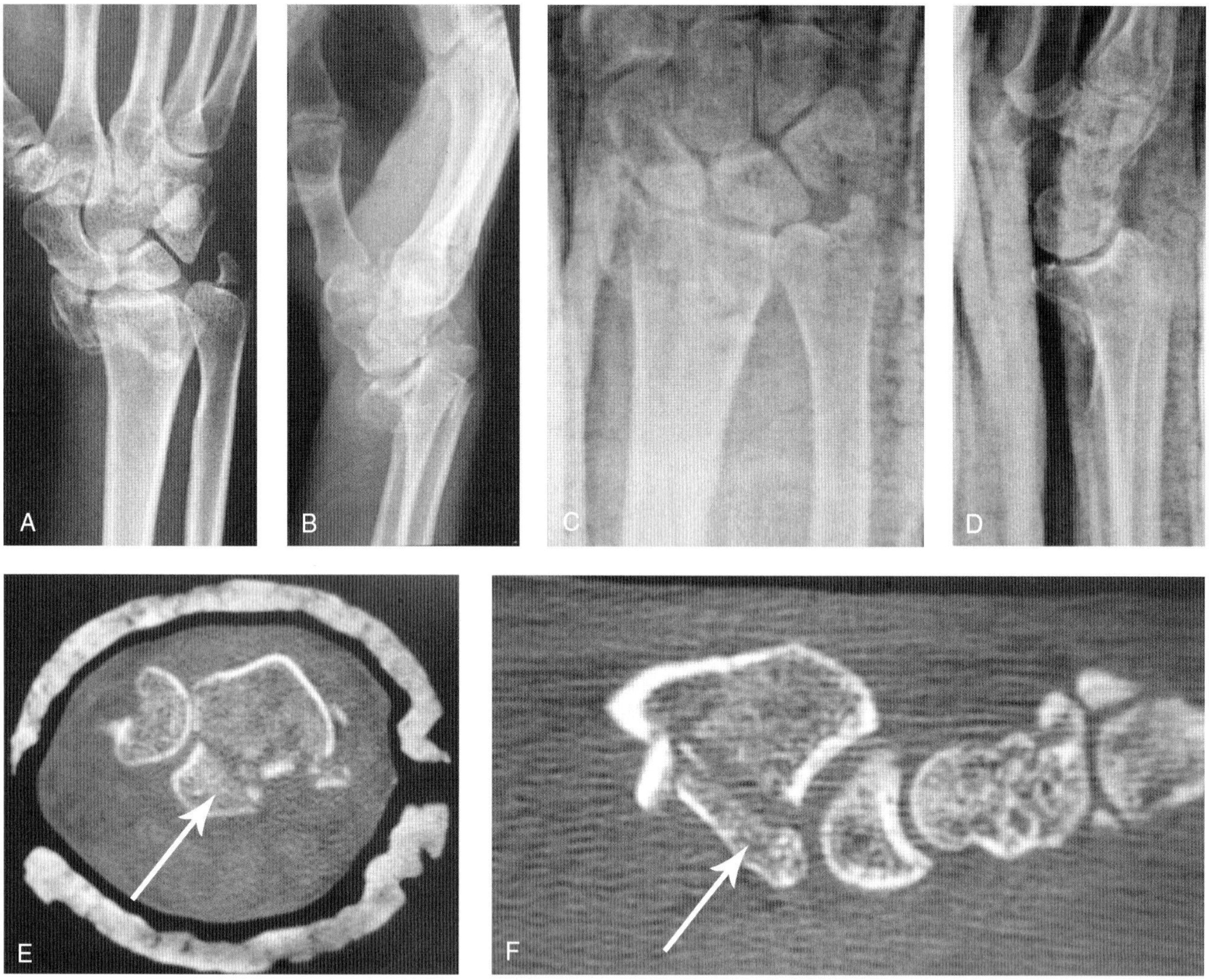

Figure 9 Radiographs and CT scans of a comminuted, unstable intra-articular fracture with residual displacement beyond acceptable limits in the right wrist of a 43-year-old, right-hand–dominant woman who fell from her bike. Prereduction PA (**A**) and lateral (**B**) radiographs of the wrist. PA (**C**) and lateral (**D**) radiographs after reduction. Axial (**E**) and sagittal (**F**) CT scans of the wrist after reduction show fracture of the volar-ulnar lunate facet (arrows).

sion. The presence of three or more of these features is predictive of fractures that are likely to displace after closed reduction and may be appropriate candidates for early surgical fixation. Other studies have suggested that patient age, which is often directly related to bone quality, is the most important factor in predicting successful maintenance of reduction.[50]

Shearing injuries, such as a volar or a dorsal Barton fracture, and some radial styloid fractures are inherently unstable and are also appropriate candidates for early fixation. The presence of a fracture of the volar-ulnar lunate facet, which is attached to the insertion of the short radiolunate ligament, warrants particular attention. These fractures can result in volar radiocarpal dislocation and are associated with a high failure rate if treated nonsurgically or if surgical stabilization is inadequate.[61,62]

Volar Plate Fixation

The patient in this case study had a comminuted, unstable, intra-articular fracture with residual displacement that was beyond acceptable limits. The patient was treated with a volar, locked plate. Open reduction and internal fixation can be performed through a dorsal or a volar surgical approach. Despite a lack of compelling clinical data proving its superiority, open reduction and volar locked-plate fixation of distal radius fractures has increased in popularity in recent years for both intra-articular and extra-articular fractures.[1] The volar approach with locked-plate fixation provides fixation that is sufficiently stable to allow early wrist rehabilitation. The construct provides stability through fixed-angle support of the subchondral bone of the distal radial articular surface and is particularly beneficial in patients with osteoporotic bone or in fractures with extensive metaphyseal comminution. Volar fixation can be performed through a relatively straightforward surgical approach, and it potentially decreases the risk of extensor tendon irritation seen with dorsal fixation as long as the screw tips are seated deep to the dorsal cortex. Indications for a volar approach and locked-plate fixation include volar shear fractures (volar Barton fractures), dorsally or volarly angulated extra-articular or intra-articular fractures, fractures with metaphyseal comminution, or malunions.

After the skin incision, the FCR tendon sheath is identified and incised, and care is taken to protect the palmar cutaneous branch of the median nerve ulnarly and the radial artery radially. The FCR is retracted and the dorsal aspect of the sheath is incised. The flexor pollicis longus is bluntly dissected ulnarly to expose the pronator quadratus, which is elevated sharply in a radial to ulnar direction. The insertion of the volar extrinsic wrist ligaments is protected. The brachioradialis can be released from the radial styloid (if necessary) to aid in reduction; care is taken to protect the first dorsal compartment tendons.[63]

The plate should be placed proximal to the watershed line to minimize the potential for flexor tendon irritation or rupture.[23] Distal screws should be placed close to the subchondral bone to minimize settling.[64] Complications can be minimized by ensuring extra-articular placement and appropriate length of distal locking screws by using multiplanar fluoroscopy, including anatomic tilt and oblique views.[2,65-67] When placing distal screws, neither the drill nor the screws should protrude beyond the dorsal cortex. Bicortical distal locked-screw fixation is unlikely to be necessary for adequate stability.

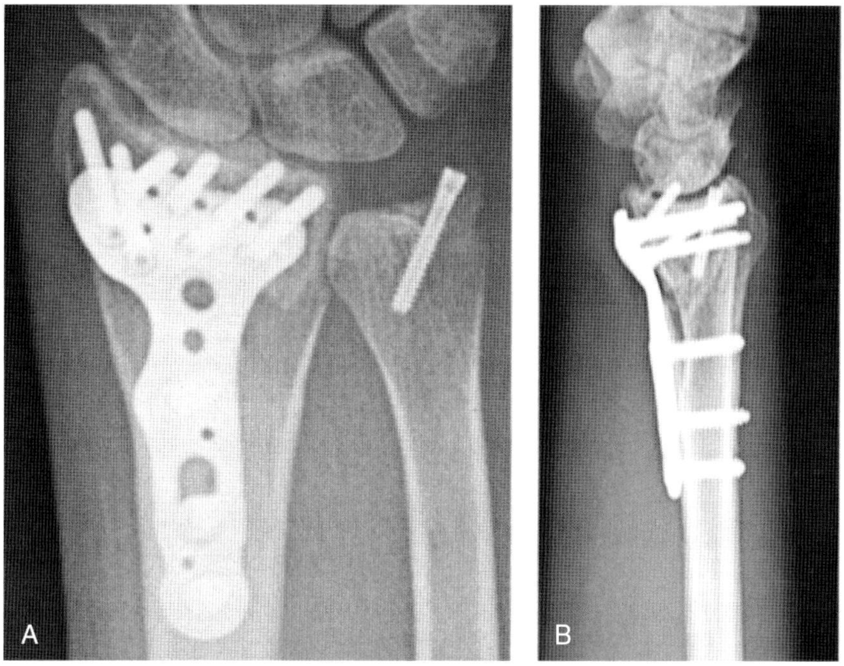

Figure 10 Postoperative PA (**A**) and lateral (**B**) radiographs of the patient in Figure 9 after open reduction and internal fixation using a volar approach with a volar locking plate. The ulnar styloid fracture was reduced and stabilized with a headless compression screw because of persistent DRUJ instability after fixation of the distal radius.

Articular reduction of intra-articular fractures is obtained indirectly by reducing the metaphyseal fragments and fluoroscopically assessing articular reduction. However, intraoperative fluoroscopy can underestimate the degree of residual intra-articular displacement.[3,68,69] Direct visualization of the articular surface can be obtained via arthroscopy or a dorsal surgical approach.

Fractures of the ulnar styloid often are seen in association with distal radius fractures. Recent literature suggests that the presence of an ulnar styloid fracture does not affect the outcome, even if it fails to unite, and may not necessarily need to be fixed regardless of its size, location, or displacement.[70-74] Nevertheless, after plate fixation, the DRUJ should be clinically assessed. If instability exists, the ulnar styloid fracture can be fixed using a variety of techniques, including K-wires with tension band wiring, suture anchors, or headless compression screws if the fragment is large enough. Alternatively, if stability can be enhanced by placing the forearm in a position of rotation that tightens the DRUJ in an anatomic position, immobilization of the forearm can be done with the expectation of a satisfactory clinical outcome. In such cases, a minimum of 3 weeks of forearm immobilization is suggested.

If there are no contraindications to below-elbow immobilization, such as proximal forearm or elbow injuries or instability of the DRUJ, patients are placed into a forearm-based plaster splint postoperatively. Provided stable fixation has been obtained, patients begin active range-of-motion exercises 7 to

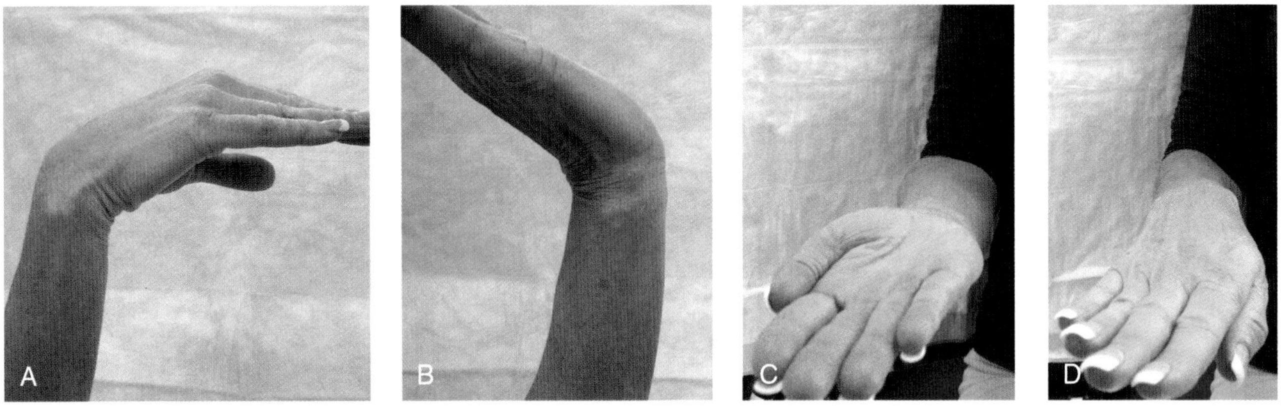

Figure 11 Clinical photographs showing final wrist range of motion for the patient described in Figure 9.

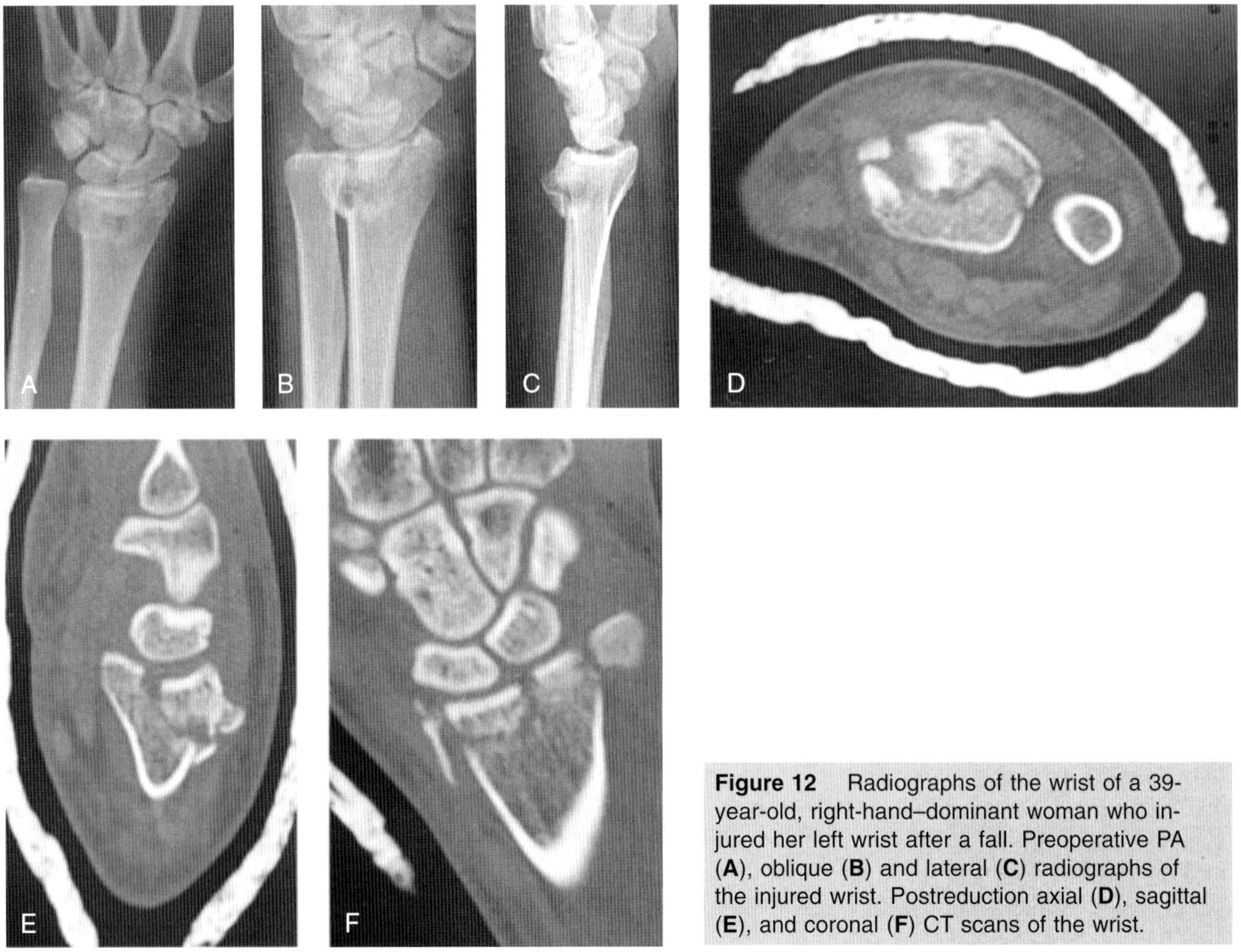

Figure 12 Radiographs of the wrist of a 39-year-old, right-hand–dominant woman who injured her left wrist after a fall. Preoperative PA (**A**), oblique (**B**) and lateral (**C**) radiographs of the injured wrist. Postreduction axial (**D**), sagittal (**E**), and coronal (**F**) CT scans of the wrist.

10 days postoperatively. In patients in whom initiation of motion is delayed, grip strength, range of motion, radiographic findings, and Disabilities of the Arm, Shoulder and Hand scores may equalize by 3 months after surgery.[75]

Outcome

The patient in this case study was treated with open reduction and internal fixation through a volar approach using a volar locking plate. The plate was positioned to support the fracture of the volar ulnar lunate facet. There was persistent DRUJ instability after fixation, and the ulnar styloid fracture was reduced and stabilized with a headless compression screw (**Figure 10**). Postoperative mobilization began after

10 days, with excellent final range of motion, comfort, and function (**Figure 11**).

Case Study 3

A 39-year-old right-hand–dominant woman sustained an isolated left wrist injury after a she tripped and fell. Radiographs and CT scans showed an impacted, displaced, intra-articular fracture of the dorsal aspect of the distal radius. The volar cortex was intact. Prereduction radiographs and postreduction CT scans are shown in **Figure 12**.

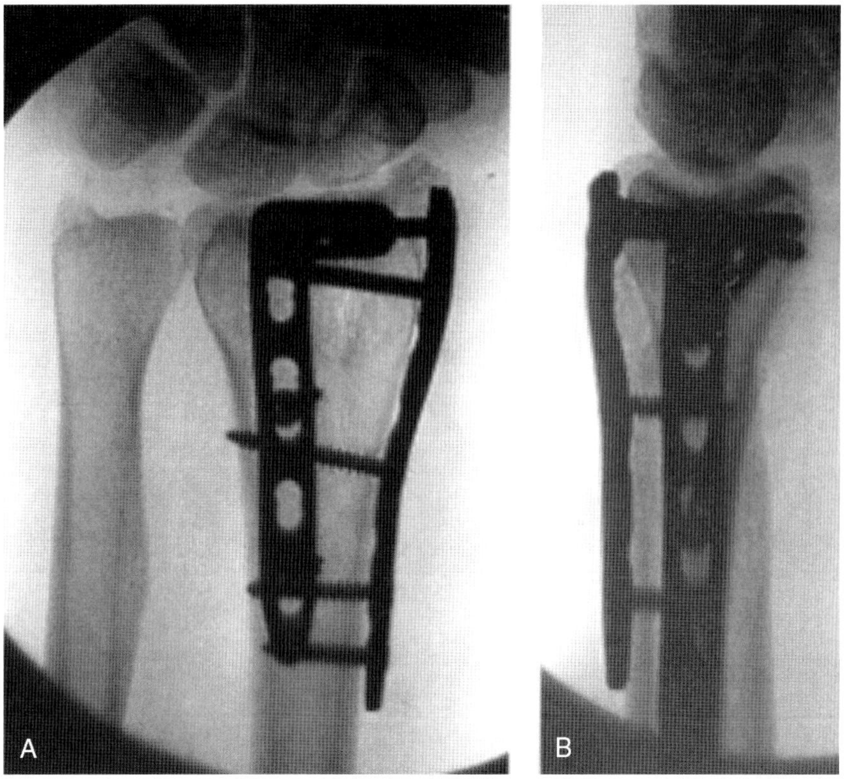

Figure 13 Postoperative PA (**A**) and lateral (**B**) radiographs of the wrist of the patient described in Figure 12 after open reduction and internal fixation using a dorsal approach and 2.4-mm locked plates.

Dorsal Plate Fixation

For intra-articular fractures, the dorsal surgical approach allows direct visualization of the articular surface and permits direct, anatomic reduction. The scapholunate and lunotriquetral ligaments, which are often injured in association with these fractures, can be directly visualized. There have been reports of extensor tendinitis or rupture following dorsal plate fixation,[25,26,76,77] although newer, low-profile implants have not been associated with the same rate of complications.[78-80] Clinical and radiographic outcomes of patients treated with volar or dorsal plating have been similar.[81,82] Indications for dorsal plate fixation include dorsal shear fractures (dorsal Barton fractures), intra-articular fractures, fractures with "die-punch" fragments, associated ligamentous injuries, dorsally angulated fractures or malunions, or other fractures in which an indirect reduction cannot be obtained.

The technique for dorsal plate fixation has been described in detail in the literature.[83] The skin incision is made ulnar to the Lister tubercle. Full-thickness skin flaps are then elevated off the extensor retinaculum. Distally, the superficial radial nerve is protected in the skin flap. The third dorsal compartment is incised proximally and distally, and the extensor pollicis longus tendon is mobilized in a radial direction. The second and fourth compartments are then elevated subperiosteally and extracompartmentally using sharp dissection or a periosteal elevator. The tendons of the fourth compartment should remain well protected by the periosteum that will, after closure, protect them from direct contact with the dorsal fixation plate(s). A longitudinal capsulotomy is performed to expose the distal radius articular surface. The scapholunate ligament is protected. The articular surface is visualized, and the fracture is mobilized and assessed. The complexity of the articular fracture lines and the degree of metaphyseal comminution determines the sequence of fixation (for example, radial-versus ulnar-sided fixation first). The least comminuted column is fixed first. In this way, a complex, complete articular fracture (AO type C fracture) is converted into a partial articular fracture (AO type B fracture). The more comminuted column and its articular surface are then reduced to this construct.

Outcome

The patient in this case study was treated with open reduction and internal fixation using a dorsal approach and 2.4-mm locked plates (**Figure 13**). At final follow-up, the patient had no pain, flexion of 60°, extension of 60°, and full pronation and supination.

Case Study 4

A 52-year-old woman presented for treatment after a fall down the stairs. The patient had an isolated injury to

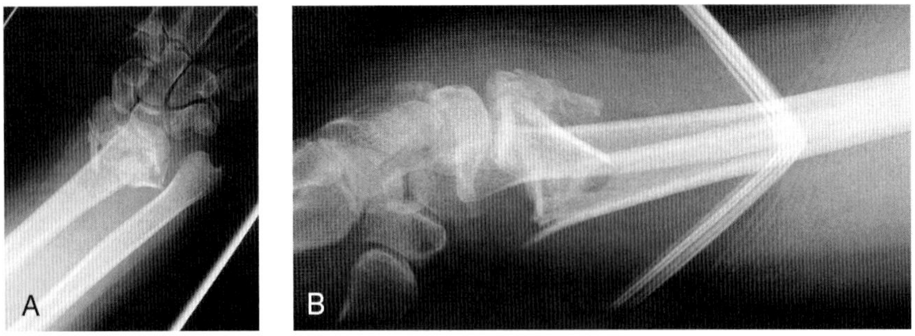

Figure 14 Preoperative PA (**A**) and lateral (**B**) radiographs of the wrist of a 52-year-old woman who fell down the stairs and injured her wrist. The patient had a large, open wound over the ulnar wrist.

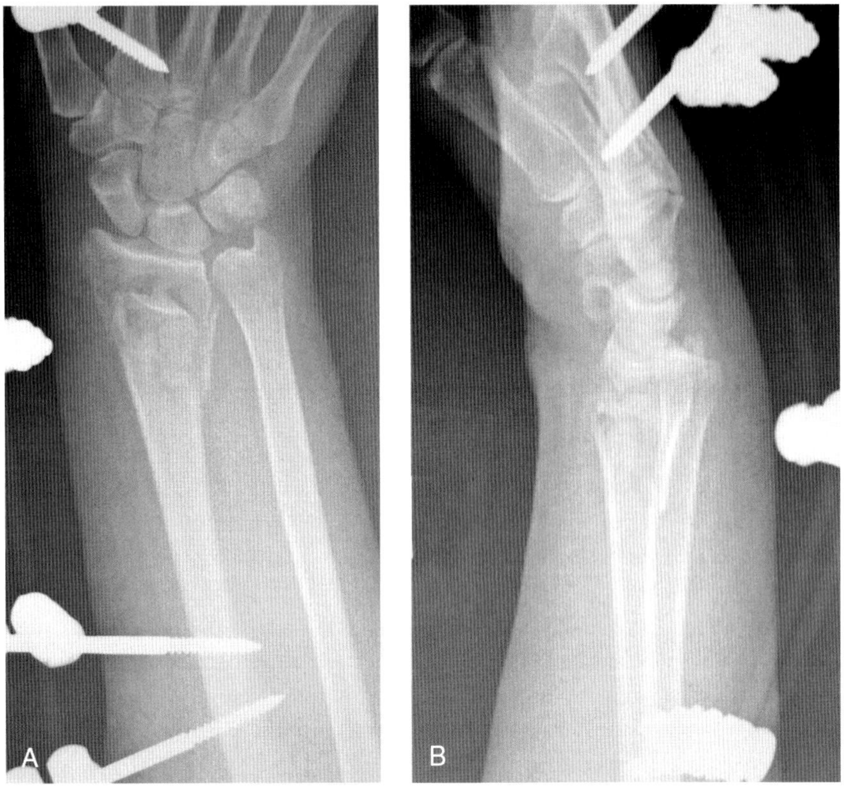

Figure 15 Postoperative PA (**A**) and lateral (**B**) radiographs of the wrist of the patient described in Figure 14 after placement of an external fixator.

the right wrist (**Figure 14**), and there was a large, open wound over the ulnar wrist. The patient's neurovascular status was intact.

External Fixation

Open fractures of the distal radius should be treated urgently, although the recent literature suggests that the degree of wound contamination is the main predictor of infection rather than the time to débridement.[84-86] Tetanus and antibiotic prophylaxis should be administered as appropriate. Standard surgical principles for open fracture management include extension of traumatic wounds; wide débridement of all nonviable and/or compromised tissue, including skin, subcutaneous tissue, muscle, and bone; and fracture stabilization.[87] Traumatic wounds are left open. Débridement and fixation should be performed as soon as the patient's medical condition permits, ideally within 6 hours of injury.[88]

External fixation can be used as temporary or definitive fixation in fractures associated with severe soft-tissue contamination or in the presence of vascular injury. It is also a useful adjunct to pin fixation, which is particularly beneficial in fractures with significant comminution in which direct fixation or buttressing of the fracture fragments cannot be obtained. Advantages of external fixation include avoidance of permanent hardware and relative ease of placement. Disadvantages include the inability to initiate early wrist motion and the potentially high complication rate.[89] External fixation requires intact soft-tissue hinges for ligamentotaxis, and it does not directly disimpact crushed cancellous bone or elevate impacted articular fragments.

In the most common configuration, half pins are placed in the index metacarpal and the radial shaft, and the fixation bridges the radiocarpal joint. Nonbridging or articulated external fixation options also are available.

Approaching half-pin insertion sites through open incisions can minimize complications by protecting the neurovascular structures and tendons with direct visualization. Distally, two pins are placed in the index metacarpal. The distal pin should have two cortices of fixation, and the more proximal pin can have two or more cortices of fixation if the half pin engages the base of the metacarpal of the long finger. Proximally, an incision is made 3 to 5 cm proximal to the fracture site. Lateral, antebrachial cutaneous nerve branches should be protected, and the superficial radial nerve should be identified and protected in the interval between the brachioradialis and the extensor carpi radialis longus while the two proximal half pins are inserted. Half-pin sites should be predrilled before insertion to minimize thermal necrosis and the potential for pin loosening or infection.

Overdistraction across the wrist must be avoided because it can be associated with acute carpal tunnel syndrome, postoperative pain, poor motion, and limited grip strength. Ensuring that the fingers can be passively flexed into the palm or evaluating the radiocarpal to midcarpal joint spaces can help assess the appropriate level of traction; however, these methods are not infallible.[90]

Supplemental K-wire fixation can significantly improve the stability of external fixation.[91] After reduction is performed, the fracture is stabilized with multiple K-wires inserted percutaneously. K-wire configurations vary; typically one or two wires are inserted through the radial styloid and, depending on the fracture configuration, one or two wires may be inserted in a dorsal-ulnar to proximal-radial direction. Small skin incisions should be made, and the soft tissues should be protected to avoid injury to the superficial radial nerve and the extensor tendons, which can be located less than 1 mm away from the pins.[27] A 14-gauge angiocatheter works well as a soft-tissue sleeve to prevent the soft tissues from being wrapped up as the wire is advanced. Although this technique is less invasive than open reduction, fracture stability in older patients with osteoporotic bone can be inadequate, and residual fracture displacement can occur despite fixation.

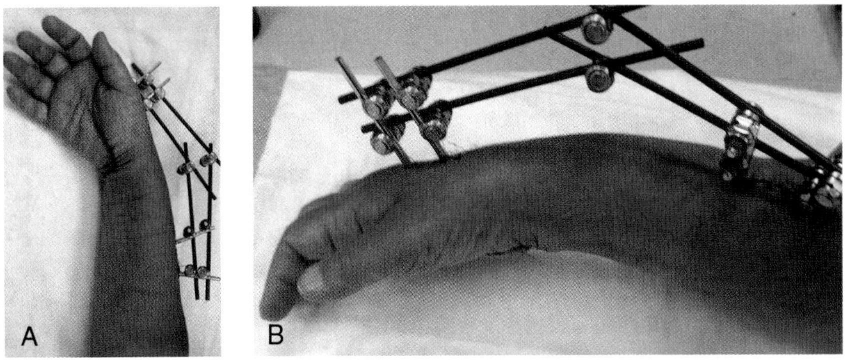

Figure 16 **A** and **B,** Clinical photographs of the wrist and hand of the patient described in Figure 14 after placement of the external fixator. The wrist was overdistracted. Note the position of the ulnar deviation and flexion of the wrist and the intrinsic minus position of the digits.

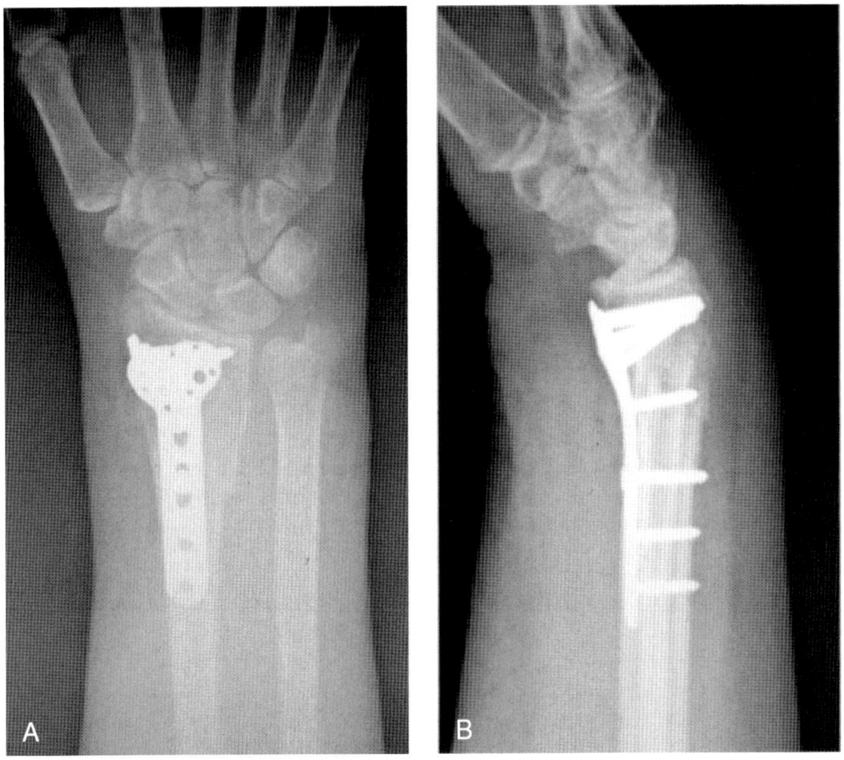

Figure 17 Postoperative PA (**A**) lateral (**B**) radiographs of the wrist of the patient described in Figure 14 after plate fixation.

Outcome

The patient in this case study was treated with an external fixator, which was applied secondary to the large open wound and the degree of metaphyseal comminution. Postoperative radiographs are shown in **Figure 15**. The wrist was overdistracted and placed in a position of flexion and ulnar deviation (**Figure 16**). The external fixator was removed and revised to a volar plate (**Figure 17**). At final follow-up, the patient had wrist motion of 70° of flexion, 65° of extension, and full supination and pronation.

Summary

The optimal treatment of patients with distal radius fractures requires an understanding of the involved anatomy, the patient evaluation findings, and options for managing the injury. The goal of treatment is to maintain or restore appropriate alignment of the distal radius to optimize outcomes. Both nonsurgical and surgical treatments can help achieve this goal. In general, no one surgical approach has shown clear superiority over another. Nonsurgical treatment is often appropriate. Volar locked plating has increased in popularity and can be used for a variety of fracture patterns. Dorsal fixation permits direct evaluation of the articular surface, allows treatment of associated intercarpal injuries, and is appropriate for dorsal shear fractures. External fixation remains a useful option, particularly for highly comminuted or contaminated open fractures. Recognizing which fracture patterns are more amenable for a particular approach and understanding the benefits and disadvantages of each approach is important in formulating a treatment plan.

References

1. Koval KJ, Harrast JJ, Anglen JO, Weinstein JN: Fractures of the distal part of the radius: The evolution of practice over time. Where's the evidence? *J Bone Joint Surg Am* 2008;90(9):1855-1861.
2. Boyer MI, Korcek KJ, Gelberman RH, Gilula LA, Ditsios K, Evanoff BA: Anatomic tilt x-rays of the distal radius: An ex vivo analysis of surgical fixation. *J Hand Surg Am* 2004;29(1):116-122.
3. Lutsky K, Boyer MI, Steffen JA, Goldfarb CA: Arthroscopic assessment of intra-articular distal radius fractures after open reduction and internal fixation from a volar approach. *J Hand Surg Am* 2008;33(4):476-484.
4. Cole RJ, Bindra RR, Evanoff BA, Gilula LA, Yamaguchi K, Gelberman RH: Radiographic evaluation of osseous displacement following intra-articular fractures of the distal radius: Reliability of plain radiography versus computed tomography. *J Hand Surg Am* 1997;22(5):792-800.
5. Harness NG, Ring D, Zurakowski D, Harris GJ, Jupiter JB: The influence of three-dimensional computed tomography reconstructions on the characterization and treatment of distal radial fractures. *J Bone Joint Surg Am* 2006;88(6):1315-1323.
6. Peh WC, Gilula LA: Normal disruption of carpal arcs. *J Hand Surg Am* 1996;21(4):561-566.
7. Levis CM, Yang Z, Gilula LA: Validation of the extensor carpi ulnaris groove as a predictor for the recognition of standard posteroanterior radiographs of the wrist. *J Hand Surg Am* 2002;27(2):252-257.
8. Medoff RJ: Essential radiographic evaluation for distal radius fractures. *Hand Clin* 2005;21(3):279-288.
9. Szabo RM: Distal radioulnar joint instability. *Instr Course Lect* 2007;56:79-89.
10. Yang Z, Mann FA, Gilula LA, Haerr C, Larsen CF: Scaphopisocapitate alignment: Criterion to establish a neutral lateral view of the wrist. *Radiology* 1997;205(3):865-869.
11. Johnston GH, Friedman L, Kriegler JC: Computerized tomographic evaluation of acute distal radial fractures. *J Hand Surg Am* 1992;17(4):738-744.
12. Pruitt DL, Gilula LA, Manske PR, Vannier MW: Computed tomography scanning with image reconstruction in evaluation of distal radius fractures. *J Hand Surg Am* 1994;19(5):720-727.
13. Rozental TD, Bozentka DJ, Katz MA, Steinberg DR, Beredjiklian PK: Evaluation of the sigmoid notch with computed tomography following intra-articular distal radius fracture. *J Hand Surg Am* 2001;26(2):244-251.
14. Katz MA, Beredjiklian PK, Bozentka DJ, Steinberg DR: Computed tomography scanning of intra-articular distal radius fractures: Does it influence treatment? *J Hand Surg Am* 2001;26(3):415-421.
15. Trumble TE, Culp RW, Hanel DP, Geissler WB, Berger RA: Intra-articular fractures of the distal aspect of the radius. *Instr Course Lect* 1999;48:465-480.
16. Frykman G: Fracture of the distal radius including sequelae: Shoulder-hand-finger syndrome, disturbance in the distal radio-ulnar joint and impairment of nerve function. A clinical and experimental study. *Acta Orthop Scand* 1967; 108(suppl):3.
17. Jupiter JB, Fernandez DL: Comparative classification for fractures of the distal end of the radius. *J Hand Surg Am* 1997;22(4):563-571.
18. Isani A, Melone CP Jr: Classification and management of intra-articular fractures of the distal radius. *Hand Clin* 1988;4(3):349-360.
19. Kreder HJ, Hanel DP, McKee M, Jupiter J, McGillivary G, Swiontkowski MF: Consistency of AO fracture classification for the distal radius. *J Bone Joint Surg Br* 1996;78(5):726-731.
20. Tavakolian JD, Jupiter JB: Dorsal plating for distal radius fractures. *Hand Clin* 2005;21(3):341-346.
21. Werner FW, Glisson RR, Murphy DJ, Palmer AK: Force transmission through the distal radioulnar carpal joint: Effect of ulnar lengthening and shortening. *Handchir Mikrochir Plast Chir* 1986;18(5):304-308.
22. Orbay JL: Volar plate fixation of distal radius fractures. *Hand Clin* 2005;21(3):347-354.
23. Cross AW, Schmidt CC: Flexor tendon injuries following locked volar plating of distal radius

fractures. *J Hand Surg Am* 2008;33(2):164-167.

24. Klug RA, Press CM, Gonzalez MH: Rupture of the flexor pollicis longus tendon after volar fixed-angle plating of a distal radius fracture: A case report. *J Hand Surg Am* 2007;32(7):984-988.
25. Ring D, Jupiter JB, Brennwald J, Büchler U, Hastings H II: Prospective multicenter trial of a plate for dorsal fixation of distal radius fractures. *J Hand Surg Am* 1997;22(5):777-784.
26. Rozental TD, Beredjiklian PK, Bozentka DJ: Functional outcome and complications following two types of dorsal plating for unstable fractures of the distal part of the radius. *J Bone Joint Surg Am* 2003;85(10):1956-1960.
27. Chia B, Catalano LW III, Glickel SZ, Barron OA, Meier K: Percutaneous pinning of distal radius fractures: An anatomic study demonstrating the proximity of K-wires to structures at risk. *J Hand Surg Am* 2009;34(6):1014-1020.
28. Nagle DJ, Santiago KJ: Anomalous palmar cutaneous branch of the median nerve in the distal forearm: Case report. *J Hand Surg Am* 2008;33(8):1329-1330.
29. Mazurek MT, Shin AY: Upper extremity peripheral nerve anatomy: Current concepts and applications. *Clin Orthop Relat Res* 2001;383:7-20.
30. Short WH, Palmer AK, Werner FW, Murphy DJ: A biomechanical study of distal radial fractures. *J Hand Surg Am* 1987;12(4):529-534.
31. Taleisnik J, Watson HK: Midcarpal instability caused by malunited fractures of the distal radius. *J Hand Surg Am* 1984;9(3):350-357.
32. Fernández DL: Malunion of the distal radius: Current approach to management. *Instr Course Lect* 1993;42:99-113.
33. Fraser GS, Ferreira LM, Johnson JA, King GJ: The effect of multiplanar distal radius fractures on forearm rotation: In vitro biomechanical study. *J Hand Surg Am* 2009;34(5):838-848.
34. Goldfarb CA, Rudzki JR, Catalano LW, Hughes M, Borrelli J Jr: Fifteen-year outcome of displaced intra-articular fractures of the distal radius. *J Hand Surg Am* 2006;31(4):633-639.
35. Knirk JL, Jupiter JB: Intra-articular fractures of the distal end of the radius in young adults. *J Bone Joint Surg Am* 1986;68(5):647-659.
36. Anzarut A, Johnson JA, Rowe BH, Lambert RG, Blitz S, Majumdar SR: Radiologic and patient-reported functional outcomes in an elderly cohort with conservatively treated distal radius fractures. *J Hand Surg Am* 2004;29(6):1121-1127.
37. Barton T, Chambers C, Bannister G: A comparison between subjective outcome score and moderate radial shortening following a fractured distal radius in patients of mean age 69 years. *J Hand Surg Eur Vol* 2007;32(2):165-169.
38. Catalano LW III, Cole RJ, Gelberman RH, Evanoff BA, Gilula LA, Borrelli J Jr: Displaced intra-articular fractures of the distal aspect of the radius: Long-term results in young adults after open reduction and internal fixation. *J Bone Joint Surg Am* 1997;79(9):1290-1302.
39. Chung KC, Kotsis SV, Kim HM: Predictors of functional outcomes after surgical treatment of distal radius fractures. *J Hand Surg Am* 2007;32(1):76-83.
40. Hoang-Kim A, Scott J, Micera G, Orsini R, Moroni A: Functional assessment in patients with osteoporotic wrist fractures treated with external fixation: A review of randomized trials. *Arch Orthop Trauma Surg* 2009;129(1):105-111.
41. Kumar S, Penematsa S, Sadri M, Deshmukh SC: Can radiological results be surrogate markers of functional outcome in distal radial extra-articular fractures? *Int Orthop* 2008;32(4):505-509.
42. Synn AJ, Makhni EC, Makhni MC, Rozental TD, Day CS: Distal radius fractures in older patients: Is anatomic reduction necessary? *Clin Orthop Relat Res* 2009;467(6):1612-1620.
43. Young BT, Rayan GM: Outcome following nonoperative treatment of displaced distal radius fractures in low-demand patients older than 60 years. *J Hand Surg Am* 2000;25(1):19-28.
44. Grewal R, MacDermid JC: The risk of adverse outcomes in extra-articular distal radius fractures is increased with malalignment in patients of all ages but mitigated in older patients. *J Hand Surg Am* 2007;32(7):962-970.
45. Jaremko JL, Lambert RG, Rowe BH, Johnson JA, Majumdar SR: Do radiographic indices of distal radius fracture reduction predict outcomes in older adults receiving conservative treatment? *Clin Radiol* 2007;62(1):65-72.
46. Trumble TE, Schmitt SR, Vedder NB: Factors affecting functional outcome of displaced intra-articular distal radius fractures. *J Hand Surg Am* 1994;19(2):325-340.
47. American Academy of Orthopaedic Surgeons: *Clinical Practice Guideline on the Treatment of Distal Radius Fractures.* Rosemont, IL, American Academy of Orthopaedic Surgeons, December 2009. http://www.aaos.org/Research/guidelines/drfguideline.pdf. Accessed February 1, 2012.
48. Gelberman RH, Szabo RM, Mortensen WW: Carpal tunnel pressures and wrist position in patients with Colles' fractures. *J Trauma* 1984;24(8):747-749.

49. Bong MR, Egol KA, Leibman M, Koval KJ: A comparison of immediate postreduction splinting constructs for controlling initial displacement of fractures of the distal radius: A prospective randomized study of long-arm versus short-arm splinting. *J Hand Surg Am* 2006;31(5):766-770.

50. Nesbitt KS, Failla JM, Les C: Assessment of instability factors in adult distal radius fractures. *J Hand Surg Am* 2004;29(6): 1128-1138.

51. Glickel SZ, Catalano LW, Raia FJ, Barron OA, Grabow R, Chia B: Long-term outcomes of closed reduction and percutaneous pinning for the treatment of distal radius fractures. *J Hand Surg Am* 2008;33(10):1700-1705.

52. Bouxsein ML, Kaufman J, Tosi L, Cummings S, Lane J, Johnell O: Recommendations for optimal care of the fragility fracture patient to reduce the risk of future fracture. *J Am Acad Orthop Surg* 2004;12(6):385-395.

53. Rozental TD, Makhni EC, Day CS, Bouxsein ML: Improving evaluation and treatment for osteoporosis following distal radial fractures: A prospective randomized intervention. *J Bone Joint Surg Am* 2008;90(5):953-961.

54. Dyer G, Lozano-Calderon S, Gannon C, Baratz M, Ring D: Predictors of acute carpal tunnel syndrome associated with fracture of the distal radius. *J Hand Surg Am* 2008;33(8):1309-1313.

55. Bauman TD, Gelberman RH, Mubarak SJ, Garfin SR: The acute carpal tunnel syndrome. *Clin Orthop Relat Res* 1981;156: 151-156.

56. Lattmann T, Dietrich M, Meier C, Kilgus M, Platz A: Comparison of 2 surgical approaches for volar locking plate osteosynthesis of the distal radius. *J Hand Surg Am* 2008;33(7):1135-1143.

57. Lichtman DM, Bindra RR, Boyer MI, et al: Treatment of distal radius fractures. *J Am Acad Orthop Surg* 2010;18(3):180-189.

58. Shah AS, Verma MK, Jebson PJ: Use of oral vitamin C after fractures of the distal radius. *J Hand Surg Am* 2009;34(9):1736-1738.

59. Zollinger PE, Tuinebreijer WE, Breederveld RS, Kreis RW: Can vitamin C prevent complex regional pain syndrome in patients with wrist fractures? A randomized, controlled, multicenter dose-response study. *J Bone Joint Surg Am* 2007;89(7):1424-1431.

60. Lafontaine M, Hardy D, Delince P: Stability assessment of distal radius fractures. *Injury* 1989; 20(4):208-210.

61. Apergis E, Darmanis S, Theodoratos G, Maris J: Beware of the ulno-palmar distal radial fragment. *J Hand Surg Br* 2002; 27(2):139-145.

62. Harness NG, Jupiter JB, Orbay JL, Raskin KB, Fernandez DL: Loss of fixation of the volar lunate facet fragment in fractures of the distal part of the radius. *J Bone Joint Surg Am* 2004;86(9):1900-1908.

63. Koh S, Andersen CR, Buford WL Jr, Patterson RM, Viegas SF: Anatomy of the distal brachioradialis and its potential relationship to distal radius fracture. *J Hand Surg Am* 2006;31(1):2-8.

64. Drobetz H, Bryant AL, Pokorny T, Spitaler R, Leixnering M, Jupiter JB: Volar fixed-angle plating of distal radius extension fractures: Influence of plate position on secondary loss of reduction. A biomechanic study in a cadaveric model. *J Hand Surg Am* 2006; 31(4):615-622.

65. Smith DW, Henry MH: The 45 degrees pronated oblique view for volar fixed-angle plating of distal radius fractures. *J Hand Surg Am* 2004;29(4):703-706.

66. Soong M, Got C, Katarincic J, Akelman E: Fluoroscopic evaluation of intra-articular screw placement during locked volar plating of the distal radius: A cadaveric study. *J Hand Surg Am* 2008; 33(10):1720-1723.

67. Maschke SD, Evans PJ, Schub D, Drake R, Lawton JN: Radiographic evaluation of dorsal screw penetration after volar fixed-angle plating of the distal radius: A cadaveric study. *Hand (NY)* 2007; 2(3):144-150.

68. Augé WK II, Velázquez PA: The application of indirect reduction techniques in the distal radius: The role of adjuvant arthroscopy. *Arthroscopy* 2000;16(8):830-835.

69. Edwards CC II, Haraszti CJ, McGillivary GR, Gutow AP: Intra-articular distal radius fractures: Arthroscopic assessment of radiographically assisted reduction. *J Hand Surg Am* 2001;26(6): 1036-1041.

70. Souer JS, Ring D, Matschke S, et al: Effect of an unrepaired fracture of the ulnar styloid base on outcome after plate-and-screw fixation of a distal radial fracture. *J Bone Joint Surg Am* 2009;91(4): 830-838.

71. Sammer DM, Shah HM, Shauver MJ, Chung KC: The effect of ulnar styloid fractures on patient-rated outcomes after volar locking plating of distal radius fractures. *J Hand Surg Am* 2009;34(9): 1595-1602.

72. Kim JK, Koh YD, Do NH: Should an ulnar styloid fracture be fixed following volar plate fixation of a distal radial fracture? *J Bone Joint Surg Am* 2010;92(1): 1-6.

73. Kim JK, Yun YH, Kim DJ, Yun GU: Comparison of united and nonunited fractures of the ulnar styloid following volar-plate fixation of distal radius fractures. *Injury* 2011;42(4):371-375.

74. Buijze GA, Ring D: Clinical impact of united versus nonunited fractures of the proximal half of the ulnar styloid following volar plate fixation of the distal radius. *J Hand Surg Am* 2010;35(2): 223-227.

75. Lozano-Calderón SA, Souer S, Mudgal C, Jupiter JB, Ring D: Wrist mobilization following volar plate fixation of fractures of the distal part of the radius. *J Bone Joint Surg Am* 2008;90(6):1297-1304.

76. Sánchez T, Jakubietz M, Jakubietz R, Mayer J, Beutel FK, Grünert J: Complications after pi plate osteosynthesis. *Plast Reconstr Surg* 2005;116(1):153-158.

77. Suckel A, Spies S, Münst P: Dorsal (AO/ASIF) pi-plate osteosynthesis in the treatment of distal intraarticular radius fractures. *J Hand Surg Br* 2006;31(6): 673-679.

78. Kamath AF, Zurakowski D, Day CS: Low-profile dorsal plating for dorsally angulated distal radius fractures: An outcomes study. *J Hand Surg Am* 2006;31(7): 1061-1067.

79. Simic PM, Robison J, Gardner MJ, Gelberman RH, Weiland AJ, Boyer MI: Treatment of distal radius fractures with a low-profile dorsal plating system: An outcomes assessment. *J Hand Surg Am* 2006;31(3):382-386.

80. Jupiter JB, Marent-Huber M; LCP Study Group: Operative management of distal radial fractures with 2.4-millimeter locking plates: A multicenter prospective case series. *J Bone Joint Surg Am* 2009;91(1):55-65.

81. Rein S, Schikore H, Schneiders W, Amlang M, Zwipp H: Results of dorsal or volar plate fixation of AO type C3 distal radius fractures: A retrospective study. *J Hand Surg Am* 2007;32(7): 954-961.

82. Ruch DS, Papadonikolakis A: Volar versus dorsal plating in the management of intra-articular distal radius fractures. *J Hand Surg Am* 2006;31(1):9-16.

83. Lutsky K, McKeon K, Goldfarb C, Boyer M: Dorsal fixation of intra-articular distal radius fractures using 2.4-mm locking plates. *Tech Hand Up Extrem Surg* 2009; 13(4):187-196.

84. Rozental TD, Beredjiklian PK, Steinberg DR, Bozentka DJ: Open fractures of the distal radius. *J Hand Surg Am* 2002;27(1): 77-85.

85. Yang EC, Eisler J: Treatment of isolated type I open fractures: Is emergent operative debridement necessary? *Clin Orthop Relat Res* 2003;410:289-294.

86. Jawa A: Open fractures of the distal radius. *J Hand Surg Am* 2010;35(8):1348-1350.

87. Zalavras CG, Marcus RE, Levin LS, Patzakis MJ: Management of open fractures and subsequent complications. *Instr Course Lect* 2008;57:51-63.

88. Werner CM, Pierpont Y, Pollak AN: The urgency of surgical débridement in the management of open fractures. *J Am Acad Orthop Surg* 2008;16(7):369-375.

89. Sanders RA, Keppel FL, Waldrop JI: External fixation of distal radial fractures: Results and complications. *J Hand Surg Am* 1991; 16(3):385-391.

90. Gupta R, Bozentka DJ, Bora FW: The evaluation of tension in an experimental model of external fixation of distal radius fractures. *J Hand Surg Am* 1999;24(1): 108-112.

91. Bindra RR: Biomechanics and biology of external fixation of distal radius fractures. *Hand Clin* 2005;21(3):363-373.

SECTION

4

Adult Reconstruction: Hip

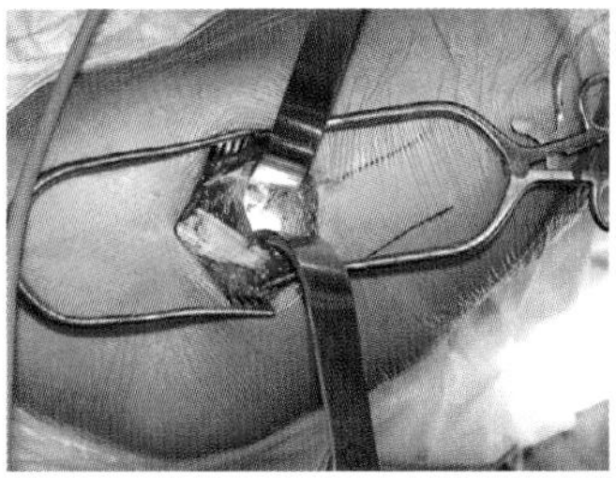

16 The Basic Science of Periprosthetic Osteolysis

17 Monitoring and Risk of Progression of Osteolysis After Total Hip Arthroplasty

18 The Changing Paradigm of Revision of Total Hip Replacement in the Presence of Osteolysis

19 Outpatient Minimally Invasive Total Hip Arthroplasty Via a Modified Watson-Jones Approach: Technique and Results

DVD 20 Total Hip Arthroplasty: The Mini-Posterior Approach

21 Total Hip Arthroplasty Using the Superior Capsulotomy Technique

22 Primary and Revision Anterior Supine Total Hip Arthroplasty: An Analysis of Complications and Reoperations

23 Patient Selection for Rotational Pelvic Osteotomy

24 Periacetabular Osteotomy: Intra-articular Work

25 Alternatives to Periacetabular Osteotomy for Adult Acetabular Dysplasia

26 Approaches and Perioperative Management in Periacetabular Osteotomy Surgery: The Minimally Invasive Transsartorial Approach

27 The Management of Acetabular Retroversion With Reverse Periacetabular Osteotomy

16

The Basic Science of Periprosthetic Osteolysis

Stuart B. Goodman, MD, PhD, FRCSC
Emmanuel Gibon, MD
Zhenyu Yao, MD, PhD

Abstract

Total joint arthroplasty has revolutionized the treatment of arthritic and degenerative conditions for many joints in the body; however, wear debris is continuously generated with day-to-day use of an artificial joint. Excessive production of wear by-products induces a foreign body and chronic inflammatory reaction that accelerates periprosthetic bone destruction and inhibits bone formation. The specific biologic reaction is dependent on the type, amount, and characteristics of the by-products of wear, along with individual genetic variations. For polymeric and ceramic particles, the inflammatory reaction is generally nonspecific and nonimmune; however, with metallic by-products, a type IV, T lymphocyte-mediated, antigen-dependent immune reaction can occur in some patients. The production of proinflammatory cytokines, chemokines, reactive oxygen species, and other mediators is upregulated by wear particles. Animal models have shown that the biologic reaction to wear particles is systemic in nature, not a localized event. Mechanical stimuli and the presence of endotoxin also appear to be important. Efficacious biologic treatments of periprosthetic osteolysis are not yet available. Research continues with the hope that viable strategies for preventing and treating particle-induced osteolysis will be introduced in the future, thus mitigating the need for revision surgery.

Instr Course Lect 2013;62:201-206.

Despite the advent of more modern implants and novel bearing surfaces for joint arthroplasty, periprosthetic osteolysis and adverse tissue responses to the by-products of wear are still of great interest to arthroplasty surgeons.[1] This statement is realistic based on several facts. (1) Highly cross-linked polyethylene was introduced in North America approximately 10 years ago. There are millions of total hip replacements with conventional polyethylene that may have to be revised because of progressive wear and osteolysis. Many total knee replacements performed during the previous decade and beyond often used very thin polyethylene inserts that were sterilized in air and had suboptimal locking mechanisms and designs; this has led to increased wear. (2) As the population ages and continues to be physically active, implants for joint arthroplasty will be subjected to higher stresses for longer periods. (3) Hard-on-hard bearings have created a new set of concerns. Metal-on-metal articulations may be associated with the increased production of metal ions, wear particulates, corrosion by-products, and adverse tissue reactions.[2] Ceramic-on-ceramic articulations may be associated with breakage, chipping, squeaking, edge loading, and stripe wear.[3] These and other tribologic-related issues underscore the continued importance of wear by-products. (4) With the increased use of larger femoral heads to decrease the dislocation rate of hip replacements, there is some evidence (although controversial) that volumetric wear of polyethylene may be increased.[4] These larger femoral heads often use thinner polyethylene liners than were previously

Dr. Goodman or an immediate family member serves as a board member, owner, officer, or committee member of the American Academy of Orthopaedic Surgeons Biologic Implants Committee and the Orthopaedic Research Society and owns stock or stock options in Accelalox, StemCor, and Tibion. Neither of the following authors nor any immediate family member has received anything of value from or owns stock in a commercial company or institution related directly or indirectly to the subject of this chapter: Dr. Gibon and Dr. Yao.

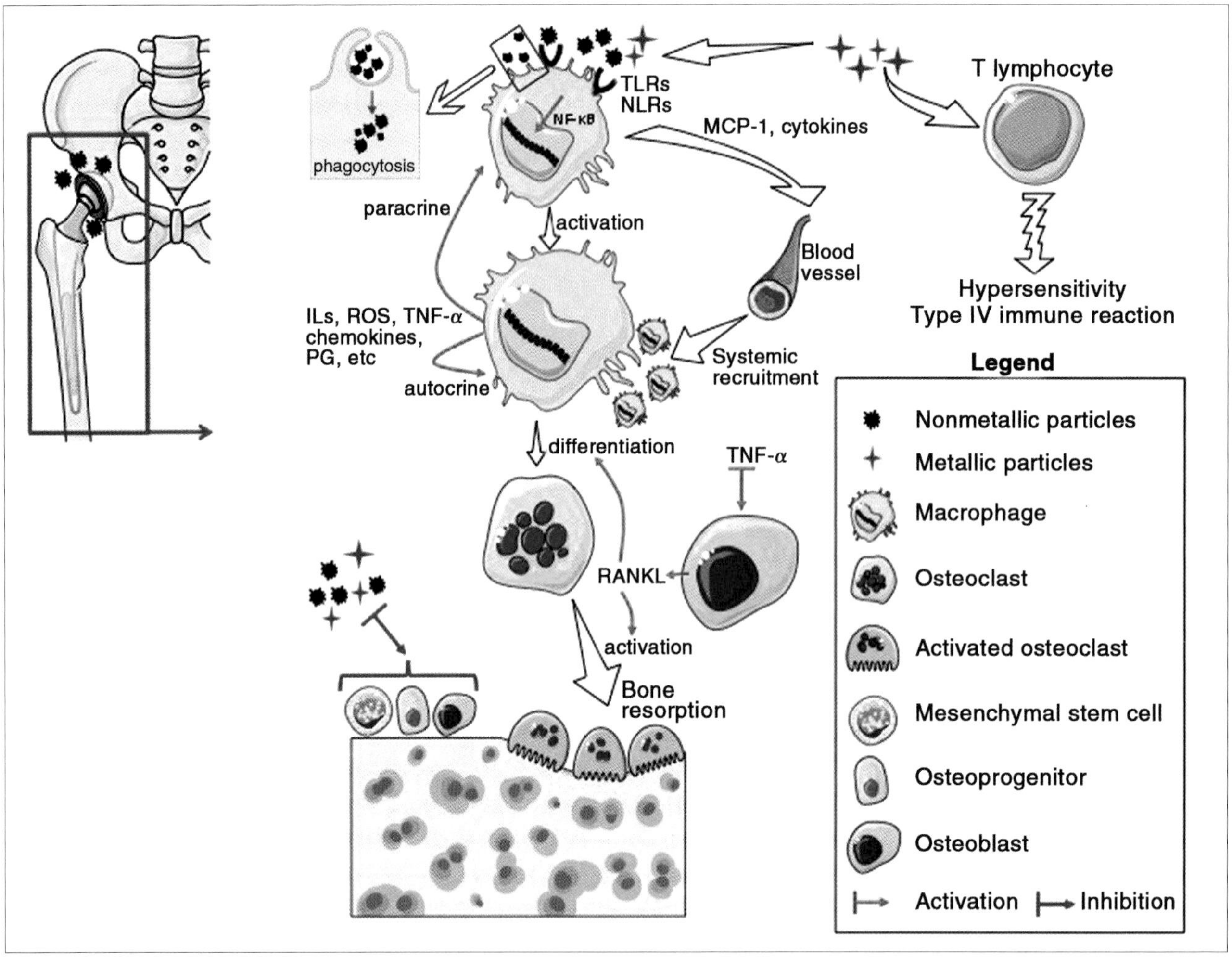

Figure 1 Illustration of the main biologic principles involved in wear particle-induced periprosthetic osteolysis. IL = interleukin, PG = prostaglandins, TLRs = toll-like receptors, NLRs = nod-like receptors, ROS = reactive oxygen species, NF-kB = nuclear factor kappaB, MCP-1 = macrophage chemotactic protein-1, TNF-α = tumor necrosis factor-α, RANKL = receptor activator of nuclear factor-kappaB ligand.

used. (5) Disk replacement in the spine and other joint replacements are in their infancy compared with hip and knee arthroplasty. Wear particle-related inflammation and osteolysis have already been noted in these joints.[5,6]

How Do Cellular By-products Activate Cells?

When wear by-products are generated, ionic moieties become solubilized and smaller particles form dispersions and aggregative complexes with serum proteins. Nearby cells are presented with small nano-sized material (up to approximately 300 nm in diameter) that can be pinocytosed (without cellular activation), particle-protein complexes that can be phagocytosed (usually smaller than 10 µm in size), or larger composites that are not phagocytosable. Particle phagocytosis leads to cellular activation; however, particle-protein complexes do not have to be phagocytosed to activate cells.[7,8] In the latter case, cell surface receptors become stimulated by larger nonphagocytosable particle-protein complexes, resulting in cellular activation. The inflammatory cascade is further stimulated by autocrine and paracrine processes resulting from released proinflammatory factors and by the stimulation of toll-like receptors and related pathways[9,10] (**Figure 1**). The presence of endotoxin on particles may also play an important exacerbating role.[11,12]

Willert and Semlitsch[13,14] were the first to recognize the importance of the biologic response to wear debris and the association with adverse tissue responses, including periprosthetic osteolysis. The local and regional biologic reaction to the presence of excessive wear debris leads to a state of decompensation or tissue dysregulation. The macrophage has traditionally been the focus of much research concerning the biology of wear particulates; however, several observations have broadened the scope of the cellular response. Tissues retrieved from revised joint arthroplasties with and without osteolysis have many different cell types, which constitute a chronic inflammatory infiltrate. These cells include monocyte/macrophage lineage cells (macrophages, foreign body giant cells, and osteoclasts), fibroblasts, lymphocytes, and cells associated with vascular structures. Histologic evidence also shows active bone remodeling in the adjacent bone bed, including the presence of osteoprogenitor cells and osteoblasts. Kadoya et al[15] reported that active bone formation was prominent in interface tissues and the adjacent bone of revised aseptically loose joint arthroplasties, indicating ongoing repair. This finding is consistent with a chronic inflammatory reaction, which consists of concurrent acute inflammation, local tissue destruction, fibrosis, and active repair. Interestingly, different cell types (in addition to cells of the monocyte/macrophage lineage) are capable of phagocytosis of wear particles, including fibroblasts and osteoblasts.

Wear particle-associated aseptic chronic inflammation is also referred to as granulomatous inflammation and may be of two general types. Nonimmune, nonspecific granulomatous inflammation is generally associated with polymeric, ceramic, and other debris and results in a histologic reaction dominated by macrophages and fibroblasts, with few lymphocytes. This reaction is believed to be dependent on the general particle characteristics, including size, shape, topography, and surface area.[16] T lymphocytes are not a prominent histologic finding.

Immune granulomas are associated with excessive metallic by-products and have a more prominent widespread lymphocytic reaction that also may be located in a perivascular location (so-called perivascular cuffing).[17] It is believed that in some patients, the metal particle-protein complex can function as a hapten, evoking a type IV T lymphocyte-mediated immune reaction. Nonmetallic wear debris (such as polymers and ceramics) primarily stimulate the innate immune system and are nonspecific, whereas metal particulates and ions can stimulate both the innate and the adaptive (T lymphocyte-mediated) immune systems.[18] Recently, it has become apparent that there are idiosyncratic, genetically based differences in an individual patient's response to different particle burdens.[19,20]

The Particle-Induced Inflammatory Cascade

After stimulation, cells of the monocyte/macrophage lineage, polymorphonuclear leukocytes, fibroblasts, osteoblasts, and other cells increase the transcription of proinflammatory substances, including cytokines, chemokines (chemotactic cytokines), reactive oxygen intermediates (nitric oxide and peroxide), prostaglandins, metalloproteinases, lysosomal enzymes, and other factors.[19,21-25] These inflammatory mediators are under direct transcriptional control of nuclear factor kappa-light-chain-enhancer of activated B cells, nuclear factor interleukin-6 (IL-6), and other factors.[8,24] In addition to activation of the innate immune system by toll-like receptors on the cell surface, some particle types (especially metals) can activate the inflammasome, a subset of the nucleotide oligomerization domain (NOD)-like receptors (NLRs). These moieties assemble into a complex multimolecular structure called NLRP (nucleotide-binding oligomerization domain, leucine-rich repeat and pyrin domain-containing), which activates the caspase-1 cascade, leading to proinflammatory factor production, especially IL-1 and IL-18.[22,26]

Particle-associated cross-talk among macrophages, fibroblasts, osteoblasts and their progenitors, and other cells leads to the production of inflammatory factors that act in an autocrine and paracrine fashion. Osteoclast differentiation, maturation, and function are upregulated by these released factors, leading to the local destruction of bone. Some of the main inflammatory factors involved in these processes include tumor necrosis factor-α, IL-1, IL-6, IL-8, receptor activator of nuclear factor-kappaB ligand (RANKL), macrophage chemotactic protein-1, and others.[27,28]

Numerous in vitro, in vivo, and tissue retrieval studies have demonstrated that wear particles stimulate acute and chronic inflammation, as well as bone destruction (osteolysis).[29,30] Recent studies have shown that retrieved interface tissues from loose implants demonstrate an imbalance in the receptor activator of nuclear factor-kappaB (RANK)-RANKL–osteoprotegerin axis, favoring bone resorption.[31] Particle-induced upregulation of the inflammatory cascade is also influenced by other factors, including mechanical forces and endotoxin.[11,32] The relative contribution of wear particles, endotoxin, mechanical forces, and other factors to the production of osteolysis is controversial; it is probably most useful to consider these factors as co-contributory, not as separate entities.[33]

Wear particles not only stimulate bone resorption but also interfere with bone formation. Recent studies have shown that both metallic and polymeric particles interfere with the proliferation, differentiation, and function of mesenchymal stem cells, osteoprogenitor cells, and osteoblasts.[34-39] These adverse effects also have been shown in animal models of bone ingrowth in the presence of wear particles.[40]

Wear Particles Induce a Systemic Immune Response

It had been surmised that wear particles from joint implants stimulate a local or perhaps a limited regional inflammatory reaction. However, based on recent animal models, it has been concluded that wear debris stimulates a systemic immune reaction, with the mobilization and trafficking of remote macrophages to the local area of particle deposition.[41-43] Macrophage chemotactic protein-1 appears to play a critical role in the chemotactic response of macrophages to wear debris. The depletion of macrophages diminishes this immune response and osteolysis.[44] These findings suggest potential opportunities for mitigation of the macrophage-associated chronic inflammatory response.

Do Wear Particles Stimulate Antigen-Specific Immune Reactions?

The subject of immune reactions to wear particles has been briefly mentioned in this chapter and reviewed in detail elsewhere.[45] However, recent evidence suggests that metallic ions and complexes may stimulate different types of tissue reactions, ranging from benign-appearing localized fibrosis and inflammation to a type IV immune reaction that can lead to severe pain, as well as bone and soft-tissue destruction.[17,18,46-48] More recent accounts of pseudotumors associated with metal-on-metal implants, especially specific types of resurfacing and total hip arthroplasties, have caused concern.[18,48] Patients with these implants should be followed closely, with serial clinical, radiographic, and laboratory examinations as indicated.

Summary

Wear in total joint arthroplasties is inevitable and dependent on the use of the joint during daily activities. Excessive wear particles stimulate a cascade of biologic events that may lead to degradation of bone and inhibition of bone formation (osteolysis). Newer, more wear-resistant bearing surfaces and implant designs have introduced new opportunities for limiting the production of particulate debris and subsequent adverse biologic reactions. However, concerns exist with some hard-on-hard bearing couples that have led to severe adverse reactions in some patients. Successful biologic treatments for managing osteolysis are not yet available. Continued mechanistic preclinical research studies may potentially yield viable strategies for prevention and treatment of particle-associated osteolysis.

Acknowledgment

This work was supported in part by NIH Grant 1R01AR055650-04 and the Ellenburg Chair in Surgery at Stanford University.

References

1. Marshall A, Ries MD, Paprosky W; Implant Wear Symposium 2007 Clinical Work Group: How prevalent are implant wear and osteolysis, and how has the scope of osteolysis changed since 2000? *J Am Acad Orthop Surg* 2008; 16(suppl 1):S1-S6.
2. Malviya A, Ramaskandhan J, Holland JP, Lingard EA: Metal-on-metal total hip arthroplasty. *J Bone Joint Surg Am* 2010;92(7): 1675-1683.
3. Walter WL, Yeung E, Esposito C: A review of squeaking hips. *J Am Acad Orthop Surg* 2010;18(6): 319-326.
4. Lachiewicz PF, Heckman DS, Soileau ES, Mangla J, Martell JM: Femoral head size and wear of highly cross-linked polyethylene at 5 to 8 years. *Clin Orthop Relat Res* 2009;467(12):3290-3296.
5. Punt IM, Austen S, Cleutjens JP, et al: Are periprosthetic tissue reactions observed after revision of total disc replacement comparable to the reactions observed after total hip or knee revision surgery? *Spine (Phila Pa 1976)* 2012;37(2): 150-159.
6. Kepler CK, Nho SJ, Bansal M, et al: Radiographic and histopathologic analysis of osteolysis after total shoulder arthroplasty. *J Shoulder Elbow Surg* 2010;19(4): 588-595.
7. Sun DH, Trindade MC, Nakashima Y, et al: Human serum opsonization of orthopedic biomaterial particles: Protein-binding and monocyte/macrophage activation in vitro. *J Biomed Mater Res A* 2003;65(2):290-298.
8. Nakashima Y, Sun DH, Trindade MC, et al: Signaling pathways for tumor necrosis factor-alpha and interleukin-6 expression in human macrophages exposed to titanium-alloy particulate debris in vitro. *J Bone Joint Surg Am* 1999;81(5): 603-615.
9. Pearl JI, Ma T, Irani AR, et al: Role of the toll-like receptor pathway in the recognition of orthopedic implant wear-debris particles. *Biomaterials* 2011;32(24):5535-5542.
10. Tamaki Y, Takakubo Y, Goto K, et al: Increased expression of toll-like receptors in aseptic loose periprosthetic tissues and septic synovial membranes around total hip implants. *J Rheumatol* 2009; 36(3):598-608.
11. Greenfield EM, Bechtold J; Implant Wear Symposium 2007 Biologic Work Group: What other biologic and mechanical factors might contribute to osteolysis? *J Am Acad Orthop Surg* 2008;16(suppl 1):S56-S62.

12. Hirayama T, Tamaki Y, Takakubo Y, et al: Toll-like receptors and their adaptors are regulated in macrophages after phagocytosis of lipopolysaccharide-coated titanium particles. *J Orthop Res* 2011; 29(7):984-992.
13. Willert HG, Semlitsch M: Reactions of the articular capsule to wear products of artificial joint prostheses. *J Biomed Mater Res* 1977;11(2):157-164.
14. Willert HG, Semlitsch M: Tissue reactions to plastic and metallic wear products of joint endoprostheses. *Clin Orthop Relat Res* 1996;333:4-14.
15. Kadoya Y, Revell PA, al-Saffar N, Kobayashi A, Scott G, Freeman MA: Bone formation and bone resorption in failed total joint arthroplasties: Histomorphometric analysis with histochemical and immunohistochemical technique. *J Orthop Res* 1996;14(3): 473-482.
16. Shanbhag AS, Jacobs JJ, Black J, Galante JO, Glant TT: Macrophage/particle interactions: Effect of size, composition and surface area. *J Biomed Mater Res* 1994;28(1):81-90.
17. Willert HG, Buchhorn GH, Fayyazi A, et al: Metal-on-metal bearings and hypersensitivity in patients with artificial hip joints: A clinical and histomorphological study. *J Bone Joint Surg Am* 2005; 87(1):28-36.
18. Jacobs JJ, Campbell PA, T Konttinen Y; Implant Wear Symposium 2007 Biologic Work Group: How has the biologic reaction to wear particles changed with newer bearing surfaces? *J Am Acad Orthop Surg* 2008;16(suppl 1): S49-S55.
19. Catelas I, Jacobs JJ: Biologic activity of wear particles. *Instr Course Lect* 2010;59:3-16.
20. Gordon A, Kiss-Toth E, Stockley I, Eastell R, Wilkinson JM: Polymorphisms in the interleukin-1 receptor antagonist and interleukin-6 genes affect risk of osteolysis in patients with total hip arthroplasty. *Arthritis Rheum* 2008;58(10):3157-3165.
21. Goodman SB, Lind M, Song Y, Smith RL: In vitro, in vivo, and tissue retrieval studies on particulate debris. *Clin Orthop Relat Res* 1998;352:25-34.
22. Hallab NJ, Jacobs JJ: Biologic effects of implant debris. *Bull NYU Hosp Jt Dis* 2009;67(2): 182-188.
23. Purdue PE, Koulouvaris P, Nestor BJ, Sculco TP: The central role of wear debris in periprosthetic osteolysis. *HSS J* 2006;2(2):102-113.
24. Purdue PE, Koulouvaris P, Potter HG, Nestor BJ, Sculco TP: The cellular and molecular biology of periprosthetic osteolysis. *Clin Orthop Relat Res* 2007;454:251-261.
25. Hukkanen M, Corbett SA, Platts LA, et al: Nitric oxide in the local host reaction to total hip replacement. *Clin Orthop Relat Res* 1998; 352:53-65.
26. Caicedo MS, Desai R, McAllister K, Reddy A, Jacobs JJ, Hallab NJ: Soluble and particulate Co-Cr-Mo alloy implant metals activate the inflammasome danger signaling pathway in human macrophages: A novel mechanism for implant debris reactivity. *J Orthop Res* 2009;27(7):847-854.
27. Granchi D, Ciapetti G, Amato I, et al: The influence of alumina and ultra-high molecular weight polyethylene particles on osteoblast-osteoclast cooperation. *Biomaterials* 2004;25(18):4037-4045.
28. Kaufman AM, Alabre CI, Rubash HE, Shanbhag AS: Human macrophage response to UHMWPE, TiAlV, CoCr, and alumina particles: Analysis of multiple cytokines using protein arrays. *J Biomed Mater Res A* 2008;84(2):464-474.
29. Bostrom M, O'Keefe R; Implant Wear Symposium 2007 Biologic Work Group: What experimental approaches (eg, in vivo, in vitro, tissue retrieval) are effective in investigating the biologic effects of particles? *J Am Acad Orthop Surg* 2008;16(suppl 1):S63-S67.
30. Tuan RS, Lee FY, Konttinen Y, Wilkinson JM, Smith RL; Implant Wear Symposium 2007 Biologic Work Group: What are the local and systemic biologic reactions and mediators to wear debris, and what host factors determine or modulate the biologic response to wear particles? *J Am Acad Orthop Surg* 2008; 16(suppl 1):S42-S48.
31. Mandelin J, Li TF, Liljeström M, et al: Imbalance of RANKL/RANK/OPG system in interface tissue in loosening of total hip replacement. *J Bone Joint Surg Br* 2003;85(8):1196-1201.
32. Bechtold JE, Kubic V, Søballe K: Bone ingrowth in the presence of particulate polyethylene: Synergy between interface motion and particulate polyethylene in periprosthetic tissue response. *J Bone Joint Surg Br* 2002;84(6): 915-919.
33. Aspenberg P, Van der Vis H: Migration, particles, and fluid pressure: A discussion of causes of prosthetic loosening. *Clin Orthop Relat Res* 1998;352:75-80.
34. Chiu R, Ma T, Smith RL, Goodman SB: Kinetics of polymethylmethacrylate particle-induced inhibition of osteoprogenitor differentiation and proliferation. *J Orthop Res* 2007;25(4):450-457.
35. Chiu R, Ma T, Smith RL, Goodman SB: Ultrahigh molecular weight polyethylene wear debris inhibits osteoprogenitor proliferation and differentiation in vitro. *J Biomed Mater Res A* 2009;89(1): 242-247.

36. Lozito TP, Tuan RS: Mesenchymal stem cells inhibit both endogenous and exogenous MMPs via secreted TIMPs. *J Cell Physiol* 2011;226(2):385-396.

37. Wang ML, Nesti LJ, Tuli R, et al: Titanium particles suppress expression of osteoblastic phenotype in human mesenchymal stem cells. *J Orthop Res* 2002;20(6): 1175-1184.

38. Ramachandran R, Goodman SB, Smith RL: The effects of titanium and polymethylmethacrylate particles on osteoblast phenotypic stability. *J Biomed Mater Res A* 2006;77(3):512-517.

39. Yao J, Cs-Szabó G, Jacobs JJ, Kuettner KE, Glant TT: Suppression of osteoblast function by titanium particles. *J Bone Joint Surg Am* 1997;79(1):107-112.

40. Goodman SB: The effects of micromotion and particulate materials on tissue differentiation: Bone chamber studies in rabbits. *Acta Orthop Scand Suppl* 1994;258: 1-43.

41. Zhang K, Jia TH, McQueen D, et al: Circulating blood monocytes traffic to and participate in the periprosthetic tissue inflammation. *Inflamm Res* 2009;58(12): 837-844.

42. Ren PG, Lee SW, Biswal S, Goodman SB: Systemic trafficking of macrophages induced by bone cement particles in nude mice. *Biomaterials* 2008;29(36): 4760-4765.

43. Ren PG, Huang Z, Ma T, Biswal S, Smith RL, Goodman SB: Surveillance of systemic trafficking of macrophages induced by UHMWPE particles in nude mice by noninvasive imaging. *J Biomed Mater Res A* 2010;94(3):706-711.

44. Ren W, Markel DC, Schwendener R, Ding Y, Wu B, Wooley PH: Macrophage depletion diminishes implant-wear-induced inflammatory osteolysis in a mouse model. *J Biomed Mater Res A* 2008;85(4):1043-1051.

45. Goodman SB: Wear particles, periprosthetic osteolysis and the immune system. *Biomaterials* 2007;28(34):5044-5048.

46. Davies AP, Willert HG, Campbell PA, Learmonth ID, Case CP: An unusual lymphocytic perivascular infiltration in tissues around contemporary metal-on-metal joint replacements. *J Bone Joint Surg Am* 2005;87(1):18-27.

47. Hallab NJ, Caicedo M, Finnegan A, Jacobs JJ: Th1 type lymphocyte reactivity to metals in patients with total hip arthroplasty. *J Orthop Surg Res* 2008;3:6.

48. Thomas P, Braathen LR, Dörig M, et al: Increased metal allergy in patients with failed metal-on-metal hip arthroplasty and peri-implant T-lymphocytic inflammation. *Allergy* 2009;64(8):1157-1165.

17

Monitoring and Risk of Progression of Osteolysis After Total Hip Arthroplasty

Michael D. Ries, MD
Thomas M. Link, MD, PhD

Abstract

Osteolysis after total hip arthroplasty (THA) develops in response to particulate wear debris and may not be associated with clinical symptoms. Osteolysis is associated with greater wear volume. Wear increases with the increased use and activity of the joint, so longer in vivo use of a THA implant increases the risk of osteolysis. Patients with non–cross-linked, ultra-high–molecular weight polyethylene implants and younger more active patients are at greater risk for the development of osteolysis.

Routine monitoring for osteolysis 5 years after THA, with radiographic imaging every 2 to 3 years thereafter, is recommended. Patients at greater risk for osteolysis should be monitored more closely. If a lesion is seen radiographically, serial radiographs are helpful to determine the relative rate of progression of the lesion. CT with metal artifact reduction can be used to effectively quantitate the lesion size and location. MRI is useful in visualizing osteolytic areas and soft-tissue pathology. Both MRI and CT with metal artifact reduction protocols have been developed to effectively visualize osteolytic lesions in proximity to THA implants and provide supplemental information to plain radiography.

Instr Course Lect 2013;62:207-214.

Osteolytic lesions may develop after total hip arthroplasty (THA) from a biologic reaction to particulate debris. Loss of bone results from osteoclastic resorption and can be seen on radiographs as cystic lesions or radiolucent regions in proximity to the femoral and acetabular components. Osteolysis may be associated with pain, particularly if bone loss results in decreased mechanical support for the prosthetic components and implant loosening. However, osteolysis may also be asymptomatic and detected only with radiographic or other imaging modalities.

Radiographs

Osteolytic lesions usually appear on radiographs as well-demarcated, scalloped areas of bone loss. Osteolysis can be differentiated from bone loss resulting from stress shielding, which causes more diffuse trabecular thinning. Stress shielding is also typically associated with an area of sclerosis and cortical thickening below the area of osteopenia or trabecular thinning. Osteolytic lesions may mimic bone loss caused by infection, which should be considered in the differential diagnosis.

Because radiographs show a two-dimensional image of a three-dimensional structure, AP and lateral views should be obtained to provide the most accurate assessment of the lesion size and location. Radiographs are useful as a screening tool to detect osteolysis but may not accurately delineate the lesion size. Shon et al,[1] using radiographs to detect periacetabular osteolysis in comparison with CT, found a sensitivity of only 57.6% but a

Dr. Ries or an immediate family member serves as a board member, owner, officer, or committee member of the Foundation for the Advancement of Research in Medicine; has received royalties from Smith & Nephew; serves as a paid consultant to or is an employee of Smith & Nephew and Stryker; and has stock or stock options in OrthAlign. Dr. Link or an immediate family member serves as a board member, owner, officer, or committee member of RSNA and ESSR; serves as a paid consultant to or is an employee of GE Healthcare and Merck; and has received research or institutional support from GE Healthcare.

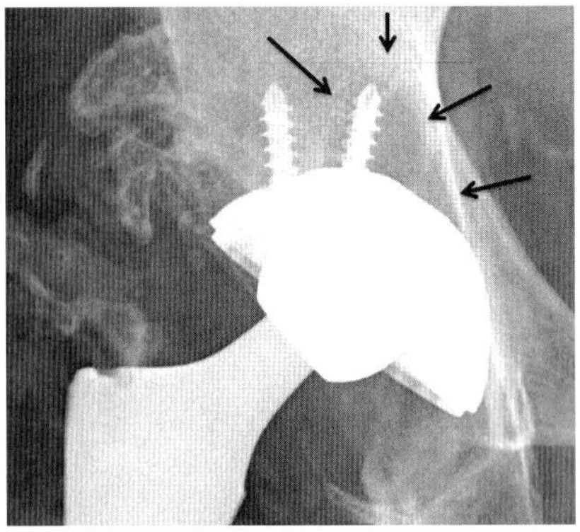

Figure 1 AP radiograph of an osteolytic lesion around a screw and dome hole (arrows).

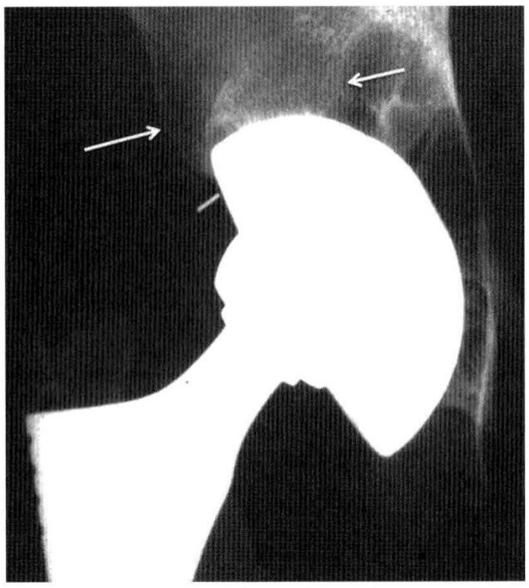

Figure 2 AP radiograph of a large osteolytic defect in the medial aspect of the acetabulum. Hip pain in association with osteolysis developed in the patient. The superior bone stock (area between the arrows) was well maintained. To treat symptomatic osteolysis and prevent further bone loss, revision was done with a cementless cup, screw fixation, and morcellized bone grafting in the medial acetabular defect.

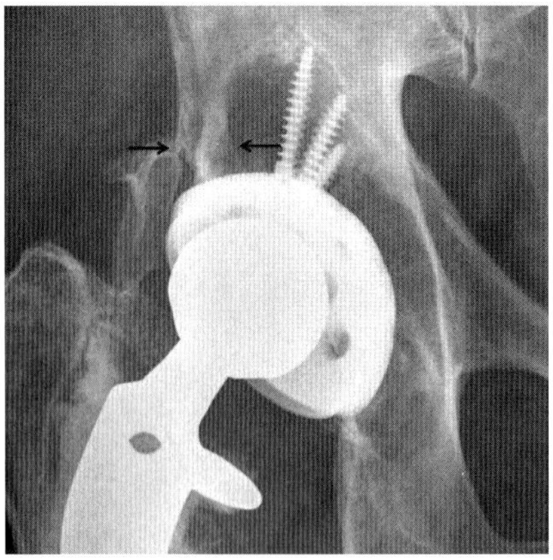

Figure 3 AP radiograph showing osteolysis in the medial aspect of the acetabulum and extending into the superior bone stock. The cup was well fixed with bone ingrowth. A narrow pillar of bone remains (between arrows), providing fixation for the cup. (Reproduced with permission from Bozic KJ, Ries MD: Wear and osteolysis in total hip arthroplasty. *Sem Arthroplasty* 2005;16:142-152.)

specificity of 92.9%. The use of oblique radiographs increased the sensitivity to 64% without changing the specificity. Other authors have similarly observed a higher specificity than sensitivity with the use of radiographs to assess osteolysis.[2,3]

Cross-sectional Imaging

CT or MRI can be used to supplement the information obtained from radiographs. These imaging modalities can provide cross-sectional images of the osteolytic lesions and are indicated when radiographs do not provide adequate visualization of the lesion size, location, or progression for clinical decision making. MRI and CT images can be distorted by metal artifact from the adjacent prosthetic components. However, metal artifact reduction protocols permit better visualization of the periprosthetic bone and soft tissues than can be obtained with conventional CT or MRI protocols. CT is faster, and acceptable visualization of osteolytic lesions is achieved by modifying standard CT protocols. MRI requires more challenging protocol changes or the use of new sequences, which are not uniformly available. In general, if this chapter's authors are more concerned with an osteolytic lesion without soft-tissue extension, a CT scan is obtained; if the lesion is primarily in soft tissue or involves soft-tissue extension of an osteolytic lesion, MRI is preferred.

Acetabular Lesions

Acetabular osteolytic lesions typically develop around the dome or screwholes of the acetabular component and in proximity to the cup rim, where particulate debris from the bearing surface tends to migrate[4,5] (**Figure 1**). The location and size of the defects affect treatment. Medial acetabular defect, which do not compromise the osseous support around the periphery of the cup, can be effectively treated with revision to a cementless hemispheric component with screw fixation and medial acetabular bone grafting (**Figure 2**). Although the cup shown in **Figure 2** was well fixed, symptoms of hip pain occurred in association with osteolysis. This is likely related to synovitis and effusion that can develop in response to ultra-high–molecular-weight polyethylene (UHMWPE) wear debris. If the shell is well fixed and in good position, liner exchange and bone grafting of the osteolytic lesions is an attractive alternative to cup revision because this does not risk additional bone loss during acetabular component removal.[6]

Superior or posterior acetabular defects that may compromise mechanical support for the acetabular component in weight-bearing regions should be treated surgically (**Figure 3**). In comparison with the osteolytic lesion shown in **Figure 2**, which is a large medial acetabular defect with relative preservation of the superior supporting bone, the lesion shown in **Figure 3** shows marked narrowing of the superior supporting bone stock. The lesion shown in **Figure 3** should be treated urgently, whereas surgical treatment of the lesion shown in **Figure 2** could be delayed if necessary. Osteolysis leading to further loss of superior or posterior

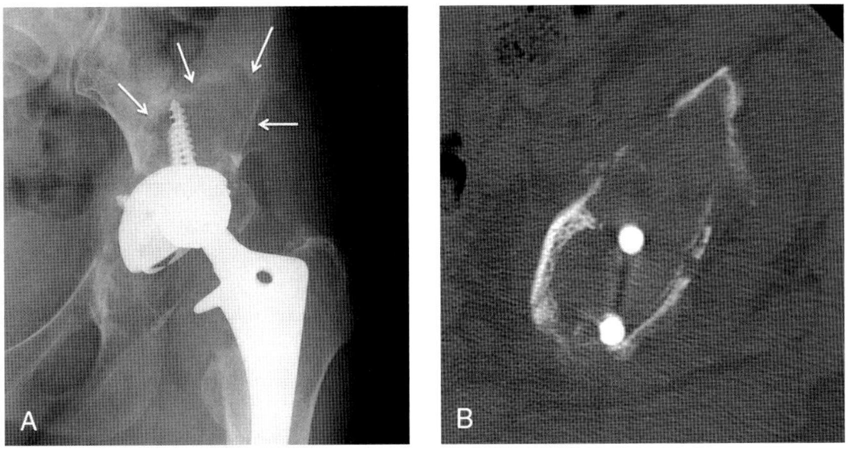

Figure 4 An active 51-year-old woman with rheumatoid arthritis presented with hip pain 20 years after THA. **A,** AP pelvic radiograph of the left hip shows extensive osteolysis with massive superior segmental acetabular bone loss (arrows) that resulted in implant loosening, superior migration of the acetabular component, and pelvic discontinuity. **B,** An axial CT section just proximal to the acetabular component shows cavitary and cortical anterior column bone loss.

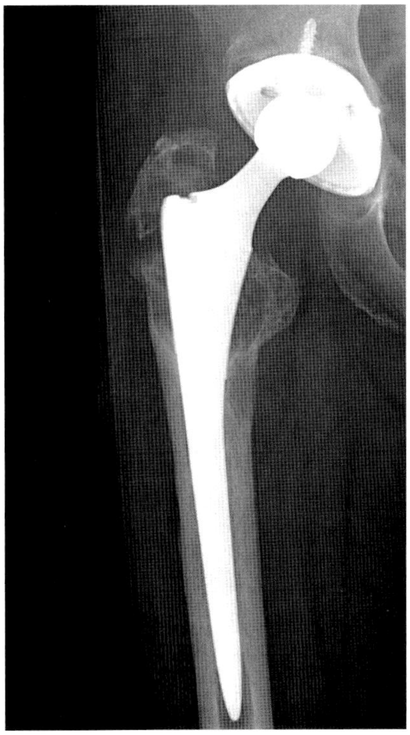

Figure 5 AP radiograph of the right hip of a 62-year-old woman, which was made 14 years after THA when she presented with lateral hip pain and abductor weakness caused by trochanteric osteolysis and spontaneous fracture of the greater trochanter.

bone stock can result in massive segmental bone loss and requires more extensive revision procedures with the use of metal augments or structural bone grafts to restore mechanical support of the acetabular component.

The decision to treat osteolytic lesions around well-fixed acetabular components surgically or to observe them is made on the basis of the presence or absence of symptoms, as well as the size, location, and rate of progression of the defect. However, the relative urgency of surgical treatment is based on the potential adverse consequences of nonsurgical treatment. Two types of catastrophic clinical problems can be encountered with prolonged observation of osteolytic periacetabular defects. These are (1) loss of superior supporting bone resulting in a segmental acetabular bone defect, which converts a contained or cavitary bone defect into a more severe, uncontained segmental defect; and (2) loss of anterior and posterior column support, which results in a pelvic discontinuity (**Figure 4**).

Superior supporting bone stock can be visualized on an AP radiograph (**Figures 2** and **3**), whereas visualization of the osseous support of the posterior and anterior columns can be obscured by the metallic acetabular shell and may not be visualized well on an AP radiograph. The use of Judet radiographs and CT or MRI should be considered to assess the integrity of the posterior and anterior columns. For patients at risk for the development of loss of superior or posterior osseous support of the acetabular cup or development of pelvic discontinuity, surgical treatment is indicated.

Femoral Lesions

Femoral lesions typically occur in proximity to the bearing surface along the calcar or greater trochanter. Trochanteric lesions may compromise the mechanical integrity of the greater trochanter, leading to fracture and loss of hip abductor muscle function (**Figure 5**). Progressive osteolysis of the greater trochanter, which weakens the bone and may lead to a fracture, is an indication for femoral head and acetabular liner exchange with bone grafting of the osteolytic lesion. If a fracture of the greater trochanter occurs and it is nondisplaced, nonsurgical treatment can result in healing.

Wear debris that reaches the distal femoral component along the bone-implant interface or the so-called effective joint space may lead to the development of periprosthetic femoral fracture.[7] Osteolysis that compromises the structural integrity of the femoral cortex in proximity to the stem tip, where stress transfer from the implant to bone is high, is a particular risk factor for fracture at or near the stem tip. This chapter's authors consider osteolysis that results in narrowing the thickness of one femoral cortex to one half

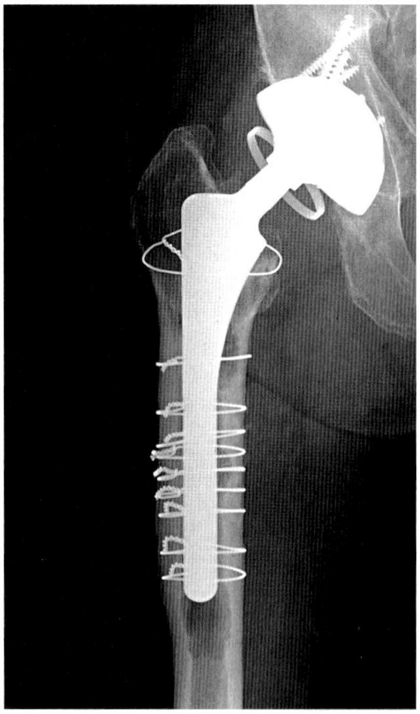

Figure 6 AP radiograph of the right hip of a 68-year-old man that was made 12 years after THA. Osteolysis developed around a cementless femoral stem. An area of cortical thinning and expansion of the medial femoral diaphysis at the stem tip represents a stress riser that can lead to periprosthetic fracture.

or less than its normal width in proximity to the stem tip to be a substantial risk for periprosthetic femoral fracture and an indication for surgery (**Figure 6**).

The rate of development and progression of osteolytic lesions is variable. The relative rate of osteolytic progression is evaluated most effectively when viewed on serial radiographic examinations (**Figure 7**). When an osteolytic lesion that may increase in size and could lead to a periprosthetic fracture or loss of structural support for the prosthetic components is detected radiographically, a follow-up radiograph is made 4 months later, and a subsequent radiograph is made 4 to 6 months after the second radiograph to determine the relative rate of progression or stability of the lesion.

Computed Tomography

Most CT scanners are now multidetector scanners and provide three-dimensional volumetric datasets that can be reconstructed in any imaging plane; coronal and sagittal reformations are standard, but three-dimensional reformations, maximum intensity projections, and other more sophisticated image reconstructions may be made. CT images are grossly distorted around cobalt-chromium and stainless steel implants, whereas artifacts around titanium implants are relatively mild.

Various techniques are available to suppress metal artifacts with CT. In a standard clinical setting, the use of a multidetector CT scanner and an increase in exposure dose (milliampere-seconds) have been advocated.[8] In addition, higher peak voltage (kilovolt peak) and narrower collimation have been used with smooth or standard reconstruction filters and thicker reconstructed sections to reduce metal artifacts.[8-10] An extended CT scale, which allows an expansion of the Hounsfield scale from a standard maximum window of 4,000 HU to 40,000 HU, is available on some scanners. This technique makes use of the fact that metals have high linear attenuation coefficients that lie outside the normal range of reconstructed CT numbers; most metallic implants are in the range of 8,000 to 20,000 HU, whereas the standard upper limit of CT scanners is 4,096 HU.[11] More advanced techniques use complicated image data processing algorithms by ignoring or interpolating the metallic objects in the raw data.[12] These techniques, however, are research applications and not established in clinical routine.

CT scans with metal artifact reduction techniques have been used successfully to quantitate the size of periacetabular osteolytic lesions.[2,13-15] Howie et al[16] used CT to assess osteolytic lesions after THA and found considerable variation in the rate of progression of osteolysis. Factors associated with progression of the lesions included high wear rate, high patient activity level, large diameter heads, and a lesion size of greater than 10 cm^3. However, in comparison with radiography, CT is associated with increased radiation exposure and cost. Therefore, CT should generally be used in addition to radiography when indicated to better delineate the extent and location of bone loss.

This chapter's authors use CT to better determine if or when surgery is indicated in the treatment of periprosthetic osteolysis. For acetabular lesions, CT is used to assess the integrity of the anterior and posterior columns and the posterior acetabular wall because this area is not well visualized on radiographs. For femoral lesions, CT is helpful in determining the structural integrity of the greater trochanter and femoral diaphysis. CT is also helpful in delineating areas of remaining bone stock when planning surgical reconstruction. CT permits three-dimensional reconstructions, which are typically used in planning for the use of custom triflange acetabular components to salvage massive acetabular bone loss and pelvic discontinuity (**Figure 4**).

Magnetic Resonance Imaging

MRI is an attractive alternative to CT because there is no ionizing radiation exposure with MRI. However, metal, particularly cobalt-chromium and stainless steel, substantially affects image quality of MRI scans because of susceptibility artifacts. Factors that affect artifacts on MRI include the composition of the metallic implant, the orientation of the implants in relation

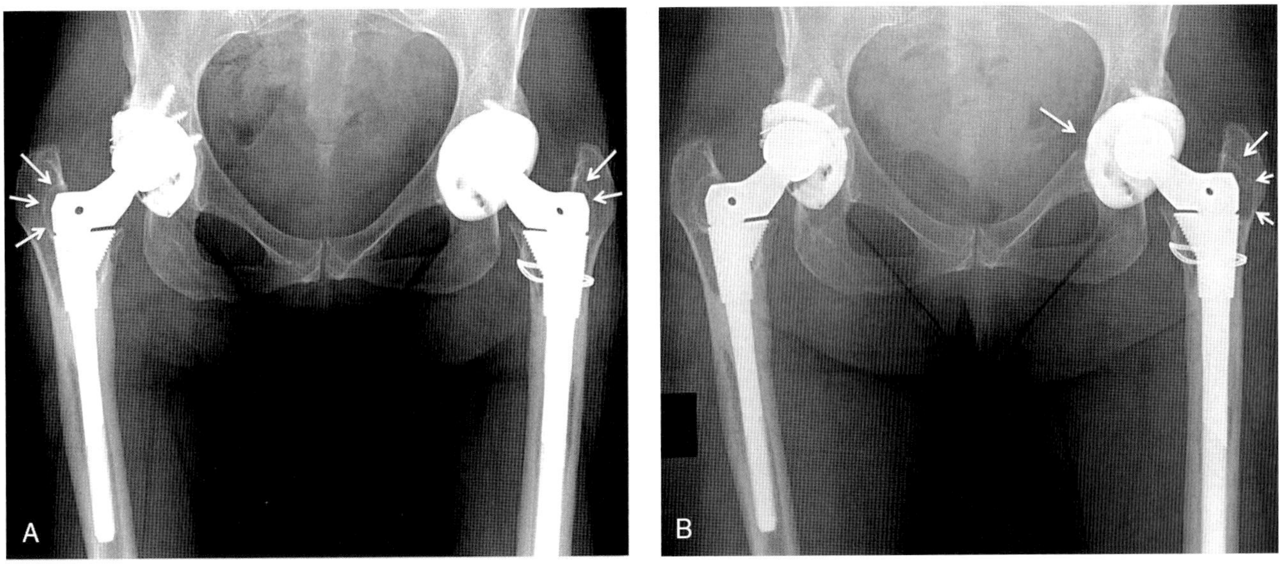

Figure 7 An active 57-year-old woman had bilateral THAs. **A,** AP radiograph made 9 years postoperatively shows small trochanteric osteolytic lesions (arrows). **B,** Fourteen years after the bilateral THAs, the patient remained active and asymptomatic, but the left trochanteric lesion had increased in size, and a medial acetabular lesion had developed (arrows).

to the direction of the main magnetic field, the strength of the magnetic field, the pulse sequence type, and other imaging parameters (mainly, voxel size, which is determined by the field of view, image matrix, section thickness, and echo train length).[8] To reduce metal artifacts, the use of lower field strength has been recommended because higher field strength increases susceptibility artifacts. Studies have used 0.2 to 0.3-T systems; this, however, affects image quality because of a low signal-to-noise-ratio, which may produce blurry images, providing limited anatomic detail.[17] With high-field systems, improvement of image quality may be achieved by increasing bandwidth. A small field of view with a high-resolution matrix, thin sections, and high gradient strength can help to reduce metal-related artifacts.[8] Instead of frequency-selective fat saturation, other techniques of fat saturation, such as short tau inversion recovery sequences, have been recommended. Recently, specific metal suppression sequences have been developed; among these, multiacquisition with variable resonance image combination (MAVRIC) hybrid sequences have shown promising results in reducing artifacts and providing high-quality images near total joint arthroplasties in a clinical setting[18,19] (**Figure 8**).

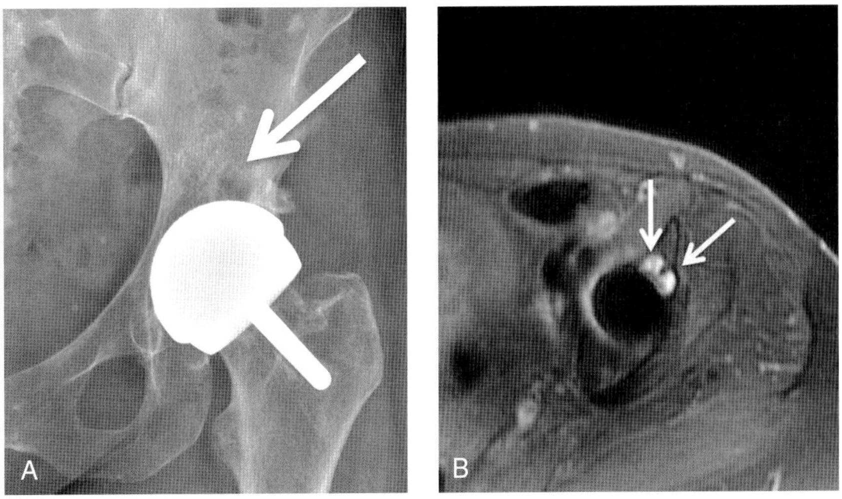

Figure 8 A 47-year-old woman was treated with metal-on-metal resurfacing of the left hip. **A,** AP radiograph of the pelvis, made 5 years postoperatively, shows osteolysis superior to the acetabular component (arrow). **B,** Axial fat-saturated metal and fat-suppressed MRI scan of the left hip acquired at the same time shows osteolytic changes anterior and superior to the acetabular component (arrows).

Potter et al[20] used metal artifact reduction protocols with MRI to assess bone and soft-tissue lesions after THA. Osteolysis, synovitis, trochanteric bursitis, and loosening have been effectively visualized on MRI with these

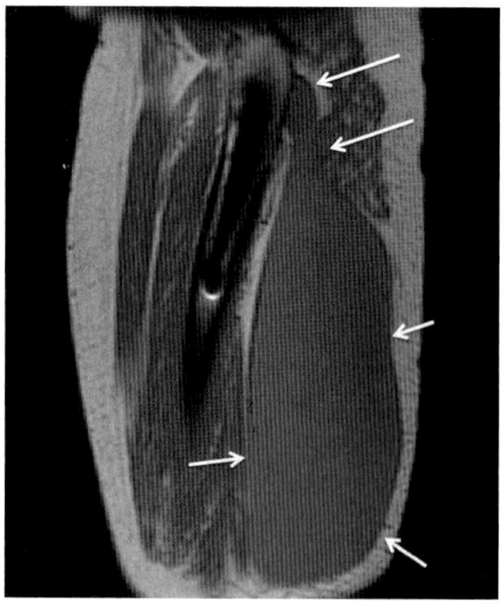

Figure 9 A 62-year-old woman presented with right hip pain and massive thigh swelling 4 years after metal-on-metal THA. Radiographs show a lucency around the acetabular component without apparent osteolysis. A sagittal T1-weighted MRI scan shows a large soft-tissue cyst originating from the hip joint and extending into the posterior aspect of the thigh (arrows).

techniques[21] (**Figure 8**). Walde et al[22] compared the accuracy of radiography, CT, and MRI in assessing periacetabular osteolytic lesions using a cadaver model. The sensitivity for detecting lesions was 51.7% for radiography, 74.7% for CT, and 95.4% for MRI. The sensitivity increased with increasing lesion size for all three methods, and MRI was the most effective in detecting small lesions.

Metal-on-metal resurfacing or THA can produce both osteolytic lesions in bone and so-called soft-tissue pseudotumors. Pseudotumors, which have been associated with an adverse local tissue reaction, can develop in soft tissue and are not well visualized on radiographs. The pseudotumors may be filled with fluid and are effectively visualized on MRI[23] (**Figure 9**). Ultrasound is also useful for detecting soft-tissue masses and can help to delineate soft-tissue pseudotumors after metal-on-metal THA.[24] However, ultrasound is not effective for detecting osteolytic bone lesions.

Monitoring Osteolysis

Osteolysis is related to many factors, but primarily it is affected by wear volume, which increases with use and patient activity. As expected, younger and more active male patients have a greater risk for the development of osteolysis.[25] It takes time to produce the wear debris, and osteolysis is uncommon before 5 years after arthroplasty, whereas the risk increases after 10 years.[26] Wear is also affected by the bearing surface materials used. Highly cross-linked UHMWPE wears less, and the risk of osteolysis is less compared with conventional UHMWPE.[26] Gamma irradiation in air of UHMWPE implants was discontinued by most manufacturers in the mid 1990s because of oxidation and increased particle debris generation, and it was replaced with non–gamma-irradiated in-air sterilization methods. Many of these implants continue to be in use and may generate higher rates of wear and osteolysis than those with highly cross-linked UHMWPE.

Highly cross-linked UHMWPE has been used in large numbers in THA for more than 10 years with excellent clinical results. However, because the long-term results with highly cross-linked UHMWPE have not been established, routine monitoring of this patient population for implant wear and osteolysis is appropriate. Patients at higher risk for the development of osteolysis, such as those with non–cross-linked UHMWPE and young, active patients, should be monitored more closely. This chapter's authors recommend that patients have a radiograph of the hip made every 2 to 3 years, beginning 5 years after THA. If osteolysis is detected, then repeat radiographs at 4 to 6 months are helpful to determine the rate of progression of the lesion and if surgical intervention is necessary. If the lesion size and location seen on radiographs suggest that clinical failure of the implant may develop or additional quantitative measurements of the lesion are needed, then CT or MRI scans with metal artifact suppression should be acquired. After the development of a lesion, the rate of progression is best determined with serial radiographs and may require serial CT scans.[14]

Summary

Osteolysis after THA develops in response to particulate wear debris and may not be associated with clinical symptoms. Osteolysis is associated with more particulate wear debris and greater wear volume. Wear increases with use and activity of the joint, so patients having longer in vivo use of their total hip replacement are at increased risk for the development of osteolysis. Patients with non–cross-linked UHMWPE and younger, more active patients are at greater risk for the development of osteolysis.

This chapter's authors recommend routine monitoring for osteolysis at 5 years after THA, with a radiograph made every 2 to 3 years thereafter. Patients at greater risk for the development of osteolysis should be monitored more closely. After a lesion is seen radiographically, serial radiographs help to determine the relative rate of progression of the lesion. CT with metal artifact reduction can be used effectively to quantitate the lesion size and location. MRI can be used to visualize osteolytic areas as well as soft-tissue pathology. Both MRI and CT with metal artifact reduction protocols have been developed to effectively visualize osteolytic lesions in proximity to THA implants and provide supplemental information to radiography.

References

1. Shon WY, Gupta S, Biswal S, Han SH, Hong SJ, Moon JG: Pelvic osteolysis relationship to radiographs and polyethylene wear. *J Arthroplasty* 2009;24(5): 743-750.
2. Puri L, Wixson RL, Stern SH, Kohli J, Hendrix RW, Stulberg SD: Use of helical computed tomography for the assessment of acetabular osteolysis after total hip arthroplasty. *J Bone Joint Surg Am* 2002;84(4):609-614.
3. Kitamura N, Pappedemos PC, Duffy PR III, et al: The value of anteroposterior pelvic radiographs for evaluating pelvic osteolysis. *Clin Orthop Relat Res* 2006;453: 239-245.
4. Stamenkov RB, Howie DW, Neale SD, McGee MA, Taylor DJ, Findlay DM: Distribution of periacetabular osteolytic lesions varies according to component design. *J Arthroplasty* 2010;25(6): 913-919.
5. Kitamura N, Naudie DD, Leung SB, Hopper RH Jr, Engh CA Sr: Diagnostic features of pelvic osteolysis on computed tomography: The importance of communication pathways. *J Bone Joint Surg Am* 2005;87(7):1542-1550.
6. Maloney WJ, Herzwurm P, Paprosky W, Rubash HE, Engh CA: Treatment of pelvic osteolysis associated with a stable acetabular component inserted without cement as part of a total hip replacement. *J Bone Joint Surg Am* 1997; 79(11):1628-1634.
7. Schmalzried TP, Jasty M, Harris WH: Periprosthetic bone loss in total hip arthroplasty: Polyethylene wear debris and the concept of the effective joint space. *J Bone Joint Surg Am* 1992;74(6): 849-863.
8. Lee MJ, Kim S, Lee SA, et al: Overcoming artifacts from metallic orthopedic implants at high-field-strength MR imaging and multi-detector CT. *Radiographics* 2007;27(3):791-803.
9. Buckwalter KA, Lin C, Ford JM: Managing postoperative artifacts on computed tomography and magnetic resonance imaging. *Semin Musculoskelet Radiol* 2011; 15(4):309-319.
10. Buckwalter KA: Optimizing imaging techniques in the postoperative patient. *Semin Musculoskelet Radiol* 2007;11(3):261-272.
11. Link TM, Berning W, Scherf S, et al: CT of metal implants: Reduction of artifacts using an extended CT scale technique. *J Comput Assist Tomogr* 2000; 24(1):165-172.
12. Prell D, Kyriakou Y, Kachelrie M, Kalender WA: Reducing metal artifacts in computed tomography caused by hip endoprostheses using a physics-based approach. *Invest Radiol* 2010;45(11): 747-754.
13. Egawa H, Ho H, Huynh C, Hopper RH Jr, Engh CA Jr, Engh CA: A three-dimensional method for evaluating changes in acetabular osteolytic lesions in response to treatment. *Clin Orthop Relat Res* 2010;468(2):480-490.
14. Goosena JH, Casteleinb RM, Verheyen CC: Silent osteolysis associated with an uncemented acetabular component: A monitoring and treatment algorithm. *Orthop Trauma* 2005;19(4): 288-293.
15. Egawa H, Ho H, Hopper RH Jr, Engh CA Jr, Engh CA: Computed tomography assessment of pelvic osteolysis and cup-lesion interface involvement with a press-fit porous-coated acetabular cup. *J Arthroplasty* 2009;24(2): 233-239.
16. Howie DW, Neale SD, Stamenkov R, McGee MA, Taylor DJ, Findlay DM: Progression of acetabular periprosthetic osteolytic lesions measured with computed tomography. *J Bone Joint Surg Am* 2007;89(8):1818-1825.
17. Guermazi A, Miaux Y, Zaim S, Peterfy CG, White D, Genant HK: Metallic artefacts in MR imaging: Effects of main field orientation and strength. *Clin Radiol* 2003;58(4):322-328.
18. Chen CA, Chen W, Goodman SB, et al: New MR imaging methods for metallic implants in the knee: Artifact correction and clinical impact. *J Magn Reson Imaging* 2011;33(5):1121-1127.
19. Hayter CL, Koff MF, Shah P, Koch KM, Miller TT, Potter HG: MRI after arthroplasty: Comparison of MAVRIC and conventional fast spin-echo techniques. *AJR Am J Roentgenol* 2011;197(3):W405-411.
20. Potter HG, Nestor BJ, Sofka CM, Ho ST, Peters LE, Salvati EA: Magnetic resonance imaging after total hip arthroplasty: Evaluation of periprosthetic soft tissue. *J Bone Joint Surg Am* 2004;86(9):1947-1954.
21. Cooper HJ, Ranawat AS, Potter HG, Foo LF, Jawetz ST, Ranawat CS: Magnetic resonance imaging in the diagnosis and management of hip pain after total hip arthroplasty. *J Arthroplasty* 2009;24(5): 661-667.
22. Walde TA, Weiland DE, Leung SB, et al: Comparison of CT, MRI, and radiographs in assessing pelvic osteolysis: A cadaveric study. *Clin Orthop Relat Res* 2005; 437:138-144.
23. Hayter CL, Potter HG, Su EP: Imaging of metal-on-metal hip resurfacing. *Orthop Clin North Am* 2011;42(2):195-205, viii.
24. Williams DH, Greidanus NV, Masri BA, Duncan CP, Garbuz DS: Prevalence of pseudotumor in asymptomatic patients after metal-on-metal hip arthroplasty. *J Bone Joint Surg Am* 2011; 93(23):2164-2171.

25. Schmalzried TP, Szuszczewicz ES, Northfield MR, et al: Quantitative assessment of walking activity after total hip or knee replacement. *J Bone Joint Surg Am* 1998; 80(1):54-59.
26. Bitsch RG, Loidolt T, Heisel C, Ball S, Schmalzried TP: Reduction of osteolysis with use of Marathon cross-linked polyethylene: A concise follow-up, at a minimum of five years, of a previous report. *J Bone Joint Surg Am* 2008;90(7): 1487-1491.

18

The Changing Paradigm of Revision of Total Hip Replacement in the Presence of Osteolysis

Vikram Chatrath, MBBS, MS, MCh (Ortho)
Paul E. Beaulé, MD, FRCSC

Abstract

Osteolysis tends to remain clinically silent and presents a treatment challenge. In the past, the progression of implant wear was used to determine the timing of interventions. Recent reports of lesions associated with metal-on-metal implants and trunnion corrosion with femoral head sizes larger than 32 mm suggest that other mechanisms of wear debris production may be present; observation alone may not provide adequate monitoring. Advanced imaging modalities, such as MRI, should be used along with routine radiography to assess soft-tissue involvement and the size of osteolytic lesions. Intraoperative mechanical stress applied to the acetabular cup helps determine if revision or retention is selected when osteolysis is present. Options for the management of acetabular osteolysis include porous metal cups, oblong cups, antiprotrusio cages, impaction grafting, structural grafts, and, more recently, versatile porous metal cups. Porous metal cups can be used with or without augments or as cup-cage constructs. Porous metal cups have shown excellent results at short-term follow-ups. Modular, uncemented, titanium stems are now more commonly used for femoral revisions. Impaction grafting and allograft-prosthesis composites are occasionally useful in femoral revision surgery. A high incidence of adverse tissue reactions has been reported with metal-on-metal bearings with large heads. Recent focus also has been directed to debris generation by the modular junctions in these bearings. Removal of all sources of debris generation should be attempted during revision of metal-on-metal hip replacements. A thorough débridement of soft-tissue masses and the use of ceramic heads should be considered.

Instr Course Lect 2013;62:215-227.

Dr. Beaulé or an immediate family member has received royalties from Wright Medical Technology; is a member of a speakers' bureau or has made paid presentations on behalf of Smith & Nephew and MEDACTA; serves as a paid consultant to or is an employee of Corin USA, Smith & Nephew, and MEDACTA; has received research or institutional support from Corin USA; and owns stock or stock options in Wright Medical Technology. Neither Dr. Chatrath nor any immediate family member has received anything of value from or owns stock in a commercial company or institution related directly or indirectly to the subject of this chapter.

The assessment and management of osteolysis after total hip replacement remains challenging.[1-4] Determining the appropriate timing of surgery and managing the associated bone loss, especially around the acetabulum, can be difficult because osteolysis is usually clinically silent.[1] Manley et al[5] suggested that the fundamental component of osteolysis is access of particulate wear debris to the fixation interface. The primary objectives of revision surgery for a failed hip replacement with associated osteolysis are to assess the integrity of the fixation area and determine the stability of the implant. This information helps the surgeon decide between revision or salvage of the components, and it is critical on the acetabular side because subsequent aseptic loosening of the retained acetabular component after isolated treatment of the osteolytic defect can be as high as 8%.[6] On the femoral side, aseptic loosening secondary to osteolysis is rare because of the larger fixation area, which usually extends fairly distally from the bearing surface.

In the past, the decision to monitor patients with known osteolysis and a metal-on-polyethylene implant was mainly based on wear progression and

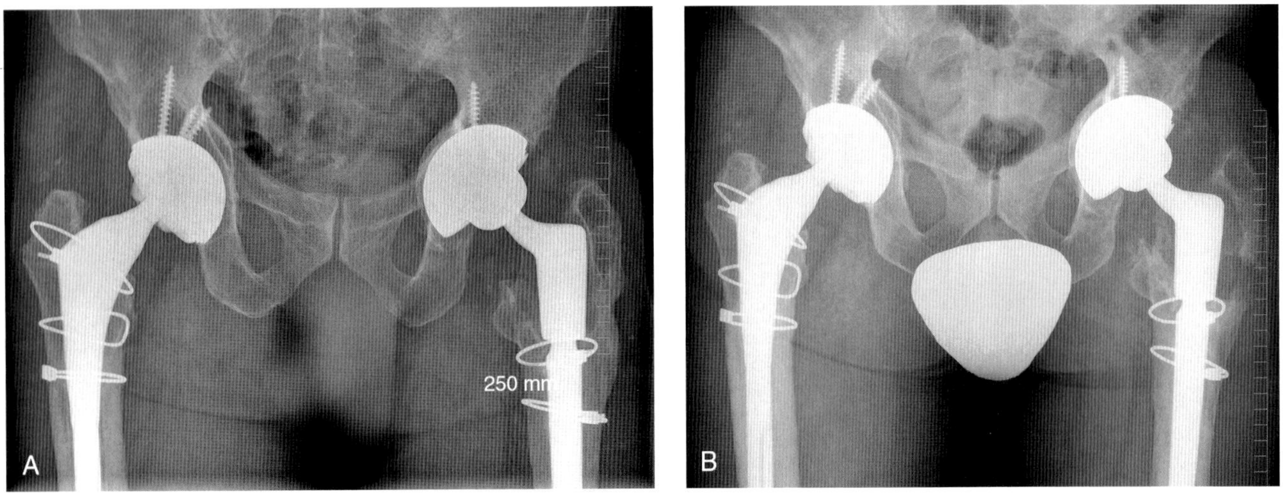

Figure 1 **A,** AP radiograph of total hip replacements in a 43-year-old man 6 years after revision for infection with a Restoration Modular Stem (Stryker, Mahwah, NJ) with a Trabecular Metal acetabular component with a Longevity liner (Zimmer, Warsaw, IN). **B,** AP radiograph taken after the patient reported increasing pain over a 6-month period. Note the progression of osteolytic defect on the femoral side.

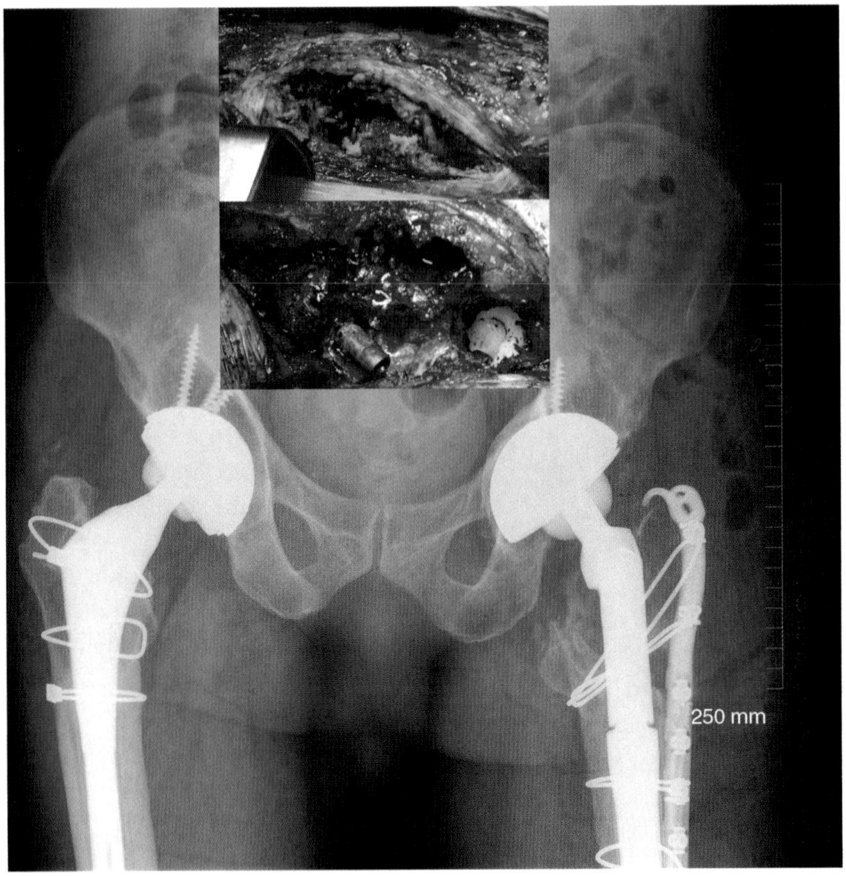

Figure 2 AP radiograph of total hip replacements. Inset shows an inflammatory pseudotumor with bone and soft-tissue destruction secondary to severe Morse taper corrosion. The hip was revised with a Link Modular Revision Stem (Waldemar Link, Hamburg, Germany) with a ceramic femoral head.

the overall thickness of the remaining polyethylene. Naudie et al[7] suggested frequent follow-up monitoring for patients with a residual polyethylene component thickness of less than 3 mm and recommended revision surgery for implants with a polyethylene thickness less than 1.5 mm and in symptomatic patients. However, in the past 5 years, there have been reports of aggressive forms of osteolysis with significant soft-tissue destruction and masses (such as pseudotumors) presenting within the first 5 years after total hip replacement or resurfacing.[8-11] Although the presence of destructive, particulate, debris-induced lesions is well documented,[12-14] it is only recently that these lesions have been reported with metal-on-metal bearings in which other mechanisms of wear debris production are involved, such as corrosive wear at modular junctions (**Figures 1** and **2**). It appears that orthopaedic surgeons are faced with a paradigm shift in the management of patients with periprosthetic osteolysis; simple observation may no longer be a satisfactory option.

Evaluation and Imaging

Evaluation should consist of a detailed patient history followed by a thorough physical examination and subsequent imaging. Pain occurring after a long interval is usually more consistent with aseptic loosening secondary to osteolysis induced by wear debris rather than early pain, which may be caused by poor initial stability and poor implant design and/or fixation.[15,16]

Radiologic evaluation helps determine the severity of osteolysis and the amount of remaining bone stock available at the time of revision surgery. In addition to standard radiographs, Judet views provide information about the integrity of the acetabular columns.[17] CT with artifact reduction is more sensitive than plain radiographs for evaluating osteolysis.[18,19] Some surgeons measure the pelvic osteolytic volume on a CT scan to guide their treatment of well-fixed acetabular components with osteolysis.[20-23] MRI has had limited use because of metallic artifacts, but metal suppression techniques are increasingly being used. In a cadaver study, Walde et al[24] reported that MRI was better for detecting periacetabular osteolytic lesions than CT or plain radiography. MRI also can detect adverse soft-tissue reactions in patients who, like those with osteolysis, are usually asymptomatic.[4,25,26] The mere presence of a small effusion or mass does not dictate the need for surgery because the natural history of these lesions in asymptomatic individuals is unknown. However, evidence of radiographic osteolysis within 5 years after implantation of a modern wear-bearing surface and/or the presence of pain warrants evaluation with high-resolution cross-sectional imaging. Some of these lesions cause rapid destruction to the soft tissues, and early revision surgery should be considered. Previous recommendations to use lesion size to determine implant stability in patients with standard metal-on-polyethylene bearings have been superseded by the importance of assessing soft-tissue involvement.[27]

A white blood cell count, erythrocyte sedimentation rate, and C-reactive protein level should be part of the standard workup before revision surgery. Considering their high sensitivity, these tests are best used to rule out infection. Spangehl et al[28] used a combination of the erythrocyte sedimentation rate and C-reactive protein level to achieve 100% specificity for excluding the diagnosis of an infected total hip arthroplasty. These tests have been combined with hip aspiration to achieve 92% sensitivity and 97% specificity in diagnosing infection.[29]

Table 1
Classification Systems for Acetabular Bone Defects

AAOS System	
Type I	Segmental
A	Peripheral
B	Central with medial wall defect
Type II	Cavitary
Type III	Combined
Type IV	Pelvic discontinuity
Type V	Arthrodesis
Paprosky System	
Type I	Intact, undistorted rim, no lysis or migration
Type II	Intact, distorted rim with < 3 cm of superomedial or superolateral migration
A	Superomedial
B	Superolateral, no superior dome, < 30% segmental rim defect
C	Anterior column and medial defect, Kohler line violated, rim intact
Type III	Superior migration > 3 cm with severe ischial and medial osteolysis
A	Kohler line intact, 30% to 60% of component supported by the graft, bone loss between the 10- and 2-o'clock positions
B	Kohler line is not intact, > 60% component supported by graft, bone loss between the 9- and 5-o'clock positions

Classification of Bone Defects

Various systems have been proposed for classifying bone defects on the acetabular side, with the American Academy of Orthopaedic Surgeons (AAOS) and Paprosky systems the most commonly used[30-32] (**Table 1**). The AAOS classification system organizes acetabular bone loss by pattern and location, with two basic categories: (1) segmental bone loss involves any complete loss of bone in the supporting hemisphere of the acetabulum, including the medial wall, and (2) cavitary defects, which are those with a volumetric loss in the acetabular cavity but with an intact rim.[30] The Paprosky system is based on anatomic landmarks and uses four criteria to predict the location and the severity of bone loss and allow appropriate planning.[31] These criteria, which can be identified on preoperative radiographs, are ischial osteolysis, teardrop osteolysis, superior migration of the hip center, and the position of the component relative to the Kohler line.

Table 2
Paprosky Femoral Defect Classification With Recommended Treatment

Type	Bone Loss	Bong Grafting Options	Femoral Fixation
I	Minimal metaphyseal bone loss, intact diaphysis	N/A	Cylindrical stem with distal fixation
II	Extensive metaphyseal bone loss, intact diaphysis	Cancellous	Tapered conical modular stem Cylindrical stem with distal fixation
III	Severe metaphyseal bone loss and nonsupportive bone		Tapered modular conical stem
A	> 4 cm proximal to isthmus intact	Strut grafting	
B	< 4 cm distal to isthmus intact	Impaction grafting	
IV	Extensive metaphyseal damage, widened canal, cortical ballooning, thin cortices	Impaction grafting Allograft prosthetic composite grafting	Tapered conical stem Long, polished stem with impaction grafting or allograft prosthetic composite grafting

On the femoral side, both D'Antonio and Paprosky have proposed classification systems for femoral defects, with the latter being the most commonly used[33] (**Table 2**). The Paprosky system is based on the integrity of the metaphysis, the size of the remaining isthmic segment, and the quality of the host cortices.

Surgical Treatment

Acetabular Side

The importance of adequate surgical exposure cannot be overstated. The posterior approach is most commonly used on the acetabular side, but this chapter's authors find that a direct anterior approach can provide sufficient exposure for simple cup revisions and liner exchanges.[34] If the femoral component is loose, it is removed first to enhance exposure. Some well-fixed cemented femoral stems can be extracted to increase exposure and then recemented into the existing mantle after treating the acetabulum.[35] If the cup has migrated and the femoral shaft is abutting the pelvis, a trochanteric slide osteotomy may be useful to allow adequate exposure.[36]

Intraoperative assessment of the acetabular component fixation involves clearing all fibrous tissue from around the shell. The liner and all screws should be removed. A mechanical stress test should be applied to all four quadrants of the acetabular shell to detect any expression of fluid between the shell and the bone. The management of stable components will not be discussed; however, in most situations, a well-positioned component can be retained. When the decision is made to remove a well-fixed component, size-specific curved-blade explant systems make it easier to remove well-fixed cups with minimal bone loss. The osteolytic defect should be débrided of all granulation tissue, and the remaining bone stock should be assessed. The primary goal of the acetabular revision is to achieve a stable construct with enough bony contact to allow osseointegration of the implant. Currently, cementless implants are the first choice for implantation when more than 50% of host bone contact is present. In a study by Lakstein et al,[37] 53 patients with acetabular defects with less than 50% of host bone contact were treated using Trabecular Metal (Zimmer) cups without structural grafts, cages, or augments. The authors reported only two failed revisions and two cases of probable loosening. These findings indicate that it may be reasonable to use porous metal shells when there is less than 50% of bony host contact; however, this chapter's authors believe that metal augments should be strongly considered in patients with less than 50% of host bone contact. **Table 3** summarizes the acetabular reconstructive options, with the most recent reports of implant survivorship.[38-48]

If a peripheral rim is present (Paprosky type I defect), fixation can be achieved with a porous, hemispheric, press-fit cup. Cancellous bone graft or bone-graft substitutes can be used to fill cavitary defects.[38,49,50] The addition of screw fixation will improve immediate stability. If the peripheral rim is incompetent, additional fixation must be used. Type IIA defects can be treated similarly to type I defects. In some instances, reaming to a larger size may be required to achieve an adequate peripheral fit. The use of jumbo cups (diameters greater than 66 mm) may be required.[39,51] Jumbo cups allow the use of a thicker acetabular liner and a larger femoral head.[52] Attempts should be made to preserve as much bone stock as possible, especially at the rim and posterior column. Type IIB defects have an uncontained defect; however, this defect is often small enough that a press-fit can be achieved

Table 3
Results of Acetabular Reconstruction

Study (Year)	Implant Design	Survivorship
Della Valle et al[48] (2005)	Porous hemispheric press-fit cup	97% at 15 years
Wasielewski et al[38] (2008)	Porous hemispheric press-fit cup ± cancellous allografts or bone substitutes	94% at 4 years
Patel et al[39] (2003)	Jumbo cups	92% at 14 years
Abeyta et al[40] (2008)	Oblong cups	76% at 11 years
	Impaction grafting	
Busch et al[42] (2011)	Traditional technique	85% at 20 years
Parratte et al[43] (2007)	With a noncemented cup	91.3% at 10 years
Sembrano and Cheng[44] (2008)	Antiprotrusio cages	81.3% at 5 years
	Structural allografts	
Woodgate et al[46] (2000)	Minor column graft	78% at 10 years
Paprosky and Martin[47] (2002)	Major column graft	55% at 5 years
Siegmeth et al[41] (2009)	Trabecular Metal ± augments	98% at 2.8 years
Kosashvili et al[45] (2009)	Cup-cage constructs (Trabecular Metal)	88.5% at 3.5 years

with a jumbo cup with screws and augments as needed. Porous metal cups have a structure that favors early osseointegration, and the lower modulus of elasticity (3 MPa) and high (70% to 80%) porosity allows for more uniform stress transfer and the potential for diminished stress shielding.[53,54] The uneven texture provides an initial scratch-fit, which enhances the initial component stability, and a range of modular porous metal augments obviate the need to contour allografts to obtain a stable construct.[53]

Oblong cups have a hemispheric inferior component that accepts a standard liner. The superior part of the cup acts like a void filler and can be secured with screws. The superior part of the defect is prepared to accept the oblong cup using a special offset reamer. Because the anteroposterior diameter of the pelvis can preclude the use of very large cups, the oblong cup provides a reasonable option.[55] In a study of acetabular defects reconstructed with an oblong prosthesis, Abeyta et al[40] reported satisfactory results at an average follow-up of 11 years. Other authors have reported mixed results with this system.[56-58]

Porous metal augments in combination with a porous metal cup provide another approach to manage acetabular defects. These components are available in a variety of shapes and sizes and provide more modularity than bilobed implants and structural allografts. With the trial implant in place, the bed for the augment is assessed and prepared. The augment can then be placed and secured with screws; the porous cup is then impacted. The space between the cup and the augment can be reinforced with cement. The early success rate of 98% reported by high-volume revision surgeons using this technique is encouraging.[41,59] Siegmeth et al[41] reported short-term results of 34 revision hip arthroplasties performed with porous metal cups supplemented with augments, with more than 50% of the surgeries performed for type IIIA acetabular defects. The authors reported only two failures, with 32 of the 34 cups requiring no further intervention at 2-year follow-up. The need for an augment was anticipated based on preoperative templating, which was confirmed intraoperatively. An augment was used if the trial implants were inherently unstable or if an oblong defect was recognized that could not support the cup without bone stock augmentation.

Impaction grafting has been used for type IIB acetabular defects as a method of restoring bone stock.[60] This method involves packing the acetabular cavity with cancellous allograft chips followed by cementing the acetabular component. In vitro studies have suggested that the optimal size of cancellous chips is 7 to 10 mm.[61] This technique also has been used with noncemented components.[62] In a study of impaction bone grafting of acetabular components in young patients, Busch et al[42] reported 85% implant survivorship at 20 years and 77% at 25 years, with revision for aseptic loosening of the cup as the end point. In a study of acetabular revisions performed with a hemispheric cup and morcellized bone grafts, Paratte et al[43] reported implant survivorship of 91.3% at 10 years. The disadvantages of the technique include its higher technical difficulty and the unknown fate of the allograft bone.[63]

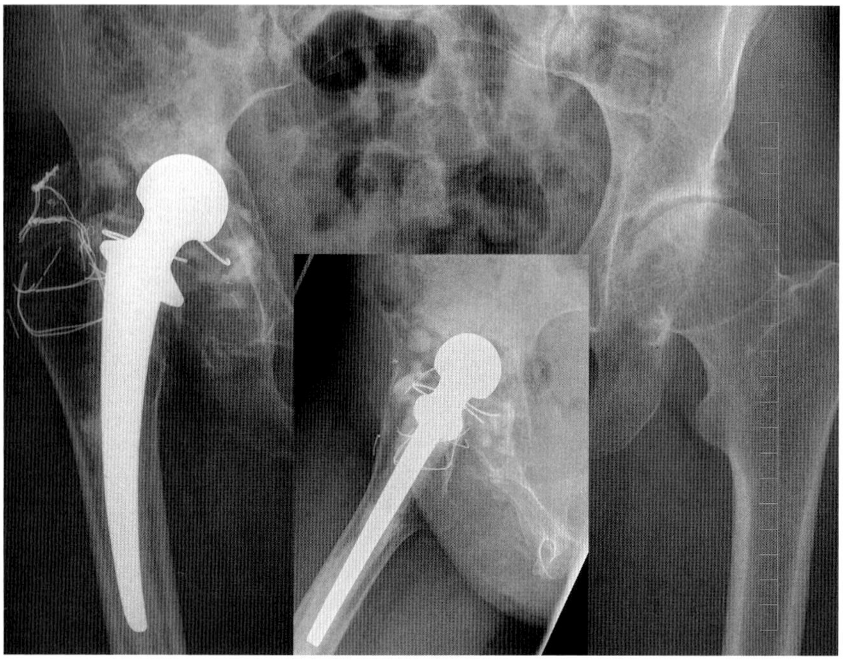

Figure 3 AP radiograph taken 20 years after a total hip replacement in a 52-year-old woman. Inset shows the lateral radiographic view. Note the failed acetabulum component.

Type IIC defects exhibit acetabular protrusio, but the peripheral rim is maintained. This enables the use of a hemispheric cup and bone grafting of the medial wall to allow lateralization. If bony contact of 50% or more is achieved, augmentation may not be necessary for structural support but may be beneficial in replenishing bone stock. If there is less than 50% bony contact, structural bone grafting or porous metal augmentation is recommended. Antiprotrusio cages can also be used in these situations. The cage is usually supported by the ilium superiorly and the pubis and the ischium inferiorly. If the posterior column is deficient, bulk allografts should be used to provide support. Current cage designs, however, do not allow for biologic fixation. Placement of the flanges requires greater soft-tissue dissection.[64] Sembrano and Cheng[44] reported an 81% survival rate at 5 years using antiprotrusio cages, whereas other authors have reported disappointing results at midterm follow-up.[65,66]

Although antiprotrusio cages with cemented liners and structural allografts have been the classic technique for treating Paprosky type IIIA and IIIB defects, porous metal acetabular components with augments are increasingly being used with good short-term results.[59] In patients with pelvic discontinuity, plating of the posterior column before reconstruction with the cup-in-cage construct has shown promising results.[45] Structural allografts are useful for restoring bone stock and providing structural support for hemispheric component stability[67] (**Figures 3** and **4**). The disadvantages of using a structural graft include the difficulty of matching the graft to the defect and unsuccessful osseointegration. Structural allograft is also called shelf graft or minor column graft when used for uncontained defects involving less then 50% of the supporting rim or wall.[46] Structural allograft is called major column graft when it supports more than 50% of the cup.[68] At 10-year follow-up, successful results have been reported in 78% of the reconstructions using minor column grafts and 55% using major column grafts.[47]

Cup-cage constructs have been used for treating massive bone loss with or without pelvic discontinuity.[45] A porous metal cup is fixed to the available bone bed. An acetabular cage is then positioned inside the cup and secured with screws above and below the cup, and, if possible, through the cup-cage construct. An acetabular liner is then cemented into the cage. The cage provides short-term stability to allow time for osseointegration of the porous cup. Early results with this technique are promising.[45,69]

Femoral Side

Revision surgery secondary to aseptic loosening from particle-induced osteolysis is a relatively rare occurrence with current cementless femoral components.[70] Poor initial stability of the femoral component with subsequent micromotion and migration is the most likely cause for revision.[71,72] Settling of the prosthesis with abnormal loading of the femur can lead to substantial remodeling and cortical erosion, which makes optimal implant placement difficult. The goal of surgery is to achieve a stable construct with sufficient bony contact and restoration of bone stock as needed.

In revision total hip arthroplasty, intimate contact between the implant and the bone in the metaphyseal area is often difficult to achieve because of bone loss or sclerosis. Maloney[73] suggested that well-fixed stems with metaphyseal osteolysis may be amenable to lesional bone grafting, whereas those with diaphyseal osteolysis and a limited area of osseointegration should be revised. It was often found to be impossible to cement a prosthesis and achieve adequate fixation with proximal bony defects;[74,75] similar findings were reported with monoblock, proximally porous-coated stems.[76] The introduction of modular revision stems has permitted the optimization of individual femoral fit and fill by the independent preparation of the proximal and the distal femur and has facilitated adjustments in leg length, version, and offset.[77] Rodriguez et al[78] reported excellent intermediate-term results with 93 of 97 hips being radiographically stable at 45 months using the Link MP Reconstruction stem (Waldemar Link), which is a modular, conical, uncemented titanium stem. Similar results have been reported at midterm follow-up.[79] Garbuz et al[71] compared modular, conical, tapered, titanium, fluted stems with nonmodular, cylindric, cobalt-chromium stems and found that modular titanium fluted stems had better function and achieved higher patient satisfaction scores. These results were attributed to the better biomechanical properties of titanium coupled with intraoperative modularity. Noncemented stems have been radiologically evaluated using a system described by Engh et al.[80-82] This system may not be applicable to modular stems. A recent study tried to define the radiographic signs of osseointegration and remodelling using a modular stem.[83] The authors evaluated the osseointegration patterns of 64 hips revised with a modular, tapered, fluted titanium stem and reported that all of the stems were well fixed if there was minimal or no radioopaque line formation at the grist-blasted surface of the distal fragment and subsidence was absent beyond the 6 weeks after full weight bearing. Importantly, the radiographic appearance of the proximal body was not a factor in the osseointegration status of the stem.

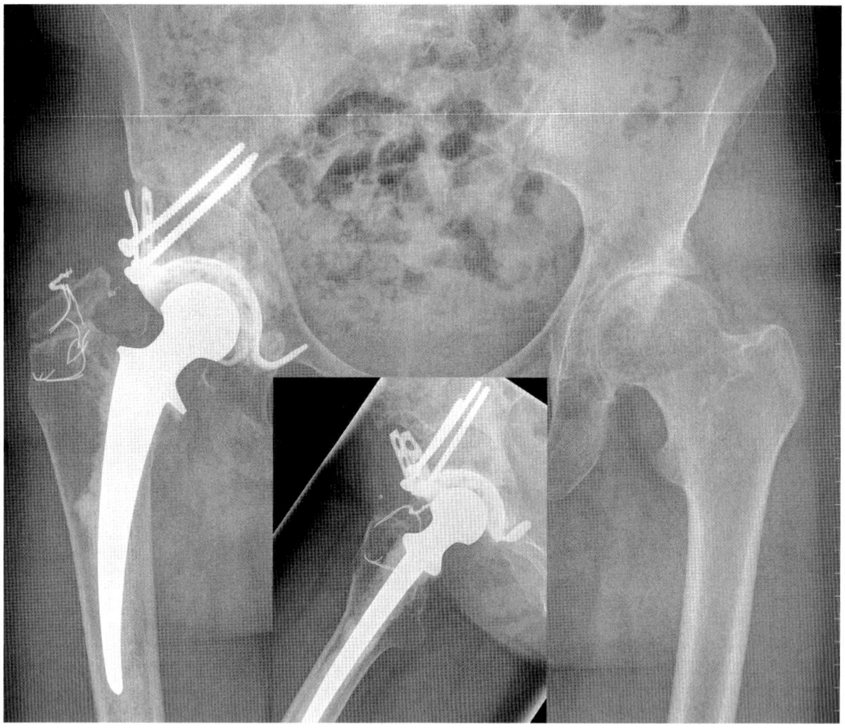

Figure 4 AP radiograph of the patient described in Figure 3 taken 2 years after acetabular reconstruction with a bulk allograft and Graft Augmentation Prosthesis cup (Stryker). Inset shows the lateral radiographic view.

For most femoral revisions, a posterior approach is chosen because of the ease of performing an extended femoral osteotomy, which is indicated to facilitate implant removal and optimize revision implant placement without breaching the intact femoral cortex. An extended femoral osteotomy may also be indicated in cases of proximal remodeling if the stem falls into varus or retroversion with significant trochanteric overhang because this can hinder extraction of the old stem and implantation of the new stem. Other specialized instruments, such as trephine reamers and flexible osteotomes, may be needed to remove the stem with minimal bone loss.

Type 1 defects are unusual and are associated with inadequate early fixation. Revision is usually relatively straightforward and can be achieved using a cylindric, straight, nonmodular stem. Proximally coated stems are less reliable in the revision situation than fully coated stems; rerevision rates of 32% at 8 years have been reported.[71] Type II defects are more common and have extensive metaphyseal loss. Insufficient contact will be achieved with proximal fixation prostheses, and fixation should be achieved with either an extensively porous-coated prosthesis or a conical tapered implant to achieve more distal fixation. Proximal cancellous grafting may improve future bone stock. Type IIIA defects have more severe metaphyseal loss but have supportive bone distally so that fixation can be achieved using a conical tapered design. Extensively coated designs allow for maximal integration and bony ongrowth. To safely remove the loosened implant and gain access to the femur for reimplantation, an extended trochanteric osteotomy is often needed. This procedure permits better access to the femur and the acetabulum and also allows incorporation of a strut graft and advancement of the trochanter if needed. Union rates are excellent.

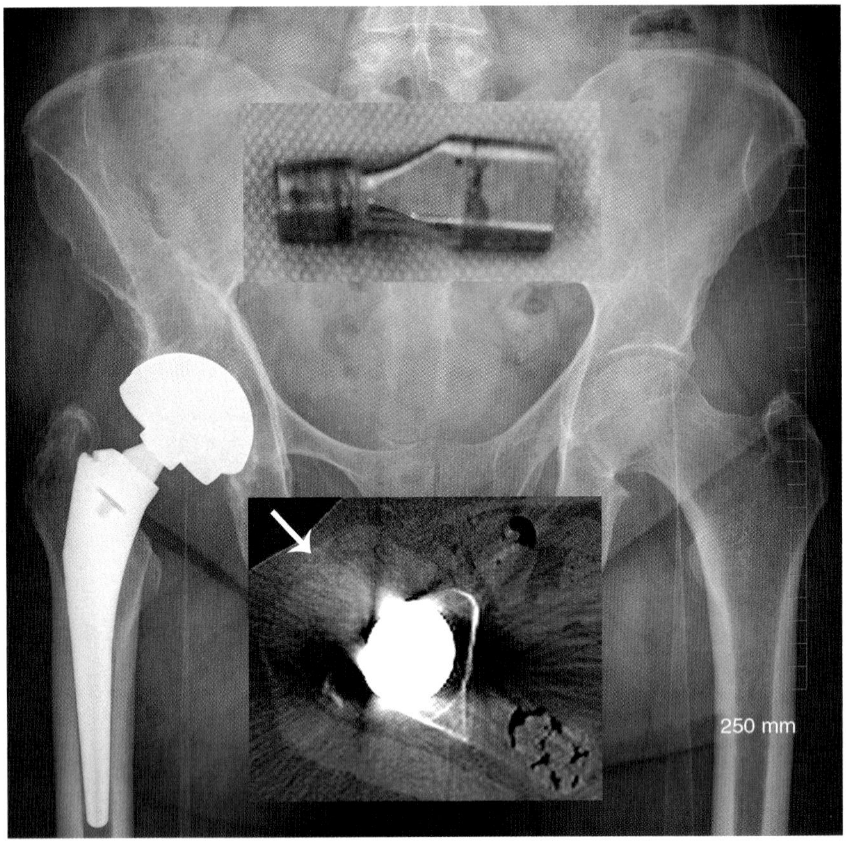

Figure 5 AP radiograph of the hip of a 67-year-old woman 2 years after primary total hip replacement using a large head metal-on-metal bearing and Conserve Plus acetabular shell and Pro-Femur TL modular stem (Wright Medical Technology, Memphis, TN). The patient presented with increasing pain. Inset (top) shows severe corrosion at the Morse taper junction within the head. Inset (bottom) shows a pseudotumor mass (white arrow) on a CT scan.

Miner et al[84] reported a union rate of 98.8%, with a mean time to union of 5 months, and an osseointegration rate of 92%. Type IIIB defects have severe deficiency and require further reconstructive techniques. If there is sufficient distal bone, a modular conical tapered stem can be used. An option for restoring bone stock is impaction grafting with reconstruction and support of the graft with struts, mesh, or plates. This technique can be especially beneficial in a younger patient who may require further intervention. Ornstein et al[85] reported a 15-year implant survival rate of 94% with impaction grafting. The major complications with this technique are surgical or perioperative femoral fracture and implant subsidence. A recent cadaver study attempted to define the appropriate force to be used during impaction grafting to prevent femoral fracture.[86] The authors reported that no femurs fractured below an impaction force of 0.5 kN.

Type IV femoral defects have extensive metaphyseal damage and a widened isthmus without support. These defects cause several problems, including early loosening because of poor fixation, stress shielding, and often poor soft-tissue attachments. If the cortical shell is intact, impaction bone grafting can be used to achieve initial fixation and restore some bone stock. With a deficient proximal cortex, more substantial reconstruction is required with a proximal allograft prosthesis composite or a proximal femoral replacement. A constrained acetabular liner can be considered in patients with minimal abductor musculature. In a systematic review, Rogers et al[87] reported an implant survival rate of 80% at 8 years with an allograft prosthesis composite.

Revision of a Low Wear-Bearing Surface for Osteolysis

Most metal-on-metal bearings used in recent years have femoral head sizes of 36 mm or greater, and severe adverse tissue reactions (pseudotumors) have been reported in some studies.[10,88] One study reported an incidence of adverse tissue reactions of 0.1%.[10] These reactions have been reported with large, highly cross-linked femoral heads and with modular stems. The exact pathomechanism is unclear, but patients with implants subject to high wear (such as a high abduction angle or poor cup design) are at higher risk for adverse reactions.[89] The Medicines and Healthcare Products Regulatory Agency has suggested a cutoff level of 7 parts per billion (ppb) to discriminate between well-functioning and failed hips.[90] Hart et al[91] reported that the cutoff level of 7 ppb has a specificity of 89% but poor sensitivity (52%).

When revising a metal-on-metal bearing because of an adverse tissue reaction, it is critical to remove all potential sources of particulate metal debris. De Smet et al[89] recently reported 113 revisions for hip resurfacings in which 20% of the revisions involved a femoral stem with a large metal-on-metal femoral head. In the latter half of the study, the practice was changed to use ceramic heads. This change contributed to a decrease in complications and rerevision rates. Gilbert et al[92] reported that isolated femoral revisions for biologic reasons (such as loosening) had poorer outcomes compared with those performed for mechanical reasons (such as a fracture or head collapse). Because biologic causes would likely persist, the authors suggested revising both components to an alternate bearing surface.

Another potential cause of adverse tissue reactions is the Morse taper junction (**Figure 5**) and the adaptor sleeve in metal-on-metal hip replacements, in which the use of a relatively large cobalt-chromium head (> 36 mm) can lead to further debris generation.[88,93]

Several studies have reported a higher level of metal ions in hip replacements compared with hip resurfacings.[94,95] Poorer outcomes have been reported in hip resurfacings that have been revised for pseudotumors compared with revisions for fractures.[96] The incidence of pseudotumors recurrence, despite the exchange to a non–metal-on-metal bearing, further indicates the need to use a ceramic femoral head or a head size of 32 mm or less in the revision procedure.[96] Thorough débridement is also needed because wear debris can remain after the first revision and contribute to pseudotumor recurrence. An increased rate of dislocations after a revision for hip resurfacing has been reported; the soft-tissue destruction is largely responsible for destroying the stabilizing structures around the hip.[96]

When revising a metal-on-metal hip, strong consideration (if not absolute) should be given in using a ceramic head to avoid further metal ion generation, the Morse taper junction should be carefully inspected, and a constrained liner should be considered if instability is detected.

Summary

The quantification of remaining bone stock is paramount when revising hip replacements with osteolysis. Current implant systems have greatly improved the quality and reliability of revision hip surgery. However, in recent years, the severe inflammatory reactions associated with the failures of metal-on-metal bearings at short-term follow-ups have changed the overall assessment and timing of interventions; simple observation may no longer be indicated.

References

1. Schmalzried TP, Guttmann D, Grecula M, Amstutz HC: The relationship between the design, position, and articular wear of acetabular components inserted without cement and the development of pelvic osteolysis. *J Bone Joint Surg Am* 1994;76(5): 677-688.
2. Holt G, Murnaghan C, Reilly J, Meek RM: The biology of aseptic osteolysis. *Clin Orthop Relat Res* 2007;460:240-252.
3. Zicat B, Engh CA, Gokcen E: Patterns of osteolysis around total hip components inserted with and without cement. *J Bone Joint Surg Am* 1995;77(3):432-439.
4. Lavernia CJ: Cost-effectiveness of early surgical intervention in silent osteolysis. *J Arthroplasty* 1998; 13(3):277-279.
5. Manley MT, D'Antonio JA, Capello WN, Edidin AA: Osteolysis: A disease of access to fixation interfaces. *Clin Orthop Relat Res* 2002;405:129-137.
6. Restrepo C, Ghanem E, Houssock C, Austin M, Parvizi J, Hozack WJ: Isolated polyethylene exchange versus acetabular revision for polyethylene wear. *Clin Orthop Relat Res* 2009;467(1):194-198.
7. Naudie DD, Engh CA Sr : Surgical management of polyethylene wear and pelvic osteolysis with modular uncemented acetabular components. *J Arthroplasty* 2004; 19(4, suppl 1):124-129.
8. Engh CA, McGovern TF, Bobyn JD, Harris WH: A quantitative evaluation of periprosthetic bone-remodeling after cementless total hip arthroplasty. *J Bone Joint Surg Am* 1992;74(7):1009-1020.
9. Engh GA, Dwyer KA, Hanes CK: Polyethylene wear of metal-backed tibial components in total and unicompartmental knee prostheses. *J Bone Joint Surg Br* 1992; 74(1):9-17.
10. Walsh AJ, Nikolaou VS, Antoniou J: Inflammatory pseudotumor complicating metal-on-highly cross-linked polyethylene total hip arthroplasty. *J Arthroplasty* 2012; 27(2):324.
11. Pandit HP, Glyn-Jones S, McLardy-Smith P, et al: Pseudotumours associated with metal-on-metal hip resurfacings. *J Bone Joint Surg Br* 2008;90(7): 847-851.
12. Svensson O, Mathiesen EB, Reinholt FP, Blomgren G: Formation of a fulminant soft-tissue pseudotumor after uncemented hip arthroplasty: A case report. *J Bone Joint Surg Am* 1988;70(8):1238-1242.
13. Griffiths HJ, Burke J, Bonfiglio TA: Granulomatous pseudotumors in total joint replacement. *Skeletal Radiol* 1987;16(2): 146-152.
14. Leigh W, O'Grady P, Lawson EM, Hung NA, Theis JC, Matheson J: Pelvic pseudotumor: An unusual presentation of an extra-articular granuloma in a well-fixed total hip arthroplasty. *J Arthroplasty* 2008;23(6):934-938.
15. White CA, Carsen SA, Rasuli K, Feibel RJ, Kim PR, Beaulé PE: High incidence of migration with poor initial fixation of the Accolade stem. *Clin Orthop Relat Res* 2011;470(2):410-417.
16. Hozack WJ, Parvizi J, Bender B: *Surgical Treatment of Hip Arthritis: Reconstruction, Replacement and Revision*. Philadelphia, PA, Saunders Elsevier, 2010.

17. Thomas A, Epstein NJ, Stevens K, Goodman SB: Utility of Judet oblique x-rays in preoperative assessment of acetabular periprosthetic osteolysis: A preliminary study. *Am J Orthop (Belle Mead NJ)* 2007;36(7):E107-E110.

18. Garcia-Cimbrelo E, Tapia M, Martin-Hervas C: Multislice computed tomography for evaluating acetabular defects in revision THA. *Clin Orthop Relat Res* 2007; 463:138-143.

19. Puri L, Lapinski B, Wixson RL, Lynch J, Hendrix R, Stulberg SD: Computed tomographic follow-up evaluation of operative intervention for periacetabular lysis. *J Arthroplasty* 2006;21(6, suppl 2):78-82.

20. Yun HH, Shon WY, Hong SJ, Yoon JR, Yang JH: Relationship between the pelvic osteolytic volume on computed tomography and clinical outcome in patients with cementless acetabular components. *Int Orthop* 2011;35(10): 1453-1459.

21. Puri L, Wixson RL, Stern SH, Kohli J, Hendrix RW, Stulberg SD: Use of helical computed tomography for the assessment of acetabular osteolysis after total hip arthroplasty. *J Bone Joint Surg Am* 2002;84(4):609-614.

22. Kitamura N, Pappedemos PC, Duffy PR III, et al: The value of anteroposterior pelvic radiographs for evaluating pelvic osteolysis. *Clin Orthop Relat Res* 2006;453: 239-245.

23. Egawa H, Powers CC, Beykirch SE, Hopper RH Jr, Engh CA Jr, Engh CA: Can the volume of pelvic osteolysis be calculated without using computed tomography? *Clin Orthop Relat Res* 2009; 467(1):181-187.

24. Walde TA, Weiland DE, Leung SB, et al: Comparison of CT, MRI, and radiographs in assessing pelvic osteolysis: A cadaveric study. *Clin Orthop Relat Res* 2005; 437:138-144.

25. Wynn-Jones H, Macnair R, Wimhurst J, et al: Silent soft tissue pathology is common with a modern metal-on-metal hip arthroplasty. *Acta Orthop* 2011; 82(3):301-307.

26. Schmalzried TP, Callaghan JJ: Wear in total hip and knee replacements. *J Bone Joint Surg Am* 1999;81(1):115-136.

27. Mehin R, Yuan X, Haydon C, et al: Retroacetabular osteolysis: when to operate? *Clin Orthop Relat Res* 2004;428:247-255.

28. Spangehl MJ, Masri BA, O'Connell JX, Duncan CP: Prospective analysis of preoperative and intraoperative investigations for the diagnosis of infection at the sites of two hundred and two revision total hip arthroplasties. *J Bone Joint Surg Am* 1999;81(5): 672-683.

29. Levitsky KA, Hozack WJ, Balderston RA, et al: Evaluation of the painful prosthetic joint: Relative value of bone scan, sedimentation rate, and joint aspiration. *J Arthroplasty* 1991;6(3):237-244.

30. Gozzard C, Blom A, Taylor A, Smith E, Learmonth ID: A comparison of the reliability and validity of bone stock loss classification systems used for revision hip surgery. *J Arthroplasty* 2003;18(5): 638-642.

31. Paprosky WG, Perona PG, Lawrence JM: Acetabular defect classification and surgical reconstruction in revision arthroplasty: A 6-year follow-up evaluation. *J Arthroplasty* 1994;9(1):33-44.

32. D'Antonio JA, Capello WN, Borden LS, et al: Classification and management of acetabular abnormalities in total hip arthroplasty. *Clin Orthop Relat Res* 1989;243: 126-137.

33. Valle CJ, Paprosky WG: Classification and an algorithmic approach to the reconstruction of femoral deficiency in revision total hip arthroplasty. *J Bone Joint Surg Am* 2003;85(suppl 4):1-6.

34. Mast NH, Laude F: Revision total hip arthroplasty performed through the Hueter interval. *J Bone Joint Surg Am* 2011; 93(suppl 2):143-148.

35. Duncan WW, Hubble MJ, Howell JR, Whitehouse SL, Timperley AJ, Gie GA: Revision of the cemented femoral stem using a cement-in-cement technique: A five- to 15-year review. *J Bone Joint Surg Br* 2009;91(5): 577-582.

36. Jando VT, Greidanus NV, Masri BA, Garbuz DS, Duncan CP: Trochanteric osteotomies in revision total hip arthroplasty: Contemporary techniques and results. *Instr Course Lect* 2005;54: 143-155.

37. Lakstein D, Backstein D, Safir O, Kosashvili Y, Gross AE: Trabecular Metal cups for acetabular defects with 50% or less host bone contact. *Clin Orthop Relat Res* 2009;467(9):2318-2324.

38. Wasielewski RC, Sheridan KC, Lubbers MA: Coralline hydroxyapatite in complex acetabular reconstruction. *Orthopedics* 2008; 31(4):367.

39. Patel JV, Masonis JL, Bourne RB, Rorabeck CH: The fate of cementless jumbo cups in revision hip arthroplasty. *J Arthroplasty* 2003;18(2):129-133.

40. Abeyta PN, Namba RS, Janku GV, Murray WR, Kim HT: Reconstruction of major segmental acetabular defects with an oblong-shaped cementless prosthesis: A long-term outcomes study. *J Arthroplasty* 2008;23(2):247-253.

41. Siegmeth A, Duncan CP, Masri BA, Kim WY, Garbuz DS: Modular tantalum augments for acetabular defects in revision hip arthroplasty. *Clin Orthop Relat Res* 2009;467(1):199-205.

42. Busch VJ, Gardeniers JW, Verdonschot N, Slooff TJ, Schreurs BW: Acetabular reconstruction with impaction bone-grafting and

a cemented cup in patients younger than fifty years old: A concise follow-up, at twenty to twenty-eight years, of a previous report. *J Bone Joint Surg Am* 2011;93(4):367-371.

43. Parratte S, Argenson JN, Flecher X, Aubaniac JM: Acetabular revision for aseptic loosening in total hip arthroplasty using cementless cup and impacted morselized allograft. *Rev Chir Orthop Reparatrice Appar Mot* 2007;93(3): 255-263.

44. Sembrano JN, Cheng EY: Acetabular cage survival and analysis of factors related to failure. *Clin Orthop Relat Res* 2008;466(7): 1657-1665.

45. Kosashvili Y, Backstein D, Safir O, Lakstein D, Gross AE: Acetabular revision using an anti-protrusion (ilio-ischial) cage and trabecular metal acetabular component for severe acetabular bone loss associated with pelvic discontinuity. *J Bone Joint Surg Br* 2009; 91(7):870-876.

46. Woodgate IG, Saleh KJ, Jaroszynski G, Agnidis Z, Woodgate MM, Gross AE: Minor column structural acetabular allografts in revision hip arthroplasty. *Clin Orthop Relat Res* 2000;371:75-85.

47. Paprosky WG, Martin EL: Structural acetabular allograft in revision total hip arthroplasty. *Am J Orthop (Belle Mead NJ)* 2002; 31(8):481-484.

48. Della Valle CJ, Shuaipaj T, Berger RA, et al: Revision of the acetabular component without cement after total hip arthroplasty: A concise follow-up, at fifteen to nineteen years, of a previous report. *J Bone Joint Surg Am* 2005;87(8): 1795-1800.

49. Blom AW, Wylde V, Livesey C, et al: Impaction bone grafting of the acetabulum at hip revision using a mix of bone chips and a biphasic porous ceramic bone graft substitute. *Acta Orthop* 2009;80(2):150-154.

50. Levai JP, Boisgard S: Acetabular reconstruction in total hip revision using a bone graft substitute: Early clinical and radiographic results. *Clin Orthop Relat Res* 1996;330:108-114.

51. Whaley AL, Berry DJ, Harmsen WS: Extra-large uncemented hemispherical acetabular components for revision total hip arthroplasty. *J Bone Joint Surg Am* 2001; 83(9):1352-1357.

52. Hendricks KJ, Harris WH: Revision of failed acetabular components with use of so-called jumbo noncemented components: A concise follow-up of a previous report. *J Bone Joint Surg Am* 2006;88(3):559-563.

53. Bobyn JD, Stackpool GJ, Hacking SA, Tanzer M, Krygier JJ: Characteristics of bone ingrowth and interface mechanics of a new porous tantalum biomaterial. *J Bone Joint Surg Br* 1999;81(5): 907-914.

54. Cohen R: A porous tantalum trabecular metal: Basic science. *Am J Orthop (Belle Mead NJ)* 2002; 31(4):216-217.

55. Moskal JT, Higgins ME, Shen J: Type III acetabular defect revision with bilobed components: Five-year results. *Clin Orthop Relat Res* 2008;466(3):691-695.

56. Berry DJ, Sutherland CJ, Trousdale RT, et al: Bilobed oblong porous coated acetabular components in revision total hip arthroplasty. *Clin Orthop Relat Res* 2000; 371:154-160.

57. Surace MF, Zatti G, De Pietri M, Cherubino P: Acetabular revision surgery with the LOR cup: Three to 8 years' follow-up. *J Arthroplasty* 2006;21(1):114-121.

58. Chen WM, Engh CA Jr, Hopper RH Jr, McAuley JP, Engh CA: Acetabular revision with use of a bilobed component inserted without cement in patients who have acetabular bone-stock deficiency. *J Bone Joint Surg Am* 2000;82(2): 197-206.

59. Weeden SH, Schmidt RH: The use of tantalum porous metal implants for Paprosky 3A and 3B defects. *J Arthroplasty* 2007;22(6, suppl 2):151-155.

60. Board TN, Rooney P, Kearney JN, Kay PR: Impaction allografting in revision total hip replacement. *J Bone Joint Surg Br* 2006; 88(7):852-857.

61. Bolder SB, Schreurs BW, Verdonschot N, van Unen JM, Gardeniers JW, Slooff TJ: Particle size of bone graft and method of impaction affect initial stability of cemented cups: Human cadaveric and synthetic pelvic specimen studies. *Acta Orthop Scand* 2003; 74(6):652-657.

62. Oakes DA, Cabanela ME: Impaction bone grafting for revision hip arthroplasty: Biology and clinical applications. *J Am Acad Orthop Surg* 2006;14(11):620-628.

63. Comba F, Buttaro M, Pusso R, Piccaluga F: Acetabular reconstruction with impacted bone allografts and cemented acetabular components: A 2- to 13-year follow-up study of 142 aseptic revisions. *J Bone Joint Surg Br* 2006;88(7):865-869.

64. Paprosky WG, Sporer SS, Murphy BP: Addressing severe bone deficiency: What a cage will not do. *J Arthroplasty* 2007;22 (4, suppl 1):111-115.

65. Udomkiat P, Dorr LD, Won Y-Y, Longjohn D, Wan Z: Technical factors for success with metal ring acetabular reconstruction. *J Arthroplasty* 2001;16(8):961-969.

66. Possai KW, Dorr LD, McPherson EJ: Metal ring supports for deficient acetabular bone in total hip replacement. *Instr Course Lect* 1996;45:161-169.

67. Deirmengian GK, Zmistowski B, O'Neil JT, Hozack WJ: Management of acetabular bone loss in revision total hip arthroplasty. *J Bone Joint Surg Am* 2011; 93(19):1842-1852.

68. Garbuz D, Morsi E, Gross AE: Revision of the acetabular component of a total hip arthroplasty with a massive structural allograft: Study with a minimum five-year follow-up. *J Bone Joint Surg Am* 1996;78(5):693-697.

69. Ballester Alfaro JJ, Sueiro Fernández J: Trabecular Metal buttress augment and the Trabecular Metal cup-cage construct in revision hip arthroplasty for severe acetabular bone loss and pelvic discontinuity. *Hip Int* 2010;20(S7):119-127.

70. Springer BD, Connelly SE, Odum SM, et al: Cementless femoral components in young patients: Review and meta-analysis of total hip arthroplasty and hip resurfacing. *J Arthroplasty* 2009; 24(6, suppl):2-8.

71. Garbuz DS, Toms A, Masri BA, Duncan CP: Improved outcome in femoral revision arthroplasty with tapered fluted modular titanium stems. *Clin Orthop Relat Res* 2006;453(12):199-202.

72. Richards CJ, Duncan CP, Masri BA, Garbuz DS: Femoral revision hip arthroplasty: A comparison of two stem designs. *Clin Orthop Relat Res* 2010;468(2):491-496.

73. Maloney WJ: The surgical management of femoral osteolysis. *J Arthroplasty* 2005;20(4, suppl 2):75-78.

74. Dohmae Y, Bechtold JE, Sherman RE, Puno RM, Gustilo RB: Reduction in cement-bone interface shear strength between primary and revision arthroplasty. *Clin Orthop Relat Res* 1988;236: 214-220.

75. Korovessis P, Repantis T: High medium-term survival of Zweymüller SLR-plus stem used in femoral revision. *Clin Orthop Relat Res* 2009;467(8):2032-2040.

76. Mulliken BD, Rorabeck CH, Bourne RB: Uncemented revision total hip arthroplasty: A 4-to-6-year review. *Clin Orthop Relat Res* 1996;325:156-162.

77. Pattyn C, Mulliez A, Verdonk R, Audenaert E: Revision hip arthroplasty using a cementless modular tapered stem. *Int Orthop* 2012; 36(1):35-41.

78. Rodriguez JA, Fada R, Murphy SB, Rasquinha VJ, Ranawat CS: Two-year to five-year follow-up of femoral defects in femoral revision treated with the link MP modular stem. *J Arthroplasty* 2009;24(5): 751-758.

79. Kwong LM, Miller AJ, Lubinus P: A modular distal fixation option for proximal bone loss in revision total hip arthroplasty: A 2- to 6-year follow-up study. *J Arthroplasty* 2003;18(3, suppl 1):94-97.

80. Engh CA, Bobyn JD, Glassman AH: Porous-coated hip replacement: The factors governing bone ingrowth, stress shielding, and clinical results. *J Bone Joint Surg Br* 1987;69(1):45-55.

81. Engh CA, Glassman AH, Suthers KE: The case for porous-coated hip implants: The femoral side. *Clin Orthop Relat Res* 1990;261: 63-81.

82. Engh CA, Massin P, Suthers KE: Roentgenographic assessment of the biologic fixation of porous-surfaced femoral components. *Clin Orthop Relat Res* 1990;257: 107-128.

83. Rodriguez JA, Deshmukh AJ, Klauser WU, Rasquinha VJ, Lubinus P, Ranawat CS: Patterns of osseointegration and remodeling in femoral revision with bone loss using modular, tapered, fluted, titanium stems. *J Arthroplasty* 2011;26(8):1409-1417.

84. Miner TM, Momberger NG, Chong D, Paprosky WL: The extended trochanteric osteotomy in revision hip arthroplasty: A critical review of 166 cases at mean 3-year, 9-month follow-up. *J Arthroplasty* 2001; 16(8, suppl 1):188-194.

85. Ornstein E, Linder L, Ranstam J, Lewold S, Eisler T, Torper M: Femoral impaction bone grafting with the Exeter stem—the Swedish experience: Survivorship analysis of 1305 revisions performed between 1989 and 2002. *J Bone Joint Surg Br* 2009;91(4): 441-446.

86. Cummins F, Reilly PO, Flannery O, Kelly D, Kenny P: Defining the impaction frequency and threshold force required for femoral impaction grafting in revision hip arthroplasty: A human cadaveric mechanical study. *Acta Orthop* 2011;82(4):433-437.

87. Rogers BA, Sternheim A, Backstein D, Safir O, Gross AE: Proximal femoral allograft for major segmental femoral bone loss: A systematic literature review. *Adv Orthop* 2011;2011:257572.

88. Langton DJ, Jameson SS, Joyce TJ, et al: Accelerating failure rate of the ASR total hip replacement. *J Bone Joint Surg Br* 2011;93(8): 1011-1016.

89. De Smet KA, Van Der Straeten C, Van Orsouw M, Doubi R, Backers K, Grammatopoulos G: Revisions of metal-on-metal hip resurfacing: Lessons learned and improved outcome. *Orthop Clin North Am* 2011;42(2):259-269.

90. Medicines and Healthcare Products Regulatory Agency: Medical Device Alert: All metal-on-metal (MoM) hip replacements. April 22, 2010. http://www.mhra.gov.uk/home/groups/dts-bs/documents/medicaldevicealert/con079162.pdf. Accessed October 4, 2012.

91. Hart AJ, Sabah SA, Bandi AS, et al: Sensitivity and specificity of blood cobalt and chromium metal ions for predicting failure of metal-on-metal hip replacement. *J Bone Joint Surg Br* 2011;93(10): 1308-1313.

92. Gilbert RE, Cheung G, Carrothers AD, Meyer C, Richardson JB: Functional results of isolated femoral revision of hip resurfacing arthroplasty. *J Bone Joint Surg Am* 2010;92(7):1600-1604.

93. Lavigne M, Belzile EL, Roy A, Morin F, Amzica T, Vendittoli PA: Comparison of whole-blood metal ion levels in four types of metal-on-metal large-diameter femoral head total hip arthroplasty: The potential influence of the adapter sleeve. *J Bone Joint Surg Am* 2011;93(suppl 2): 128-136.
94. Garbuz DS, Tanzer M, Greidanus NV, Masri BA, Duncan CP: Metal-on-metal hip resurfacing versus large-diameter head metal-on-metal total hip arthroplasty: A randomized clinical trial. *Clin Orthop Relat Res* 2010;468(2): 318-325.
95. Beaulé PE, Kim PR, Hamdi A, Fazekas A: A prospective metal ion study of large-head metal-on-metal bearing: A matched-pair analysis of hip resurfacing versus total hip replacement. *Orthop Clin North Am* 2011;42(2):251-257.
96. Grammatopolous G, Pandit H, Kwon YM, et al: Hip resurfacings revised for inflammatory pseudotumour have a poor outcome. *J Bone Joint Surg Br* 2009;91(8): 1019-1024.

19

Outpatient Minimally Invasive Total Hip Arthroplasty Via a Modified Watson-Jones Approach: Technique and Results

Darwin Chen, MD
Richard A. Berger, MD

Abstract

A variety of minimally invasive approaches to hip surgery in combination with multimodal anesthesia techniques and rapid rehabilitation can facilitate early discharge after total hip arthroplasty (THA). Hip replacement can be performed as outpatient surgery using the surgical technique of THA through a modified abductor-sparing Watson-Jones (anterolateral) approach, along with a comprehensive clinical pathway. One hundred thirteen sequential patients were treated with primary THA completed by noon by a single surgeon from January to August 2011. Eighty-seven of the 113 patients agreed to be placed in an outpatient protocol, and 26 were treated with an in-patient protocol. Eighty-six of the 87 patients (98.9%) in the outpatient group were successfully discharged home the day of surgery. The remaining patient was discharged home the next morning (postoperative day 1). No patients had significant medical complications, and there were no readmissions within the acute 2-week postoperative period. A deep hip infection developed in one patient at 3 weeks postoperatively. That patient was readmitted to the hospital and treated with a one-stage reimplantation procedure. This study confirmed that outpatient THA can be successfully and safely performed through a modified, minimally invasive Watson-Jones (anterolateral) approach coupled with a comprehensive clinical pathway.

Instr Course Lect 2013;62:229-236.

Modern total hip arthroplasty (THA) faces a challenging new era in health care. Orthopaedic surgeons are confronted by a medical landscape influenced by high patient expectations, direct marketing to consumers, and pressure from insurers and hospital administrators to minimize the patient's length of stay.[1-3] Patients want a highly functioning hip, a rapid recovery, and a postoperative course that minimizes pain. The orthopaedic surgeon is challenged to meet these demands while executing a safe and well-performed hip replacement. Minimally invasive THA, in combination with multimodal anesthesia techniques, rapid rehabilitation, and proper patient education, can help surgeons achieve these goals and make THA an outpatient procedure for many patients.[4]

The surgical approach is one of the main components of the outpatient minimally invasive THA procedures discussed in this chapter. The original Watson-Jones anterolateral approach to the hip was described through the interval between the tensor fascia lata and the gluteus medius.[5] The anterior aspect of the abductor complex was taken off the wing of the ilium, allowing the hip to dislocate anteriorly and providing excellent exposure of the acetabulum after the neck osteotomy. The main advantage to this approach is a lower dislocation rate secondary to preservation of the posterior structures, and

Dr. Berger or an immediate family member has received royalties from Zimmer and serves as a paid consultant to or is an employee of Salient Surgical. Neither Dr. Chen nor any immediate family member has received anything of value from or owns stock in a commercial company or institution related directly or indirectly to the subject of this chapter.

the main disadvantage is violation of the abductor musculature, potentially leading to a limp and weakness. Bertin and Röttinger[6] described a modified, minimally invasive, anterolateral approach through the same muscular interval as the Watson-Jones approach with preservation of the abductors. They concluded that less muscle damage from this approach could allow for more rapid rehabilitation and recovery. This chapter's authors have further modified and incorporated this approach as a part of an outpatient THA pathway.

Specialized anesthesia and rapid rehabilitation protocols play important roles in enabling a minimally invasive outpatient approach to THA.[4,7,8] Regional anesthesia allows for less narcotic administration, which leads to decreased postoperative nausea and hypotension.[9] Initiation of preemptive oral analgesia and antiemetics early in the recovery phase also aid in pain management and nausea control.[10-12] Physical therapy on the day of surgery allows patients to ambulate independently and facilitates early discharge. Preoperative education and discharge planning are critical in managing the patient's expectations and ensuring adequate care at home.[13]

Currently, the only reported experiences with outpatient THA have been with the two-incision and mini-posterior techniques.[7,14,15] In those studies, the authors demonstrated that outpatient hip replacement is both possible and safe in appropriately selected patients. In the current study, this chapter's authors describe outpatient THA using a minimally invasive, abductor-sparing, Watson-Jones (anterolateral) approach, coupled with a rapid rehabilitation and recovery protocol. The purpose of this study is to evaluate the effectiveness of such a pathway for outpatient hip replacement and assess its feasibility and safety in a group of patients chosen with less stringent criteria.

Materials and Methods

Of 113 consecutive patients who were treated by this chapter's senior author (RAB) with primary THA between January 2011 and August 2011 (only surgeries completed by noon are included), 87 patients agreed to be in the study described in this chapter and were placed on a protocol for outpatient THA surgery. The remaining 26 patients were treated with an in-patient THA protocol by the same surgeon. A prospective review was performed on the 87 patients in this institutional review board–approved study.

Of the 87 patients enrolled in this study, 53 (59.8%) were men and 34 (40.2%) were women. The average age of the patients was 56 years (range, 38 to 73 years). Fifteen patients (17.2%) were younger than 50 years, 65 patients (74.7%) were 50 to 65 years of age, and 7 patients (8.1%) were older than 65 years. The average weight of all the study patients was 85.7 kg (range, 47.2 to 145.2 kg). The average weight of the men was 94.2 kg (range, 63.5 to 145.2 kg), and the average weight of the women was 73.0 kg (range, 47.2 to 113.4 kg). The average overall body mass index (BMI) was 27.9 (range, 18.5 to 43.3). The average BMI for the men was 29 (range, 22.5 to 43.3), and the average BMI for the women was 26.8 (range, 18.5 to 40.2). Patients with an important history of cardiac or pulmonary disease who would need prolonged monitoring after surgery were excluded. Aside from these exclusion criteria, all other patients were eligible to choose the outpatient protocol. A family support system was not necessary for inclusion in the study.

Perioperative Care

All patients in this study were enrolled in a comprehensive clinical pathway, which included preoperative, intraoperative, and postoperative care. This pathway resulted from a collaborative effort between the surgeon, anesthesiologist, physical therapists, nurses, and discharge planners. The pathway specifically addressed pain management, postoperative nausea and hypotension, and home aftercare.

Preoperative Care

Preoperatively, all patients attended a class taught by a clinical nurse and a physical therapist. Patients were informed about what to expect before, during, and after surgery, including all aspects of their hospital course of treatment. Pain management was specifically outlined to reassure patients that their pain would be well controlled. Patients were encouraged to ask questions, and adequate time was allotted to provide answers. The patients participated in a physical therapy session, which provided instruction in gait training with crutches and weight bearing as tolerated. Each patient was medically cleared for surgery by an internist and preoperatively donated one unit of blood. A discharge planner assisted the patients in arranging postoperative care, including transportation home, home aftercare, and physical therapy administered at the patient's home for 1 to 2 weeks.

On the morning of surgery, the patients were instructed to take 10 mg of controlled-release oxycodone hydrochloride (OxyContin; Purdue Pharma, Stamford, CT) just prior to coming to the hospital. In the preoperative holding area, an epidural catheter was inserted before the patient was brought to the operating room.

Surgical Care

In the operating room, a Foley catheter was inserted, and intravenous antibiotics were started. The patients were given a titrated dose of propofol (Diprivan;

AstraZeneca Pharmaceuticals, Wilmington, DE) for sedation during the procedure at the discretion of the anesthesiologist. Care was taken to give the minimum amount of sedation necessary to perform the surgery. Nausea prophylaxis was achieved with 4 mg of ondansetron hydrochloride (Zofran; Glaxo SmithKline, Philadelphia, PA) and 10 mg of metoclopramide (Reglan; Wyeth Pharmaceuticals, Madison, NJ) given intravenously. Patients were given adequate intravenous hydration and a transfusion of one unit of autologous blood. Intravenous and epidural narcotics were avoided during surgery.

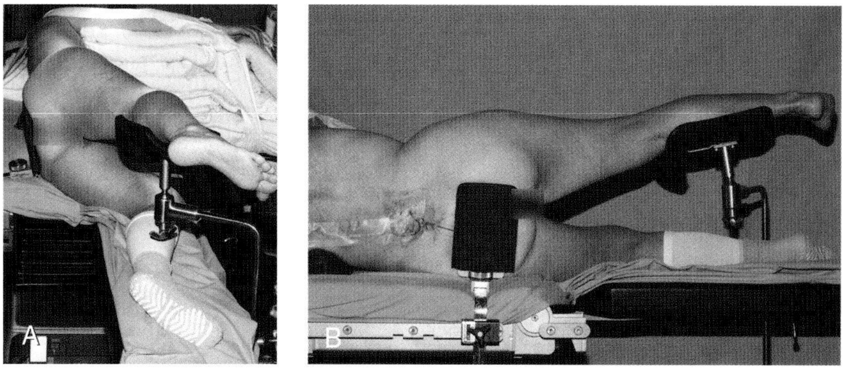

Figure 1 **A,** The patient is positioned in the lateral decubitus position with standard pelvic positioners. The posterior lower half of the operating table is removed. The operative extremity is positioned in a leg holder in slight abduction. **B,** Posterior view of the setup of the surgical table and patient positioning.

Postoperative Care

In the recovery room, a second dose of Zofran was administered. A 500-mL bolus of hydroxyethyl starch (Hespan; B. Braun Medical, Melsungen, Germany) was given intravenously as a volume expander, and intravenous fluids were maintained with 125 mL/hour of lactated Ringer solution. The epidural was dosed with 10 μg/mL fentanyl plus 0.1% bupivacaine at 6 mL, 1 mL per 15 minutes with 40 mL for a 4-hour lockout interval. Two hours after surgery, the Foley urinary catheter was removed. Patients were given either 10 mg or 20 mg of OxyContin (10 mg for patients older than 70 years or weighing less than 54.431 kg) and 10/325 Norco (Watson Pharmaceuticals, Corona, CA) as needed every 4 hours for breakthrough pain. Four hours after surgery, the epidural was discontinued, and the intravenous line was heparin locked. Physical therapy began 5 to 6 hours after surgery, and patients were allowed to bear weight as tolerated with crutches, a cane, or independently. Patients were encouraged to ambulate either with a cane or unassisted if possible.

To address postoperative problems, a clinical nurse was available and checked all same-day surgery patients on rounds. In general, nausea was treated with additional Reglan, hypotension was treated with additional fluid boluses, and breakthrough pain was treated with intravenous morphine and/or OxyContin or Norco administered by mouth. Patients were discharged when they were able to independently transfer out of bed to a standing position and vice versa, ambulate 100 feet, and ascend and descend one flight of stairs. Before discharge, patients had to have stable vital signs, adequately controlled pain, the ability to tolerate a regular diet, and a willingness to go home.

After discharge, patients were told to take 325 mg aspirin twice a day for prophylaxis against venous thromboembolism for 3 weeks. Patients continued taking OxyContin 10 mg or 20 mg twice daily; they were weaned from the drug over 5 days. Patients also took 10/325 Norco every 6 hours as needed for breakthrough pain for a few weeks. Diclofenac (75 mg; Voltaren; Norvartis, Parsippany, NJ) twice a day was added as an anti-inflammatory medication for 3 months, and 20 mg omeprazole (Prilosec; Proctor & Gamble, Cincinnati, OH) was given for gastroesophageal reflux protection. Patients participated in home physical therapy for 1 to 2 weeks, followed by outpatient physical therapy for an additional 3 to 6 weeks. Clinical and radiographic follow-up occurred at 2 weeks, 6 weeks, and 1 year postoperatively.

Surgical Technique

Positioning

The patient is positioned in the lateral decubitus position using standard table-mounted pelvic positioners. The pubic symphysis and contralateral anterosuperior iliac spine are supported anteriorly, and the sacrum is supported posteriorly. A Universal Jupiter Table (Trumpf Inc, Farmington, CT) allows the removal of the leg sections independently. Removing the posterior lower half of the table allows the operative leg to be placed in a position of extension, adduction, and external rotation and facilitates femoral exposure. A leg holder is used to support the operative leg in a position of 15° of abduction during the approach and acetabular exposure (**Figure 1**). The extremity is prepared and draped in the standard fashion using a hip drape with side pouches.

Approach

A modified, abductor-sparing anterolateral approach through the Watson-Jones interval was used for the THA.

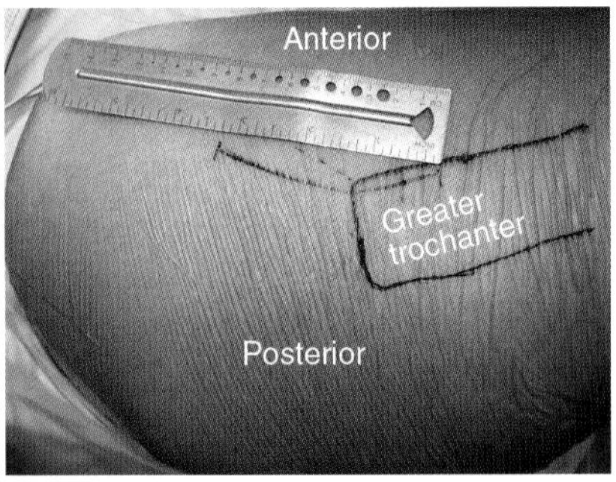

Figure 2 Using a modified, abductor-sparing anterolateral approach, a curvilinear incision is placed bordering the Watson-Jones interval.

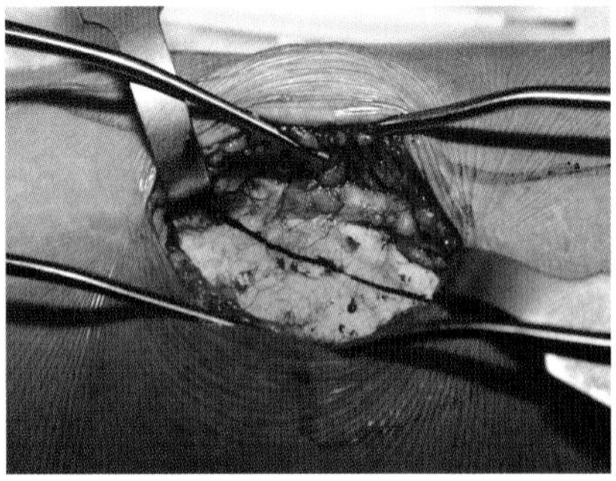

Figure 3 The fascial incision is based over the anterior border of the gluteus medius.

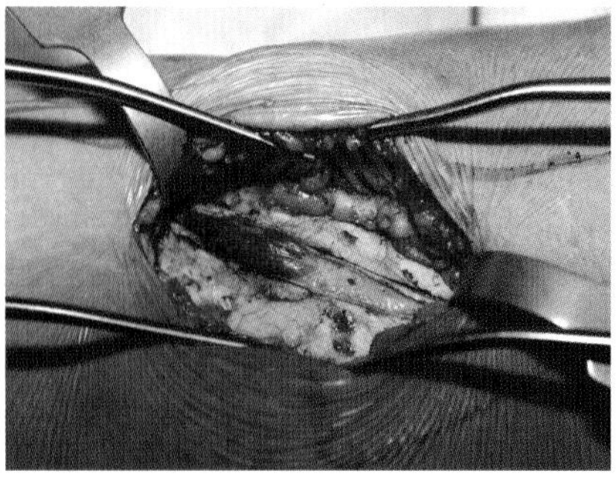

Figure 4 The interval between the tensor fascia lata and the gluteus medius is split gently.

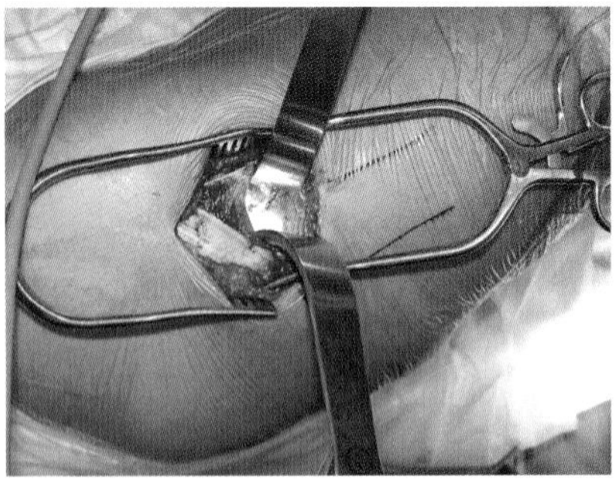

Figure 5 Retractors are placed around the femoral neck, further opening the interval.

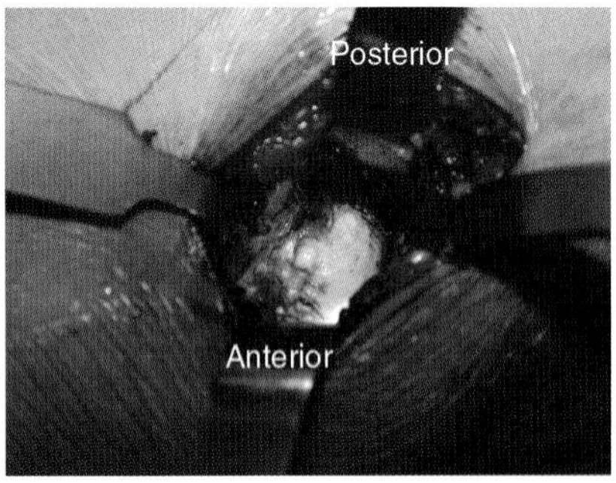

Figure 6 Intraoperative photograph of exposure of the femoral head and neck after anterior capsulotomy.

The anterior border of the femur and the superior border of the greater trochanter are identified with a spinal needle and marked. The interval between the tensor fascia lata and the gluteus medius is palpated, and the proximal end of the incision begins slightly posterior to this interval. The incision then curves gently toward and is centered over the anterosuperior corner of the greater trochanter. The distal end of the incision parallels and is slightly posterior to the anterior border of the femur. The total incision length is approximately 3.5 to 4 inches (**Figure 2**).

After the incision is made, electrocautery is used to maintain hemostasis and dissect the subcutaneous fat down to the level of the fascia, in line with the incision. The fascial border between the tensor fascia lata and the gluteus medius is identified. Frequently, a perforating vessel is evident through the tensor fascia that can be used as a landmark. The bluish hue of the tensor muscle through its thin fascia also can aid in identification. The fascial incision is made over the anterior border of the gluteus medius, anterior to the greater trochanter (**Figure 3**). The interval between the tensor and the gluteus medius is then split gently, paying careful attention to maintain hemostasis because of the perforating vessels in this fatty interval (**Figure 4**). A lit, curved Hohmann retractor is then placed extracapsularly over the superior aspect of the femoral neck underneath the gluteus medius and minimus, protecting the abductor complex. Another lit retractor is placed along the inferior femoral neck (**Figure 5**). The retractors are spread, identifying the anterior capsule. A capsulotomy is performed, resecting a capsular flap along the anterosuperior femoral neck, the intertrochanteric ridge, the inferior neck, and the acetabular rim. The saddle point between the inner aspect of the greater trochanter and the base of the superior femoral neck must be identified and cleared of capsular remnants because this marks the superolateral border of the femoral neck osteotomy. The retractors are then repositioned intracapsularly over the acetabular rim in preparation for the femoral head and neck osteotomy (**Figure 6**).

Femoral Head and Neck Osteotomy

The femoral head and neck are cut in situ without dislocating the hip. The femoral head is cut sequentially into thin wafer slices using an oscillating saw. The first cut is thin (3 to 5 mm) and made underneath the acetabular rim along the superior dome of the femoral head (**Figure 7**). Two to three additional cuts of increasing thickness are then made (**Figure 8**), and the fragments are removed with a flat osteotome and Kocher clamp, decreasing the tension in the hip joint as each

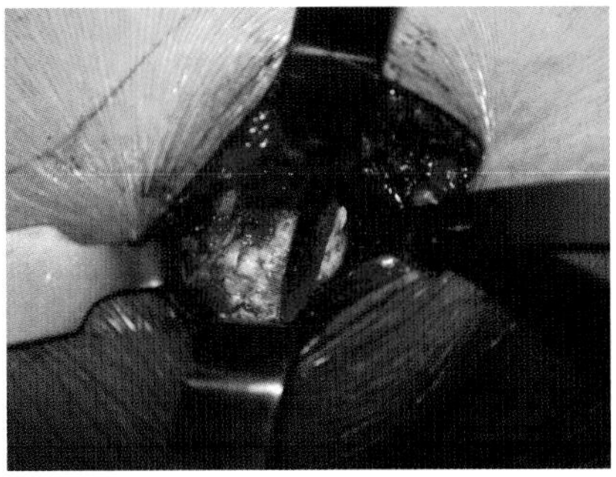

Figure 7 The first cut of the femoral neck osteotomy is made just under the superior dome of femoral head.

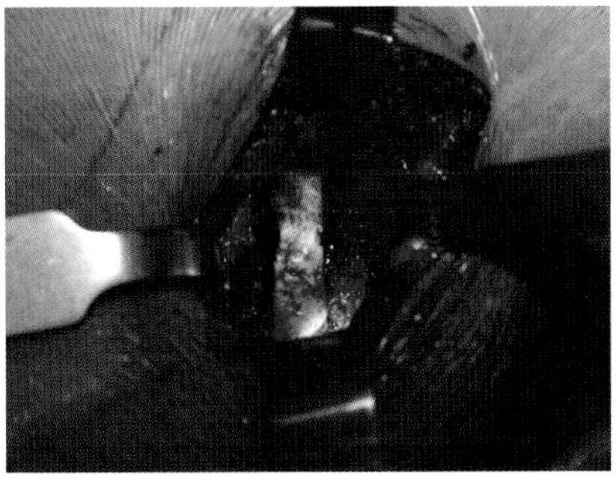

Figure 8 Sequential cuts of the femoral neck are performed.

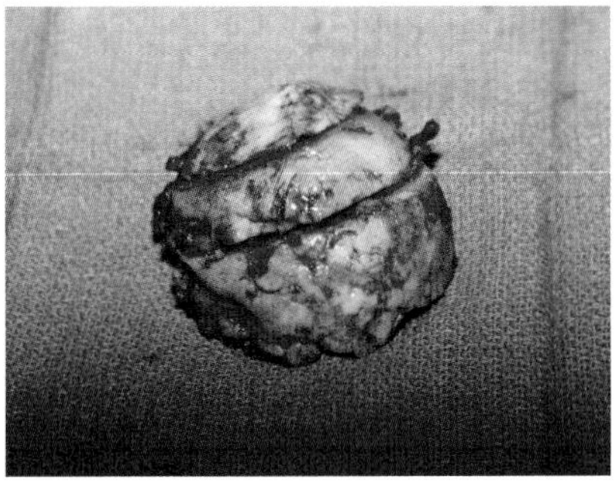

Figure 9 The femoral head is removed after sequential cuts.

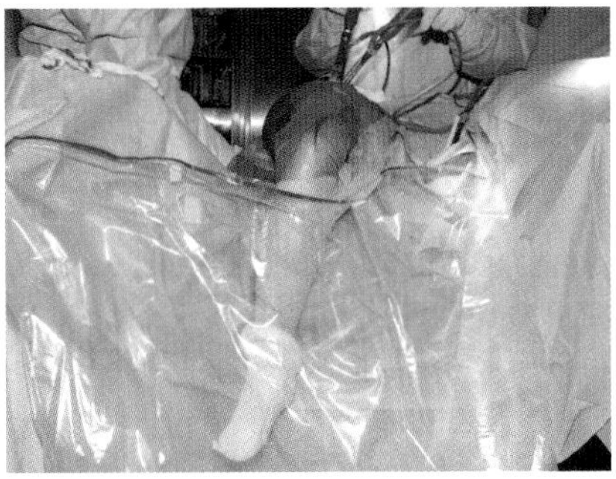

Figure 10 The leg placed is placed in a figure-of-4 position to facilitate exposure of the inferior femoral neck and the lesser trochanter.

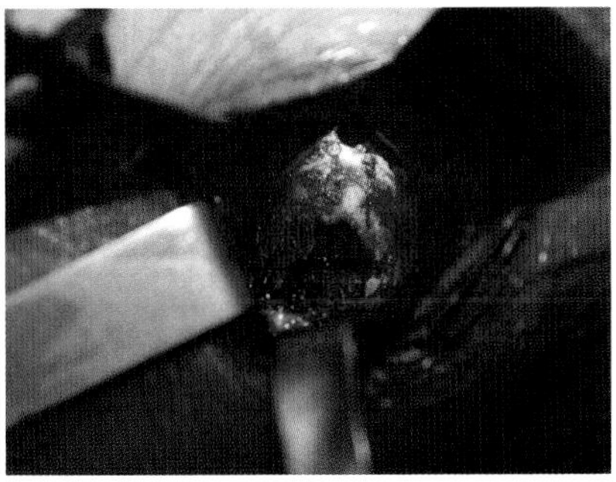

Figure 11 Intraoperative photograph showing 360° acetabular exposure.

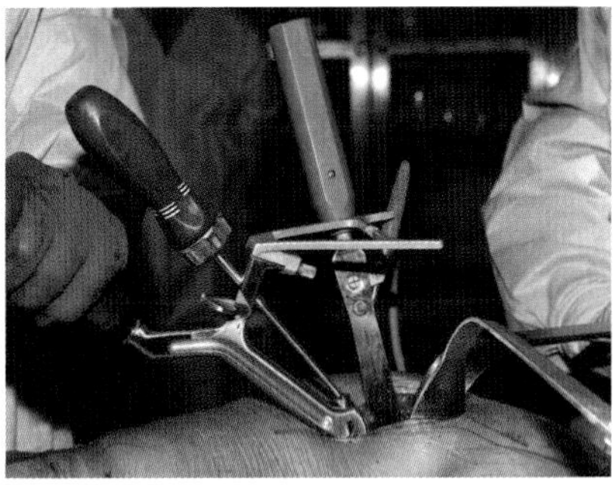

Figure 12 The acetabular shell is impacted with an offset handle.

fragment is removed (**Figure 9**). Care must be taken to prevent plunging the oscillating saw into the acetabulum.

After the head is completely removed, the remainder of the neck cut must be performed down to the preoperatively templated level. A lit, double-pronged Mueller-type retractor is placed under the lesser trochanter. The leg is placed in the figure-of-4 position, with the foot placed into the sterile hip pouch, allowing the hip to be flexed and externally rotated (**Figure 10**). The curved Hohmann retractor remains over the anterosuperior rim of the acetabulum, retracting the abductors during the neck osteotomy. An oscillating saw is used to perform the neck cut, extending from the saddle point to the templated level above the lesser trochanter.

Acetabular Preparation

The leg is taken out of the hip pouch and placed into the leg holder. The double-pronged retractor is placed posteriorly behind the acetabular wall, retracting the femur posteriorly. A cobra retractor is placed anteroinferiorly into the obturator foramen. A lit, wide, curved Hohmann retractor is placed posterosuperiorly to retract the abductor complex. After 360° visualization of the acetabulum is achieved, the pulvinar and labrum are excised (**Figure 11**). Acetabular reaming is then performed with cutout reamers, first reaming medially to the floor of the cotyloid fossa and then widening the acetabular rim until a good press fit is achieved. Offset reamer handles can be used, but straight reamers are usually adequate with the hip flexed and abducted. The final implant is then impacted into place in the appropriate abduction and anteversion (**Figure 12**), with or without adjunctive screw fixation, followed by placement of the acetabular liner (**Figure 13**).

Femoral Preparation

The leg is placed into a sterile kangaroo pouch attached to an assistant's gown, allowing the hip to be extended, adducted, and externally rotated (**Figure 14**). A thin, curved, single-pronged Hohmann retractor is placed in the piriformis fossa or over the greater trochanter to simultaneously elevate the femur anteriorly and retract the abductors posteriorly. A double-pronged retractor is placed around the

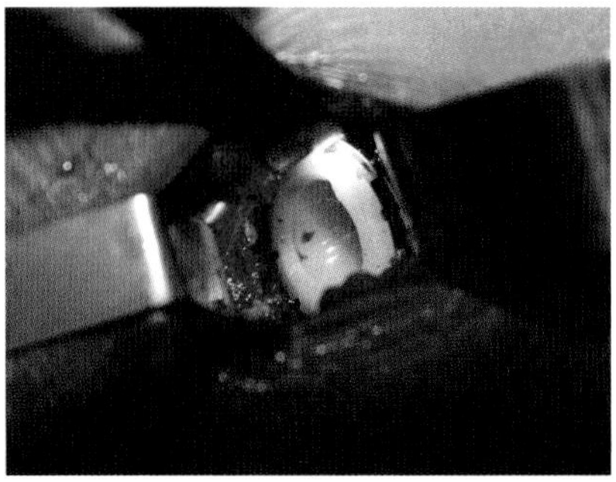

Figure 13 The acetabular liner is placed.

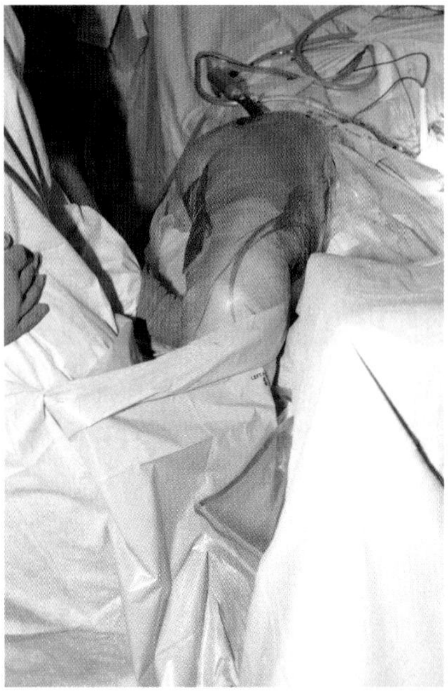

Figure 14 The leg is placed into a sterile kangaroo pouch attached to an assistant's gown, allowing the hip to be extended, adducted, and externally rotated.

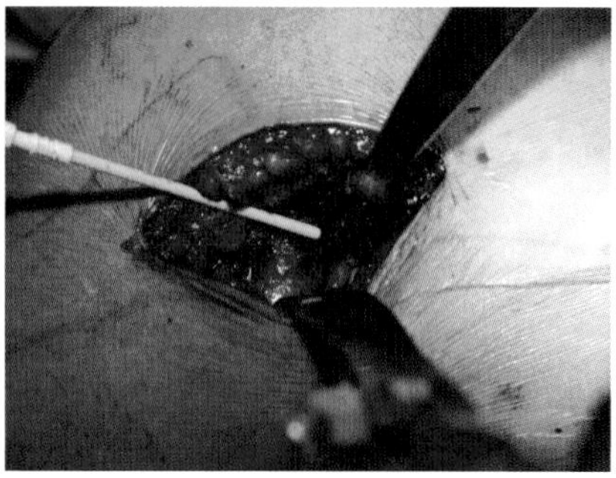

Figure 15 The superior capsule is released from the saddle point.

calcar. Another thin, curved, Hohmann retractor is placed along the lateral aspect of the femur and is used to push the femur anteriorward over the acetabulum. Release of the posterior superior capsule from the saddle point and the inner aspect of the greater trochanter (**Figure 15**) is often necessary to further present the femur anteriorly for instrumentation (**Figure 16**). After exposure is achieved, a curved awl is used to enter the femoral canal. A large motorized burr is useful to ream out the inner aspect of the greater trochanter, preventing varus positioning of the femoral stem. A tapered femoral stem design facilitates instrumentation; however, straight cylindrical stems also can be used with this approach with additional femoral exposure. Broaching is performed with offset handles until adequate fit, depth, and version are achieved (**Figure 17**). The final stem is inserted (**Figure 18**) and trial reduction is then performed with varying neck lengths until adequate hip stability, soft-tissue tension, and leg length are achieved. The trial head is then removed, and the final head is impacted into place. The hip is reduced for a final time.

Closure

The wound is thoroughly irrigated with dilute povidone-iodine solution, followed by normal saline pulsatile lavage. Typically, a drain is not placed. The fascial interval is closed in an interrupted fashion. The deep fat layer is closed with running suture, and the deep dermal layer is closed with an interrupted suture. Running subcuticular closure is then performed, and a skin adhesive is used to seal the wound.

Results

Of the 87 patients who were scheduled for outpatient THA and had surgery completed by noon, 86 (98.9%) were discharged home the same day. One patient (1.1%) was unable to complete the required elements of physical therapy and was discharged home on the day following surgery (postoperative day 1) when the required regimen could be completed. Mean surgical time was 59 minutes (range, 38 to 91 minutes). Mean estimated blood loss was 250 mL (range, 50 to 1,500 mL). All 87 patients received epidural anesthesia. All 87 patients were discharged home with home physical therapy services and without nursing services.

All patients received uncemented acetabular and femoral THA components. A DePuy Pinnacle Porocoat (DePuy, Warsaw, IN) acetabular shell was used in 34 patients (39.1%), and a Zimmer Trilogy (Zimmer, Warsaw, IN) fiber metal mesh acetabular shell was used in 53 patients (60.92%). Twenty-seven patients (31%) had a Zimmer VerSys Beaded FullCoat stem, 26 patients (29.9%) had a Zimmer M/L Taper Kinectiv modular tapered stem, 33 patients (37.9%) had a DePuy Tri-Lock tapered stem, and 1 patient (1.2%) had a Zimmer VerSys fiber metal tapered stem.

None of the patients had substantial medical complications in the acute postoperative period (less than 2 weeks after surgery). There were no deep venous thromboses, pulmonary embolisms, cardiopulmonary events, deaths, or other serious medical complications. There were no readmissions for postoperative complications during this period. A deep hip infection occurred in one patient at 3 weeks postoperatively. The patient was treated with a one-stage exchange revision hip arthroplasty and intravenous antibiotics. To date, the hip infection has not recurred in that patient.

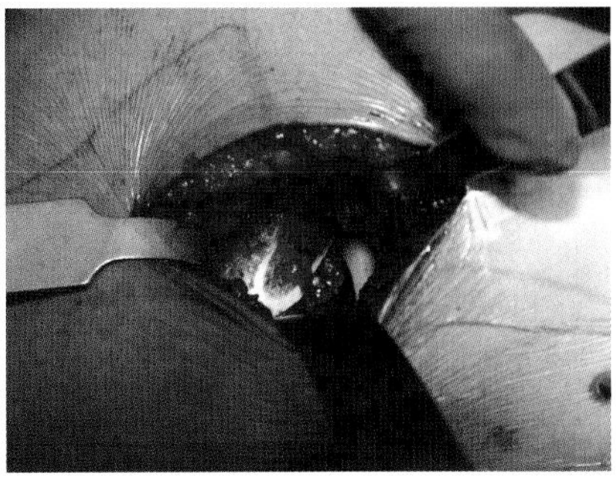

Figure 16 The final femoral exposure is shown.

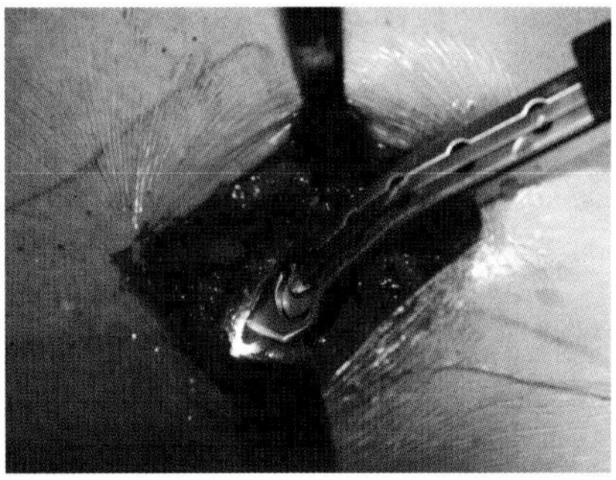

Figure 17 Femoral broaching using offset handles.

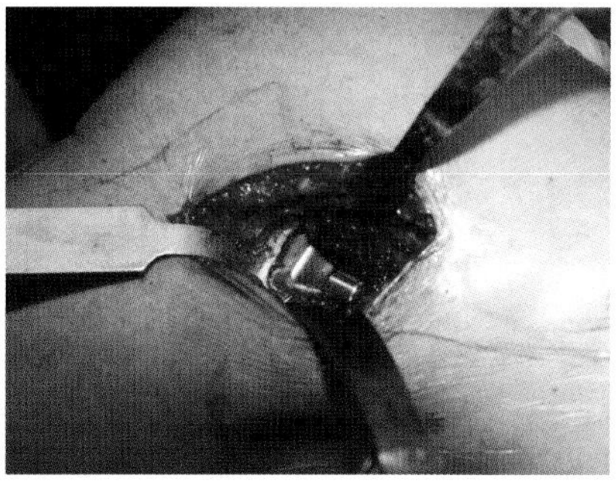

Figure 18 The femoral component is placed.

Discussion

The purpose of this study was to describe the technique of minimally invasive THA through a modified Watson-Jones (anterolateral) approach coupled with a comprehensive clinical pathway and demonstrate the efficacy and safety of such an outpatient surgery protocol for THA in a subgroup of patients. Prior studies have shown that outpatient hip replacement is both feasible and safe with the mini-posterior and two-incision techniques;[7,15] this study confirms similar results with a modified Watson-Jones (anterolateral) approach.

Ninety-nine percent of the patients in this study (86 of 87) were successfully discharged home on the same day of surgery. This represents a higher success rate than previously reported studies on outpatient total joint replacement by the senior author.[4,7,8,14] This success can be attributed to small iterative refinements of an established outpatient pathway and increased institutional support and acceptance of the protocol. There were no readmissions within the first 2 weeks after surgery, and there were no medical complications in this period. There was one deep infection at 3 weeks postoperatively, which was treated with a one-stage exchange revision arthroplasty.

This study had a few noteworthy limitations. Although the patients included in the study were not selected specifically as outpatient THA candidates, there was an element of self-selection. Because these patients chose the senior author—a well-known proponent of outpatient joint replacement—for their THA surgery, it is likely that they were motivated to participate in outpatient surgery with a goal of rapid rehabilitation. Preoperatively, all the THA candidates were given a choice between outpatient surgery or an overnight hospital stay. The patients who chose the outpatient pathway were probably more likely to possess the motivation necessary to complete same-day discharge requirements. Because most patients (87 of 113 sequential patients) undergoing THA performed by the senior author agreed to be placed in this outpatient protocol, the patient selection for this protocol was mitigated.

The demographics of the study population reflect the senior author's practice and the institutional bias toward younger patients. The average age of the patients in this study was 56 years, and the average BMI was 27.9; these statistics are likely lower than the averages of many typical arthroplasty practices. This study did not assess any radiographic or functional outcomes; such analyses were beyond the scope of the study and should be the subject of further investigation.

The length of a hospital stay after THA has dramatically decreased in the past 20 years. The average stay has decreased from more than 1 week to 3 to 4 days, with some procedures done with an overnight stay or as same-day surgery. Detractors of outpatient THA argue that such early discharge may not be medically safe, and complications are more likely to arise in the first few postoperative days.[16] However, many studies have validated the safety of early discharge in select patient populations.[7,14,15] With decreasing reimbursements and healthcare spending cuts, there may be a financial incentive to perform outpatient THA in the future. In a matched cohort study, Bertin[17] reported that the average hospital bill was $4,000 less for patients treated with outpatient THA compared with inpatient THA.

Summary

Outpatient THA can be performed successfully and safely. Although minimally invasive surgery plays a role in outpatient THA, multimodal anesthesia techniques, rapid rehabilitation, and preoperative patient education are at least equally important factors. When these factors are combined with a comprehensive clinical pathway, outpatient THA can achieve safe, effective, and reproducible outcomes.

References

1. Mason JB: The new demands by patients in the modern era of total joint arthroplasty: A point of view. *Clin Orthop Relat Res* 2008; 466(1):146-152.
2. Booth RE Jr: Truth in advertising: The ethical limits of direct-to-consumer marketing. *Orthopedics* 2006;29(9):780-781.
3. Bozic KJ, Smith AR, Hariri S, et al: The impact of direct-to-consumer advertising in orthopaedics. *Clin Orthop Relat Res* 2007; 458:202-219.
4. Berger RA, Sanders SA, Thill ES, Sporer SM, Della Valle C: Newer anesthesia and rehabilitation protocols enable outpatient hip replacement in selected patients. *Clin Orthop Relat Res* 2009; 467(6):1424-1430.
5. Watson-Jones R: Fractures of the neck of the femur. *Br J Surg* 1936; 23:787-808.
6. Bertin KC, Röttinger H: Anterolateral mini-incision hip replacement surgery: A modified Watson-Jones approach. *Clin Orthop Relat Res* 2004;429:248-255.
7. Berger RA, Jacobs JJ, Meneghini RM, Della Valle C, Paprosky W, Rosenberg AG: Rapid rehabilitation and recovery with minimally invasive total hip arthroplasty. *Clin Orthop Relat Res* 2004;429: 239-247.
8. Berger RA: A comprehensive approach to outpatient total hip arthroplasty. *Am J Orthop (Belle Mead NJ)* 2007;36(suppl 9):4-5.
9. Macfarlane AJ, Prasad GA, Chan VW, Brull R: Does regional anaesthesia improve outcome after total hip arthroplasty? A systematic review. *Br J Anaesth* 2009; 103(3):335-345.
10. Dorr LD, Raya J, Long WT, Boutary M, Sirianni LE: Multimodal analgesia without parenteral narcotics for total knee arthroplasty. *J Arthroplasty* 2008;23(4):502-508.
11. DiIorio TM, Sharkey PF, Hewitt AM, Parvizi J: Antiemesis after total joint arthroplasty: Does a single preoperative dose of aprepitant reduce nausea and vomiting? *Clin Orthop Relat Res* 2010; 468(9):2405-2409.
12. Duellman TJ, Gaffigan C, Milbrandt JC, Allan DG: Multimodal, pre-emptive analgesia decreases the length of hospital stay following total joint arthroplasty. *Orthopedics* 2009;32(3):167.
13. Kearney M, Jennrich MK, Lyons S, Robinson R, Berger B: Effects of preoperative education on patient outcomes after joint replacement surgery. *Orthop Nurs* 2011; 30(6):391-396.
14. Berger RA: Total hip arthroplasty using the minimally invasive two-incision approach. *Clin Orthop Relat Res* 2003;417:232-241.
15. Dorr LD, Thomas DJ, Zhu J, Dastane M, Chao L, Long WT: Outpatient total hip arthroplasty. *J Arthroplasty* 2010;25(4): 501-506.
16. Parvizi J, Mui A, Purtill JJ, Sharkey PF, Hozack WJ, Rothman RH: Total joint arthroplasty: When do fatal or near-fatal complications occur? *J Bone Joint Surg Am* 2007;89(1):27-32.
17. Bertin KC: Minimally invasive outpatient total hip arthroplasty: A financial analysis. *Clin Orthop Relat Res* 2005;435:154-163.

20

Total Hip Arthroplasty: The Mini-Posterior Approach

John G. Ginnetti, MD
Jill Erickson, PA-C
Christopher L. Peters, MD

Abstract

A successful surgical exposure during total hip arthroplasty must not only provide adequate visualization of both the acetabulum and the proximal femur but also avoid injury to critical neurovascular structures and minimize dissection of soft-tissue hip stabilizers. Numerous surgical approaches to the hip have been described and subsequently modified since the advent of modern total hip arthroplasty. Descendent from the standard posterolateral approach, the mini-posterior approach not only satisfies the prerequisites for a successful total hip arthroplasty exposure but also exemplifies a utilitarian approach to the hip, which is applicable to the entire spectrum of reconstructive cases.

Instr Course Lect 2013;62:237-243.

In 1962, John Charnley performed his first "low-friction" hip arthroplasty using high-density polyethylene placed through a transtrochanteric approach.[1] Despite Charnley's strict guidelines for trochanteric advancement and reattachment, complications, including malunion, nonunion, trochanteric bursitis, and symptomatic hardware, were reported.[2,3] Consequently, a decade later, the posterolateral hip approach was introduced as an alternative to the Charnley trochanteric osteotomy.[4] Although new to the realm of total hip arthroplasty (THA) in the 1970s, the posterolateral hip approach was far from a novel concept given its 19th century European origins.

Bernhard Von Langenbeck developed a posterior approach to the hip joint for the treatment of suppurative arthritis and other war wounds while serving as Surgeon General of the Prussian Army during periods of military conflict (Schieswig-Holstein Wars, the Austrian War, and the Franco Prussian War).[5] First described in 1867, Langenbeck's longitudinal incision was later modified in 1907 by the Swiss surgeon Theodore Kocher, who extended the approach caudally in line with the femur to gain improved acetabular exposure for the treatment of tuberculosis.[5] In the mid 20th century, a Canadian surgeon, Alexander Gibson, promoted the advantages of posterior hip exposure for numerous infirmities and described his modification of the Kocher approach.[6] In the United States, while employed at the Columbia State Hospital for the mentally ill, Austin Moore placed femoral prostheses for the treatment of femoral neck fractures using his "southern exposure," a posterior approach that divided the short external rotators, the piriformis, and part of the quadratus femoris while sparing the hip abductor musculature.[7] Several years later, Judet further popularized the work of Langenbeck, Kocher, and Gibson through his published report on the treatment of acetabular fractures, and Letournel coined the term Kocher-Langenbeck approach in his classic paper describing acetabular fractures.[8,9]

The 21st century brought further modification to the posterolateral approach. Enticed by the prospect of

Dr. Peters or an immediate family member serves as a board member, owner, officer, or committee member of the American Academy of Orthopaedic Surgeons; has received royalties from Biomet; is a member of a speakers' bureau or has made paid presentations on behalf of Biomet; and serves as a paid consultant to or is an employee of Biomet. Neither of the following authors or any immediate family member has received anything of value from or owns stock in a commercial company nor institution related directly or indirectly to the subject of this chapter: Dr. Ginnetti and Dr. Erickson.

decreased tissue damage resulting in improved postoperative pain and abbreviated recovery times, Dorr, Hartzband, and Sculco became advocates of minimally invasive arthroplasty.[10-12] The standard posterolateral approach was modified into the mini-posterior approach with encouraging results. In contrast with the classic posterolateral approach, which involved dissection of the posterior soft-tissue structures (including the gluteal sling, short external rotators, quadratus femoris, and hip capsule), the mini-posterior hip approach in its purest form is characterized by a skin incision of less than 10 cm, preservation of the gluteus maximus tendon, and minimal disruption of the quadratus femoris.[13]

Advantages and Disadvantages

In general, proponents of minimally invasive surgical techniques believe that compact incisions provide adequate exposure and have the added benefits of reduced soft-tissue trauma, improved cosmesis, decreased blood loss, improved postoperative pain, and faster recovery.[14-16] However, these assertions are controversial.[17,18] To date, convincing evidence proving the superiority of minimally invasive THA approaches is lacking. Nevertheless, minimally invasive surgical techniques, including the anterior supine, the modified Watson-Jones, and mini-posterior approaches, have gained support in large part because of patient education and demand.

Each minimally invasive approach has a unique profile of benefits and shortcomings that must be weighed by the treating surgeon. Foremost among the advantages afforded by the mini-posterior approach is the preservation of the hip abductor musculature. Similar to muscle-sparing anterior approaches, the mini-posterior approach does not violate the gluteus medius and gluteus minimus muscles, which are vital to THA soft-tissue balance, hip stability, and gait mechanics.

Surgeon familiarity is also a critical advantage. Because of the many applications of the posterolateral approach in trauma, reconstructive, and pediatric surgical procedures, most surgeons are well acquainted with the posterior hip approach and the involved anatomy. An enhanced surgical comfort level translates into more efficient and expeditious THA surgery. Familiarity with the posterior anatomy also shortens the learning curve for the mini-posterior approach, an important advantage considering the complications reported during early experience with alternative minimally invasive approaches.[19]

The mini-posterior approach is also quite versatile. Unlike other minimally invasive approaches, such as the anterior supine and modified Watson-Jones approaches, the mini-posterior approach is easily extended cephalad or caudad to address acute THA complications, such as iatrogenic femoral and acetabular fractures, and is useful in treating hip infection and performing revision procedures. Difficulties resulting from patient-specific variables, such as increased body mass index, increased quadriceps size, retained hardware, aberrant acetabular/proximal femoral morphology, congenital hip dislocation, slipped capital femoral epiphysis, and Legg-Calvé-Perthes disease can be successfully managed using the mini-posterior approach or an extension of the approach.

Opponents of minimally invasive THA cite component malpositioning, increased complication rates, and the potential for increased soft-tissue damage caused by excessive retractor force applied to smaller soft-tissue windows as disadvantages of the techniques and as evidence supporting a more generous exposure.[18,20] However, the literature does not universally confirm these disadvantages.[21-24] There are several specific criticisms regarding the mini-posterior approach. One perceived limitation is an increased risk of postoperative hip instability. Dislocation rates after primary THA range from 0.3% to 10%. Several studies have associated higher dislocation rates with the posterolateral approach;[25-30] however, these studies involved approaches with more comprehensive posterior soft-tissue dissections, the placement of small femoral heads, and inconsistent soft-tissue repair techniques after implantation of the prostheses.

At 10-year follow-up, Berry et al[31] reported dislocation rates of 6.9%, 3.4%, and 3.1% using 28-mm heads for posterolateral, transtrochanteric, and anterolateral approaches, respectively. However, when comparing 32-mm head sizes, the reported dislocation rates at 10-year follow-up were 3.8%, 2.8%, and 2.4% for posterolateral, transtrochanteric, and anterolateral approaches, respectively.[31] These results are consistent with recent reports associating larger femoral head diameters with lower dislocation rates after primary and revision THAs using the posterolateral approach.[32,33] The personal experience of the senior author (CLP) with large femoral head diameters is consistent with previous reports.[31-33] In 136 primary THAs, patients who received a 38-mm head through a posterior approach had no dislocations in the early postoperative period (average follow-up, 52 months).[34] In 469 patients who received large diameter metal-on-metal heads through a posterolateral approach, 2 dislocations (0.4%) were identified.[34] An unpublished recent comprehensive review of the senior author's database, including the placement of all femoral head diameters through a posterolateral approach, showed 10 dislocations in 883 THAs (1.1%).

In addition to a larger femoral head diameter, Kwon et al[25] suggested that adequate soft-tissue repair after THA enhances hip stability. The authors performed a meta-analysis comparing dislocation rates after using the posterior approach with and without soft-tissue repair. The dislocation rate using the posterior approach was dramatically reduced after soft-tissue repair (4.46% to 0.49%). The relative risk of dislocation was 8.21 times greater in the absence of soft-tissue repair. When accompanied by soft-tissue repair, comparable dislocation rates associated with the anterolateral (0.70%), the direct lateral (0.43%), and the posterior approach (1.01%) were identified.[25] When using a standard or mini-posterior THA approach, concern over postoperative hip instability is alleviated by using larger diameter femoral heads and routine posterior soft-tissue repair.[35-38]

In addition to instability, critics of the mini-posterior approach focus on the potential for sciatic nerve injury and the technical aspect of intraoperative limb-length determination. Although there is only a low incidence of nerve injury (0.6%) associated with posterolateral THA,[39] permanent sciatic nerve injury represents a devastating complication and is more prevalent with the posterolateral approach.[40]

Because lateral decubitus positioning is required with the mini-posterior approach, opponents suggest that accurate limb-length measurement is more difficult and less accurate compared with measurements taken using supine positioning, which allows for direct side-to-side comparisons. Intraoperative fluoroscopy to assess limb length and component positioning is often more difficult to accomplish in the lateral decubitus position. Postoperative limb-length inequality after THA is a common source of litigation.[41]

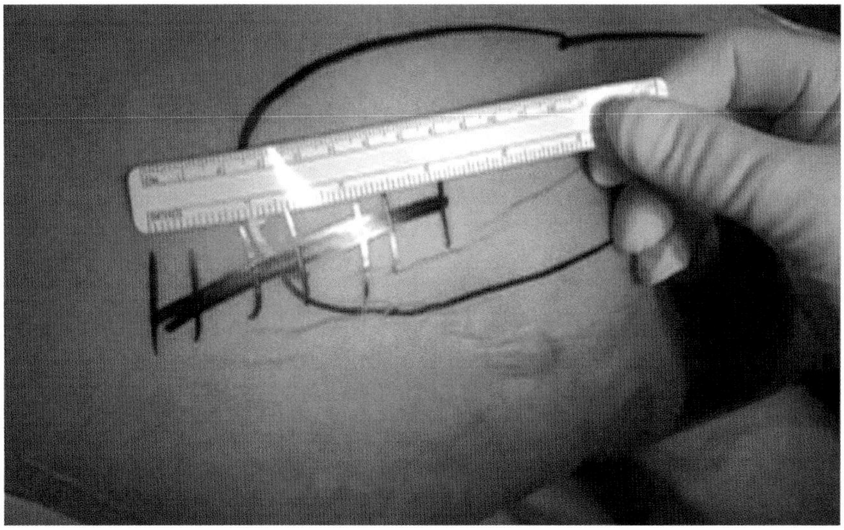

Figure 1 The placement of incision (7.5 cm in this instance) for the mini-posterior approach is shown.

These drawbacks may be overemphasized. More anterior-directed minimally invasive approaches spare the sciatic nerve at the expense of other neurovascular structures, such as the femoral nerve and the lateral femoral cutaneous nerve. In the senior author's experience, intraoperative Steinmann pin referencing of limb length has proven to be both an accurate and a reliable measure of leg length.

Senior Author's Preferred Technique

The patient is positioned in the lateral decubitus position in the operating room. The pelvis is stabilized perpendicular to the floor with the assistance of the Montreal Lateral Positioning Device (Schaerer Mayfield, Cincinnati, OH). The patient is prepped and draped in a sterile fashion, the greater trochanter is palpated, and the outline of the proximal femur is drawn with a marking pen. The surgical incision is oriented parallel to the femoral shaft with the hip in slight flexion and is placed over the posterior one third of the greater trochanter. The incision ranges in length from 7.5 to 12 cm depending on the patient's body habitus, and it is centered over the tip of the greater trochanter (**Figure 1**). After the skin in incised, self-retaining retractors are placed, and sharp dissection is carried down to the level of the fascia lata and gluteus maximus fascia while maintaining meticulous hemostasis. After the fascial level is reached, the surgical assistant abducts the leg, and the fascia is incised distally over the midshaft of the femur. A finger is placed inside the fascial window to apply gentle pressure while Bovie electrocautery is used to extend the fascial incision proximally and distally. A Charnley retractor is then placed at the level of the greater trochanter in the standard fashion, with one arm under the anterior fascial layer and the second arm placed into the gluteus maximus; care is taken to avoid injury to the sciatic nerve. The assistant then internally rotates and extends the hip to facilitate deep surgical exposure. Peritrochanteric bursal tissue is incised in line with the posterior femur at the level of the greater trochanter and bluntly dissected posteriorly with the

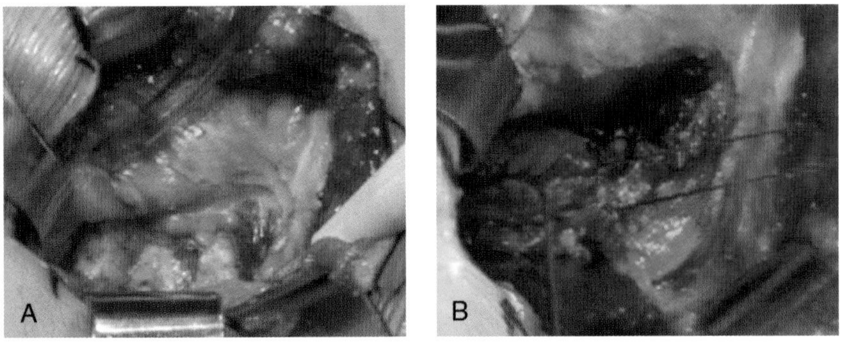

Figure 2 Intraoperative photographs showing capsular exposure and preparation. **A,** The gluteus minimus/piriformis interval is exposed with a Hibbs retractor superiorly (on the left), with exposure to the quadratus femoris distally (on the right). **B,** Two tag stitches are placed in the posterior capsule and the external rotators, the first through the piriformis tendon and the capsule superiorly (on the left) and the second through the external rotators and capsule 1 to 2 cm distal to the piriformis tendon (on the right).

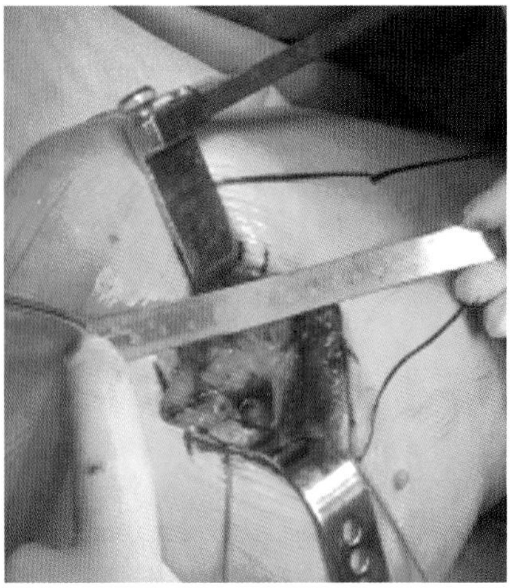

Figure 3 A limb-length pin is placed in the pelvis (on the left), and a metal ruler is used to measure limb length to a point on the femur (on the right).

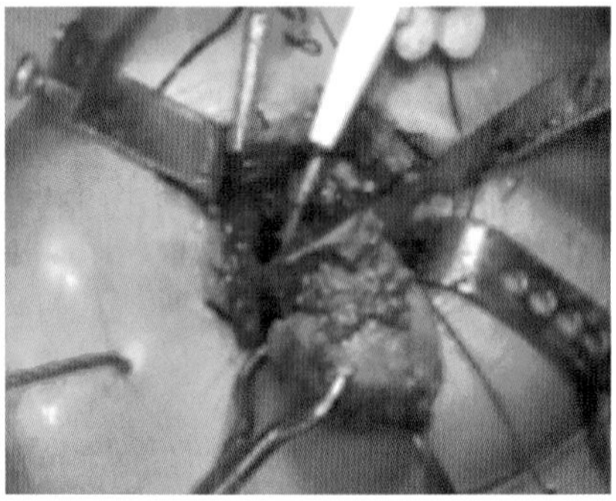

Figure 4 The femoral head and neck are removed after osteotomy.

assistance of a surgical lap sponge to uncover the short external rotators. Careful attention is given to cauterize blood vessels residing on the posterior surface of the short external rotators. A Hibbs retractor is placed deep to the gluteus medius in the interval between the gluteus medius and the gluteus minimus. Gentle anterosuperior retraction of the gluteus medius uncovers the interval between the gluteus minimus and piriformis tendon (**Figure 2, A**). After identifying the piriformis tendon, a full-thickness capsulotendinous flap is raised. The full-thickness arthrotomy begins at the level of the acetabular rim and proceeds distally along the posterosuperior femoral neck using the superior border of the piriformis as a surgical landmark before coursing slightly anterior under the greater trochanter to fully release the piriformis and conjoint tendon from their respective osseous insertions. The arthrotomy continues distally and posteriorly along the femoral neck to include the superior one third of the quadratus femoris. To facilitate exposure and later closure, two No. 2 nonabsorbable sutures are placed as full-thickness tag stitches incorporating the capsule and the piriformis tendon, and the capsule and conjoint tendon, respectively (**Figure 2, B**). The leg is placed back into a neutral position, and a limb-length Steinmann pin (0.14 inch) is placed into the ilium from an entry point outside the surgical incision (approximately 2 cm anterior and 2 cm proximal to the proximal apex of the incision) in line with the femoral diaphysis, unless the surgical incision is long enough to accommodate the pin. The pin is malleted in place until bicortical purchase is achieved and is bent 90° away from the surgical incision. A discernible transverse mark is made in the middle of the greater trochanter with Bovie electrocautery, and the distance between the Steinmann pin and greater trochanter marking is measured with a flat metal ruler (**Figure 3**). After measuring the limb length, both the surgical assistant and surgeon palpate the apparent limb lengths at the inferior pole of the patellae. The surgical assistant gently dislocates the hip in the standard fashion, and the surgeon monitors for potential tearing of the quadratus femoris, which indicates the need for additional release with electrocautery. A Homan retractor is placed under the inferior femoral neck, and the level of the neck osteotomy is marked according to the preoperative template. The neck osteotomy is completed with an oscillating saw, and the femoral head is removed (**Figure 4**).

Video 20.1: The Mini-Posterior Approach: Exposure. Christopher L. Peters, MD (4 min)

Adequate acetabular exposure is achieved by mobilizing the femur to an anterior position and placing tension on the unsupported hip capsule, which overhangs the acetabulum, ob-

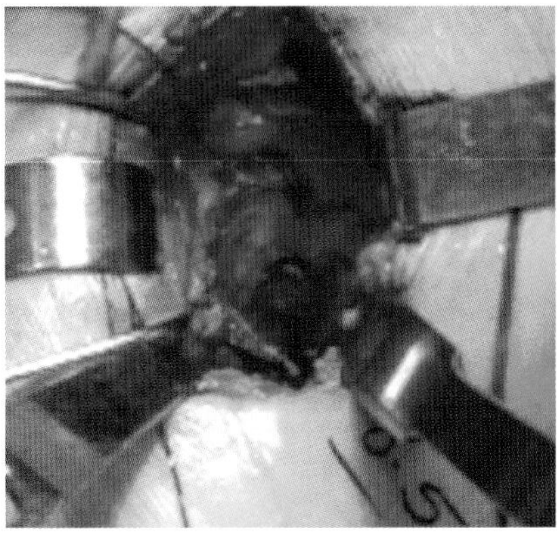

Figure 5 Adequate acetabular exposure is seen in this photograph with retractor placement (anterior on the right), Steinmann pins posteriorly (on the left), and Homan retractors inferiorly (bottom).

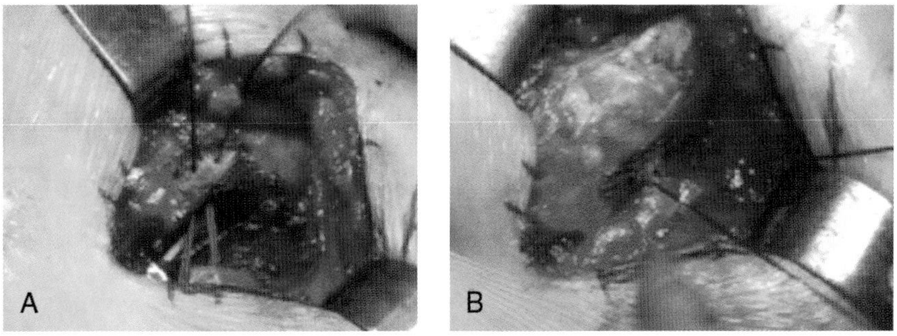

Figure 6 **A,** Two nonabsorbable tag stitches are passed through two drill holes in the posterior greater trochanter (superior, on the left) for a posterior repair. **B,** The capsule and the external rotators are repaired back to the trochanter for a tight posterior repair.

scuring the surgeon's view of the osseous anatomy. This can be accomplished through numerous techniques; however, a combination of strategically placed 0.14-inch Steinmann pins and specialized retractors is preferred. With the leg at 90° of internal rotation, a Wagner retractor is placed at the level of the greater trochanter/resected neck junction and inserted through the anterior capsule at approximately the 3-o'clock position (anterior in the right hip), over the anterior acetabular wall deep to the iliopsoas muscle. Gentle retraction with the limb resting in slight internal rotation on a padded elevated Mayo stand mobilizes the femur to a more anterior position. To retract the superior capsule and gluteus minimus overhang, a Steinmann pin is placed at the 12-o'clock position into the ilium outside the acetabular labrum deep to the capsule. Care is taken to orient this pin in a cephalad direction to avoid joint penetration and subsequent impedance to acetabular reaming. As described previously, the pin is malleted into a secure position and bent away from the surgical incision. A second Steinmann pin is then placed into the pelvic ischium to place tension on the posteroinferior capsule. It is critical to place the pin deep to the capsule outside the labrum with a cephalad orientation. To retract the posterior capsule, a third pin is placed in the posterior column at the 10-o'clock position (posterior in the right hip) engaging only a single cortex. Acetabular exposure is completed by placing a Homan retractor inferiorly under the transverse acetabular ligament at the 6-o'clock position (**Figure 5**). With the exposure complete, the acetabular labrum is excised, and the cotyloid fossa is cleared of extraneous soft tissue. The acetabulum is sequentially reamed, and a press-fit component is impacted. All Steinmann pins are then removed (except the limb-length pin).

Exposure of the proximal femur for implant preparation is achieved by placing a femoral elevating retractor around the lesser trochanter/posterior femoral neck to deliver the proximal femur into the surgical field. The surgical assistant facilitates this maneuver by flexing, adducting, and internally rotating the limb and applying counter-force to the patient's knee. The femur can then be reamed and/or broached. Trial femoral heads are placed on the final femoral stem. Limb length is assessed by remeasuring the distance between the Steinmann pin and the greater trochanter, marking the distance with the hip reduced, comparing the palpation of the limb lengths at the inferior pole of the patellae, and comparing the offset of the capsulotendinous flap to the trochanter distance by pulling up on the tag stitches. The neck length is then adjusted based on the limb-length measurement and soft-tissue balance. After placement of the final implants, an augmented capsular closure is performed by placing two drill holes with a 2.0 drill through the posterior aspect of greater trochanter. A Hoffee Blue Lasso Suture Retriever (Beatty, Redman, WA) is used to pass the previously placed tag stitches through the respective drill holes (**Figure 6, A**). The suture is tied over the greater trochanter after tensioning the capsulotendinous flap with the leg resting in a neutral position (**Figure 6, B**). The iliotibial band, the subcutaneous tissue, and the skin are then closed with the hip slightly abducted.

DVD **Video 20.2:** The Mini-Posterior Approach: Repair. Christopher L. Peters, MD (1 min)

Postoperative Management

The first physical therapy session routinely occurs the day of surgery or within the first 24 hours after surgery.

Patients begin ambulation with an assistive device but are allowed to progress with weight bearing as tolerated. Posterior hip precautions are still encouraged for the first 6 weeks when the implanted femoral head diameter is 36 mm or larger. The senior author requires all patients to use an elevated toilet seat for 6 weeks. Active abduction and quadriceps strengthening activities are encouraged. The average length of stay after THA at the University of Utah Orthopaedic Center/University Hospital is 2.7 days (range, 1 to 4 days). During the first 2 weeks, patients receive home physical therapy for gait training, hip exercises against gravity only, and activities of daily living. Outpatient physical therapy is initiated after home physical therapy at the patient's request or at the 6-week visit if the patient has a positive Trendelenburg limp. Patients return for routine postoperative visits at 2 weeks, 6 weeks, 6 months, 1 year, and biannually thereafter.

Summary

Based on the senior author's experience, the mini-posterior approach most effectively satisfies the prerequisites required for a successful surgical hip exposure in a classic academic referral practice. The mini-posterior approach not only provides safe and sufficient exposure for implantation of femoral and acetabular components but also affords the flexibility to successfully address complications and complexities across a wide spectrum of reconstructive situations.

References

1. Charnley J: The long-term results of low-friction arthroplasty of the hip preformed as primary intervention. *J Bone Joint Surg Br* 1972;54(1):61-76.
2. Frankel A, Booth RE Jr, Balderston RA, Cohn J, Rothman RH: Complications of trochanteric osteotomy: Long-term implications. *Clin Orthop Relat Res* 1993;288:209-213.
3. Hodgkinson JP, Shelley P, Wroblewski BM: Re-attachment of the un-united trochanter in Charnley low friction arthroplasty. *J Bone Joint Surg Br* 1989;71(3):523-525.
4. Gristina AG, Rovere GD, Nicastro JF, Burke JG: Posterior approach for total hip arthroplasty. *South Med J* 1980;73(1):51-54.
5. Mehlman CT, Meiss L, DiPasquale TG: Hyphenated-history: The Kocher-Langenbeck surgical approach. *J Orthop Trauma* 2000;14(1):60-64.
6. Gibson A: Posterior exposure of the hip joint. *J Bone Joint Surg Br* 1950;32(2):183-186.
7. Moore AT: The self-locking metal hip prosthesis. *J Bone Joint Surg Am* 1957;39(4):811-827.
8. Judet R, Judet J, Letournel E: Fractures of the acetabulum: Classification and surgical approaches for open reduction preliminary report. *J Bone Joint Surg Am* 1964;46(8):1615-1646.
9. Letournel E: Acetabulum fractures: Classification and management. *Clin Orthop Relat Res* 1980;151:81-106.
10. Hartzband MA: Posterolateral minimal incision for total hip replacement: Technique and early results. *Orthop Clin North Am* 2004;35(2):119-129.
11. Sculco TP: Minimally invasive total hip arthroplasty: In the affirmative. *J Arthroplasty* 2004;19(4, suppl 1):78-80.
12. Berry DJ, Berger RA, Callaghan JJ, et al: Minimally invasive total hip arthroplasty: Development, early results, and a critical analysis. Presented at the Annual Meeting of the American Orthopaedic Association, Charleston, South Carolina, USA, June 14, 2003. *J Bone Joint Surg Am* 2003;85(11):2235-2246.
13. Sculco TP, Boettner F: Minimally invasive total hip arthroplasty: The posterior approach. *Instr Course Lect* 2006;55:205-214.
14. Meneghini RM, Smits SA: Early discharge and recovery with three minimally invasive total hip arthroplasty approaches: A preliminary study. *Clin Orthop Relat Res* 2009;467(6):1431-1437.
15. Berger RA, Jacobs JJ, Meneghini RM, Della Valle C, Paprosky W, Rosenberg AG: Rapid rehabilitation and recovery with minimally invasive total hip arthroplasty. *Clin Orthop Relat Res* 2004;429:239-247.
16. Wenz JF, Gurkan I, Jibodh SR: Mini-incision total hip arthroplasty: A comparative assessment of perioperative outcomes. *Orthopedics* 2002;25(10):1031-1043.
17. Cheng T, Feng JG, Liu T: Minimally invasive total hip arthroplasty: A systemic review. *Int Orthop* 2009;33(6):1473-1481.
18. Graw BP, Woolson ST, Huddleston HG, Goodman SB, Huddleston JI: Minimal incision surgery as a risk factor for early failure of total hip arthroplasty. *Clin Orthop Relat Res* 2010;468(9):2372-2376.
19. Seng BE, Berend KR, Ajluni AF, Lombardi AV Jr: Anterior-supine minimally invasive total hip arthroplasty: Defining the learning curve. *Orthop Clin North Am* 2009;40(3):343-350.
20. Jewett BA, Collis DK: High complication rate with anterior total hip arthroplasties on a fracture table. *Clin Orthop Relat Res* 2011;469(2):503-507.
21. Pagnano MW, Trousdale RT, Meneghini RM, Hanssen AD: Patients preferred a mini-posterior THA to a contralateral two-

incision THA. *Clin Orthop Relat Res* 2006;453:156-159.

22. Fink B, Mittelstaedt A, Schulz MS, Sebena P, Singer J: Comparison of a minimally invasive posterior approach and the standard posterior approach for total hip arthroplasty: A prospective and comparative study. *J Orthop Surg Res* 2010;5:46.
23. Kennon RE, Keggi JM, Wetmore RS, Zatorski LE, Huo MH, Keggi KJ: Total hip arthroplasty through a minimally invasive anterior surgical approach. *J Bone Joint Surg Am* 2003;85(suppl 4):39-48.
24. Goldstein WM, Branson JJ, Berland KA, Gordon AC: Minimal-incision total hip arthroplasty. *J Bone Joint Surg Am* 2003; 85(suppl 4):33-38.
25. Kwon MS, Kuskowski M, Mulhall KJ, Macaulay W, Brown TE, Saleh KJ: Does surgical approach affect total hip arthroplasty dislocation rates? *Clin Orthop Relat Res* 2006;447:34-38.
26. Eftekhar NS: Dislocation and instability complicating low friction arthroplasty of the hip joint. *Clin Orthop Relat Res* 1976;121: 120-125.
27. Woo RY, Morrey BF: Dislocations after total hip arthroplasty. *J Bone Joint Surg Am* 1982;64(9):1295-1306.
28. Lewinnek GE, Lewis JL, Tarr R, Compere CL, Zimmerman JR: Dislocations after total hip-replacement arthroplasties. *J Bone Joint Surg Am* 1978;60(2): 217-220.
29. Masonis JL, Bourne RB: Surgical approach, abductor function, and total hip arthroplasty dislocation. *Clin Orthop Relat Res* 2002;405: 46-53.
30. Sierra RJ, Raposo JM, Trousdale RT, Cabanela ME: Dislocation of primary THA done through a posterolateral approach in the elderly. *Clin Orthop Relat Res* 2005;441:262-267.
31. Berry DJ, von Knoch M, Schleck CD, Harmsen WS: Effect of femoral head diameter and operative approach on risk of dislocation after primary total hip arthroplasty. *J Bone Joint Surg Am* 2005; 87(11):2456-2463.
32. Lachiewicz PF, Soileau ES: Dislocation of primary total hip arthroplasty with 36 and 40-mm femoral heads. *Clin Orthop Relat Res* 2006;453:153-155.
33. Hummel MT, Malkani AL, Yakkanti MR, Baker DL: Decreased dislocation after revision total hip arthroplasty using larger femoral head size and posterior capsular repair. *J Arthroplasty* 2009; 24(6, suppl):73-76.
34. Peters CL, McPherson E, Jackson JD, Erickson JA: Reduction in early dislocation rate with large-diameter femoral heads in primary total hip arthroplasty. *J Arthroplasty* 2007;22(6, suppl 2): 140-144.
35. Chiu FY, Chen CM, Chung TY, Lo WH, Chen TH: The effect of posterior capsulorrhaphy in primary total hip arthroplasty: A prospective randomized study. *J Arthroplasty* 2000;15(2): 194-199.
36. Pellicci PM, Bostrum M, Poss R: Posterior approach to total hip replacement using enhanced posterior soft tissue repair. *Clin Orthop Relat Res* 1998;355:224-228.
37. Suh KT, Park BG, Choi YJ: A posterior approach to primary total hip arthroplasty with soft tissue repair. *Clin Orthop Relat Res* 2004;418:162-167.
38. Weeden SH, Paprosky WG, Bowling JW: The early dislocation rate in primary total hip arthroplasty following the posterior approach with posterior soft-tissue repair. *J Arthroplasty* 2003;18(6): 709-713.
39. Navarro RA, Schmalzried TP, Amstutz HC, Dorey FJ: Surgical approach and nerve palsy in total hip arthroplasty. *J Arthroplasty* 1995;10(1):1-5.
40. Edwards BN, Tullos HS, Noble PC: Contributory factors and etiology of sciatic nerve palsy in total hip arthroplasty. *Clin Orthop Relat Res* 1987;218:136-141.
41. Upadhyay A, York S, Macaulay W, McGrory B, Robbennolt J, Bal BS: Medical malpractice in hip and knee arthroplasty. *J Arthroplasty* 2007;22(6, suppl 2): 2-7.

Video References

20.1: Peters CL: Video. *Total Hip Arthroplasty: The Mini-Posterior Approach Exposure.* Salt Lake City, UT, 2012.

20.2: Peters CL: Video. *Total Hip Arthroplasty: The Mini-Posterior Approach Repair.* Salt Lake City, UT, 2012.

21

Total Hip Arthroplasty Using the Superior Capsulotomy Technique

Stephen B. Murphy, MD

Abstract

Dislocation of the native hip during total hip arthroplasty has traditionally been an integral part of all surgical exposures. However, dislocation of the native hip may require greater soft-tissue release than surgical excision of the femoral head during total hip arthroplasty. The superior capsulotomy technique allows preparation of the femur in situ, with excision of the femoral head after femoral component preparation has been completed. The advantages of this technique include preservation of the hip joint capsule and less tissue dissection during surgery; special traction equipment or fluoroscopy is not needed. This technique allows immediate mobilization of patients without motion or weight-bearing precautions, little parental narcotic use, and discharge home within 24 hours of surgery for most patients.

Instr Course Lect 2013;62:245-250.

Less invasive surgical techniques for total hip arthroplasty (THA) are typically more limited versions of traditional surgical hip exposures. Less invasive anterior, lateral, anterolateral, and posterior exposures represent refined versions of long-established surgical exposures. The superior capsulotomy technique or exposure was developed a decade ago by defining specific design goals and asking fundamental questions at the outset.[1] For example, if the hip joint capsule is essential for hip joint stability, why is it released or excised? If dislocation of the native femoral head requires more soft-tissue dissection and release, why is the head dislocated rather than excised? If the femur is stronger and more resistant to fracture with the full head and neck in place, why is the femur broached after the head is removed instead of before removal?[2] The fundamental design principles established for superior capsulotomy techniques are listed in **Table 1**. These design principles were aimed at ensuring that patients would be exposed to decreased risks from the outset of the procedure. The superior capsulotomy technique is performed with the patient in the lateral position, allows for proper trial reduction, does not require traction or intraoperative fluoroscopy, and can easily be transitioned into a more extensile exposure if necessary.[3]

Surgical Method

The patient is placed in the lateral position. The foot is placed on a padded Mayo stand, and the hip is flexed about 45° (**Figure 1**). The incision is placed laterally and in line with the longitudinal axis of the femur and begins just distal to the tip of the greater trochanter and extends proximally approximately 8 cm (**Figure 2**). The fascia is incised, and the fibers of the gluteus maximus are spread 8 cm. The posterior border of the gluteus medius is retracted anteriorly to expose the piriformis tendon. The tendon can be retracted posteriorly or incised distally, with reattachment as desired (**Figure 3**). A spiked Hohmann retractor is placed through the hip joint capsule and into the posterior femoral head to maintain the posterior side of the exposure and retract the piriformis tendon. The posterior border of the gluteus minimus becomes visible with the

Dr. Murphy or an immediate family member serves as a board member, owner, officer, or committee member of the International Society of Computer Assisted Orthopedic Surgery; has received royalties from Wright Medical Technology; serves as a paid consultant to or is an employee of Ceramtec and AG; and has stock or stock options in Surgical Planning Associates.

Table 1
Design Principles and Rationale for the Superior Capsulotomy Technique

Principle	Rationale
Lateral position	Easily converted to an extensile posterior exposure if necessary; away from the hip flexion crease because concave flexion creases are more prone to wound complications and infection
Leg draped free without traction	Better assessment of range of motion; no need for specialized operating tables
Preserve abductors	Rapid and reliable recovery of strength
Preserve posterior capsule and short external rotators	Improved hip joint stability allows motion without restriction, reduces patient fear, and simplifies the physical therapy education process
Prepare femur in situ	The femur is stronger before neck transection than after; the prosthetic femoral version is known before acetabular component implantation
Enable easily performed trial reduction	Trial reduction to assess tissue tension, range of motion, and stability is a fundamental principle of hip replacement surgery
No need for fluoroscopic imaging	Routine fluoroscopic imaging increases the equipment needs, occupies space that an assistant could occupy, and increases the volume of people entering and exiting the operating room
Direct longitudinal access to the femur	Direct longitudinal access to the femur allows the surgeon to use any implant design and does not limit the type of design that can be used with the surgery

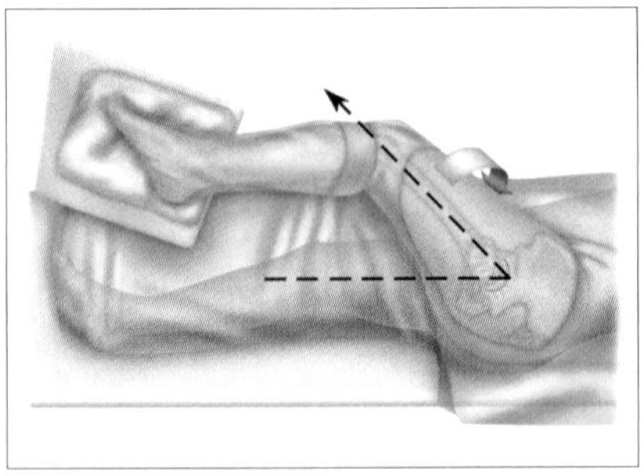

Figure 1 In the superior capsulotomy technique, the patient is placed in the lateral position with the leg draped free, the hip flexed and internally rotated, and the foot placed on a padded Mayo stand. The dashed line shows the angle of hip flexion.

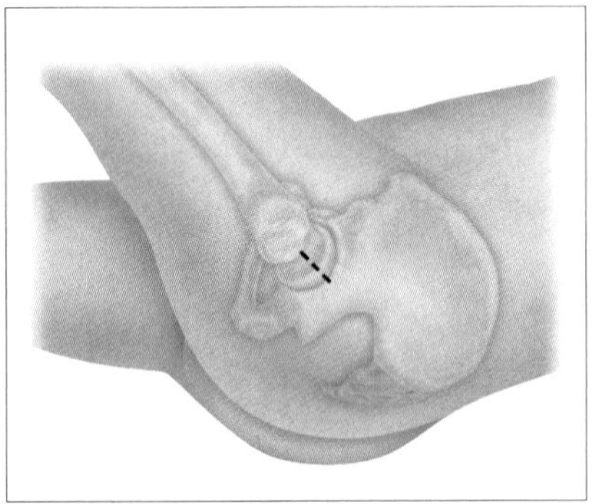

Figure 2 The incision (dashed line) is placed in line with the longitudinal axis of the femur, starting just distal to the tip of the greater trochanter and extending proximally.

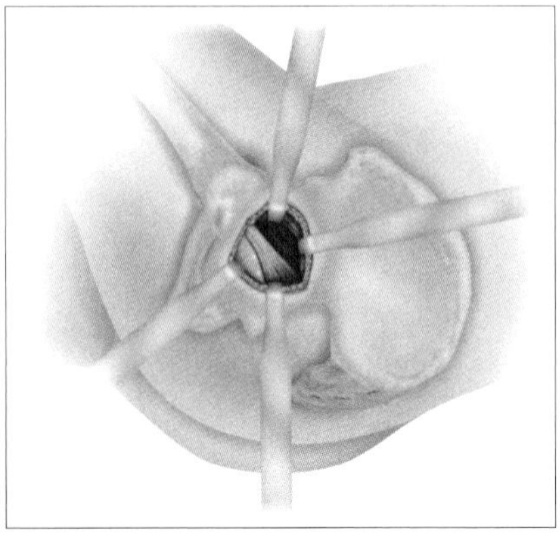

Figure 3 The piriformis tendon is identified and either retracted posteriorly or incised.

piriformis tendon retracted posteriorly (**Figure 4**). The posterior border of the gluteus minimus is carefully mobilized anteriorly to exposure the superior hip joint capsule. A blunt retractor is placed anteriorly in the interval between the gluteus minimus tendon and the anterior hip joint capsule. The hip joint capsule is then incised in line with the course of the piriformis tendon from the acetabular rim into the trochanteric fossa (**Figure 5**). The anterior capsule is tagged, and blunt Hohmann retractors are placed inside the capsule around the anterior and posterior femoral head (**Figure 6**). A spiked Hohmann retractor is placed into the superior femoral head at the acetabular rim to provide longitudinal access to the femur. The femoral canal is then entered with a reamer through the top of the femoral neck in a manner that is reminiscent of femoral nailing procedures (**Figure 7**). The superior head and neck are opened with an osteotome to allow access for femoral broaches (**Figure 8**). The femur is then prepared with broaches (**Figure 9**). The depth of the broaches is gauged relative to the tip of the greater trochanter. After the femur is prepared, the final broach is left in place and used as an internal neck resection guide. An oscillating saw is then used to transect the femoral neck (**Figure 10**). A Shanz pin is placed into the femoral head, and the head is excised (**Figure 11**).

Spiked Hohmann retractors are placed at the anterior and posterior rims of the acetabulum to allow for the

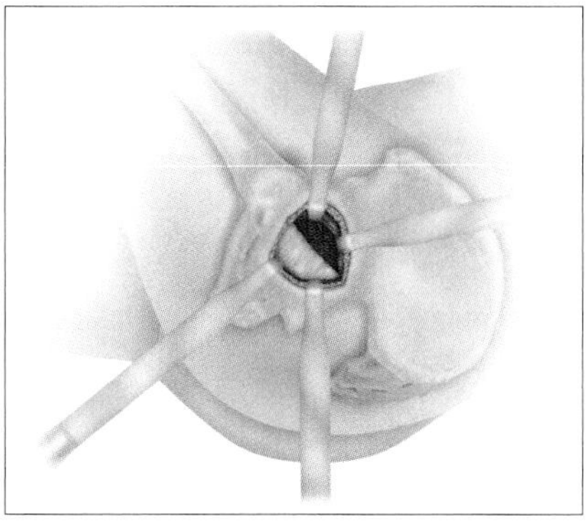

Figure 4 With the piriformis retracted posteriorly, the posterior border of the gluteus minimus muscle is carefully and sharply mobilized anteriorly to reveal the hip joint capsule.

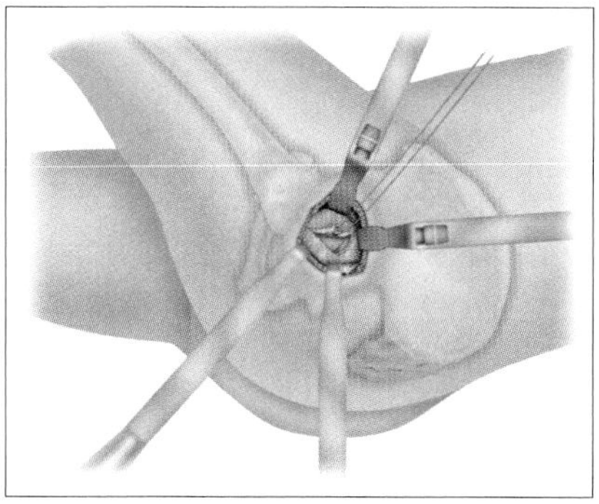

Figure 5 The hip joint capsule is incised longitudinally with a short turn anteriorly at the acetabular rim and tagged for later anatomic closure.

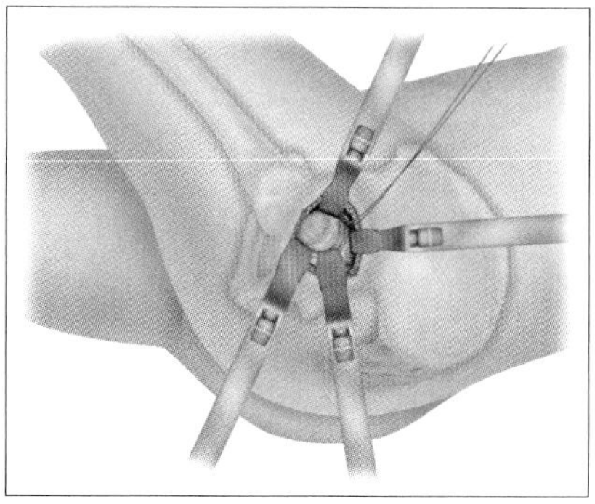

Figure 6 Blunt Hohmann retractors are placed inside the capsule around the anterior and posterior femoral neck with spiked Hohmann retractors placed anterosuperiorly in the ilium and superiorly in the femoral head.

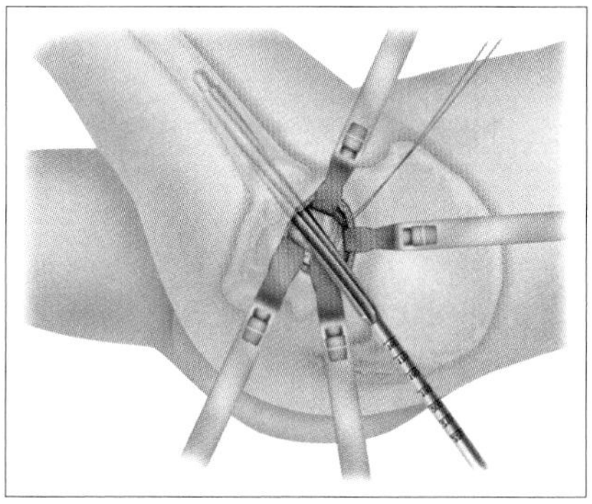

Figure 7 The femoral canal is entered using a reamer.

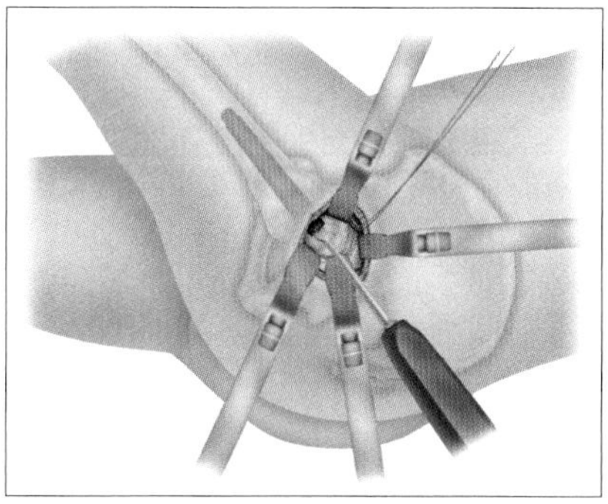

Figure 8 The superior head and neck are opened with an osteotome to allow for broaching with the head in situ.

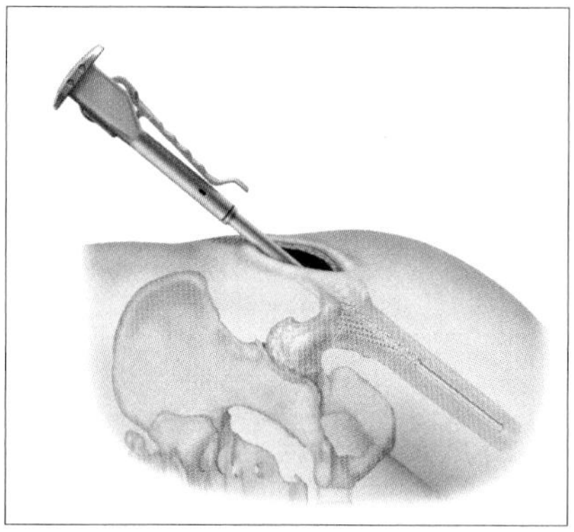

Figure 9 Femoral broaching is done with the head intact.

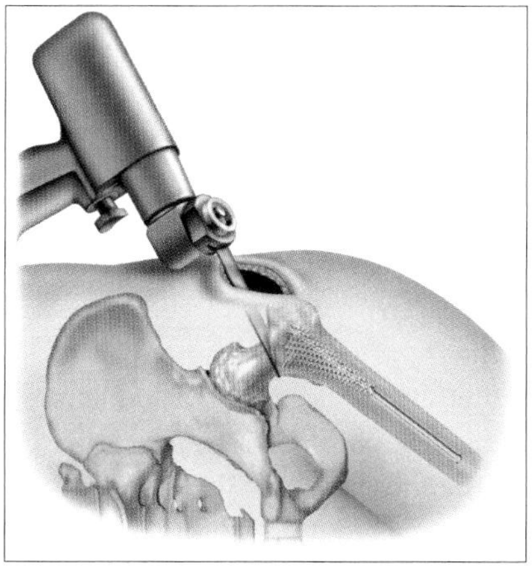

Figure 10 The femoral neck is transected with an oscillating saw, with the broach used as an internal neck-cutting guide.

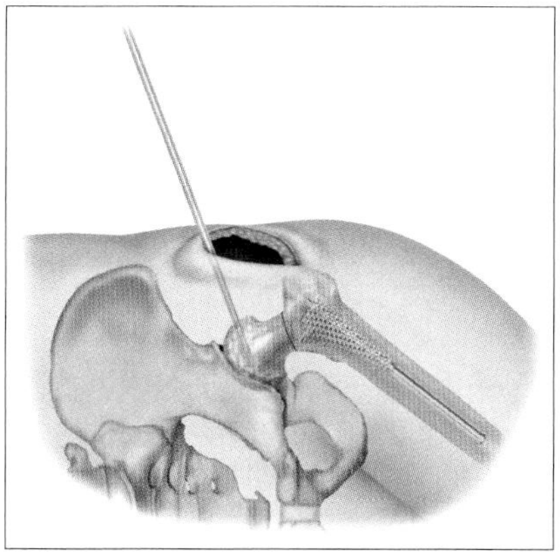

Figure 11 A Shanz pin is placed into the head to facilitate femoral head excision.

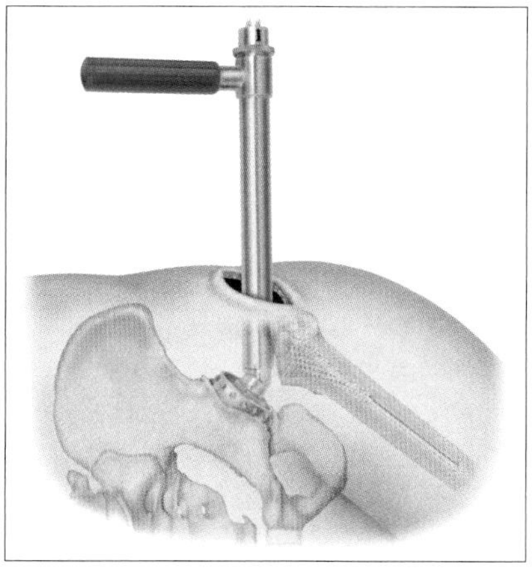

Figure 12 The acetabulum is prepared with a 45° reamer.

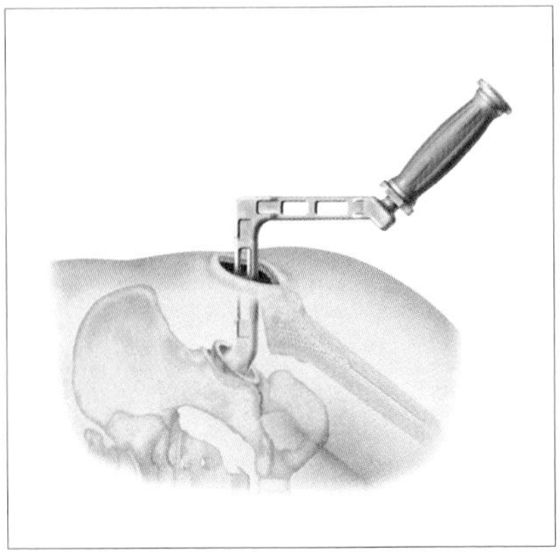

Figure 13 The cup is impacted with a double-angled cup impactor.

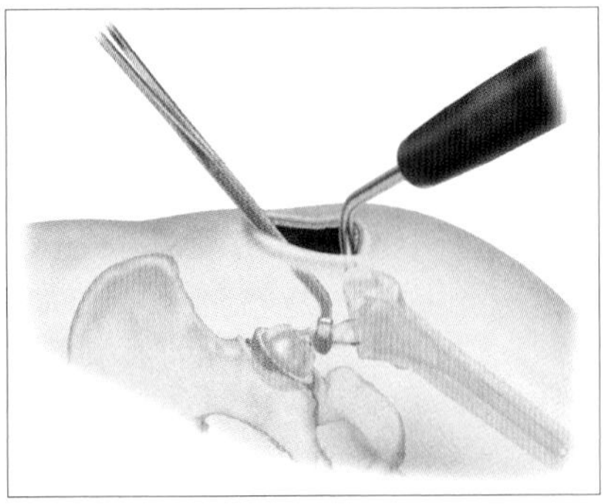

Figure 14 The femoral head is placed into the socket, and the neck is reduced into the head to minimize distortion of the soft-tissue envelope.

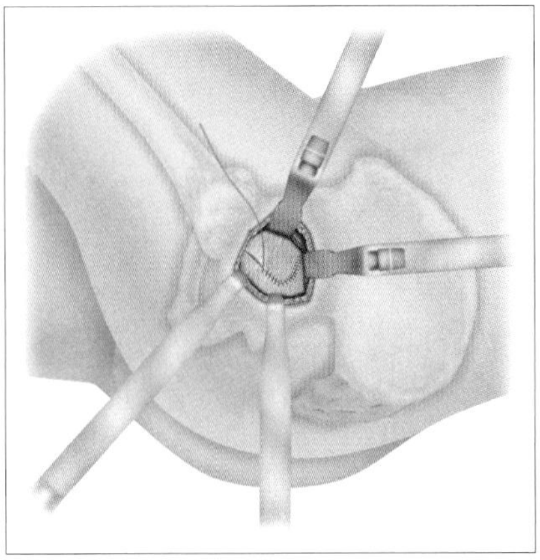

Figure 15 After final assembly, the hip joint capsule is closed anatomically.

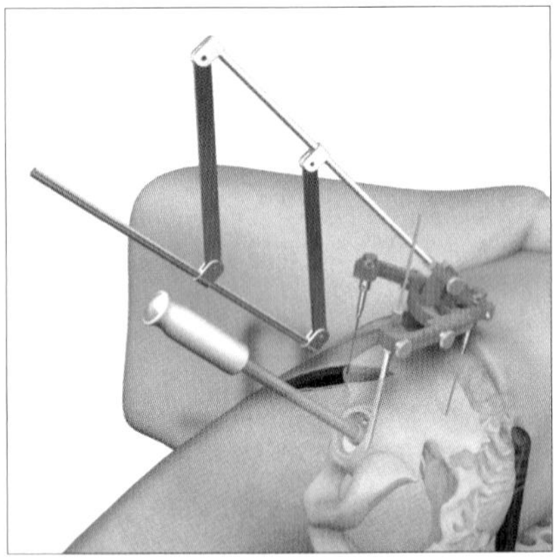

Figure 16 Illustration showing a mechanical navigation instrument, which is adjusted on a patient-specific basis, for cup placement.

excision of the labrum, preparation of the acetabulum, and the excision of osteophytes. A 45° reamer is used to prepare the acetabulum (**Figure 12**), and a double-angled cup impactor is used to implant the acetabular component (**Figure 13**). Standard screw insertion instruments can be used if screws are necessary. This process is facilitated if the fascial incision is made a bit more distally.

A trial reduction is performed by placing the trial femoral head into the trial acetabular liner and then assembling the trial femoral neck into the trial femoral head (**Figure 14**). This maneuver minimizes any soft-tissue dissection necessary to perform the surgery. Proper trial reduction is then performed to assess stability, impingement, tissue tension, offset, and leg length. When satisfactory, the trial components are removed, and the actual implants are assembled in situ in the same manner. The hip joint capsule is closed anatomically from the acetabular rim to the trochanteric fossa (**Figure 15**), and the superficial fascia is closed in the usual manner.

Postoperative Management

Patients who have donated autologous blood receive the donated blood preemptively in the operating room before transfer to the postanesthesia care unit (PACU). Patients are placed on a stretcher, and the head of the stretcher is elevated before the patient leaves the PACU. Patients then stand, typically with the assistance of a physical therapist and a nurse, and walk from the hallway to the hospital bed. Patients are encouraged to walk several times on the day of surgery and progress to a normal full diet immediately if possible. Urinary catheters are rarely used, even in patients with a history of prostatectomy or benign prostatic hyperplasia. Pneumatic compression is discontinued as soon as the patient is ambulatory. Parenteral narcotics are used, if needed, with transition to oral medications typically within a few hours of surgery. The discharge criteria are typical. Patients are allowed unrestricted progression of motion and weight bearing.

Experience of This Chapter's Author

Since October 2002, this chapter's author had experience with 1,454 THAs performed using the superior capsulotomy technique, of which 1,026 THAs have been followed for a minimum of 2 years. For the first 28 procedures, only the femoral component was implanted through the superior capsulotomy interval, and the cup was implanted through the anterolateral interval. Thereafter, all components were implanted through the incision in the superior capsule. Canal-filling components were used to reduce the risk of component subsidence associated with tapered components.[4] Surgical navigation of cup implantation was used for 1,367 of these 1,454 procedures (94%). Navigation systems included Brainlab (Munich, Germany) CT-based navigation (513 THAs) and 710 THAs performed with patient-specific mechanical navigation techniques[5] (HipSextant; Surgical

Table 2
Incidence of Surgical Complications in 1,454 Hips Treated With the Superior Capsulotomy Technique From October 2002 to June 2012

Complication	Number	Incidence
Dislocation	3	0.21%
Intraoperative greater trochanteric fracture	1	0.07%
Postoperative greater trochanteric fracture treated nonsurgically	1	0.07%
Partial peroneal palsy	2	0.14%
Calcar fracture, intraoperative, treated by cerclage	2	0.14%
Calcar fracture, occult intraoperative or postoperative, treated nonsurgically	2	0.14%
Failure of osseointegration of femur	2	0.14%
Failure of osseointegration of acetabulum	3	0.21%
Death within 90 days	2	0.14%

Table 3
Length of Hospital Stay Based on the THA Exposure Used

Exposure	Mean Length of Stay	Range
Anterior	3.00 (± 0.784) days	2 to 4 days
Anterolateral	3.11 (± 1.12) days	1 to 9 days
Posterior	2.97 (± 1.26) days	1 to 23 days
Superior capsulotomy	1.64 (± 0.983) days	0 to 9 days

Planning Associates, Boston, MA) (**Figure 16**). Of the last 300 THAs performed, 298 procedures were done using the superior capsulotomy technique. Perioperative complications are listed in **Table 2**.

All primary THAs performed at the New England Baptist Hospital from January 1, 2011, to April 20, 2012, were studied. The discharge criteria were identical. The THA procedures included 14 anterior exposures, 228 anterolateral exposures, 2,058 posterior exposures, and 256 superior capsulotomy exposures. Patients received preoperative acetaminophen, celecoxib (unless contraindicated), and local anesthetic infiltration.[6-8] No postoperative pain catheters were used.[9] Postoperative rehabilitation protocols varied slightly between surgeons but generally involved immediate mobilization. Comparison of the length of hospital stay was tested using the two-sample Wilcoxon rank-sum (Mann-Whitney) test and is summarized in **Table 3**. The length of stay for patients treated with the superior capsulotomy technique was lower than the anterolateral ($P < 0.0001$), posterior ($P < 0.0001$), and anterior ($P < 0.0001$) approaches. Ninety-eight percent of the patients treated with the superior capsulotomy technique were discharged directly home, whereas 68% of the patients treated by the posterior exposure were discharged directly home.

Summary

The superior capsulotomy technique for THA is a reliable method of maximally preserving the periarticular soft tissues and hip joint capsule. This technique has low dislocation, calcar, and trochanteric fracture rates and a shorter length of hospital stay compared with other THA techniques used at the New England Baptist Hospital. Ninety-eight percent of the unselected patients treated with the technique are discharged directly home. The superior capsulotomy technique is performed with the patient in the lateral position, allows for proper trial reduction of components, does not require traction or intraoperative fluoroscopy, and can easily be transitioned into a more extensile exposure.

Acknowledgments

The author acknowledges the contributions to this chapter by Diane Gulczynski, RN, and Dan Casey, RPT, for collaboration on rehabilitation development and William S. Murphy, BA, for data interpretation and analysis.

References

1. Murphy SB, Ecker TM, Tannast M: THA performed using conventional and navigated tissue-preserving techniques. *Clin Orthop Relat Res* 2006;453:160-167.
2. Kurtz W, Timmerman I, Nambu S, et al: Abstract No. 2093. Comparison of load to failure and calcar strain for two press-fit femoral stem implantation techniques in matched cadaver femora during simulated impaction. *Transactions of the 56th Annual Meeting* of the *Orthopedic Research Society.*

CD-ROM Rosemont, IL, Orthopaedic Research Society, 2010.

3. Jewett BA, Collis DK: High complication rate with anterior total hip arthroplasties on a fracture table. *Clin Orthop Relat Res* 2011; 469(2):503-507.
4. Jacobs CA, Christensen CP: Progressive subsidence of a tapered, proximally coated femoral stem in total hip arthroplasty. *Int Orthop* 2009;33(4):917-922.
5. Steppacher SD, Kowal JH, Murphy SB: Improving cup positioning using a mechanical navigation instrument. *Clin Orthop Relat Res* 2011;469(2):423-428.
6. Maund E, McDaid C, Rice S, Wright K, Jenkins B, Woolacott N: Paracetamol and selective and non-selective non-steroidal anti-inflammatory drugs for the reduction in morphine-related side-effects after major surgery: A systematic review. *Br J Anaesth* 2011;106(3):292-297.
7. Buvanendran A, Kroin JS, Tuman KJ, et al: Effects of perioperative administration of a selective cyclooxygenase 2 inhibitor on pain management and recovery of function after knee replacement: A randomized controlled trial. *JAMA* 2003;290(18):2411-2418.
8. Kehlet H, Andersen LØ: Local infiltration analgesia in joint replacement: The evidence and recommendations for clinical practice. *Acta Anaesthesiol Scana* 2011; 55(7):778-784.
9. Horlocker TT, Kopp SL, Pagnano MW, Hebl JR: Analgesia for total hip and knee arthroplasty: A multimodal pathway featuring peripheral nerve block. *J Am Acad Orthop Surg* 2006;14(3):126-135.

22

Primary and Revision Anterior Supine Total Hip Arthroplasty: An Analysis of Complications and Reoperations

Keith R. Berend, MD
Joseph J. Kavolus, BA
Michael J. Morris, MD
Adolph V. Lombardi Jr, MD, FACS

Abstract

Anterior total hip arthroplasty (THA) has been touted by some as a muscle-sparing, less invasive procedure. Reports have focused on the high intraoperative and postoperative complication rates, the increased transfusion risk, and its questionable clinical benefits. The senior author's experience regarding complications and reoperations that occurred after primary and revision THA using an anterior supine intermuscular approach has been generally favorable. An electronic database was used to identify 906 patients treated with 1,035 consecutive anterior supine intermuscular THAs performed by a single surgeon between January 2007 and December 2010, which included 986 primary THAs, 2 resurfacings, 2 conversions of failed open reduction and internal fixation for fracture, and 45 revision THAs. The surgical technique used an anterior approach with a modified Smith-Petersen interval and was performed with the patient supine on a standard operating table without traction. The transfusion rate was 5%. There were three intraoperative calcar cracks and one canal perforation, which was treated with cerclage cables. Four wound complications required débridement, four hips had substantial lateral femoral cutaneous nerve paresthesias that had not resolved by the 12-month follow-up, and one femoral nerve palsy was reported. At up to 40 month's follow-up, there have been 25 revisions (2.4%), including 9 periprosthetic femoral fractures; 1 stem subsidence; 4 hips with aseptic loosening; 5 metal-on-metal bearing complications; 1 cup malpositioning, which was corrected the same day; 4 dislocations; and 1 infection. This 4-year experience with primary and revision anterior THAs has showed acceptable rates of perioperative transfusion, complications, and revisions.

Instr Course Lect 2013;62:251-263.

Smith-Petersen[1] first described the anterior approach to the hip joint in 1917. In the 1940s and 1950s, Smith-Petersen[2] and Judet and Judet[3] were the first to advocate the anterior approach for total hip arthroplasty (THA). The technique was further refined during the 1960s in France, where it is known as the Hueter approach.[4] Since that time, many other techniques (including direct lateral, anterolateral, posterolateral, and posterior approaches) have been used in THA, with the posterolateral approach being the most commonly used current approach.[5] Increasing interest in the benefits of minimally invasive surgery and the pressure to stay competitive in the current consumer-driven medical market have encouraged orthopaedic surgeons to seek a definitively superior approach. This has led to surgical innovations, such as the two-incision technique and a renewed interest in the anterior approach.

The reported advantages of minimally invasive THA include less blood loss, less pain, and a shorter hospital stay, which may provide a faster recovery peroid.[6-9] However, a comparable number of studies have failed to show any important advantages over standard approaches, with findings showing essentially identical gait and function at 6-month follow-up.[10-15] Some surgeons believe that minimally invasive techniques are unsatisfactory because of the significant learning curve and the increased risk of early complications.[16-21] The long-term outcomes of these minimally invasive procedures, in terms of fixation and implant longevity, remain unproven. Some of this chapter's authors (KRB and AVL) have broad experience with less invasive modifications of the direct lateral approach and have reported less blood loss and a shorter hospital stay.[22] Other authors have suggested that the less invasive direct lateral approach does not provide an advantage over the traditional approach.[10,13,23] Importantly, soft-tissue dissection requires the removal and repair of the abductor musculature and disruption of the tensor fascia lata.

In contrast to these less invasive approaches, which may or may not offer substantial benefits, multiple reports have detailed various techniques of minimally invasive THA performed through a single anterior incision via the Smith-Petersen interval.[24-45] The anterior interval is both intermuscular and internervous, and the muscle-sparing aspect of the approach provides the theoretic and clinical benefits of greater stability and easier recovery, making this technique truly minimally invasive.[46-48] These anterior-based approaches, like most other less invasive or minimally invasive approaches, are aided by specialized instrumentation. One such approach is the anterior supine intermuscular technique using Microplasty Anterior Supine Intramuscular instrumentation (Biomet, Warsaw, IN).

Anterior supine intermuscular THA is a muscle-sparing, less invasive procedure. It is versatile, with reported use expanding beyond the primary realm to revision and resurfacing THAs, as well as the treatment of acute fractures in elderly patients, who may benefit more from the muscle-sparing nature of the anterior approach because of their diminished regenerative capacity.[49-55] The reported risks and complications of anterior THA have focused on the high intraoperative and postoperative complication rates, increased transfusion risk, and questionable clinical benefits.[14,19,21,56] The literature on anterior approach THA has dissenting opinions, with some surgeons focusing on the lack of demonstrable benefit in the face of proven costs and risks, whereas others focus on the need for cautious innovation because of the practical advantages of the anterior approach.[37,56] This chapter will report on early complications and reoperations after primary, revision, and resurfacing anterior supine intramuscular THA.

Surgical Technique

At Joint Implant Surgeons, New Albany, Ohio, THA via the anterior supine intermuscular approach is performed using a standard radiolucent operating table (with the table extender at the foot of the bed) and fluoroscopic assistance. The patient is positioned supine on the operating table, with the pubic symphysis aligned at the table break for subsequent repositioning during preparation of the femur and insertion of the femoral component (**Figure 1**). Both lower extremities are prepped and draped in a standard fashion with sterile stockinettes. A bilateral lower extremity drape is placed over both limbs and is cut on the surgical side to expose the anterior superior iliac spine (ASIS) and the anterior thigh. The contralateral limb is exposed free to be later placed onto a padded Mayo stand. A sterile iodoform sticky drape is applied posteriorly as a mesentery to seal off the buttocks and groin, and a second iodoform drape is applied anteriorly to the thigh up to the ASIS (**Figure 2**). The surgical extremity is then covered with three additional stockinettes, which will be removed later during relocation and dislocation maneuvers with femoral preparation.

After prepping and draping are completed, the surgical landmarks are identified. The ASIS and the center of the knee are marked, and a line is drawn between the two points. The incision generally commences proximally from two finger breadths distal and two finger breadths lateral to the ASIS and extends distally toward the center of the knee, from 8 to 10 cm in most patients (**Figure 3**). Using fluoroscopic guidance, the location of the anterior aspect of the femoral neck is confirmed (**Figure 4**). The incision is placed approximately over the center of the lateral aspect of the greater trochanter. This lateral placement of the incision avoids the lateral femoral cutaneous nerve and contrasts with the two-incision technique that places the anterior incision more medially.

Dr. Berend or an immediate family member serves as a board member, owner, officer, or committee member of the American Association of Hip and Knee Surgeons; has received royalties from Biomet; serves as a paid consultant to or is an employee of Biomet; and has received research or institutional support from Biomet. Dr. Morris or an immediate family member serves as a paid consultant to or is an employee of Biomet and has received research or institutional support from Biomet. Dr. Lombardi or an immediate family member serves as a board member, owner, officer, or committee member of the Hip Society, the Knee Society, and New Albany Surgical Hospital; has received royalties from Biomet and Innomed; is a member of a speakers' bureau or has made paid presentations on behalf of Biomet; serves as a paid consultant to or is an employee of Biomet; and has received research or institutional support from Biomet and Stryker. Neither Mr. Kavolus nor any immediate family member has received anything of value from or has stock or stock options in a commercial company or institution related directly or indirectly to the subject of this chapter.

The skin is incised, and the incision is carried down through the subcutaneous tissues to identify the tensor fascia lata, which has a distinctive purple hue (**Figure 5**). The fibers of the tensor fascia lata are incised, and the tensor fascia lata muscle is dissected free from the intermuscular septum lateral to the sartorius and the rectus muscles. Using blunt dissection, the tensor fascia lata muscle is pulled laterally. The deep, investing aponeurosis of the tensor fascia lata is split using a tonsil. Just below this fascia lie the lateral circumflex vessels. These should be identified and ligated or cauterized (**Figure 6**). Two veins and one artery course across the anterior hip capsule in this location. A retractor is placed superior to the femoral neck over the top of the superior hip capsule. Blunt dissection is again performed to open this interval. A blunt cobra-type retractor is then placed along the inferior femoral neck, deep to the rectus muscle and tendon. A sharp retractor is used to peel the rectus tendon off the anterior capsule and place it over the anterior rim of the acetabulum.

An anterior capsulectomy is then performed, splitting the capsule to the rim of the acetabulum. With the femoral neck exposed, the saw blade is positioned for resection at a level based on preoperative templating and confirmed with fluoroscopy (**Figure 7**). A subcapital resection is performed to create a "napkin ring" slice of the femoral neck, and a threaded Steinmann pin on a drill is used to remove the napkin ring slice and then the femoral head (**Figure 8**). A sharp retractor is placed superiorly right (at the 3-o'clock position on a left hip or the 6-o'clock position on a right hip), a double-pronged posterior retractor is placed on the ischium (at approximately the 7-o'clock position for a left hip or the 5-o'clock position for a right hip), and an anterior retractor is

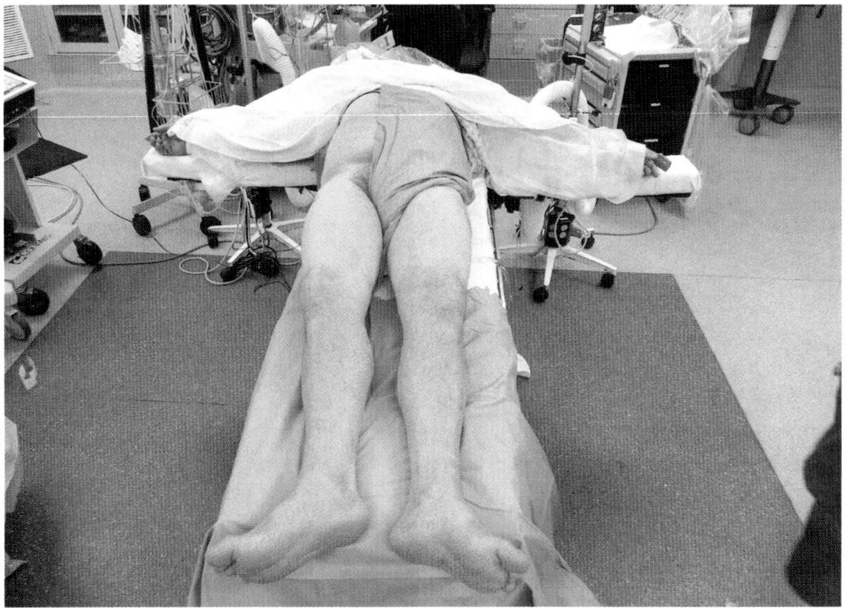

Figure 1 The patient is positioned supine on a standard radiolucent operating table with a table extender at the foot of the bed. The pubic symphysis is aligned at the table break for subsequent repositioning during preparation of the femur and insertion of the femoral component. (Courtesy of Joint Implant Surgeons, New Albany, OH.)

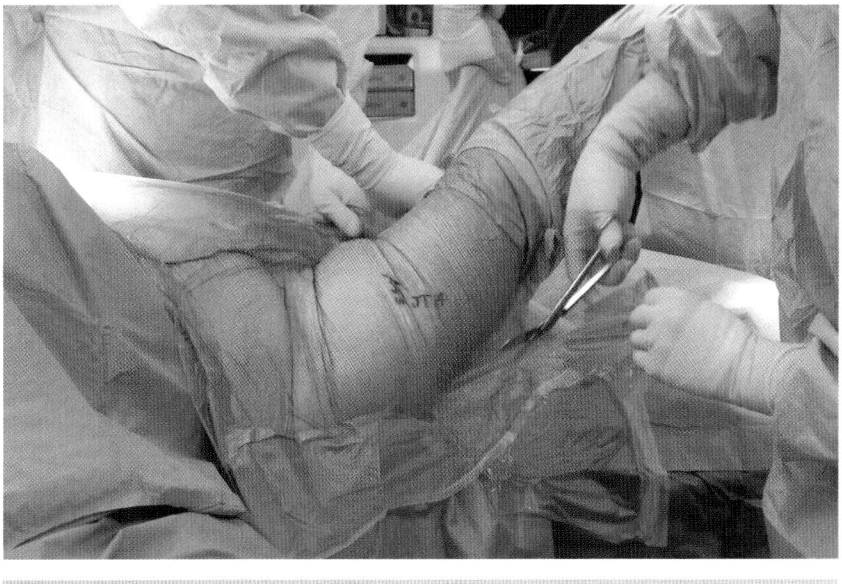

Figure 2 A bilateral lower extremity drape is placed over both limbs and cut on the surgical side to expose the ASIS and the anterior thigh. The contralateral limb is exposed free to be later placed onto a padded Mayo stand. A sterile iodoform sticky drape is applied posteriorly as a mesentery to seal off the buttocks and groin, and a second iodoform drape is applied anteriorly to the thigh up to the ASIS. (Courtesy of Joint Implant Surgeons, New Albany, OH.)

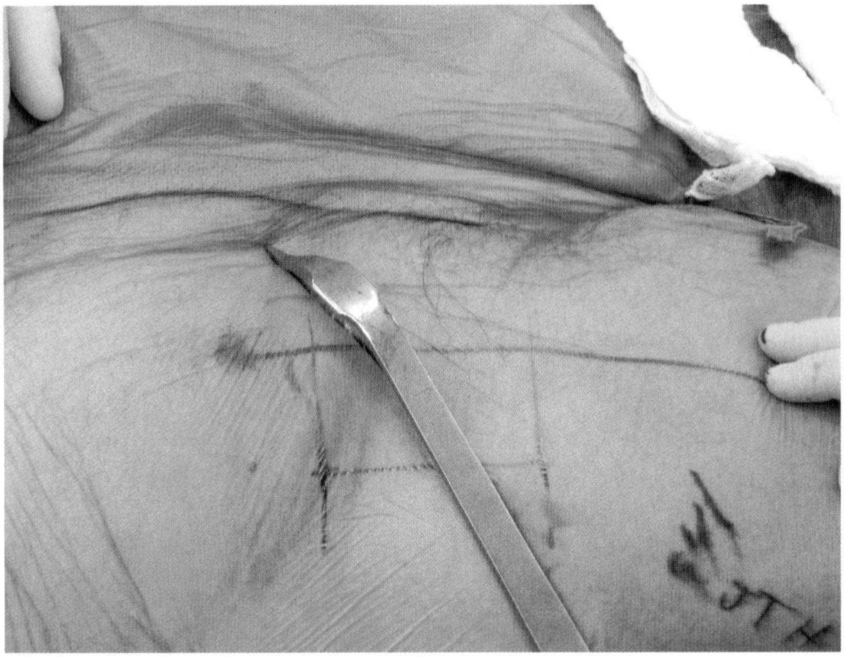

Figure 3 After prepping and draping, the surgical landmarks are identified. The ASIS and the center of the knee are marked, and a line is drawn between the two points. The incision generally commences proximally from two finger breadths distal and two finger breadths lateral to the ASIS and will extend distally toward the center of the knee from 8 to 10 cm in most patients. (Courtesy of Joint Implant Surgeons, New Albany, OH.)

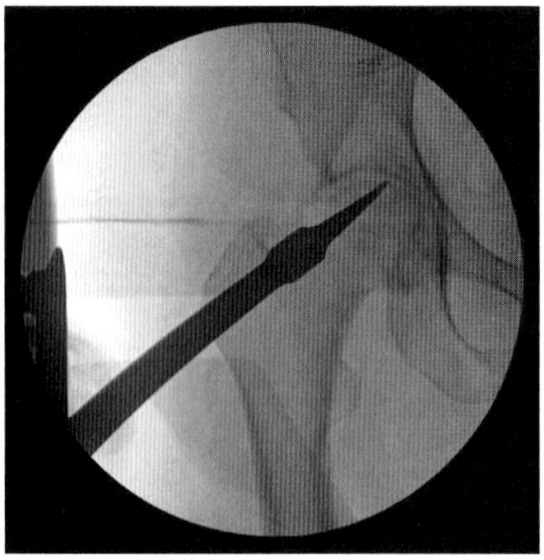

Figure 4 The location of the anterior aspect of the femoral neck is confirmed with fluoroscopy. The incision is placed approximately over the center of the lateral aspect of the greater trochanter. Lateral placement of the incision avoids disrupting the lateral femoral cutaneous nerve. (Courtesy of Joint Implant Surgeons, New Albany, OH.)

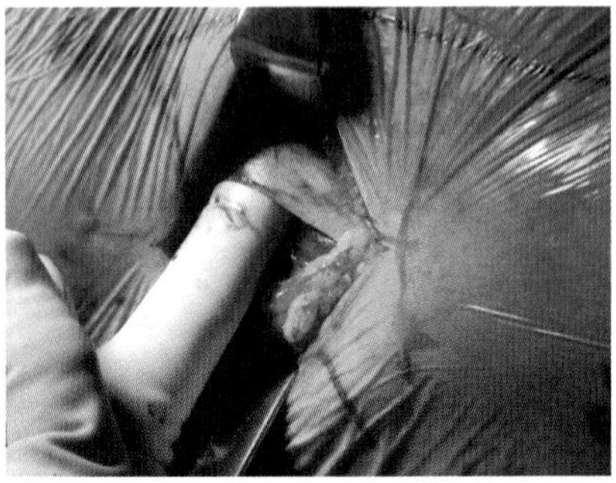

Figure 5 The skin is incised, and the incision is carried down through the subcutaneous tissues to identify the tensor fascia lata, which has a distinctive purple hue. The fibers of the tensor fascia lata are incised, and the tensor fascia lata muscle is dissected free from the intermuscular septum lateral to the sartorius and the rectus muscles. Using blunt dissection, the tensor fascia lata muscle is pulled laterally. (Courtesy of Joint Implant Surgeons, New Albany, OH.)

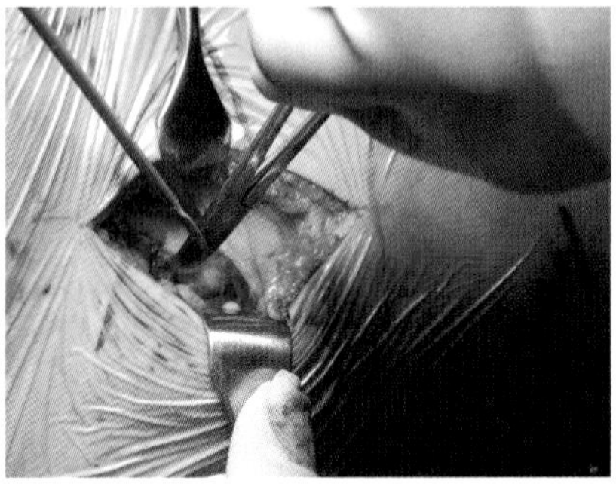

Figure 6 The deep, investing aponeurosis of the tensor fascia is split using a tonsil; just below are the lateral circumflex vessels. Two veins and one artery course across the anterior hip capsule in this location. These vessels should be identified and either ligated or cauterized, as shown in this figure. (Courtesy of Joint Implant Surgeons, New Albany, OH.)

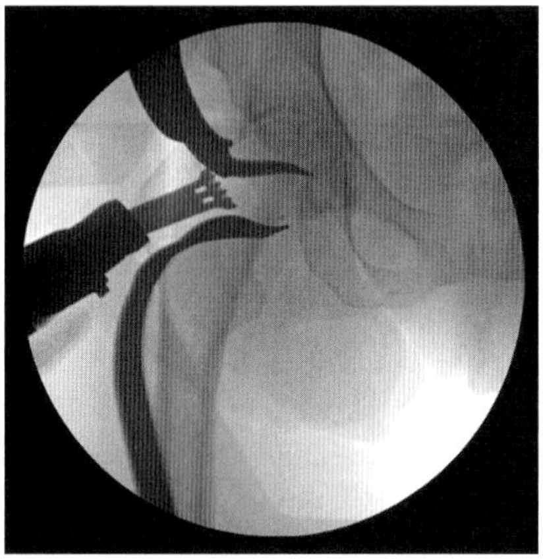

Figure 7 Fluoroscopy is used to confirm correct positioning of the saw blade for resection of the exposed femoral neck at a level based on preoperative templating. (Courtesy of Joint Implant Surgeons, New Albany, OH.)

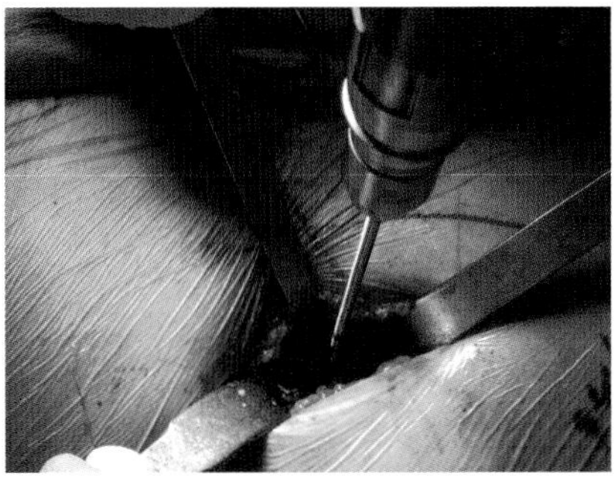

Figure 8 Femoral neck resection and a second subcapital resection are performed to create a "napkin ring" slice of the femoral neck. A threaded Steinmann pin on a drill is used to remove the napkin ring slice and then the femoral head. (Courtesy of Joint Implant Surgeons, New Albany, OH.)

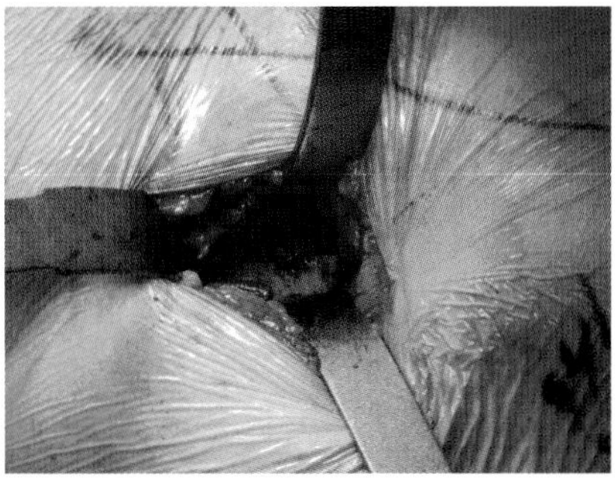

Figure 9 The acetabulum is exposed with a sharp retractor and is placed superiorly right (at the 3-o'clock position on a left hip and the 6-o'clock position on a right hip). A double-pronged posterior retractor is placed on the ischium (at approximately the 7-o'clock position for a left hip and the 5-o'clock position for a right hip), and an anterior retractor is replaced. The labrum, osteophytes, and any capsule that lie in the way of acetabular preparation are removed. (Courtesy of Joint Implant Surgeons, New Albany, OH.)

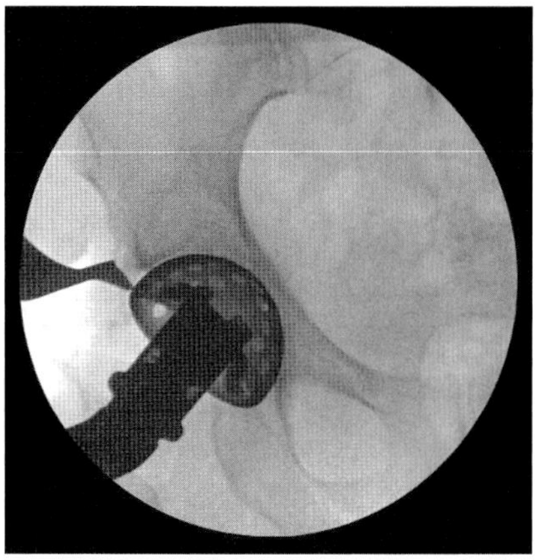

Figure 10 Fluoroscopy is used to confirm appropriate reaming of the acetabulum, which is performed with only one or two sequential reamers, with underreaming by 1 mm from the templated size. (Courtesy of Joint Implant Surgeons, New Albany, OH.)

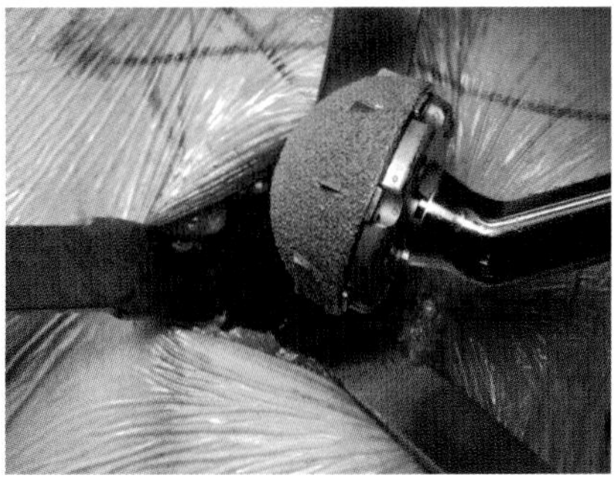

Figure 11 A porous, hemispheric acetabular shell is placed, followed by a polyethylene liner. (Courtesy of Joint Implant Surgeons, New Albany, OH.)

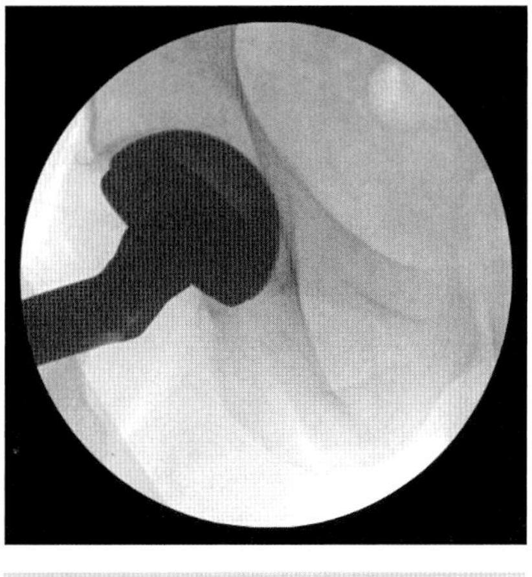

Figure 12 Correct positioning of the acetabular component is confirmed with fluoroscopy. (Courtesy of Joint Implant Surgeons, New Albany, OH.)

replaced (**Figure 9**). The surgeon palpates medially to locate a tight band of capsule, and blunt dissection is performed to prevent damage to the insertion of the iliopsoas muscle.

The labrum, the osteophytes, and any capsule that lie in the way of acetabular preparation are removed. Acetabular reaming is performed using only one or two sequential reamers, with underreaming by 1 mm from the templated size; fluoroscopic guidance is used as needed (**Figure 10**). The acetabular component is then placed (**Figure 11**), and its position is confirmed with fluoroscopy (**Figure 12**).

On the femoral side, the surgeon palpates underneath and around the tensor, around the lateral aspect of the femur, proximal to the gluteus maximus tendon, and places a bone hook around the proximal femur. Femoral preparation and stem insertion require maneuvering the operating table and adjusting the patient's position. The table is jackknifed by lowering the foot of the table to approximately 45° and placing the bed into approximately 15° of the Trendelenburg position. The contralateral leg is placed on the padded Mayo stand. A table-mounted femur elevator (Omni-Tract Surgical, St. Paul, MN) is attached to the bed (**Figure 13**) (requiring a change in surgical gloves) and attached to the traction hook around the proximal femur (**Figure 14**).

Gentle retraction is placed on the femur to tension the capsule. A retractor is placed around the cut femoral neck, and a retractor is placed over the anterosuperior corner of the greater trochanter to expose the trochanter

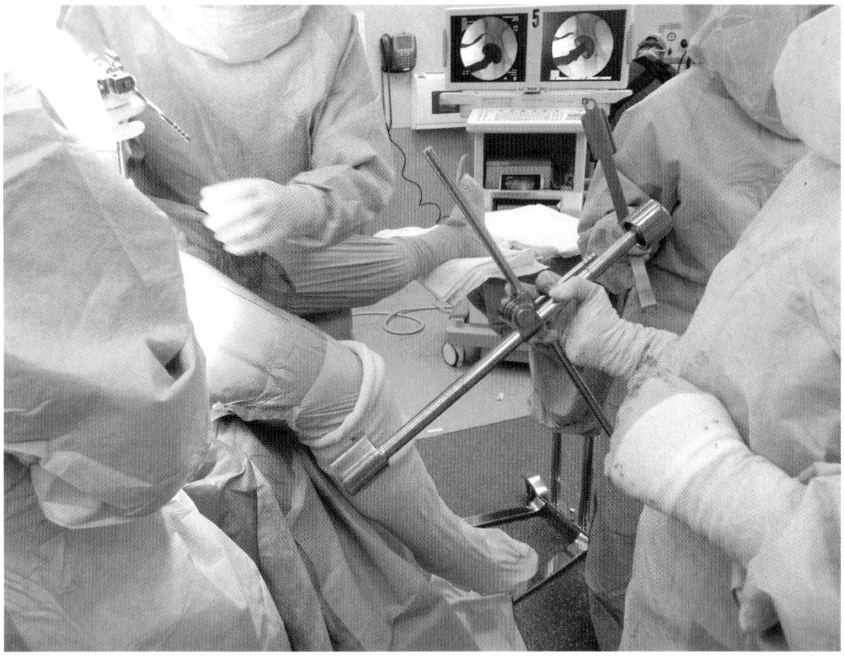

Figure 13 The operating table is jackknifed by lowering the foot of the table to approximately 45°, and the bed is placed into approximately 15° of the Trendelenburg position to accomplish femoral preparation and stem insertion. The contralateral leg has been placed on a padded Mayo stand. A table-mounted femur elevator is attached to the bed, requiring a change in surgical gloves. (Courtesy of Joint Implant Surgeons, New Albany, OH.)

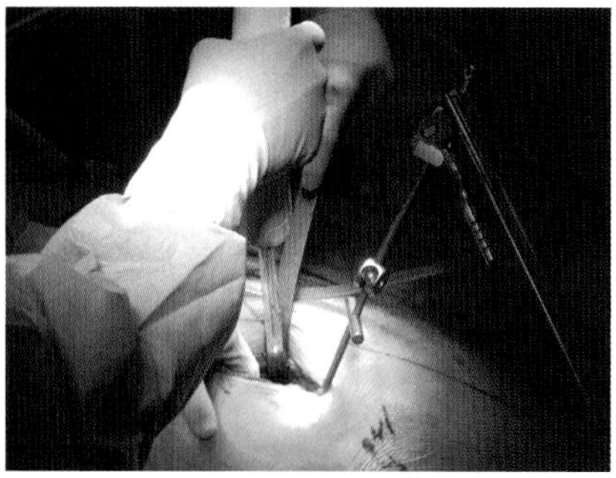

Figure 14 A traction bone hook is carefully placed around the proximal femur. After the femur elevator has been attached to the bed, the other end of the apparatus is attached to the traction hook around the proximal femur, and gentle retraction is applied to tension the capsule. (Courtesy of Joint Implant Surgeons, New Albany, OH.)

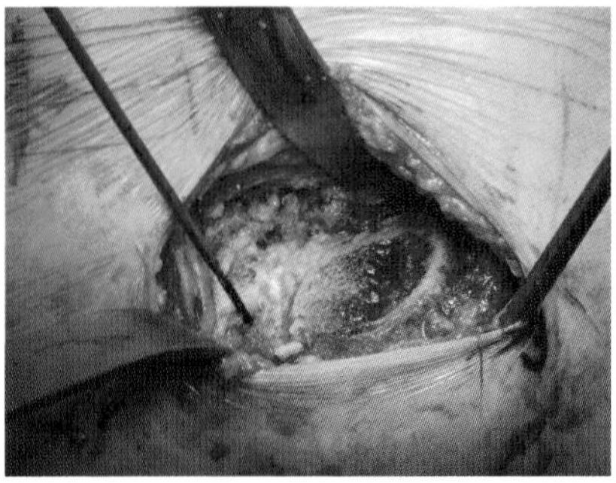

Figure 15 The hip capsule fibers are dissected from anterior to the posteriormost superior tip of the trochanter. As the capsule is released, the femur comes up and out of the wound and into view. (Courtesy of Joint Implant Surgeons, New Albany, OH.)

and further excise the proximal superior capsule. The retractor is then repositioned in a manner so that the tip is placed laterally over the greater trochanter to laterally expose the saddle or the shoulder. The surgeon then dissects from anterosuperiorly to the posteriormost superior tip of the trochanter. As the capsule is released, the femur will begin to come up and out of the wound and into view (**Figure 15**). With increasing gentle retraction via the table-mounted hook, the femur is elevated. Simultaneously, the surgical limb is externally rotated by the assistant and adducted underneath the contralateral leg in a lazy figure-of-4 position (**Figure 16**).

Broaching begins with a canal finder and moves laterally. The use of a broach-only stem design is preferred because direct, straight reaming of the femur is difficult in most cases. Specialized offset broaches and broach handles may facilitate femoral preparation (**Figure 17**). The final broach is left in place, trial components are placed, traction is unhooked, the outermost stockinette is removed, and the hip is relocated and maneuvered to assess offset and stability. Fluoroscopic images are obtained to confirm femoral implant positioning, offset, and neck and limb length. The surgeon can directly measure limb length in the supine position through direct comparison of the medial malleoli (**Figure 18**) and fluoroscopy (**Figure 19**). The hip is then dislocated, the traction hook is reattached, and the final femoral component is inserted (**Figure 20**). Final trial reduction for limb length can then be performed, again detaching the traction hook; removing another stockinette layer; relocating the hip; assessing offset, length, and stability; and confirming the trial reduction with final fluoroscopic images (**Figure 21**). If satisfactory, the final head component is implanted, and final reduction is performed (**Figure 22**). The operating table is returned to the flat position, the wound is irrigated, a deep drain is placed (**Figure 23**), and the wound is closed in layers.

A standardized hospitalization and rehabilitation protocol was used for all patients[57,58] and included preemptive pain and nausea medications, intrathe-

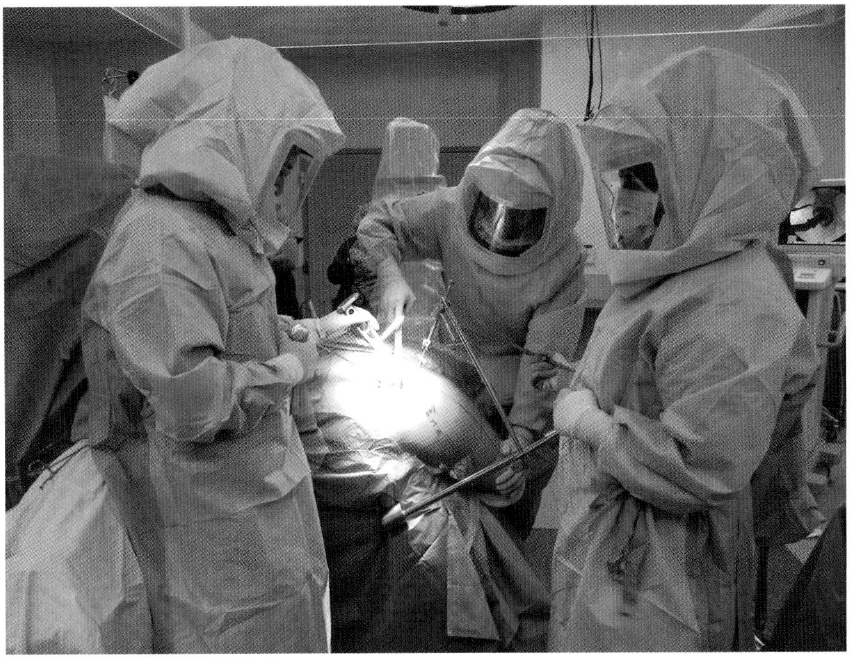

Figure 16 As the femur is elevated from the wound by dissection of capsular fibers and gentle retraction, the surgical limb is externally rotated by the assistant and adducted underneath the nonsurgical limb in a lazy figure-of-4 position. (Courtesy of Joint Implant Surgeons, New Albany, OH.)

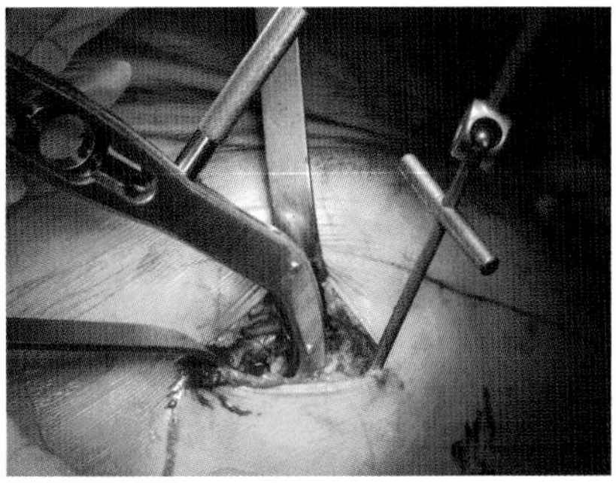

Figure 17 The use of a broach-only stem design is preferred because direct straight reaming of the femur is usually difficult. Specialized offset broaches and broach handles may facilitate femoral preparation, with attention given to clearing the lateral aspect of the proximal femur. (Courtesy of Joint Implant Surgeons, New Albany, OH.)

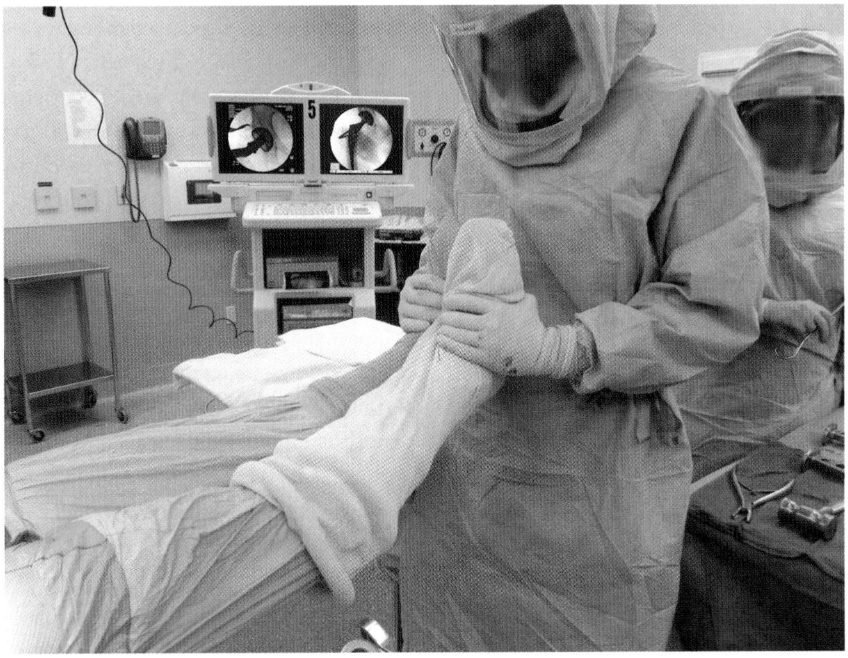

Figure 18 With the final broach left in place, trial neck and head components are inserted. Traction is unhooked, the outermost stockinette is removed, and the hip is relocated and maneuvered to assess offset and stability. The surgeon can readily measure limb length in the supine position through direct comparison of the medial malleoli. (Courtesy of Joint Implant Surgeons, New Albany, OH.)

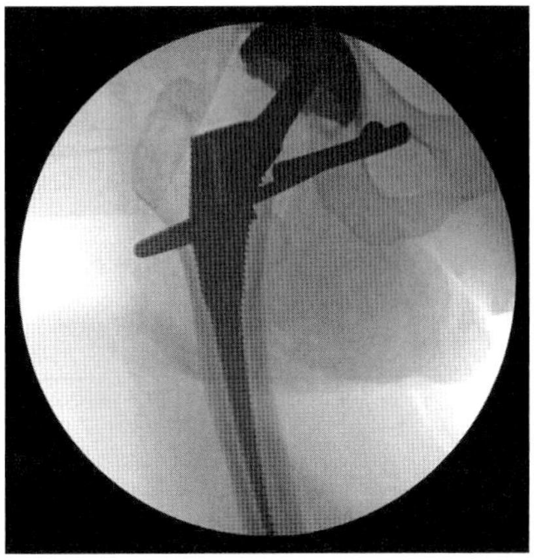

Figure 19 Fluoroscopic images are obtained to confirm femoral implant positioning, offset, and neck and limb length. (Courtesy of Joint Implant Surgeons, New Albany, OH.)

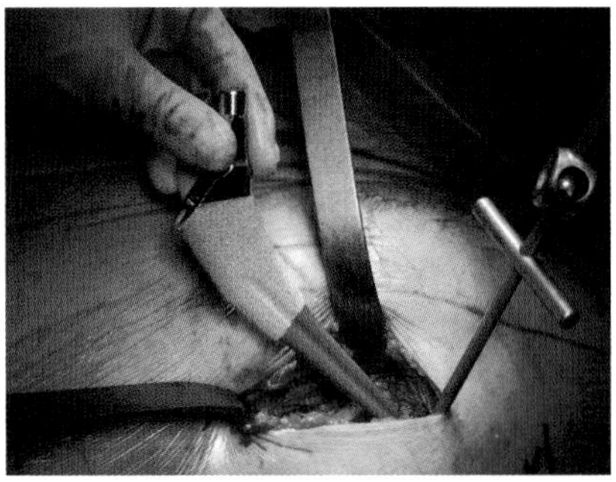

Figure 20 With satisfactory stability, limb length, and offset obtained, the hip is dislocated, the traction hook is reattached, and the final femoral component is inserted. (Courtesy of Joint Implant Surgeons, New Albany, OH.)

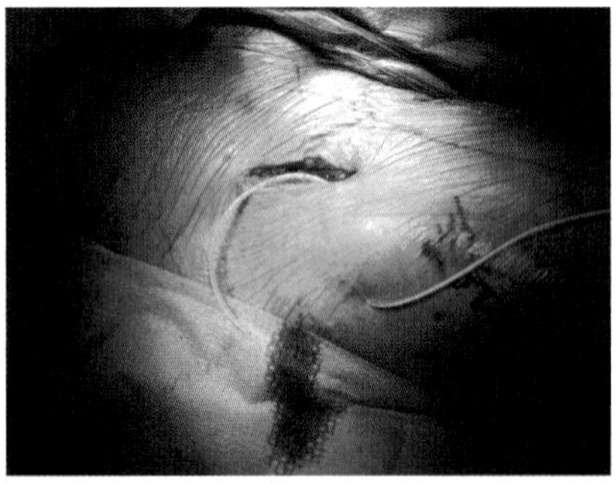

Figure 23 With all implants inserted, the table is returned to the flat position, the wound is irrigated, and a deep drain is placed. The wound will be closed in layers. (Courtesy of Joint Implant Surgeons, New Albany, OH.)

cal spinal anesthetic and a long-acting narcotic, and a periarticular soft-tissue injection cocktail. Patients ambulate on the day of surgery with a walker and are discharged from the hospital when the physical therapy goals are accomplished. Patients use a walker or cane for 2 weeks and then progress to unassisted walking when able. Routine follow-up is performed at 6 weeks and involves a standard physical and radiographic evaluation. Patients are instructed to return for annual follow-up examinations or for evaluation if problems occur.

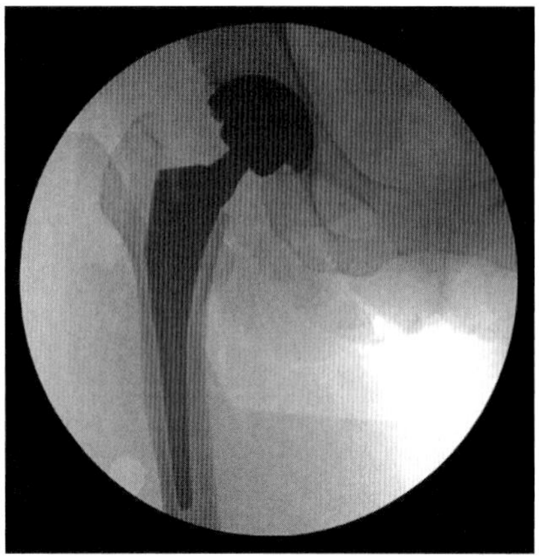

Figure 21 Final trial reduction for limb length is performed, again detaching the traction hook; removing another stockinette layer; relocating the hip; and assessing for offset, limb length, and stability. Fluoroscopy is used to confirm final positioning. (Courtesy of Joint Implant Surgeons, New Albany, OH.)

Author's Experience

From January 2007 to December 2010, 906 patients (432 men [48%] and 474 women [52%]) were treated with 1,035 consecutive anterior supine intermuscular THAs performed by a single surgeon (KRB). Follow-up averaged 14.6 months (SD = 12.9; range, 0.4 to 56.1 months). Average age at the time of surgery was 62.7 years (SD = 12.4; range, 27 to 92 years). Body mass index averaged 29.7 kg/m² (SD = 6.1; range, 17 to 57 kg/m²).

The retrospective case series included 45 revision procedures (4.3%); 2 resurfacing arthroplasties for osteoarthritis (0.2%); 2 conversions of failed open reduction and internal fixation for femoral fractures (0.2%), which also required hardware removal; and 986 primary THAs (95.3%). The most common underlying diagnosis for primary THA was osteoarthritis in 861 patients, which accounted for 87% of the patients in the study. Other diagnoses were osteonecrosis in 65 patients (6.6%), congenital dysplasia in 19 patients (1.9%), rheumatoid

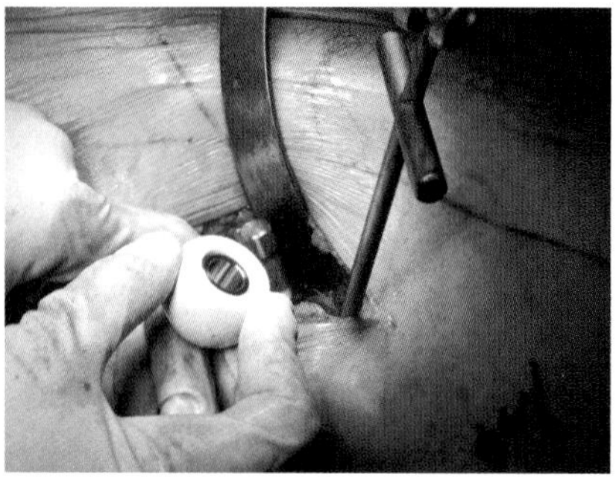

Figure 22 With appropriate neck length determined to achieve optimal stability, the final femoral head component is inserted, and final reduction is performed. (Courtesy of Joint Implant Surgeons, New Albany, OH.)

arthritis in 10 patients (1.0%), acute femoral fracture in 10 patients (1.0%), posttraumatic arthritis in 9 patients (0.9%), Legg-Calvé-Perthes disease in 6 patients (0.6%), and slipped capital femoral epiphysis in 6 patients (0.6%). For revision cases, the underlying diagnoses were polyethylene wear in 31 patients (68.9%), metal-on-metal bearing complications in 5 patients (11%), recurrent dislocation in 3 patients (6.7%), aseptic loosening of the acetabular component in 3 patients (6.7%), loosening of the femoral component in 1 patient (2%), and periprosthetic femoral fracture in 2 patients (4%).

Perioperative data, including information on the average prosthesis size, surgical time, blood loss, and the length of the hospital stay is summarized in **Table 1**. Intraoperatively, there were four complications (0.4%), including three calcar cracks (0.3%) and one canal perforation (0.1%), all of which were treated with cerclage cables. Postoperative complications included six nonhealing wounds (0.6%) requiring débridement, four lateral femoral cutaneous nerve paresthesias (0.4%) not resolved at 12 months, and one femoral nerve palsy (0.1%). At up to 56 months' follow-up, there have been 25 revisions (2.4%) (**Table 2**). The most common reason for revision was periprosthetic femoral fracture occurring nine times (0.9%), followed by metal-on-metal bearing complications that occurred in five patients (0.5%), and dislocation in four patients (0.4%). Other reasons for revision were cup and stem loosening in two patients (0.2%); isolated cup loosening in two patients (0.2%); and one incident each of infection, cup malposition, and femoral subsidence (0.1%).

Table 1
Perioperative Factors

Characteristic	Result
Stem length	Mean = 114.4 mm (range, 95-165 mm)
Cup diameter	Mean = 54.6 mm (range, 36-70 mm)
Head diameter	Mean = 36.3 mm (range, 28-58 mm)
Surgical time	Mean = 63.6 min (range, 10-143 min)
Estimated blood loss	Mean = 145.3 mL (range, 25-1,000 mL)
Intraoperative transfusions	10 patients (1.0%)
Hemoglobin at discharge	Mean = 10.5 g/dL (range, 7.2-16.2 g/dL)
Inpatient transfusions	53 patients (5.3%)
Length of hospital stay	Mean = 1.7 days (range, 1-12 days)

Table 2
Revision of Any Component

Reason for Revision	Incidence
Infection	1 (0.1%)
Malposition of cup (corrected same day)	1 (0.1%)
Metal-on-metal bearing complications	5 (0.5%)
Dislocation	4 (0.4%)
Loosening, cup	2 (0.2%)
Loosening, cup and stem	2 (0.2%)
Femoral subsidence	1 (0.1%)
Periprosthetic femoral fracture	9 (0.9%)
Total	**25 (2.4%)**

Discussion

The Joint Implant Surgeons' study investigated the early complications and reoperations associated with primary, conversion, and revision THA and hip resurfacing performed via a muscle-sparing, anterior supine intermuscular approach performed on a standard operating table with fluoroscopy. Study weaknesses included the performance of all the procedures by a single, experienced arthroplasty surgeon at a high-volume center; the absence of a control group treated with traditional approaches; and the retrospective study design. The strength of the study was the systematic analysis of the complications and reoperations on a continuous series of patients.

The results showed a 2.4% reoperation or revision rate and an equally low rate of perioperative complications. Primary and revision THA can be safely performed using this muscle-sparing approach.[24-45,48-51] Many complications and drawbacks have been associated with anterior hip surgery, including high blood loss and transfusion rates, intraoperative femoral and trochanteric fractures, and high percentages of meralgia paresthetica.[16,21] In this series, the rate of complications was not alarmingly high. Instead, rapid recovery and quick return to function were observed, with an average hospital stay of 1.7 days.

Other authors have reported improved early recovery after anterior hip surgery.[24-45] Goebel et al[30] reported that patients treated with anterior supine intermuscular THA had less postoperative pain, required less pain medication, had a shorter length of hospital stay, and had a quicker time to full recovery than those treated with more traditional approaches. Less soft-tissue disruption, as evidenced on MRI, also has been reported with the anterior supine intermuscular approach.[29] This was confirmed by the work of Bergin et al[28] who reported substantially less muscle damage than with a minimally invasive posterior approach. The anterior approach is the only truly internervous and intermuscular approach that can be used for THA.[32,40]

In this series, the most common mode of failure or complication was postoperative periprosthetic femoral fracture (rate, 0.9%). This chapter's authors believe that exposure for preparing the femur is technique dependent and a concern when learning the anterior supine intermuscular approach. Sariali et al[59] reported seven false reamings of the proximal femur caused by increased difficulty with femoral exposure; all were noted intraoperatively and without consequence. This chapter's authors believe that difficulty with femoral exposure and the resultant implant malpositioning can lead to early perioperative femoral fracture. Tight anterior soft tissues, bulky muscle, and obesity can cause incorrect anteversion of the stem (despite adequate positioning on intraoperative fluoroscopy), resulting in early subsidence and rotational instability. In a patient with a high body mass index, special care is needed when considering this approach. A body mass index greater than 30 may be considered a relative contraindication to anterior supine intermuscular THA.[39,42,43] Of the remaining procedures requiring revision, five were related to complications of metal-on-metal articulations, which could potentially be avoided by using highly cross-linked polyethylene bearings.

Revision THA procedures have a higher complication rate than primary procedures.[49,60] The complication rate in this study appears to be acceptable when compared with findings in other revision THA studies. The recovery advantages included less scar tissue and decreased risks of injury to the sciatic and femoral nerves afforded by the anterior supine intermuscular THA.[60]

Four clinically significant lateral femoral cutaneous nerve paresthesias (0.4%) were noted at final follow-up. This rate is somewhat lower and less concerning than that reported in several earlier studies. Bhargava et al[61] reported a 15% rate of paresthesias, with 2 of 81 (2.4%) unresolved at 2-year follow-up. Goulding et al[62] reported that 88% of hips had neurapraxia, and only 6% of these completely resolved.

In contrast to other studies, this chapter's authors did not specifically query patients regarding paresthesias. At the time of data collection, four patients had unresolved and symptomatic meralgia paresthetica. It is not known if this significant difference in the rate of nerve paresthesia resulted from the more lateral placement of skin and fascial incisions or the failure to specifically question patients about symptoms indicative of paresthesia. However, only one patient in this study required further treatment with lateral femoral cutaneous nerve resection, and only three additional patients continue to report this complication. This chapter's authors strongly suggest a lateral incision location as distal to the ASIS as possible, with careful attention to a lateral fascial incision over the tensor fascia lata to help protect the lateral femoral cutaneous nerve.[63]

The risk of complications and revisions per 1,000 cases was reviewed. This chapter's authors found the intraoperative risks in our series to be 0.3% for a calcar crack, 0.1% for femoral perforation, 0.1% for cup malpositioning, 0% for stem malpositioning, 0.4% for lateral femoral cutaneous nerve paresthesia, and 0.1% for femoral nerve palsy. Postoperative risks were 0.9% for periprosthetic femur fracture requiring stem revision, 0.1% for femoral subsidence, 0.4% for dislocation, 0.6% for delayed wound healing requiring incision and débridement, and 0.1% for deep infection requiring two-stage treatment of radical débridement and delayed reimplantation. It is important to remember that these results were obtained from the practice of a single surgeon with more than 4 years of experience at a very high- volume center. There is a learning curve for the anterior approach, with approximately 40 cases or 6 months of experience required for proficiency.[21,27] It would be prudent for the novice surgeon to have one-on-one training sessions on cadavers before performing the procedure on patients.[43]

Apart from the learning curve, one of the other primary criticisms of the anterior approach is the cost of implementation.[56] Most often, this cost is attributed to the specialized fracture table used during the procedure.[36,42,45] The technique used by this chapter's authors, a modification of the approach popularized by Kennon et al,[9] uses a standard operating table. This method has been shown to be efficacious, with good outcomes.[24,27]

Summary

Anterior supine intermuscular THA appears to be a safe procedure with a proven recovery advantage for the patient. The complication rate, most notably for periprosthetic femoral fractures, appears to be low and decreases with the increased experience of the surgeon. No special surgical or fracture table is needed. As with any surgical technique, care must be taken as a surgeon becomes comfortable with the approach. Thoughtful patient selection and patience are encouraged during the early phases of implementation. Further research is needed to compare various anterior techniques and assess the long-term outcomes of the approaches.

References

1. Smith-Petersen M: A new supra-articular subperiosteal approach to the hip joint. *Am J Orthop Surg* 1917;15:592-595.
2. Smith-Petersen MN: Approach to and exposure of the hip joint for mold arthroplasty. *J Bone Joint Surg Am* 1949;31(1):40-46.
3. Judet J, Judet R: The use of an artificial femoral head for arthroplasty of the hip joint. *J Bone Joint Surg Br* 1950;32(2):166-173.
4. Lowell JD, Aufranc OE: The anterior approach to the hip joint. *Clin Orthop Relat Res* 1968;61: 193-198.
5. Palan J, Beard DJ, Murray DW, Andrew JG, Nolan J: Which approach for total hip arthroplasty: Anterolateral or posterior? *Clin Orthop Relat Res* 2009;467(2): 473-477.
6. Berger RA: Total hip arthroplasty using the minimally invasive two-

incision approach. *Clin Orthop Relat Res* 2003;417:232-241.

7. Berry DJ, Berger RA, Callaghan JJ, et al: Minimally invasive total hip arthroplasty: Development, early results, and a critical analysis. Presented at the Annual Meeting of the American Orthopaedic Association, Charleston, South Carolina, USA, June 14, 2003. *J Bone Joint Surg Am* 2003; 85(11):2235-2246.
8. Chimento GF, Pavone V, Sharrock N, Kahn B, Cahill J, Sculco TP: Minimally invasive total hip arthroplasty: A prospective randomized study. *J Arthroplasty* 2005;20(2):139-144.
9. Kennon RE, Keggi JM, Wetmore RS, Zatorski LE, Huo MH, Keggi KJ: Total hip arthroplasty through a minimally invasive anterior surgical approach. *J Bone Joint Surg Am* 2003;85(suppl 4):39-48.
10. Asayama I, Kinsey TL, Mahoney OM: Two-year experience using a limited-incision direct lateral approach in total hip arthroplasty. *J Arthroplasty* 2006;21(8):1083-1091.
11. Klausmeier V, Lugade V, Jewett BA, Collis DK, Chou LS: Is there faster recovery with an anterior or anterolateral THA? A pilot study. *Clin Orthop Relat Res* 2010; 468(2):533-541.
12. Ogonda L, Wilson R, Archbold P, et al: A minimal-incision technique in total hip arthroplasty does not improve early postoperative outcomes: A prospective, randomized, controlled trial. *J Bone Joint Surg Am* 2005;87(4): 701-710.
13. Pagnano MW, Leone J, Lewallen DG, Hanssen AD: Two-incision THA had modest outcomes and some substantial complications. *Clin Orthop Relat Res* 2005;441: 86-90.
14. Wayne N, Stoewe R: Primary total hip arthroplasty: A comparison of the lateral Hardinge approach to an anterior mini-invasive approach. *Orthop Rev (Pavia)* 2009;1(2):e27.
15. Woolson ST, Mow CS, Syquia JF, Lannin JV, Schurman DJ: Comparison of primary total hip replacements performed with a standard incision or a mini-incision. *J Bone Joint Surg Am* 2004;86(7):1353-1358.
16. Archibeck MJ, White RE Jr: Learning curve for the two-incision total hip replacement. *Clin Orthop Relat Res* 2004;429: 232-238.
17. Bal BS, Haltom D, Aleto T, Barrett M: Early complications of primary total hip replacement performed with a two-incision minimally invasive technique. *J Bone Joint Surg Am* 2005; 87(11):2432-2438.
18. Fehring TK, Mason JB: Catastrophic complications of minimally invasive hip surgery: A series of three cases. *J Bone Joint Surg Am* 2005;87(4):711-714.
19. Jewett BA, Collis DK: High complication rate with anterior total hip arthroplasties on a fracture table. *Clin Orthop Relat Res* 2011; 469(2):503-507.
20. Kim YH: Comparison of primary total hip arthroplasties performed with a minimally invasive technique or a standard technique: A prospective and randomized study. *J Arthroplasty* 2006;21(8):1092-1098.
21. Woolson ST, Pouliot MA, Huddleston JI: Primary total hip arthroplasty using an anterior approach and a fracture table: Short-term results from a community hospital. *J Arthroplasty* 2009; 24(7):999-1005.
22. Berend KR, Lombardi AV Jr: Total hip arthroplasty via the less invasive direct lateral abductor splitting approach. *Semin Arthroplasty* 2004;15:87-93.
23. Noble PC, Johnston JD, Alexander JA, et al: Making minimally invasive THR safe: Conclusions from biomechanical simulation and analysis. *Int Orthop* 2007; 31(suppl 1):S25-S28.
24. Alecci V, Valente M, Crucil M, Minerva M, Pellegrino CM, Sabbadini DD: Comparison of primary total hip replacements performed with a direct anterior approach versus the standard lateral approach: Perioperative findings. *J Orthop Traumatol* 2011; 12(3):123-129.
25. Bhandari M, Matta JM, Dodgin D, et al: Outcomes following the single-incision anterior approach to total hip arthroplasty: A multicenter observational study. *Orthop Clin North Am* 2009;40(3): 329-342.
26. Bender B, Nogler M, Hozack WJ: Direct anterior approach for total hip arthroplasty. *Orthop Clin North Am* 2009;40(3):321-328.
27. Berend KR, Lombardi AV Jr, Seng BE, Adams JB: Enhanced early outcomes with the anterior supine intermuscular approach in primary total hip arthroplasty. *J Bone Joint Surg Am* 2009; 91(suppl 6):107-120.
28. Bergin PF, Doppelt JD, Kephart CJ, et al: Comparison of minimally invasive direct anterior versus posterior total hip arthroplasty based on inflammation and muscle damage markers. *J Bone Joint Surg Am* 2011;93(15):1392-1398.
29. Bremer AK, Kalberer F, Pfirrmann CW, Dora C: Soft-tissue changes in hip abductor muscles and tendons after total hip replacement: Comparison between the direct anterior and the transgluteal approaches. *J Bone Joint Surg Br* 2011;93(7):886-889.
30. Goebel S, Steinert AF, Schillinger J, et al: Reduced postoperative pain in total hip arthroplasty after minimal-invasive anterior approach. *Int Orthop* 2012;36(3): 491-498.

31. Horne PH, Olson SA: Direct anterior approach for total hip arthroplasty using the fracture table. *Curr Rev Musculoskelet Med* 2011;4(3):139-145.
32. Lesch DC, Yerasimides JG, Brosky JA Jr: Rehabilitation following anterior approach total hip arthroplasty in a 49-year-old female: A case report. *Physiother Theory Pract* 2010;26(5):334-341.
33. Lovell TP: Single-incision direct anterior approach for total hip arthroplasty using a standard operating table. *J Arthroplasty* 2008; 23(7):64-68.
34. Lugade V, Wu A, Jewett B, Collis D, Chou LS: Gait asymmetry following an anterior and anterolateral approach to total hip arthroplasty. *Clin Biomech (Bristol, Avon)* 2010;25(7):675-680.
35. Masonis J, Thompson C, Odum S: Safe and accurate: Learning the direct anterior total hip arthroplasty. *Orthopedics* 2008;31(12).
36. Matta JM, Shahrdar C, Ferguson T: Single-incision anterior approach for total hip arthroplasty on an orthopaedic table. *Clin Orthop Relat Res* 2005;441:115-124.
37. Moskal JT: Anterior approach in THA improves outcomes: Affirms. *Orthopedics* 2011;34(9): e456-e458.
38. Nakata K, Nishikawa M, Yamamoto K, Hirota S, Yoshikawa H: A clinical comparative study of the direct anterior with mini-posterior approach: Two consecutive series. *J Arthroplasty* 2009; 24(5):698-704.
39. Oinuma K, Eingartner C, Saito Y, Shiratsuchi H: Total hip arthroplasty by a minimally invasive, direct anterior approach. *Oper Orthop Traumatol* 2007;19(3): 310-326.
40. Rachbauer F, Kain MS, Leunig M: The history of the anterior approach to the hip. *Orthop Clin North Am* 2009;40(3):311-320.
41. Restrepo C, Mortazavi SM, Brothers J, Parvizi J, Rothman RH: Hip dislocation: Are hip precautions necessary in anterior approaches? *Clin Orthop Relat Res* 2011;469(2):417-422.
42. Restrepo C, Parvizi J, Pour AE, Hozack WJ: Prospective randomized study of two surgical approaches for total hip arthroplasty. *J Arthroplasty* 2010;25(5):671-679, e1.
43. Seng BE, Berend KR, Ajluni AF, Lombardi AV Jr: Anterior-supine minimally invasive total hip arthroplasty: Defining the learning curve. *Orthop Clin North Am* 2009;40(3):343-350.
44. Siguier T, Siguier M, Brumpt B: Mini-incision anterior approach does not increase dislocation rate: A study of 1037 total hip replacements. *Clin Orthop Relat Res* 2004;426:164-173.
45. Yerasimides JG: Use of the Fitmore hip stem bone-preserving system for the minimally invasive anterior-supine approach in hip replacement. *Am J Orthop (Belle Mead NJ)* 2010;39(10):13-16.
46. Mayr E, Nogler M, Benedetti MG, et al: A prospective randomized assessment of earlier functional recovery in THA patients treated by minimally invasive direct anterior approach: A gait analysis study. *Clin Biomech (Bristol, Avon)* 2009;24(10):812-818.
47. Meneghini RM, Pagnano MW, Trousdale RT, Hozack WJ: Muscle damage during MIS total hip arthroplasty: Smith-Petersen versus posterior approach. *Clin Orthop Relat Res* 2006;453:293-298.
48. van Oldenrijk J, Hoogland PV, Tuijthof GJ, Corveleijn R, Noordenbos TW, Schafroth MU: Soft tissue damage after minimally invasive THA. *Acta Orthop* 2010; 81(6):696-702.
49. Cogan A, Klouche S, Mamoudy P, Sariali E: Total hip arthroplasty dislocation rate following isolated cup revision using Hueter's direct anterior approach on a fracture table. *Orthop Traumatol Surg Res* 2011;97(5):501-505.
50. Kołodziej Ł, Bohatyrewicz A, Zietek P: Minimally invasive direct anterior approach for revision total hip arthroplasty. *Chir Narzadow Ruchu Ortop Pol* 2008;73(6): 359-362.
51. Mast NH, Laude F: Revision total hip arthroplasty performed through the Hueter interval. *J Bone Joint Surg Am* 2011; 93(suppl 2):143-148.
52. Benoit B, Gofton W, Beaulé PE: Hueter anterior approach for hip resurfacing: Assessment of the learning curve. *Orthop Clin North Am* 2009;40(3):357-363.
53. Kreuzer S, Leffers K, Kumar S: Direct anterior approach for hip resurfacing: Surgical technique and complications. *Clin Orthop Relat Res* 2011;469(6):1574-1581.
54. Ossendorf C, Scheyerer MJ, Wanner GA, Simmen HP, Werner CM: Treatment of femoral neck fractures in elderly patients over 60 years of age: Which is the ideal modality of primary joint replacement? *Patient Saf Surg* 2010; 4(1):16.
55. Müller M, Tohtz S, Dewey M, Springer I, Perka C: Age-related appearance of muscle trauma in primary total hip arthroplasty and the benefit of a minimally invasive approach for patients older than 70 years. *Int Orthop* 2011;35(2): 165-171.
56. Sculco TP: Anterior approach in THA improves outcomes: Opposes. *Orthopedics* 2011;34(9): e459-e461.
57. Berend KR, Lombardi AV Jr, Mallory TH: Rapid recovery protocol for peri-operative care of total hip and total knee arthroplasty patients. *Surg Technol Int* 2004;13:239-247.
58. Berend KR, Lombardi AV Jr: Multimodal venous thromboem-

bolic disease prevention for patients undergoing primary or revision total joint arthroplasty: The role of aspirin. *Am J Orthop (Belle Mead NJ)* 2006;35(1):24-29.

59. Sariali E, Leonard P, Mamoudy P: Dislocation after total hip arthroplasty using Hueter anterior approach. *J Arthroplasty* 2008;23(2): 266-272.

60. Kennon R, Keggi J, Zatorski LE, Keggi KJ: Anterior approach for total hip arthroplasty: Beyond the minimally invasive technique. *J Bone Joint Surg Am* 2004; 86(suppl 2):91-97.

61. Bhargava T, Goytia RN, Jones LC, Hungerford MW: Lateral femoral cutaneous nerve impairment after direct anterior approach for total hip arthroplasty. *Orthopedics* 2010;33(7):472.

62. Goulding K, Beaulé PE, Kim PR, Fazekas A: Incidence of lateral femoral cutaneous nerve neuropraxia after anterior approach hip arthroplasty. *Clin Orthop Relat Res* 2010;468(9):2397-2404.

63. Ropars M, Morandi X, Huten D, Thomazeau H, Berton E, Darnault P: Anatomical study of the lateral femoral cutaneous nerve with special reference to minimally invasive anterior approach for total hip replacement. *Surg Radiol Anat* 2009;31(3):199-204.

23

Patient Selection for Rotational Pelvic Osteotomy

Cara Beth Lee, MD
Michael B. Millis, MD

Abstract

Acetabular dysplasia is a common cause of hip pain and can lead to premature osteoarthritis. Preserving the native hip is the first choice in young, active patients with minimal arthrosis. Techniques in rotational pelvic osteotomy have evolved to offer long-term benefits, but appropriate patient selection is an important determinant of success. Applying a stepwise approach when evaluating adult patients with acetabular dysplasia and understanding current outcomes and predictive data will allow the orthopaedic surgeon to choose appropriate candidates for pelvic osteotomy.

Instr Course Lect 2013;62:265-277.

Background

Appropriate patient selection is an important factor in the success of any surgical intervention. Many factors, both clinical and nonclinical, contribute to good patient outcomes after periacetabular osteotomy (PAO). Acetabular dysplasia is a common cause of hip pain in young adults. In some regions of the world, it is the single most common cause of osteoarthritis (OA).[1,2] The association between acetabular dysplasia and early OA has been observed for decades. In 1939, Wiberg[3] described the center-edge (CE) angle and reported a direct relationship between low femoral head coverage and the earlier development of OA. Subsequent authors reported acetabular dysplasia in 25% to 50% of patients with so-called primary OA.[2,4,5] In a recent retrospective report, Clohisy et al[6] reported that in 162 of 337 patients (48%) younger than 50 years treated with total hip arthroplasty, acetabular dysplasia was the predisposing factor in their OA. The strong correlation between bony deformity and OA led Harris[7] to question the existence of idiopathic OA and to suggest that if the condition does exist, it is rare.

Few studies describe the natural history of untreated dysplasia. In a series of 286 patients, Murphy et al[8] reported that no patient older than 65 years with a CE angle less than 16° and an acetabular roof index greater than 15° had a well-functioning hip. In contrast, Cooperman et al[9] found no radiographic parameters that were predictive for OA progression in patients with CE angles less than 20°.

Acetabular dysplasia is characterized by a shallow and oblique acetabular weight-bearing zone that provides insufficient coverage to the femoral head. Weight-bearing forces borne by the dysplastic acetabulum result in chondral and rim overload, which can lead to OA. Although this condition primarily affects females, acetabular dysplasia also occurs in males and may have a familial predisposition. Acetabular dysplasia can be a residual finding in patients treated for childhood developmental dysplasia of the hip or a new diagnosis in patients with hip pain in the absence of known childhood hip disease.

The term rotational pelvic osteotomy (RPO) is used to describe several surgical procedures, including PAO, triple pelvic osteotomy, and rotational acetabular osteotomy, which reorient the acetabulum.[10,11] RPOs are technically complex procedures, but the results can dramatically improve the quality of life for well-selected patients. The clinical goals of RPO are to relieve pain, normalize function, and improve the longevity of the native

Neither of the following authors nor any immediate family member has received anything of value from or has stock or stock options in a commercial company or institution related directly or indirectly to the subject of this chapter: Dr. Lee and Dr. Millis.

hip. The anatomic goals are to correct acetabular position and femoral head coverage, increase the weight-bearing area, and improve stability without creating femoroacetabular impingement. The guiding principle is that improvement in hip mechanics will serve to resolve symptoms.

Long-term follow-up studies ranging from 10 to 23 years suggest that good results can be achieved and maintained in younger patients who have minimal arthrosis at the time of surgery.[12-14] Several series have documented that RPO also can be effective in many patients who were previously believed to be at high risk for treatment failure, including older patients and those with severe preoperative pain.[13,15-17] A systematic approach to evaluation and a solid understanding of the variables that can influence outcomes are essential in selecting an optimal treatment program for the patient with symptomatic acetabular dysplasia.

Patient Evaluation

History

In addition to obtaining a general medical, surgical, and social history, the patient interview should screen for systemic symptoms that may indicate a neuromuscular cause of dysplasia, such as Charcot-Marie-Tooth disease or myelomeningocele, which can alter the prognosis. It is beneficial to review prior treatments, particularly physical therapy regimens and injections. A standardized hip questionnaire can yield essential clinical information, which can be supplemented with direct questions from the interviewer. This chapter's authors use a combination of functional outcome instruments, including the University of California Los Angeles (UCLA) activity score, the hip disability and osteoarthritis outcomes score (HOOS), EuroQol-5D, and the Medical Outcomes Study 12-Item Short Form. Regardless of the instrument chosen, it should be validated in the patient population measured and used consistently to assess the response to treatment. It is critical to document the current level of hip function, overall physical function, and the patient's professional and social functional needs, which are the primary factors affecting patient expectations. Because patient satisfaction is largely determined by whether expectations are met (irrespective of the surgeon's assessment of clinical results), early clarification of expectations is essential. It is also beneficial to query patients about their fears and concerns and explain realistic goals for hip preservation. Patients should be counseled that a pelvic osteotomy will not reverse existing joint damage. This procedure improves but often cannot normalize the mechanical environment of the hip. The risk of future joint deterioration and some degree of pain may persist after surgery.

In a study of the clinical presentation of 57 patients (65 hips) with symptomatic acetabular dysplasia, Nunley et al[18] reported that most patients experienced an insidious onset of pain that was exacerbated with activities, and 77% rated their daily pain as moderate to severe. Groin pain was present in 72% of the patients and lateral hip pain in 66%. Because of the combination of abductor weakness and fatigue, patients may report episodes of the hip giving way that accompany lateral hip pain. Groin pain evolves as the labrum becomes stressed and can be associated with locking or catching from an unstable tear, although this is rare. Catching and popping sensations are more commonly caused by extra-articular sources, such as the iliopsoas riding over the iliopectineal eminence or the iliotibial band at the greater trochanter. Buttock pain is rarely caused by dysplasia, although femoroacetabular impingement may be associated with buttock or posterior hip symptoms.

Physical Examination

A general physical examination should be performed in every patient with hip pain, with particular attention paid to the neurologic, circulatory, and skin evaluations, as well as the overall musculoskeletal assessment. This screening process may reveal systemic disorders that affect results, such as Ehlers-Danlos syndrome, Charcot-Marie-Tooth disease, or spinal deformity.

Having the patient wear shorts for the physical examination enables direct visualization and freedom of movement of the lower extremities and pelvis. The hip examination begins by assessing gait; any limp must be characterized. Abductor weakness may be present, or the gait may be truly antalgic. Standing alignment should be observed in coronal and sagittal planes. Pelvic obliquity suggests scoliosis, limb-length discrepancy, or abductor weakness. A delayed positive Trendelenburg test, observed when the patient is unable to hold the pelvis level for 30 seconds, indicates subtle abductor weakness that may not be appreciable with gait assessment.[19]

Passive range of hip motion is measured supine in full extension and at 90° of hip flexion. Motion evaluation should be performed slowly. Subtle compensatory pelvic or lumbar spine motion can falsely increase the apparent motion of the hip joint. Limited motion suggests mechanical or joint congruity issues that may compromise the result. RPOs routinely involve anterior and lateral redirection of the acetabulum, which may reduce flexion and abduction.

Several special tests are used to screen for impingement, dysplasia, and abductor fatigue. The anterior impingement test assesses pain with compression of the anterior rim structures by the anterior femoral head-neck junction. The maneuver involves flexion beyond 90° and adduction and internal rotation; a positive test is indicated by pain in the groin. This test is not specific for labral tears, but it is usually positive if the labrum or rim are damaged.[20,21] In a study of 57 skeletally mature patients with acetabular dysplasia, Nunley et al[18] reported that 97% of the patients had a positive impingement sign, nearly 50% had a limp, and almost 40% had a positive Trendelenburg sign. Steppacher et al[13] identified preoperative limp and a positive anterior impingement test as factors predictive of a poor outcome after PAO.

The anterior apprehension test maneuver uses passive extension, adduction, and external rotation to stress the anterior rim structures with the anteriorly directed femoral head while the contralateral hip is hyperflexed to the chest. The test is positive if the patient experiences anterior hip pain or a sense of apprehension. This test is nonspecific, but it is useful for detecting rim damage. If the discomfort is located in the posterior hip or buttock, posterior impingement is suggested. With the contralateral hip hyperflexed to the chest, the examiner can use the Thomas test to evaluate for hip flexion contracture of the symptomatic hip; this flexion contracture may be present in the dysplastic hip with advanced OA.

With the patient in a side-lying position, the Ober test is performed to assess iliotibial band tightness, and the bicycle test can identify subtle abductor weakness or inefficiency. For this test, the upper leg is moved actively with a bicycle-riding motion while in slight abduction and with downward resistance applied to the midthigh by the examiner. A positive test is indicated by either pain in the groin or the lateral hip or local tenderness at the posterior greater trochanter. The side-lying position is the most valid and reliable placement to perform manual assessment of hip abductor strength.[22] The physical examination assessments for a patient with symptomatic acetabular dysplasia are summarized in **Table 1**.

Table 1
Physical Examination of a Patient With Dysplasia

Patient Position	Assessment
Standing	Assessment of gait and stance (pelvic obliquity, leg lengths, and spine evaluation) Trendelenburg test Toe-touch and other hypermobility tests
Supine	Hip range of motion Anterior impingement test Anterior apprehension test Lower extremity neurologic and circulatory examination
Side-lying	Trochanteric and piriformis palpation Manual hip abduction strength testing Ober test Bicycle test

It can be challenging to differentiate intra-articular hip pain from periarticular soft-tissue sources or referred pain from the lumbar spine. In equivocal cases, differential injections can be useful in determining the source of pain. Increasingly, this can be accomplished with in-office ultrasound.[23] The differential injection technique is used at Children's Hospital of Boston by asking the patient to grade his or her pain on a scale of 0 to 10 while performing provocative tests of the hip, such as the impingement test. With ultrasound guidance, a combination of short- and long-acting local anesthetic is injected in an area that is suspected of being a source of pain, typically the iliopsoas sheath. After 15 minutes, the provocative tests and pain scoring are reported. If a patient has complete pain relief from the first injection, the procedure is stopped. If pain relief is incomplete, the patient is given an intra-articular injection followed by a repeat examination after 15 minutes.

Imaging

Radiography

Appropriate imaging is critical to assess a patient with acetabular dysplasia who is being considered for pelvic osteotomy.[24] Radiographic evaluation begins with a well-centered, AP pelvic view with proper pelvic tilt.[25] The center of the sacrum and coccyx should be in line with the pubic symphysis. Siebenrock et al[26] reported an average distance from the superior border of the pubic symphysis to the sacrococcygeal joint of 32 mm in men and 47 mm in women. Most clinicians consider distances of 2 to 5 cm within an acceptable range for pelvic tilt on an AP radiograph. Moving from supine to standing, the pelvis extends (reclines), which can alter measurements of acetabular coverage and joint space width on plane radiographs.[27] Troelsen et al[28] recommended standing AP pelvic images to assess functional joint space width and quantify acetabular parameters in dysplasia.

Two measures obtained from the AP pelvic view are the lateral CE angle and the acetabular roof or Tönnis angle.[3,29] Normal lateral CE values are 25° to 35°, with less than 20° considered dysplastic. A normal Tönnis angle

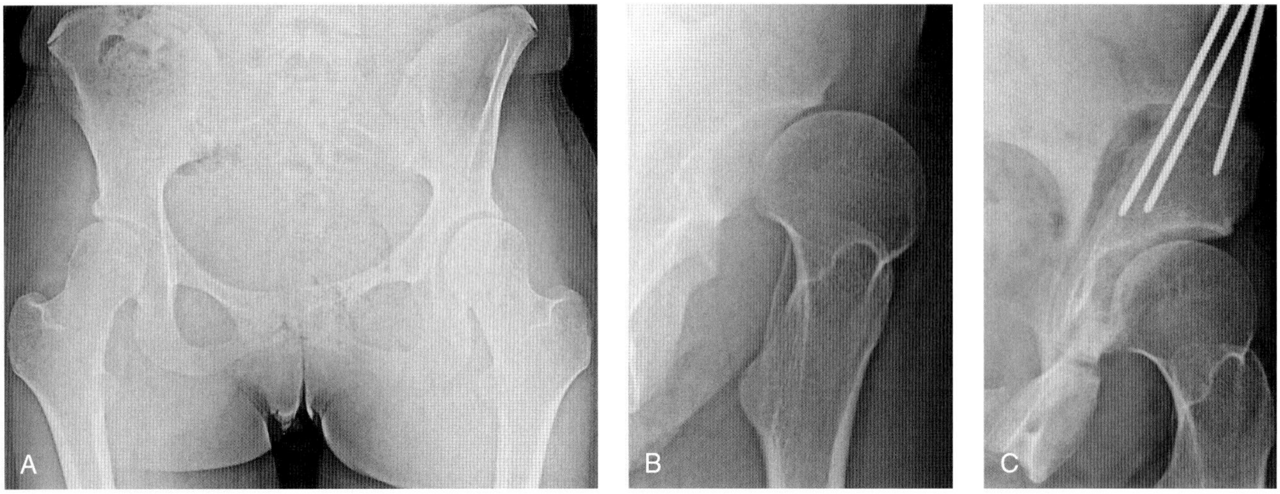

Figure 1 **A,** AP radiograph of the pelvis of a 16-year-old girl with mild bilateral acetabular dysplasia. **B,** False profile view of the same patient shows severe anterior acetabular deficiency with subluxation. **C,** False profile view after PAO showing correction of subluxation and anterior coverage.

is between 0° to 10°. Dysplastic hips have a steeper roof, with Tönnis angles greater than 10°. The Shenton line, which describes the arc from the superior obturator foramen to the medial inferior femoral neck, should retain a smooth contour in the normal hip.[30] Disruption of the Shenton line of greater than 5 mm indicates dysplasia with femoral head subluxation. On a well-positioned AP image, a positive crossover sign or ischial spine sign may indicate acetabular retroversion.[31,32] The ischial spine sign is less affected by tilt.[33] In a normal hip, the posterior wall of the acetabulum aligns with the center of the femoral head on an AP image. The posterior wall sign is considered positive if the rim of the wall is medial to the center of the femoral head.[31] This reflects inadequate posterior coverage that can be associated with retroversion or a globally dysplastic acetabulum.

In addition to decreased lateral femoral head coverage, acetabular dysplasia can involve isolated anterior deficiency, which is detected on a false profile view[34] (**Figure 1**). This image is a lateral view of the acetabulum, tangential to the anterior rim, that is sensitive for identifying mild dysplasia or decreased joint space not evident on the AP view.[35] The image is taken with the patient standing, with the affected hip against the cassette and the ipsilateral foot parallel to it. The pelvis is rotated 65° away from the cassette, and the beam is centered on the femoral head with a tube-to-film distance of 40 inches (90 cm). In a properly positioned false profile view, the center of the femoral head and the axes of the femoral neck and shaft are in the same vertical plane, and the distance between the two femoral heads is equivalent to two thirds up to the full diameter of the affected femoral head.[35] The intersection of a vertical line through the center of the femoral head and a second line from the center of the head to the anterior edge of the sclerotic weight-bearing zone of the acetabulum determines the anterior (or vertical) CE angle. Comparable to the lateral CE angle, the normal anterior CE angle ranges between 25° to 35°, with less than 20° considered dysplastic.[34]

Functional radiographs simulate the position of the hip and joint congruence after acetabular reorientation. The abduction-internal rotation or von Rosen view,[36] an AP image taken with the patient supine and both legs in maximum abduction and internal rotation, shows lateral coverage and congruence (**Figure 2**). A false profile view obtained with the hip in flexion shows the expected anterior coverage. Incongruity or joint space narrowing on functional views predicts a poor result after PAO.[37] Radiographic joint congruence is graded as poor, fair, good, or excellent based on the curvature of the femoral head and acetabulum.[38] The congruence is graded excellent if the two surfaces are identical and there is no joint space narrowing; good if the joint space is maintained, although the curvature is not identical; fair if there is narrowing; and poor if joint space obliteration is present.

Acetabular dysplasia is commonly associated with proximal femoral abnormalities such as coxa valga, femoral anteversion, and femoral head deformity. With increased awareness of femoroacetabular impingement, it is now recognized that more than 70% of patients with acetabular dysplasia also have an aspheric femoral head or decreased femoral head-neck offset.[39] Increased anterior coverage after a pelvic

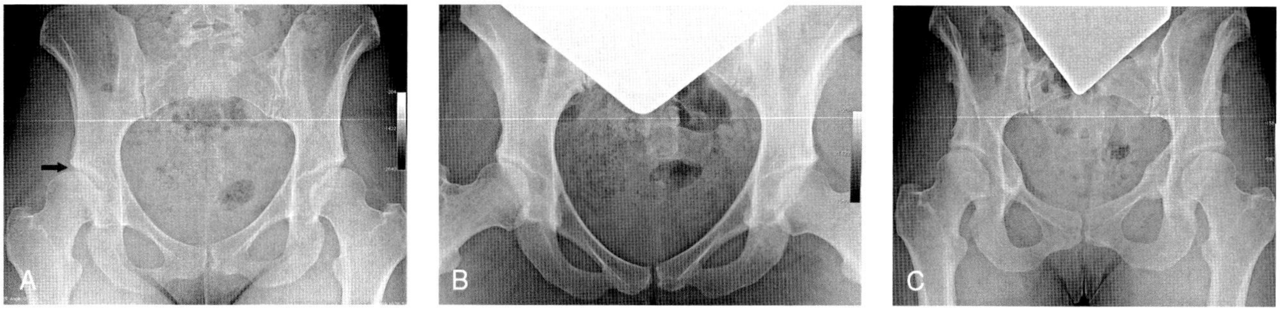

Figure 2 **A,** AP radiograph of a 29-year-old woman with symptomatic bilateral acetabular dysplasia. Note the joint-space narrowing (arrow). **B,** Abduction internal radiograph showing increased joint space on the right and good congruence bilaterally. **C,** AP radiograph 2.2 years after a right PAO and 1.5 years after a left PAO; the patient is symptom free.

osteotomy can lead to impingement.[40] It is important to assess the femoral morphology of the dysplastic hip. A lateral radiograph is best able to detect femoral head-neck deformities, although the diagnostic superiority of particular views is debated.[41,42] The frog-leg lateral and cross-table lateral views are commonly obtained, but the false profile and 45° Dunn lateral views are also helpful in detecting abnormal femoral head-neck offset. The 45° Dunn lateral radiograph is taken supine with the affected hip positioned in 45° flexion with 20° abduction and neutral rotation. The beam is directed at a point midway between the pubic symphysis and the anterior superior iliac spine with a tube-to-cassette distance of 40 inches (90 cm). Using MRI radial views as the standard, Domayer et al[43] found that the 45° Dunn view had more than 96% sensitivity for detecting a cam lesion in the superior-anterior femoral head-neck junction where most cam lesions occur. Based on their results, the authors recommended that the 45° Dunn view be included as first-line imaging for impingement. Imaging recommendations for a patient with symptomatic acetabular dysplasia are listed in **Table 2**.

Table 2
Radiographic Evaluation Before Rotational Pelvic Osteotomy

Supine and standing AP pelvic radiographs
False profile view(s)
Functional radiographs (abduction-internal rotation view, false profile view with hip flexion)
45° Dunn lateral (alternatively, cross-table or frog-leg lateral) view
MRI with femoral versional assessment and radial views
If early arthrosis present, consider dGEMRIC study, if available

Computed Tomography

CT has greatly improved the understanding of normal and dysplastic pelvic anatomy. CT scans can be reformatted in various planes to yield a more accurate and comprehensive depiction of bony structure compared with two-dimensional radiographs.

Klaue et al[44] were the first investigators to use CT to simulate surgical correction of femoral head coverage as a component of surgical planning for pelvic and femoral osteotomies. The authors used a three-dimensional graphics program to create a topographic map of the acetabulum and femoral head from overlapping contours on serial axial images. Murphy et al[45] similarly depicted femoral head coverage with surface contour maps and established that dysplasia involves global rather than isolated anterolateral acetabular deficiency, as had previously been believed. Janzen et al[46] described a CT method to measure CE angles in 10° increments circumferentially around the acetabular rim, and Haddad et al[47] used the technique to generate a graphic comparison of femoral head coverage before and after PAO. Ito et al[48] reported good correlation of the CE and acetabular roof angles measured with three-dimensional CT and conventional radiographs. However, because of the wide range in the degree and location of acetabular deficiency, the authors recommended three-dimensional CT over conventional CT to individualize the surgical plan.

CT is a powerful tool for assessing bony anatomy, but errors similar to those seen with plane radiography can occur. The patient's position in the gantry determines pelvic obliquity and tilt, which can alter measurements of the acetabulum.[49] Positional correction after image acquisition requires three-dimensional reformatting, which is not routinely performed with standard CT studies.[50,51] Radiation exposure and the risk of radiation-associated cancers are the principal

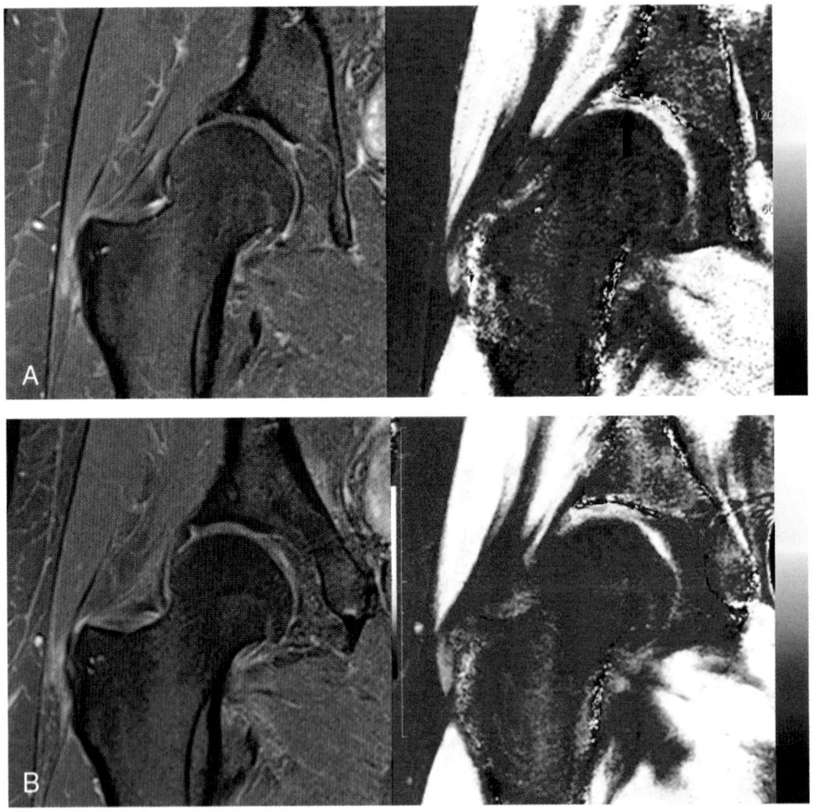

Figure 3 **A,** Preoperative, coronal, fat-saturated MRI scan (left) and corresponding dGEMRIC T1 map image (right) of the right hip of the patient described in Figure 2. Note the zone of low GAG content (arrow). **B,** Postoperative MRI (left) and dGEMRIC images (right) at 2.2 years after PAO. The GAG content values have improved.

deterrents to CT for patients with acetabular dysplasia.[52] This is a particular concern in the population of young, predominantly female patients for whom the risks are highest.[53] At Children's Hospital of Boston, CT is not routinely used in the preoperative analysis of hip dysplasia or femoroacetabular impingement.

Magnetic Resonance Imaging

MRI provides a comprehensive evaluation of bony anatomy as well as excellent detail of soft tissues and intra-articular structures.[54] Radial views are useful to measure femoral head-neck offset and may detect subtle deformities and labral pathology not evident on radiographs.[55-58] Although subject to positional errors similar to CT, acetabular version can be measured with axial views through the roof of the acetabulum. Femoral version can be determined from axial cuts through the center of the femoral neck and at the level of the femoral condyles.[59]

Magnetic resonance arthrography is the gold standard for detecting labral damage but must be interpreted with caution because of a higher false-positive rate than noncontrast MRI.[60-63] Although newer techniques using higher field resolution and small pixel size enable visualization of labral and cartilage pathology without contrast, the sensitivity to identify early cartilage damage and acetabular chondral delamination is lacking.[64-68]

Biochemical MRI

A key factor in the success of RPO is the degree of arthrosis at the time of surgery. Techniques in biochemical MRI are improving the ability to detect cartilage degeneration before it is evident with standard MRI or plain radiography. Delayed gadolinium-enhanced MRI of cartilage (dGEMRIC), T2 mapping, and T1rho mapping are currently the three most clinically used modalities for assessing cartilage in the hip. In general, biochemical MRI reflects the layered structure and molecular composition of cartilage.[69]

Delayed Gadolinium-Enhanced MRI of Cartilage

A decrease in proteoglycan concentration is one of the first events in articular cartilage degeneration.[70] In a dGEMRIC study, gadolinium pentetate was used as an intravenously administered ion probe to measure the concentration of the highly negatively charged glycosaminoglycan (GAG) molecules that compose proteoglycan.[71] After image acquisition, a T1 map was created that enabled quantitative assessment of GAG content reported as a dGEMRIC index (**Figure 3**). Thus, dGEMRIC is sensitive to early changes of OA as reflected by lower dGEMRIC values. Both hips can be imaged with one intravenous contrast injection. This is helpful for patients with bilateral involvement, which commonly occurs in dysplasia. The primary disadvantage of dGEMRIC compared with T2 and T1rho mapping is the risk associated with a gadolinium injection, which is contraindicated in patients with renal impairment.

Kim et al[72] found that dGEMRIC is a better indicator of early OA than plain radiographs in patients with acetabular dysplasia, and the dGEMRIC index correlates with pain and the severity of dysplasia. In a subsequent report, the dGEMRIC index was the most important predictor of short-term to midterm outcomes after PAO compared with standard MRI, radiography, and clinical measures.[73] Of the biochemical MRI modalities in clinical use, dGEMRIC has been the most widely studied, particularly for hip disorders. It can identify early cartilage degeneration and demonstrate patterns of articular damage in femoral acetabular impingement, Legg-Calvé-Perthes disease, and slipped capital femoral epiphysis.[74-77]

T2 and T2 Mapping*

T2 relaxation times reflect the interaction between water molecules and collagen; T2 mapping is a visual depiction of the layered architecture of articular cartilage.[78] As cartilage degrades, there is an increase in water content and disruption of the highly organized structure that corresponds with an increased T2 signal and alteration of the normal zonal gradation of the T2 map.[79,80] T2* mapping is a newer technique with the benefits of a shorter imaging time and the ability to obtain three-dimensional images. The drawback of T2* mapping is that there is a higher susceptibility to foreign body particles and artifacts at the bone-cartilage border compared with standard T2 mapping.[81] Because T2 mapping is unaffected by changes in proteoglycan content, it does not detect the earliest stages of OA.[82]

T1rho Mapping

T1rho is sensitive to changes in collagen structure and water content, as well as the proteoglycan concentration.[83] Because T1rho is influenced by alterations in multiple tissues, these competing effects make accurate interpretation of T1rho values difficult and prone to error.[84] Nevertheless, T1rho mapping is a promising, noninvasive modality that has increasingly been shown to provide an accurate measure of early OA.[85,86]

Predictors of Outcome: Identifying the Ideal Patient

Long-Term Results

Siebenrock et al[87] reported the outcomes of 71 hips at an average follow-up of 11.3 years from an original cohort of 75 dysplastic hips (63 patients) treated with PAO. The native hip was preserved in 58 of 71 hips (82%), with good-to-excellent results in 52 of 58 retained hips (90%). Older patient age (≥ 30 years) at surgery and increasing grades of arthritis and labral pathology were preoperative predictors of poor results. In a 20-year follow-up of this patient group, Steppacher et al[13] reported that 60% of the hips were preserved. The mean Merle d'Aubigné and Postel scores (measures of pain, hip flexion, and walking ability)[88] had decreased relative to the 10-year average and were comparable to preoperative values. In addition to older patient age, which was noted in the 10-year follow-up, four preoperative variables correlated with worse outcomes: limp, a preoperative OA Tönnis grade of 2 or more,[29] a positive anterior impingement sign,[1] and lower preoperative Merle d'Aubigné and Postel scores. Preoperative measures that were not predictive of outcome were sex, range of motion, and walking ability. Body mass index also was not correlated with outcomes in this series, but it was a risk factor for the development of OA at a mean of 5 years after eccentric rotational acetabular osteotomy in another report.[89]

Nakamura et al[14] reviewed the long-term outcomes of rotational acetabular osteotomy in 145 hips in 131 patients with a mean age of 28 years (at the time of surgery) at an average follow-up of 13 years. The authors reported good-to-excellent results in 90 of 112 hips (80%) that had early-stage preoperative OA, compared with 9 of 33 hips (27%) that had advanced preoperative OA.

In a study of 109 patients (135 hips) at an average follow-up of 9 years after PAO, Matheney et al[90] reported that 102 of 135 hips (76%) were preserved, whereas 33 (24%) met the criteria for failure as defined by a Western Ontario and McMaster Universities Osteoarthritis Index pain score of 10 or greater or the need for total hip arthroplasty. The two independent predictors of failure were preoperative age older than 35 years and poor to fair preoperative joint congruency. The probability of failure was 95% for patients who were older than 35 years and had less than good joint congruency, whereas the probability was 36% with one factor, and 14% if neither factor was present.

Discussion

The ideal candidate for RPO is younger than 30 years; does not have severe pain; and has a body mass index less than 25, good range of motion, a negative impingement sign, no limp, minimal or no radiographic arthrosis, good to excellent congruence on functional imaging, and less severe dysplastic measurements. The ideal patient also should have reasonable postoperative functional expectations and a clear understanding concerning the demands of the procedure. The patient must be willing to comply with the prolonged use of crutches, be committed to a rehabilitation program that may require 1 year to regain preoperative hip strength,[91] and accept that hip motion may be decreased after surgery.[92] The variables predictive of good outcomes after RPO are listed in **Table 3**.

The Less-Than-Ideal Patient

Rarely will a patient meet all the criteria to be considered an ideal candidate for RPO. The orthopaedic surgeon

Table 3
Criteria Predictive of Good Results After RPO

Age younger than 30 years
Body mass index less than 25
No severe pain
No limp
Negative anterior impingement sign
Good range of motion (flexion > 90°, abduction > 25°)
Minimal radiographic arthrosis (Tönnis grade 0 to 1)
Less severe dysplasia (lateral CE angle > 0°, anterior CE angle > 5°)
Good or excellent congruence on functional views
Absence of femoral head deformity and os acetabulum

also must formulate a treatment plan for those patients whose clinical parameters are borderline for success, such as older patients and those with moderate OA.

Older Age

In the reports associating poor results with older patients, age may be a proxy for joint damage. Three studies that specifically address age and outcome indicate that RPO can be successful in older patients with minimal arthrosis. Millis et al[17] reported improved pain and function in patients older than 40 years (mean, 43.6 years) with OA (Tönnis grades 0 to 1) at the time of surgery. The risk of conversion to total hip arthroplasty was 27% for patients with Tönnis grade 2 changes compared with 12% for those with grades 0 or 1 at 5 years after PAO. Yasunaga et al[15] compared the results of rotational acetabular osteotomy between a group of patients older than 45 years and a group 45 years or younger. Improvement in radiographic and clinical measures occurred in both groups at a mean 8.2 years after surgery. Survivorship analysis predicted a 10-year survival rate of 70.0% in the older group and 93.7% in the younger group. Yamaguchi et al[16] reported similar findings in a comparison of a group of patients older than 50 years with a group younger than 50 years. The two groups had similar improvement in functional scores, but 15-year hip survivorship was 71% in the older group compared with 81% in the younger group.

Osteoarthritis

Many patients present with early stages of arthrosis or labral deterioration because this damage precipitates the symptoms that prompt patients to seek care. A minimum joint space width greater than 2 mm is essential to consider RPO.[93] Functional radiographs and specialized tests, such as biochemical MRI, can guide the prognosis in patients with established OA.[37,73]

Okano et al[94] evaluated 90 hips in patients with early OA and an average age of 32.5 years at the time of rotational acetabular osteotomy; 76 hips had no change in OA grade, and 14 hips had OA progression at a mean of 12 years after surgery. Only 6 of 82 hips with good or excellent preoperative congruency showed radiographic progression of OA, and 5 of these 6 hips had a femoral head deformity. OA progressed in all 8 hips with only fair congruence. Measurements of the CE angle and acetabular head index on the preoperative abduction-internal rotation views showed substantial differences between the two groups. The patients with no progression of OA had an average CE angle of 34.8° and an acetabular head index of 88.6% compared with 24.3° and 79.9%, respectively, in the group with OA progression.

Although their study was limited by a small number of patients, Murphy and Deshmukh[37] reported similar success in patients with OA in whom joint space narrowing (evident on the AP radiograph) improved in the von Rosen view taken in abduction-internal rotation, which simulates the relationship between the femoral head and the acetabulum after osteotomy. There was one failure in eight hips with Tönnis grade 3 OA at a minimum 2-year follow-up after PAO. The one failure showed joint space narrowing on the preoperative von Rosen view, whereas the remaining seven hips had retained joint space on this image. Four of 43 hips with Tönnis grades 1 or 2 OA failed, 2 of which had limited preoperative motion.

Of the available biochemical MRI techniques, only dGEMRIC has been investigated with RPO. In a prospective cohort study of 47 patients treated with PAO for hip dysplasia, Cunningham et al[73] reported lower preoperative dGEMRIC scores and joint subluxation (> 5 mm break in the Shenton line) to be important predictors of failure as defined by a Western Ontario and McMaster Universities Osteoarthritis Index pain score greater than 10 or a minimum joint space less than 3 mm. There were no differences between the groups in preoperative or postoperative anterior or lateral CE angles or the Tönnis angle. Multivariate analysis identified the dGEMRIC index as the most important predictor of osteotomy failure. The authors suggested that MRI has little benefit for patients with no radiographic evidence of OA (Tönnis grade 0) because there were no failures in this group. How-

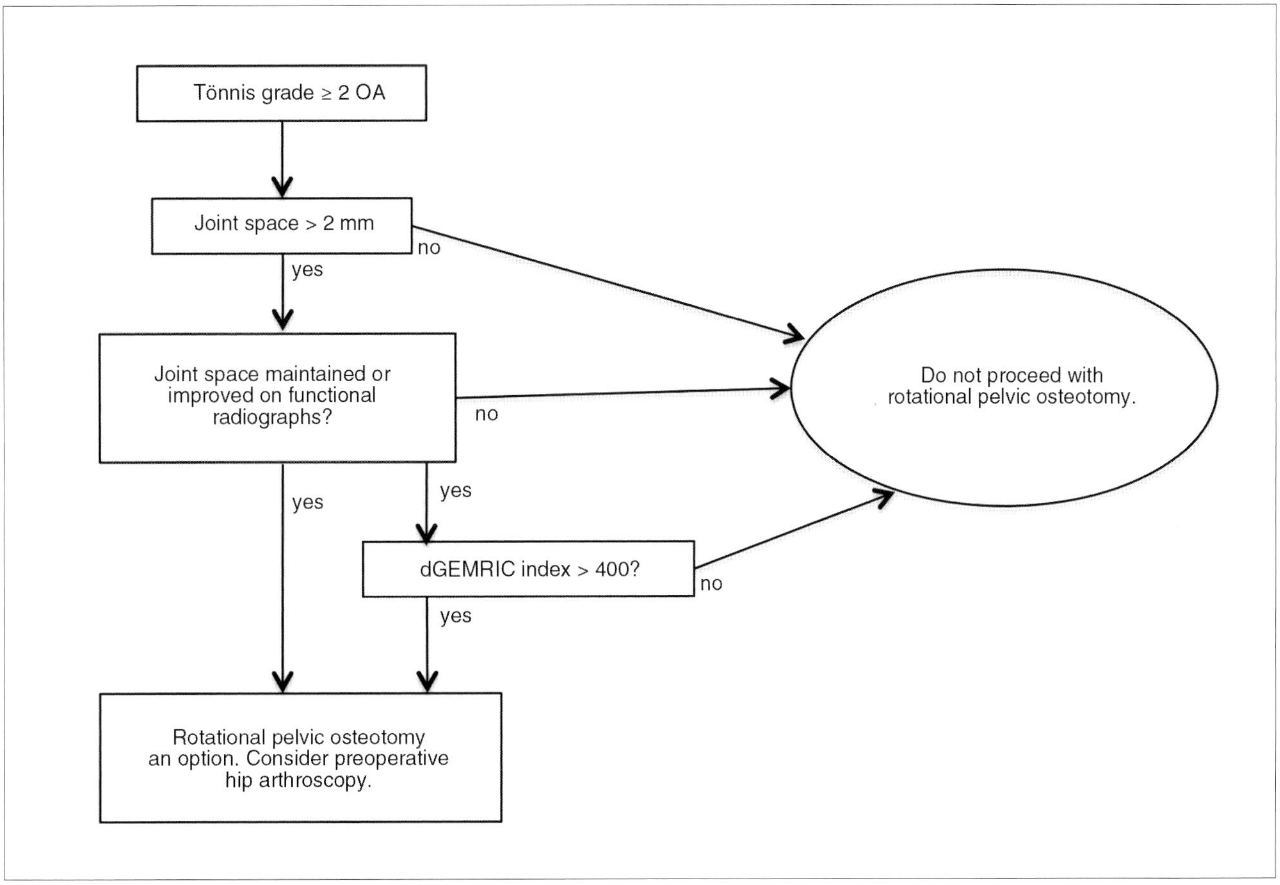

Figure 4 Algorithm for assisting decision making for RPO in patients with established OA.

ever, they advocated the role of dGEMRIC for hips with mild OA on plain radiographs because it may identify patients who are likely to have a poor outcome based on the dGEMRIC scores.

Increasingly, arthroscopy is used in conjunction with RPO[95] and may be beneficial in patients with borderline OA. If joint damage is more severe than expected, the pelvic osteotomy can be aborted. Yasunaga et al[38] reported radiographic progression of OA at short-term follow-up in 4 of 12 hips with arthroscopically observed Outerbridge grade 4 damage at the time of the rotational acetabular osteotomy. At a mean follow-up of 9.9 years, Fujii et al[96] reported on 121 patients (121 hips) who had rotational acetabular osteotomy combined with arthroscopy at an average age of 40.2 years. The authors reported that advanced intra-articular lesions, particularly exposure of femoral subchondral bone, were an independent risk factor for progression of OA, even in hips with only early stages of radiographic OA. **Figure 4** is an algorithm to assist decision making for RPO in patients with established OA.

Summary

Preserving the native hip is the first choice in the young, active patient with correctable dysplasia before the onset of moderate to severe arthrosis. Appropriate realignment can often yield decades of good hip function. The best long-term results are reported for patients with congruous dysplasia who are younger than 35 years with mild to moderate pain. Free motion, no anterior impingement sign, and no limp are favorable findings on physical examination. Radiographic imaging should include supine and standing AP pelvic, false profile, 45° Dunn lateral, and functional abduction-internal rotation views. In many instances, a dedicated hip MRI with radial imaging and cuts through the acetabulum and femoral condyles is useful to assess the labrum, articular cartilage, and version.

Favorable imaging findings include spherically congruous acetabular dysplasia with anterior and lateral CE angles not less than 0°, reduction of any subluxation on the abduction view, and minimal to no arthrosis. Favorable MRI findings include the absence of labral tear and normal cartilage structure and health. If factors predictive of poor outcome are present, alternative therapies can be considered. In the patient with questionable indications and early radiographic arthrosis, biochemical MRI may be useful, with techniques such as dGEMRIC allowing more accurate assessment of the prognosis than radiography. Arthroscopy, either staged or at the time of the planned RPO, can be done to determine the status of the articular cartilage in borderline cases.

References

1. Inoue K, Wicart P, Kawasaki T, et al: Prevalence of hip osteoarthritis and acetabular dysplasia in french and Japanese adults. *Rheumatology (Oxford)* 2000;39(7):745-748.
2. Aronson J: Osteoarthritis of the young adult hip: Etiology and treatment. *Instr Course Lect* 1986; 35:119-128.
3. Wiberg G: Studies on dysplastic acetabula and congenital subluxation of the hip joint with special reference to the complication osteoarthritis. *Acta Chir Scand* 1939;83(suppl 58):5-135.
4. Murray RO: The aetiology of primary osteoarthritis of the hip. *Br J Radiol* 1965;38(455): 810-824.
5. Stulberg SC: A major cause of idiopathic osteoarthritis of the hip, in Cordell LD, Harris WH, Ramsey PL, MacEwen GD, eds: *The Hip: Proceedings of the Third Open Scientific Meeting of the Hip Society*. St. Louis, MO, CV Mosby, 1975, pp 212-228.
6. Clohisy JC, Dobson MA, Robison JF, et al: Radiographic structural abnormalities associated with premature, natural hip-joint failure. *J Bone Joint Surg Am* 2011; 93(suppl 2):3-9.
7. Harris WH: Etiology of osteoarthritis of the hip. *Clin Orthop Relat Res* 1986;213:20-33.
8. Murphy SB, Ganz R, Müller ME: The prognosis in untreated dysplasia of the hip: A study of radiographic factors that predict the outcome. *J Bone Joint Surg Am* 1995;77(7):985-989.
9. Cooperman DR, Wallensten R, Stulberg SD: Acetabular dysplasia in the adult. *Clin Orthop Relat Res* 1983;175:79-85.
10. Ganz R, Klaue K, Vinh TS, Mast JW: A new periacetabular osteotomy for the treatment of hip dysplasias: Technique and preliminary results. *Clin Orthop Relat Res* 1988;232:26-36.
11. Ninomiya S, Tagawa H: Rotational acetabular osteotomy for the dysplastic hip. *J Bone Joint Surg Am* 1984;66(3):430-436.
12. van Hellemondt GG, Sonneveld H, Schreuder MH, Kooijman MA, de Kleuver M: Triple osteotomy of the pelvis for acetabular dysplasia: Results at a mean follow-up of 15 years. *J Bone Joint Surg Br* 2005;87(7):911-915.
13. Steppacher SD, Tannast M, Ganz R, Siebenrock KA: Mean 20-year followup of Bernese periacetabular osteotomy. *Clin Orthop Relat Res* 2008;466(7):1633-1644.
14. Nakamura S, Ninomiya S, Takatori Y, Morimoto S, Umeyama T: Long-term outcome of rotational acetabular osteotomy: 145 hips followed for 10-23 years. *Acta Orthop Scand* 1998;69(3): 259-265.
15. Yasunaga Y, Takahashi K, Ochi M, et al: Rotational acetabular osteotomy in patients forty-six years of age or older: Comparison with younger patients. *J Bone Joint Surg Am* 2003;85(2): 266-272.
16. Yamaguchi J, Hasegawa Y, Kanoh T, Seki T, Kawabe K: Similar survival of eccentric rotational acetabular osteotomy in patients younger and older than 50 years. *Clin Orthop Relat Res* 2009; 467(10):2630-2637.
17. Millis MB, Kain M, Sierra R, et al: Periacetabular osteotomy for acetabular dysplasia in patients older than 40 years: A preliminary study. *Clin Orthop Relat Res* 2009; 467(9):2228-2234.
18. Nunley RM, Prather H, Hunt D, Schoenecker PL, Clohisy JC: Clinical presentation of symptomatic acetabular dysplasia in skeletally mature patients. *J Bone Joint Surg Am* 2011;93(suppl 2):17-21.
19. Hardcastle P, Nade S: The significance of the Trendelenburg test. *J Bone Joint Surg Br* 1985;67(5): 741-746.
20. Klaue K, Durnin CW, Ganz R: The acetabular rim syndrome: A clinical presentation of dysplasia of the hip. *J Bone Joint Surg Br* 1991;73(3):423-429.
21. Macdonald SJ, Garbuz D, Ganz R: Clinical evaluation of the symptomatic young adult hip. *Semin Arthroplasty* 1997;8:3-9.
22. Widler KS, Glatthorn JF, Bizzini M, et al: Assessment of hip abductor muscle strength: A validity and reliability study. *J Bone Joint Surg Am* 2009;91(11):2666-2672.
23. Smith J, Hurdle MF: Office-based ultrasound-guided intra-articular hip injection: Technique for physiatric practice. *Arch Phys Med Rehabil* 2006;87(2):296-298.
24. Clohisy JC, Carlisle JC, Beaulé PE, et al: A systematic approach to the plain radiographic evaluation of the young adult hip. *J Bone Joint Surg Am* 2008; 90(suppl 4):47-66.
25. Tannast M, Zheng G, Anderegg C, et al: Tilt and rotation correction of acetabular version on pelvic radiographs. *Clin Orthop Relat Res* 2005;438:182-190.
26. Siebenrock KA, Kalbermatten DF, Ganz R: Effect of pelvic tilt on acetabular retroversion: A study of pelves from cadavers. *Clin Orthop Relat Res* 2003;407: 241-248.

27. Fuchs-Winkelmann S, Peterlein C-D, Tibesku CO, Weinstein SL: Comparison of pelvic radiographs in weightbearing and supine positions. *Clin Orthop Relat Res* 2008; 466(4):809-812.
28. Troelsen A, Jacobsen S, Rømer L, Søballe K: Weightbearing anteroposterior pelvic radiographs are recommended in DDH assessment. *Clin Orthop Relat Res* 2008; 466(4):813-819.
29. Tonnis D: *Congenital Dysplasia and Dislocation of the Hip in Children and Adults*. New York, NY, Springer, 1987.
30. Shenton E: *Disease in Bone and Its Detection by X-Rays*. London, England, Macmillan, 1911.
31. Reynolds D, Lucas J, Klaue K: Retroversion of the acetabulum: A cause of hip pain. *J Bone Joint Surg Br* 1999;81(2):281-288.
32. Kalberer F, Sierra RJ, Madan SS, Ganz R, Leunig M: Ischial spine projection into the pelvis: A new sign for acetabular retroversion. *Clin Orthop Relat Res* 2008; 466(3):677-683.
33. Kakaty DK, Fischer AF, Hosalkar HS, Siebenrock KA, Tannast M: The ischial spine sign: Does pelvic tilt and rotation matter? *Clin Orthop Relat Res* 2010;468(3): 769-774.
34. Lequesne M, de SEZE: False profile of the pelvis: A new radiographic incidence for the study of the hip. Its use in dysplasias and different coxopathies. *Rev Rhum Mal Osteoartic* 1961;28:643-652.
35. Lequesne MG, Laredo JD: The faux profil (oblique view) of the hip in the standing position: Contribution to the evaluation of osteoarthritis of the adult hip. *Ann Rheum Dis* 1998;57(11):676-681.
36. Andren L, Von Rosen S: The diagnosis of dislocation of the hip in newborns and the primary results of immediate treatment. *Acta Radiol* 1958;49(2):89-95.
37. Murphy S, Deshmukh R: Periacetabular osteotomy: Preoperative radiographic predictors of outcome. *Clin Orthop Relat Res* 2002; 405:168-174.
38. Yasunaga Y, Ikuta Y, Kanazawa T, Takahashi K, Hisatome T: The state of the articular cartilage at the time of surgery as an indication for rotational acetabular osteotomy. *J Bone Joint Surg Br* 2001;83(7):1001-1004.
39. Clohisy JC, Nunley RM, Carlisle JC, Schoenecker PL: Incidence and characteristics of femoral deformities in the dysplastic hip. *Clin Orthop Relat Res* 2009; 467(1):128-134.
40. Myers SR, Eijer H, Ganz R: Anterior femoroacetabular impingement after periacetabular osteotomy. *Clin Orthop Relat Res* 1999;363:93-99.
41. Clohisy JC, Nunley RM, Otto RJ, Schoenecker PL: The frog-leg lateral radiograph accurately visualized hip cam impingement abnormalities. *Clin Orthop Relat Res* 2007;462:115-121.
42. Meyer DC, Beck M, Ellis T, Ganz R, Leunig M: Comparison of six radiographic projections to assess femoral head/neck asphericity. *Clin Orthop Relat Res* 2006;445: 181-185.
43. Domayer SE, Ziebarth K, Chan J, Bixby S, Mamisch TC, Kim YJ: Femoroacetabular cam-type impingement: Diagnostic sensitivity and specificity of radiographic views compared to radial MRI. *Eur J Radiol* 2011;80(3):805-810.
44. Klaue K, Wallin A, Ganz R: CT evaluation of coverage and congruency of the hip prior to osteotomy. *Clin Orthop Relat Res* 1988;232:15-25.
45. Murphy SB, Kijewski PK, Millis MB, Harless A: Acetabular dysplasia in the adolescent and young adult. *Clin Orthop Relat Res* 1990; 261:214-223.
46. Janzen DL, Aippersbach SE, Munk PL, et al: Three-dimensional CT measurement of adult acetabular dysplasia: Technique, preliminary results in normal subjects, and potential applications. *Skeletal Radiol* 1998; 27(7):352-358.
47. Haddad FS, Garbuz DS, Duncan CP, Janzen DL, Munk PL: CT evaluation of periacetabular osteotomies. *J Bone Joint Surg Br* 2000;82(4):526-531.
48. Ito H, Matsuno T, Hirayama T, Tanino H, Yamanaka Y, Minami A: Three-dimensional computed tomography analysis of non-osteoarthritic adult acetabular dysplasia. *Skeletal Radiol* 2009; 38(2):131-139.
49. van Bosse HJ, Lee D, Henderson ER, Sala DA, Feldman DS: Pelvic positioning creates error in CT acetabular measurements. *Clin Orthop Relat Res* 2011;469(6): 1683-1691.
50. Dandachli W, Ul Islam S, Tippett R, Hall-Craggs MA, Witt JD: Analysis of acetabular version in the native hip: Comparison between 2D axial CT and 3D CT measurements. *Skeletal Radiol* 2011;40(7):877-883.
51. Abel MF, Sutherland DH, Wenger DR, Mubarak SJ: Evaluation of CT scans and 3-D reformatted images for quantitative assessment of the hip. *J Pediatr Orthop* 1994;14(1):48-53.
52. Berrington de González A, Mahesh M, Kim KP, et al: Projected cancer risks from computed tomographic scans performed in the United States in 2007. *Arch Intern Med* 2009;169(22):2071-2077.
53. Smith-Bindman R, Lipson J, Marcus R, et al: Radiation dose associated with common computed tomography examinations and the associated lifetime attributable risk of cancer. *Arch Intern Med* 2009;169(22):2078-2086.

54. Lang P, Genant HK, Jergesen HE, Murray WR: Imaging of the hip joint: Computed tomography versus magnetic resonance imaging. *Clin Orthop Relat Res* 1992; 274:135-153.
55. Plötz GM, Brossmann J, von Knoch M, Muhle C, Heller M, Hassenpflug J: Magnetic resonance arthrography of the acetabular labrum: Value of radial reconstructions. *Arch Orthop Trauma Surg* 2001;121(8): 450-457.
56. Kubo T, Horii M, Yamaguchi J, et al: Acetabular labrum in hip dysplasia evaluated by radial magnetic resonance imaging. *J Rheumatol* 2000;27(8):1955-1960.
57. Dudda M, Albers C, Mamisch TC, Werlen S, Beck M: Do normal radiographs exclude asphericity of the femoral head-neck junction? *Clin Orthop Relat Res* 2009; 467(3):651-659.
58. Rakhra KS, Sheikh AM, Allen D, Beaulé PE: Comparison of MRI alpha angle measurement planes in femoroacetabular impingement. *Clin Orthop Relat Res* 2009; 467(3):660-665.
59. Koenig JK, Pring ME, Dwek JR: MR evaluation of femoral neck version and tibial torsion. *Pediatr Radiol* 2012;42(1):113-115.
60. Czerny C, Hofmann S, Neuhold A, et al: Lesions of the acetabular labrum: Accuracy of MR imaging and MR arthrography in detection and staging. *Radiology* 1996; 200(1):225-230.
61. Leunig M, Werlen S, Ungersböck A, Ito K, Ganz R: Evaluation of the acetabular labrum by MR arthrography. *J Bone Joint Surg Br* 1997;79(2):230-234.
62. Petersilge CA: MR arthrography for evaluation of the acetabular labrum. *Skeletal Radiol* 2001; 30(8):423-430.
63. Byrd JW, Jones KS: Diagnostic accuracy of clinical assessment, magnetic resonance imaging, magnetic resonance arthrography, and intra-articular injection in hip arthroscopy patients. *Am J Sports Med* 2004;32(7):1668-1674.
64. Sundberg TP, Toomayan GA, Major NM: Evaluation of the acetabular labrum at 3.0-T MR imaging compared with 1.5-T MR arthrography: Preliminary experience. *Radiology* 2006; 238(2):706-711.
65. Mintz DN, Hooper T, Connell D, Buly R, Padgett DE, Potter HG: Magnetic resonance imaging of the hip: Detection of labral and chondral abnormalities using noncontrast imaging. *Arthroscopy* 2005;21(4):385-393.
66. Keeney JA, Peelle MW, Jackson J, Rubin D, Maloney WJ, Clohisy JC: Magnetic resonance arthrography versus arthroscopy in the evaluation of articular hip pathology. *Clin Orthop Relat Res* 2004;429: 163-169.
67. Schmid MR, Nötzli HP, Zanetti M, Wyss TF, Hodler J: Cartilage lesions in the hip: Diagnostic effectiveness of MR arthrography. *Radiology* 2003;226(2):382-386.
68. Mamisch TC, Bittersohl B, Hughes T, et al: Magnetic resonance imaging of the hip at 3 Tesla: Clinical value in femoroacetabular impingement of the hip and current concepts. *Semin Musculoskelet Radiol* 2008;12(3): 212-222.
69. Ulrich-Vinther M, Maloney MD, Schwarz EM, Rosier R, O'Keefe RJ: Articular cartilage biology. *J Am Acad Orthop Surg* 2003; 11(6):421-430.
70. Venn M, Maroudas A: Chemical composition and swelling of normal and osteoarthrotic femoral head cartilage: I. Chemical composition. *Ann Rheum Dis* 1977; 36(2):121-129.
71. Gray ML, Burstein D, Kim YJ, Maroudas A: Magnetic resonance imaging of cartilage glycosaminoglycan: Basic principles, imaging technique, and clinical applications. *J Orthop Res* 2008;26(3): 281-291.
72. Kim YJ, Jaramillo D, Millis MB, Gray ML, Burstein D: Assessment of early osteoarthritis in hip dysplasia with delayed gadolinium-enhanced magnetic resonance imaging of cartilage. *J Bone Joint Surg Am* 2003;85(10):1987-1992.
73. Cunningham T, Jessel R, Zurakowski D, Millis MB, Kim YJ: Delayed gadolinium-enhanced magnetic resonance imaging of cartilage to predict early failure of Bernese periacetabular osteotomy for hip dysplasia. *J Bone Joint Surg Am* 2006;88(7):1540-1548.
74. Bittersohl B, Steppacher S, Haamberg T, et al: Cartilage damage in femoroacetabular impingement (FAI): Preliminary results on comparison of standard diagnostic vs delayed gadolinium-enhanced magnetic resonance imaging of cartilage (dGEMRIC). *Osteoarthritis Cartilage* 2009;17(10): 1297-1306.
75. Mamisch TC, Kain MS, Bittersohl B, et al: Delayed gadolinium-enhanced magnetic resonance imaging of cartilage (dGEMRIC) in femoacetabular impingement. *J Orthop Res* 2011;29(9):1305-1311.
76. Zilkens C, Holstein A, Bittersohl B, et al: Delayed gadolinium-enhanced magnetic resonance imaging of cartilage in the long-term follow-up after Perthes disease. *J Pediatr Orthop* 2010;30(2): 147-153.
77. Zilkens C, Miese F, Bittersohl B, et al: Delayed gadolinium-enhanced magnetic resonance imaging of cartilage (dGEMRIC), after slipped capital femoral epiphysis. *Eur J Radiol* 2011; 79(3):400-406.
78. Mosher TJ, Dardzinski BJ: Cartilage MRI T2 relaxation time mapping: Overview and applications. *Semin Musculoskelet Radiol* 2004; 8(4):355-368.

79. Dunn TC, Lu Y, Jin H, Ries MD, Majumdar S: T2 relaxation time of cartilage at MR imaging: Comparison with severity of knee osteoarthritis. *Radiology* 2004; 232(2):592-598.

80. David-Vaudey E, Ghosh S, Ries M, Majumdar S: T2 relaxation time measurements in osteoarthritis. *Magn Reson Imaging* 2004; 22(5):673-682.

81. Bittersohl B, Hosalkar HS, Hughes T, et al: Feasibility of T2* mapping for the evaluation of hip joint cartilage at 1.5T using a three-dimensional (3D), gradient-echo (GRE) sequence: A prospective study. *Magn Reson Med* 2009; 62(4):896-901.

82. Regatte RR, Akella SV, Borthakur A, Kneeland JB, Reddy R: Proteoglycan depletion-induced changes in transverse relaxation maps of cartilage: Comparison of T2 and T1rho. *Acad Radiol* 2002;9(12): 1388-1394.

83. Regatte RR, Akella SV, Borthakur A, Kneeland JB, Reddy R: In vivo proton MR three-dimensional T1rho mapping of human articular cartilage: Initial experience. *Radiology* 2003;229(1):269-274.

84. Burstein D, Gray ML: Is MRI fulfilling its promise for molecular imaging of cartilage in arthritis? *Osteoarthritis Cartilage* 2006; 14(11):1087-1090.

85. Tsushima H, Okazaki K, Takayama Y, et al: Evaluation of cartilage degradation in arthritis using T1ρ magnetic resonance imaging mapping. *Rheumatol Int* 2012;32(9):2867-2875.

86. Wang L, Chang G, Xu J, et al: T1rho MRI of menisci and cartilage in patients with osteoarthritis at 3T. *Eur J Radiol* 2011.

87. Siebenrock KA, Schöll E, Lottenbach M, Ganz R: Bernese periacetabular osteotomy. *Clin Orthop Relat Res* 1999;363:9-20.

88. Merle D'Aubigné R: Numerical classification of the function of the hip: 1970. *Rev Chir Orthop Reparatrice Appar Mot* 1990; 76(6):371-374.

89. Hasegawa Y, Masui T, Yamaguchi J, Kawabe K, Suzuki S: Factors leading to osteoarthritis after eccentric rotational acetabular osteotomy. *Clin Orthop Relat Res* 2007;459:207-215.

90. Matheney T, Kim YJ, Zurakowski D, Matero C, Millis M: Intermediate to long-term results following the Bernese periacetabular osteotomy and predictors of clinical outcome. *J Bone Joint Surg Am* 2009;91(9):2113-2123.

91. Sucato DJ, Tulchin K, Shrader MW, DeLaRocha A, Gist T, Sheu G: Gait, hip strength and functional outcomes after a Ganz periacetabular osteotomy for adolescent hip dysplasia. *J Pediatr Orthop* 2010;30(4):344-350.

92. Crockarell J Jr, Trousdale RT, Cabanela ME, Berry DJ: Early experience and results with the periacetabular osteotomy: The Mayo Clinic experience. *Clin Orthop Relat Res* 1999;363:45-53.

93. Hasegawa Y, Kanoh T, Seki T, Matsuoka A, Kawabe K: Joint space wider than 2 mm is essential for an eccentric rotational acetabular osteotomy for adult hip dysplasia. *J Orthop Sci* 2010; 15(5):620-625.

94. Okano K, Yamada K, Takahashi K, Enomoto H, Osaki M, Shindo H: Joint congruency in abduction before surgery as an indication for rotational acetabular osteotomy in early hip osteoarthritis. *Int Orthop* 2010;34(1):27-32.

95. Kim KI, Cho YJ, Ramteke AA, Yoo MC: Peri-acetabular rotational osteotomy with concomitant hip arthroscopy for treatment of hip dysplasia. *J Bone Joint Surg Br* 2011;93(6):732-737.

96. Fujii M, Nakashima Y, Noguchi Y, et al: Effect of intra-articular lesions on the outcome of periacetabular osteotomy in patients with symptomatic hip dysplasia. *J Bone Joint Surg Br* 2011;93(11): 1449-1456.

24

Periacetabular Osteotomy: Intra-articular Work

John G. Ginnetti, MD
Jill Erickson, PA-C
Christopher L. Peters, MD

Abstract

The goal of periacetabular osteotomy (PAO) is to correct acetabular pathomorphology and restore a more normal interplay between the acetabulum and proximal femur. After PAO, the biomechanically improved hip joint is presumed to better resist the progression of degenerative joint disease. Isolated PAO without intra-articular inspection often will underestimate the extent of hip disease in young adults. If intra-articular inspection is not performed at the time of PAO, chondrolabral injuries and dysplastic hip pathologies associated with femoroacetabular impingement will not be detected. The interaction of the acetabulum with the proximal femur is critical, and the presence of iatrogenic femoroacetabular impingement can be assessed with intra-articular inspection at the time of PAO.

Instr Course Lect 2013;62:279-286.

An expanding body of evidence implicates abnormal hip morphologies as the overriding cause of hip osteoarthritis in young adults.[1-7] Such abnormal hip morphologies exist along a continuum of hip pathomorphology anchored at one end by the dysplastic or undercovered hip and at the opposing end by femoroacetabular impingement (FAI) or the overcovered hip. The goal of current hip preservation surgery is to interrupt the process of degenerative joint disease by correcting the pathomorphologic characteristics of the acetabulum and/or the proximal femur. Periacetabular osteotomy (PAO) improves hip biomechanics by reorienting the acetabulum, with the intent of postponing degenerative progression. In this regard, PAO has yielded encouraging results.[8-11] However, early experience with PAO failed to include routine intra-articular inspection of the hip joint.[8-10] Two notable caveats have been identified. PAO in the setting of hip dysplasia has been implicated in overcoverage of the femoral head, which results in iatrogenic FAI.[12,13] Chondrolabral pathology associated with dysplastic and FAI-afflicted hip articulations has been initially overlooked.[9] Together, these findings provide the basis for routine intra-articular inspection and subsequent targeted intervention based on intraoperative findings at the time of PAO.

Background

Historically, routine hip arthrotomy was not preformed at the time of PAO.[8-10] As the understanding of hip pathology in young adults has expanded over the past two decades, intra-articular hip inspection in conjunction with PAO has become more commonplace. This change in surgical routine was largely the result of two major findings: (1) the revelation that chondrolabral injury is quite common and is associated with the entire spectrum of hip pathomorphology, and (2) iatrogenic FAI is a potential complication of PAO.

A retrospective review of the senior author's (CLP) database over a 6-year period showed that acetabular cartilage delamination was present in 28 of 64 hips (44%) treated with a surgical

Dr. Peters or an immediate family member serves as a board member, owner, officer, or committee member of the American Academy of Orthopaedic Surgeons; has received royalties from Biomet; is a member of a speakers' bureau or has made paid presentations on behalf of Biomet; and serves as a paid consultant to or is an employee of Biomet. Neither of the following authors nor any immediate family member has received anything of value from or has stock or stock options in a commercial company or institution related directly or indirectly to the subject of this chapter: Dr. Ginnetti and Ms. Erickson.

dislocation procedure for FAI.[14] A 22% incidence of labral injury at the time of PAO for dysplastic pathomorphology also has been reported[9] and is consistent with a report by Siebenrock et al.[15] Ross et al[16] retrospectively reviewed 71 patients (73 hips) with hip dysplasia who underwent hip arthroscopy secondary to mechanical symptoms before PAO. The authors reported that 63 of 73 hips (86.3%) had labral tearing and/or degeneration, whereas 46 of 73 hips (63%) had a hypertrophied labrum. Chondromalacia was reported in two thirds of the patients, whereas chondral surface debonding and cleavage was verified in 11 and 7 patients, respectively.

Iatrogenic FAI or overcoverage was found to be a potential pitfall of PAO, as reported by Myers et al[12] who identified posterior FAI after PAO correction of acetabular retroversion. In a retrospective analysis of acetabular version after Salter and LeCoeur osteotomies, Dora et al[13] found that 25 of 95 osteotomies (26%) resulted in acetabular retroversion and its resultant anterior femoral head overcoverage. From a technical standpoint, the orthopaedic surgeon must negotiate a delicate balance between the desire for improved acetabular orientation and the potential for overcorrection that will cause iatrogenic pincer-type FAI. This balance cannot be fully appreciated or successfully accomplished without intra-articular inspection to examine the dynamic interplay between the acetabulum and proximal femur at the time of PAO.

The practice of examining both sides of the hip articulation is critical because most symptomatic young adult hips do not fit neatly into defined morphologic entities such as dysplasia or FAI. Rather, afflicted hips often demonstrate complex pathomorphologies combining features of hip dysplasia along with FAI, acetabular retroversion, and/or sequela of childhood hip conditions (such as Legg-Calvé-Perthes disease or slipped capital femoral epiphysis).[17] Intraoperative dynamic tests of impingement should be performed to determine if further correction of the femoral head-neck offset is warranted after reorientation of the acetabulum.

Intra-articular Work

Labral Pathology

Labral pathology is frequently encountered during PAO and has been characterized according to hip pathomorphologic subtypes.[2,4,9,10,15,16] In cross-sectional views, the acetabular labrum is a triangular structure with a basilar attachment to the osseous acetabular rim, a capsular insertion along the external surface, and a free intra-articular apical margin.[18] In young adults with dysplastic hip pathomorphology, labral tissue is distinctly hypertrophic with myxoid degeneration and/or detachment from the osseous acetabular rim.[19,20] In contrast, patients with FAI-type morphology have undersurface labral tearing in the absence of hypertrophy.[19] From a gross histologic perspective, labral tearing caused by a pincer-type mechanism extends perpendicular to the labral surface, whereas cam-type tearing occurs at the transition zone (the zone between the fibrocartilaginous labrum and the articular hyaline cartilage) perpendicular to the articular surface.[21]

Despite the previous identification and characterization of labral pathology, the management of labral injury associated with hip disease in young adults is controversial. When contemplating surgical options at the time of PAO, several questions arise. Does labral injury alone generate sufficient pain to require intervention? The answer appears to be yes based on the discovery of nerve endings within histologic tissue samples taken from the acetabular labrum,[22] the body of arthroscopic literature replete with positive outcomes in terms of pain relief after débridement and/or fixation of labral tears,[23] and the findings of Matheny et al[10] who identified labral pathology as a source of hip pain after PAO.

Another topic of uncertainty is whether function of the acetabular labrum is critical to long-term hip survival, and, if so, can function be properly preserved or restored through surgical intervention? The answers to these questions are more elusive. The precise function of the acetabular labrum has not been completely delineated. Surprisingly, the labrum does not appear to have a major load-sharing role in the normal adult hip.[24,25] Instead, it is generally believed that the labrum derives its anatomic importance from its ability to create a seal that promotes fluid-film lubrication of the hip joint and chondrocyte nutrition by limiting the rate of fluid egression from articular cartilage.[26,27] Unlike knee meniscectomy, the literature lacks natural history studies that evaluate the long-term outcomes of partial acetabular labrectomy. Older clinical reports critical of partial acetabular labrectomy indirectly support débridement and fixation when possible; however, the reported poor outcomes are confounded by the presence of concomitant chondral injury and untreated FAI.[5,28-30] More recently, Espinosa et al[31] reported that in the short term, patients with labral injury who were treated with surgical dislocation and osteochondroplasty for FAI fared better with labral repair compared with partial labrectomy. Despite clinical evidence favoring preservation or repair of the labrum, this chapter's authors are not aware of any studies that have examined the ability of a repaired labrum to reconstitute a functional seal or that quantified the minimum

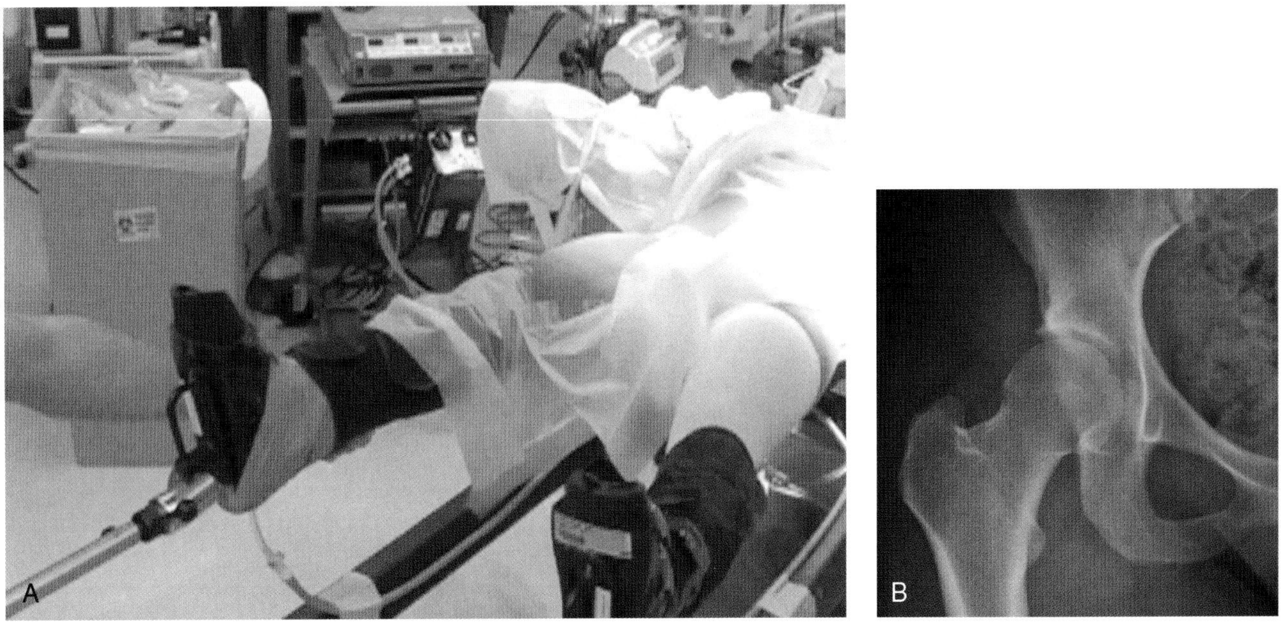

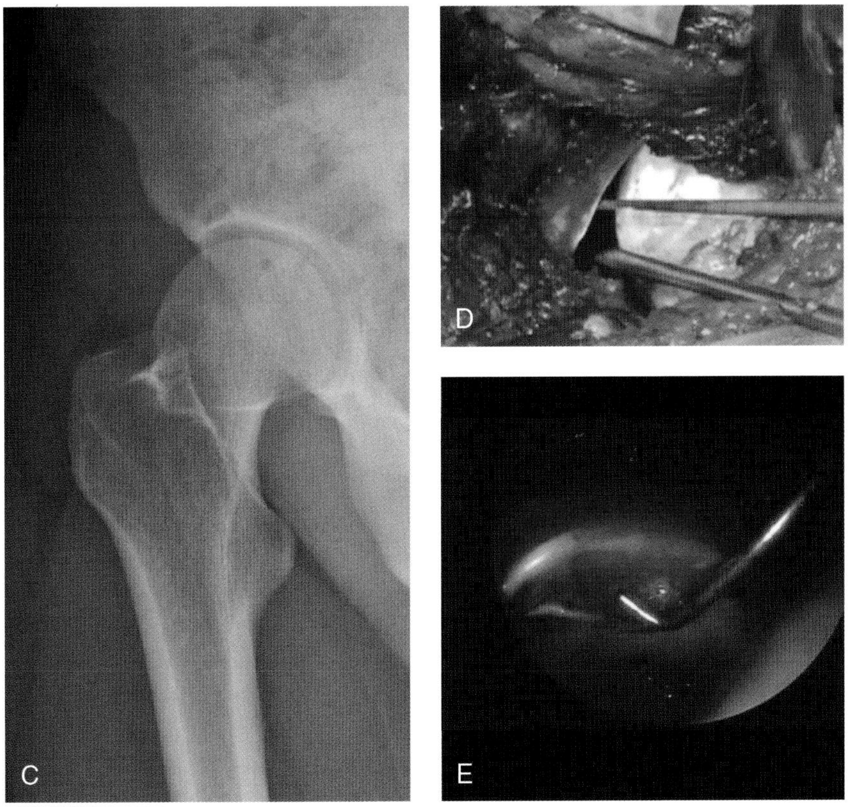

Figure 1 **A,** A traction table may be used to facilitate exposure for intra-articular work, as illustrated in this photograph. **B**, Preoperative AP pelvic view showing acetabular dysplasia of the right hip and a cam lesion on the femoral head. MRI confirmed chondral damage in the acetabulum. **C,** Preoperative false profile lateral view of right hip shows lack of femoral head-neck offset and mild joint space narrowing anteriorly. **D,** Intraoperative photograph showing dry arthroscopy approach to inspect the undersurface of the acetabular labral and chondral surfaces. **E,** Dry arthroscopy photograph showing acetabular chondral delamination and undersurface labral detachment.

amount of labrum required to maintain function. No randomized trials have evaluated the clinical outcomes of labral management options in the setting of PAO.

Despite controversy regarding chondrolabral injury, the senior author of this chapter uses the following practices for labral pathology identified at the time of PAO. Anterior hip arthrotomy is routinely preformed with PAO. As part of the modified Smith-Petersen approach used for Bernese PAO, the indirect head of the rectus femoris is tagged and mobilized for improved visualization of the hip capsule.[9] Capsular incision is then preformed along the long axis of the femoral neck. The capsular incision is extended in an anterior-posterior direction at the level of the acetabular rim (forming a T

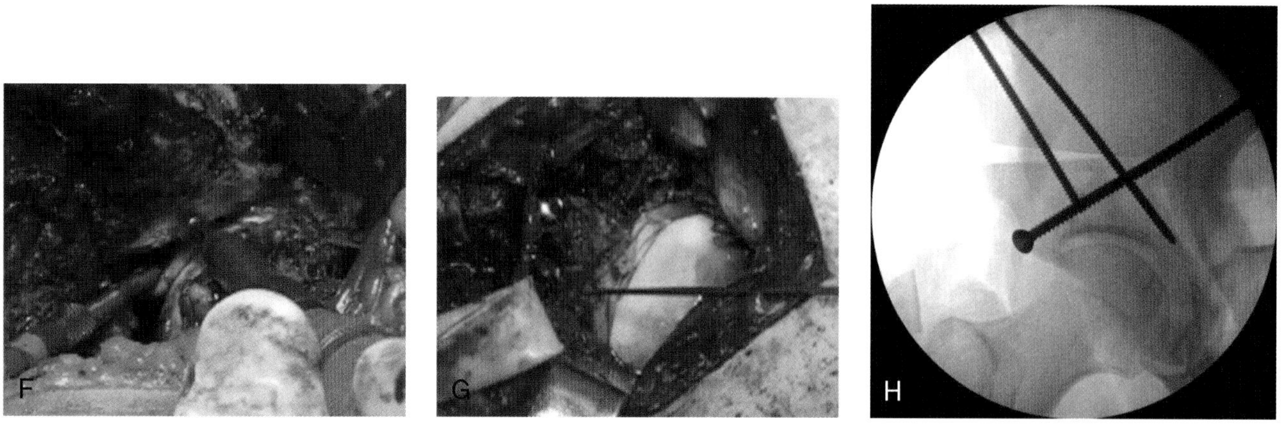

Figure 1 (continued) **F,** Intraoperative photograph showing labral takedown and rim resection with a high-speed rotating burr to allow adequate chondral treatment. **G,** Intraoperative photograph showing labral refixation with suture anchors fixed to the new acetabular rim. **H,** Intraoperative fluoroscopic image (simulated dynamic false-profile view, hip flexion of 90° with 15° to 20° of internal rotation) illustrating the correction achieved with PAO after intra-articular work was completed.

with the longitudinal incision). Care is taken to avoid injury to the underlying labral tissue. The management strategy is predicated on intraoperative findings. Simple débridement is used to address ganglion cysts and degenerative labral tears. Labral repair using a suture anchor technique is used for labral detachment at the extra-articular osseous insertion.[32] Detachment at this anatomic location theoretically maintains the greatest healing potential given the preservation of the blood supply through the capsular insertion, which supplies the external one third of the acetabular labrum[18,33] (**Figure 1**). Debulking or labral takedown with reduction of the proximal surface of the labrum accompanied by labral repair with suture anchors is the treatment of choice for the unstable hypertrophied labrum that is frequently encountered with dysplastic pathomorphology.

Chondral Pathology

Similar to labral pathology, chondral injury is associated with the full spectrum of hip pathomorphology. In a retrospective review of arthroscopic findings before PAO, Ross et al[16] reported on the extent of chondral damage associated with the dysplastic hip. The authors reported that 49 of 71 patients had arthroscopically verified chondral lesions, which were characterized as chondromalacic, cleavage, or debonding injuries. When present, the chondral lesions were preferentially located at the anterior and superolateral aspect of the acetabulum, with an average size of 171.7 mm².

This chapter's senior author has identified and characterized acetabular chondral lesions linked to the FAI end of the pathomorphologic spectrum. Cam-type impingement is frequently accompanied by anterosuperior acetabular cartilage injury in the form of full-thickness delamination. Conversely, pincer-type impingement alone results in global sparing of acetabular articular hyaline cartilage.[14]

In contrast with labral pathology, the preoperative diagnosis of chondral injury has implications for preoperative planning. An anterior arthrotomy provides limited access to the acetabular cartilage and is typically used to evaluate intra-articular hip structures. Traction and/or hip arthroscopy may be required in conjunction with PAO in the setting of acetabular chondral injury. Hip magnetic resonance arthrography, the mainstay of soft-tissue hip diagnostic imaging, achieves excellent specificity but lacks sufficient sensitivity. A study by Anderson et al[14] reported that only 8 of 28 hips with intraoperative findings of acetabular delamination were identified with magnetic resonance arthrography; this represents a sensitivity of 22% and a specificity of 100%. These results are consistent with the findings Kim et al.[34]

As with the treatment of labral pathology at the time of PAO, the management of chondral injuries remains controversial. The natural history of these lesions and whether chondral lesions are an independent source of pain have not been determined. Unlike labral tissue, hyaline articular cartilage lacks innervation, although subchondral bone exposure in instances of full-thickness delamination implicates chondral lesions in the complex pain pathway. If the known poor outcomes of untreated dysplasia are considered and the theory that altered hip pathomorphology initiates articular cartilage injury that results in arthritis is believed, then nascent chondral lesions identified at the time of PAO represent an opportunity to alter the degenerative cascade.[35]

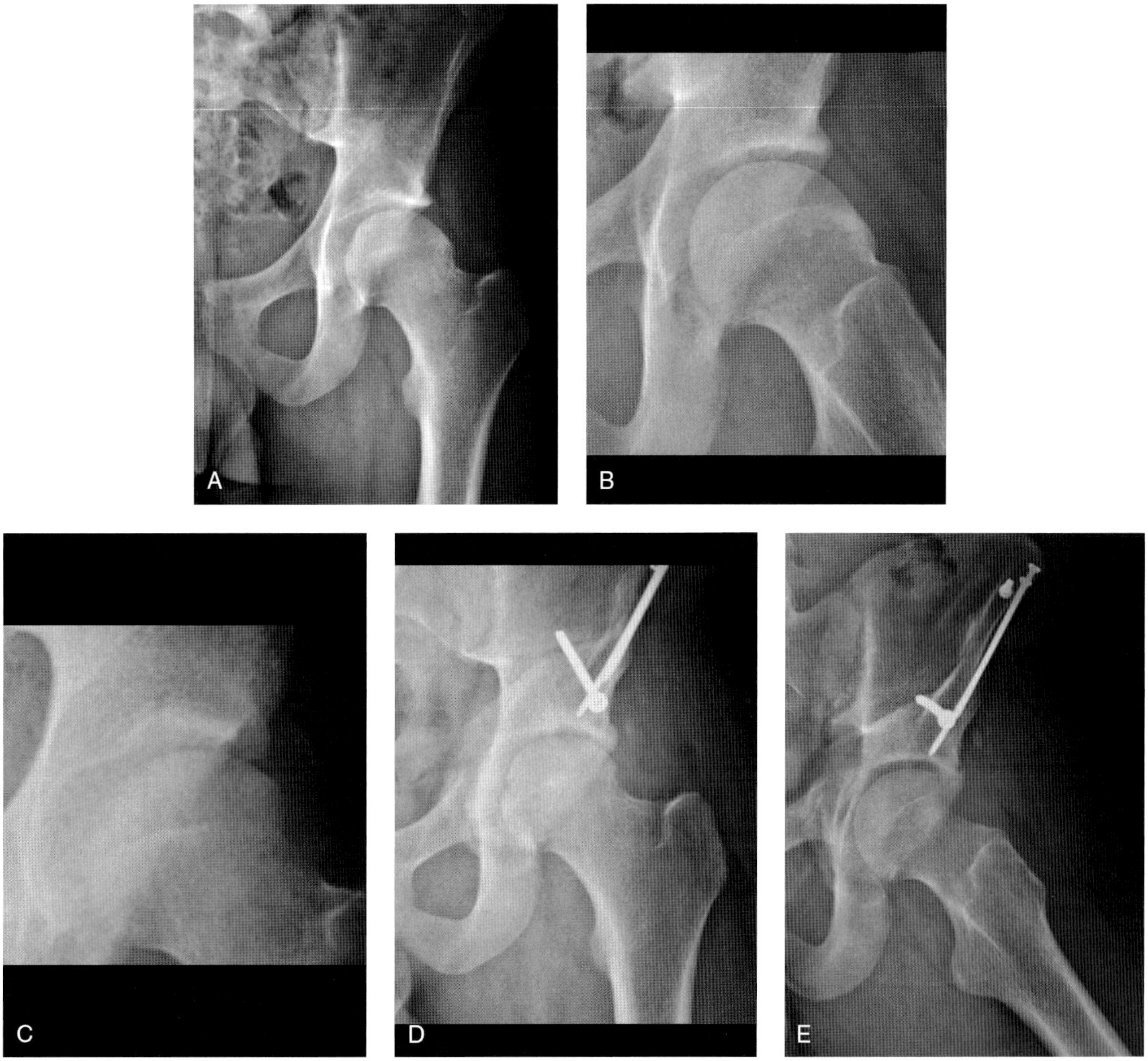

Figure 2 Radiographs showing complex left hip pathomorphology with acetabular and femoral contributions requiring acetabular rim resection and subsequent PAO. **A,** Preoperative AP pelvic radiograph showing the left hip before anterior rim débridement (on a traction table). **B,** Preoperative frog-lateral view of the left hip. **C,** Intraoperative fluoroscopic image of the left hip confirming that the rim resection that was required to treat the chondral damage in the acetabulum now required PAO to ensure adequate coverage. **D,** Postoperative AP pelvic radiograph showing adequate lateral acetabular coverage after rim débridement and PAO. **E,** Postoperative lateral view after PAO showing adequate femoral head-neck osteochondroplasty and PAO coverage.

Despite a sound theoretic basis, there are few evidence-based clinical data to direct the optimal management of chondral injuries at the time of PAO. Treatment options ranging from isolated débridement, microfracture, and acetabular rim resection of the cartilage flap with labral refixation have been reported in the literature.[14,31,36-38] This chapter's authors use traction and dry arthroscopy (based on the preoperative index of suspicion for the presence of chondral lesions) to examine the acetabular articular surface at the time of PAO. This is done in approximately 10% of patients. This clinical suspicion is based on the patient's specific hip pathomorphology and the results of available diagnostic imaging (**Figure 1**). After inspection, the senior author of this chapter believes that rim resection with labral advancement and refixation is a promising technique.[36]

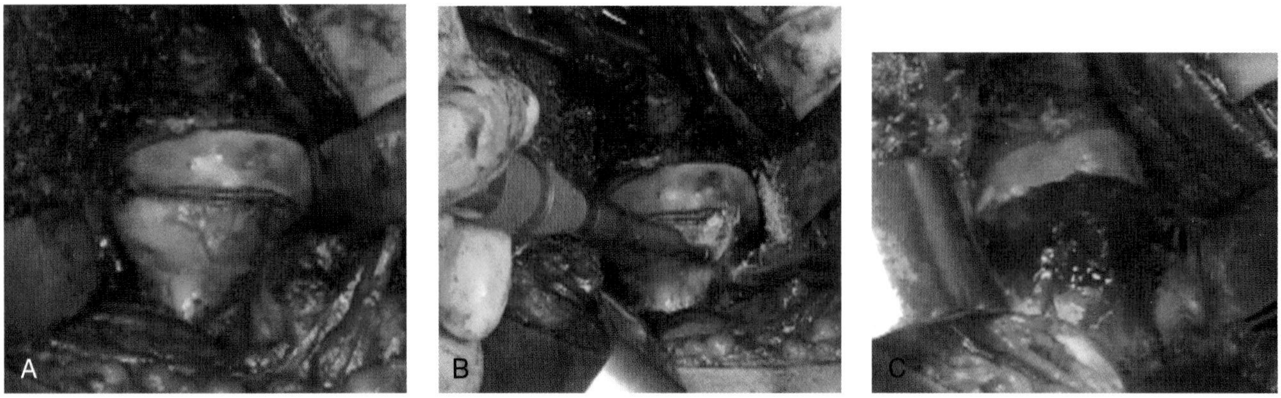

Figure 3 Femoral head-neck osteochondroplasty was performed through anterior arthrotomy at the time of PAO. **A,** Intraoperative photograph of a small cam lesion on the femoral head-neck junction where it abuts the newly corrected PAO fragment in 80° flexion. **B,** A high-speed rotating burr allows adequate restoration of the femoral head-neck offset to prevent iatrogenic FAI after PAO. **C,** Intraoperative photograph showing adequate offset achieved through this approach.

From a technical standpoint, the amount of rim resection required to properly address the chondral lesion may influence the magnitude of redirection. If rim resection is used to treat predominantly cam-type impingement, the potential exists to iatrogenically uncover and destabilize the femoral head. Therefore, the routine practice of this chapter's authors is to plan for a staged surgical dislocation followed by PAO at a later date, or, after a full discussion with the patient, to obtain consent for a possible simultaneous PAO depending on the intraoperative findings and the amount of rim resection required to successfully manage the chondral lesion (**Figure 2**).

Femoral Head-Neck Offset

To categorize symptomatic young adult hip pathomorphology as either hip dysplasia or FAI oversimplifies a complex disease entity. In reality, hip pathomorphology exists along a spectrum of disease, with most cases combining pathomorphologic elements of dysplasia, FAI, acetabular retroversion, and the sequelae of childhood hip diseases.[17,39-41] When treating acetabular pathomorphology with PAO, there is a high likelihood of concomitant pathologic femoral head-neck offset (**Figure 3**). The senior author of this chapter believes that more than 90% of patients treated with PAO require some degree of femoral head-neck offset correction. Iatrogenic FAI represents a real clinical concern after PAO.[12,13] A 2006 study reported that 35 of 49 hips (71%) treated with anterior arthrotomy required osteochondroplasty to correct the abutment of the femoral head-neck-junction against the reoriented anterior acetabular rim with the hip positioned in 90° or less of hip flexion and 20° or less of internal rotation.[9] For these reasons, it is customary to use intraoperative C-arm fluoroscopy to obtain a simulated false-profile view and a dynamic impingement view (90° of hip flexion and 15° to 20° of internal rotation). With this imaging protocol, the intended acetabular correction, femoral head-neck offset, and the potential exacerbation of FAI by the newly positioned acetabulum can be accurately assessed (**Figure 1, G**).

Summary

A wide spectrum of acetabular and proximal femoral pathomorphology has been implicated as the root cause of hip osteoarthritis in young adults. To preserve hip function, PAO remains a useful treatment option to correct acetabular pathomorphology. Historically, PAO was performed without routine intra-articular inspection of the hip joint. However, a unilateral acetabular-sided approach to hip preservation without intra-articular inspection ignores preexisting chondrolabral derangement, underestimates the complexity of the disease process, and overlooks the physiologic interplay between the acetabulum and proximal femur. Routine intra-articular hip assessment through an anterior arthrotomy at the time of PAO is simple and prudent.

References

1. Bardakos NV, Villar RN: Predictors of progression of osteoarthritis in femoroacetabular impingement: A radiological study with a minimum of ten years follow-up. *J Bone Joint Surg Br* 2009;91(2):162-169.
2. Ganz R, Parvizi J, Beck M, Leunig M, Nötzli H, Siebenrock KA: Femoroacetabular impingement: A cause for osteoarthritis of the hip. *Clin Orthop Relat Res* 2003;417:112-120.
3. Tannast M, Goricki D, Beck M, Murphy SB, Siebenrock KA: Hip

damage occurs at the zone of femoroacetabular impingement. *Clin Orthop Relat Res* 2008; 466(2):273-280.

4. Beck M, Kalhor M, Leunig M, Ganz R: Hip morphology influences the pattern of damage to the acetabular cartilage: Femoroacetabular impingement as a cause of early osteoarthritis of the hip. *J Bone Joint Surg Br* 2005;87(7): 1012-1018.
5. Tanzer M, Noiseux N: Osseous abnormalities and early osteoarthritis: The role of hip impingement. *Clin Orthop Relat Res* 2004; 429:170-177.
6. Leunig M, Beck M, Dora C, Ganz R: Femoroacetabular impingement: Trigger for the development of coxarthrosis. *Orthopade* 2006;35(1):77-84.
7. Leunig M, Ganz R: Femoroacetabular impingement: A common cause of hip complaints leading to arthrosis. *Unfallchirurg* 2005;108(1):9-10, 12-17.
8. Ganz R, Klaue K, Vinh TS, Mast JW: A new periacetabular osteotomy for the treatment of hip dysplasias: Technique and preliminary results. *Clin Orthop Relat Res* 1988;232:26-36.
9. Peters CL, Erickson JA, Hines JL: Early results of the Bernese periacetabular osteotomy: The learning curve at an academic medical center. *J Bone Joint Surg Am* 2006; 88(9):1920-1926.
10. Matheny T, Kim YJ, Zurakowski D, Matero C, Millis M: Intermediate to long-term results following the Bernese periacetabular osteotomy and predictors of clinical outcome. *J Bone Joint Surg Am* 2009;91(9):2113-2123.
11. Clohisy JC, Nunley RM, Curry MC, Schoenecker PL: Periacetabular osteotomy for the treatment of acetabular dysplasia associated with major aspherical femoral head deformities. *J Bone Joint Surg Am* 2007;89(7):1417-1423.
12. Myers SR, Eijer H, Ganz R: Anterior femoroacetabular impingement after periacetabular osteotomy. *Clin Orthop Relat Res* 1999;363:93-99.
13. Dora C, Mascard E, Mladenov K, Seringe R: Retroversion of the acetabular dome after Salter and triple pelvic osteotomy for congenital dislocation of the hip. *J Pediatr Orthop B* 2002;11(1):34-40.
14. Anderson LA, Peters CL, Park BB, Stoddard GJ, Erickson JA, Crim JR: Acetabular cartilage delamination in femoroacetabular impingement: Risk factors and magnetic resonance imaging diagnosis. *J Bone Joint Surg Am* 2009; 91(2):305-313.
15. Siebenrock KA, Schoeniger R, Ganz R: Anterior femoroacetabular impingement due to acetabular retroversion: Treatment with periacetabular osteotomy. *J Bone Joint Surg Am* 2003;85(2): 278-286.
16. Ross JR, Zaltz I, Nepple JJ, Schoenecker PL, Clohisy JC: Arthroscopic disease classification and interventions as an adjunct in the treatment of acetabular dysplasia. *Am J Sports Med* 2011; 39(suppl):72S-78S.
17. Peters CL, Erickson JA, Anderson L, Anderson AA, Weiss J: Hip-preserving surgery: Understanding complex pathomorphology. *J Bone Joint Surg Am* 2009;91(suppl 6): 42-58.
18. Seldes RM, Tan V, Hunt J, Katz M, Winiarsky R, Fitzgerald RH Jr: Anatomy, histologic features, and vascularity of the adult acetabular labrum. *Clin Orthop Relat Res* 2001;382:232-240.
19. Leunig M, Podeszwa D, Beck M, Werlen S, Ganz R: Magnetic resonance arthrography of labral disorders in hips with dysplasia and impingement. *Clin Orthop Relat Res* 2004;418:74-80.
20. Klaue K, Durnin CW, Ganz R: The acetabular rim syndrome: A clinical presentation of dysplasia of the hip. *J Bone Joint Surg Br* 1991;73(3):423-429.
21. Beaulé PE, O'Neill M, Rakhra K: Acetabular labral tears. *J Bone Joint Surg Am* 2009;91(3): 701-710.
22. Kim YT, Azuma H: The nerve endings of the acetabular labrum. *Clin Orthop Relat Res* 1995;320: 176-181.
23. Robertson WJ, Kadrmas WR, Kelly BT: Arthroscopic management of labral tears in the hip: A systematic review of the literature. *Clin Orthop Relat Res* 2007;455: 88-92.
24. Henak CR, Ellis BJ, Harris MD, Anderson AE, Peters CL, Weiss JA: Role of the acetabular labrum in load support across the hip joint. *J Biomech* 2011;44(12): 2201-2206.
25. Konrath GA, Hamel AJ, Olson SA, Bay B, Sharkey NA: The role of the acetabular labrum and the transverse acetabular ligament in load transmission in the hip. *J Bone Joint Surg Am* 1998; 80(12):1781-1788.
26. Ferguson SJ, Bryant JT, Ganz R, Ito K: The acetabular labrum seal: A poroelastic finite element model. *Clin Biomech (Bristol, Avon)* 2000;15(6):463-468.
27. Ferguson SJ, Bryant JT, Ganz R, Ito K: An in vitro investigation of the acetabular labral seal in hip joint mechanics. *J Biomech* 2003; 36(2):171-178.
28. Farjo LA, Glick JM, Sampson TG: Hip arthroscopy for acetabular labral tears. *Arthroscopy* 1999; 15(2):132-137.
29. Santori N, Villar RN: Acetabular labral tears: Result of arthroscopic partial limbectomy. *Arthroscopy* 2000;16(1):11-15.
30. Kim KC, Hwang DS, Lee CH, Kwon ST: Influence of femoroacetabular impingement on results

of hip arthroscopy in patients with early osteoarthritis. *Clin Orthop Relat Res* 2007;456:128-132.

31. Espinosa N, Rothenfluh DA, Beck M, Ganz R, Leunig M: Treatment of femoro-acetabular impingement: Preliminary results of labral refixation. *J Bone Joint Surg Am* 2006;88(5):925-935.

32. Espinosa N, Beck M, Rothenfluh D, Ganz R, Leunig M: Treatment of femoro-acetabular impingement: Preliminary results of labral fixation. Surgical technique. *J Bone Joint Surg Am* 2007; 89(suppl 2, pt 1):36-53.

33. Kelly BT, Shapiro GS, Digiovanni CW, Buly RL, Potter HG, Hannafin JA: Vascularity of the hip labrum: A cadaveric investigation. *Arthroscopy* 2005;21(1):3-11.

34. Kim YJ, Jaramillo D, Millis MB, Gray ML, Burstein D: Assessment of early osteoarthritis in hip dysplasia with delayed gadolinium-enhanced magnetic resonance imaging of cartilage. *J Bone Joint Surg Am* 2003;85(10):1987-1992.

35. Murphy SB, Ganz R, Müller ME: The prognosis in untreated dysplasia of the hip: A study of radiographic factors that predict the outcome. *J Bone Joint Surg Am* 1995;77(7):985-989.

36. Peters CL, Erickson J: The etiology and treatment of hip pain in the young adult. *J Bone Joint Surg Am* 2006;88(suppl 4):20-26.

37. Haviv B, Singh PJ, Takla A, O'Donnell J: Arthroscopic femoral osteochondroplasty for cam lesions with isolated acetabular chondral damage. *J Bone Joint Surg Br* 2010;92(5):629-633.

38. McCarthy JC: The diagnosis and treatment of labral and chondral injuries. *Instr Course Lect* 2004;53: 573-577.

39. Rab GT: The geometry of slipped capital femoral epiphysis: Implications for movement, impingement, and corrective osteotomy. *J Pediatr Orthop* 1999;19(4): 419-424.

40. Stulberg SD, Cordell LD, Harris WH, Ramsey PL, MacEwen GD: A major cause of idiopathic osteoarthritis of the hip, in *The Hip: Proceedings of the Third Open Scientific Meeting of the Hip Society.* St. Louis, MO, CV Mosby, 1975, pp 212-228.

41. Steppacher SD, Tannast M, Werlen S, Siebenrock KA: Femoral morphology differs between deficient and excessive acetabular coverage. *Clin Orthop Relat Res* 2008; 466(4):782-790.

25

Alternatives to Periacetabular Osteotomy for Adult Acetabular Dysplasia

Cara Beth Lee, MD
Michael B. Millis, MD

Abstract

Pelvic osteotomy is a powerful tool for improving the mechanical forces in a dysplastic hip. Multiple techniques have evolved over the past 70 years to treat the symptomatic adult patient with acetabular dysplasia. Although the Bernese periacetabular osteotomy is commonly used in the United States, several other types of osteotomies, including the rotational (spheric or dial) acetabular osteotomy, the triple pelvic osteotomy, and the Chiari medial displacement pelvic osteotomy, have demonstrated good success and are used in many parts of the world.

Instr Course Lect 2013;62:287-295.

Salter[1] made the seminal observation that instability in the dysplastic hip is caused by inadequate anterior and lateral femoral head coverage, and, in 1957, he pioneered the technique of innominate osteotomy to reorient the face of the acetabulum. Prior to Salter's work, dysplasia had primarily been managed by techniques that augmented acetabular coverage, including shelf arthroplasties and the Chiari medial displacement pelvic osteotomy. Modifications of Salter's osteotomy technique have led to improvements in correcting the components of the dysplastic hip.

In the United States, periacetabular osteotomy (PAO) is currently the most commonly used reorientation procedure for adult acetabular dysplasia. PAO was first performed in 1984 and subsequently described by Ganz et al[2] in 1988. The authors articulated five advantages of PAO over other available procedures to treat dysplasia. PAO is a single surgical approach; has the ability to obtain a large, multiplanar correction; preserves the acetabular blood supply; maintains posterior column integrity; and conserves the true pelvis.[2] With modifications in the original technique, there is now the additional advantage of an abductor-sparing[3] or, more recently, a limited incision approach.[4] PAO demonstrated good midterm to long-term results and can achieve substantial correction, even in patients with severe dysplasia with femoral head subluxation.[5-8]

In the years between the introduction of Salter's innovative osteotomy technique and the development of PAO, many alternative techniques emerged to treat dysplasia; several of these techniques are still in common use throughout the world. This chapter reviews the rotational acetabular osteotomy, the triple pelvic osteotomy, and the Chiari medial displacement pelvic osteotomy. The advantages and disadvantages of each pelvic osteotomy procedure are summarized in **Table 1**.

Rotational Acetabular Osteotomy

Spheric osteotomy adjacent to the acetabulum was first described by Blavier and Blavier[9] in 1962. Similar rotational or dial osteotomies were later reported by Wagner[10] in Germany, Eppright[11] in the United States, and Ninomiya and Tagawa[12] in Japan, where this technique remains in common use. Using specially curved osteotomes that follow its circumference, the rotational acetabular osteotomy is made approximately 1.5 cm proximal

Neither of the following authors nor any immediate family member has received anything of value from or owns stock in a commercial company or institution related directly or indirectly to the subject of this chapter: Dr. Lee and Dr. Millis.

Table 1
Advantages and Disadvantages of Current Pelvic Osteotomy Procedures

Procedure	Advantages	Disadvantages
Periacetabular osteotomy	Large, multiplanar corrections Maintains true pelvis Maintains posterior column Preserves acetabular blood supply Abductor sparing	Violates triradiate cartilage
Rotational acetabular osteotomy	Large, multiplanar corrections Maintains true pelvis	Fragment medialization difficult Intra-articular fracture risk Acetabular osteonecrosis risk Abductor dissection Violates triradiate cartilage
Triple pelvic osteotomy	Large multiplanar corrections Effective with open triradiate cartilage Abductor sparing	Disrupts true pelvis Higher nonunion rate in adults
Chiari pelvic osteotomy	Improves coverage in incongruent hip Improves coverage with very small weight-bearing zone	Disrupts true pelvis Articulation with capsule rather than hyaline cartilage

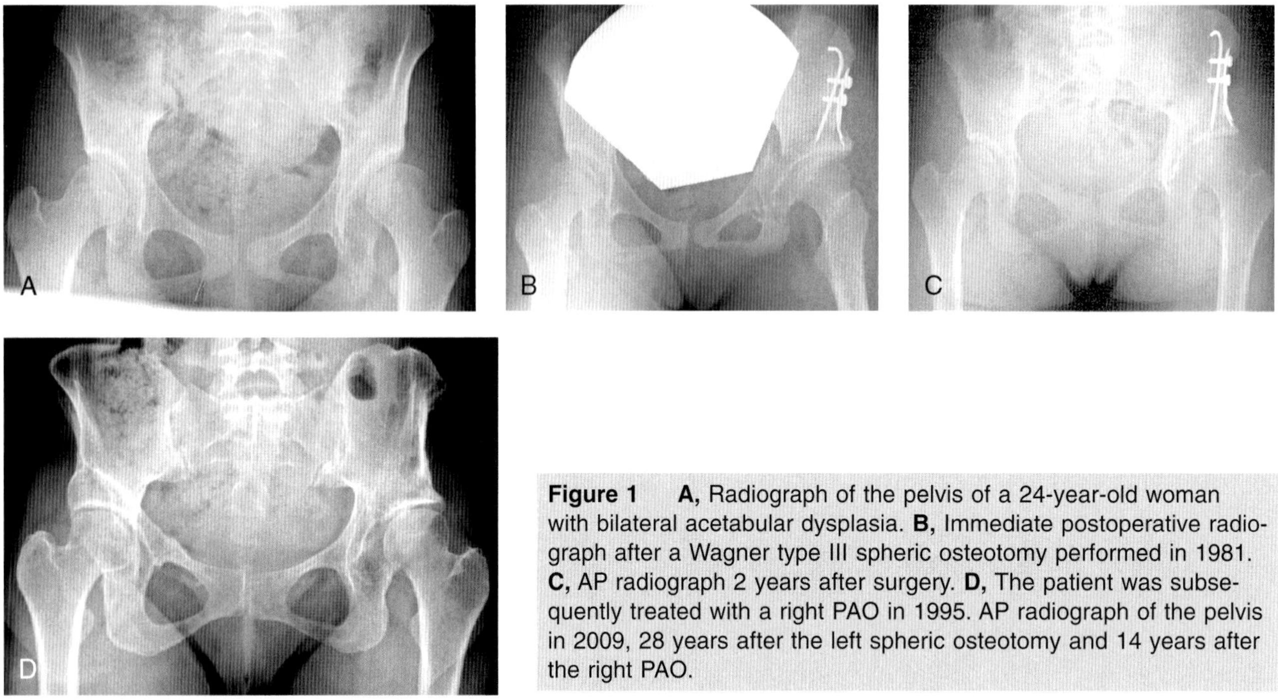

Figure 1 **A,** Radiograph of the pelvis of a 24-year-old woman with bilateral acetabular dysplasia. **B,** Immediate postoperative radiograph after a Wagner type III spheric osteotomy performed in 1981. **C,** AP radiograph 2 years after surgery. **D,** The patient was subsequently treated with a right PAO in 1995. AP radiograph of the pelvis in 2009, 28 years after the left spheric osteotomy and 14 years after the right PAO.

to the acetabular roof. Wagner's method uses an extensive anterior iliofemoral approach to expose the pelvis. He described three variations of correction.[10] In a type I correction, the acetabular fragment is rotated anteriorly and laterally to improve coverage, and bone graft is placed proximal to the overhanging acetabular bone. In type II, iliac crest graft is inserted into the osteotomy site, which allows the fragment to be moved distally up to 2 cm to increase leg length. The type III acetabular osteotomy is performed for hips that require medialization of the acetabular fragment. The rotational osteotomy is combined with a complete cut of the ilium, similar to a Chiari osteotomy (**Figure 1**). The proximal ilium is shifted laterally while the distal acetabular fragment moves medially. All three variations of the procedure are stabilized with internal fixation, and the joint capsule remains intact.

The technique of Ninomiya and Tagawa[12] resembles Wagner's type II osteotomy, except the procedure is carried out with the patient in the lateral position and uses both anterior iliofemoral and posterior approaches to the hip to expose the medial and lateral pelvic cuts, respectively. Two

2.0-mm Kirschner wires are used for fixation and are removed through small skin incisions at 6 weeks postoperatively. Other surgeons have modified the procedure to a transtrochanteric approach with bioabsorbable fixation.[13-15]

Advantages and Disadvantages

There are several advantages of the rotational acetabular osteotomy compared with other innominate osteotomies. Because this osteotomy is performed close to the acetabular deformity, major correction can be achieved without altering the shape of the true pelvis; thus, childbirth is unaffected.[16]

There are also several disadvantages of this procedure. Because of the proximity of the osteotomy to the joint, vascularity to the acetabulum is at risk, and the fragment can be difficult to stabilize adequately enough to allow early weight bearing.[17-19] In patients with sclerotic bone, or if the osteotomy is performed too close to the acetabulum, there is risk of fracture into the hip joint.[20,21] Ninomiya and Tagawa[12] recommended against using this technique in patients with an open triradiate cartilage and joint incongruity. They also considered abductor muscle weakness a relative contraindication because prolonged limp can be a sequela from the abductor dissection in the surgical exposure.

Results

Good success rates in well-selected patients have been reported with rotational acetabular osteotomy.[22,23] Schramm et al[22] reported on 20-year follow-up of 22 patients treated with spheric osteotomies using Wagner's technique. Kaplan-Meier survivorship was 86% at 20 years, with conversion to total hip arthroplasty as the end point. Postoperative joint congruence was a key factor in preserving the native hip. Nakamura et al[23] reported 80% good-to-excellent long-term results in 112 hips with minimal or no arthrosis at the time of surgery. Even in patients with advanced osteoarthritis secondary to acetabular dysplasia, rotational acetabular osteotomy can decrease pain at 8- to 12-year follow-ups.[21,24-27] A minimum of 2.5 mm of joint space is recommended to consider rotational acetabular osteotomy, and results are better if there is joint congruence on preoperative imaging.[27,28] Successful outcomes have been reported in patients with major deformities and in older patients in the absence of severe osteoarthritis.[29-34] Undercorrection and persistent lateralization of the femoral head are risk factors for progressive osteoarthritis.[35,36]

Triple Pelvic Osteotomy

The single innominate osteotomy described by Salter[1] divides the pelvis from just proximal to the anterior inferior iliac spine transversely to the sciatic notch. With the pubic symphysis as a hinge, the distal fragment is rotated anteriorly and laterally to increase femoral head coverage. This procedure was initially developed to treat persistent dislocation and subluxation in children. Its value can be restricted by stiffness at the symphysis, which limits its effectiveness in adolescents and adults. In 1965, LeCoeur[37] described a triple pelvic osteotomy that involved a transverse innominate osteotomy performed through an anterior iliofemoral incision, with superior and inferior pubic ramus cuts via a medial incision.[38] In 1966, Hopf[39] described a method for performing a triple osteotomy through an anterior iliofemoral approach, and Steel[40] described a triple osteotomy using an anterior iliofemoral incision along with a posterior, transverse incision just distal to the ischial tuberosity to complete the ischial cut. The double innominate osteotomy of Sutherland and Greenfield[41] also uses two incisions, but it osteotomizes the pubis just lateral to the symphysis and medial to the obturator foramen. The authors believe that this approach allows better correction and improved ability to medialize the fragment compared with the Salter osteotomy and offers simpler intraoperative positioning than the Steel osteotomy.

Carlioz et al[42] and Tönnis et al[43] modified prior techniques by performing the cuts closer to the acetabulum, particularly the ischial cut, which is made proximal to the ischial spine. This method eliminates the tethering effect of the sacrospinous and sacrotuberous ligaments that constrained correction in previous innominate osteotomies. Tönnis described a two-stage procedure starting with the patient prone for the ischial osteotomy and then turned supine for the iliac and pubic ramus cuts. Subsequent modifications included medial rather than posterior incision for the ischial osteotomy and single-incision techniques, with an abductor-sparing approach as initially described for PAO.[3,44]

Advantages and Disadvantages

A key advantage of the triple osteotomy as modified by Tönnis et al[43] is the ability to medialize the joint and achieve a much larger correction than is possible with other innominate osteotomies. The procedure can be effective in patients with persistent subluxation and dislocation. Unlike rotational acetabular osteotomy and PAO, triple pelvic osteotomy is safe for patients with an open triradiate cartilage, if performed with extraperiosteal dissection of the superior public ramus[44,45] (**Figure 2**).

A drawback of the triple pelvic osteotomy is that it lacks intrinsic stability because both columns of the pelvis are disrupted. In hips requiring

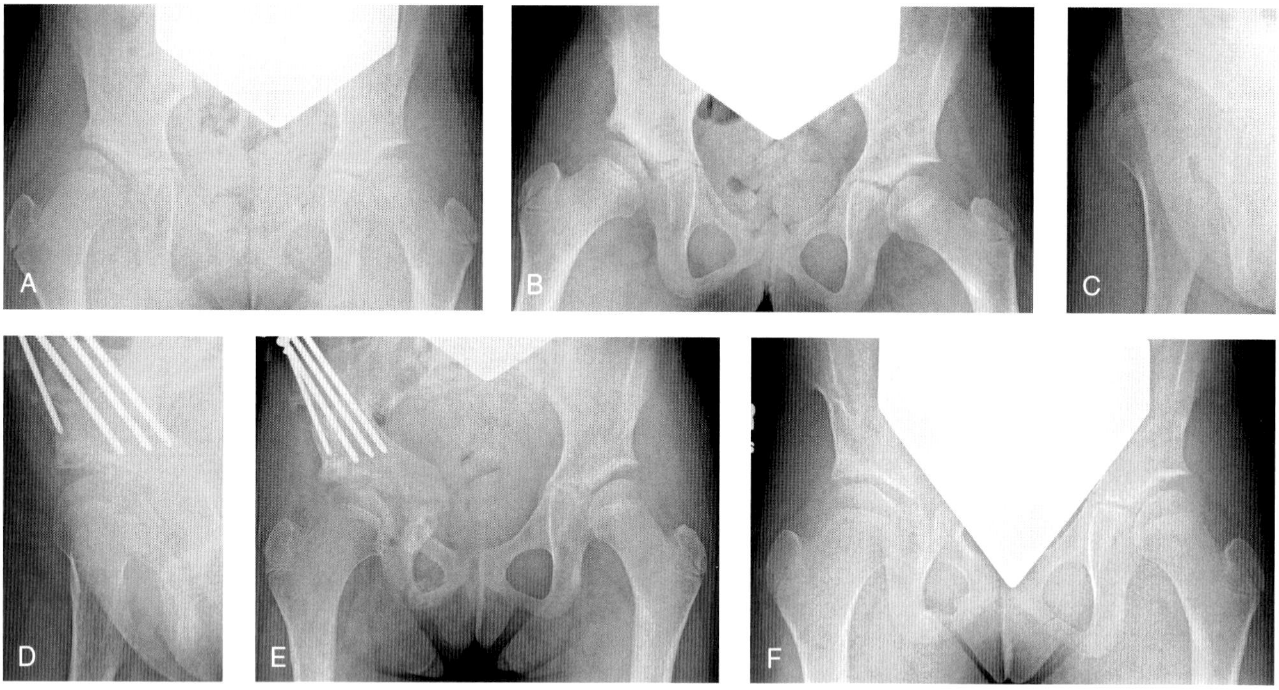

Figure 2 **A,** AP radiograph of the pelvis of an 11-year-old patient with developmental dysplasia of the hip and residual right hip dysplasia after Dega acetabuloplasty and varus intertrochanteric osteotomy performed at age 3 years. **B,** Von Rosen view shows excellent congruence of the right hip. **C,** False profile view shows insufficient anterior coverage with an acetabular cyst. **D,** False profile view 6 months after treatment with a triple pelvic osteotomy shows healing of the osteotomy and excellent anterior coverage. **E,** AP radiograph 6 months after the triple pelvic osteotomy shows the joint center is well medialized, and the osteotomy is healed and remodeling well. **F,** AP radiograph 18 months after surgery. The acetabular cyst has resolved.

substantial correction, large gaps at the osteotomy sites can result in nonunion.[46-48] This technique also alters the morphology of the true pelvis, which can impede childbirth.

Results

A study by van Hellemondt et al[49] reported that 42 of 48 hips (88%) were preserved at an average of 15 years after triple pelvic osteotomy. Based on Merle d'Aubigné and Postel functional scores, 64% of hips were rated good to excellent; 31 of 41 hips (76%) that had no osteoarthritis at the time of surgery showed no osteoarthritis over the 15-year interval. Peters et al[50] reported on outcomes for 60 hips with acetabular dysplasia treated with triple innominate osteotomy. Forty-nine of 50 patients (98%) were satisfied with the procedure at a mean follow-up of 9 years; however, 16 of the 60 osteotomies (27%) were considered failures because of the need to convert to a total hip arthroplasty or the presence of intractable hip pain. When nonunion occurs, patients are less satisfied with the procedure.[48]

Chiari Pelvic Osteotomy

With advances in reorienting osteotomies, the Chiari medial displacement osteotomy is currently considered a salvage augmentation procedure. The Chiari osteotomy is primarily indicated for a dysplastic hip with incongruity or to supplement coverage in an acetabulum with an exceedingly small weight-bearing zone.[51] Chiari[51] began performing the medial displacement osteotomy in 1950 and published details of his technique and early results in 1953. The osteotomy is performed through an anterior iliofemoral approach and involves division of the ilium from just inferior to the anterior inferior iliac spine and curving in a semicircle to exit posteriorly through the sciatic notch.[52] The osteotomy is directed approximately 15° laterally to medially to allow medial displacement of the distal fragment. The lateralized ilium serves as the augmented bony coverage of the femoral head with the capsule interposed. In the initial series, patients were immobilized in an abduction spica cast for 4 weeks; immobilization is now accomplished with internal fixation.

Advantages and Disadvantages

Unlike osteotomies that redirect the native acetabulum to increase coverage of the femoral head, the Chiari osteotomy abducts the distal fragment,

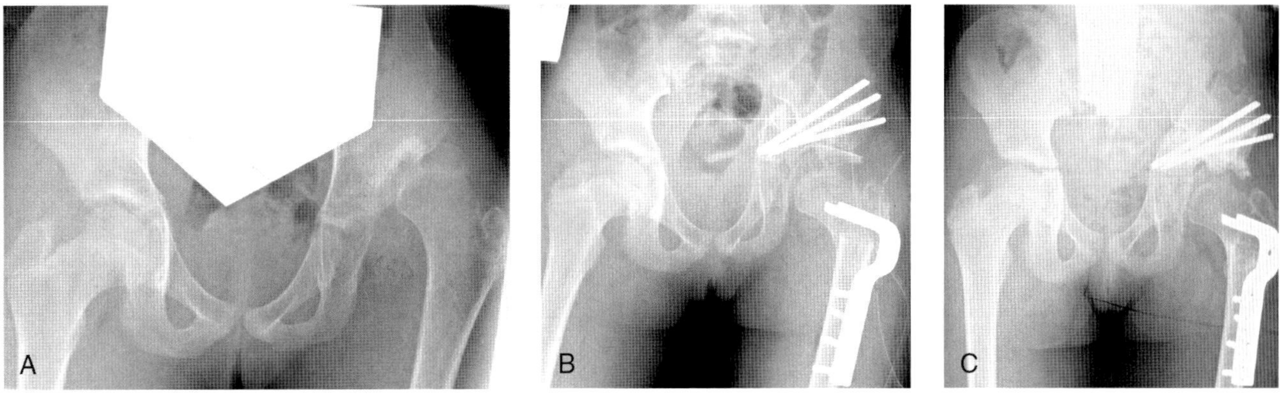

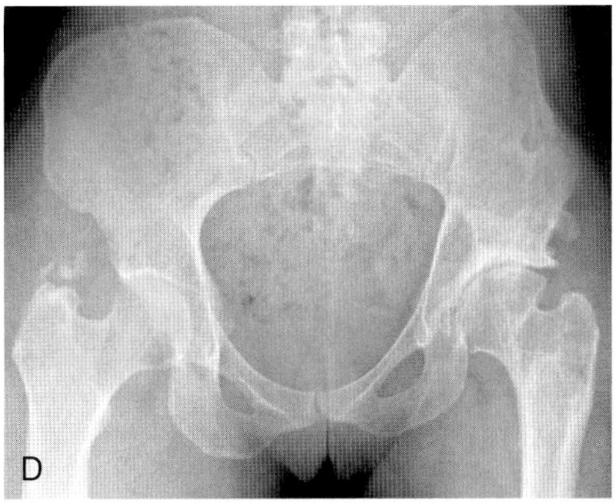

Figure 3 **A,** Radiograph of the pelvis of a 13-year-old girl with left hip dislocation. **B,** Immediate postoperative radiograph after Chiari and femoral shortening osteotomies performed in 1982. **C,** AP radiograph taken 5 months postoperatively shows the healed femoral and pelvic osteotomies. The femoral head remains reduced, with good joint space. **D,** AP radiograph 21 years after surgery shows narrowing—but still present—hip joint space.

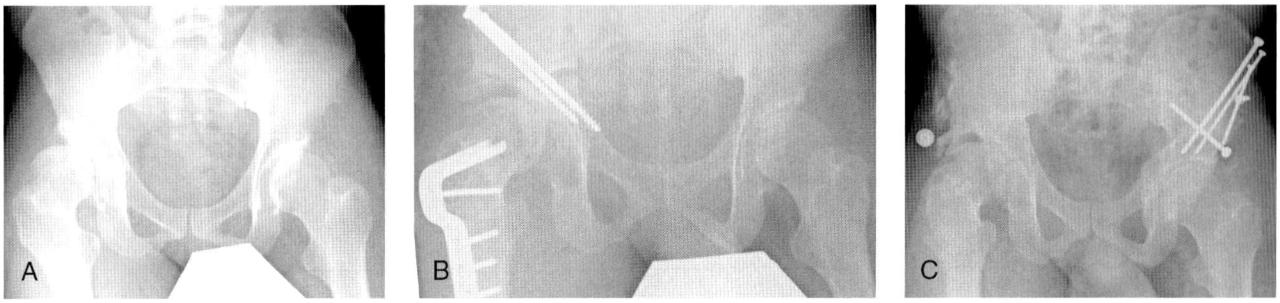

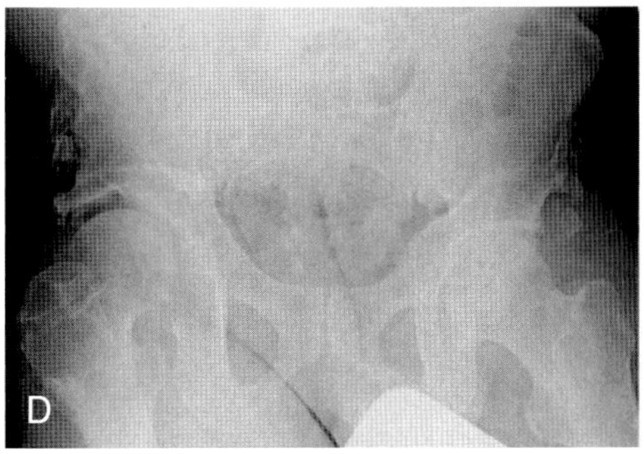

Figure 4 **A,** Radiograph of the pelvis of a 30-year-old man with polio and bilateral acetabular dysplasia. **B,** Immediate postoperative radiograph after right Chiari and shortening intertrochanteric osteotomies performed in 1991. A left PAO was subsequently performed. **C,** AP radiograph taken 5 years after the right Chiari osteotomy and 7 months after a left PAO show the femoral heads are well covered bilaterally, and the left PAO has healed. **D,** AP radiograph taken 18 years after the right and 14 years after the left hip procedures show maintenance of excellent coverage and good cartilage space in both hips.

which results in a more vertical orientation of the true acetabulum and may be beneficial in unstable hips with anterolateral impingement. The hip joint reaction forces are decreased, and the mechanical environment of the hip is improved because of the increased weight-bearing area and medialization of the femoral head.[52,53] From a technical standpoint, greater than 100% displacement of the osteotomy is desirable to achieve adequate coverage of the femoral head by the iliac shelf (**Figures 3** and **4**). This displacement often leaves an anterior gap above the femoral head between the lateralized proximal fragment and the medialized distal fragment. This gap is best filled with interposition of corticocancellous graft, which can be easily obtained from the anteromedial surface of the ilium.

The primary disadvantage of the Chiari osteotomy is that the femoral head articulates with the capsule and labrum rather than the native articular cartilage. There is evidence that the capsule may undergo metaplasia to form fibrocartilage,[54,55] but this is less desirable than the shifting of hyaline cartilage into the weight-bearing zone, which is done with redirectional osteotomies. Labral pathology is common in patients with dysplasia, and labral tears and detachment compromise the result of a Chiari osteotomy.[56,57] Abductor weakness with a persistent Trendelenburg sign can occur, although less abductor dysfunction was reported when the procedure was done through a transtrochanteric approach with trochanteric advancement when needed.[58-60] Similar to other innominate osteotomies, the Chiari osteotomy alters the true pelvis and narrows the birth canal.[59]

Results

Overall, results of the Chiari osteotomy are positive with consistent pain improvement.[52,58,61,62] Several studies have reported on the long-term follow-ups of patients treated with the procedure.[63-66] Windhager et al[64] reviewed 236 hips in 208 patients from Chiari's early studies performed from 1953 to 1967. Twenty-one of 236 hips (9%) had revision procedures (19 total hip arthroplasties and 2 arthrodeses) at a mean 15 years after the osteotomy. The remaining 215 hips (91%) were assessed at an average 24.8 years (range, 20 to 34.2 years) after surgery. Fifty-four percent of the hips had good-to-excellent results based on measures of pain, walking distance, Trendelenburg sign, and range of motion; 60% of patients were able to walk unlimited distances. Kotz et al[66] reported that 38 of 70 native hips (54%) in 66 patients were preserved at a mean follow-up of 32 years. In the 32 hips that were converted to total hip arthroplasty, hip replacement was performed an average of 26 years after the Chiari procedure, which corresponded with the 25-year hip longevity reported by Ohashi et al.[67] An expanded evaluation of Chiari's patients reported that, at 32 years follow-up (range, 21 to 53 years), 305 hips (238 patients) had 49% survivorship of the native hip, with a mean Harris hip score of 82.[63] Older age and more severe arthrosis at the time of surgery correlated with poorer outcomes.[58,64-66,68-71]

Lack et al[65] reported that when total hip arthroplasty was required, the Chiari osteotomy improved the bone stock that supports the acetabular implant. Tokunaga et al[72] reported that survivorship of arthroplasty at 8 years was no different between patients with previous Salter and/or Chiari osteotomies compared with patients with osteoarthritis caused by dysplasia who had no prior surgery.

Summary

Pelvic osteotomies are complex, technically demanding procedures that offer mechanical correction and symptom improvement in properly selected patients with acetabular dysplasia. The Chiari medial displacement pelvic osteotomy is reserved for dysplastic hips with an incongruent articulation and rare cases in which the acetabular weight-bearing surface is exceedingly small and requires augmentation. Reorientation osteotomies are preferable in patients with congruent dysplasia and minimal arthrosis. PAO is a single surgical approach that can obtain a large multiplanar correction among other advantages. The primary drawback of PAO is that it disrupts the triradiate cartilage in skeletally immature patients. The rotational acetabular and triple pelvic osteotomies share some but not all of the benefits and weaknesses of PAO. All of the techniques can achieve major corrections and have demonstrated good results at long-term follow-up. The triple pelvic osteotomy can be performed through a single, abductor-sparing incision with extraperiosteal dissection, making it an option for patients with open triradiate cartilage. Disadvantages of a triple pelvic osteotomy are instability from disruption of both columns of the pelvis, which alters the true pelvis and can lead to a higher nonunion rate. The rotational acetabular osteotomy maintains the true pelvis but requires abductor muscle dissection that can result in a prolonged limp or Trendelenburg sign. Rotational acetabular osteotomy also risks acetabular fragment osteonecrosis and intra-articular fracture in sclerotic bone; medialization can be difficult without innominate osteotomy.

At Boston Children's Hospital, adult patients with symptomatic acetabular dysplasia are managed with PAO, and skeletally immature patients are treated with a triple pelvic osteotomy. The rotational acetabular osteotomy has been widely used in Japan with good long-term success, and the Chiari pelvic osteotomy is used to treat the rare patient who requires augmentation rather than reorientation of the dysplastic acetabulum.

References

1. Salter RB: Innominate osteotomy in the treatment of congenital dislocation and subluxation of the hip. *J Bone Joint Surg Br* 1961;43: 518-539.

2. Ganz R, Klaue K, Vinh TS, Mast JW: A new periacetabular osteotomy for the treatment of hip dysplasias: Technique and preliminary results. *Clin Orthop Relat Res* 1988;232:26-36.
3. Murphy SB, Millis MB: Periacetabular osteotomy without abductor dissection using direct anterior exposure. *Clin Orthop Relat Res* 1999;364:92-98.
4. Troelsen A, Elmengaard B, Søballe K: A new minimally invasive transsartorial approach for periacetabular osteotomy. *J Bone Joint Surg Am* 2008;90(3):493-498.
5. Steppacher SD, Tannast M, Ganz R, Siebenrock KA: Mean 20-year followup of Bernese periacetabular osteotomy. *Clin Orthop Relat Res* 2008;466(7):1633-1644.
6. Matheney T, Kim YJ, Zurakowski D, Matero C, Millis M: Intermediate to long-term results following the Bernese periacetabular osteotomy and predictors of clinical outcome. *J Bone Joint Surg Am* 2009;91(9):2113-2123.
7. Clohisy JC, Schutz AL, St John L, Schoenecker PL, Wright RW: Periacetabular osteotomy: A systematic literature review. *Clin Orthop Relat Res* 2009;467(8): 2041-2052.
8. Clohisy JC, Barrett SE, Gordon JE, Delgado ED, Schoenecker PL: Periacetabular osteotomy for the treatment of severe acetabular dysplasia. *J Bone Joint Surg Am* 2005;87(2):254-259.
9. Blavier L, Blavier J: Treatment of subluxation of the hip. *Rev Chir Orthop Reparatrice Appar Mot* 1962;48:208-213.
10. Wagner H: *Osteotomies for Congenital Hip Dislocation*. St. Louis, MO, CV Mosby, 1976.
11. Eppright R: Dial osteotomy of the acetabulum in the treatment of dysplasia of the hip. *J Bone Joint Surg Am* 1975;57:1172.
12. Ninomiya S, Tagawa H: Rotational acetabular osteotomy for the dysplastic hip. *J Bone Joint Surg Am* 1984;66(3):430-436.
13. Ito H, Matsuno T, Minami A: Rotational acetabular osteotomy through an Ollier lateral u approach. *Clin Orthop Relat Res* 2007;459:200-206.
14. Nakamura S, Takatori Y, Morimoto S, et al: Rotational acetabular osteotomy using biodegradable internal fixation. *Int Orthop* 1999;23(3):148-149.
15. Maezawa K, Nozawa M, Matsuda K, et al: Radiographic and magnetic resonance imaging findings of polylevolactic acid screws after rotational acetabular osteotomy. *Arch Orthop Trauma Surg* 2004; 124(7):455-460.
16. Masui T, Hasegawa Y, Yamaguchi J, Kanoh T, Ishiguro N: Childbirth and sexual activity after eccentric rotational acetabular osteotomy. *Clin Orthop Relat Res* 2007;459:195-199.
17. Kalhor M, Beck M, Huff TW, Ganz R: Capsular and pericapsular contributions to acetabular and femoral head perfusion. *J Bone Joint Surg Am* 2009;91(2): 409-418.
18. Leunig M, Siebenrock KA, Ganz R: Rationale of periacetabular osteotomy and background work. *Instr Course Lect* 2001;50: 229-238.
19. Tönnis D, Arning A, Bloch M, Heinecke A, Kalchschmidt K: Triple pelvic osteotomy. *J Pediatr Orthop B* 1994;3:54-67.
20. Wagner H: Experiences with spherical acetabular osteotomy for the correction of the dysplastic acetabulum, in Weil UH, ed: *Progress in Orthopaedic Surgery 2: Acetabular Dysplasia—Skeletal Dysplasias in Childhood.* Berlin, Germany, Springer-Verlag, 1978, pp 131-145.
21. Millis MB, Kaelin AJ, Schluntz K, Curtis B, Hey L, Hall JE: Spherical acetabular osteotomy for treatment of acetabular dysplasia in adolescents and young adults. *J Pediatr Orthop B* 1994;3:47-53.
22. Schramm M, Hohmann D, Radespiel-Troger M, Pitto RP: Treatment of the dysplastic acetabulum with Wagner spherical osteotomy: A study of patients followed for a minimum of twenty years. *J Bone Joint Surg Am* 2003;85(5):808-814.
23. Nakamura S, Ninomiya S, Takatori Y, Morimoto S, Umeyama T: Long-term outcome of rotational acetabular osteotomy: 145 hips followed for 10-23 years. *Acta Orthop Scand* 1998;69(3): 259-265.
24. Nozawa M, Maezawa K, Matsuda K, Kim S, Shitoto K, Kurosawa H: Rotational acetabular osteotomy for advanced osteoarthritis of the hip joint with acetabular dysplasia. *Int Orthop* 2009;33(6): 1549-1553.
25. Okano K, Enomoto H, Osaki M, Shindo H: Rotational acetabular osteotomy for advanced osteoarthritis secondary to developmental dysplasia of the hip. *J Bone Joint Surg Br* 2008;90(1):23-26.
26. Yasunaga Y, Ochi M, Terayama H, Tanaka R, Yamasaki T, Ishii Y: Rotational acetabular osteotomy for advanced osteoarthritis secondary to dysplasia of the hip. *J Bone Joint Surg Am* 2006;88(9): 1915-1919.
27. Hasegawa Y, Kanoh T, Seki T, Matsuoka A, Kawabe K: Joint space wider than 2 mm is essential for an eccentric rotational acetabular osteotomy for adult hip dysplasia. *J Orthop Sci* 2010; 15(5):620-625.
28. Okano K, Enomoto H, Osaki M, Shindo H: Joint congruency as an indication for rotational acetabular osteotomy. *Clin Orthop Relat Res* 2009;467(4):894-900.

29. Nozawa M, Shitoto K, Hirose T, et al: Rotational acetabular osteotomy for severely dysplastic acetabulum. *Arch Orthop Trauma Surg* 2000;120(7-8):376-379.
30. Hartofilakidis G, Stamos K, Ioannidis TT: Rotational acetabular osteotomy for severe dysplasia of the hip. *J Bone Joint Surg Br* 1997; 79(3):510.
31. Shindo H, Igarashi H, Taneda H, Azuma H: Rotational acetabular osteotomy for severe dysplasia of the hip with a false acetabulum. *J Bone Joint Surg Br* 1996;78(6): 871-877.
32. Ninomiya S: Rotational acetabular osteotomy for the severely dysplastic hip in the adolescent and adult. *Clin Orthop Relat Res* 1989; 247:127-137.
33. Yamaguchi J, Hasegawa Y, Kanoh T, Seki T, Kawabe K: Similar survival of eccentric rotational acetabular osteotomy in patients younger and older than 50 years. *Clin Orthop Relat Res* 2009; 467(10):2630-2637.
34. Yasunaga Y, Takahashi K, Ochi M, et al: Rotational acetabular osteotomy in patients forty-six years of age or older: Comparison with younger patients. *J Bone Joint Surg Am* 2003;85(2): 266-272.
35. Koga H, Matsubara M, Suzuki K, Morita S, Muneta T: Factors which affect the progression of osteoarthritis after rotational acetabular osteotomy. *J Bone Joint Surg Br* 2003;85(7):963-968.
36. Hasegawa Y, Masui T, Yamaguchi J, Kawabe K, Suzuki S: Factors leading to osteoarthritis after eccentric rotational acetabular osteotomy. *Clin Orthop Relat Res* 2007;459:207-215.
37. LeCoeur P: Correction des dé fants d'orientation de l'articulation coxofémorale par ostéotomie de l'ishtme iliaque. *Rev Chir Orthop Reparatrice Appar Mot* 1965;51:211-212.
38. Lehman WB, Atar D, Grant AD: Pelvic osteotomies in children. *Bull N Y Acad Med* 1992;68(4): 483-496.
39. Hopf A: Hip acetabular displacement by double pelvic osteotomy in the treatment of hip joint dysplasia and subluxation in young people and adults. *Z Orthop Ihre Grenzgeb* 1966;101(4):559-586.
40. Steel HH: Triple osteotomy of the innominate bone: A procedure to accomplish coverage of the dislocated or subluxated femoral head in the older patient. *Clin Orthop Relat Res* 1977;122:116-127.
41. Sutherland DH, Greenfield R: Double innominate osteotomy. *J Bone Joint Surg Am* 1977;59(8): 1082-1091.
42. Carlioz H, Khouri N, Hulin P: Triple juxtacotyloid osteotomy. *Rev Chir Orthop Reparatrice Appar Mot* 1982;68(7):497-501.
43. Tönnis D, Behrens K, Tscharani F: A modified technique of the triple pelvic osteotomy: Early results. *J Pediatr Orthop* 1981;1(3): 241-249.
44. Zaltz I: *Pediatric Orthopaedic Surgery.* Philadelphia, PA, Elsevier-Saunders, 2011, pp 159-171.
45. Rebello G, Kim YJ: *Pediatric Orthopaedic Surgery.* Philadelphia, PA, Elsevier-Saunders, 2011, pp 149-158.
46. Tschauner C, Sylkin A, Hofmann S, Graf R: Painful nonunion after triple pelvic osteotomy: Report of five cases. *J Bone Joint Surg Br* 2003;85(7):953-955.
47. Vukasinovic Z, Pelillo F, Spasovski D, Seslija I, Zivkovic Z, Matanovic D: Triple pelvic osteotomy for the treatment of residual hip dysplasia: Analysis of complications. *Hip Int* 2009; 19(4):315-322.
48. Hailer NP, Soykaner L, Ackermann H, Rittmeister M: Triple osteotomy of the pelvis for acetabular dysplasia: Age at operation and the incidence of nonunions and other complications influence outcome. *J Bone Joint Surg Br* 2005;87(12):1622-1626.
49. van Hellemondt GG, Sonneveld H, Schreuder MH, Kooijman MA, de Kleuver M: Triple osteotomy of the pelvis for acetabular dysplasia: Results at a mean follow-up of 15 years. *J Bone Joint Surg Br* 2005;87(7):911-915.
50. Peters CL, Fukushima BW, Park TK, Coleman SS, Dunn HK: Triple innominate osteotomy in young adults for the treatment of acetabular dysplasia: A 9-year follow-up study. *Orthopedics* 2001;24(6):565-569.
51. Chiari K: Pelvic osteotomy in hip arthroplasty. *Wien Med Wochenschr* 1953;103(38):707-709.
52. Chiari K: Medial displacement osteotomy of the pelvis. *Clin Orthop Relat Res* 1974;98:55-71.
53. Giuzio E, Costa L, Servodio Iammarrone C, Nastro M: The biomechanics of pelvic osteotomy according to the Chiari method. *Chir Organi Mov* 1991;76(1): 77-82.
54. Hiranuma S, Higuchi F, Inoue A, Miyazaki M: Changes in the interposed capsule after Chiari osteotomy: An experimental study on rabbits with acetabular dysplasia. *J Bone Joint Surg Br* 1992; 74(3):463-467.
55. Moll FK Jr : Capsular change following Chiari innominate osteotomy. *J Pediatr Orthop* 1982; 2(5):573-576.
56. Nishina T, Saito S, Ohzono K, Shimizu N, Hosoya T, Ono K: Chiari pelvic osteotomy for osteoarthritis: The influence of the torn and detached acetabular labrum. *J Bone Joint Surg Br* 1990;72(5): 765-769.
57. Nakano S, Nishisyo T, Hamada D, et al: Treatment of dysplastic osteoarthritis with labral tear by Chiari pelvic osteotomy: Outcomes after more than 10 years

follow-up. *Arch Orthop Trauma Surg* 2008;128(1):103-109.

58. Calvert PT, August AC, Albert JS, Kemp HB, Catterall A: The Chiari pelvic osteotomy: A review of the long-term results. *J Bone Joint Surg Br* 1987;69(4):551-555.
59. Rejholec M, Stryhal F, Rybka V, Popelka S: Chiari osteotomy of the pelvis: A long-term study. *J Pediatr Orthop* 1990;10(1):21-27.
60. Ito H, Matsuno T, Minami A: Comparison of the surgical approaches for a Chiari pelvic osteotomy. *J Bone Joint Surg Br* 2003;85(2):204-208.
61. Zlatić M, Radojević B, Lazović C, Lupulović I: Late results of Chiari's pelvic osteotomy: A follow-up of 171 adult hips. *Int Orthop* 1988;12(2):149-154.
62. Høgh J, Macnicol MF: The Chiari pelvic osteotomy: A long-term review of clinical and radiographic results. *J Bone Joint Surg Br* 1987;69(3):365-373.
63. Chiari C, Hofmann H, Hofstätter J, Lunzer A, Peloschek P, Kotz R: Long-term results of the Chiari pelvic osteotomy. *Proceedings: 2010 Annual Meeting*. CD. Rosemont, IL, American Academy of Orthopaedic Surgeons, 2010, pp 370-371.
64. Windhager R, Pongracz N, Schönecker W, Kotz R: Chiari osteotomy for congenital dislocation and subluxation of the hip: Results after 20 to 34 years follow-up. *J Bone Joint Surg Br* 1991;73(6):890-895.
65. Lack W, Windhager R, Kutschera HP, Engel A: Chiari pelvic osteotomy for osteoarthritis secondary to hip dysplasia: Indications and long-term results. *J Bone Joint Surg Br* 1991;73(2):229-234.
66. Kotz R, Chiari C, Hofstaetter JG, Lunzer A, Peloschek P: Long-term experience with Chiari's osteotomy. *Clin Orthop Relat Res* 2009;467(9):2215-2220.
67. Ohashi H, Hirohashi K, Yamano Y: Factors influencing the outcome of Chiari pelvic osteotomy: A long-term follow-up. *J Bone Joint Surg Br* 2000;82(4):517-525.
68. Macnicol MF, Lo HK, Yong KF: Pelvic remodelling after the Chiari osteotomy: A long-term review. *J Bone Joint Surg Br* 2004;86(5):648-654.
69. Ito H, Tanino H, Yamanaka Y, Nakamura T, Minami A, Matsuno T: The Chiari pelvic osteotomy for patients with dysplastic hips and poor joint congruency: Long-term follow-up. *J Bone Joint Surg Br* 2011;93(6):726-731.
70. Migaud H, Chantelot C, Giraud F, Fontaine C, Duquennoy A: Long-term survivorship of hip shelf arthroplasty and Chiari osteotomy in adults. *Clin Orthop Relat Res* 2004;418:81-86.
71. Rush J: Chiari osteotomy in the adult: a long-term follow-up study. *Aust N Z J Surg* 1991;61(10):761-764.
72. Tokunaga K, Aslam N, Zdero R, Schemitsch EH, Waddell JP: Effect of prior Salter or Chiari osteotomy on THA with developmental hip dysplasia. *Clin Orthop Relat Res* 2011;469(1):237-243.

26

Approaches and Perioperative Management in Periacetabular Osteotomy Surgery: The Minimally Invasive Transsartorial Approach

Kjeld Søballe, MD, PhD
Anders Troelsen, MD, PhD

Abstract

In the early days of periacetabular osteotomy (PAO), surgical approaches were characterized by extensive soft-tissue dissection. The Smith-Petersen approach (and iliofemoral modifications) and the ilioinguinal approach have traditionally been used for PAO. The optimal surgical approach for PAO, or any surgical procedure, should be characterized by few complications, minimized surgical trauma, and no compromise of long-term surgical results. A minimally invasive transsartorial approach using fluoroscopy and an approximately 7-cm skin incision has been developed for performing PAO. No muscles are detached, and the femoral nerve and vessels are protected by the iliopsoas and sartorius muscles. This approach is safe, minimizes blood loss and transfusion requirements, is associated with a short duration of surgery, and allows for optimal correction of the acetabular fragment. Follow-ups (range, 3.9 to 8.1 years) of 209 PAOs performed using this approach have shown Kaplan-Meier survivorship rates of 94.7% at 5 years and 88.6% at 8.1 years, with conversion to total hip arthroplasty as the end point. Perioperative management includes a patient education program, optimized pain treatment strategies (local infiltration analgesia), and a progressive mobilization and exercise program. The transsartorial approach coupled with a specific perioperative management program has proved successful for PAO surgery.

Instr Course Lect 2013;62:297-303.

This chapter presents a brief overview of the surgical approaches for performing periacetabular osteotomy (PAO) to treat symptomatic developmental dysplasia of the hip. Perioperative management, including patient education methods, pharmacologic prophylaxis, postoperative pain management, and postoperative mobilization, is also reviewed.

Dr. Søballe or an immediate family member has received research or institutional support from Zimmer and Biomet. Neither Dr. Troelsen nor any immediate family member has received anything of value from or owns stock in a commercial company or institution related directly or indirectly to the subject of this chapter.

Background

In the early days of PAO, surgical approaches were characterized by extensive dissection and soft-tissue trauma. Whereas the five steps for performing a PAO, including leaving the posterior column intact, have remained the same since its development, some advances have been introduced to minimize soft-tissue trauma. The optimal surgical approach for PAO, or any surgical procedure, should be characterized by few complications, minimized surgical trauma, and no compromise of long-term results.

The choice of surgical approach should be thoroughly evaluated because each approach has benefits as well as the risk for complications. Patients should be informed about the risks and frequency of complications. The orientation of the incision and the soft-tissue dissection is associated with varying complications, especially neurovascular complications. The amount of blood loss, the transfusion requirements, the duration of surgery, and the ability to perform optimal redirection of the acetabular fragment are affected by the chosen surgical approach.[1-10]

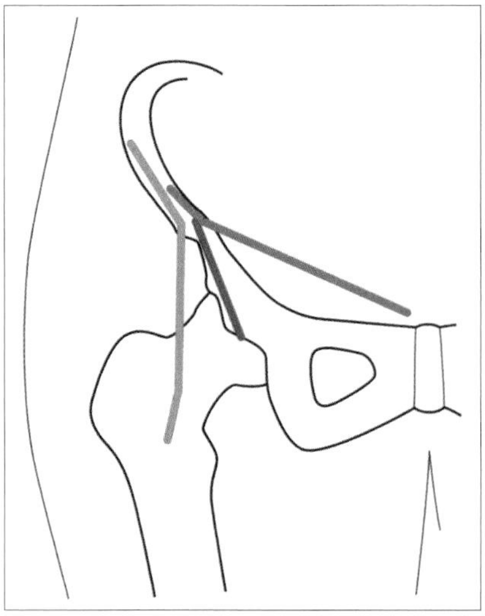

Figure 1 Incisions of the modified Smith-Petersen (green line), ilioinguinal (blue line), and minimally invasive approach (red line) are shown.

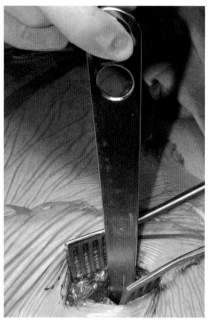

Figure 2 The use of proper instruments and fluoroscopy are of paramount importance when using the minimally invasive approach. Access to perform the osteotomies is obtained by placing a blunt retractor along the medial aspect of the ilium to retract the iliopsoas and the medial part of the split sartorius muscles medially.

The Smith-Petersen approach (and iliofemoral modifications) together with the ilioinguinal approach have been traditionally favored for PAOs.[1-5] These approaches allow for optimal acetabular fragment reorientation; however, because of the soft-tissue dissection involved, a less invasive approach for PAO surgery was developed.[11]

Surgical Approaches

At the Aarhus University Hospital in Denmark, the senior author (KS) of this chapter has used the ilioinguinal, modified Smith-Petersen, and new minimally invasive transsartorial approaches in succession. The transsartorial approach has been used since April 2003.

Ilioinguinal Approach

The ilioinguinal approach was adapted from acetabular fracture surgery and is performed as described by Letournel[12] but without lateral extension along the iliac crest. The skin incision extends from the anterior superior iliac spine, along the inguinal ligament, and terminates at the level of the pubic symphysis near the midline. The inguinal ligament is incised, leaving the origins of the abdominal musculature and fascia attached to the proximal part of the split ligament. Further access is created by incising the iliopectineal fascia that separates the lacuna musculorum and lacuna vasorum. This allows mobilization of the iliopsoas muscle, which, combined with medial retraction of the external iliac vessels, creates access to perform the osteotomies through two windows—one medial and one lateral to the iliopsoas muscle (**Figure 1**).

Smith-Petersen Approach

Specific modifications of the Smith-Petersen approach have been reported.[5] The approach used at the Aarhus University Hospital includes a skin incision along the anterior third of the iliac crest to the anterosuperior iliac spine. The incision is then curved distally and continued vertically along the tensor fasciae latae for approximately 10 cm. The internervous planes between the tensor fasciae latae and sartorius muscle and between the gluteus medius and rectus femoris are developed. In contrast to the previously described modification of the Smith-Petersen approach, the rectus femoris is not detached. In some of the first cases treated at Aarhus University Hospital, the origin of the sartorius muscle was detached by means of an osteotomy.

Minimally Invasive Transsartorial Approach

Because of complications described for classic PAO approaches, especially the risk of vascular complications associated with the previously favored ilioinguinal approach,[13] the senior author of this chapter developed a new, minimally invasive transsartorial approach for PAO surgery. The goals of this approach were to introduce a safe surgical technique; reduce surgical trauma, blood loss, and the duration of surgery; ensure that optimal acetabular reorientation was not compromised; and improve rehabilitation.

The surgical technique for the approach has been previously described together with instructions for performing the five osteotomies using fluoroscopy.[11] Audiovisual material detailing the approach also is available.[14]

Fluoroscopy is necessary throughout the performance of the osteotomies and reorientation of the acetabular fragment. A radiolucent operating table is used, and fluoroscopic images are obtained in the AP and 60° (false profile) views. Patients are placed supine on the operating room table. Draping should allow for full mobilization of the lower extremity on the

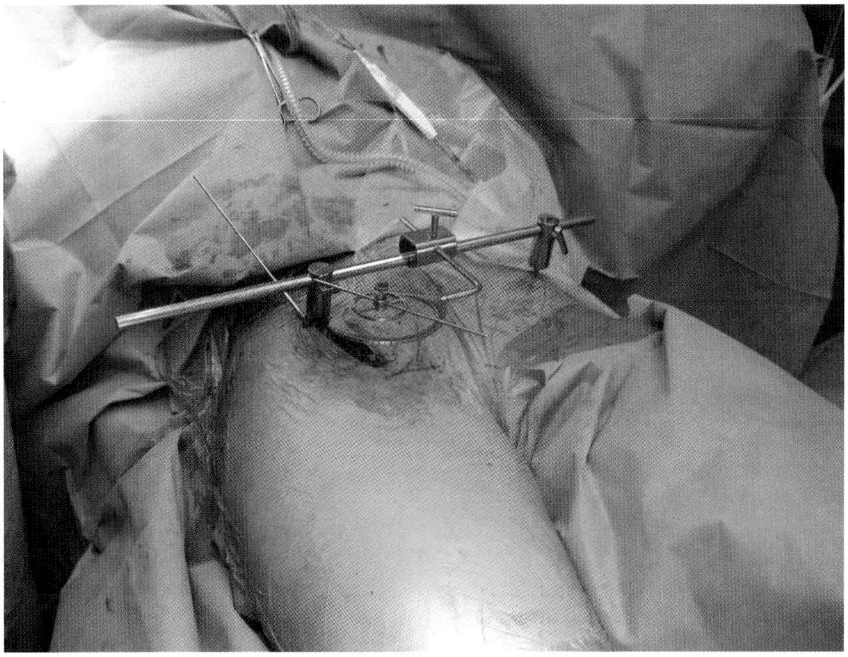

Figure 3 A novel measuring device is used to perform intraoperative assessment of the center-edge and acetabular index angles. The device is mounted bilaterally at the anterosuperior iliac spines using spikes. The measuring disk for the center-edge angle measurement is mounted on the alignment road connecting the spikes. Adjustments of the disk and the final measurement are made under fluoroscopy. (Reproduced with permission from Troelsen A, Elmengaard B, Romer L, Søballe K: Reliable angle assessment during periacetabular osteotomy with a Novel device. *Clin Orthop Relat Res* 2008;466:1169-1176.)

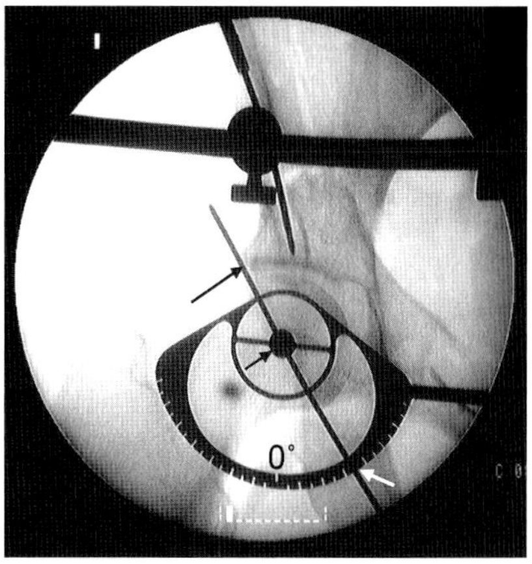

Figure 4 Fluoroscopic image showing measurement of the center-edge angle. The disk is positioned in relation to the center of the femoral head (short arrow) and the lateral point of the acetabular sclerotic roof (long arrow). The measured angle is 35° (white arrow). (Reproduced with permission from Troelsen A, Elmengaard B, Romer L, Søballe K: Reliable angle assessment during periacetabular osteotomy with a Novel device. *Clin Orthop Relat Res* 2008; 466:1169-1176.)

operated side. In the minimally invasive transsartorial approach, an approximately 7 cm skin incision begins at the anterior superior iliac spine and runs distally along the sartorius muscle. After incising the skin and subcutaneous layers, the fascia is incised. Care is taken to isolate and gently retract the lateral femoral cutaneous nerve, which is very sensitive to traction. During the next steps of the approach, the hip is positioned on a splint, which leaves the joint semiflexed. This allows easier transverse retraction of the soft tissues. A periosteal elevator is placed subperiosteally along the medial aspect of the ilium, starting at the anterior superior iliac spine, and it is advanced until it lies just below the linea terminalis. To allow further soft-tissue mobilization, the inguinal ligament is cut and released from the attachment at the anterior superior iliac spine. By pushing the periosteal elevator medially, the sartorius muscle is split in the direction of muscle fibers, and the deep fascia is cut and split in the same direction. A blunt retractor replaces the periosteal elevator at its position along the medial aspect of the ilium, and the iliopsoas muscle and the medial part of the split sartorius are retracted medially. At this point in the procedure, the stepwise osteotomies are performed using instruments and fluoroscopy as have been previously described[11] (**Figure 2**).

The time spent on the approach is approximately 5 minutes. Direct visualization of the osteotomies is limited, and the use of fluoroscopy is an integral part of performing the transsartorial approach for PAO surgery. The average duration of radiation exposure is 35 seconds.[15] To ensure that optimal reorientation has been achieved, intraoperative assessment of the center-edge and acetabular index angles is done using a novel, validated measuring device[16] (**Figure 3**). The measuring device is simple and reliable, and measurements are made using adjustable measuring disks under fluoroscopy in the anteroposterior plane. The device is mounted bilaterally at the anterior superior iliac spine using spikes. The disks are mounted on an alignment rod connecting the spikes. The disk for the center-edge angle measurement is adjusted until a correct position has been achieved in relation to the center of the femoral head and the most lateral point of the acetabular sclerotic roof (**Figure 4**). A correct position of the disk for acetabular index

Table 1

Overview of Studies Reporting Duration of Surgery, Blood Loss, Transfusion Requirements, or Length of Hospital Stay After PAO Surgery

Study (Year)	No. of Hips	Mean Age (Range)	Simultaneous Femoral Osteotomy No. of Hips	Surgical Approach	Mean Duration of Surgery (Range)	Mean Blood Loss (Range)	Transfusion-Percentage of Procedures; No. of Ports (Range)
Siebenrock et al[22] (1999)	75	29.3 years (13-56 years)	16	Modified Smith-Petersen	3.5 hours (2-5 hours)	2,000 mL (750-4,500 mL)	100% 4 ports (1-11)
Trumble et al[2] (1999)	123	32.9 years (14-54 years)	33	56 Modified Smith-Petersen	4.5 hours (NA)	800 mL (NA)	NA
				67 ilioinguinal	6.5 hours (NA)	1,400 mL (NA)	NA
Matta et al[1] (1999)	66	33.6 years (19-51 years)	NA	Modified Smith-Petersen	No femoral osteotomy: 3.1 hours (2-5 hours)	939 mL (400-2,000 mL)	NA
					Femoral osteotomy: 4.1 hours (3.2-6 hours)	980 mL (500-1,800 mL)	NA
Davey and Santore[6] (1999)	70	36.5 years (16-53 years)	NA	Modified Smith-Petersen	3.4 hours (NA)	NA	NA
Pogliacomi et al[4] (2005)	36	35 years[a] (15-55 years)	0	4 Modified Smith-Petersen 32 ilioinguinal	3.3 hours (1.8-7 hours)	2,300 mL (800-6,900 mL)	NA
Kralj et al[23] (2005)	26	34 years (18-50 years)	NA	NA	NA	1,400 mL (NA)	NA
Peters et al[8] (2006)	83	28 years (25-47 years)	14	Modified Smith-Petersen	NA	715 mL (NA)	NA
Atwal et al[24] (2008)	122	23.6 years (18-28 years)	NA	NA	NA	2,191 mL (1,200-4,021 mL)	NA
Troelsen et al[11] (2008)	94	37 years (14-58 years)	0	Minimally invasive	1.2 hours (0.8-2.0 hours)	250 mL[a] (150-350 mL)[b]	3% 2 ports (2-3)
Troelsen et al[13] (2008)	263	31 years[a] (22-40 years)[b]	0	98 ilioinguinal	1.7 hours[a] (1.3-2.0 hours)[b]	500 mL[a] (350-700 mL)[b]	18% 2 ports (1-7)
		35 years[a] (26-44 years)[b]	0	165 minimally invasive	1.2 hours[a] (1.0-1.3)[b]	250 mL[a] (200-350 mL)[b]	4% 2 ports (1-3)

[a]Median.
[b]Interquartile range
NA = not available

angle measurements relates to the most medial and lateral points of the acetabular sclerotic roof. The surgeon also should ascertain proper anteversion of the fragment by assessing the anterior and posterior acetabular rims, verifying that the crossover is not present.[8,9,16-18] The posterior acetabular rim should be lateral to the anterior rim and the femoral head center; the anterior rim should be medial to the femoral head center.

Outcomes and Complications Associated With PAO Approaches

Inherent characteristics of the surgical approach will affect the rate of complications, intraoperative blood loss, the duration of surgery, transfusion requirements, the ability to obtain an optimal acetabular reorientation, and the length of hospital stay.[2,5-10] An overview of blood loss, duration of surgery, and transfusion requirements after PAO surgery reported in 10 studies is summarized in **Table 1**. It is clear that the outcome measures of the transsartorial approach compare favorably with those of other surgical approaches.

The classic Smith-Petersen and ilioinguinal approaches have been used extensively. These approaches result in extensive trauma to the soft tissues; historically, detachment of muscles, including the sartorius, rectus femoris, gluteus medius, and tensor fascia latae, has been performed as part of the procedure. Complications associated with these approaches include femoral nerve palsy, peroneal nerve palsy, obturator nerve palsy, femoral artery and vein lesions/thrombosis, intra-articular osteotomy, secondary displacement, malpositioning of the acetabulum, nonunion, infection, and deep venous thrombosis.[5-10]

In a previous report of the initial experience with the new minimally invasive transsartorial approach, no moderate or severe complications were reported.[11] With the minimally invasive approach, no muscles are detached, and the sartorius is split in line with the muscle fibers. The femoral nerve and vessels are protected by the iliopsoas and sartorius muscles. This approach spares the abductor muscle, and the acetabular blood supply remains intact.

Good results in terms of the absence of complications, minimized blood loss, and the short duration of surgery can be achieved when using the minimally invasive approach. Hip joint survival rates also are encouraging. Kaplan-Meier survivorship data, with conversion to total hip replacement as the end point, for 209 hips treated using the minimally invasive approach between April 2003 and May 2007 are shown in **Figure 5**. Hip joint survivorship for 87 of these hips was reported at 2 and 4.3 years postoperatively.[11] Complete follow-ups were secured by inquiry to the National Registry of Patients. The mean follow-up period was 6.2 years (range, 3.9 to 8.1 years). The joint survivorship rate at 5 years was 94.7% and 88.6% at 8.1 years. It should be acknowledged that the good survivorship results also can be attributed to the accumulated experience of the surgeon (this chapter's senor author) with the procedure.

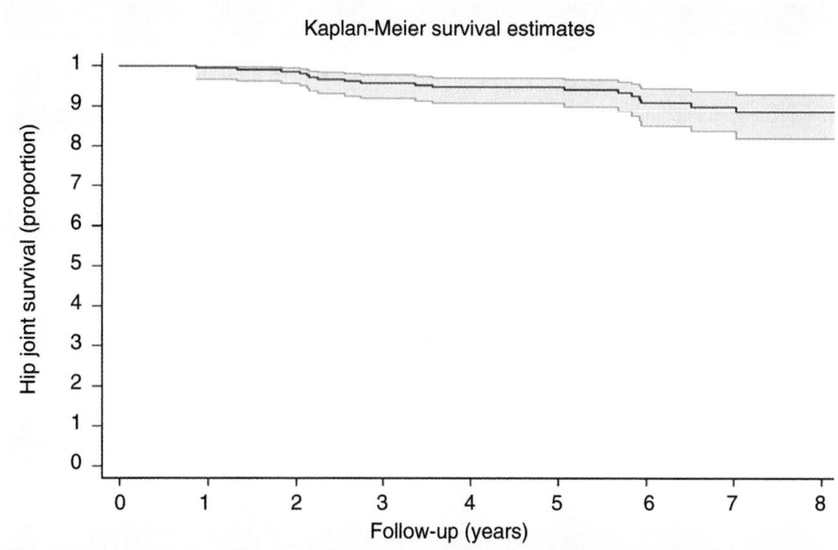

Figure 5 Kaplan-Meier hip joint survival curve from the Aarhus University Hospital, with conversion to total hip replacement as the end point. Inquiry to the National Registry of Patients allowed complete follow-up of 209 PAOs performed between April 2003 and May 2007. Follow-up ranged from 3.9 to 8.1 years.

Perioperative Management

Patient Education Program

All patients are offered a preoperative education program regarding the PAO surgery. Groups of 8 to 10 patients attend a seminar approximately 2 weeks before surgery. A nurse, physiotherapist, anesthesiologist, and the surgeon use lectures and slides to inform patients about the surgical procedure and the postoperative mobilization and exercise program. Patients also are given a video about the PAO treatment and receive written information with illustrations of the procedure, a detailed description of potential complications, and a description of exercises to be performed after surgery.[19]

General Management

Spinal anesthesia is administered to all patients undergoing the PAO procedure. To reduce blood loss, 10 mg/kg of tranexamic acid is given at the beginning of surgery and repeated at 3 hours postoperatively. No bladder catheter is used. For thromboprophylaxis, an injection of 2.5 mg fondaparinux is administered subcutaneously for 2 days, beginning on the day after surgery.

Pain Management

All patients receive 1 g paracetamol orally four times a day, starting in the postanesthesia care unit. In cases of insufficient analgesia (pain exceeding 30 mm on a visual analog scale, maximum 100 mm), the patient is given supplemental oxycodone (5 to 10 mg orally). A local infiltration analgesia is administered before the wound is closed. A solution of 50 mL ropivacaine (2 mg/mL), 1 mL ketorolac (30 mg/mL), and 0.5 mL epinephrine (1 mg/mL) is prepared and loaded into a 100 mL syringe and infiltrated in deep tissues (iliopsoas muscle, tensor fascia latae muscle) and subcutaneous tissues.

A multihole, 20-gauge epidural catheter is tunneled under direct visualization before closure of the fascia into deep layers in the wound with the tip

Table 2
Timetable of Progress and Allowed Activities After PAO Surgery

Activities	Time After PAO Surgery
Stationary biking, ride as passenger in automobile, sleep on operated or nonoperated side, sleep on stomach, intercourse	Immediately after hospital discharge
Swimming	4 weeks
Recreational dancing, crawling, squatting, driving automobile, on-road biking	6 to 8 weeks
Horseback riding, badminton, tennis, gymnastics, yoga, running, jumping	3 to 4 months
Skiing, roller-skating, high-impact sports	Individual recommendations

sited along the iliopsoas muscle. The catheter is connected to a bacterial filter and stitched to the skin. The catheter is connected to a pump and bolus injections of 20 mL ropivacaine (7.5 mg/mL), 1 mL ketorolac (30 mg/mL), and 0.5 mL epinephrine (1 mg/mL) are administered through the 20-G catheter 8, 16, and 24 hours postoperatively.[20]

Mobilization and Exercise Program

The patient walks with crutches if possible 6 to 8 hours after surgery. The next day, under the supervision of the physiotherapist, the mobilization program is continued with the patient using two crutches and allowed 30 kg of weight bearing for the first 6 weeks. This regimen has proven safe in a study using radiographic stereophotogrammetric analysis; fixation of the acetabular fragment was obtained with two screws.[21] Before discharge, patients train on stair climbing. Patients participate in an extensive rehabilitation program that includes muscle strengthening and joint motion exercises; periodically, the exercises are performed in a heated swimming pool. Patients are given instructions for performing a well-defined rehabilitation program with clearly defined weekly goals. The exercises are performed twice daily. Immediately after hospital discharge, the patient is allowed to exercise on a stationary bike, can ride as a passenger in an automobile, and can sleep on the operated side. Progress and allowed activities follow a specific timetable (**Table 2**).

After 6 to 8 weeks, radiographs are obtained at an outpatient clinic. If pain has decreased, there is good callus formation, and no radiographic changes have occurred in the position of the acetabulum compared with the initial postoperative results, progressive weight bearing is allowed, with full weight bearing after 8 weeks.

Summary

The surgeon performing a PAO should be aware that the choice of surgical approach will affect the nature and rate of complications and parameters such as blood loss and the duration of surgery. The transsartorial approach has been developed with the specific goals of minimizing tissue trauma (abductor muscle and rectus femoris sparing) and allowing optimal acetabular reorientation. This minimally invasive, fluoroscopically guided approach is a safe procedure. Hip joint survivorship at medium-term follow-up has been encouraging. The transsartorial approach coupled with a specific perioperative management regimen has been a successful method of performing PAO surgery.

References

1. Matta JM, Stover MD, Siebenrock K: Periacetabular osteotomy through the Smith-Petersen approach. *Clin Orthop Relat Res* 1999;363:21-32.
2. Trumble SJ, Mayo KA, Mast JW: The periacetabular osteotomy: Minimum 2 year followup in more than 100 hips. *Clin Orthop Relat Res* 1999;363:54-63.
3. Søballe K: Pelvic osteotomy for acetabular dysplasia. *Acta Orthop Scand* 2003;74(2):117-118.
4. Pogliacomi F, Stark A, Wallensten R: Periacetabular osteotomy: Good pain relief in symptomatic hip dysplasia, 32 patients followed for 4 years. *Acta Orthop* 2005; 76(1):67-74.
5. Hussell JG, Mast JW, Mayo KA, Howie DW, Ganz R: A comparison of different surgical approaches for the periacetabular osteotomy. *Clin Orthop Relat Res* 1999;363:64-72.
6. Davey JP, Santore RF: Complications of periacetabular osteotomy. *Clin Orthop Relat Res* 1999;363: 33-37.
7. Ganz R, Klaue K, Vinh TS, Mast JW: A new periacetabular osteotomy for the treatment of hip dysplasias: Technique and preliminary results. *Clin Orthop Relat Res* 1988;232:26-36.
8. Peters CL, Erickson JA, Hines JL: Early results of the Bernese periacetabular osteotomy: The learning curve at an academic medical center. *J Bone Joint Surg Am* 2006; 88(9):1920-1926.
9. Trousdale RT, Cabanela ME: Lessons learned after more than 250 periacetabular osteotomies. *Acta Orthop Scand* 2003;74(2): 119-126.
10. Hussell JG, Rodriguez JA, Ganz R: Technical complications of the Bernese periacetabular osteotomy. *Clin Orthop Relat Res* 1999;363: 81-92.

11. Troelsen A, Elmengaard B, Søballe K: A new minimally invasive transsartorial approach for periacetabular osteotomy. *J Bone Joint Surg Am* 2008;90(3):493-498.
12. Letournel E: The treatment of acetabular fractures through the ilioinguinal approach. *Clin Orthop Relat Res* 1993;292:62-76.
13. Troelsen A, Elmengaard B, Søballe K: Comparison of the minimally invasive and ilioinguinal approaches for periacetabular osteotomy: 263 single-surgeon procedures in well-defined study groups. *Acta Orthop* 2008;79(6):777-784.
14. Troelsen A: A new minimally invasive transsartorial approach for periacetabular osteotomy. *Video Journal of Orthopaedics.* http://www.vjortho.com/streaming/jbjs.cfm?c=4075&b=783617706001&m=s. Accessed February 20, 2012.
15. Mechlenburg I, Daugaard H, Søballe K: Radiation exposure to the orthopaedic surgeon during periacetabular osteotomy. *Int Orthop* 2009;33(6):1747-1751.
16. Troelsen A, Elmengaard B, Rømer L, Søballe K: Reliable angle assessment during periacetabular osteotomy with a novel device. *Clin Orthop Relat Res* 2008;466(5):1169-1176.
17. Troelsen A, Jacobsen S, Rømer L, Søballe K: Weightbearing anteroposterior pelvic radiographs are recommended in DDH assessment. *Clin Orthop Relat Res* 2008;466(4):813-819.
18. Troelsen A, Rømer L, Jacobsen S, Ladelund S, Søballe K: Cranial acetabular retroversion is common in developmental dysplasia of the hip as assessed by the weight bearing position. *Acta Orthop* 2010;81(4):436-441.
19. Kjeld Søballe website. Minimally invasive surgery for hip dysplasia. http://www.soballe.com/default.asp?MainMenuId=104&PageId=104&Desc=English. Accessed January 5, 2012.
20. Andersen KV, Pfeiffer-Jensen M, Haraldsted V, Søballe K: Reduced hospital stay and narcotic consumption, and improved mobilization with local and intraarticular infiltration after hip arthroplasty: A randomized clinical trial of an intraarticular technique versus epidural infusion in 80 patients. *Acta Orthop* 2007;78(2):180-186.
21. Mechlenburg I, Kold S, Rømer L, Søballe K: Safe fixation with two acetabular screws after Ganz periacetabular osteotomy. *Acta Orthop* 2007;78(3):344-349.
22. Siebenrock KA, Schöll E, Lottenbach M, Ganz R: Bernese periacetabular osteotomy. *Clin Orthop Relat Res* 1999;363:9-20.
23. Kralj M, Mavcic B, Antolic V, Iglic A, Kralj-Iglic V: The Bernese periacetabular osteotomy: Clinical, radiographic and mechanical 7-15-year follow-up of 26 hips. *Acta Orthop* 2005;76(6):833-840.
24. Atwal NS, Bedi G, Lankester BJ, Campbell D, Gargan MF: Management of blood loss in periacetabular osteotomy. *Hip Int* 2008;18(2):95-100.

27

The Management of Acetabular Retroversion With Reverse Periacetabular Osteotomy

Rafael J. Sierra, MD

Abstract

Retroversion of the acetabulum is a structural disorder in which the acetabulum opens in a posterolateral direction instead of an anterolateral direction in the sagittal plane. The limitations in range of motion (flexion and internal rotation) conferred by sectorial overcoverage resulting from retroversion may predispose patients to femoroacetabular impingement. If left untreated in a symptomatic patient, femoroacetabular impingement can lead to early hip arthritis. In a symptomatic patient with preserved articular cartilage, treatment of the structural disorder may be warranted to alleviate pain and limit the progression of hip disease. It is helpful to review the clinical diagnosis, radiographic interpretation, and management of acetabular retroversion, including treatment with reverse periacetabular osteotomy.

Instr Course Lect 2013;62:305-313.

In a normal hip, the opening of the acetabulum points anterolaterally in the sagittal plane and progresses in a reverse spiral from caudal to cranial. In a retroverted hip socket, the opening is directed in a more posterolateral fashion, the spiral is lost, and cranial version is often lacking[1] (**Figure 1**). Acetabular retroversion was reported in 20% of patients undergoing total hip arthroplasty for osteoarthritis and in 5% of the general population.[2] Acetabular retroversion is present in as many as 50% of patients with Legg-Calvé-Perthes disease[3,4] (**Figure 2**) and in patients with bladder exstrophy,[5] a neuromuscular disease,[6] or proximal femoral focal deficiency.[7] Acetabular retroversion is present in one in six patients (17%) with developmental hip dysplasia.[8,9] The condition also can result from an improperly done pelvic osteotomy[10] or a traumatic closure of the triradiate cartilage in a patient younger than 5 years.[11]

Dr. Sierra or an immediate family member serves as a board member, owner, officer, or committee member of the Midamerica Orthopaedic Association, the Maurice Mueller Foundation, and the American Association of Hip and Knee Surgeons; is a member of a speakers' bureau or has made paid presentations on behalf of Biomet and Arthrex; serves as a paid consultant to or is an employee of Biomet; and has received research or institutional support from Zimmer, Stryker, and DePuy.

The Patient With Acetabular Retroversion

The typical patient with acetabular retroversion is an adolescent or a young adult who reports groin pain. On physical examination, an anterior impingement sign (pain with flexion, adduction, and internal rotation) usually is positive.[12] In a patient with marked acetabular retroversion, it is often possible for the physician to trace the anterior acetabular contour on physical examination. As the hip is passively brought into progressive flexion, the femur externally rotates as the femoral neck contacts the prominent anterior acetabular rim. A patient with long-standing acetabular retroversion may have posterior acetabular or femoral head cartilage damage (a so-called coup-contrecoup lesion), and posterior pain can be reproduced with a posterior impingement test. Limitation of internal rotation at 90° of hip flexion suggests the severity of retroversion and whether a concomitant cam lesion is present. Range of motion in the prone position should be checked because acetabular retroversion can be present with concomitant femoral retrotorsion. It is important to observe exactly how much internal rotation exists at 90° of flexion because this

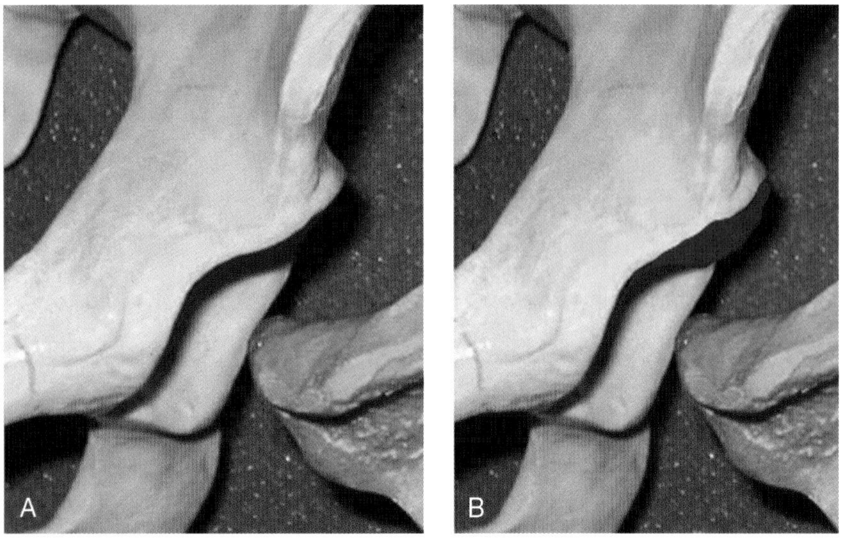

Figure 1 Photographs of a bone model showing cephalad retroversion. **A,** Normal opening of the acetabulum. **B,** Sectorial overcoverage as a result of cephalad retroversion.

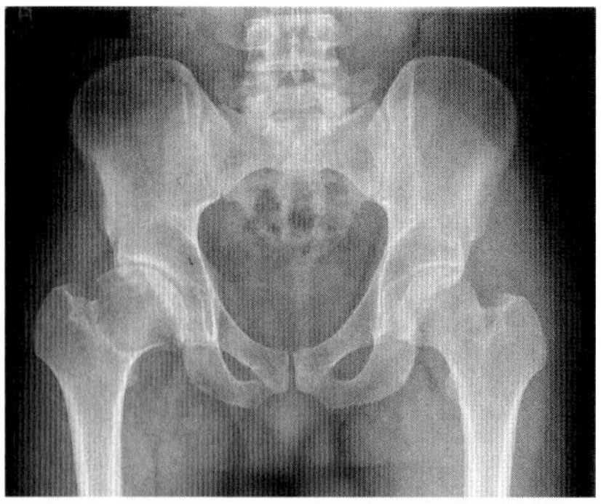

Figure 2 AP radiograph showing Legg-Calvé-Perthes disease in the right hip of a 28-year-old man. The crossover sign can be seen.

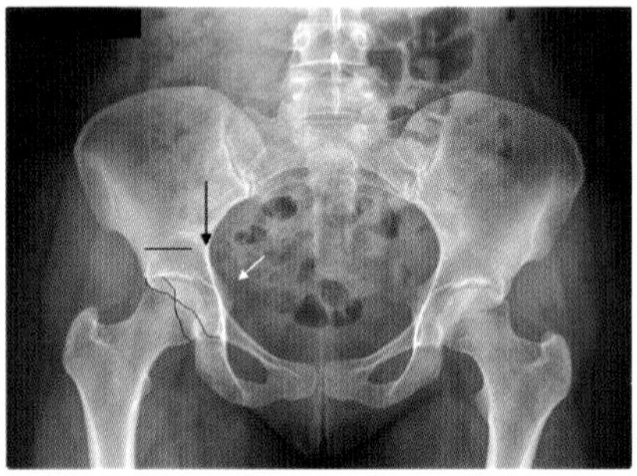

Figure 3 AP radiograph showing bilateral acetabular retroversion in a 30-year-old woman. The PRIS sign is shown by the white arrow; roof length, by the black line; and fossa height, by the black arrow. The two red lines outline anterior and posterior contours depicting the crossover sign and, therefore, acetabular retroversion.

measurement is used intraoperatively to determine the postcorrection improvement in range of motion.

Radiographic Assessment

A standard AP radiograph of a normal hip usually shows that the contours of the anterior and posterior acetabular wall edges meet superolaterally, indicating acetabular anteversion. Reynolds et al[1] described a more distal meeting of the contours of the anterior and posterior wall edges, called the crossover sign, which indicates acetabular retroversion. Kalberer et al[13] developed the prominence of the ischial spine (PRIS) sign to also measure acetabular retroversion. In this study, a positive crossover sign was used as the gold standard for measuring retroversion (**Figure 3**). The PRIS sign was 98% sensitive and 73% specific, and it had a 94% positive predictive value and an 88% negative predictive value for the diagnosis of acetabular retroversion. Both the crossover sign and the PRIS sign are highly sensitive to radiographic pelvic tilt and rotation. Jamali et al[14] validated the crossover sign as a measure of retroversion in anatomic studies. Recently, Larson et al[3] showed the validity of the PRIS sign in patients with early-onset Legg-Calvé-Perthes disease. One advantage of the PRIS sign is that it allows retroversion to be diagnosed in young patients in whom the acetabular walls have not yet ossified.

Several other radiographic measurements are commonly used in the assessment of patients with femoral acetabular impingement. The posterior wall sign is present when the center of rotation of the femoral head is lateral to the contour of the posterior wall. This sign is useful in deciding whether the hip is better suited for treatment with reverse periacetabular osteotomy (PAO) or rim trimming. The roof (acetabular sourcil) length, fovea height, and lateral center-edge angle are used in determining how much rim can be trimmed, if trimming is chosen. A combined cam lesion and pincer impingement must be corrected during surgery.

MRI arthrography and CT can be used as ancillary resources for diagnosis or surgical planning in patients with acetabular retroversion. MRI is particularly helpful in identifying the presence of concomitant labral pathology, especially if the labrum is torn or thin and may require repair or reconstruction. MRI also is useful in determining whether the cartilage is damaged and may require treatment during surgery. MRI or CT of the hip can be combined with MRI or CT of the knee to allow measurement of femoral version (**Figure 4**). Femoral derotational osteotomies occasionally must be combined with treatment of the acetabulum; the amount of rotation required can be estimated before surgery, but intraoperative assessment is required.

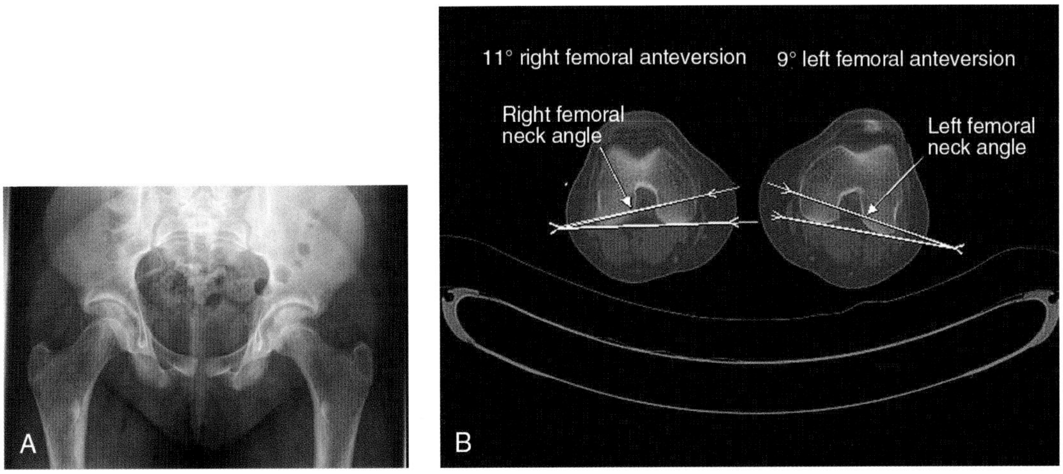

Figure 4 AP radiograph (**A**) and CT scan (**B**) showing acetabular retroversion and decreased femoral anteversion in a 13-year-old girl. Both abnormalities required surgical correction.

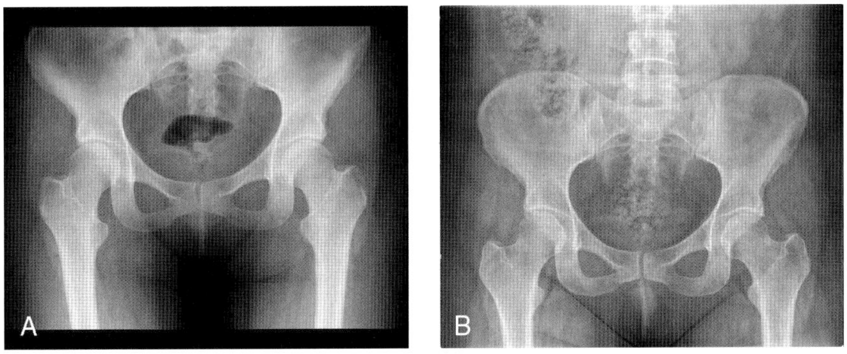

Figure 5 AP radiographs over a 10-year span, showing bilateral acetabular retroversion in a woman at age 24 years (**A**) and age 34 years (**B**). Increasing ossification of the anterosuperior rim can be seen, with worsening sectorial overcoverage.

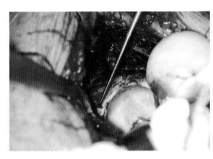

Figure 6 Intraoperative photograph showing severe rim ossification and rim chondromalacia in a 50-year-old woman with global overcoverage.

The Treatment of Acetabular Retroversion

Reasons for Treatment

In patients with symptoms, untreated acetabular retroversion can lead to early degenerative joint disease. Activity-related contact of the femur with the prominent anterior acetabular rim (called a pincer impingement) leads to labral degeneration and tearing.[15-17] Repetitive contact leads to rim changes and additional bony deposition at the rim, causing worsening sectorial overcoverage (**Figure 5**). Damage to the acetabular cartilage in the area of impaction leads to focal chondromalacia[17] (**Figure 6**). Recurrent abutment of the femoral head-neck junction against the anterior acetabular rim may increase the contact pressure of the posterior femoral head against the socket posteriorly during the impingement and can lead to posterior acetabular cartilage damage. Relative undercoverage of the head posteriorly may lead to abnormal stresses subject to the posterior aspect of the acetabulum because of the high loads in this area during activities of daily living.

The Decision-Making Tree

The decision to proceed with surgical treatment of acetabular retroversion hinges on the patient's symptoms and the radiographic findings (**Figure 7**). The initial treatment should be nonsurgical. Activities that put the hip at risk of impingement, such as those that lead to high flexion with loading, should be limited. If surgical treatment is warranted, several issues should be considered.

Acetabular retroversion is not always the primary source of symptoms. Patients with severe pistol grip deformity may have mild acetabular retroversion, with a borderline lateral center-edge angle, a short roof, and a posterior wall sign. In select patients, it is best to not treat the retroversion unless there is severe cartilage damage to the rim. Instead, decompressing the cam lesion may have the greatest effect on the results of treatment (**Figure 8**).

In addition to acetabular retroversion, other pathology may be present, such as femoral retroversion, cam mor-

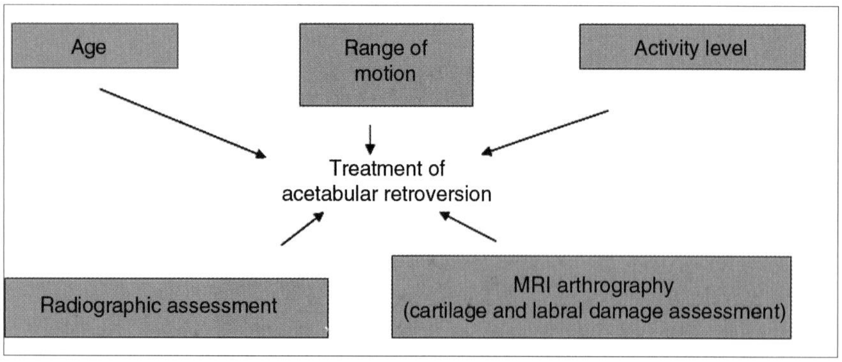

Figure 7 Schematic diagram of the factors that determine the treatment of acetabular retroversion.

phology, or psoas tendinitis (internal snapping hip). These other disorders may require treatment alone or in combination with reverse PAO or rim trimming. If psoas tendinitis is suspected, ultrasound-guided iliopsoas sheath injection and physical therapy are recommended before surgery is considered; the patient's symptoms occasionally can be resolved through these nonsurgical treatments. Femoral retroversion and cam morphology may require treatment at the time of surgery. Acetabular cartilage damage may be seen on MRI. Substantial anterior rim damage or a coup-contrecoup lesion may be contraindications to joint-preserving surgery, except in the very young patient in whom osteotomy may be warranted as a salvage procedure.

The Treatment Options

If the cam morphology and acetabular cartilage damage are more consistent with cam-type impingement than with acetabular retroversion, it may be possible to treat only the damage with a femoral-sided head-neck junction osteoplasty (**Figure 8**).

Acetabular Osteochondroplasty

Acetabular osteochondroplasty (labral takedown, refixation, or reconstruction) can be used to treat retroversion in a patient with no posterior wall sign and with good coverage (more than 35° at the lateral center edge). Acetabular osteochondroplasty also can be used to resect damaged cartilage in a patient with cranial retroversion and good acetabular coverage. The ideal candidate is younger than 40 years and has both impingement and an acetabular chondrolabral injury. The retroverted rim can be resected in its entirety. However, the lateral coverage and roof width must be measured to determine how much resection can be performed while maintaining a lateral center-edge angle of at least 25°. Open or arthroscopic acetabular osteochondroplasty can be performed, depending on the patient's age, the length of the retroverted segment, the extent of underlying cartilage damage, the labral status, and the surgeon's expertise.

The younger the patient and the more severe the cartilage damage or labral pathology (such as thinning or maceration), the more inclined the surgeon should be to do an open surgical procedure (such as a surgical hip dislocation). An open approach allows all anatomic abnormalities to be precisely corrected, and cartilage and labral damage to be treated, occasionally with precise resection of the damaged cartilage, if possible, and with reconstruction of the labral defect.

Reverse PAO

Reverse PAO is indicated for correcting retroversion in patients with femoroacetabular impingement if the patient has a positive anterior impingement test as well as MRI arthrographic findings of an acetabular rim lesion with insufficient posterior coverage.[18] A reverse PAO (reorientation osteotomy) should not be performed if the posterior wall coverage is excessive because correction could lead to impingement in extension and external rotation. In addition, if severe articular cartilage damage is present, that would move the advanced anterior cartilage degeneration into the weight-bearing zone. If the posterior wall sign is present, indicating a lack of posterior coverage, and the patient has decreased internal rotation at 90°, a reverse PAO is the treatment of choice. Rim trimming alone in this setting could lead to global hip instability.

The ideal candidate for correction of acetabular retroversion is younger than 40 years, is not obese, has symptomatic hip pathology (**Figure 9**), a radiographic Tönnis grade of 0 or 1, a posterior wall sign, and no cartilage degeneration on MRI in the area of acetabular overcoverage.

Surgical Planning and Technique

The surgeon should critically evaluate the radiographs to determine the appropriate correction of a retroverted hip. The goal should be to correct the crossover sign while maintaining a horizontal roof. The review of MRI or CT should include particular attention to posterior cartilage degeneration, the location of the acetabular fossa, and the shape of the femoral head-neck junction because reshaping may be required.

Surgery is performed with the patient supine on an imaging table. A spinal or general anesthetic is used. An

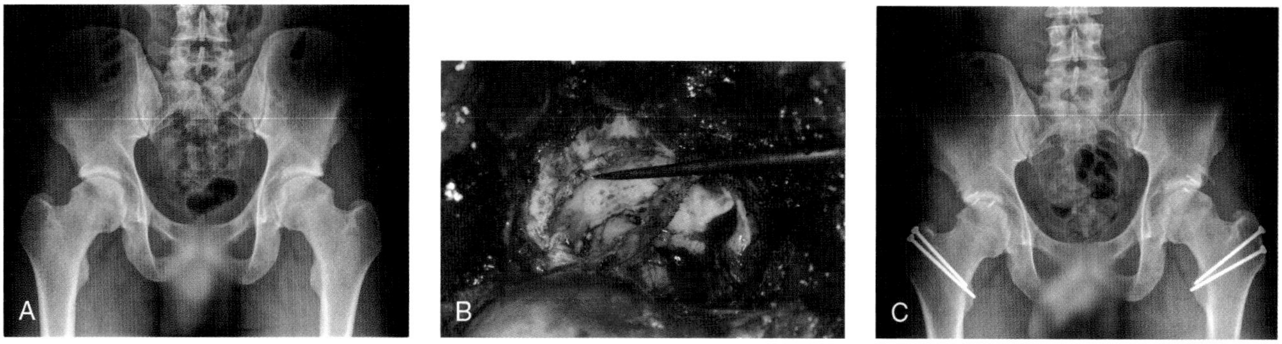

Figure 8 **A,** AP radiograph showing cephalad acetabular retroversion in a 20-year-old man with substantial femoroacetabular impingement. **B,** Intraoperative photograph of the acetabulum showing severe cartilage damage occurring in the area of retroversion. **C,** AP radiograph showing 2-year results after resection of the retroverted segment as part of the treatment of the articular cartilage rim damage.

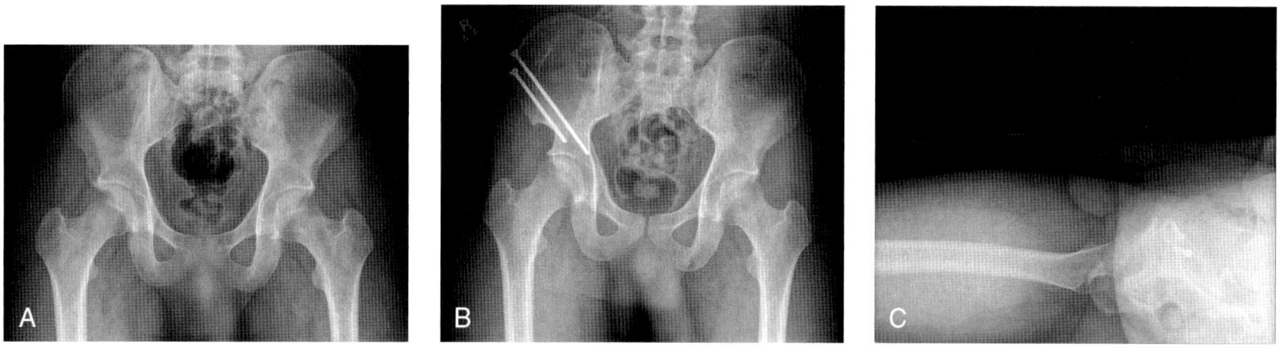

Figure 9 **A,** AP radiograph showing acetabular retroversion, a short roof, and a borderline lateral center-edge angle in an 18-year-old man who had undergone two unsuccessful hip arthroscopic procedures. AP **(B)** and lateral **(C)** radiographs at 2-year follow-up after reverse PAO. The patient was pain free and returned to high-impact activities.

epidural catheter can be placed for pain control during the 48 hours after surgery. AP and iliac oblique radiographs are obtained before surgery, and fluoroscopy is used during surgery. A blood-salvage device may be useful because blood loss is a concern in some patients. Most patients are young and healthy, and the need for an allogeneic blood transfusion is unlikely; therefore, preoperative autologous donation is not recommended.

Intraoperative electromyography is used to monitor the nerves to the affected extremity. Some data suggest that using electromyographic monitoring during surgery can prevent nerve injury; however, electromyographic monitoring is not a replacement for a precise and atraumatic surgical technique.[19]

The surgery is performed through a C-shaped incision centered over the anterior superior iliac spine. The distal superficial exposure requires an incision of the fascia over the tensor. The medial fascia should be retracted, and the tensor fascia muscle should be separated and retracted laterally. Slight abduction of the leg makes this separation easier. The interval is then extended proximally between the sartorius and the tensor fascia laterally. The sartorius is released from bone and retracted medially. Flexion of the hip on a triangle or bump is recommended throughout the surgery except when radiographs are being obtained or femoral osteochondroplasty is being performed.

The proximal exposure includes an incision of the fascia and periosteum over the iliac crest, with a subperiosteal exposure medially elevating the abdominal oblique musculature and iliacus from the inner pelvis downward past the pelvic rim. An Eva retractor is placed onto the inner aspect of the iliac crest. Exposure of the crest is limited medially to prevent constant bleeding in the iliac fossa, most commonly where the iliolumbar artery penetrates the iliac crest 2 cm from the sacroiliac joint. Usually this bleeding can be stopped by slightly enlarging the hole and adding bone wax. The deep distal exposure is done by visualizing the rectus femoris tendon and retracting it medially. Every attempt should be made to preserve the pedicle of the ascending branch of the lateral circumflex artery.

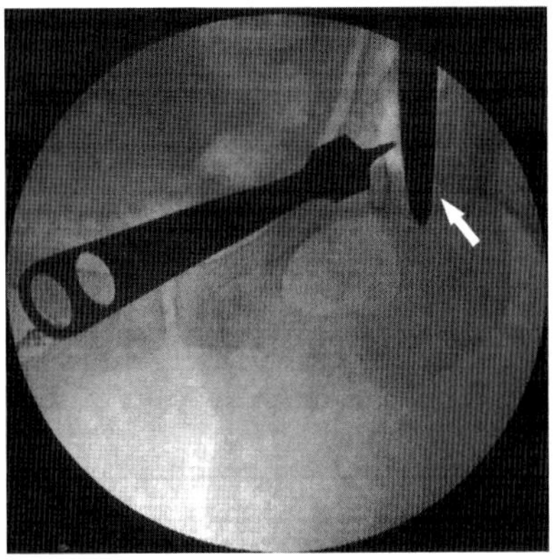

Figure 10 Fluoroscopic AP image showing scissors (arrow) held over the ischium to identify ischial osteotome placement.

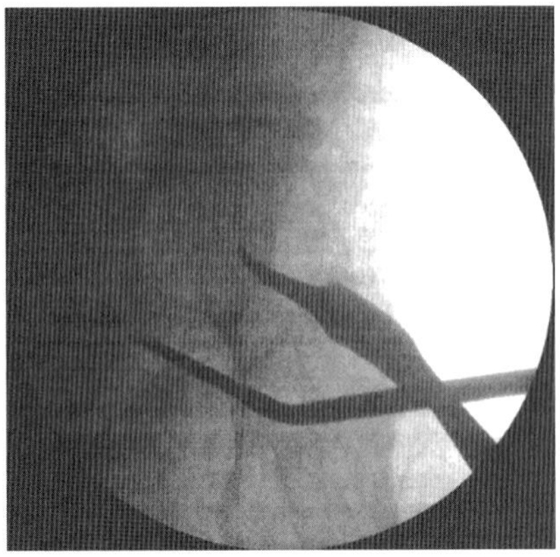

Figure 11 Fluoroscopic iliac oblique image showing position of the Ganz osteotome in ischial osteotomy. The osteotomy should be inferior to the infracotyloid groove.

A decision should be made before surgery as to whether the joint requires opening for the treatment of intra-articular pathology or a femoral head-neck junction osteochondroplasty. The head-neck junction may need to be reshaped, and therefore it is likely that the rectus femoris will need to be taken down at the time of the PAO. The reflected head of the rectus femoris tendon can be seen proximally as it dives posteriorly to its insertion in the superolateral acetabular area. This insertion is divided transversely, and the direct head of the rectus femoris is released from the anterior inferior iliac spine. The release is performed circumferentially around the anterior inferior iliac spine toward its medial border to provide good exposure of the iliocapsularis muscle. The iliocapsularis is dissected from the capsule laterally to medially, proximally from its origin on the undersurface of the anterior inferior iliac spine. Completing the dissection between the iliocapsularis, especially at the inferolateral border, allows the calcar femoris to be palpated through the capsule. Medially, this dissection exposes the iliopectineal bursa. Placing a Hohmann retractor into the pubis medial to the iliopectineal eminence allows the medial tissues to be properly retracted and the medial extent of the pubic osteotomy to be visualized.

The ischial osteotomy should be done first, followed by the pubic, iliac, and retroacetabular osteotomies. The inferomedial capsule is palpated for the ischial osteotomy. The psoas tendon usually is distal. The space is opened with scissors. Deep in this area, the scissors should be kept proximal to the obturator externus muscle. The ischium is triangular in shape, with the base posterior. The position of the scissors on the ischium can be verified on an AP radiograph (**Figure 10**). The space made by the scissors is used to place the Ganz osteotome onto the ischium. Proximally, the infracotyloid groove should be felt with the osteotome. The infracotyloid groove usually indicates the inferior border of the acetabulum. The position of the osteotome can be verified on the iliac oblique radiograph (**Figure 11**). The osteotome should be aimed toward the patient's ipsilateral shoulder and inclined with the hand toward the patient's abdomen at approximately 20° to 30°. When the osteotome is placed over the lateral border of the ischium, the leg should be abducted to bring the sciatic nerve more lateral. The osteotome should be side wiggled to confirm it is fully in bone or exiting lateral or medial. The osteotome is slowly retrieved while palpating to determine that the lateral aspect of the ischium is fully osteotomized. Most commonly, the lateral aspect of the ischium still requires an osteotomy; if this is the case, the osteotome should be translated laterally, and the osteotomy should be repeated in the medial aspect of the ischium. The ischial osteotomy is an incomplete osteotomy that should not be completed through the posterior column. A depth of 2.5 cm is sufficient. It is more important to osteotomize the hard medial cortex than the thinner lateral cortex, which may eventually break at the end after the posterior column is osteotomized.

The osteotomy of the pubic bone requires splitting the periosteum with a knife in line with the pubis toward the tip of the Hohmann retractor. Repositioning the Hohmann retractor more medially is commonly required. The periosteum should be elevated superoinferiorly to expose bone, while protecting the soft tissues by placing retractors superiorly and inferiorly medial to the iliopectineal eminence. The use of an oscillating saw is recommended to osteotomize the pubis at an approximate 45° angle in a superomedial direction away from the joint, so as to prevent trapping the pubic bones at the time of correction. The limb should be flexed during this osteotomy to relieve tension on the femoral nerve.

The transverse iliac osteotomy now can be performed. The level and starting point of this osteotomy can be assessed on both AP and iliac oblique fluoroscopic views (**Figure 12**). The osteotomy should be as high as possible for three reasons: to lessen the risk of injury to the gluteus minimus, which contains the supra-acetabular branch of the superior gluteal artery

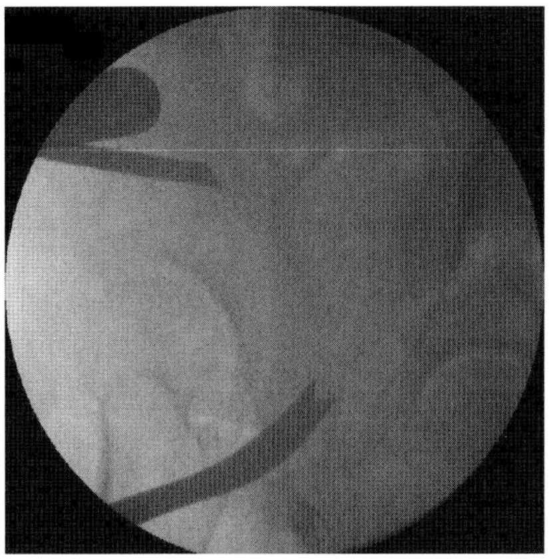

Figure 12 Fluoroscopic iliac oblique image showing the saw at the time of the horizontal iliac osteotomy.

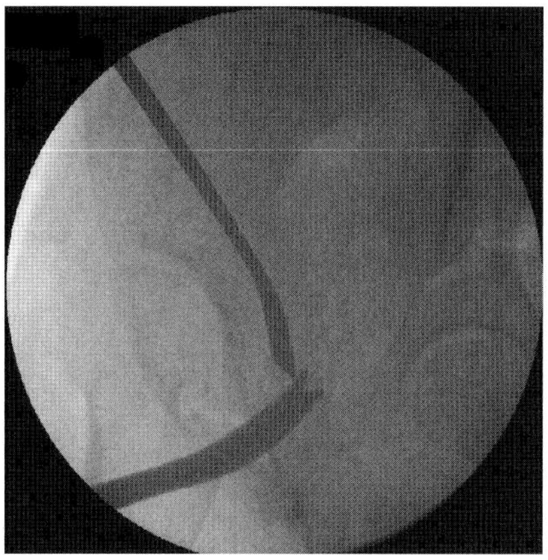

Figure 13 Fluoroscopic iliac oblique image showing the retroacetabular osteotomy connecting the horizontal iliac osteotomy with the ischial osteotomy.

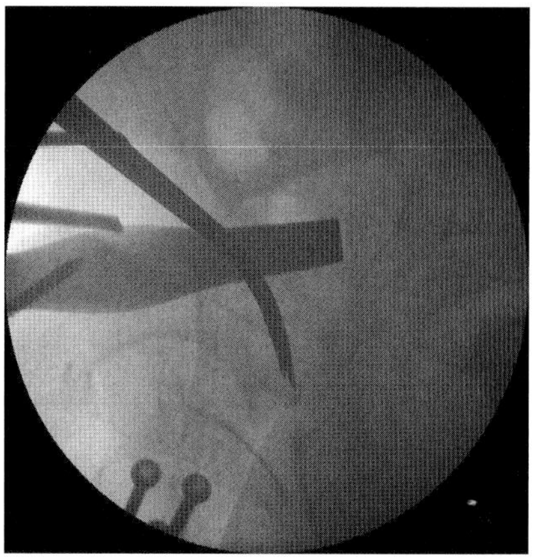

Figure 14 Fluoroscopic iliac oblique image showing the Ganz osteotome in the posterolateral corner to relieve hinging bone.

that provides vascularity to the fragment; to retain a large bone bridge between the osteotomy and the joint for better purchase of the Schanz screw that will be used for reorienting the fragment; and to lessen the risk of breaking into the joint during the retroacetabular osteotomy. The iliac osteotomy starts at the distal edge of the anterior superior iliac spine and proceeds in a slightly proximal direction toward the rim distal to the sacroiliac joint. The direction and depth of the osteotomy should be verified on the iliac oblique fluoroscopic view (**Figure 12**). The soft tissues about the lateral aspect of the pelvis should be protected before this osteotomy. The tensor fascia insertion on the pelvis is released minimally for access to the outer table. A periosteal elevator is used to palpate and elevate the muscles from the outside, aiming slightly distal toward and into the sciatic notch. A second retractor is then placed laterally. The steps of the osteotomy are as follows: the osteotomy is marked out; the corner of the osteotomy is determined, usually 1 cm lateral from the pelvic brim, and is marked out (a pencil tip burr can be used to mark the turning point and give the osteotome support and direction); and the transverse iliac osteotomy is performed while directly visualizing the edge of the saw blade within the inner table.

The retroacetabular osteotomy is done after subperiosteal preparation of the quadrilateral surface 4 cm beneath the iliopectineal line (**Figure 13**). A curved narrow osteotomy from medial to lateral is used to make the corner. The iliac oblique radiograph is used with fluoroscopic guidance. The osteotome should be carried from superior to inferior in a medial-to-lateral fashion, taking care to osteotomize both medial and lateral cortices. The fluoroscopic image guides the osteotome so it is in line with the posterior column and away from the joint and the posterior column border itself. The osteotome should not be brought deep into the column until it is removed and repositioned because it can become trapped in the column and is difficult to remove. When the osteotomy is complete, the fragment will translate.

A 5.0 Schanz screw is placed, beginning proximal to the anterior inferior iliac spine and continuing toward the osteotomy corner. A laminar spreader is placed into the iliac osteotomy and splayed open. A larger laminar spreader should be placed between the posterior column and fragment. If the fragment does not fully open, usually the posterior column osteotomy is incomplete, and the larger angulated osteotome should be placed by sliding it over the posterior column remnant. This move can be done under fluoroscopic control, and impinging bone should be removed (**Figure 14**). When the posteroinferior aspect of the osteotomy is completed, the osteotomy fragment should be free to move in the desired location. In pure acetabular retroversion, the fragment also can be hinged using the posterolateral aspect as the axis point. If correction is required in several directions, the fragment must be totally free.

Before the acetabular fragment is repositioned, it must be completely free. The junction of the posteroinferior column and the ischial osteotomy may prevent impingement-free motion of the fragment. It is also important to access the pubic ramus to allow the fragment to tilt anterolaterally to ensure complete displacement. For acetabular retroversion, reorientation is achieved by combined flexion and internal rotation of the acetabular fragment, usually at approximately 10° to

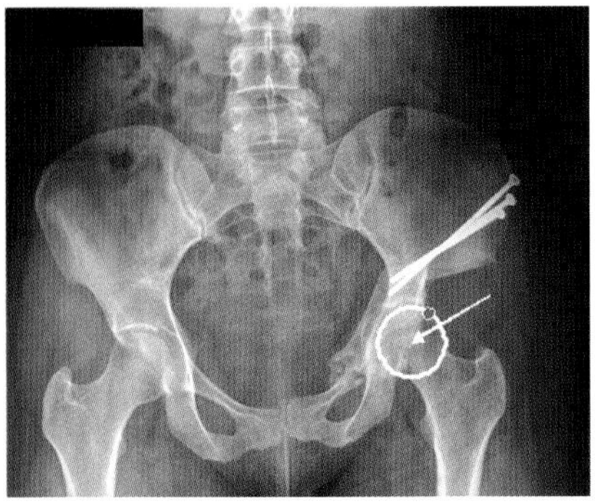

Figure 15 Postoperative AP radiograph showing correction of acetabular retroversion with a reverse PAO in the patient shown in **Figure 3**. The patient was pain free at 3-year follow-up. The large circle outlines the femoral head. The arrow shows the connection of the posterior wall and the solid red circle shows the meeting of the anterior and posterior walls, which is indicative of acetabular anteversion.

20° each[18] (**Figure 15**). The goal is to eliminate the crossover sign and allow sufficient impingement-free range of motion and internal rotation. Intraoperative radiographs should allow assessment of the anteroposterior walls as well as the posterior wall sign. The posterior wall sign will determine whether excessive posterior overcoverage is a concern. After the fragment is temporarily positioned and fixed in the chosen position with two smooth Steinmann pins, the hip should be brought to 90°, and internal rotation should be measured. The improvement in internal rotation with fragment repositioning should be at least 25°, if there is no evidence of posterior wall prominence. It is common to obtain an additional 10° of internal rotation with a femoral head-neck junction osteochondroplasty, for a combined improvement of approximately 35°. Under fluoroscopic guidance, the hip is brought through a range of motion, and areas of impingement are noted. The inferior iliac spine can be a source of extra-articular impingement and is trimmed down if it is impinging.

Postoperative Rehabilitation

The schedule for postoperative rehabilitation depends on whether the reverse PAO has been performed alone or as an adjunct to other procedures. Most commonly, the patient is maintained on toe-touch, flat foot weight bearing for 4 weeks. Passive range of motion of the hip is used through the first 4 weeks, and active range of motion is allowed thereafter. After 4 to 6 weeks, when bony union is well underway, patients are allowed to use a stationary bicycle and begin abduction strengthening exercises, first standing and then lying on the opposite hip.

Complete bony union requires several months. Most patients have pain-free range of motion 8 weeks to 3 months after surgery, depending on their age, bone quality, and extent of correction. The use of crutches can be discontinued at this time. Complete rehabilitation may require as long as 1 year if the hip had severe preexisting abductor weakness.

Research

Siebenrock et al[18] described the results of reverse PAO for isolated correction of acetabular retroversion. Between 1997 and August 1999, 29 PAOs were performed in 22 patients (average age, 23 years) to reorient a retroverted acetabulum. In 24 of the hips, a concomitant femoral head-neck offset reshaping was performed through an anterior capsulotomy. The goal of the surgery was to obtain internal rotation of 30° at 90° of flexion. At an average 30-month follow-up (range, 24 to 49 months), the average Merle D'Aubigné hip score had improved from 14 to 16.9 points, and 28 hips had a good or an excellent result. None of the patients had signs of osteoarthritis on postoperative radiographs. Three patients required additional surgery. In one of these patients, a second reverse PAO was required because of partial loss of correction, with screw bending noticed at 8 weeks. The second patient had a posterior impingement resulting from the PAO, which was treated with surgical hip dislocation and trimming of the posterior rim, with excellent results. The third patient had an incomplete correction, as evidenced by a persistent crossover sign on postoperative radiographs and poor correction of the anterior center-edge angle. This patient underwent surgical revision for improvement of the anterior head-neck offset, which had not been treated during the PAO. The authors stressed the importance of assessing the correction at the time of surgery by reviewing well-centered intraoperative pelvic radiographs and evaluating hip range of motion. Excessive posterior wall coverage can lead to posterior acetabular impingement in extension and external rotation. An acetabular index less than 0° also can compromise the clinical outcome secondary to impingement. A persistent femoral deformity can compromise the surgical results, and therefore it is important to assess the labrum and anterior femoral head-neck junction through an anterior capsulotomy for signs of impingement at the time of surgery.

Summary

Retroversion of the acetabulum has been associated with femoroacetabular impingement. Patients usually have limited range of motion and an anterior impingement sign on physical examination. A symptomatic patient with minimal cartilage degeneration may benefit from surgical treatment if nonsurgical management is unsuccessful. The decision to proceed with surgery should be based on a thorough review of the clinical scenario, including the patient's age, activity level, and physical examination findings, as well as a precise review of radiographs and MRI and a frank discussion about surgical expectations and return to sports. In symptomatic patients with limited range of motion and a posterior wall sign, a reverse PAO often is the treatment of choice. The reverse PAO allows patient-specific three-dimensional reorientation of the acetabulum, resulting in objective improvement in range of motion, pain, and function.

References

1. Reynolds D, Lucas J, Klaue K: Retroversion of the acetabulum: A cause of hip pain. *J Bone Joint Surg Br* 1999;81(2):281-288.
2. Giori NJ, Trousdale RT: Acetabular retroversion is associated with osteoarthritis of the hip. *Clin Orthop Relat Res* 2003;417:263-269.
3. Larson AN, Stans AA, Sierra RJ: Ischial spine sign reveals acetabular retroversion in Legg-Calvé-Perthes disease. *Clin Orthop Relat Res* 2011;469(7):2012-2018.
4. Ezoe M, Naito M, Inoue T: The prevalence of acetabular retroversion among various disorders of the hip. *J Bone Joint Surg Am* 2006;88(2):372-379.
5. Sponseller PD, Bisson LJ, Gearhart JP, Jeffs RD, Magid D, Fishman E: The anatomy of the pelvis in the extrophy complex. *J Bone Joint Surg Am* 1995;77(2): 177-189.
6. Kim HT, Wenger DR: Location of acetabular deficiency and associated hip dislocation in neuromuscular hip dysplasia: Three-dimensional computed tomographic analysis. *J Pediatr Orthop* 1997;17(2):143-151.
7. Dora C, Bühler M, Stover MD, Mahomed MN, Ganz R: Morphologic characteristics of acetabular dysplasia in proximal femoral focal deficiency. *J Pediatr Orthop B* 2004;13(2):81-87.
8. Li PL, Ganz R: Morphologic features of congenital acetabular dysplasia: One in six is retroverted. *Clin Orthop Relat Res* 2003;416: 245-253.
9. Mast JW, Brunner RL, Zebrack J: Recognizing acetabular version in the radiographic presentation of hip dysplasia. *Clin Orthop Relat Res* 2004;418:48-53.
10. Dora C, Mascard E, Mladenov K, Seringe R: Retroversion of the acetabular dome after Salter and triple pelvic osteotomy for congenital dislocation of the hip. *J Pediatr Orthop B* 2002;11(1):34-40.
11. Dora C, Zurbach J, Hersche O, Ganz R: Pathomorphologic characteristics of posttraumatic acetabular dysplasia. *J Orthop Trauma* 2000;14(7):483-489.
12. Klaue K, Durnin CW, Ganz R: The acetabular rim syndrome: A clinical presentation of dysplasia of the hip. *J Bone Joint Surg Br* 1991;73(3):423-429.
13. Kalberer F, Sierra RJ, Madan SS, Ganz R, Leunig M: Ischial spine projection into the pelvis: A new sign for acetabular retroversion. *Clin Orthop Relat Res* 2008; 466(3):677-683.
14. Jamali AA, Mladenov K, Meyer DC, et al: Anteroposterior pelvic radiographs to assess acetabular retroversion: High validity of the "cross-over-sign." *J Orthop Res* 2007;25(6):758-765.
15. Ganz R, Leunig M, Leunig-Ganz K, Harris WH: The etiology of osteoarthritis of the hip: An integrated mechanical concept. *Clin Orthop Relat Res* 2008;466(2): 264-272.
16. Ganz R, Parvizi J, Beck M, Leunig M, Nötzli H, Siebenrock KA: Femoroacetabular impingement: A cause for osteoarthritis of the hip. *Clin Orthop Relat Res* 2003; 417:112-120.
17. Beck M, Kalhor M, Leunig M, Ganz R: Hip morphology influences the pattern of damage to the acetabular cartilage: Femoroacetabular impingement as a cause of early osteoarthritis of the hip. *J Bone Joint Surg Br* 2005;87(7): 1012-1018.
18. Siebenrock KA, Schoeniger R, Ganz R: Anterior femoro-acetabular impingement due to acetabular retroversion: Treatment with periacetabular osteotomy. *J Bone Joint Surg Am* 2003;85(2): 278-286.
19. Pring ME, Trousdale RT, Cabanela ME, Harper CM: Intraoperative electromyographic monitoring during periacetabular osteotomy. *Clin Orthop Relat Res* 2002;400:158-164.

SECTION

5

Adult Reconstruction: Knee

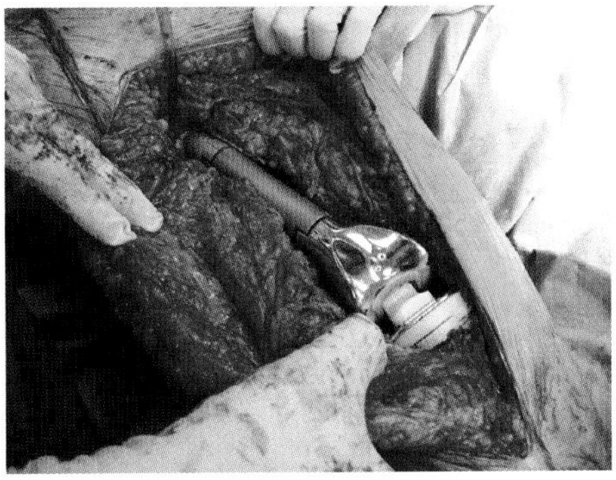

DVD marks chapter 30.

28 Contemporary Internal Fixation Techniques for Periprosthetic Fractures of the Hip and Knee

29 Revision for Periprosthetic Fractures of the Hip and Knee

DVD 30 Management of Bone Defects in Revision Total Knee Arthroplasty

31 Evaluation and Management of the Infected Total Knee Arthroplasty

32 Patellofemoral Arthroplasty: The Other Unicompartmental Knee Replacement

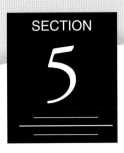

28

Contemporary Internal Fixation Techniques for Periprosthetic Fractures of the Hip and Knee

Frank A. Liporace, MD
Derek J. Donegan, MD
Joshua R. Langford, MD
George J. Haidukewych, MD

Abstract

The volume of total hip and knee arthroplasties continues to increase as the US population ages. The number of prosthetic complications, specifically those involving periprosthetic fractures, is also increasing. Periprosthetic fractures can be difficult to manage. Reduction and fixation of these fractures is a complex undertaking, primarily because the preexisting implants can obstruct the reduction and placement of fixation devices. It is crucial to consider the fracture location, implant stability, and bone quality when determining a treatment plan. Expertise in both fracture management and joint reconstruction is often necessary to provide the best care and outcomes for patients. Although periprosthetic fractures are challenging, advancements in surgical techniques and available implants offer the surgeon tools to provide good outcomes and patient satisfaction.

Instr Course Lect 2013;62:317-332.

Total hip arthroplasty (THA) and total knee arthroplasty (TKA) are highly effective treatments for disabling degenerative joint disease, with high success rates and low complication rates. When complications such as periprosthetic fractures occur, they can be devastating to the patient and challenging for the surgeon. Reduction and fixation of these fractures is a complex undertaking, primarily because preexisting implants can obstruct the reduction and placement of fixation devices.[1] It is crucial to take into consideration fracture location, implant stability, and bone quality when determining a treatment plan. Expertise in both fracture management and joint reconstruction is often necessary to provide the best care and outcomes for these patients.

Epidemiology

The incidence of periprosthetic fractures for THA is variable, with studies reporting rates from 0.1% to 18%.[2-6] The incidence is greater for revision arthroplasty. The largest reported series from the Mayo Clinic joint arthroplasty database identified an incidence of periprosthetic fractures of 1% (238 in 23,980) in primary THAs and 4% (252 in 6,349) in revision THAs.[2] Lindahl et al[7] reported a higher risk of death after a periprosthetic fracture compared with similar patients who had uncomplicated THAs.

The rates of periprosthetic fractures for TKA also vary. Rates of 0.3% to 5.5% have been reported for primary TKAs and up to 30% for revision TKAs.[8-11] Supracondylar femoral frac-

Dr. Liporace or an immediate family member has received royalties from DePuy; is a member of a speakers' bureau or has made paid presentations on behalf of DePuy, Synthes, Smith & Nephew, Stryker, and Medtronic; serves as a paid consultant to or is an employee of DePuy, Medtronic, Synthes, Smith & Nephew, and Stryker; serves as an unpaid consultant to AO; and has received research or institutional support from Synthes, Smith & Nephew, and Accumed. Dr. Langford or an immediate family member serves as a paid consultant to or is an employee of Stryker and Internal Fixation Systems and owns stock or stock options in Internal Fixation Systems. Dr. Haidukewych or an immediate family member serves as a board member, owner, officer, or committee member of the American Academy of Orthopaedic Surgeons; has received royalties from DePuy; serves as a paid consultant to or is an employee of Smith & Nephew and Synthes; and owns stock or stock options in Surmodics and Orthopediatrics. Neither Dr. Donegan nor any immediate family member has received anything of value from or owns stock in a commercial company or institution related directly or indirectly to the subject of this chapter.

tures are the most common type, with an incidence of 0.3% to 2.5% for primary TKAs and 1.6% to 38% for revision TKAs.[8-10,12] Periprosthetic tibial fractures are less common than periprosthetic femoral fractures. The Mayo Clinic database reported an incidence of 0.1% intraoperative and 0.4% postoperative fractures, with a higher incidence after revision TKA.[13] Periprosthetic fractures of the patella occur more often in knees without patellar resurfacing than in knees with resurfacing. A large study by Ortiguera and Berry[14] reported a 0.68% rate of periprosthetic fracture of the patella after TKA. Fractures of the patella are more common after revision TKA, with one study reporting a six times higher frequency of patellar fractures after revision TKA compared with primary TKA.[15] The true incidence of patellar fractures is unknown because many of these fractures are asymptomatic.[14]

Risk Factors and Etiology

Periprosthetic fractures about a THA or TKA typically result from a low-energy fall in an elderly patient or a high-energy injury in a young patient.[2] In high-energy traumatic injuries, formal Advanced Trauma Life Support protocol should be followed because it is necessary to rule out other potential injuries.

The absolute number of periprosthetic THA fractures has increased over time as the number of patients being treated with THA has grown.[16] Surgical technique is a risk factor because revision arthroplasty techniques often involve implant constructs that transfer forces to the tip of the stem and increase the risk of fracture.[16-18] Patient characteristics, such as female sex and older age, have been cited as independent risk factors.[19] Inflammatory arthropathies, including rheumatoid arthritis, have been suggested as risk factors for periprosthetic THA fractures; however, all of these factors can be confounded by the presence of osteopenia or osteoporosis.[20,21] The change in the geometry of the femur with age, such as increasing femoral bow, canal dilation, thinning cortices, and alteration in bone morphology, may increase the risk of a periprosthetic THA fracture.

Multiple risk factors have been identified for periprosthetic TKA fractures. Metabolic disorders (such as osteoporosis) are known risk factors. Studies have reported decreased bone mineral density after TKA.[22,23] One study reported that 30 of 41 patients with a periprosthetic TKA fracture had a preexisting disease, including 16 patients with osteoporosis; 7 with rheumatoid arthritis, which required long-term steroid use; and 2 with neurologic disorders.[22] Wang et al[23] demonstrated decreased periprosthetic bone loss in patients treated with TKA and alendronate. Rheumatoid arthritis also has been identified as an independent risk factor. It is unclear whether it is the inflammatory disease process or the commonly used treatment regimens that contribute more to the development of these fractures. Multiple studies have shown that most patients with rheumatoid arthritis who sustained a periprosthetic fracture were being treated with steroids.[12,24]

Surgical technique has also been implicated; specifically, notching of the distal femur. Some studies have shown that violation of the anterior cortex of the distal femur is an important risk factor for periprosthetic distal femoral fracture after TKA, whereas others have found no correlation.[10,22,25] Culp et al[25] reported that a 3-mm anterior cortical notch decreased torsional strength by 29.2%. Platzer et al[22] reported the presence of anterior femoral notching in 11 of 41 patients with periprosthetic distal femoral fractures. Other studies have questioned this relationship. A large clinical series of 660 patients treated with TKA reported that only 2 of 180 patients who had anterior femoral notching sustained a fracture.[10] There is a theoretic increased risk of periprosthetic fracture because of the change in the geometry of the femur and the decreased radius of curvature, which can lead to higher stresses on the distal femur.

Clinical Evaluation

In elderly patients, approximately 90% of periprosthetic fractures are caused by low-energy mechanisms and 10% by high-energy mechanisms.[26] A patient history should be obtained, including any preexisting symptoms that could indicate a loose implant. Prior medical records are helpful in identifying the surgical approach used and the type of implant. If infection is suspected based on symptoms or if radiographs indicate a loose implant, further investigation is needed. If the findings of the infection workup are suspicious, an intraoperative biopsy or staged procedures should be planned. After a general medical examination, a comprehensive examination of the affected limb should be performed. The condition of the skin and the neurovascular status should be documented, including the ankle-brachial index. Further investigation is warranted if the ankle-brachial index is less than 0.90. Mills et al[27] found that 11 of 11 patients with an ankle-brachial index of less then 0.90 had an arterial injury requiring surgical intervention.

Standard AP and lateral radiographs of the affected extremity should be obtained, with imaging of the joint above and below the injury. AP pelvic radiographs, with full-length radiographs of the injured bone, should be obtained for all hip-related disorders. Plain radiographs can be used to determine the entire extent of the fracture, assess components for loosening, and evaluate available bone stock. This information also allows classification of the fracture and facilitates preoperative planning.[28,29] A series of mechanical axis radiographs is beneficial in some instances. Routine use of advanced imaging is unnecessary. It is important to obtain preinjury radiographs to help determine the stability of the implant and assess if an obvious mechanical situation contributed to the fracture.

Classification

The accurate classification of periprosthetic fractures helps to direct treatment. Periprosthetic THA fractures about the femoral stem are classified using the Vancouver system, which is based on fracture location, implant stability, and bone quality[28,29] (**Figure 1**). Brady et al[30] demonstrated its reliability and validity. The Vancouver system divides the femur into three zones: A, the trochanteric region; B, the diaphysis, including the region just distal to the tip of the prosthesis; and C, the region well distal to the tip of the prosthesis. Type A fractures are subclassified into type A_G, for fractures about the greater trochanter and type A_L, for fractures about the lesser trochanter. Type B fractures are subclassified based on the stability of the implant and bone quality. Type B1 are fractures around a stable implant; type B2 are fractures with a loose implant but good bone stock; and type B3 are fractures with a loose implant and poor bone stock. Type C fractures are well distal to the prosthesis and do not affect the stability of the implant.

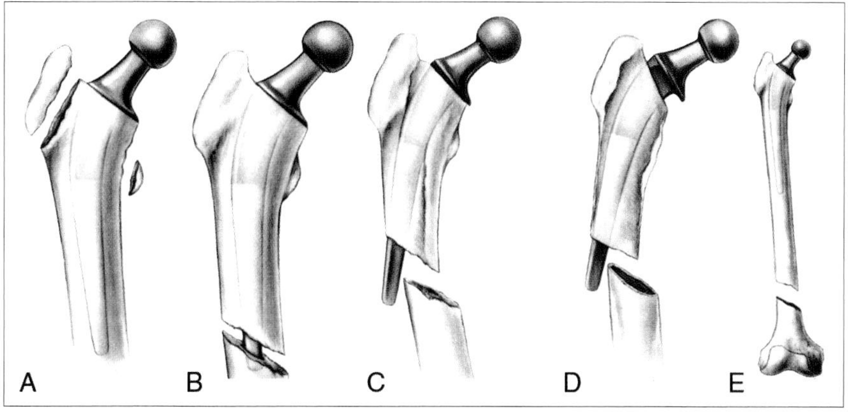

Figure 1 Illustration of the Vancouver classification of femoral fractures about a THA. **A,** Type A fracture. **B,** Type B1 fracture. **C,** Type B2 fracture. **D,** Type B3 fracture. **E,** Type C fracture. (Adapted with permission from Garbuz DS, Masri BA, Duncan CP: Fracture of the femur following total joint arthroplasty, in Steinberg ME, Garino JP, eds: *Revision Total Hip Arthroplasty.* Philadelphia, PA, Lippincott-Raven, 1998, p 497.)

Periprosthetic fractures about a TKA are classified based on anatomic location and component involvement. Multiple classification schemes have been proposed for supracondylar femoral fractures after TKA[31-34] (**Table 1**). Kim et al[35] recently suggested a new

Table 1
Supracondylar Periprosthetic Fractures: Classification Systems

Study	Type/Group	Description
Neer et al[31]	Type I	Nondisplaced (< 5 mm displacement and/or < 5° angulation)
	Type II	Displaced > 1 cm
	Type IIa	With lateral femoral shaft displacement
	Type IIb	With medial femoral shaft displacement
	Type III	Displaced and comminuted
DiGioia and Rubash[32]	Group I	Extra-articular, nondisplaced (< 5 mm displacement and < 5° angulation)
	Group II	Extra-articular, displaced (> 5 mm displacement or > 5° angulation)
	Group III	Severely displaced (loss of cortical contact) or angulated (> 10°); may have intercondylar or T-shaped component
Chen et al[33]	Type I	Nondisplaced (Neer type I)
	Type II	Displaced and/or comminuted (Neer types II and III)
Lewis and Rorabeck[34]	Type I	Nondisplaced fracture; prosthesis intact
	Type II	Displaced fracture; prosthesis intact
	Type III	Displaced or nondisplaced fracture; prosthesis loose or failing

(Reproduced from Su ET, DeWal H, Di Cesare PE: Periprosthetic femoral fractures above total knee replacements. *J Am Acad Orthop Surg* 2004;12(1):12-20.)

Table 2
Classification of Periprosthetic Fractures About a TKA

Type	Fracture Reducible	Bone Stock in Distal Fragment	Component Well Positioned and Well Fixed	Treatment
IA	Yes	Good	Yes	Conservative
IB	No	Good	Yes	Surgical fixation
II	Yes/no	Good	No	Revision with long-stem component
III	Yes/no	Poor	No	Prosthetic replacement

(Reproduced with permission from Kim KI, Egol KA, Hozack WJ, Parvizi J: Periprosthetic fractures after total knee arthroplasties. *Clin Orthop Relat Res* 2006;446:167-175.)

Table 3
Classification of Periprosthetic Patellar Fractures

Type of Fracture	Characteristics
I	Stable implant; intact extensor mechanism
II	Disrupted extensor mechanism
IIIa	Loose patellar component; reasonable bone stock
IIIb	Loose patellar component; poor bone stock

(Reproduced with permission from Ortiguera CJ, Berry DJ: Patellar fracture after total knee arthroplasty. *J Bone Joint Surg Am* 2002;84:532-540.)

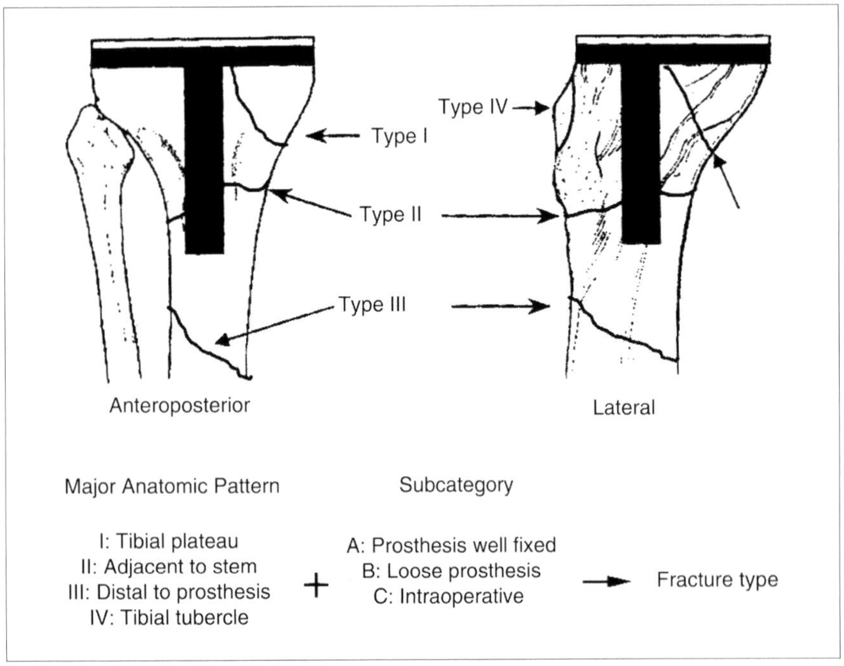

Figure 2 Mayo classification of periprosthetic tibial fractures around a TKA. (Reproduced with permission from Stuart MJ, Hanssen AD: Total knee arthroplasty: Periprosthetic tibial fractures. *Orthop Clin North Am* 1999;30(2):279-286.)

classification system that lends itself to treatment regimens (**Table 2**). Type I fractures consist of supracondylar femoral fractures with good bone stock and a well-fixed component. Type II are fractures with a loose component and good bone stock, and type III fractures have loose components and poor bone stock.

Periprosthetic tibial fractures are classified using the Mayo classification system, which is based on the location of the fracture, component stability, and intraoperative occurrence[36] (**Figure 2**). Type I fractures occur around the tibial plateau, type II fractures are adjacent to the tibial stem, type III fractures are distal to the stem, and type IV fractures involve the tibial tubercle. Each fracture pattern is subclassified into three subtypes: A, those with a well-fixed component; B, those with a loose component; and C, intraoperative fractures.

Periprosthetic patellar fractures have been classified based on disruption of the extensor mechanism, component stability, and bone stock. Ortiguerra and Berry[14] proposed a classification system that would help guide treatment (**Table 3**). Type I fractures involve an intact extensor mechanism and a stable implant, type II fractures have a disrupted extensor mechanism, and type III fractures have a loose patellar component and are subdivided into type IIIa (with good

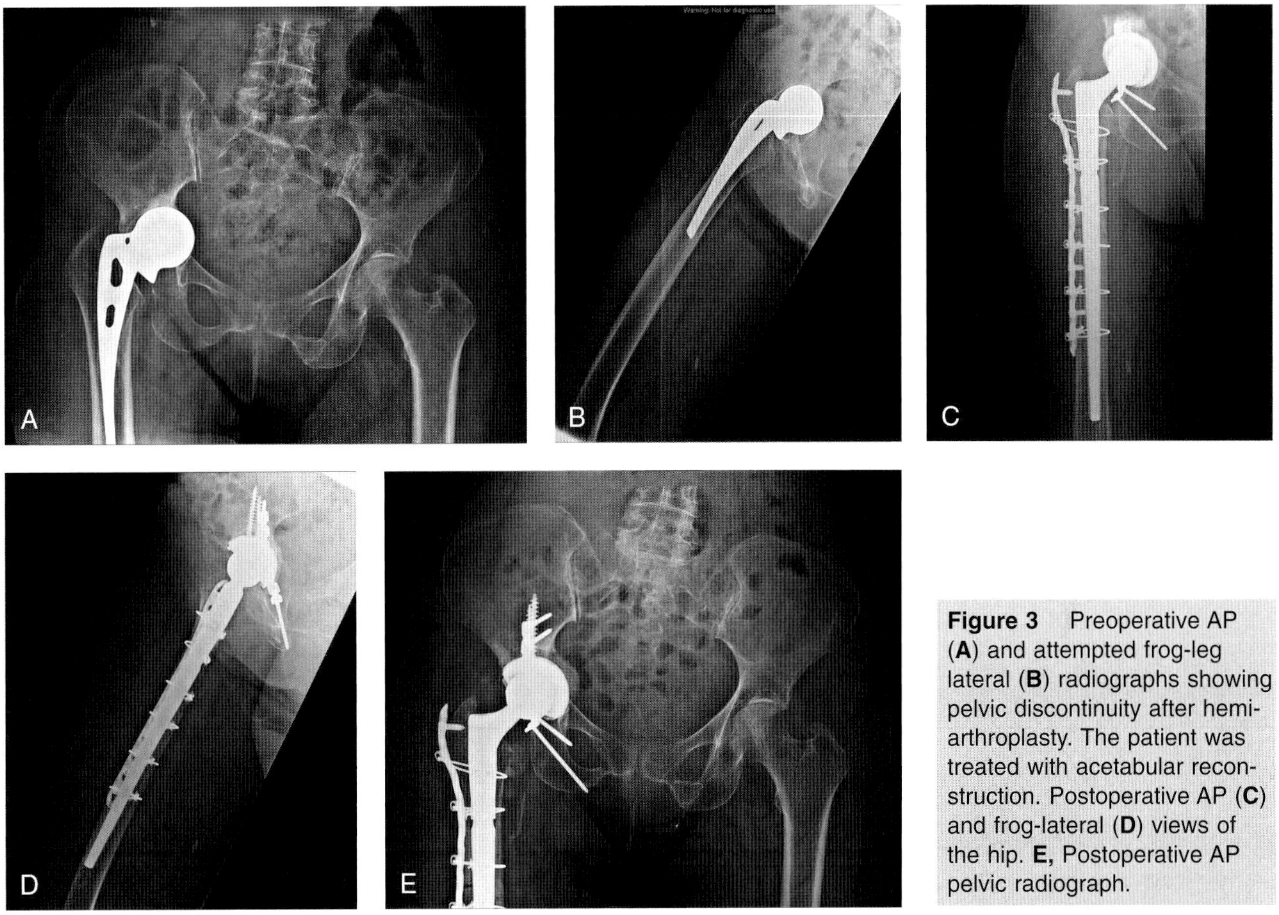

Figure 3 Preoperative AP (**A**) and attempted frog-leg lateral (**B**) radiographs showing pelvic discontinuity after hemiarthroplasty. The patient was treated with acetabular reconstruction. Postoperative AP (**C**) and frog-lateral (**D**) views of the hip. **E,** Postoperative AP pelvic radiograph.

bone stock) and type IIIb (with poor bone stock).

Although classification systems provide a means for communication about and documentation of periprosthetic fractures, it is necessary to establish answers to the following questions to guide treatment: (1) Is the fracture within the area of the implant? (2) Is the implant stable? and (3) What is the status of the surrounding bone quality?

Management

The goals of treatment for periprosthetic fractures are to provide stable fixation, restore alignment, minimize surgical trauma, avoid complications, and allow early movement. It is imperative to consider the stability of the implant and the quality of the bone stock when planning and treating these fractures.

Total Hip Arthroplasty

Periprosthetic fractures of the acetabulum are relatively rare but can be challenging to treat. Pelvic discontinuity, which can be particularly difficult to manage, is more commonly associated with female sex and the presence of inflammatory arthritis and may occur with THA or hemiarthroplasty. Concomitant vertical migration of the femur is common.[37] After identification, preoperative planning is essential to adequately manage this disorder. Treatment strategies include prophylactically plating the posterior column to help prevent propagation of the fracture pattern before removing the prosthesis. An extended trochanteric osteotomy can facilitate the removal of the femoral prosthesis and the reconstruction of the acetabulum. Bone graft can be used to help fill the acetabular defect, and a revision-type femoral stem prosthesis can be used to reconstruct the proximal femur (**Figure 3**).

Type A Fractures

Periprosthetic fractures about a THA can be treated based on the Vancouver classification system. Type A fractures involving the trochanteric region are usually treated nonsurgically. Type A_G fractures are typically treated surgically if displacement is greater than 2.5 cm because of compromised abductor function. Treatment consists of trochanteric plates and heavy suture placed into the abductor tendons if bone quality is poor. Type A_L fractures are surgically treated when they extend into the calcar and affect the stability of the implant. If discovered intraoperatively, treatment can consist of cerclage wiring with or without bone

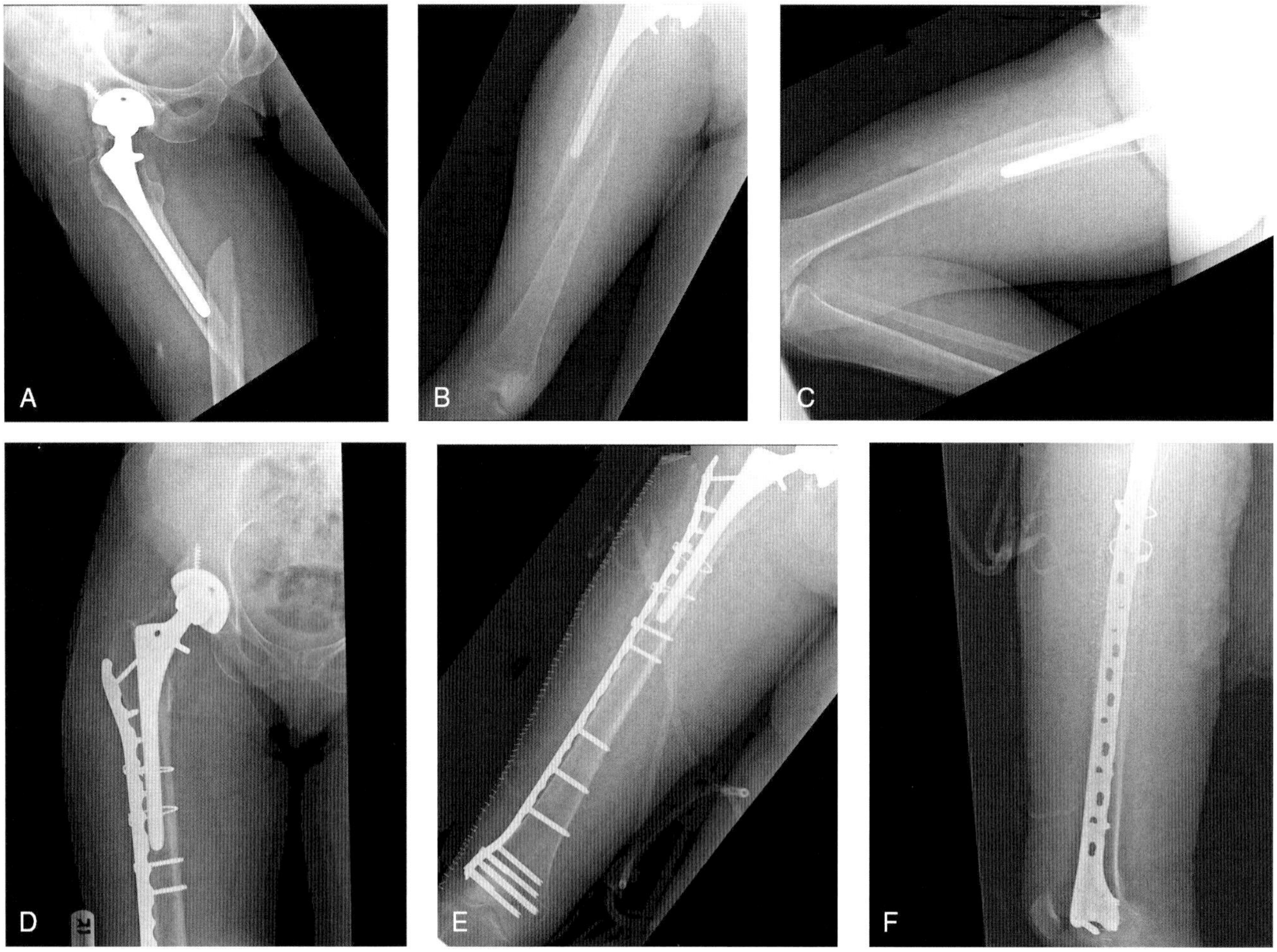

Figure 4 AP (**A**), AP femoral (**B**), and lateral (**C**) radiographs of a Vancouver type B1 periprosthetic fracture of the hip. The patient was treated with ORIF with a long, lateral locking plate with nonlocking screws, locking screws, and cables. Postoperative AP hip (**D**), AP femoral (**E**), and lateral femoral (**F**) radiographs.

grafting.[38] If discovered postoperatively, protected weight bearing is often sufficient. When either type of fracture results from underlying wear and osteolysis, revision arthroplasty may be needed to address the wear (with polyethylene liner change or acetabular component revision) and possibly treat the fracture.[39]

Type B1 Fractures

Vancouver type B1 fractures involve a fracture around a stable implant. It is critical to establish that the stem is well fixed. A periprosthetic fracture with a loose component should not be treated with internal fixation. In treating type B1 fractures, proximal fixation is of the utmost importance. Most of these fractures are treated with a laterally based locked plate construct with a combination of locking screws, nonlocking screws, and cables (**Figure 4**). In general, a combination of screws (unicortical locked and nonlocked) and cables is used proximally with multiple screws distally in a long, well-balanced plate construct. The use of three cables and three unicortical locked screws proximally and four bicortical screws distally to achieve balanced fixation above and below the fracture has been suggested.[40] Dennis et al[41] reported that a plate construct with proximal unicortical screws and distal bicortical screws or with proximal unicortical screws, proximal cables, and distal bicortical screws was substantially more stable in axial compression, lateral bending, and torsional loading. When possible, compression across the fracture site should be obtained. Hybrid fixation techniques with nonlocking and locking screws distally can aid in compressing and balancing the rigidity of the proximal and distal fixation. Some authors have recommended the placement of a nonlocked screw close to the fracture site, whereas others have recommended a nonlocked screw at the distal aspect of the fixation furthest from the fracture to allow a gradual transition of modulus between the construct and surrounding osteopenic bone.[42,43] Screw fixation strength in osteoporotic bone can be improved by augmentation with tricalcium phosphate bone cement or polymethyl methacrylate.[44]

The fracture pattern will ultimately determine the amount and type of fixation achieved. With the goals of minimizing surgical trauma and preserving blood supply to the femur, minimally percutaneous plating has gained popularity for treating type B1 fractures. This technique relies on limited direct or indirect reduction techniques. Abhaykumar and Elliott[45] reported a 100% union rate and full mobility after 5 months in a series of seven periprosthetic femoral fractures managed with a minimally invasive submuscular technique. Ricci et al[46] suggested that the plate be of sufficient length to allow as much overlap of the prosthesis as possible and should bypass the implant by a minimum of six screws; stress risers should be avoided at the proximal and distal ends of the plate; locked plates should be used whenever possible in osteoporotic bone; and cables can be combined with the fixation construct, particularly if linked to the plate with eyelet attachments. These techniques may be more appropriate for comminuted fractures because the strain can be distributed between multiple fracture lines to promote secondary bone healing.

Open reduction and internal fixation (ORIF) augmented with supplementary allograft has been described for the treatment of Vancouver type B1 fractures. There are limited data suggesting that combining lateral plating with an anterior cortical allograft is the most stable construct;[47] however, the added stability comes at the cost of additional soft-tissue disruption and insult to the vascularity of the fracture, and it can take up to 7 years for the allograft to incorporate. Positive results have been reported with the use of long plates and stable hybrid fixation without strut allograft.

Type B2 Fractures

Vancouver type B2 fractures involve a fracture around the stem with a loose implant and good bone stock. Diagnosis of the loose component should be attempted preoperatively; however, it is sometimes difficult to determine, and the diagnosis is often made intraoperatively. When the implant is loose, revision of the femoral component is the preferred treatment. A cementless revision femoral stem that bypasses the fracture site by two cortical diameters is recommended.[48] A cemented stem is not ideal because the cement can interdigitate with the fracture and lead to a nonunion.[49] In certain situations, however, the use of cement is necessary. For example, a cemented stem may be appropriate in an elderly patient with osteopenia if distal fixation of the implant would be precarious or if passing the fracture site by two cortical diameters would not allow at least 6 cm of the diaphyseal long-stem component to be in contact with the diaphysis. Alternatively, a fluted, tapered, Wagner-type stem could be used. In some cases, provisional reconstruction of the "tube" of the femur can be done with limited fixation, and the revision stem then can be introduced. The construct can be augmented by adding a laterally based locked plate while abiding by the same fixation principles used for treating Vancouver type B1 fractures. If the previous stem was cemented, it can be challenging to remove the retained component and the residual cement without damaging the remaining femoral bone. An extended trochanteric osteotomy often is useful to facilitate cement removal, exposure, and implantation of the revision component and can allow better access to the canal, especially if there is concomitant curvature or deformity, for reaming and trial implantation.[50,51]

Type B3 Fractures

Vancouver type B3 fractures involve a loose implant and poor bone stock. Although these fractures have been successfully treated using the techniques described for B2 fractures, success has recently been reported with proximal femoral replacements. Klein at al[52] reported on the treatment of type B3 periprosthetic fractures with proximal femoral replacement over a 7-year period and found excellent short-term results in 20 of 21 patients. Because proximal femoral replacement typically leads to abductor deficiency and instability, a constrained liner should be used. Other options include impaction bone grafting in combination with a revision stem or a Wagner-type implant. Lee et al[53] described good to excellent results for impaction grafting in seven patients with Vancouver type B3 fractures; full incorporation of the bone graft occurred at an average of 56 weeks in all patients.

Type C Fractures

Vancouver type C fractures are distal to the tip of the prosthesis and do not affect the stability of the implant. Treatment principles are similar to those used to manage an osteopenic distal femoral fracture, with the addition of a potential stress riser proximally from the femoral stem. It is usually recommended that a long plate be used to bypass the femoral stem by at least two cortical diameters (**Figure 5**). Modern technology allows the minimally invasive insertion of long, locked plates to preserve the biology around the fracture and limit surgical trauma. Ricci et al[54] reported high union rates with plates inserted submuscularly and stabilized with locked screws proximally and distally. Although plates are

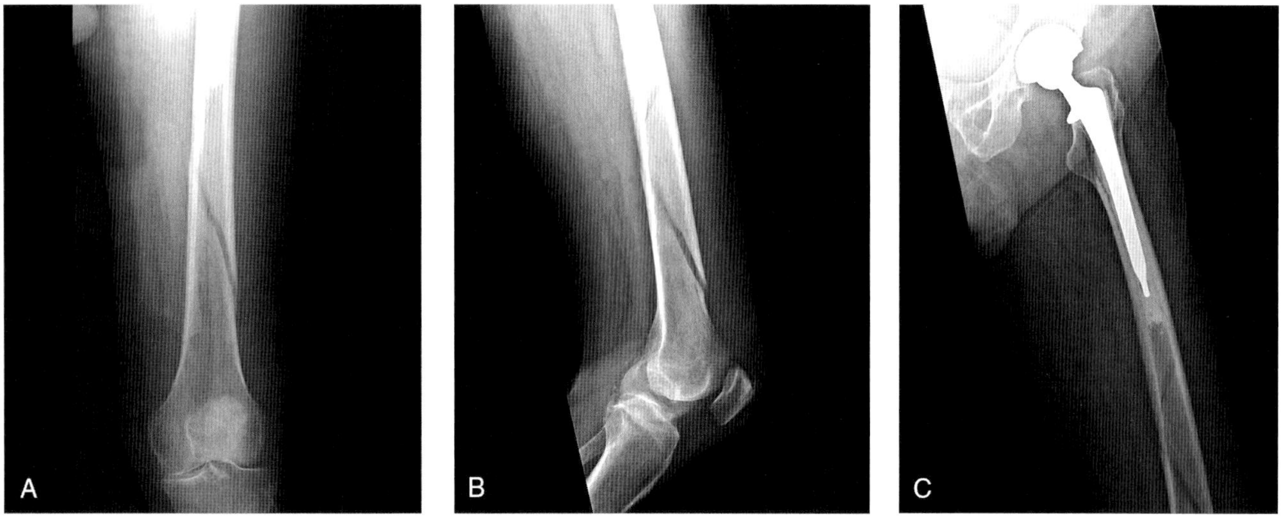

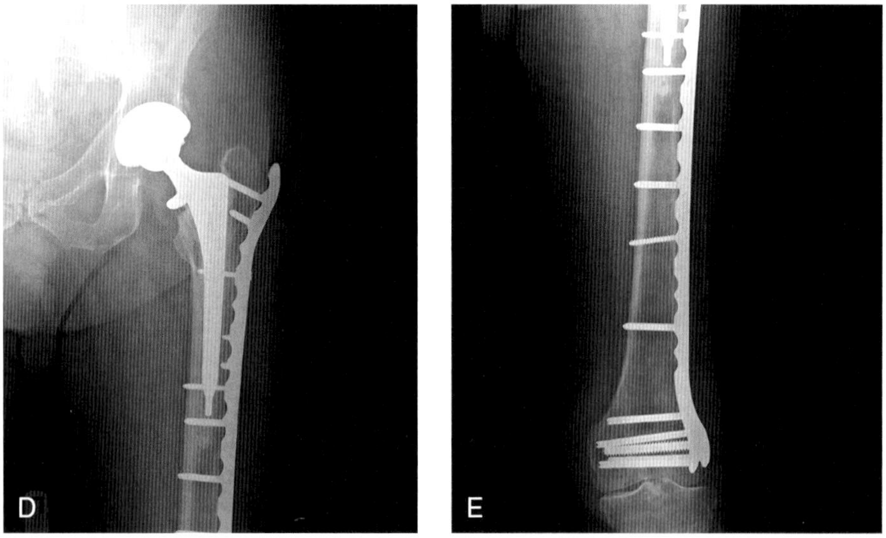

Figure 5 AP femoral (**A**), lateral femoral (**B**), and AP hip (**C**) radiographs of a Vancouver type C periprosthetic fracture. The patient was treated with ORIF using a laterally based locking plate and nonlocking screws, locking screws, and cables. Postoperative AP (**D**) and AP femoral (**E**) radiographs.

not routinely used, a recent biomechanical study reported that plate constructs with greater than 10 cm interdevice distance and intramedullary nails with less than 2 cm interdevice distance exhibited similar axial load-bearing capacities as those of control specimens.[55]

Total Knee Arthroplasty

Femoral Fractures

Femoral fractures about a TKA are managed with many of the same principles as fractures about a THA. Loose implants require revision for successful treatment. Fractures about a stable femoral component are typically treated with intramedullary nailing or laterally based locked plating. Retrograde intramedullary nailing, which limits soft-tissue disruption and allows the use of a previously placed incision for the TKA, is a good option when there is adequate distal bone stock. In a cadaver model of periprosthetic fractures of the distal femur, Bong et al[56] reported nailing to be biomechanically superior to locked plating. The disadvantages of retrograde intramedullary nailing are that it can be performed only in cruciate-retaining total knee replacements that allow access to the notch and are not hindered by a "box." The location of the femoral box can alter the starting point of the retrograde nail and lead to sagittal plane deformity. Multiplanar distal interlocking screws in retrograde nails can be used to enhance the stability of the construct. High union rates, satisfactory functional outcomes, and low revision rates have been reported in several studies.[57-59] Occasionally, antegrade femoral nailing can be used for periprosthetic distal femoral fractures if there is a long distal segment that can provide stable distal fixation (**Figure 6**).

Locked plates are an important advance in the treatment of periprosthetic fractures of the distal femur; the use of traditional plate fixation has been virtually abandoned (**Figure 7**). Locked plating allows multiple, fixed-

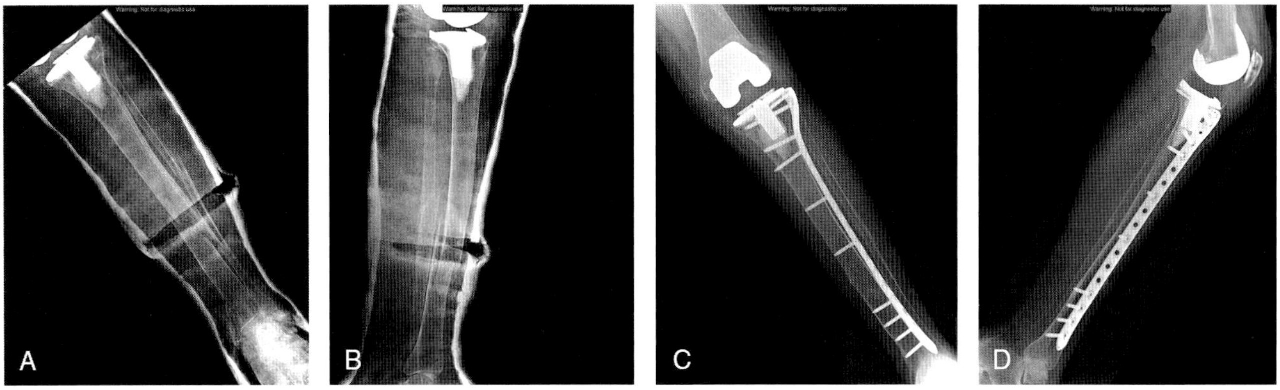

Figure 8 AP tibial (**A**) and lateral tibial (**B**) radiographs of a tibial shaft fracture distal to a TKA. The patient was treated with a laterally based locking plate using hybrid fixation. Postoperative AP tibial (**C**) and lateral tibial (**D**) radiographs.

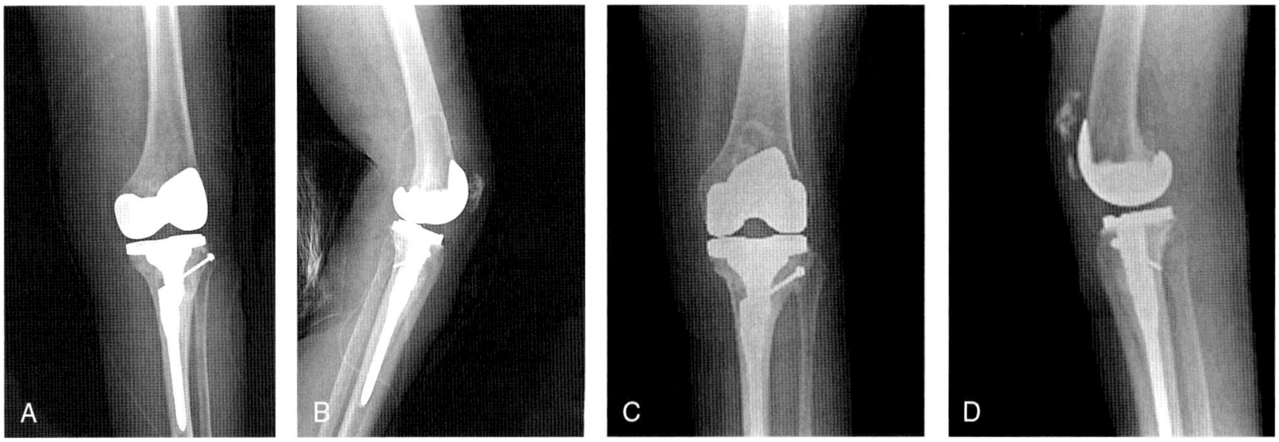

Figure 9 Immediate postoperative AP supine (**A**) and cross-table lateral (**B**) radiographs of a patient with a TKA who fell 2 months postoperatively and sustained a patella fracture. The patella fracture was treated nonsurgically. AP (**C**) and lateral (**D**) radiographs taken 6 months after the fracture show a stable implant.

and passive flexion for 4 more weeks; progressive strengthening with closed-chain exercises is then started. With a stable implant and extensor mechanism, nonsurgical treatment of type I fractures has a high success rate (> 97%).[14]

Type II fractures involve a disrupted extensor mechanism. The fixation of periprosthetic patellar fractures is challenging because of the patellar component. Fixation strategies often require the use of a circumferential cerclage wire instead of the typical tension band construct. If the displaced fragment is small or otherwise irreparable to the main body of the patella, excision of the fragment with primary soft-tissue repair of the extensor mechanism can be performed.[40]

Type III fractures involve a loose component with an intact extensor mechanism. Surgical management involves component revision if there is good remaining bone stock. If bone stock is inadequate, patellar component removal with patelloplasty or complete removal of the patella polyethylene component is recommended. Nelson et al[73] described the use of a trabecular metal patella for marked patella bone loss during revision TKA and reported good or excellent results in 17 of 20 patients; however, further research is needed on the role of porous metal patellar components in the setting of periprosthetic fracture.

Interprosthetic Fractures

The interprosthetic fracture between a THA and a TKA (**Figure 10**) or a TKA and a proximal ORIF presents a unique challenge. Treatment goals for interprosthetic fractures are the same as for periprosthetic fractures: restoring axial limb alignment with stable fixation to allow early range of motion, fracture healing, and long-term stabil-

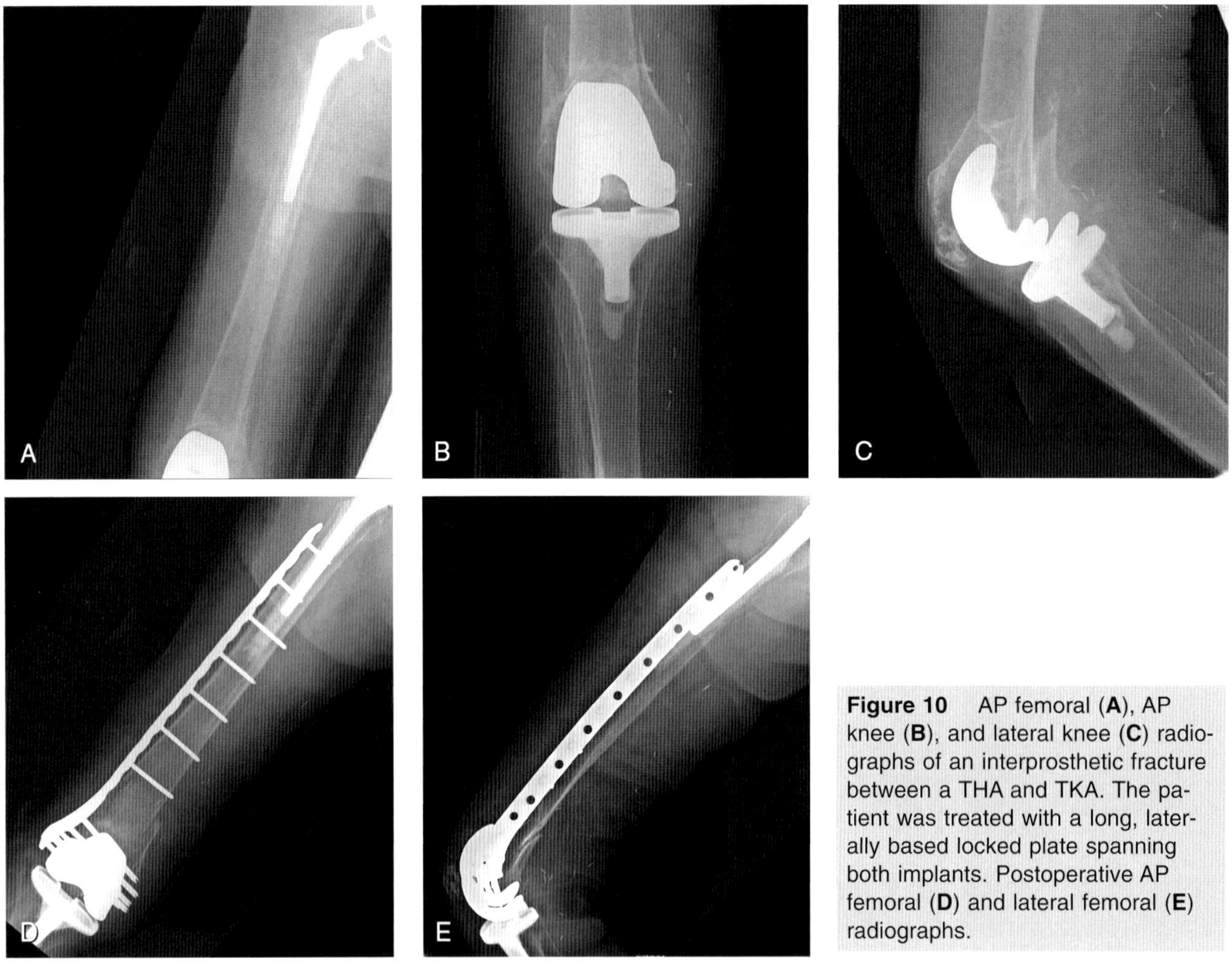

Figure 10 AP femoral (**A**), AP knee (**B**), and lateral knee (**C**) radiographs of an interprosthetic fracture between a THA and TKA. The patient was treated with a long, laterally based locked plate spanning both implants. Postoperative AP femoral (**D**) and lateral femoral (**E**) radiographs.

ity of both prostheses without the need for secondary surgeries. In general, fixation devices should be long, span both prostheses, and avoid stress risers. Mamczak et al[74] reported on 20 consecutive patients with interprosthetic fractures treated with a common surgical protocol of plate fixation that spanned the entire interprosthetic zone and the use of biologic tissue-preserving plating techniques without supplemental bone grafts. All of the fractures healed after the index procedure. Fractures between a TKA and ORIF proximally (**Figure 11**) are treated in a similar manner; however, the proximal fixation devices often must be removed, and the defect must be filled with cement to augment screw fixation above the position of the previous device. The greatest stability may be achieved with bicortical locked screws, but often this is not possible based on the positioning of the implant stem. Therefore, spanning the entire available femur and using balanced fixation is optimal, if possible. In situations that preclude the use of bicortical locked or nonlocked screws, this chapter's authors prefer to use at least two to three cables in conjunction with two to three unicortical locked screws.

Future Directions

Although the advent of locked plating technology has advanced the ability for orthopaedic surgeons to treat periprosthetic fractures, all problems associated with these challenging fractures have not yet been solved. Some potential areas of progress in fixation strategies include more locking options in retrograde nails to increase distal fixation, and the development of a combined nail-plate device. Current arthroplasty designs may be modified to facilitate the treatment of these fractures. A tibial base plate of a TKA could be designed to accommodate the insertion of a tibial nail, or the distal stem of a THA could be changed to accommodate a Morse taper with a retrograde femoral nail.

Summary

As the population continues to age and more arthroplasties are performed, it is likely that the number of periprosthetic fractures will increase. The ap-

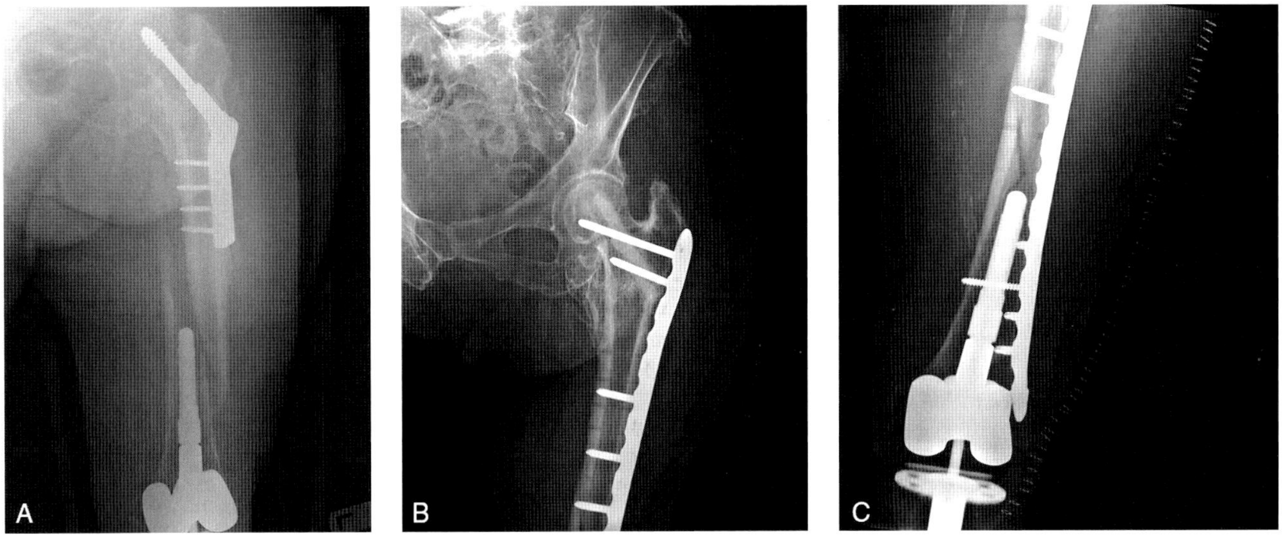

Figure 11 **A,** AP femoral radiograph of an interprosthetic fracture between a sliding hip screw and a TKA. The patient was treated with the removal of the sliding hip screw and the placement of a long, laterally based locking plate spanning the entire femur with screws placed into the femoral head and supplemented with cement. Postoperative AP hip (**B**) and AP femoral (**C**) radiographs.

plication of the basic tenets of fracture fixation and a thorough understanding of implants, anatomy, fracture patterns, and potential pitfalls contribute to successful treatment. The goals of providing stable fixation, avoiding complications, and allowing early movement regardless of the type of periprosthetic fracture remain the same. Orthopaedic surgeons should strive to restore alignment and minimize surgical trauma. A basic treatment algorithm, taking into account bone stock and implant stability, can facilitate care. If the bone stock is good and the implant is stable, nail or plate fixation can be used. If the bone stock is good but the implant is unstable, the prosthesis should be revised. If the bone stock is poor and the implant is stable, revision or ORIF with augmentation should be considered. If the bone stock is very poor and the implant is unstable, the prosthesis should be revised.

When treating a periprosthetic fracture, the orthopaedic surgeon should obtain a complete radiographic workup, including a mechanical axis series; consider indirect reduction techniques if implants are stable; check the box status and not leave reamings in the joint when using retrograde intramedullary nailing; consider polyaxial implants and bone substitutes for augmentation; and span both implants in interprosthetic fractures. The surgeon should not accept axis deviation, leave loose implants, use incompetent fixation, delay postoperative range of motion, or delay surgery in elderly patients.

References

1. Della Rocca GJ, Leung KS, Pape HC: Periprosthetic fractures: Epidemiology and future projections. *J Orthop Trauma* 2011; 25(suppl 2):S66-S70.
2. Berry DJ: Epidemiology: Hip and knee. *Orthop Clin North Am* 1999;30(2):183-190.
3. Schwartz JT Jr, Mayer JG, Engh CA: Femoral fracture during noncemented total hip arthroplasty. *J Bone Joint Surg Am* 1989;71(8): 1135-1142.
4. Beals RK, Tower SS: Periprosthetic fractures of the femur: An analysis of 93 fractures. *Clin Orthop Relat Res* 1996;327:238-246.
5. Lewallen DG, Berry DJ: Periprosthetic fracture of the femur after total hip arthroplasty: Treatment and results to date. *Instr Course Lect* 1998;47:243-249.
6. Lindahl H, Malchau H, Herberts P, Garellick G: Periprosthetic femoral fractures classification and demographics of 1049 periprosthetic femoral fractures from the Swedish National Hip Arthroplasty Register. *J Arthroplasty* 2005;20(7):857-865.
7. Lindahl H, Oden A, Garellick G, Malchau H: The excess mortality due to periprosthetic femur fracture: A study from the Swedish national hip arthroplasty register. *Bone* 2007;40(5):1294-1298.
8. Healy WL, Siliski JM, Incavo SJ: Operative treatment of distal femoral fractures proximal to total knee replacements. *J Bone Joint Surg Am* 1993;75(1):27-34.
9. Inglis AE, Walker PS: Revision of failed knee replacements using fixed-axis hinges. *J Bone Joint Surg Br* 1991;73(5):757-761.

10. Ritter MA, Faris PM, Keating EM: Anterior femoral notching and ipsilateral supracondylar femur fracture in total knee arthroplasty. *J Arthroplasty* 1988;3(2): 185-187.
11. Figgie MP, Goldberg VM, Figgie HE III, Sobel M: The results of treatment of supracondylar fracture above total knee arthroplasty. *J Arthroplasty* 1990;5(3):267-276.
12. Merkel KD, Johnson EW Jr: Supracondylar fracture of the femur after total knee arthroplasty. *J Bone Joint Surg Am* 1986; 68(1):29-43.
13. Felix NA, Stuart MJ, Hanssen AD: Periprosthetic fractures of the tibia associated with total knee arthroplasty. *Clin Orthop Relat Res* 1997;345:113-124.
14. Ortiguera CJ, Berry DJ: Patellar fracture after total knee arthroplasty. *J Bone Joint Surg Am* 2002; 84(4):532-540.
15. Grace JN, Sim FH: Fracture of the patella after total knee arthroplasty. *Clin Orthop Relat Res* 1988; 230:168-175.
16. Garbuz DS, Masri BA, Duncan CP: Periprosthetic fractures of the femur: Principles of prevention and management. *Instr Course Lect* 1998;47:237-242.
17. Mitchell PA, Greidanus NV, Masri BA, Garbuz DS, Duncan CP: The prevention of periprosthetic fractures of the femur during and after total hip arthroplasty. *Instr Course Lect* 2003;52: 301-308.
18. Greidanus NV, Mitchell PA, Masri BA, Garbuz DS, Duncan CP: Principles of management and results of treating the fractured femur during and after total hip arthroplasty. *Instr Course Lect* 2003;52:309-322.
19. Franklin J, Malchau H: Risk factors for periprosthetic femoral fracture. *Injury* 2007;38(6): 655-660.
20. Lindahl H, Garellick G, Regnér H, Herberts P, Malchau H: Three hundred and twenty-one periprosthetic femoral fractures. *J Bone Joint Surg Am* 2006;88(6):1215-1222.
21. Lindahl H: Epidemiology of periprosthetic femur fracture around a total hip arthroplasty. *Injury* 2007;38(6):651-654.
22. Platzer P, Schuster R, Aldrian S, et al: Management and outcome of periprosthetic fractures after total knee arthroplasty. *J Trauma* 2010;68(6):1464-1470.
23. Wang CJ, Wang JW, Ko JY, Weng LH, Huang CC: Three-year changes in bone mineral density around the knee after a six-month course of oral alendronate following total knee arthroplasty: A prospective, randomized study. *J Bone Joint Surg Am* 2006;88(2): 267-272.
24. Bogoch E, Hastings D, Gross A, Gschwend N: Supracondylar fractures of the femur adjacent to resurfacing and MacIntosh arthroplasties of the knee in patients with rheumatoid arthritis. *Clin Orthop Relat Res* 1988;229: 213-220.
25. Culp RW, Schmidt RG, Hanks G, Mak A, Esterhai JL Jr, Heppenstall RB: Supracondylar fracture of the femur following prosthetic knee arthroplasty. *Clin Orthop Relat Res* 1987;222: 212-222.
26. Cooke PH, Newman JH: Fractures of the femur in relation to cemented hip prostheses. *J Bone Joint Surg Br* 1988;70(3): 386-389.
27. Mills WJ, Barei DP, McNair P: The value of the ankle-brachial index for diagnosing arterial injury after knee dislocation: A prospective study. *J Trauma* 2004; 56(6):1261-1265.
28. Brady OH, Garbuz DS, Masri BA, Duncan CP: Classification of the hip. *Orthop Clin North Am* 1999;30(2):215-220.
29. Duncan CP, Masri BA: Fractures of the femur after hip replacement. *Instr Course Lect* 1995;44: 293-304.
30. Brady OH, Garbuz DS, Masri BA, Duncan CP: The reliability and validity of the Vancouver classification of femoral fractures after hip replacement. *J Arthroplasty* 2000;15(1):59-62.
31. Neer CS II, Grantham SA, Shelton ML: Supracondylar fracture of the adult femur: A study of one hundred and ten cases. *J Bone Joint Surg Am* 1967;49:591-613.
32. DiGioia AM III, Rubash HE: Periprosthetic fractures of the femur after total knee arthroplasty: A literature review and treatment algorithm. *Clin Orthop Relat Res* 1991;271:135-142.
33. Chen F, Mont MA, Bachner RS: Management of ipsilateral supracondylar femur fractures following total knee arthroplasty. *J Arthroplasty* 1994;9:521-526.
34. Lewis PL, Rorabeck CH: *Revision Total Knee Arthroplasty*. Baltimore, MD, Williams & Wilkins, 1997, pp 275-295.
35. Kim KI, Egol KA, Hozack WJ, Parvizi J: Periprosthetic fractures after total knee arthroplasties. *Clin Orthop Relat Res* 2006;446: 167-175.
36. Stuart MJ, Hanssen AD: Total knee arthroplasty: Periprosthetic tibial fractures. *Orthop Clin North Am* 1999;30(2):279-286.
37. Paprosky WG, Perona PG, Lawrence JM: Acetabular defect classification and surgical reconstruction in revision arthroplasty: A 6-year follow-up evaluation. *J Arthroplasty* 1994;9(1):33-44.
38. Parvizi J, Rapuri VR, Purtill JJ, Sharkey PF, Rothman RH, Hozack WJ: Treatment protocol for proximal femoral periprosthetic

fractures. *J Bone Joint Surg Am* 2004;86(suppl 2):8-16.

39. Parvizi J, Vegari DN: Periprosthetic proximal femur fractures: Current concepts. *J Orthop Trauma* 2011;25(suppl 2): S77-S81.
40. Della Valle CJ, Haidukewych GJ, Callaghan JJ: Periprosthetic fractures of the hip and knee: A problem on the rise but better solutions. *Instr Course Lect* 2010;59: 563-575.
41. Dennis MG, Simon JA, Kummer FJ, Koval KJ, DiCesare PE: Fixation of periprosthetic femoral shaft fractures occurring at the tip of the stem: A biomechanical study of 5 techniques. *J Arthroplasty* 2000;15(4):523-528.
42. Freeman AL, Tornetta P III, Schmidt A, Bechtold J, Ricci W, Fleming M: How much do locked screws add to the fixation of "hybrid" plate constructs in osteoporotic bone? *J Orthop Trauma* 2010;24(3):163-169.
43. Doornink J, Fitzpatrick DC, Boldhaus S, Madey SM, Bottlang M: Effects of hybrid plating with locked and nonlocked screws on the strength of locked plating constructs in the osteoporotic diaphysis. *J Trauma* 2010;69(2): 411-417.
44. Collinge C, Merk B, Lautenschlager EP: Mechanical evaluation of fracture fixation augmented with tricalcium phosphate bone cement in a porous osteoporotic cancellous bone model. *J Orthop Trauma* 2007;21(2): 124-128.
45. Abhaykumar S, Elliott DS: Percutaneous plate fixation for periprosthetic femoral fractures: A preliminary report. *Injury* 2000;31(8): 627-630.
46. Ricci WM, Bolhofner BR, Loftus T, Cox C, Mitchell S, Borrelli J Jr: Indirect reduction and plate fixation, without grafting, for periprosthetic femoral shaft fractures about a stable intramedullary implant: Surgical technique. *J Bone Joint Surg Am* 2006; 88(suppl 1 pt 2):275-282.
47. Wilson D, Frei H, Masri BA, Oxland TR, Duncan CP: A biomechanical study comparing cortical onlay allograft struts and plates in the treatment of periprosthetic femoral fractures. *Clin Biomech (Bristol, Avon)* 2005;20(1):70-76.
48. Biggi F, Di Fabio S, D'Antimo C, Trevisani S: Periprosthetic fractures of the femur: The stability of the implant dictates the type of treatment. *J Orthop Traumatol* 2010;11(1):1-5.
49. Fink B, Fuerst M, Singer J: Periprosthetic fractures of the femur associated with hip arthroplasty. *Arch Orthop Trauma Surg* 2005;125(7):433-442.
50. Levine BR, Della Valle CJ, Lewis P, Berger RA, Sporer SM, Paprosky W: Extended trochanteric osteotomy for the treatment of Vancouver B2/B3 periprosthetic fractures of the femur. *J Arthroplasty* 2008;23(4):527-533.
51. Stiehl JB: Extended osteotomy for periprosthetic femoral fractures in total hip arthroplasty. *Am J Orthop (Belle Mead NJ)* 2006;35(1): 20-23.
52. Klein GR, Parvizi J, Rapuri V, et al: Proximal femoral replacement for the treatment of periprosthetic fractures. *J Bone Joint Surg Am* 2005;87(8):1777-1781.
53. Lee GC, Nelson CL, Virmani S, Manikonda K, Israelite CL, Garino JP: Management of periprosthetic femur fractures with severe bone loss using impaction bone grafting technique. *J Arthroplasty* 2010;25(3):405-409.
54. Ricci WM, Bolhofner BR, Loftus T, Cox C, Mitchell S, Borrelli J Jr: Indirect reduction and plate fixation, without grafting, for periprosthetic femoral shaft fractures about a stable intramedullary implant. *J Bone Joint Surg Am* 2005;87(10):2240-2245.
55. Peindl RD, Mazurek MT, Bosse MJ, Kellam JF, Masonis JL, Coley ER: A biomechanical assessment. *Orthopaedic Trauma Association 19th Annual Meeting Book*. Rosemont, IL, Orthopaedic Trauma Association, 2003, pp 259-260.
56. Bong MR, Egol KA, Koval KJ, et al: Comparison of the LISS and a retrograde-inserted supracondylar intramedullary nail for fixation of a periprosthetic distal femur fracture proximal to a total knee arthroplasty. *J Arthroplasty* 2002; 17(7):876-881.
57. Gliatis J, Megas P, Panagiotopoulos E, Lambiris E: Midterm results of treatment with a retrograde nail for supracondylar periprosthetic fractures of the femur following total knee arthroplasty. *J Orthop Trauma* 2005;19(3):164-170.
58. Chettiar K, Jackson MP, Brewin J, Dass D, Butler-Manuel PA: Supracondylar periprosthetic femoral fractures following total knee arthroplasty: Treatment with a retrograde intramedullary nail. *Int Orthop* 2009;33(4):981-985.
59. El-Kawy S, Ansara S, Moftah A, Shalaby H, Varughese V: Retrograde femoral nailing in elderly patients with supracondylar fracture femur: Is it the answer for a clinical problem? *Int Orthop* 2007;31(1):83-86.
60. Nauth A, Ristevski B, Bégué T, Schemitsch EH: Periprosthetic distal femur fractures: Current concepts. *J Orthop Trauma* 2011; 25(suppl 2):S82-S85.
61. Haidukewych GJ: Innovations in locking plate technology. *J Am Acad Orthop Surg* 2004;12(4): 205-212.
62. Ricci WM, Borrelli J Jr: Operative management of periprosthetic femur fractures in the elderly using biological fracture reduction and fixation techniques. *Injury* 2007;38(suppl 3):S53-S58.

63. Kolb W, Guhlmann H, Windisch C, Marx F, Koller H, Kolb K: Fixation of periprosthetic femur fractures above total knee arthroplasty with the less invasive stabilization system: A midterm follow-up study. *J Trauma* 2010; 69(3):670-676.

64. Streubel PN, Gardner MJ, Morshed S, Collinge CA, Gallagher B, Ricci WM: Are extreme distal periprosthetic supracondylar fractures of the femur too distal to fix using a lateral locked plate? *J Bone Joint Surg Br* 2010;92(4): 527-534.

65. Bobak P, Polyzois I, Graham S, Gamie Z, Tsiridis E: Nailed cementoplasty: A salvage technique for Rorabeck type II periprosthetic fractures in octogenarians. *J Arthroplasty* 2010;25(6): 939-944.

66. Rorabeck CH, Taylor JW: Periprosthetic fractures of the femur complicating total knee arthroplasty. *Orthop Clin North Am* 1999;30(2):265-277.

67. Berend KR, Lombardi AV Jr: Distal femoral replacement in nontumor cases with severe bone loss and instability. *Clin Orthop Relat Res* 2009;467(2):485-492.

68. Rand JA, Coventry MB: Stress fractures after total knee arthroplasty. *J Bone Joint Surg Am* 1980; 62(2):226-233.

69. Parvizi J, Jain N, Schmidt AH: Periprosthetic knee fractures. *J Orthop Trauma* 2008;22(9): 663-671.

70. Keating EM, Haas G, Meding JB: Patella fracture after post total knee replacements. *Clin Orthop Relat Res* 2003;416:93-97.

71. Parvizi J, Kim KI, Oliashirazi A, Ong A, Sharkey PF: Periprosthetic patellar fractures. *Clin Orthop Relat Res* 2006;446:161-166.

72. Sheth NP, Pedowitz DI, Lonner JH: Periprosthetic patellar fractures. *J Bone Joint Surg Am* 2007; 89(10):2285-2296.

73. Nelson CL, Lonner JH, Lahiji A, Kim J, Lotke PA: Use of a trabecular metal patella for marked patella bone loss during revision total knee arthroplasty. *J Arthroplasty* 2003;18(7, suppl 1):37-41.

74. Mamczak CN, Gardner MJ, Bolhofner B, Borrelli J Jr, Streubel PN, Ricci WM: Interprosthetic femoral fractures. *J Orthop Trauma* 2010;24(12):740-744.

29

Revision for Periprosthetic Fractures of the Hip and Knee

George J. Haidukewych, MD
Joshua R. Langford, MD
Frank A. Liporace, MD

Abstract

Many periprosthetic fractures about the hip and knee can be managed successfully with modern internal fixation techniques; however, there are particular circumstances when revision arthroplasty is a better choice. These revision cases often require a substantial amount of preoperative planning and resources. Knowledge of the indications, techniques, and implants needed for managing these complex conditions is paramount for success.

Instr Course Lect 2013;62:333-340.

Although most of the available literature on periprosthetic fractures after hip and knee arthroplasty has focused on internal fixation techniques, many of these fractures require arthroplasty revision. These cases require familiarity with internal fixation and revision arthroplasty techniques. Typically, revision is indicated for fractures around loose components, nonunions, or fractures for which internal fixation attempts are likely to fail.[1] This chapter discusses indications, techniques, and results of revision for periprosthetic fractures of the hip and knee.

Fractures Around the Femoral Component of a Total Hip Arthroplasty

Fractures around the femoral component of a total hip arthroplasty become more common as patients age. These patients usually present to the emergency department and are often managed by trauma surgeons with varying amounts of revision experience. Osteopenic bone, a femoral component that is often loose, and an elderly patient with medical comorbidities all complicate management. Most periprosthetic fractures around the stem of a femoral component are associated with a loose femoral implant, for which revision arthroplasty is preferable to internal fracture fixation.[2-6] It is important to understand the fundamental decision making and technical aspects of managing periprosthetic fractures of the femur associated with a loose femoral component.

The Vancouver classification system helps to guide treatment and is based on the location of the fracture, the fixation status of the femoral component, and the quality of the remaining bone stock[1] (**Table 1**). Vancouver type A fractures involve the greater or lesser trochanter and are generally associated with osteolysis-related avulsion fractures (**Figure 1**). The mainstay of treatment of these fractures is to address the underlying osteolysis, typically with polyethylene liner exchange. Lytic lesions are bone grafted with allograft, and unstable fractures of the greater trochanter are stabilized with internal fixation. Tension-band techniques using wires or heavy braided suture have been recommended. The

Dr. Haidukewych or an immediate family member serves as a board member, owner, officer, or committee member of the American Academy of Orthopaedic Surgeons; has received royalties from DePuy; serves as a paid consultant to or is an employee of Smith & Nephew and Synthes; and has stock or stock options in Surmodics and Orthopediatrics. Dr. Langford or an immediate family member serves as a paid consultant to or is an employee of Stryker and Internal Fixation Systems and has stock or stock options in Internal Fixation Systems. Dr. Liporace or an immediate family member has received royalties from DePuy; is a member of a speakers' bureau or has made paid presentations on behalf of DePuy, Synthes, Smith & Nephew, Stryker, and Medtronic; serves as a paid consultant to or is an employee of DePuy, Medtronic, Synthes, Smith & Nephew, and Stryker; serves as an unpaid consultant to AO; and has received research or institutional support from Synthes, Smith & Nephew, and Acumed.

Table 1
Vancouver Classification System for Periprosthetic Fractures Around the Hip

Type	Fracture Location	Implant Status	Bone Quality
A_G	Proximal greater trochanter	Stable	
A_L	Proximal lesser trochanter	Stable	
B1	Around stem	Stable	
B2	Around stem	Loose	Good
B3	Around stem	Loose	Poor
C	Distal to stem	Stable	

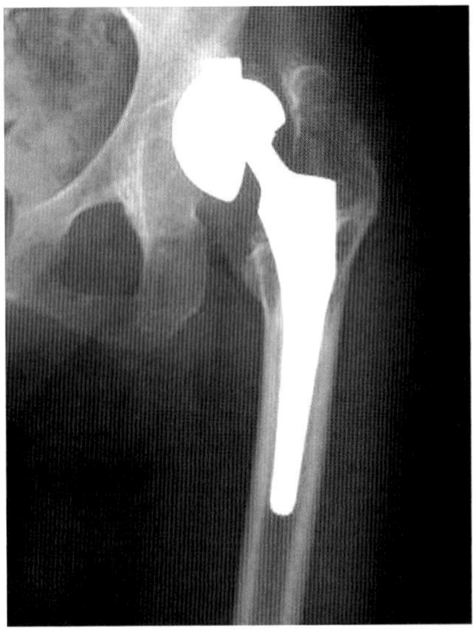

Figure 1 AP radiograph of a hip with a Vancouver type A periprosthetic fracture of the greater trochanter related to osteolysis.

bone quality is typically extremely poor because the trochanter has been "hollowed out" by the lytic process. If the greater trochanter fracture fragment is displaced and unstable, this chapter's authors prefer to suture into the abductor tendon with a heavy braided nonabsorbable suture, which provides more robust fixation than suturing into the remaining bone. This technique is analogous to the fixation of tuberosities of proximal humeral fractures in osteopenic patients. Often, wires or cables will slice through the bone. Newer cable plates may offer an advantage by providing broader support to osteopenic greater trochanters. Postoperative abduction bracing and a period of protected weight bearing are recommended.

Vancouver type B fractures occur around the tip of the femoral stem and are the most common fractures encountered. Type B1 fractures occur around a well-fixed implant; type B2 fractures, around a loose implant with good remaining bone stock; and type B3 fractures, around a loose implant with poor remaining proximal bone stock. For fractures around a well-fixed implant (type B1), internal fixation with a plate with or without an allograft strut is recommended.

For fractures around a loose implant (Vancouver types B2 and B3), revision of the femoral component is recommended. This strategy addresses both the loose component and the fracture and provides intramedullary stability by virtue of the long femoral stems typically used for revision. Attempting plate fixation of fractures around a loose implant typically leads to fracture nonunion. Knowledge of specific revision techniques is necessary to effectively treat these challenging cases.

Thorough medical optimization is recommended preoperatively. Good-quality orthogonal radiographs are needed to evaluate the status of the acetabular component and the remaining acetabular and femoral bone stock. If possible, the surgical notes from the original arthroplasty should be reviewed to determine the manufacturer of the component so that the surgeon is prepared to place a new acetabular liner or revise the acetabular components. If the radiographs are equivocal for loosening, prefracture symptoms, such as thigh or groin pain, suggest that the components are loose. Radiographic signs of femoral component loosening include subsidence, cement mantle fractures, and complete or progressive radiolucencies at the bone-cement interface. Erythrocyte sedimentation rates and C-reactive protein levels are of unknown assistance in the presence of an acute fracture. Preoperative aspiration is recommended if there is any concern about infection. Generally, a culture result can be obtained within 48 hours, while medical optimization is taking place. Skeletal traction may be required for more unstable fracture patterns in some patients. A tibial traction pin is preferred. When infection is not suspected, an intraoperative frozen section histologic evaluation can be obtained from the membrane around the loose femoral component, not the fracture site itself. With suspicion of infection, all components and residual cement are removed, and an antibiotic cement spacer is placed to provide some stability. This chapter's authors prefer the use of a metal guide pin with a so-called cement nail made with bone cement impregnated with 3 g of vancomycin and 2.4 g of tobramycin per 40 g batch of cement. Cerclage wires can be placed around the fracture fragments and a so-called spacer nail to allow satisfactory alignment of the fracture fragments. If infection is present, organism-specific intravenous antibiotics are given, and the revision arthroplasty is performed in a staged fashion, typically 6 weeks after explantation.

The specific femoral revision strategy chosen depends on the quality of the remaining bone stock, the diameter of the femoral canal distal to the fracture, and patient factors, such as age. Many surgical exposures can be used for revision. This chapter's authors prefer a posterior approach because it is widely extensile. The cement, implants, and cement restrictors can generally be removed through the fracture site. If necessary, the proximal fracture fragment is split coronally to access the stem and allow direct visualization of the distal part of the canal for accurate reaming. The acetabular component is exposed after the femoral component is removed. The liner is removed, if modular, and the acetabular component is manually tested for stability. If the acetabular component is loose, revision is required. A full discussion of acetabular revision methods is beyond the scope of this chapter; however, in general, the use of a larger uncemented hemispheric acetabular component with multiple screw augmentation is recommended. If the acetabular component is well fixed, the liner is changed and the femoral head size is increased, if possible, to improve hip stability. Anecdotally, this chapter's authors have noted that the acetabular component is stable in most patients. When the manufacturer cannot be identified preoperatively and the proper acetabular liner is not available, a liner from another manufacturer can be cemented into a well-fixed shell with good results.

After the acetabulum has been repaired, the femur is reconstructed. Several strategies are effective, but all rely on obtaining secure distal fixation. Most often, an uncemented reconstruction is done.

Several preoperative radiographic findings help to guide the selection of the appropriate uncemented reconstruction, including the endosteal diameter and morphology of the distal femoral fragment. When the distal fragment has parallel endosteal cortices with 5 cm or more of tubular diaphysis (usually with a diameter of less than 18 mm), an extensively coated, uncemented, monoblock long-stemmed prosthesis is appropriate, and these reconstructions have a good track record.[7,8] This stem has an excellent long-term survivorship when used for revision arthroplasty or a periprosthetic fracture. The distal canal is reamed, and a trial stem is inserted into the distal fragment. In general, slight underreaming (0.5 to 1 mm) is appropriate for such stems; however, for longer, curved stems, a line-to-line ream, which provides sufficient prosthetic stability, is recommended because there is inevitably a slight mismatch in the femoral bow. The proximal fragments can then be reduced using the trial implant as a template. This chapter's authors prefer to select a trial implant one size smaller than the definitive implant and to use that trial implant as a guide to proximal fracture reduction. Essentially, the proximal part of the femur is reconstructed around a trial implant a few millimeters smaller than the real implant, after which the slightly larger final trial implant is impacted to obtain a distal press fit. Cerclage cables are applied, and a trial reduction is performed. If the limb length and stability are acceptable, the trial implant is removed and the final femoral component is impacted. The cerclage cables are then retensioned, crimped, and cut. The appropriate femoral head size and femoral head-neck offset are selected, and the reconstruction is completed.

If the distal diaphysis has divergent endosteal morphology, less than 5 cm of parallel endosteal cortex, or large endosteal diameters (typically larger than 18 mm), a fluted, grit-blasted, titanium tapered modular stem can be used effectively. These stems are available in diameters of 30 mm or less and can be useful in large femoral intramedullary canals. It is wise to ream with the use of fluoroscopy and by hand (not with a powered reamer), especially in osteopenic bone, to avoid anterior femoral cortical perforation. It is helpful to remember that a straight cone is being reamed into a bowed canal, and varus malalignment and anterior cortical impingement or perforation may occur. When axial stability is obtained by diaphyseal reaming, the implant is impacted into place. It is wise to place prophylactic cerclage cables at the mouth of the distal fragment before stem impaction. The proximal bodies of the modular implants are then chosen to restore appropriate limb length, offset, and hip stability.

After the trial reconstruction is complete, the components are assembled, and the hip is reduced. The proximal fragments are then reduced with cerclage cables around the body of the implant (**Figures 2** and **3**). Essentially, the stem serves as an endoskeleton for the fragments while providing stable distal fixation. This strategy is effective for type B2 and even most type B3 fractures; however, concerns remain about the durability of the modular junction of such stems without proximal osseous support. The advantages of these modular constructs include the independent control of the distal diameter, limb length, offset, and femoral anteversion that make such reconstructions very time efficient and clini-

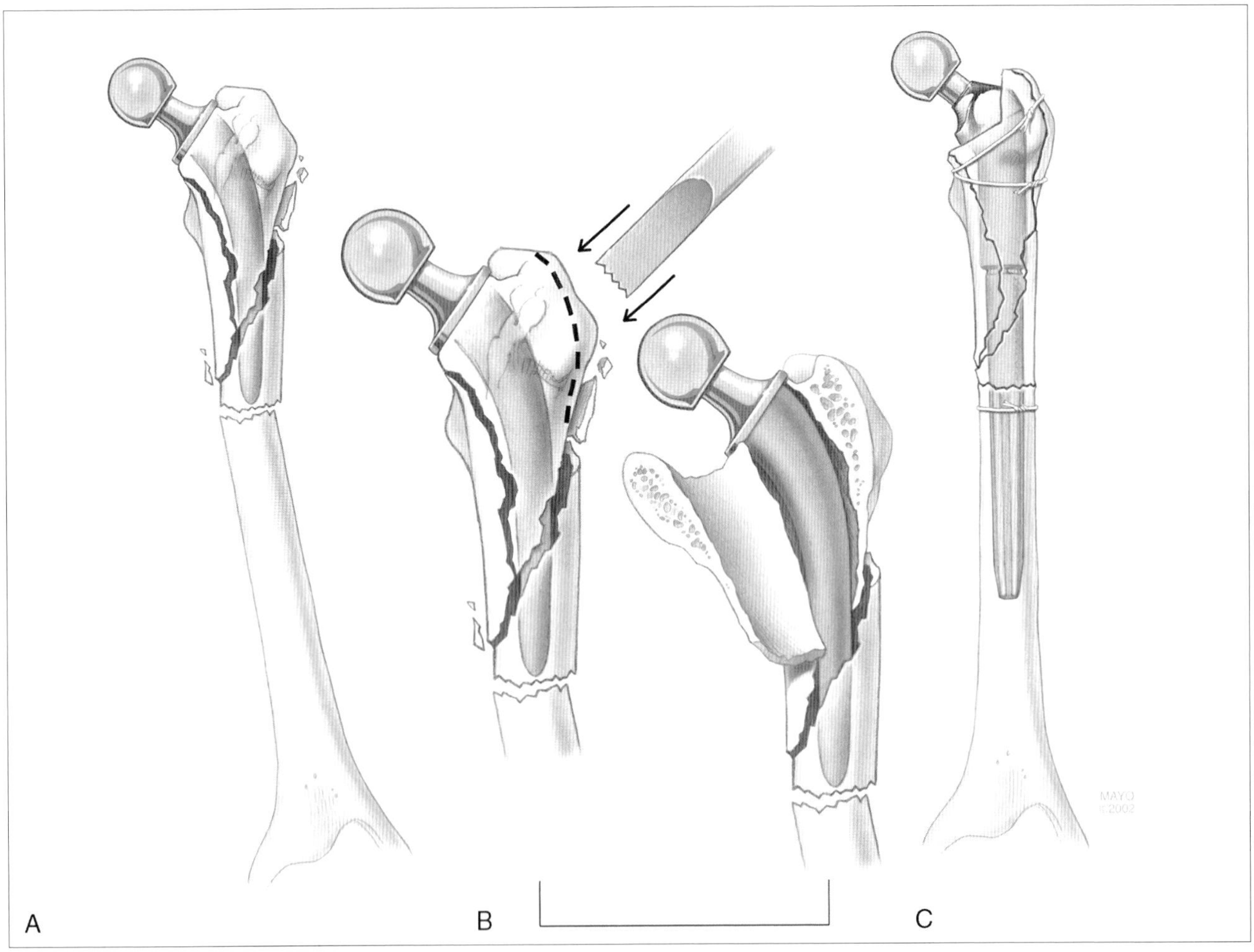

Figure 2 Illustrations of the so-called endoskeleton technique using a modular, fluted, tapered stem with cerclage fixation of the proximal fragments. **A,** Periprosthetic fracture around a loose stem. **B,** An osteotomy is performed to allow component removal and revision stem implantation. **C,** Final construct with good distal fixation and cerclage fixation of proximal fragments. (Reproduced with permission from the Mayo Foundation for Medical Education and Research, Rochester, MN.)

cally effective. Berry[7] demonstrated excellent results and favorable proximal osseous remodeling with this technique.

A cemented long-stemmed femoral component is rarely recommended for revisions, but it can be used when the patient has extremely osteopenic bone with a large femoral intramedullary canal because obtaining press-fit stability in such hips is difficult. When a cemented long-stemmed femoral component is used, the fracture is initially reduced and fixed with cerclage cables. The polymethyl methacrylate is pressurized gently to minimize extravasation. After cementation, intraoperative radiographs are made to determine if any problematic cement extravasation has occurred, and extravasated cement is removed.

Rarely, the proximal femoral bone is extremely osteoporotic such that a modular proximal femoral replacement (a so-called tumor prosthesis or megaprosthesis) is necessary. Cemented distal fixation is recommended in this situation. Preserving a sleeve of remaining proximal bone can provide some soft-tissue attachment and assist in maintaining a stable hip. A coronal split of the proximal part of the bone facilitates femoral stem removal. The implant is cemented into the distal fragment, and the proximal sleeve of remaining bone and soft tissue can be circumferentially fixed around the body of the prosthesis with cable or heavy braided suture. If the hip abductors are deficient, the construct should generally include a constrained acetabular liner to minimize the risk of postoperative dislocation. If the acetabular component is of sufficient diameter and a compatible constrained liner is

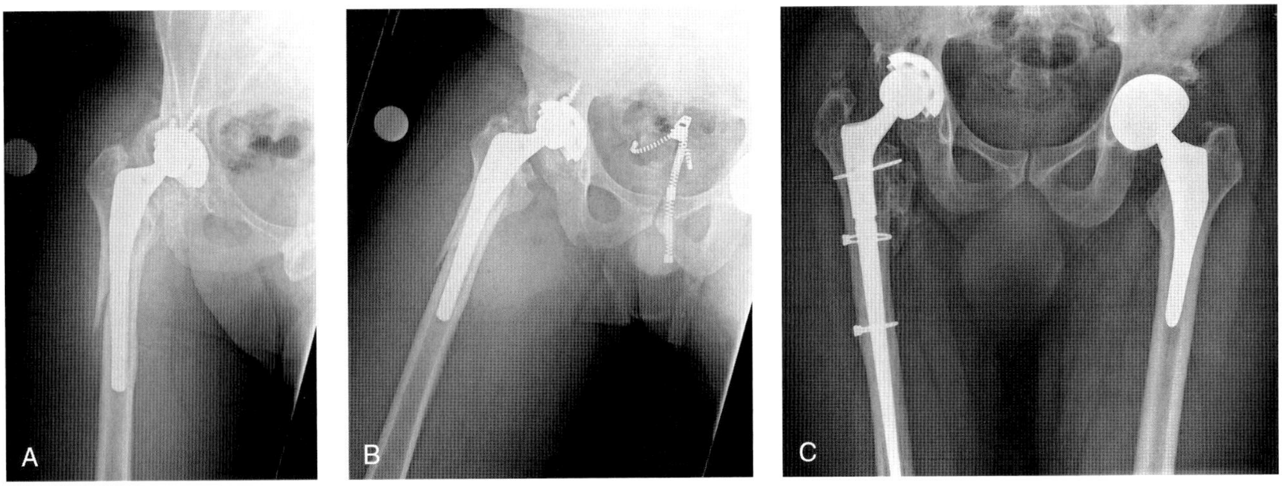

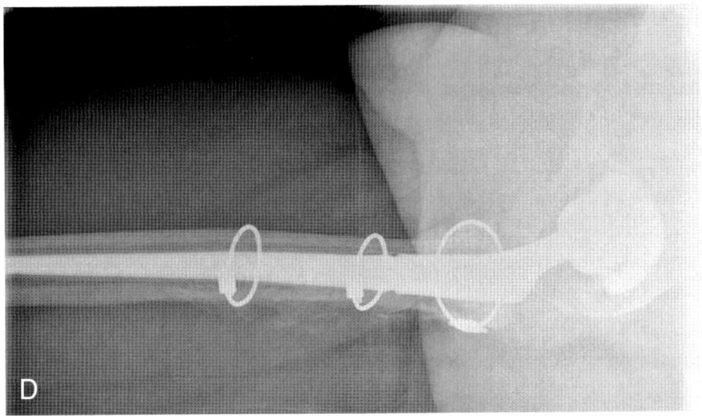

Figure 3 Periprosthetic fracture around a loose femoral component. AP (**A**) and lateral (**B**) radiographs show subsidence of the femoral component. AP (**C**) and lateral (**D**) radiographs made after revision to a tapered, fluted stem. Radiographs show remodeling of the proximal femoral bone stock.

not available, some surgeons have recommended cementing a constrained liner into a well-fixed acetabular component.[9] Adequate containment of the constrained liner by the acetabular component is required, and cup position should be acceptable to prevent impingement. Contouring the backside of a smooth liner to be cemented is recommended to allow cement interdigitation. This chapter's authors routinely add antibiotics to any cemented reconstructions in this setting, using 1 g of vancomycin powder for 40 g of cement.

After revision or internal fixation, patients are mobilized as soon as possible. Initial partial weight bearing with a walker is allowed, and, at 6 weeks, the patient progresses to full weight bearing. After revision arthroplasty, an abduction brace with a 70° flexion stop is used if necessary to avoid hyperflexion and adduction, which may compromise greater trochanteric fixation.

Orthopaedic complications include dislocation, infection, limb-length discrepancy, abductor muscle deficiency, limp, and mechanical failure or nonunion of proximal fragments. With modern modular stems, limb length and stability can be optimized by adjusting proximal body height, femoral head-neck offset, and version. Abductor mechanism problems, however, have no good solution. Careful attention to detail and understanding the principles of revision arthroplasty are necessary for optimal outcomes.

Periprosthetic Fractures of the Acetabulum

Acetabular fractures are rare compared with femoral fractures. They occur in two general scenarios: early, during cup impaction, and late, as a result of osteolytic involvement of the underlying bone with loss of cup fixation and fracture.

Intraoperative Acetabular Fractures

Various risk factors have been documented for intraoperative acetabular fractures, including poor bone quality, posttraumatic arthritis, underreaming, and the use of elliptical monoblock components. In general, this chapter's authors prefer to ream by 1 or 2 mm less than the true size of the shell to be impacted. It is important to know true diameters because some manufacturers "build in" some press fit by the elliptical nature of the shell. For example, a shell labeled as 54 mm may actually measure 55.5 mm at the rim. If a fracture occurs, acute revision to a so-called multihole shell is recommended

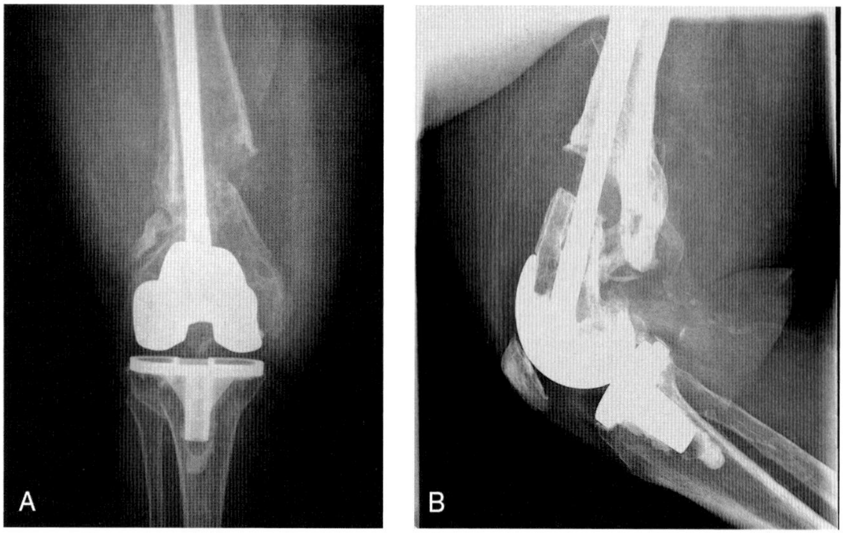

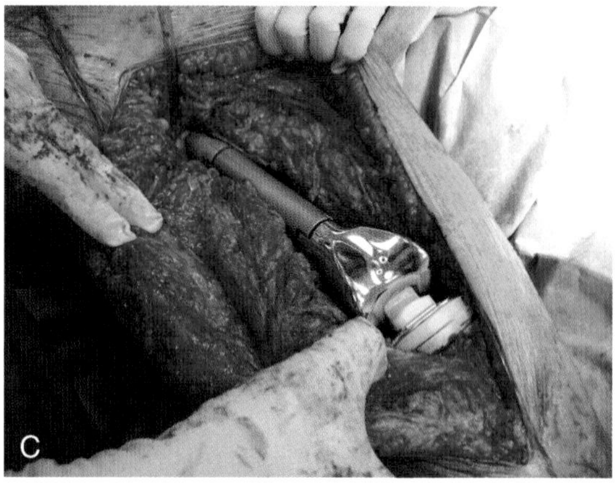

Figure 4 A periprosthetic distal femoral fracture in an 85-year-old woman who had multiple surgeries. AP (**A**) and lateral (**B**) radiographs show the poor remaining bone stock. **C,** Intraoperative photograph made after revision to a modular distal femoral replacement.

if the component is unstable. If the impacted cup is stable, no further treatment is necessary. Multiple screws are used to improve fixation, and bone obtained from reaming is placed along the fracture line. The outcomes of such a strategy have been generally satisfactory.[10-16] For more unstable fractures, the addition of a posterior column plate may be necessary.

Late Periprosthetic Fractures of the Acetabulum

These fractures are generally associated with severe osteolysis of the acetabulum.[14] If a preoperative CT scan leads to this diagnosis, a jumbo cup with allograft bone and multiple screws generally is used. For more severe defects or discontinuities, a posterior column plate may be necessary. Modular porous metal augments are available and can be customized to fill defects and improve component stability. Rarely, so-called custom triflange components are necessary for massive combined osseous deficiencies.

Revision for Periprosthetic Fractures of the Knee

Supracondylar Distal Femoral Fractures

Although most periprosthetic fractures around a femoral stem require revision because the femoral component is loose, most fractures of the distal part of the femur occur above a total knee replacement that is well fixed and has been functioning well before the fracture. Internal fixation is therefore indicated for most periprosthetic distal femoral fractures. Both locked plates and retrograde intramedullary nails can provide good outcomes. The amount of available distal bone stock and the intercondylar notch access influence the selection of the fixation device. Regardless of the device chosen, secure distal fragment fixation must be achieved for predictable healing.[1,17-21]

Revision arthroplasty is recommended for fractures around loose implants. In the experience of this chapter's authors, loose implants are rare, occurring primarily in elderly patients with massive distal osteolysis who sustain a distal femoral fracture. An effective way to manage this problem is to use a distal femoral replacement megaprosthesis.[1] These patients can be mobilized immediately without protected weight bearing. The role of such prostheses in fractures above a well-fixed total knee replacement is controversial. Most periprosthetic fractures above a total knee replacement heal with internal fixation; therefore, such megaprostheses should probably be reserved for fractures above a loose total knee replacement, nonunion, or patients in whom internal fixation is likely to fail because of very poor distal bone stock (**Figure 4**). An alternative strategy for the management of a fracture and a loose femoral prosthesis is to use a long-stemmed femoral component to stabilize the fracture. This chapter's authors have not found this strategy to be effective because the distal bone stock typically is insufficient after component removal, so the femoral stem carries an excessive load. If revision arthroplasty is contemplated, traditional revision implants and distal femoral replacements should be available.

Fractures Around a Tibial Component

Periprosthetic fractures around a tibial component almost always occur around a loose tibial component, so revision arthroplasty is usually indi-

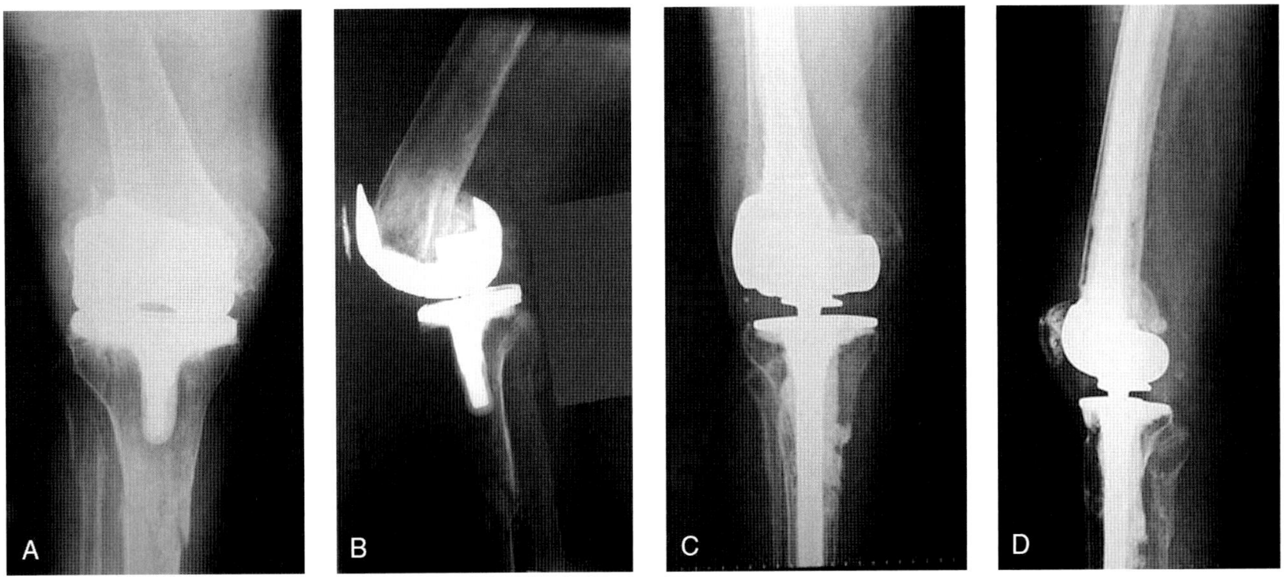

Figure 5 Radiographs of a patient with a periprosthetic distal femoral fracture and a periprosthetic fracture around a loose tibial component. Preoperative AP (**A**) and lateral (**B**) radiographs. Postoperative AP (**C**) and lateral (**D**) radiographs. Note the use of metal augmentation and long stems. (Reproduced with permission from Jeong GK, Pettrone SK, Liporace FA, Meere PA: "Floating total knee": Ipsilateral periprosthetic fractures of the distal femur and proximal tibia after total knee arthroplasty. *J Arthroplasty* 2006;21(1):138-40.)

cated.[1,22,23] Poor bone quality and varus malalignment are risk factors for periprosthetic tibial fracture. Felix et al[22] proposed a classification for tibial periprosthetic fractures. Metal augmentations, stepped sleeves, or porous metal cones can be used to manage osseous defects. A tibial component that has a stem long enough to extend distal to the fracture should be used in all cases. Both cemented and press-fit stems are effective and have good long-term data to support their use[23] (**Figure 5**). Restoration of a neutral mechanical axis is important.

Fractures of the Patella

Patellar fractures remain the most challenging periprosthetic fractures to manage because poor results and complications are common.[1] Ortiguera and Berry[24] proposed a classification system to guide treatment on the basis of the integrity of the extensor mechanism and the stability of the patellar component. Revision is indicated for loose components. Often, the residual bone stock will not support a new patellar button; therefore, simple resection of the loose component and patelloplasty are indicated. If the button is loose and the extensor mechanism is disrupted, some form of fixation is necessary to restore extensor mechanism integrity. The preferred fixation depends on the quality of the remaining bone and soft tissue. For example, if sufficient patellar bone stock remains, tension-band techniques or cannulated screw techniques can be effective. If remaining bone stock is poor, partial patellectomy may be considered. In some patients, the remaining tissues are too attenuated and cannot be repaired effectively. In these situations, an extensor mechanism allograft is used. This chapter's authors prefer an Achilles tendon allograft with a calcaneal bone block that is press fit and wired into the proximal part of the tibia. It is wise to evaluate the fixation status and rotational relationships of the femoral and tibial components concurrently because a malrotation may have contributed to patellar fracture. Complication rates remain high, and patients should be counseled about the generally poor outcomes of treatment of this fracture. Nonunion, loss of fixation, and hardware-related problems are common.[24]

Summary

Although most periprosthetic fractures around the hip and knee can be managed effectively with internal fixation, it is important to recognize the specific indications for revision arthroplasty in this setting. Familiarity with biologically friendly techniques of internal fixation and revision is important to minimize complications and improve outcomes.

References

1. Della Valle CJ, Haidukewych GJ, Callaghan JJ: Periprosthetic fractures of the hip and knee: A problem on the rise but better solutions. *Instr Course Lect* 2010;59: 563-575.

2. Lindahl H: Epidemiology of periprosthetic femur fracture around a total hip arthroplasty. *Injury* 2007;38(6):651-654.
3. Lindahl H, Garellick G, Regnér H, Herberts P, Malchau H: Three hundred and twenty-one periprosthetic femoral fractures. *J Bone Joint Surg Am* 2006;88(6):1215-1222.
4. Lindahl H, Malchau H, Herberts P, Garellick G: Periprosthetic femoral fractures classification and demographics of 1049 periprosthetic femoral fractures from the Swedish National Hip Arthroplasty Register. *J Arthroplasty* 2005;20(7):857-865.
5. Lindahl H, Malchau H, Odén A, Garellick G: Risk factors for failure after treatment of a periprosthetic fracture of the femur. *J Bone Joint Surg Br* 2006;88(1):26-30.
6. Lindahl H, Oden A, Garellick G, Malchau H: The excess mortality due to periprosthetic femur fracture: A study from the Swedish national hip arthroplasty register. *Bone* 2007;40(5):1294-1298.
7. Berry DJ: Treatment of Vancouver B3 periprosthetic femur fractures with a fluted tapered stem. *Clin Orthop Relat Res* 2003;417: 224-231.
8. Springer BD, Berry DJ, Lewallen DG: Treatment of periprosthetic femoral fractures following total hip arthroplasty with femoral component revision. *J Bone Joint Surg Am* 2003;85(11):2156-2162.
9. Callaghan JJ, Parvizi J, Novak CC, et al: A constrained liner cemented into a secure cementless acetabular shell. *J Bone Joint Surg Am* 2004;86(10):2206-2211.
10. Berry DJ, Lewallen DG, Hanssen AD, Cabanela ME: Pelvic discontinuity in revision total hip arthroplasty. *J Bone Joint Surg Am* 1999;81(12):1692-1702.
11. Haidukewych GJ, Jacofsky DJ, Hanssen AD, Lewallen DG: Intraoperative fractures of the acetabulum during primary total hip arthroplasty. *J Bone Joint Surg Am* 2006;88(9):1952-1956.
12. Kim YS, Callaghan JJ, Ahn PB, Brown TD: Fracture of the acetabulum during insertion of an oversized hemispherical component. *J Bone Joint Surg Am* 1995; 77(1):111-117.
13. Peterson CA, Lewallen DG: Periprosthetic fracture of the acetabulum after total hip arthroplasty. *J Bone Joint Surg Am* 1996; 78(8):1206-1213.
14. Sánchez-Sotelo J, McGrory BJ, Berry DJ: Acute periprosthetic fracture of the acetabulum associated with osteolytic pelvic lesions: A report of 3 cases. *J Arthroplasty* 2000;15(1):126-130.
15. Sharkey PF, Hozack WJ, Callaghan JJ, et al: Acetabular fracture associated with cementless acetabular component insertion: A report of 13 cases. *J Arthroplasty* 1999;14(4):426-431.
16. Springer BD, Berry DJ, Cabanela ME, Hanssen AD, Lewallen DG: Early postoperative transverse pelvic fracture: A new complication related to revision arthroplasty with an uncemented cup. *J Bone Joint Surg Am* 2005; 87(12):2626-2631.
17. Bong MR, Egol KA, Koval KJ, et al: Comparison of the LISS and a retrograde-inserted supracondylar intramedullary nail for fixation of a periprosthetic distal femur fracture proximal to a total knee arthroplasty. *J Arthroplasty* 2002; 17(7):876-881.
18. Figgie MP, Goldberg VM, Figgie HE III, Sobel M: The results of treatment of supracondylar fracture above total knee arthroplasty. *J Arthroplasty* 1990;5(3):267-276.
19. Gliatis J, Megas P, Panagiotopoulos E, Lambiris E: Midterm results of treatment with a retrograde nail for supracondylar periprosthetic fractures of the femur following total knee arthroplasty. *J Orthop Trauma* 2005;19(3):164-170.
20. Kenny P, Rice J, Quinlan W: Interprosthetic fracture of the femoral shaft. *J Arthroplasty* 1998; 13(3):361-364.
21. Krettek C, Schandelmaier P, Miclau T, Tscherne H: Minimally invasive percutaneous plate osteosynthesis (MIPPO) using the DCS in proximal and distal femoral fractures. *Injury* 1997; 28(suppl 1):A20-A30.
22. Felix NA, Stuart MJ, Hanssen AD: Periprosthetic fractures of the tibia associated with total knee arthroplasty. *Clin Orthop Relat Res* 1997;345:113-124.
23. Haidukewych GJ, Hanssen AD, Jones RD: Metaphyseal fixation in revision total knee arthroplasty: Indications and techniques. *J Am Acad Orthop Surg* 2011;19(6): 311-318.
24. Ortiguera CJ, Berry DJ: Patellar fracture after total knee arthroplasty. *J Bone Joint Surg Am* 2002; 84(4):532-540.

30

Management of Bone Defects in Revision Total Knee Arthroplasty

Brian K. Daines, MD
Douglas A. Dennis, MD

Abstract

Many treatment options are available to manage bone loss associated with revision total knee arthroplasty. Selection of the best treatment method is based on many factors, including defect size and location and the patient's age, health, and ability to participate in the necessary postoperative rehabilitation. Metaphyseal sleeves and cones appear to be a promising addition in dealing with large, central, contained and noncontained defects. The use of stem extensions in cases of bone deficits is helpful in enhancing fixation and lessening stresses to weakened condylar bone.

Instr Course Lect 2013;62:341-348.

Managing substantial bone loss is a challenge in revision total knee arthroplasty. The etiology of bone loss is usually multifactorial and can range from subsidence of loose implants, stress shielding, and periprosthetic osteolysis to osteonecrosis and even infection.[1] Goals of revision total knee arthroplasty include preservation of host bone, correction of sagittal and coronal alignment, restoration of flexion-extension balance, optimization of ligamentous stability, and establishment of a stable bone-implant interface. Selection of reconstructive methods, such as bone cement and screws, block augments, impaction or bulk allografts, or metaphyseal sleeves and cones, is determined by the location and quantity of osseous defects in the femur and tibia. This chapter reviews the different surgical methods for dealing with bone loss in revision total knee arthroplasty.

Preoperative Assessment

The goal of preoperative assessment is to precisely determine the mechanism of failure and thereby decrease the risk of repeating mistakes that may have led to the initial failure of the total knee replacement. Because the results of revision total knee arthroplasty in patients with unexplained pain are often unsatisfactory, it is mandatory to determine the mechanism of failure, what is deficient, and what must be reconstructed in terms of both bone and soft-tissue deficits.[2] The surgeon must determine whether the patient's symptoms are consistent with a failed total knee replacement and are not related to extrinsic causes of knee pain such as spine or hip pathology. Conditions in which revision total knee arthroplasty may be contraindicated, such as infection, Charcot arthropathy, neuromuscular disease, or adverse medical conditions, must be ruled out.

The preoperative evaluation of the patient begins with a detailed history and clinical examination. Surgical reports should be reviewed to assess the previous surgical approach used, the soft-tissue releases performed, and the size and type of present prosthetic components. To rule out an infection, a complete blood count with differential, erythrocyte sedimentation rate, and C-reactive protein should be

Dr. Dennis or an immediate family member serves as a board member, owner, officer, or committee member of the American Academy of Orthopaedic Surgeons, the Hip Society, Joint Vue, and the International Congress for Joint Reconstruction; has received royalties from DePuy and Innomed; is a member of a speakers' bureau or has made paid presentations on behalf of DePuy; serves as a paid consultant to or is an employee of DePuy; has received research or institutional support from DePuy and Porter Adventist Hospital; and owns stock or stock options in Joint Vue. Neither Dr. Daines nor any immediate family member has received anything of value from or owns stock in a commercial company or institution related directly or indirectly to the subject of this chapter.

obtained. This chapter's authors also recommend routine knee aspiration to obtain specimens for culture as well as cell count with differential. Synovial fluid aspirates with leukocyte counts of 2,500/mm³ or more in conjunction with a neutrophil percentage of 60% are highly suggestive of infection.[3] A critical review of radiographs helps to direct preoperative planning. Weight-bearing radiographs with AP, lateral, and Merchant patellar views allow evaluation of femoral and tibial implant size, assessment of current bone stock, review of implant position and fixation, and critique of patellar height and coronal position. Radiographs often underestimate the true magnitude of bone loss. Full-length AP radiographs from hip to ankle provide information regarding coronal limb alignment and the presence of diaphyseal deformities. CT can be used preoperatively to more accurately assess bone loss and component rotation.[4]

Bone Loss Classification

Multiple classification systems have been designed to assess bone loss and guide treatment.[1,5,6] The size, symmetry, and extent of bone loss are ultimately determined intraoperatively after removal of the failed implants. Bone defects can be classified as contained or uncontained. A contained defect has an intact peripheral cortical rim that allows treatment with morcellized bone graft or cement and screws. In an uncontained defect, the peripheral cortical rim is absent and typically requires reconstruction with modular block augments, bulk allograft, or metal metaphyseal sleeves or cones.

The Anderson Orthopaedic Research Institute (AORI) system is a currently accepted classification for categorizing bone loss during a revision total knee arthroplasty.[6-8] Bone loss of the distal part of the femur or the proximal aspect of the tibia is divided into three types. AORI type I bone defects are minor osseous deficiencies that typically have an intact cortical rim, a nearly normal joint line, and limited or no component subsidence. Treatment options for AORI type I defects include removing the bone defect with a thicker bone resection, shifting the component away from the defect, or filling the defect with particulate bone graft or bone cement and screws.[9-14] AORI type II defects are more extensive and are subdivided into involvement of one condyle (type IIA) or both condyles (type IIB). The cortical rim may be intact or partially absent and is typically associated with some loss of both central and peripheral metaphyseal bone. Loss of metaphyseal bone is often associated with joint-line alteration or implant subsidence. Collateral ligament origins and insertions are preserved in type II defects. Many of the surgical strategies previously mentioned for minor defects can also be used for lesser type II defects. Additional treatment options available for these defects include structural bone graft, prosthetic augments, or metaphyseal sleeves or cones to restore the joint line. AORI type III defects involve extensive loss of metaphyseal bone. Associated cortical loss is substantial and may result in the loss of collateral ligament attachments. For this reason, the use of constrained prosthetic devices is often required. Management options for type III defects include reconstruction with structural allograft, metaphyseal sleeves or cones, condyle-replacing hinged components, or amputation.

Bone Defect Treatment Options

Increased Resection or Component Shift

Increasing the bone resection from the proximal part of the tibia or the distal end of the femur theoretically is a simple strategy to remove the bone deficiency. However, it must be realized that bone was already removed at the time of the initial knee replacement, additional bone loss occurred because of the failure of the primary total knee replacement, and more bone is typically lost during component removal. Aggressive bone resection further decreases the strength of supporting cancellous bone and may require a decrease in the size of the tibial component selected. Harada et al[15] reported an abrupt decrease in tibial bone strength over the first 5 mm of resection. Smaller tibial components lead to a decreased surface area for fixation and a corresponding increase in the unit load across the tibial tray and fixation interface. For these reasons, removing substantial bone in revision total knee arthroplasty should be avoided. This chapter's authors recommend that no more than 1 to 2 mm from the most prominent femoral or tibial condyle be removed; any remaining deficits of the contralateral condyle are then managed with other methods.

Shifting the tibial component in the coronal plane away from an osseous defect to an area of greater osseous support is another option for dealing with small (< 5 mm) defects. Component shift can be detrimental if it leads to a smaller tibial component. The risk of subsidence increases if the tibial tray is supported by more cancellous bone. Shifting the tray also affects ligament kinetics. For example, shifting the tibial tray medially to avoid a lateral tibial defect lateralizes the tibial tubercle and increases the risk of patellofemoral instability. Shifting the tibial tray should be limited to no more than 3 mm.[16] This chapter's authors reserve shifting the tibial tray to the lateral direction and limit this shift to no more than 2 mm. Decreasing the size of the tray to accommodate this shift is not recommended. Because of the risk of patellar instability and collateral ligament irritation, femoral component shift is rarely indicated. Downsizing the femoral component creates a larger flexion gap and can elevate the joint line.

Cement and Screw Reconstruction

Small defects in the knees of elderly patients can be filled with polymethyl methacrylate (PMMA) and screws.[13,14] The defect construct is strengthened by the addition of screws to the PMMA. Filling a bone deficiency with PMMA is indicated for a peripheral deficiency of 10% or less of the condylar area or for small central defects.[5] Filling with PMMA is simple, economical, and easily contoured to the osseous defect. Large masses of PMMA, however, can lead to the potential for osseous thermal necrosis secondary to the heat of polymerization. It can also be difficult to pressurize PMMA in the setting of sclerotic uncontained defects. As PMMA cures, it can lose approximately 2% of its volume, leading to decreased support.[17] Although PMMA has inferior load transfer compared with custom implants or metal augments, the use of PMMA has led to favorable clinical results, at least in primary total knee arthroplasty.[17] Ritter[13] reported that 13 of 47 total knee replacements (28%) treated with PMMA and screws and observed for an average of 6.1 years had radiolucent lines, but the lines did not progress, and there was no prosthetic loosening. A 1993 study by Ritter et al[14] evaluated 125 total knee replacements in which PMMA and screws were used to fill large medial tibial defects. In this group, there were two failures with varus collapse at a mean of 7.9 years but no loosening in the remainder of the patients. PMMA with screws can be considered in type I or II defects involving less than 50% of condylar width and less than 10 mm in depth.

Localized Autograft or Particulate Allograft

Particulate allograft or local autograft can easily be molded to fit cystic and small contained areas of bone deficiency.[9-12] Bone grafting is an attractive option for younger patients who may need further revision because of its potential to restore bone stock.[12] Bone grafts are a cost-effective option compared with metal augments, are useful in large defects, and have increased physiologic load transfer compared with PMMA.[18] Donor site options for autograft include the resected condyles, intercondylar notch, and iliac crest. There are numerous sources for allograft, such as the femoral head, the distal end of the femur, or the proximal part of the tibia.[19] Allograft material can be fresh-frozen, frozen with radiation, or freeze-dried. There is a risk of nonunion, malunion, or late collapse with the use of bone graft. Allograft also has a minimal risk of disease transmission.[20]

Whiteside[21] reported on the use of morcellized femoral head allograft in 56 cementless revision total knee arthroplasties over 2 years. He observed new osseous trabeculation in 15 knees with femoral grafting and in 21 knees with tibial grafting and reported that 47 of 56 knees (84%) had mild to no pain, and 9 of 56 (16%) had moderate to severe pain. In a prospective study of 48 patients treated with impaction allograft for substantial bone loss, Lotke et al[11] reported that all radiographs showed incorporation and remodeling of bone graft with no mechanical failures. Six complications, including two infections and two periprosthetic fractures, were noted. Morcellized cancellous bone grafts are best used for contained type I or II defects in which the graft can be captured and, when compacted, provides some degree of structural support. Extensive type II contained defects can be managed with impaction bone graft as long as stem extensions are used[7] (**Figure 1**). The addition of wire mesh can also be used to create a contained defect when the peripheral rim is not intact.[11]

Prosthetic Augments

Prosthetic augments are most commonly selected for noncontained unicondylar (type IIA) or bicondylar (type IIB) defects of moderate size. Tibial augments are available in various shapes, including hemiplateau rectangular blocks, hemiplateau angular wedges, or a full plateau angular wedge.[22-26] Chen and Krackow[27] reported that alterations in defect configuration can affect the rigidity of the construct. They observed that block augments were more stable than wedge augments because of a reduction in shear forces. Fehring et al[28] also found that block augments compared with angular wedge augments resulted in superior strain distribution to the supporting bone. Bilateral block tibial augmentations can restore the anatomic joint line in type IIB defects and avoid the use of excessively thick modular tibial polyethylene inserts. Peripheral defects between 5 and 15 mm in depth that extend over most of the width of the medial or lateral tibial condyle are ideally managed with tibial augments. Femoral prosthetic augments range from approximately 5 to 15 mm in thickness, are typically block shaped, and can be used for both distal and posterior femoral bone defects. Unlike bone allografts, prosthetic augments have no risk of disease transmission, malunion, nonunion, or augment collapse. They have demonstrated good load transmission to underlying bone and provide immediate support and stability.[17] However, pros-

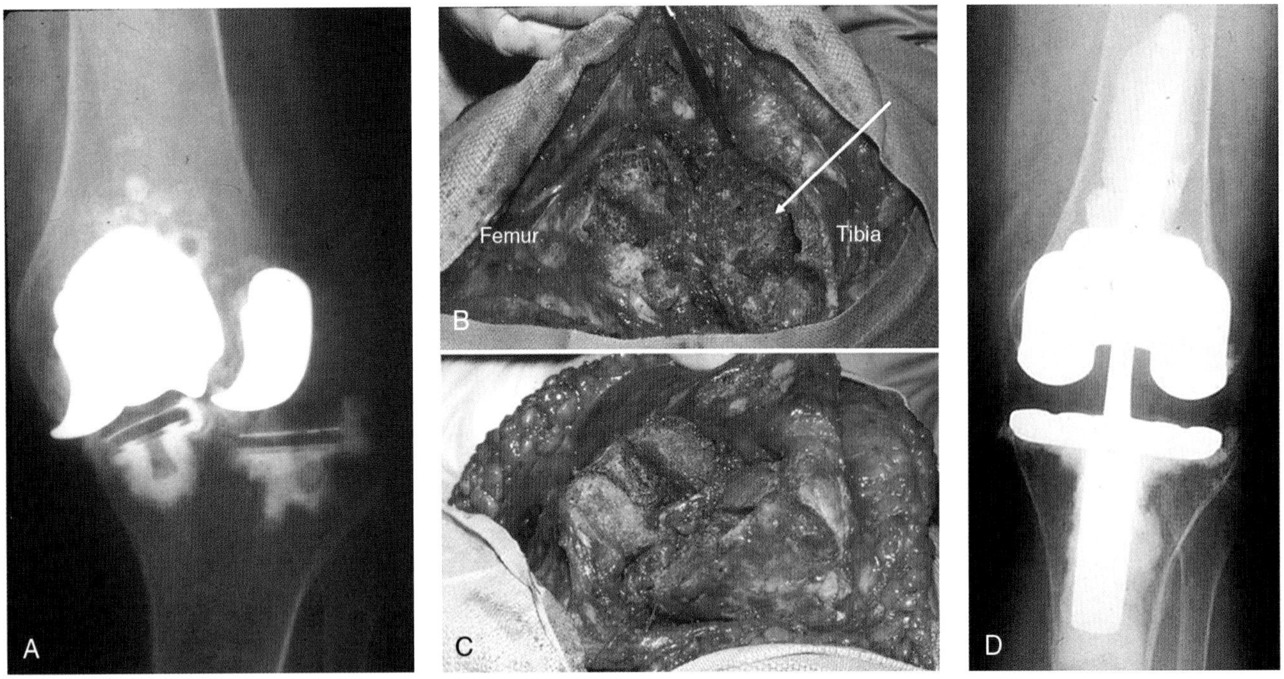

Figure 1 **A,** Preoperative AP radiograph of a knee replacement that failed because of component loosening and subsidence. Intraoperative photographs showing (**B**) an extensive cavitary defect (arrow) managed with particulate allografting (**C**). **D,** AP radiograph made 13 years postoperatively.

thetic augments are expensive and are limited in size and shape. There is a potential for debris creation from their modular attachment to the main component, and they can loosen if the bone supporting the augment is poor. The use of stem extensions can protect weakened condylar bone and enhance fixation. Because augments are often combined with other treatment modalities, such as bone grafting and stem extensions, the results of augmentation in revision total knee arthroplasty are somewhat difficult to precisely interpret. Patel et al[22] reported on 79 revision total knee replacements in knees with AORI type II defects that were followed for a mean of 7 years. One hundred seventy-six augments were implanted into the femur and tibia. Nonprogressive radiolucent lines were observed in 14% of the knees and were unassociated with clinical results. The survival rate of the implants at 11 years was 92%.

Structural Allografts

For noncontained type II defects that are too large to be managed with prosthetic augments and for type III deficits, structural allografts may be considered (**Figure 2**). Dorr et al[12] suggested that tibial defects involving more than 50% of the osseous support of either tibial plateau would benefit from allograft reconstruction. Preoperatively, it is critical to match the specimen with the host defect size. Femoral head, distal femoral, or proximal tibial allografts can be used. The technical keys of bone grafting include developing a healthy, bleeding, host recipient site; maximizing allograft-host and prosthesis-host contact; optimizing the mechanical interlock between the graft and the host; restoring the anatomic joint line; and supplying rigid implant fixation with no instability or malalignment. The addition of stem extensions to enhance implant fixation and offload the structural allograft during incorporation is recommended.

Advantages of structural allograft reconstruction include the biologic potential for bone stock restoration and versatility because the graft can be shaped to fit the host defect. The structural allografts can be used to restore the joint line and have the potential for ligament reattachment. Disadvantages include a minimal risk of disease transmission (< 1 per 1,000,000 risk of HIV transmission)[20] and risks of allograft nonunion, malunion, collapse, or resorption.

Although complications are frequent in complex cases requiring allograft reconstruction, multiple studies have demonstrated high union rates if rigid fixation is achieved.[29-31] Clatworthy et al[29] reported on revision total knee arthroplasty in 50 patients (52 knees) with large, noncontained osseous defects treated with structural allografts. Thirty-seven of the 52 knee revisions were classified as a success,

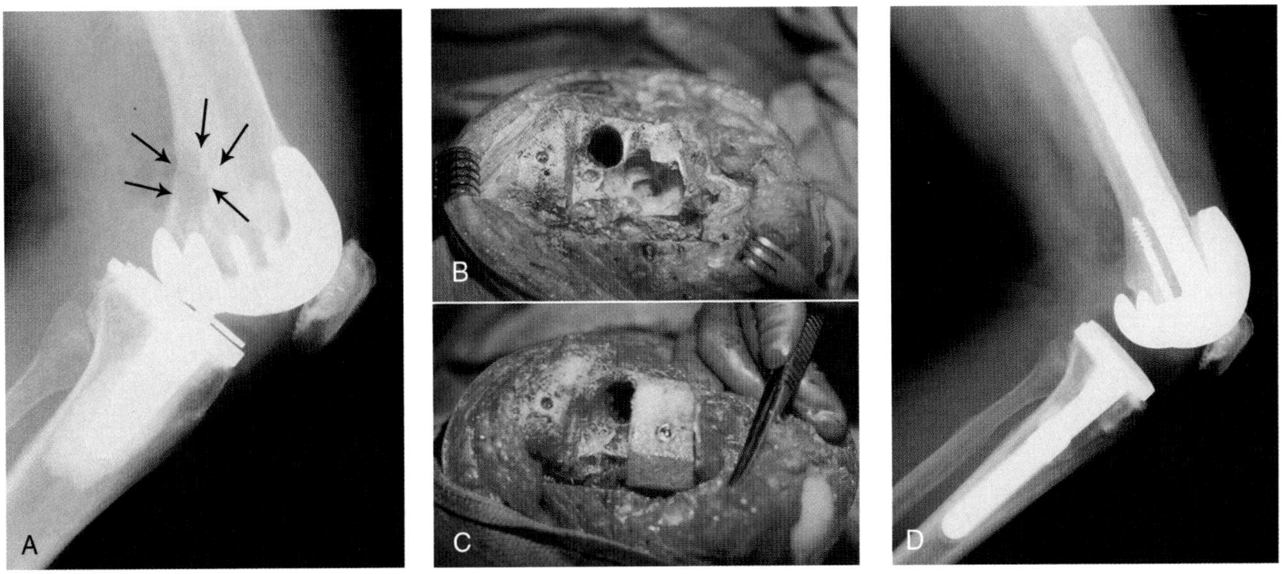

Figure 2 **A,** Preoperative lateral radiograph showing an osseous defect (arrows) in a total knee replacement that failed because of polyethylene wear and distal femoral osteolysis. Intraoperative photographs showing a type IIA osseous defect of the lateral femoral condyle (**B**) managed with a structural femoral head allograft (**C**). **D,** Postoperative lateral radiograph obtained 8 years after reconstruction of the structural allograft.

with 46 of 50 grafts surviving at 5 years and 36 at 10 years. The authors reported 11 failures because of infection (4), graft resorption (5), and allograft nonunion (2). Engh and Ammeen[30] evaluated 46 patients who had revision total knee arthroplasty with use of structural allografts. At a mean duration of follow-up of 95 months, they noted only four failed allografts, two of which were secondary to infection. No allograft collapse was observed. Bauman et al[31] reviewed 70 revision total knee replacements with structural allograft repair that were followed for a minimum of 5 years. Eight failures related to the allograft were found, and they observed a revision-free survival rate of 75.9% (95% confidence interval, 65.6 to 87.8) at 10 years.

Metaphyseal Sleeves or Cones

Contained cavitary and combined cavitary-segmental metaphyseal defects in the femur and tibia can be filled with metaphyseal sleeves or porous cones. These allografts provide metaphyseal implant support and fixation and are ideal for managing large, central, cone-shaped deficiencies in the femoral or tibial metaphysis. Additional fixation is obtained on condylar bone or via diaphyseal-engaging stems. Unlike bulk allograft reconstructions, the metaphyseal sleeves and cones avoid the risk of nonunion and resorption. Porous metal cones achieve peripheral osseous ingrowth, and any prosthetic device can be cemented into their inner central surface.

Long and Scuderi[32] reported on 16 patients who were treated with tibial tantalum cones and followed for 31 months. There were no revisions for aseptic loosening, and all patients showed evidence of osseointegration on follow-up radiographs. Meneghini et al[25] reported on 15 patients who had revision knee arthroplasties with implantation of porous metal metaphyseal tibial cones and were followed for a mean of 2 years. On radiographs, all of the tibial cones demonstrated evidence of osseointegration, and there were no reported failures.

Metaphyseal sleeves are designed for cementless fixation via a porous ingrowth surface and are implant specific (**Figure 3**). Progressive metaphyseal loading is achieved through a step design. The metaphyseal bone is prepared similar to broaching for a cementless femoral component in total hip arthroplasty. Progressively larger broaches are implanted until rigid fixation of the broach is obtained. This creates a precisely engineered cavity for later sleeve insertion. To increase the rigidity of fixation, attaching a diaphyseal-engaging stem extension to the metaphyseal sleeve is recommended (**Figure 4**). Disadvantages of sleeve and cone use include the expense and potential removal difficulties.[33] Clinical results with metaphyseal sleeve use are currently short term but favorable. Jones et al,[34] in a study with a mean follow-up of 49 months, described a combined series of 30 knee revisions in which press-fit diaphyseal-engaging stems and metaphyseal sleeves were used. All of the implants showed bone apposition and positive

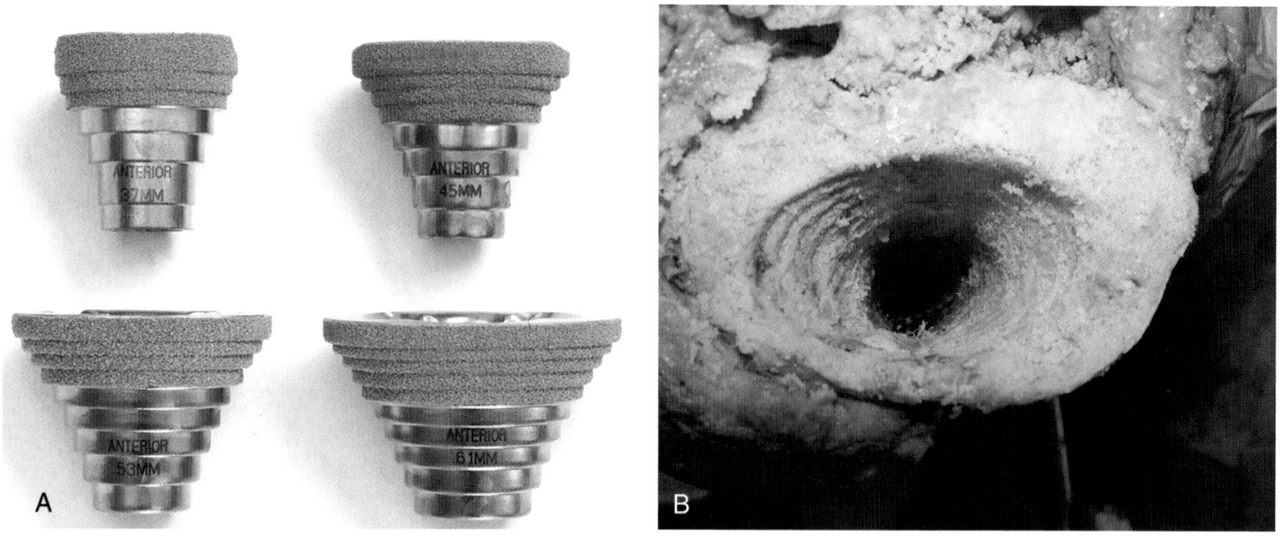

Figure 3 **A,** Photograph of the various tibial metaphyseal sleeves available to treat type II and III osseous defects. **B,** Intraoperative photograph of the proximal part of the tibia after broaching for a metaphyseal sleeve, showing precise defect preparation. (Part B reproduced with permission from Dennis DA: A stepwise approach to revision total knee arthroplasty. *J Arthroplasty* 2007;22(4 suppl 1):32-38.)

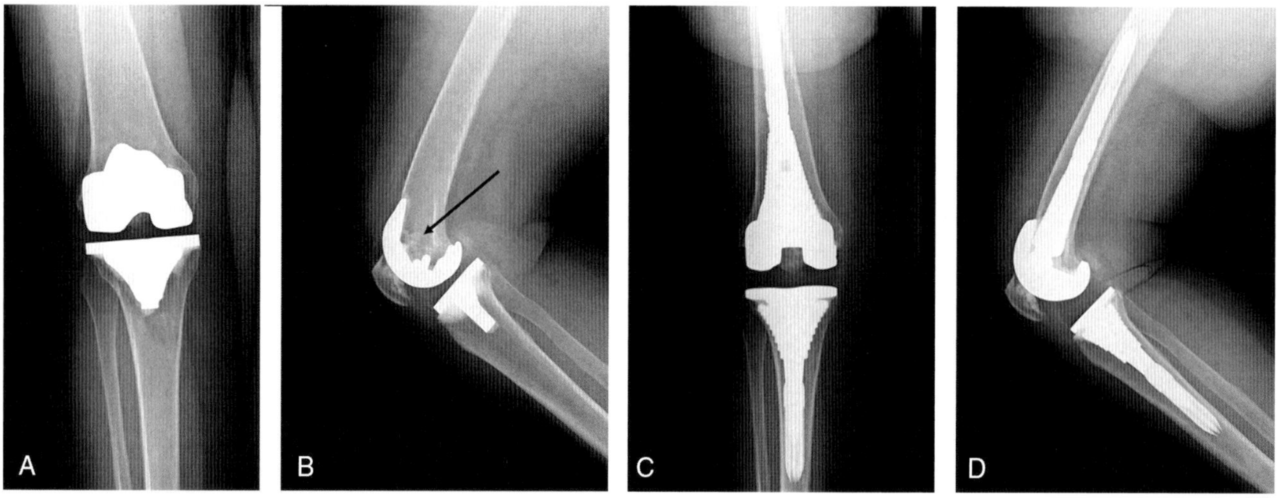

Figure 4 Preoperative AP (**A**) and lateral (**B**) radiographs showing many 8-mm cement plugs in the femur (arrow) and tibia of a total knee replacement that failed because of flexion instability. Postoperative AP (**C**) and lateral (**D**) radiographs after reconstruction with a diaphyseal-engaging stem and femoral and tibial metaphyseal sleeves.

remodeling of bone adjacent to the metaphyseal sleeves on follow-up radiographs with no mechanical failures.

Video 30.1: Management of Large Bone Defects in Revision Total Knee Arthroplasty With Metallic Implants. Daniel J. Berry, MD (20 min)

Condyle-Replacing Hinged Prosthesis

In massive type III defects with loss of collateral ligamentous support, a condyle-replacing hinged prosthesis should be considered, especially in low-demand, elderly patients. The surgical procedure is relatively simple and efficient and allows rapid rehabilitation and weight bearing (**Figure 5**). The most prominent disadvantage of this treatment option is that there are few remaining reconstructive options if this method fails.

Summary

Numerous treatment options are available to manage bone loss associated with revision total knee arthroplasty.

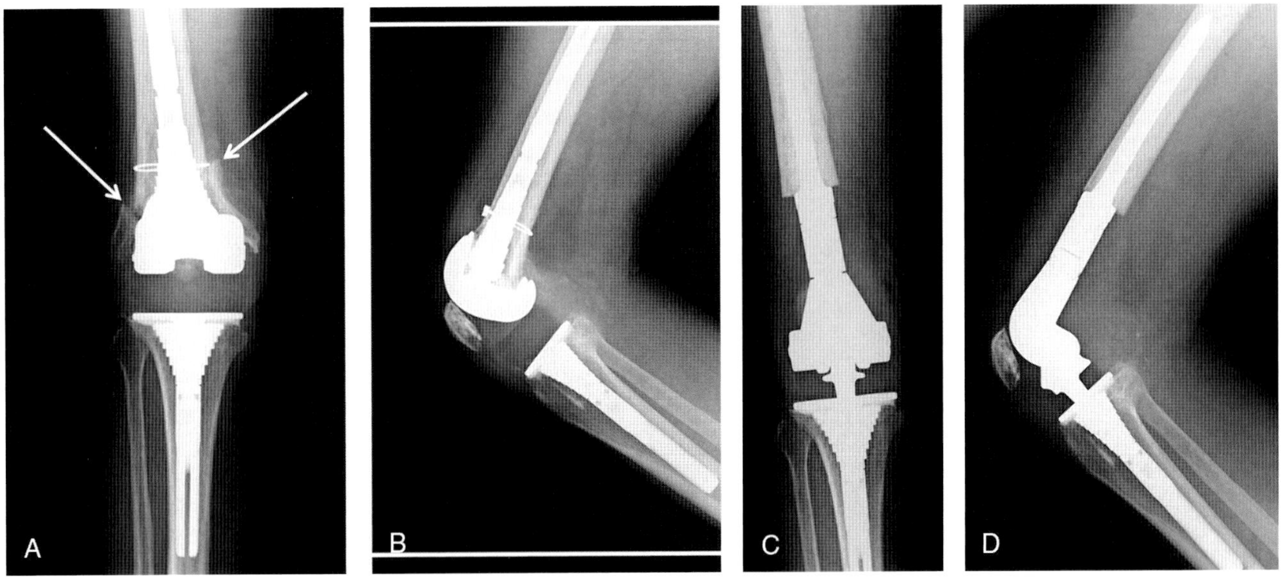

Figure 5 A revision total knee replacement failed in an 82-year-old man because of femoral component loosening and fractures of the medial and lateral condyles. **A,** Preoperative AP radiograph showing fractures of the medial and lateral condyles (arrows). **B,** Preoperative lateral radiograph. Postoperative AP (**C**) and lateral (**D**) radiographs after reconstruction with a distal femoral condyle-replacing hinged prosthesis.

Selection of the treatment method is based on many factors, including the defect size and location in addition to the age, health, and ability of the patient to participate in the necessary postoperative rehabilitation.

References

1. Engh GA, Ammeen DJ: Bone loss with revision total knee arthroplasty: Defect classification and alternatives for reconstruction. *Instr Course Lect* 1999;48:167-175.
2. Mont MA, Serna FK, Krackow KA, Hungerford DS: Exploration of radiographically normal total knee replacements for unexplained pain. *Clin Orthop Relat Res* 1996;331:216-220.
3. Mason JB, Fehring TK, Odum SM, Griffin WL, Nussman DS: The value of white blood cell counts before revision total knee arthroplasty. *J Arthroplasty* 2003; 18(8):1038-1043.
4. Gonzalez MH, Mekhail AO: The failed total knee arthroplasty: Evaluation and etiology. *J Am Acad Orthop Surg* 2004;12(6): 436-446.
5. Rand JA: Bone deficiency in total knee arthroplasty: Use of metal wedge augmentation. *Clin Orthop Relat Res* 1991;271:63-71.
6. Engh GA, Ammeen DJ: Classification and preoperative radiographic evaluation: Knee. *Orthop Clin North Am* 1998;29(2):205-217.
7. Mabry TM, Hanssen AD: The role of stems and augments for bone loss in revision knee arthroplasty. *J Arthroplasty* 2007; 22(4, suppl 1):56-60.
8. Engh GA, Parks NL: The management of bone defects in revision total knee arthroplasty. *Instr Course Lect* 1997;46:227-236.
9. Lonner JH, Lotke PA, Kim J, Nelson C: Impaction grafting and wire mesh for uncontained defects in revision knee arthroplasty. *Clin Orthop Relat Res* 2002;404:145-151.
10. Lotke PA, Carolan GF, Puri N: Technique for impaction bone grafting of large bone defects in revision total knee arthroplasty. *J Arthroplasty* 2006;21(4, suppl 1): 57-60.
11. Lotke PA, Carolan GF, Puri N: Impaction grafting for bone defects in revision total knee arthroplasty. *Clin Orthop Relat Res* 2006; 446:99-103.
12. Dorr LD, Ranawat CS, Sculco TA, McKaskill B, Orisek BS: Bone graft for tibial defects in total knee arthroplasty. *Clin Orthop Relat Res* 1986;205:153-165.
13. Ritter MA: Screw and cement fixation of large defects in total knee arthroplasty. *J Arthroplasty* 1986;1(2):125-129.
14. Ritter MA, Keating EM, Faris PM: Screw and cement fixation of large defects in total knee arthroplasty: A sequel. *J Arthroplasty* 1993;8(1):63-65.
15. Harada Y, Wevers HW, Cooke TD: Distribution of bone strength in the proximal tibia. *J Arthroplasty* 1988;3(2):167-175.

16. Lee JG, Keating EM, Ritter MA, Faris PM: Review of the all-polyethylene tibial component in total knee arthroplasty: A minimum seven-year follow-up period. *Clin Orthop Relat Res* 1990;260:87-92.
17. Brooks PJ, Walker PS, Scott RD: Tibial component fixation in deficient tibial bone stock. *Clin Orthop Relat Res* 1984;184:302-308.
18. Shrivastava SC, Ahmed AM, Shirazi-Adl A, Burke DL: Effect of a cement-bone composite layer and prosthesis geometry on stresses in a prosthetically resurfaced tibia. *J Biomed Mater Res* 1982;16(6):929-949.
19. Lyall HS, Sanghrajka A, Scott G: Severe tibial bone loss in revision total knee replacement managed with structural femoral head allograft: A prospective case series from the Royal London Hospital. *Knee* 2009;16(5):326-331.
20. Buck BE, Malinin TI, Brown MD: Bone transplantation and human immunodeficiency virus: An estimate of risk of acquired immunodeficiency syndrome (AIDS). *Clin Orthop Relat Res* 1989;240:129-136.
21. Whiteside LA: Cementless revision total knee arthroplasty. *Clin Orthop Relat Res* 1993;286:160-167.
22. Patel JV, Masonis JL, Guerin J, Bourne RB, Rorabeck CH: The fate of augments to treat type-2 bone defects in revision knee arthroplasty. *J Bone Joint Surg Br* 2004;86(2):195-199.
23. Sah AP, Scott RD, Springer BD, Bono JV, Deshmukh RV, Thornhill TS: Custom-made angled inserts for tibial coronal malalignment in total knee arthroplasty. *J Arthroplasty* 2009;24(2):288-296.
24. Radnay CS, Scuderi GR: Management of bone loss: Augments, cones, offset stems. *Clin Orthop Relat Res* 2006;446:83-92.
25. Meneghini RM, Lewallen DG, Hanssen AD: Use of porous tantalum metaphyseal cones for severe tibial bone loss during revision total knee replacement. *J Bone Joint Surg Am* 2008;90(1):78-84.
26. Meneghini RM, Lewallen DG, Hanssen AD: Use of porous tantalum metaphyseal cones for severe tibial bone loss during revision total knee replacement: Surgical technique. *J Bone Joint Surg Am* 2009;91(suppl 2 pt 1):131-138.
27. Chen F, Krackow KA: Management of tibial defects in total knee arthroplasty: A biomechanical study. *Clin Orthop Relat Res* 1994;305:249-257.
28. Fehring TK, Peindl RD, Humble RS, Harrow ME, Frick SL: Modular tibial augmentations in total knee arthroplasty. *Clin Orthop Relat Res* 1996;327:207-217.
29. Clatworthy MG, Ballance J, Brick GW, Chandler HP, Gross AE: The use of structural allograft for uncontained defects in revision total knee arthroplasty: A minimum five-year review. *J Bone Joint Surg Am* 2001;83-A(3):404-411.
30. Engh GA, Ammeen DJ: Use of structural allograft in revision total knee arthroplasty in knees with severe tibial bone loss. *J Bone Joint Surg Am* 2007;89(12):2640-2647.
31. Bauman RD, Lewallen DG, Hanssen AD: Limitations of structural allograft in revision total knee arthroplasty. *Clin Orthop Relat Res* 2009;467(3):818-824.
32. Long WJ, Scuderi GR: Porous tantalum cones for large metaphyseal tibial defects in revision total knee arthroplasty: A minimum 2-year follow-up. *J Arthroplasty* 2009;24(7):1086-1092.
33. Haidukewych GJ, Hanssen A, Jones RD: Metaphyseal fixation in revision total knee arthroplasty: Indications and techniques. *J Am Acad Orthop Surg* 2011;19(6):311-318.
34. Jones RE, Barrack RL, Skedros J: Modular, mobile-bearing hinge total knee arthroplasty. *Clin Orthop Relat Res* 2001;392:306-314.

Video Reference

30.1: Berry DJ: Video. Excerpt. *Cones/Wedges/Augments/Bone Grafting/Stems.* Rosemont, IL, American Academy of Orthopaedic Surgeons, 2011.

31

Evaluation and Management of the Infected Total Knee Arthroplasty

Bryan D. Springer, MD
Giles R. Scuderi, MD

Abstract

Infection after total knee arthroplasty (TKA) remains a difficult complication to treat. The risk of infection ranges from 0.5% to 2% for primary TKAs and 2% to 4% for revision TKAs. Several demographic studies indicate that more infections are occurring after these procedures, and infection is one of the most common reasons for TKA failure. Prevention remains the key to minimizing the risk of infection; however, little evidence-based literature exists to establish the optimal approach.

Every patient with a painful TKA should be suspected of having an infection until proven otherwise. An algorithmic approach to these patients should include standard laboratory screening tests to rule out infection. Synovial fluid aspiration remains the best test for diagnosing infection. Synovial fluid white blood cell counts greater than 1,700 cells/μL and a differential greater than 69% polymorphonuclear cells should raise a high index of suspicion for infection.

Several options are available to treat deep periprosthetic infection. The timing of the infection as it relates to surgery and the onset of symptoms are critical in determining treatment success. Prosthetic retention is indicated only in patients with an acute onset of infection, but its limited success reported in recent literature brings into question its role in infected TKAs. A two-stage exchange arthroplasty remains the gold standard for treatment of infection following TKA.

Instr Course Lect 2013;62:349-361.

Infection after total knee arthroplasty (TKA) remains one of the most difficult complications to treat. The overall incidence of infection ranges between 0.5% to 2% for primary TKAs and 2% to 4% for revision TKAs.[1-3] In 2005, 16.8% of all revision TKAs were done because of infection. It is estimated that by the year 2030, 65% of all revision procedures will be done because of infection; this represents an estimated 52,000 infected total knee replacements.[4] The economic impact of treating a patient with an infection after TKA is substantial. Treatment of an infected TKA costs from $60,000 to $100,000, in part because of long hospital stays and a high complication rate.[5-7] Treating a TKA infection is one of the most resource-consumptive procedures in orthopaedic surgery. This chapter will focus on the diagnosis and management of the infected TKA.

Diagnosis of the Infected TKA

Several tools, including plain radiographs, laboratory tests, joint aspiration, advanced imaging techniques, and intraoperative testing, can assist in the diagnosis of a patient with a suspected infected TKA. There is currently no standard of care for either the diagnosis or perioperative workup that should be done to evaluate a patient with a suspected periprosthetic joint infection. Recently, the American

Dr. Springer or an immediate family member is a member of a speakers' bureau or has made paid presentations on behalf of DePuy and serves as a paid consultant to or is an employee of Stryker and Convatec Surgical. Dr. Scuderi or an immediate family member serves as a board member, owner, officer, or committee member of the Knee Society and ICJR; has received royalties from Zimmer and Salient Surgical; is a member of a speakers' bureau or has made paid presentations on behalf of Zimmer and Salient Surgical; and serves as a paid consultant to or is an employee of Zimmer and Salient Surgical.

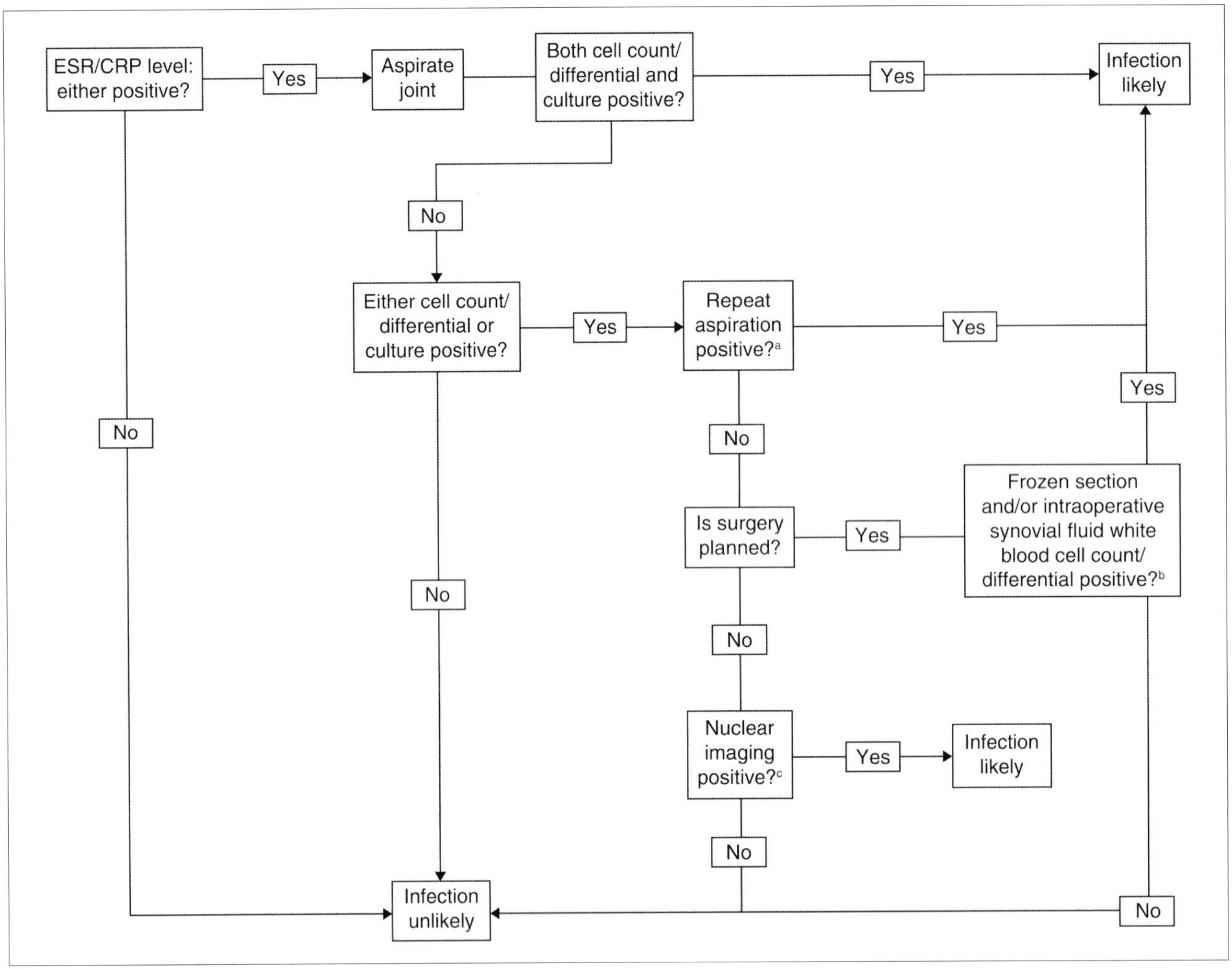

Figure 1 Algorithm for the diagnosis of patients with a higher probability of hip or knee periprosthetic joint infection. [a]Perform repeat aspiration when a discrepancy exists between the probability of infection and the result of the initial aspiration culture. [b]Perform frozen section when the diagnosis has not been established at the time of surgery; synovial fluid WBC count and differential may also be obtained intraoperatively. [c]Nuclear imaging modalities: labeled-leukocyte imaging combined with bone or bone marrow imaging, F-18 fluorodeoxyglucose–positron emission tomography, gallium imaging, or label-leukocyte imaging. (Reproduced from Della Valle C, Parvizi J, Bauer T, et al: AAOS Clinical Practice Guideline Summary: Diagnosis of Preprosthetic Joint Infection of the Hip and Knee. *J Am Acad Orthop Surg* 2010;18(12):760-770.)

Academy of Orthopaedic Surgeons workgroup evaluated the available evidence for each diagnostic modality and proposed algorithms that can be used by clinicians in diagnosing infection[8] (**Figures 1** and **2**).

A thorough clinical history and physical examination is the mainstay of the initial evaluation. In general, infection should be suspected in every patient with a painful TKA until proven otherwise. The location and character of pain should be noted. Sources of referred pain, such as the hip and the lumbar spine, must be ruled out. The timing of the onset of pain should be determined. Has the pain persisted since the TKA or did the patient have a pain-free interval? Does the level of pain change with activity? Is there substantial warmth or erythema around the knee? Were there wound healing or drainage problems after the initial surgery? Were antibiotics administered for a suspected infection? Did the patient have a procedure that could have resulted in a bacteremic episode, such as dental work, a colonoscopy, or urologic procedures?

Plain radiographs can provide useful information in diagnosing infection. Obtaining the patient's initial postoperative radiographs and comparing them to the most recent studies is often helpful. If infection is present, plain radiographs may show periosteal

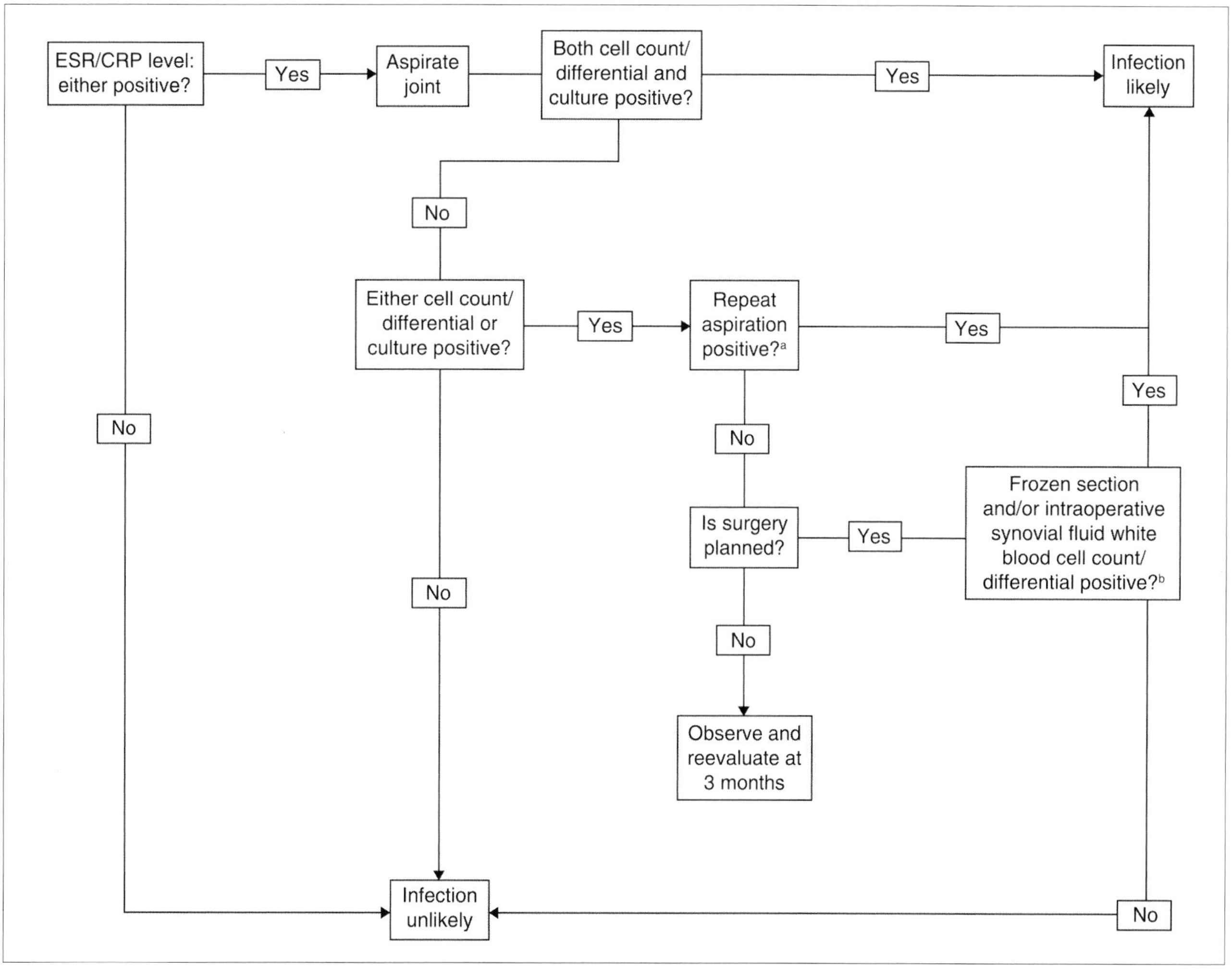

Figure 2 Algorithm for the diagnosis of patients with a lower probability of hip or knee periprosthetic joint infection. [a]Perform repeat aspiration when a discrepancy exists between the probability of infection and the result of the initial aspiration culture. [b]Perform frozen section when the diagnosis has not been established at the time of surgery; synovial fluid WBC count and differential may also be obtained intraoperatively. (Reproduced from Della Valle C, Parvizi J, Bauer T, et al: AAOS Clinical Practice Guideline Summary: Diagnosis of Preprosthetic Joint Infection of the Hip and Knee. *J Am Acad Orthop Surg* 2010;18(12):760-770.)

lamination, subchondral bony resorption, progressive radiolucencies, or localized osteolysis. It is important to remember that bony destruction and lytic lesions are typically seen only after a 30% to 50% loss of bone.

Hematologic tests include the systemic white blood cell (WBC) count, the erythrocyte sedimentation rate (ESR), the C-reactive protein (CRP) level, and, more recently, an analysis of the interleukin-6 (IL-6) level. It is important to remember that no test is 100% specific for infection. These tests generally have a high sensitivity and a low specificity for infection, making them good screening tests rather than accurate predictors of infection. The AAOS workgroup recommends that a serum ESR and CRP level be performed at the initial screening test in all patients with a suspected infection.[8]

The systemic WBC count is not a reliable indicator of a TKA infection. Studies have shown that up to 70% of patients with infection have a normal WBC count.[9,10] The ESR generally peaks 5 to 7 days after surgery and will return to normal slowly in approximately 3 months. The CRP level rises within 6 hours of surgery, generally peaks 2 to 3 days after surgery, and will return to normal within 3 weeks. Neither the ESR or the CRP level alone or in combination are sufficient to make a diagnosis of infection; the tests have a specificity of only 56%.[11] However, when used in combination, the tests are reasonably accurate for ruling out the presence of infection, with a sensitivity of 96% and a negative predictive value of 95%.[11,12] Analysis of the serum IL-6 level has recently gained in popularity. It generally peaks within 6 hours of surgery but can return to normal within 72 hours after surgery. The IL-6 level has been shown to have a sensitivity of 100% and a specificity of 95% for predicting the presence of infection.[13] IL-6 analysis is not readily available in all clinical settings.

Joint aspiration remains one of the most effective tools for diagnosing infection; however, it can be associated with false-negative results. To minimize false-negative culture findings, the patient should not have used antibiotics within 2 to 3 weeks before the joint aspiration. If necessary, aspiration in patients who have recently used antibiotics may still yield a useful cell count and differential analysis; however, culture results will be unreliable.

Mason et al[14] showed that a WBC count of greater than 2,500 cells/μL with greater than 60% polymorphonuclear cells had a sensitivity of 98%, a specificity of 95%, and a positive predictive value of 91% in the diagnosis of infection. Leone and Hanssen[15] reported that an aspirate of less than 2,000 cells/ μL with a differential of less than 50% had a 98% negative predictive value in ruling out infection. More recently, the literature has supported a variable range of synovial WBC counts and differentials to diagnose periprosthetic joint infection.[14,16,17] In general, suspicion should be high when the synovial fluid WBC count is greater than 1,760 cells/μL with greater than 69% polymorphonuclear cells present in the differential.[18]

In the acute postoperative period, the synovial fluid cell count and differential may be elevated as a response to surgery and may not accurately reflect the presence of infection. If traditional cell counts and differentials are used to diagnose infection in the acute postoperative period, there is concern that these values may lead to unnecessary surgery. A recent study by Bedair et al[19] provided information on the use of synovial fluid in the diagnosis of acute postoperative infection after TKA. In 146 patients who had a knee aspiration within 6 weeks of TKA, infection was diagnosed in 19 patients. Using receiver operating curves to determine the optimal cutoff, the authors concluded that a synovial fluid WBC count of 27,800 cells/μL had a positive predictive value of 94% and a negative predictive value of 98%. The optimal cutoff for polymorphonuclear cells was 89%.

Radionuclide scanning tests may be useful in diagnosing infection, particularly in equivocal situations; however, these tests are expensive, cumbersome for the patient, and lack specificity for diagnosing infection. A technetium Tc-99m scan is a measure of osteoblastic activity. Although it may be positive in the presence of infection, several other factors, including trauma, degenerative joint disease, and tumor, can cause a positive result. Most importantly, Tc-99m scans can remain positive for up to 12 months after surgery; they have sensitivity and a positive predictive value in the range of 30% to 38%. Indium In-111–labeled leukocyte scanning will show radionuclide accumulation in areas of WBCs. This test has been shown to have a sensitivity of 77% and a specificity of 86%.[20] Combining these two scanning tests will improve specificity and is generally recommended.[21]

Recently, there has been growing interest in the use of molecular genetics for diagnosing infection. This can include the use of polymerase chain reaction analysis after sonication of implants. Many of these tests allow rapid processing within 4 to 6 hours, and the tests can be effective in the presence of antibiotics. The disadvantage of molecular genetic tests for infection is that they do not provide information on antibiotic sensitivity. The technology is also complex and somewhat expensive, and the tests are oversensitive, which can result in false-positive findings.

Intraoperative testing includes the use of Gram staining and frozen-section histopathology. In general, a Gram stain is unreliable and has poor sensitivity; it should not be used alone to rule out infection.[22] The AAOS workgroup recommends against the use of Gram stains to rule out periprosthetic joint infection.[8]

Frozen-section histopathology produces variable results.[23-25] It is technique-dependent and relies on the experience of the pathologist to determine the presence of acute inflammation. Sampling errors often occur. Various tests show that 5 to 10 WBCs per high-power field has adequate sensitivity and specificity for diagnosing infection. The AAOS workgroup strongly recommends frozen-section peri-implant tissue analysis in patients who are undergoing revision surgery when the diagnosis of infection has not been established or excluded.[8] The AAOS workgroup was not able to establish the best threshold (5 or 10 WBC in a field) because the literature contains insufficient data to distinguish between the two counts.

A New Definition for Diagnosing Infection

Although there are many tests to evaluate patients with a suspected periprosthetic joint infection, there is no single accepted diagnostic criterion. Recently, a workgroup of the Musculoskeletal Infection Society analyzed all the available evidence and proposed a new definition for periprosthetic joint infection.[26] These criteria should allow for a wide adoption of the definition of periprosthetic joint infection among clinicians.

Table 1
Periprosthetic Infection

Type	Description	Definition	Treatment
I	Positive intraoperative culture	Two or more positive cultures obtained at surgery	Appropriate antibiotic-directed therapy
II	Early postoperative infection	Infection within first 4 weeks after surgery	Attempted irrigation and débridement
III	Acute hematogenous infection	Seeding of a previously well-functioning joint	Attempted irrigation and débridement versus prosthesis removal
IV	Chronic (late) infection	Symptoms present for more than 1 month	Prosthesis removal with two-stage exchange arthroplasty

Based on the proposed criteria, a periprosthetic joint infection exists when (1) there is a sinus tract communicating with the joint, (2) a pathogen is isolated by culture from two separate tissue or fluid samples for the affected joint, or (3) four of six criteria are met. These six criteria are elevated ESR or CRP level, elevated synovial leukocyte count, elevated synovial leukocyte percentage, the presence of purulence in the affected joint, the isolation of a microorganism in one culture of tissue or fluid, and greater than five neutrophils per high-power field in five high-powered fields from the analysis of periprosthetic tissue (×400).

Surgical Management

The treatment of a patient with an infected TKA can include retention of the prosthesis with antibiotic suppression, open irrigation and débridement with polyethylene exchange, or prosthesis removal. Prosthesis removal can involve resection arthroplasty, arthrodesis, single-stage exchange arthroplasty, two-stage exchange arthroplasty, or amputation. Several factors should be considered when choosing a treatment option, including the depth and timing of the infection, the status of the soft tissues, the fixation of the prosthesis, the involved pathogenic organism, the ability of the host to fight the infection, the resources of the physician, and the patient's expectations.

Based on the Tsukayama et al[27] classification system for infected total knee joints, a type I infection is characterized by a positive culture at the time of surgery, and a type II infection is an early infection that occurs within the first month after surgery. A type III infection is a late, acute, hematogenous infection that occurs after the TKA, with symptoms of less than 4 weeks' duration. A type IV infection is a late, chronic infection with symptoms that have persisted for more than 4 weeks. **Table 1** describes the classification system and provides recommended treatment options based on the type of infection.

Antibiotic Suppression

Antibiotic suppression without surgical débridement is recommended only in a patient who is medically debilitated and unable to tolerate surgery. The infectious agent should be a low-virulence organism, the patient should be in stable condition, the components should be well fixed, and a suitable oral antibiotic agent must be available. The success rate of antibiotic suppression without surgical débridement is approximately 20%.[17,28]

Irrigation and Débridement

It is generally agreed that open irrigation and débridement for an infected TKA should be reserved for patients with an acute onset of infection. Irrigation, débridement, and component retention for treatment of a chronic infection (signs and symptoms for more than 4 weeks) has a high failure rate and should not be considered.[29,30]

Arthroscopic Technique

Arthroscopic irrigation and débridement has been described as an attractive and expeditious treatment alternative to open irrigation and débridement. It is done through small arthroscopic portals with minimal disruption of the soft tissues. The current literature on arthroscopic irrigation and débridement is limited to a few studies with small numbers of patients. Waldman et al[31] reported on 16 patients with acute periprosthetic infections. All patients treated with arthroscopic irrigation and débridement had symptoms for less than 7 days. At a mean follow-up of 56 months, the rate of successful eradication of infection was 38%. In a 2004 study, Dixon et al[32] reported an infection eradication rate of 60% in 15 patients treated with arthroscopic irrigation and débridement at a mean follow-up of 55 months.

In addition to the limited outcomes data, there are several other concerns with arthroscopic irrigation and débridement. Arthroscopic examination of the joint is inferior to an open procedure because it allows only limited evaluation of the bone-cement and prosthetic interfaces. The polyethylene cannot be exchanged, which precludes débridement in the posterior aspect of the knee. A complete and thorough synovectomy cannot be performed. It is also more difficult to remove debris through arthroscopic portals than with an open procedure. For these reasons, as well as the inferior results that have been reported in the literature, arthroscopic irrigation and debridement should be performed only in rare circumstances for an infected TKA.

Open Technique

The results of open irrigation and débridement for the treatment of acute periprosthetic joint infections have varied[29,33-46] (**Table 2**). Based on an evaluation of more than 20 published articles, the success rate of this procedure ranges from 19% to 83%, with most studies reporting success rates less than 60%. A 2002 meta-analysis by Silva et al[33] evaluated 530 patients treated with open irrigation and débridement for an acute periprosthetic joint infection. This study included acute postoperative infections and late acute hematogenous infections. The overall success rate was 33.6%. Several variables clearly affect outcomes, including the timing of surgery, patient risk factors, the surgical technique, and the type of infecting organism (**Table 3**).

The timing of surgery appears to be a critical factor in the success of treatment using irrigation, débridement, and polyethylene exchange. Irrigation and débridement with polyethylene exchange has a high failure rate for patients with an onset of symptoms of more than 4 weeks' duration. Schoifet and Morrey[29] reported an overall failure rate of 77% for irrigation and débridement for the treatment of periprosthetic TKA infections. All treatment failures occurred in patients with symptoms of more than 28 days' duration. Although several studies have reported that the time from the onset of symptoms to surgical irrigation and débridement was not a factor in the outcome (< 4 weeks), some authors have shown improved success rates when treatment is initiated after a shorter duration of symptoms.[34,47,48] Brandt et al[47] reported a higher probability of treatment failure for patients treated with irrigation and débridement more than 2 days after the onset of symptoms. Marculescu et al[34] reported that a duration of symptoms of more than 8 days was associated with a two times greater risk of treatment failure. Hsieh et al[48] found that a short duration of symptoms (< 5 days) before surgery was the only identifiable factor associated with the success of irrigation and débridement for patients with a gram-negative prosthetic joint infection.

A methicillin-resistant *Staphylococcus aureus* (MRSA) infection poses a particular challenge because of its virulent nature and the limited options for antibiotic therapy. Reports suggest that the overall incidence of MRSA infections in total joint arthroplasty is increasing. Bradbury et al[35] reported on 19 acute periprosthetic MRSA knee infections treated with open irrigation, débridement, and component retention. At a minimum 2-year follow-up, the failure rate was 84%. The authors also reported on 34 studies in the current literature in which 13 patients were identified with an acute MRSA infection and treated with open irrigation, débridement, and component retention. The reported failure rate was 77%.

Primary Exchange Arthroplasty

Primary exchange arthroplasty involves the removal of all components and the reinsertion of a new prosthesis in a single surgery. Although this is an attractive treatment option, there are currently limited outcome data based on a small number of patients. The largest and second largest published studies involved 22 and 18 patients, respectively.[49,50] The authors reported success rates ranging from 89% to 91%. Only patients with optimal characteristics may be appropriate candidates for this procedure in the current era of drug-resistant organisms.[49,50] Factors associated with successful outcomes include patients with limited comorbidities, the use of appropriate antibiotics in the cement directed at the infecting organism, a gram-positive infecting organism, the absence of a draining sinus, and a prolonged course (12 weeks) of intravenous antibiotics.

Two-Stage Exchange Arthroplasty

Two-stage exchange arthroplasty is considered the gold standard for the treatment of a chronic periprosthetic THA infection. The procedure involves the removal of the infected prosthesis and thorough débridement to remove any necrotic and foreign material, including all cement. A high-dose antibiotic cement spacer is placed at the time of the initial surgery, and the patient is treated with a course of intravenous antibiotics tailored to treat the infecting organism. Treatment variables include the amount and type of antibiotics used in the spacer, the type of spacer (static versus articulating), the length of intravenous antibiotic therapy, and the chosen interval between resection and reimplantation.

Antibiotics: Type and Amount

Data show that the inclusion of antibiotics in the cement spacer is an important variable in the treatment of infection. Leone and Hanssen[15] reported that the addition of antibiotic-loaded bone cement improved the success rate of direct exchange from 58% to 74%

Table 2
Study Results for Irrigation and Débridement for the Treatment of Acute Periprosthetic Joint Infections

Study (Year)	No. of Patients	Follow-up	Success Rate	Comments
Koyonos et al[36] (2011)	136	54 months	35%	
Choi et al[37] (2011)	32	36 months	31%	
Odum et al[38] (2011)	150 (THA/TKA)		31%	No difference with organism or timing of irrigation and débridement
Zmistowski et al[39] (2011)			Gram-negative = 70% MSSA = 33% MRSA = 49%	
Azzam et al[40] (2010)	104 (THA/TKA)	5.7 years	44%	No relationship to timing; increased risk with elevated American Society of Anesthesiologists scores, gross purulence, or *S aureus*
Bradbury et al[35] (2009)	19	Minimum 2 years	16%	Average time to irrigation and débridement was 5 days; all MRSA infections
Salgado et al[41] (2007)	20		33%	Average duration to irrigation and débridement was 14 days; included hip and knee replacements (meta-analysis of the literature)
Marculescu et al[34] (2006)	99	24 months	60%	
Deirmengian et al[42] (2003)	31	4 years	35%	92% failure rate with any *Staphylococcus* infection; 44% failure rate with any other gram-positive infection; older age was a risk factor; no difference with time to débridement
Silva et al[33] (2002)	530		33.6%	Factors in successful treatment: < 4 months to surgery, < 4-week symptom duration, antibiotic-sensitive gram-positive organism, young age Factors in failed treatment: presence of sinus tracts at time of débridement, wound drainage > 2 weeks, hinged components, immunocompromised patient
Segawa et al[43] (1999)	10 acute postoperative	3.7 years	50%	No difference in time to irrigation and débridement, four of five failures occurred in immunocompromised patients
Wasielewski[44] (1996)	10	32 months	75% acute 50% chronic	Eight patients with acute infection (< 2 weeks symptom duration) Two patients with chronic infection (> 2 weeks symptom duration)
Kramhøft et al[45] (1994)	27	NR	19%	All successful outcomes had débridement within 1 week of symptoms
Teeny et al[46] (1990)	21	4 years	29%	Patients with symptoms of more than 2 weeks' duration had higher failure rates
Schoifet and Morrey[29] (1990)	31	3 years	23%	Average time to irrigation and débridement for failed treatment was 32 days and for successful treatment was 21 days

TKA = total knee arthroplasty, THA = total hip arthroplasty, MSSA = methicillin-susceptible *S aureus*, MRSA = methicillin-resistant *S aureus*, NR = not reported.

Table 3
Risk Factors for the Treatment Failure of Irrigation, Débridement, and Polyethylene Exchange

Increasing age
Duration of symptoms (> 2 weeks)
Prolonged wound drainage
S aureus
Resistant organisms
Immunocompromised host
Rheumatoid arthritis
Diabetes mellitus
Malnourishment
Presence of sinus tracts
Radiographic evidence of osteitis
Radiographic evidence of component loosening

and two-stage exchange from 88% to 92%.

The amount and type of antibiotics used in the spacer remain controversial. In general, a high-dose antibiotic spacer has between 2 g and 8 g of antibiotic per batch of cement. The most commonly available powdered antibiotics that are heat stable are vancomycin, gentamicin, and tobramycin. It is important to remember that different types of cement elute antibiotics differently.[51-53] Higher doses of antibiotics create greater porosity and voids in the cement. This promotes antibiotic elution and results in higher levels of local antibiotic than are obtained with intravenous administration. Although there are variable reports of systemic toxicity from antibiotics in cement, high local concentrations of antibiotics in cement are generally well tolerated with minimal systemic risks.[54,55]

Static Versus Articulating Spacers

Static antibiotic spacers preserve the joint space and minimize the generation of cement debris but do not allow motion during the interval period. Static, preformed block spacers have been associated with increased bone loss, migration, and extensor mechanism necrosis and generally should be avoided.[56] In a molded static spacer, the cement is placed in a doughy state to allow the cement to mold to the bony surfaces. This can prevent many of the problems associated with preformed block spacers (**Figure 3**).

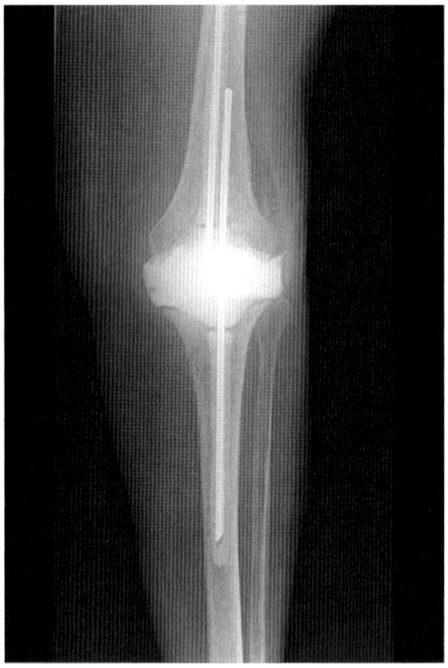

Figure 3 AP radiograph of a molded, static, antibiotic cement spacer.

Articulating spacers maintain soft-tissue pliability and can reduce bone loss in the interval period. These types of spacers facilitate range of motion during the period prior to reimplantation. This allows for improved patient mobility as well as easier exposure at the time of the revision surgery. However, wound healing must remain the top priority, and motion should be restricted if there are concerns about wound healing.

Several types of articulating spacers are available, including cemented articulating spacers in which both the femoral and the tibial components are created using cement molds (**Figure 4**). Recently, the process of sterilizing the explanted prosthesis or using new, low cost, femoral and all-polyethylene tibial components with high-dose antibiotic cement has been described to create a mobile articulating spacer.[57] Regardless of the type of spacer used, débridement of the intramedullary canals of the femur and tibia and the placement of antibiotic dowels into the canals should be done routinely.[58] Data have shown that infection exists in the intramedullary canals in up to one third of patients with an infected TKA.[59]

Limited conclusive results are available concerning the advantages of articulating spacers compared with static spacers. Emerson et al[60] reported no difference in infection rates in a comparison of 26 static spacers with 22 articulating spacers at 36-month follow-up. However, the group with the articulating spacers showed better overall range of motion at final follow-up compared with the group with a static spacer. In a comparative study of static versus articulating spacers, Freeman et al[61] reported a comparable infection eradication rate; however, the group with the articulating spacers had better functional results compared with the group with static spacers.

Duration of Antibiotic Therapy

The optimal duration of intravenous antibiotic administration after resection arthroplasty and the amount of time off antibiotics prior to reimplantation have not been clearly defined. In general, a 6-week course of intravenous antibiotics is typically administered followed by a 2- to 6-week period off antibiotics, at which time patients are clinically evaluated.

Readiness for Reimplantation

Prior to reimplantation, patients should be evaluated for the presence of persistent infection. Clinical and serologic examinations are performed to evaluate the status of infection eradication. The serological markers—ESR and CRP level—are useful tools to evaluate the effect of treatment prior to reimplantation. Although these markers may not return to normal levels prior to reimplantation, they should demonstrate improvement. In a study by Kusuma et al,[62] the ESR remained elevated in 54% of patients, and the CRP level remained elevated in 21% of patients who were proven to be free of infection at the time of reimplantation. The authors were unable to identify an optimum cutoff value for the ESR or the CRP level prior to reimplantation. More important than absolute values, a trend toward normalization of the values over the treatment period may be the best indicator of the response to treatment. Although aspiration analysis prior to reimplantation may be the most useful tool to evaluate persistent infection, strict cell count and differential values have yet to be determined to guide treatment, and aspiration results have been associated with false-negative results.

At the time of reimplantation, the presence of infection must be evaluated in concert with the preoperative information. A frozen section may be used as an indicator of persistence of infection, but results are subject to sampling errors and the experience of the pathologist. Prosthesis reimplantation is contraindicated in patients with evidence of persistent infection. Relative contraindications to reimplantation include patients with a poor or absent extensor mechanism, poor bone stock, and inadequate soft tissue to allow for appropriate coverage

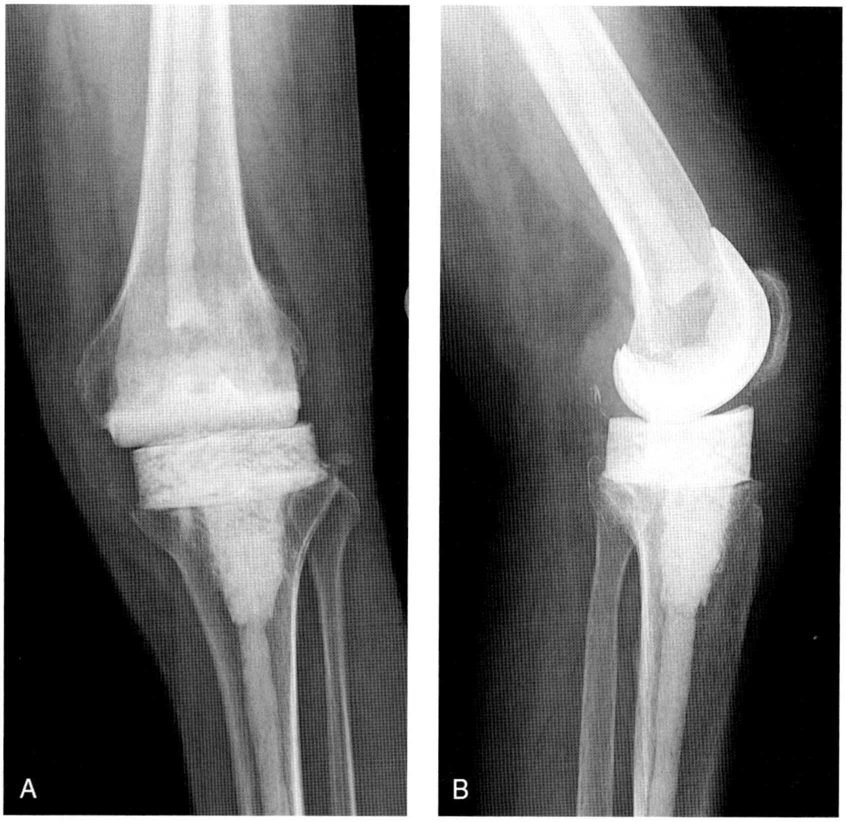

Figure 4 AP (**A**) and lateral (**B**) radiographs of an articulating antibiotic cement spacer.

Table 4

Results of Two-Stage Exchange for Infected Total Knee Arthroplasty

Study (Year)	No. of Knees	Spacer Type	Follow-up	Results
Macheras et al[63] (2011)	34	Mobile and static	12.1 years	91.1% rate of eradication of infection
Westrich et al[64] (2010)	72	Mobile and static	52.4 months	90.7% rate of eradication of infection
Mittal et al[65] (2009)	37	Mobile and static	51 months	All resistant organisms 10% reinfection rate with same organism 14% reinfection rate with new organism
Hoffman et al[57] (2005)	50	Mobile	67 months	88% rate of eradication of infection
Haleem et al[66] (2004)	96	Static	68 months	85% rate of survival free of infection at 10 years
Haddad et al[67] (2000)	45	Mobile (PROSTALAC; DePuy, Warsaw, IN)	48 months	91% rate of successful eradication of infection

Outcomes

Table 4 lists data from the past decade on the success of two-stage exchange arthroplasty for the treatment of chronically infected TKAs.[57,63-67] Multiple studies in the literature have reported clinical success in the eradication of infection, with rates between 85% and 91%. A recent study by Mortazavi et al[68] attempted to identify predictors of failure for two-stage exchange arthroplasty. The authors evaluated 117 patients who had a two-stage exchange for periprosthetic TKA infection. At a minimum 2-year follow-up, there were 33 failures (28%) that required further surgery for continued treatment of infection. Fifteen presurgical and 11 surgical factors were studied that could be related to treatment failure. Despite the high failure rate, the authors identified only culture-negative infections, infection with methicillin-resistant organisms, and increased surgical time during reimplantation as risk factors for failure. ESR and CRP values at the time of reimplantation were not predictors of failure.

Arthrodesis

Arthrodesis may be indicated if no reconstructive salvage options remain. Arthrodesis may be indicated in younger patients who have single joint disease, extensor mechanism disruption, a poor soft-tissue envelope, and those with a highly virulent organism that cannot be adequately controlled with antibiotics. Relative contraindications include ipsilateral hip and ankle disease, severe segmental bone loss, and contralateral extremity amputation.

The most common techniques for knee arthrodesis include using external fixation, intramedullary rod fixation, and dual-plating techniques. A comparative study of external fixation versus intramedullary fusion reported similar fusion and reinfection rates with both techniques.[69] Intramedullary nailing had a trend toward better fusion rates than external fixation but was also associated with a trend toward higher infection rates. Overall, complications occurred in 40% of patients.

The most common complications associated with arthrodesis are nonunion at the arthrodesis site, recurrent infection, and hardware breakage and migration.[28] Despite a relatively high complication rate, arthrodesis remains a reasonable salvage option.

Amputation

Amputation may be required in patients who had multiple revisions for sepsis or life-threatening sepsis, a previous segmental hinge prosthesis, severe bone loss, or intractable pain. Because above-knee amputation is required to eradicate the infection, many patients are unable to ambulate successfully, and functional outcomes are often poor. The patient and family should be counseled on this potential outcome prior to surgery.[70]

Summary

The possibility of infection should be considered in all patients with a painful TKA until proven otherwise. Before surgery, information that includes the ESR, the CRP level, aspirate analysis results, and a thorough history and physical examination should be obtained. The timing of the infection is critical when deciding between prosthesis retention versus resection. It is important to use a team approach, including an infectious disease specialist. Two-stage exchange arthroplasty with a high-dose antibiotic cement spacer remains the gold standard for treating patients with chronic, deep periprosthetic TKA infections.

References

1. Grogan TJ, Dorey F, Rollins J, Amstutz HC: Deep sepsis following total knee arthroplasty: Ten-year experience at the University of California at Los Angeles Medical Center. *J Bone Joint Surg Am* 1986;68(2):226-234.
2. Poss R, Thornhill TS, Ewald FC, Thomas WH, Batte NJ, Sledge CB: Factors influencing the incidence and outcome of infection following total joint arthroplasty. *Clin Orthop Relat Res* 1984;182: 117-126.
3. Salvati EA, Robinson RP, Zeno SM, Koslin BL, Brause BD, Wilson PD Jr: Infection rates after 3175 total hip and total knee replacements performed with and without a horizontal unidirectional filtered air-flow system. *J Bone Joint Surg Am* 1982;64(4): 525-535.
4. Kurtz SM, Lau E, Schmier J, Ong KL, Zhao K, Parvizi J: Infection burden for hip and knee arthroplasty in the United States. *J Arthroplasty* 2008;23(7):984-991.
5. Bozic KJ, Ries MD: The impact of infection after total hip arthroplasty on hospital and surgeon resource utilization. *J Bone Joint Surg Am* 2005;87(8):1746-1751.
6. Kurtz SM, Ong KL, Schmier J, et al: Future clinical and economic impact of revision total hip and knee arthroplasty. *J Bone Joint Surg Am* 2007;89(suppl 3): 144-151.
7. Lavernia C, Lee DJ, Hernandez VH: The increasing financial burden of knee revision surgery in the United States. *Clin Orthop Relat Res* 2006;446:221-226.
8. Della Valle C, Parvizi J, Bauer TW, et al; American Academy of Orthopaedic Surgeons: Diagnosis of periprosthetic joint infections of the hip and knee. *J Am Acad Orthop Surg* 2010;18(12): 760-770.
9. Morrey BF, Westholm F, Schoifet S, Rand JA, Bryan RS: Long-term results of various treatment op-

tions for infected total knee arthroplasty. *Clin Orthop Relat Res* 1989;248:120-128.

10. Della Valle CJ, Sporer SM, Jacobs JJ, Berger RA, Rosenberg AG, Paprosky WG: Preoperative testing for sepsis before revision total knee arthroplasty. *J Arthroplasty* 2007;22(6, suppl 2):90-93.
11. Austin MS, Ghanem E, Joshi A, Lindsay A, Parvizi J: A simple, cost-effective screening protocol to rule out periprosthetic infection. *J Arthroplasty* 2008;23(1): 65-68.
12. Greidanus NV, Masri BA, Garbuz DS, et al: Use of erythrocyte sedimentation rate and C-reactive protein level to diagnose infection before revision total knee arthroplasty: A prospective evaluation. *J Bone Joint Surg Am* 2007;89(7): 1409-1416.
13. Di Cesare PE, Chang E, Preston CF, Liu CJ: Serum interleukin-6 as a marker of periprosthetic infection following total hip and knee arthroplasty. *J Bone Joint Surg Am* 2005;87(9):1921-1927.
14. Mason JB, Fehring TK, Odum SM, Griffin WL, Nussman DS: The value of white blood cell counts before revision total knee arthroplasty. *J Arthroplasty* 2003; 18(8):1038-1043.
15. Leone JM, Hanssen AD: Management of infection at the site of a total knee arthroplasty. *Instr Course Lect* 2006;55:449-461.
16. Trampuz A, Hanssen AD, Osmon DR, Mandrekar J, Steckelberg JM, Patel R: Synovial fluid leukocyte count and differential for the diagnosis of prosthetic knee infection. *Am J Med* 2004;117(8): 556-562.
17. Garvin KL, Cordero GX: Infected total knee arthroplasty: Diagnosis and treatment. *Instr Course Lect* 2008;57:305-315.
18. Ghanem E, Parvizi J, Burnett RS, et al: Cell count and differential of aspirated fluid in the diagnosis of infection at the site of total knee arthroplasty. *J Bone Joint Surg Am* 2008;90(8):1637-1643.
19. Bedair H, Ting N, Jacovides C, et al: Diagnosis of early postoperative TKA infection using synovial fluid analysis. *Clin Orthop Relat Res* 2011;469(1):34-40.
20. Palestro CJ, Swyer AJ, Kim CK, Goldsmith SJ: Infected knee prosthesis: Diagnosis with In-111 leukocyte, Tc-99m sulfur colloid, and Tc-99m MDP imaging. *Radiology* 1991;179(3):645-648.
21. Joseph TN, Mujtaba M, Chen AL, et al: Efficacy of combined technetium-99m sulfur colloid/indium-111 leukocyte scans to detect infected total hip and knee arthroplasties. *J Arthroplasty* 2001; 16(6):753-758.
22. Morgan PM, Sharkey P, Ghanem E, et al: The value of intraoperative Gram stain in revision total knee arthroplasty. *J Bone Joint Surg Am* 2009;91(9):2124-2129.
23. Lonner JH, Desai P, Dicesare PE, Steiner G, Zuckerman JD: The reliability of analysis of intraoperative frozen sections for identifying active infection during revision hip or knee arthroplasty. *J Bone Joint Surg Am* 1996; 78(10):1553-1558.
24. Feldman DS, Lonner JH, Desai P, Zuckerman JD: The role of intraoperative frozen sections in revision total joint arthroplasty. *J Bone Joint Surg Am* 1995; 77(12):1807-1813.
25. Della Valle CJ, Bogner E, Desai P, et al: Analysis of frozen sections of intraoperative specimens obtained at the time of reoperation after hip or knee resection arthroplasty for the treatment of infection. *J Bone Joint Surg Am* 1999; 81(5):684-689.
26. Parvizi J, Zmistowski B, Berbari EF, et al: New definition for periprosthetic joint infection: From the Workgroup of the Musculoskeletal Infection Society. *Clin Orthop Relat Res* 2011;469(11): 2992-2994.
27. Tsukayama DT, Goldberg VM, Kyle R: Diagnosis and management of infection after total knee arthroplasty. *J Bone Joint Surg Am* 2003;85(suppl 1):S75-S80.
28. Rand JA: Evaluation and management of infected total knee arthroplasty. *Semin Arthroplasty* 1994;5(4):178-182.
29. Schoifet SD, Morrey BF: Treatment of infection after total knee arthroplasty by débridement with retention of the components. *J Bone Joint Surg Am* 1990;72(9): 1383-1390.
30. Rasul AT Jr, Tsukayama D, Gustilo RB: Effect of time of onset and depth of infection on the outcome of total knee arthroplasty infections. *Clin Orthop Relat Res* 1991;273:98-104.
31. Waldman BJ, Hostin E, Mont MA, Hungerford DS: Infected total knee arthroplasty treated by arthroscopic irrigation and débridement. *J Arthroplasty* 2000; 15(4):430-436.
32. Dixon P, Parish EN, Cross MJ: Arthroscopic debridement in the treatment of the infected total knee replacement. *J Bone Joint Surg Br* 2004;86(1):39-42.
33. Silva M, Tharani R, Schmalzried TP: Results of direct exchange or debridement of the infected total knee arthroplasty. *Clin Orthop Relat Res* 2002;404:125-131.
34. Marculescu CE, Berbari EF, Hanssen AD, et al: Outcome of prosthetic joint infections treated with debridement and retention of components. *Clin Infect Dis* 2006; 42(4):471-478.
35. Bradbury T, Fehring TK, Taunton M, et al: The fate of acute methicillin-resistant *Staphylococcus aureus* periprosthetic knee infections treated by open debridement and retention of components. *J Arthroplasty* 2009;24(6, suppl): 101-104.

36. Koyonos L, Zmistowski B, Della Valle CJ, Parvizi J: Infection control rate of irrigation and débridement for periprosthetic joint infection. *Clin Orthop Relat Res* 2011;469(11):3043-3048.
37. Choi H-R, von Knoch F, Zurakowski D, Nelson SB, Malchau H: Can implant retention be recommended for treatment of infected TKA? *Clin Orthop Relat Res* 2011;469(4):961-969.
38. Odum SM, Fehring TK, Lombardi AV, et al; Periprosthetic Infection Consortium: Irrigation and debridement for periprosthetic infections: does the organism matter? *J Arthroplasty* 2011; 26(6, suppl):114-118.
39. Zmistowski B, Fedorka CJ, Sheehan E, Deirmengian G, Austin MS, Parvizi J: Prosthetic joint infection caused by gram-negative organisms. *J Arthroplasty* 2011; 26(6, suppl):104-108.
40. Azzam KA, Seeley M, Ghanem E, Austin MS, Purtill JJ, Parvizi J: Irrigation and debridement in the management of prosthetic joint infection: Traditional indications revisited. *J Arthroplasty* 2010; 25(7):1022-1027.
41. Salgado CD, Dash S, Cantey JR, Marculescu CE: Higher risk of failure of methicillin-resistant Staphylococcus aureus prosthetic joint infections. *Clin Orthop Relat Res* 2007;461:48-53.
42. Deirmengian C, Greenbaum J, Stern J, et al: Open debridement of acute gram-positive infections after total knee arthroplasty. *Clin Orthop Relat Res* 2003;416: 129-134.
43. Segawa H, Tsukayama DT, Kyle RF, Becker DA, Gustilo RB: Infection after total knee arthroplasty: A retrospective study of the treatment of eighty-one infections. *J Bone Joint Surg Am* 1999; 81(10):1434-1445.
44. Wasielewski RC, Barden RM, Rosenberg AG: Results of different surgical procedures on total knee arthroplasty infections. *J Arthroplasty* 1996;11(8):931-938.
45. Kramhøft M, Bødtker S, Carlsen A: Outcome of infected total knee arthroplasty. *J Arthroplasty* 1994; 9(6):617-621.
46. Teeny SM, Dorr L, Murata G, Conaty P: Treatment of infected total knee arthroplasty: Irrigation and debridement versus two-stage reimplantation. *J Arthroplasty* 1990;5(1):35-39.
47. Brandt CM, Sistrunk WW, Duffy MC, et al: *Staphylococcus aureus* prosthetic joint infection treated with debridement and prosthesis retention. *Clin Infect Dis* 1997; 24(5):914-919.
48. Hsieh P-H, Lee MS, Hsu K-Y, Chang Y-H, Shih H-N, Ueng SW: Gram-negative prosthetic joint infections: risk factors and outcome of treatment. *Clin Infect Dis* 2009;49(7):1036-1043.
49. Buechel FF, Femino FP, D'Alessio J: Primary exchange revision arthroplasty for infected total knee replacement: A long-term study. *Am J Orthop (Belle Mead NJ)* 2004;33(4): 190-198.
50. Göksan SB, Freeman MA: One-stage reimplantation for infected total knee arthroplasty. *J Bone Joint Surg Br* 1992;74(1):78-82.
51. van de Belt H, Neut D, Uges DR, et al: Surface roughness, porosity and wettability of gentamicin-loaded bone cements and their antibiotic release. *Biomaterials* 2000;21(19):1981-1987.
52. Sterling GJ, Crawford S, Potter JH, Koerbin G, Crawford R: The pharmacokinetics of Simplex-tobramycin bone cement. *J Bone Joint Surg Br* 2003;85(5): 646-649.
53. Anagnostakos K, Wilmes P, Schmitt E, Kelm J: Elution of gentamicin and vancomycin from polymethylmethacrylate beads and hip spacers in vivo. *Acta Orthop* 2009;80(2):193-197.
54. Springer BD, Lee G-C, Osmon D, Haidukewych GJ, Hanssen AD, Jacofsky DJ: Systemic safety of high-dose antibiotic-loaded cement spacers after resection of an infected total knee arthroplasty. *Clin Orthop Relat Res* 2004;427: 47-51.
55. Dovas S, Liakopoulos V, Papatheodorou L, et al: Acute renal failure after antibiotic-impregnated bone cement treatment of an infected total knee arthroplasty. *Clin Nephrol* 2008;69(3):207-212.
56. Jacobs C, Christensen CP, Berend ME: Static and mobile antibiotic-impregnated cement spacers for the management of prosthetic joint infection. *J Am Acad Orthop Surg* 2009;17(6):356-368.
57. Hofmann AA, Goldberg T, Tanner AM, Kurtin SM: Treatment of infected total knee arthroplasty using an articulating spacer: 2- to 12-year experience. *Clin Orthop Relat Res* 2005;430:125-131.
58. Hanssen AD, Spangehl MJ: Practical applications of antibiotic-loaded bone cement for treatment of infected joint replacements. *Clin Orthop Relat Res* 2004;427: 79-85.
59. Mont MA, Waldman BJ, Hungerford DS: Evaluation of preoperative cultures before second-stage reimplantation of a total knee prosthesis complicated by infection: A comparison-group study. *J Bone Joint Surg Am* 2000; 82(11):1552-1557.
60. Emerson RH Jr, Muncie M, Tarbox TR, Higgins LL: Comparison of a static with a mobile spacer in total knee infection. *Clin Orthop Relat Res* 2002;404:132-138.
61. Freeman MG, Fehring TK, Odum SM, Fehring K, Griffin WL, Mason JB: Functional advantage of articulating versus static spacers in 2-stage revision for total knee arthroplasty infection. *J Arthroplasty* 2007;22(8): 1116-1121.

62. Kusuma SK, Ward J, Jacofsky M, Sporer SM, Della Valle CJ: What is the role of serological testing between stages of two-stage reconstruction of the infected prosthetic knee? *Clin Orthop Relat Res* 2011; 469(4):1002-1008.

63. Macheras GA, Kateros K, Galanakos SP, Koutsostathis SD, Kontou E, Papadakis SA: The long-term results of a two-stage protocol for revision of an infected total knee replacement. *J Bone Joint Surg Br* 2011;93(11):1487-1492.

64. Westrich GH, Walcott-Sapp S, Bornstein LJ, Bostrom MP, Windsor RE, Brause BD: Modern treatment of infected total knee arthroplasty with a 2-stage reimplantation protocol. *J Arthroplasty* 2010;25(7):1015-1021, e1-e2.

65. Mittal Y, Fehring TK, Hanssen A, Marculescu C, Odum SM, Osmon D: Two-stage reimplantation for periprosthetic knee infection involving resistant organisms. *J Bone Joint Surg Am* 2007;89(6): 1227-1231.

66. Haleem AA, Berry DJ, Hanssen AD: Mid-term to long-term followup of two-stage reimplantation for infected total knee arthroplasty. *Clin Orthop Relat Res* 2004; 428:35-39.

67. Haddad FS, Masri BA, Campbell D, McGraw RW, Beauchamp CP, Duncan CP: The PROSTALAC functional spacer in two-stage revision for infected knee replacements: Prosthesis of antibiotic-loaded acrylic cement. *J Bone Joint Surg Br* 2000;82(6):807-812.

68. Mortazavi SM, Vegari D, Ho A, Zmistowski B, Parvizi J: Two-stage exchange arthroplasty for infected total knee arthroplasty: Predictors of failure. *Clin Orthop Relat Res* 2011;469(11):3049-3054.

69. Mabry TM, Jacofsky DJ, Haidukewych GJ, Hanssen AD: Comparison of intramedullary nailing and external fixation knee arthrodesis for the infected knee replacement. *Clin Orthop Relat Res* 2007; 464:11-15.

70. Pring DJ, Marks L, Angel JC: Mobility after amputation for failed knee replacement. *J Bone Joint Surg Br* 1988;70(5):770-771.

32

Patellofemoral Arthroplasty: The Other Unicompartmental Knee Replacement

Torrance Walker, MD
Brian Perkinson, MD
William M. Mihalko, MD, PhD

Abstract

Many patients with signs and symptoms of patellofemoral arthritis do not respond well to conservative treatment modalities. Patients with isolated patellofemoral arthritis with severe anterior knee pain may be candidates for patellofemoral arthroplasty. The success of the procedure and the long-term survivorship of the implant rely on good surgical technique and adherence to strict indications and contraindications in patient selection. Newer implant designs have also contributed to improved outcomes.

Instr Course Lect 2013;62:363-371.

Patellofemoral arthritis is a relatively common condition, affecting up to 24% of women and 11% of men older than 55 years who have symptomatic osteoarthritis of the knee.[1] Isolated patellofemoral arthritis is not as prevalent and has reportedly been seen in 9% of radiographs of symptomatic knees in individuals older than 40 years.[2] Approximately 75% of all patellofemoral arthroplasties are done in women,[3-6] and the increased frequency of patellofemoral disease may be related to the frequency of knee malalignment and dysplasia in women, although some studies have noted no sex-specific differences in knee kinematics.[7]

Total knee arthroplasty has been successful in treating isolated patellofemoral arthritis in older patients, but anterior knee pain persists in 7% to 19% of patients.[8,9] The desire to have a reliable, conservative surgical option that retains tibiofemoral knee kinematics for a relatively young patient population has driven the development of more modern patellofemoral arthroplasty implants and techniques. Although the clinical results of patellofemoral arthroplasty depend primarily on implant design and surgical technique, careful patient selection, with strict inclusion and exclusion criteria, is necessary for good outcomes and long-term survivorship.

Historical Perspectives

Although historically controversial because of poor survivorship with first-generation patellofemoral arthroplasty implant designs, enthusiasm for patellofemoral arthroplasty has been renewed by improved clinical outcomes associated with contemporary implant designs.[10,11] First-generation designs failed primarily because of tracking problems, patellar catching, continued anterior knee pain, and disease progression in other knee compartments. These designs were too conforming, with a narrow trochlear implant that was too deep, unforgiving, and overconstrained.[12] The most common reason for the failure of the second-generation designs is the progression of

Dr. Mihalko or an immediate family member serves as a board member, owner, officer, or committee member of ASTM International and the Orthopaedic Research Society; has received royalties from Aesculap/B. Braun; is a member of a speaker's bureau or has made paid presentations on behalf of Aesculap/B. Braun; serves as a paid consultant to or is an employee of Aesculap/B. Braun; serves as an unpaid consultant to Blue Belt Technology; has received research or institutional support from Aesculap/B. Braun; and has received nonincome support (such as equipment or services), commercially derived honoraria, or other non–research-related funding (such as paid travel) from Aesculap/B. Braun. Neither of the following authors nor any immediate family member has received anything of value from or has stock or stock options in a commercial company or institution related directly or indirectly to the subject of this chapter: Dr. Walker and Dr. Perkinson.

tibiofemoral arthritis. This design-specific improvement refocuses the patellofemoral arthroplasty debate away from implant design flaws and toward the importance of careful patient selection, which is a key determinant of success in patellofemoral arthroplasty. Recently described treatment strategies combine patellofemoral arthroplasty with cartilage restoration procedures or multicompartment arthroplasty.[13]

Indications and Contraindications

At present, patellofemoral arthroplasty usually is done only after failure of a lengthy period of nonsurgical treatment or failure of more conservative surgical procedures. Pain localized to the patellofemoral articulation that occurs during daily activities and is unresponsive to nonsteroidal anti-inflammatory drugs, injection therapy, and activity modification is a good indication for patellofemoral arthroplasty. The ideal candidate for patellofemoral arthroplasty is typically a patient in the fifth decade of life with debilitating, isolated patellofemoral arthritis refractory to conservative treatment and no patellar malalignment. Older patients with isolated patellofemoral arthritis may fare better with a total knee arthroplasty, but this chapter's authors know of no published data showing age-dependent outcomes of patellofemoral arthroplasty.

Improved outcomes have been reported with patellofemoral arthroplasty for posttraumatic arthritis, primary patellofemoral osteoarthritis, and patellofemoral dysplasia without malalignment. Patients with posttraumatic arthritis for whom patellectomy is considered should be evaluated for patellofemoral arthroplasty. Primary patellofemoral arthritis includes Outerbridge type IV chondromalacia of the patella and/or trochlea. It is important to note that tibiofemoral arthritis progresses more commonly in patients with primary osteoarthritis than with posttraumatic arthritis or dysplasia.[14] Malalignment is most often determined with use of the quadriceps angle (Q angle). The Q angle is the angle formed by the intersection of a line drawn from the anterior superior iliac spine to the center of the patella and the projection of a line drawn from the tibial tubercle to the center of the patella. Angles greater than 15° in men and 20° in women are considered abnormal. Any condition that increases the Q angle increases the lateral displacement forces on the patella and possibly leads to subluxation or dislocation. Patellofemoral arthroplasty alone cannot be expected to correct patellar malalignment, which is not an indication for the procedure. Mild patellar tilt or subluxation can be corrected at the time of patellofemoral arthroplasty with lateral retinacular release, medialization of the patellar component, and partial lateral facetectomy. If malalignment exists, it should be corrected before patellofemoral arthroplasty. No particular patellar or trochlear wear pattern has been identified as a contraindication to patellofemoral arthroplasty, but the prosthesis should address lesions in their entirety without extending into the femoral condyles.

The progression of tibiofemoral arthritis is the most common cause of revision to total knee arthroplasty, emphasizing the fact that tibiofemoral arthritis is a principal contraindication to patellofemoral arthroplasty. Inflammatory arthropathies by nature involve the entire joint, and patellofemoral arthroplasty currently is contraindicated in patients with these conditions, including patients with chondrocalcinosis, because of progressive tibiofemoral arthritis and painful synovitis. Because one purposed benefit of patellofemoral arthroplasty is retention of normal tibiofemoral kinematics, intact ligaments and menisci without tibiofemoral instability are reasonable prerequisites to patellofemoral arthroplasty; however, there is no consensus that cruciate deficiency or previous meniscectomy causes poor outcomes. Patellofemoral arthroplasty is not indicated in severe coronal plane deformity of the knee (valgus > 8° or varus > 5°) unless the deformity is corrected with an osteotomy before patellofemoral arthroplasty.[15] In the sagittal plane, 120° of free flexion with less than 10° of flexion contracture is recommended. Knee stiffness must be critically assessed because these patients have a high rate of previous surgical procedures, which increases the prevalence of arthrofibrosis or patellar height aberrations. Patients with patella baja from quadriceps muscle atrophy or patellar tendon scarring are not good candidates for patellofemoral arthroplasty.

Experimental models have shown that patellofemoral joint reaction forces are up to 3.3 times body weight at 60° of knee flexion and 7.8 times body weight at 130°.[16] Although there are few data correlating patellofemoral arthroplasty with body mass index (BMI), a general consensus is that patellofemoral arthroplasty should be avoided in obese patients to prevent overloading the implant. Recently, van Jonbergen et al[17] showed a higher rate of revision to total knee arthroplasty in obese patients (BMI > 30) than in those with a lower BMI. Primary diagnosis, age, and sex did not significantly affect the revision rate in their series.

Clinical Evaluation

Patient History

Patients with patellofemoral arthritis typically describe anterior or retropatellar knee pain that is exacerbated with activities that preferentially load the patellofemoral articulation. These provocative activities usually involve ascending or descending stairs, walking on uneven surfaces, and kneeling or squatting. Patients often describe preferring to sit with the legs extended rather than flexed. Frequently, patients do not recognize the association of their pain with knee posture, but they report pain with long car rides or prolonged sitting and activities associated with lengthy periods of knee flexion. Often there is a history of crepitus and effusions, but it also is important to inquire about subluxation or dislocation events that could indicate patellar malalignment.

Physical Examination

It is critical to evaluate both lower extremities from the pelvis to the feet. Limb length, alignment, quadriceps muscle atrophy, and foot alignment should be evaluated. Particularly, assessing the Q angle and patellar tracking quickly determines whether patellofemoral arthroplasty should be included in the treatment algorithm. Patients with large Q angles (> 15° in men and > 20° in women) or signs of patellar instability will need corrective surgery before or in conjunction with patellofemoral arthroplasty. A positive patellar apprehension test and the J sign are indicative of patellar instability, malalignment, or muscle imbalances. A positive J sign is visible when the knee is actively extended, and lateral patellar subluxation occurs in the terminal 20° of extension. Excessive femoral internal torsion or tibial external torsion can lead to malalignment as well. A planovalgus foot can be associated with patellar maltracking, and symptoms may resolve with orthotic treatment alone.

Palpation of the patella during tracking can help to localize pain. Pain elicited with the patellar grind or patellar tap test is indicative of patellofemoral pathology. Any tenderness to palpation at the medial or lateral joint lines usually indicates tibiofemoral involvement, a contraindication to patellofemoral arthroplasty. Although anterior or posterior cruciate ligament insufficiency is not a strict contraindication to patellofemoral arthroplasty, it is important to evaluate all knee ligaments and consider reconstruction before patellofemoral arthroplasty to avoid progressive tibiofemoral arthritis caused by instability.

The neurovascular status, skin integrity and previous scars, hip motion, and the lumbar spine should always be evaluated. Referred pain from the hip to the knee region, as well as L3-L4 nerve root radiculopathy, can produce anterior knee pain and should be considered during the examination.

Preoperative Imaging

Weight-bearing AP and lateral radiographs should be made to avoid underestimation of tibiofemoral abnormality. Lateral radiographs allow assessment of the patella, and occasionally arthritic patellofemoral changes are visible (**Figure 1**). Patella baja should be corrected before patellofemoral arthroplasty.[18] Standing PA 45° flexion radiographs (Rosenberg views) are used to assess the extent of abnormality of the posterior femoral condyle. Axial radiographs demonstrate the extent of patellofemoral arthritis, trochlear dysplasia, and patellar tilt or subluxation. Full-length standing radiographs are useful for evaluating the mechanical alignment of the entire limb (**Figure 2**).

CT is used to evaluate posttraumatic osseous architecture, rotational abnormalities, and trochlear dysplasia but has little role in assessing patellofemoral arthritis. MRI with use of delayed gadolinium-enhanced imaging for cartilage (dGEMRIC) and T1rho are being studied and may prove useful in assessing articular cartilage.[19,20] Bone scans help to determine the extent of abnormality in the medial and lateral compartments of the knee.

Images from any prior arthroscopic procedure should be reviewed. This chapter's authors know of no published data to support routine arthroscopic examination before patellofemoral arthroplasty, but, if the surgeon believes he or she can better assess the lateral compartment, then it may be advantageous.

Advantages of Patellofemoral Arthroplasty

Emerging surgical procedures combining patellofemoral arthroplasty with the treatment of osteochondral lesions bridge the gap between sports medicine and adult reconstructive patient groups; however, most advantages of patellofemoral arthroplasty are relative to total knee arthroplasty, the gold standard for the treatment of degenerative osteoarthritis of the knee. Compared with total knee arthroplasty, patellofemoral arthroplasty conserves more bone, allows shorter postoperative rehabilitation, and maintains more normal knee kinematics because of the preservation of the tibiofemoral articulation, ligaments, and menisci. Specifically, in vivo sagittal plane kinematics after patellofemoral arthroplasty closely resembles that of a normal knee.[21] Patellofemoral arthroplasty uses a medial parapatellar arthrotomy, which allows direct observation of all joint compartments to determine whether patellofemoral arthroplasty needs to be abandoned for total knee arthroplasty or combined with a cartilage restoration procedure. The medial parapatellar approach is the most common approach used for total knee arthroplasty if subsequent revision is performed. Most modern patellofemoral arthroplasties allow retention of the patellar component for ease of revision surgery. One small series found that the outcome scores after revision total

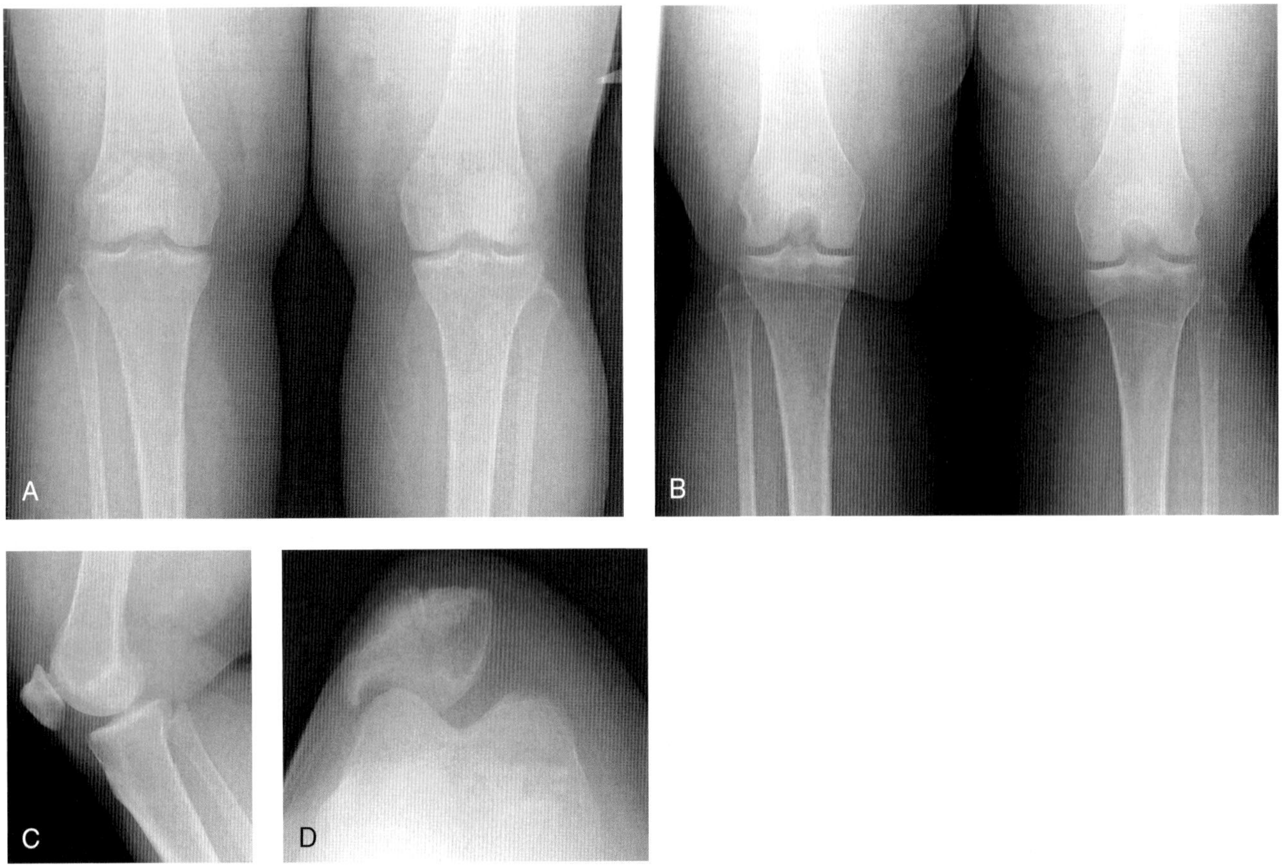

Figure 1 Radiographic examination before patellofemoral arthroplasty should include AP standing (**A**), PA flexion (**B**), lateral (**C**), and Merchant (**D**) views of the knee.

knee arthroplasty after patellofemoral arthroplasty were equal to those after primary total knee arthroplasty.[22]

Design Features

The evolution of the implant design has led to increased patient satisfaction and survivorship of patellofemoral replacements. Design attributes that have improved results include onlay prosthetic design with a broad trochlear surface, a valgus tracking angle, and a congruous articulation throughout the range of motion.[12] An onlay design removes the entire trochlea and eliminates the need to set the prosthesis flush with the remaining trochlear bone, which can be technically challenging. The prosthesis should extend proximal enough to prevent catching, snapping, or popping of the patellar component during knee flexion. The trochlear component should allow free movement of the patella in extension and should also be broad enough to cover the entire medial and lateral aspects of the anterior distal end of the femur without overhang of the implant, which can lead to retinacular irritation and pain. An asymmetric or valgus tracking angle should help with patellar tracking, especially in patients with a high Q angle. An all-polyethylene patellar component and congruous articulation promotes accurate patellar tracking. The patellar button should also be retainable and compatible if revision to a total knee arthroplasty is necessary. These types of design features result in less frequent patellar snapping, maltracking, catching, and subluxation, as well as less frequent need for concomitant or subsequent surgery to improve extensor mechanism alignment.[19]

Alternative Treatments

Conservative measures should be exhausted before proceeding with surgical treatment of patellofemoral arthritis. The usual nonsurgical modalities include rest, activity modification, nonsteroidal anti-inflammatory medicines, weight reduction, physical therapy, taping and bracing, periodic intra-articular corticosteroid injection, and viscosupplementation.[23,24] These treatments may provide adequate relief to avoid or postpone surgical treatment. A systematic review by van Jonbergen et al[24] resulted in recommendations in support of or against treatments on the basis of the best available evidence in the litera-

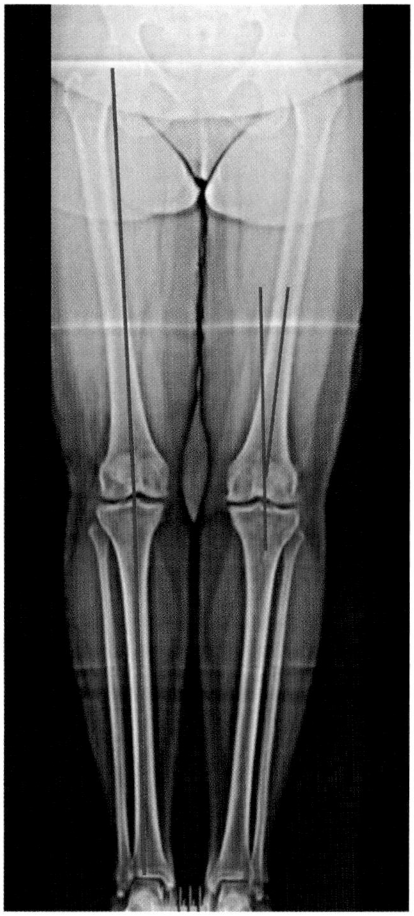

Figure 2 A full-length hip-to-ankle standing AP radiograph is made to assess for lower extremity deformity (as shown on the right lower extremity) at the knee and to determine the Q angle (as shown on the left lower extremity).

ture. There was high-quality evidence for using physical therapy, although this treatment was given a weak recommendation for use. Taping was weakly recommended on the basis of moderate-quality evidence. Corticosteroid injection therapy also was weakly recommended because of low-quality evidence. Despite the relative lack of published data, an adequate period of nonsurgical treatment should be tried before considering surgical alternatives.

Alternative surgical approaches that have been used to treat isolated patellofemoral arthritis include arthroscopic débridement, with or without lateral release; chondroplasty; autologous osteochondral chondrocyte implantation; osteochondral allografts; lateral facetectomy; anteromedial tibial tubercle transfer; patellectomy; and total knee arthroplasty.[18,23-28] Most of these treatment options do not have long-term, durable results. On the basis of moderate-quality evidence, there was a strong recommendation against the use of arthroscopy with débridement. In contrast, there was a weak recommendation for the use of osteochondral allografts and partial lateral facetectomy. There has been more success with cartilage transplantation to the trochlea than with patellar resurfacing. Lateral retinacular release should provide temporary relief and reduction in symptoms when a patient has lateral patellar tilt and arthritis. Patients with lateral facet arthritis associated with patellar subluxation may benefit from anteromedial tibial tubercle transfer if there is healthy proximal and medial articular cartilage (**Figure 3**). Patellectomy may lead to poor results and patient dissatisfaction because of inconsistent pain relief, loss of extension power, extension lag, and instability.[23]

Total knee arthroplasty has long been considered a reliable treatment option for isolated patellofemoral arthritis.[25,27] Mont et al,[8] in a study of 30 total knee replacements done for the treatment of patellofemoral arthritis, reported 28 excellent results, 1 good result, and 1 poor result at a mean follow-up interval of 81 months. The mean Knee Society Score improved from 50 points preoperatively to 93 points postoperatively. The poor result was in a patient who sustained a patellar tendon rupture as the result of a fall. Parvizi et al[9] reported a 94% survival rate for 31 total knee replacements for patellofemoral osteoarthritis in 24 patients with a mean age of 73 years and a mean follow-up interval of 5.2 years. The mean Knee Society objective and functional scores were 88.9 and 89.5 points, respectively.

Patellofemoral Arthroplasty Outcomes

Many studies have shown good to excellent results at 3 to 17 years of follow-up for 66% to 100% of patients.[3-9,29-33] Fifty-five of 65 patients with a first-generation patellofemoral arthroplasty were reported to have good to excellent results at an average of 4 years.[29] Soft-tissue realignments and tibial tubercle transfers were done concomitantly to improve patellar tracking. Early complications in first-generation implants were attributed to the higher constraint of the implant and patellar maltracking problems.[12,30] Ackroyd and Chir[3] reported 2- to 5-year follow-up results for 306 second-generation Avon (Stryker, Kalamazoo, MI) patellofemoral arthroplasties in 240 patients. The median outcome scores improved for the Bristol Pain Score, the Melbourne Patellofemoral Score, and the Oxford Knee Score. Nine patients had slight maltracking, leading to one revision of the trochlear component and one distal soft-tissue realignment. Revision to total knee arthroplasty was required in 3.6% of the patients because of progression of tibiofemoral arthritis.

Leadbetter et al[4] reported the results of a multicenter study with 79 patellofemoral arthroplasties in 70 patients with a mean follow-up of 3 years (range, 2 to 6 years). Ninety percent functioned without pain in daily activities and stair climbing, 84% achieved Knee Society Scores of greater than 80 points, and the overall mean Knee Society Score improved from 56 to 83 points. There were 13 clinical failures: 6 knees were revised to total knee arthroplasty, 5 had persistent pain

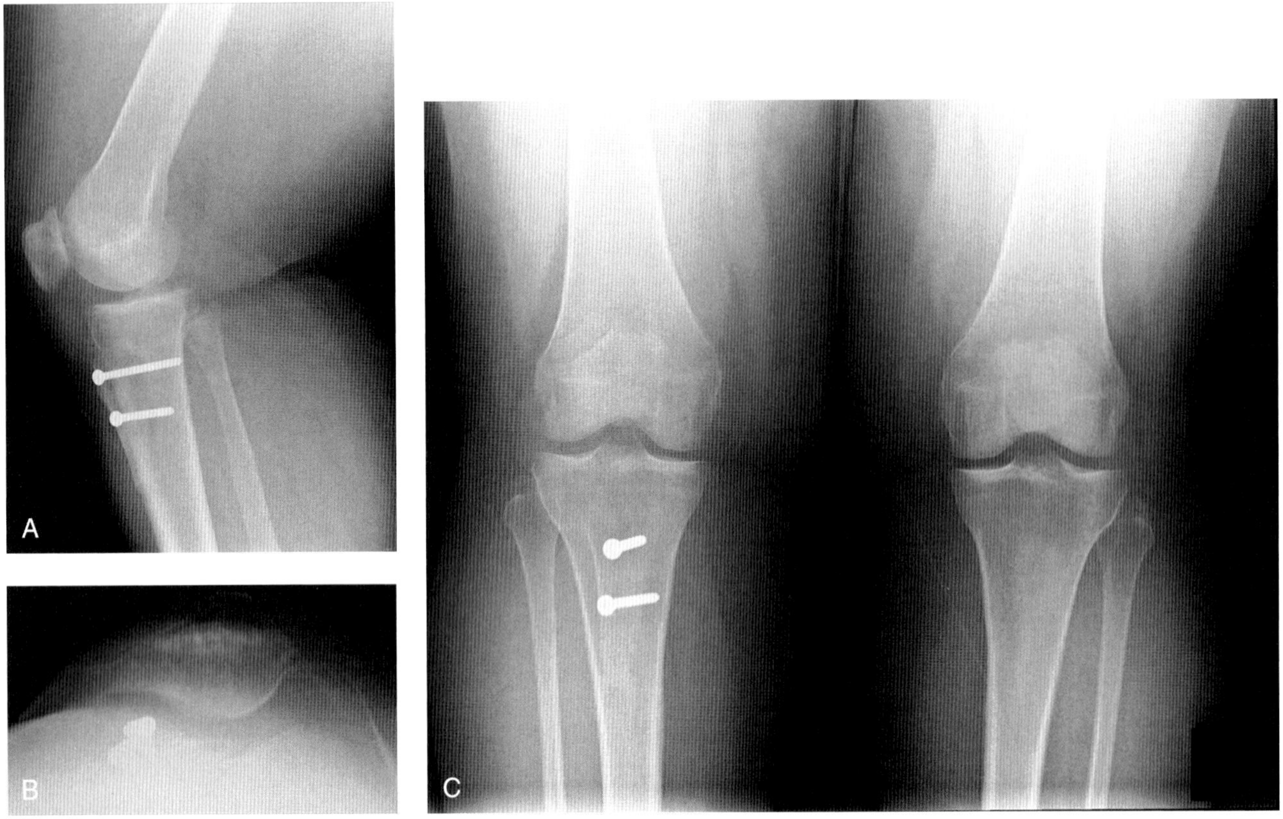

Figure 3 Radiographs of the patient in Figure 1 made after an anteromedialization of the tibial tubercle was done to correct the maltracking and alleviate the inferolateral osteoarthritic area of the patella.

and/or recurrent effusions, and arthrofibrosis developed in 2 knees.

Sisto and Sarin[5] reported 18 excellent and 7 good results at a mean follow-up of 73 months after 25 custom patellofemoral arthroplasties in 22 patients with a mean age of 45 years. The mean Knee Society functional score improved from 49 to 89 points, and the mean Knee Society objective score improved from 52 to 91 points. The authors reported no additional surgical procedures or evidence of component loosening.

On the basis of clinical failure of the primary arthroplasty, survivorship of 185 Richards type II patellofemoral arthroplasties was estimated by van Jonbergen et al[17] to be 84% at 10 years and 69% at 20 years. Their 161 patients had isolated involvement of the patellofemoral joint, with diagnoses that included primary patellofemoral osteoarthritis, posttraumatic patellofemoral osteoarthritis, and patellofemoral osteoarthritis with a previous realignment procedure for patellar subluxation or trochlear dysplasia. Primary diagnosis, sex, or age at the time of patellofemoral arthroplasty did not significantly affect the rate of revision ($P = 0.35$, $P = 0.24$, and $P = 0.65$, respectively). The rate of revision in obese patients (BMI > 30 kg/m^2) was higher than that in nonobese patients ($P = 0.02$). Six percent of patients required manipulation for stiffness, and 43% required additional surgery. Loosening and/or wear of the patellar component occurred in 4%. Tibiofemoral arthritis was observed in 45% of knees and resulted in conversion to total knee arthroplasty in 13%.

Dahm et al[25] compared 23 patellofemoral arthroplasties with 22 total knee arthroplasties at the Mayo Clinic and concluded that patellofemoral arthroplasty yields clinical outcomes comparable with those of total knee arthroplasty as treatment of isolated patellofemoral arthritis. The mean postoperative Knee Society Scores were 89 and 90 points in the patellofemoral arthroplasty and total knee arthroplasty cohorts, respectively. The mean University of California Los Angeles scores were 6.6 and 4.2 points, respectively, and the mean blood loss and hospital stay were significantly lower among patients who had patellofemoral arthroplasty. The authors considered patellofemoral arthroplasty to be a less invasive option for this select subgroup of patients.

Patellofemoral Arthroplasty Complications

Early problems usually stem from implant or technique-related issues and include malalignment and implant malposition leading to catching, instability, and maltracking. Late problems are loosening and/or wear of the patellar component, loosening of the trochlear component, and the development of tibiofemoral disease.

Early implant designs led to problems with patellar tracking and instability. Newer designs are more accommodating and have reduced these complications. Malposition of the implant also can cause patellar catching and instability. Placing the implant in flexion can lead to catching of the patellar component on initiation of flexion. Malrotation of the trochlea or a laterally placed patellar component can cause subluxation or dislocation with recurrent instability. A trochlear component that is too large may irritate the peripatellar retinaculum.

Some studies have described the need for manipulation with the patient under anesthesia in the early postoperative period for 3% to 14% of patients, and noted that it may be required to achieve 90° of flexion by 6 weeks postoperatively.[3,14,17] Prior surgery may have an effect on the need for manipulation under anesthesia; however, it also can result from overstuffing of the patellofemoral joint. Measuring the patellar thickness before resection and restoring it should reduce the chance for overstuffing.

Loosening and/or wear of the patellar component in 4% of patients was reported by van Jonbergen et al[17] These patients may be candidates for revision patellofemoral arthroplasty rather than conversion to total knee arthroplasty.[34] Hendrix et al[34] reported mixed results in a small series (14 knees) in which a failed first-generation inlay patellofemoral replacement was revised to a second-generation onlay patellofemoral arthroplasty. With long-term outcome data up to 20 years now available, the development of femorotibial osteoarthritis has been determined to be the most common reason for failure and conversion to total knee arthroplasty. Conversion rates of one in five have been reported after an average of 7 to 16 years.[14,31] Tibiofemoral arthritis was observed in 45% of knees and resulted in conversion to total knee arthroplasty in 13% in the study by van Jonbergen et al.[17] It has been suggested that patients presenting with idiopathic patellofemoral arthritis may be more prone to progression to generalized tibiofemoral arthritis than patients with other types of arthritis, and caution should be used when considering these patients for patellofemoral arthroplasty.[25] However, van Jonbergen et al[17] reported that primary diagnosis and age did not significantly affect the conversion rate.

van Jonbergen et al[22] reported the results of conversion of 14 patellofemoral replacements to total knee arthroplasties in 13 patients (average age, 67 years; range, 50 to 77 years) because of tibiofemoral arthritis. At a mean follow-up of 5.7 years (range, 2 to 13 years), there were no significant differences in Knee Society Scores and Western Ontario and McMaster Universities Osteoarthritis Index scores when this group of patients was compared with a matched cohort. Three knees in three patients required manipulation under anesthesia, and two of those knees also required manipulation after the previous patellofemoral arthroplasty. They concluded that patellofemoral arthroplasty does not have a negative effect on the outcome of total knee arthroplasty.[22] On the basis of their experience with a small group of 12 patients, Lonner et al[35] agreed, concluding that the results of total knee arthroplasty do not appear to be compromised after revision of a failed patellofemoral component.

Surgical Pearls and Pitfalls

The procedure is done through a midline or parapatellar incision and is easily done with a minimally invasive approach. Care must be taken not to injure the anterior horn of the medial meniscus or the anterior transverse meniscal ligament (**Figure 4**). The medial and lateral compartments of the knee should be carefully inspected to ensure that the patient does not have articular cartilage changes that would preclude patellofemoral arthroplasty. Most implant systems involve an anterior trochlear femoral cutting block attachment, which is comparable with the anterior cut during a total knee arthroplasty. If the patient has a hypoplastic trochlear groove, flexing the cutting block slightly will allow a deeper cut and trochlear groove without overstuffing the anterior compartment of the knee. When seating a trial implant to determine the appropriate size of the femoral-trochlear component, adequate coverage should be ensured, and any overhanging edge of the femoral component should be avoided. With a symmetric trochlear implant, the surgeon needs to be aware that the normal trochlear groove lies approximately 7° to 16° lateral from the joint line. Care should be taken during the procedure to keep the femoral and tibial compartments moist with irrigation fluid to prevent desiccation intraoperatively. After the intercondylar preparation is made, the trochlear implant should have a smooth transition with the medial and lateral aspects of the lateral and medial femoral condyles. It should be remembered that the quadriceps tendon articulates with the trochlear groove, and an increase in the length of the arc of the groove can increase tension in the tendon with knee flexion and ultimately decrease postoperative knee motion; the thickness of the trochlear

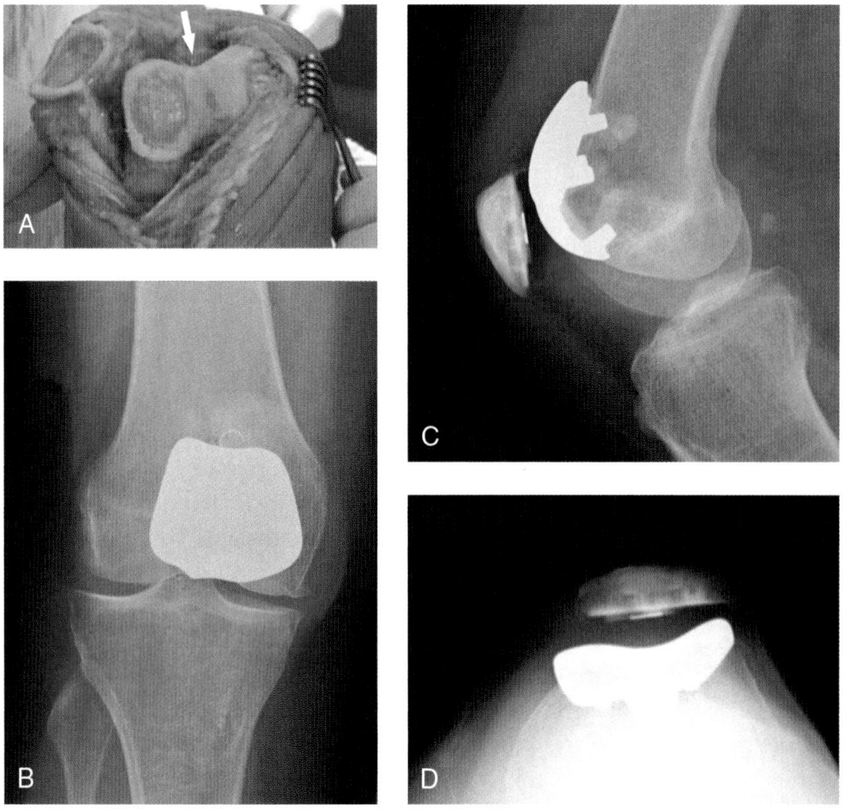

Figure 4 Intraoperative photograph (**A**), taken from the head of the surgical table, showing the intact anterior transverse meniscal ligament (arrow). It should also be noted that the patella does not need to be everted to perform the patellofemoral arthroplasty. AP (**B**), lateral (**C**), and Merchant (**D**) radiographs of the knee made after the patellofemoral arthroplasty.

groove or the patella must not be increased after the procedure is finished. The patellar resection is performed just as for a primary total knee arthroplasty, with a medialized button placement to mimic the peak height of the native patella and allow symmetric tracking.

Summary

The current generation of patellofemoral arthroplasty implant designs, when used in properly selected patients on the basis of clear history, physical examination, and radiographic criteria, provides a sound option for the treatment of isolated osteoarthritis of the patellofemoral joint. Determining which patients may not be good candidates is difficult but is essential to ensure long-term implant survivorship and patient satisfaction. Correcting any patellar maltracking before or at the time of patellofemoral arthroplasty is mandatory, and patellofemoral arthroplasty should never be used alone to treat patellar instability.

References

1. McAlindon TE, Snow S, Cooper C, Dieppe PA: Radiographic patterns of osteoarthritis of the knee joint in the community: The importance of the patellofemoral joint. *Ann Rheum Dis* 1992;51(7): 844-849.
2. Davies AP, Vince AS, Shepstone L, Donell ST, Glasgow MM: The radiologic prevalence of patellofemoral osteoarthritis. *Clin Orthop Relat Res* 2002;402:206-212.
3. Ackroyd CE, Chir B: Development and early results of a new patellofemoral arthroplasty. *Clin Orthop Relat Res* 2005;436:7-13.
4. Leadbetter WB, Kolisek FR, Levitt RL, et al: Patellofemoral arthroplasty: A multi-centre study with minimum 2-year follow-up. *Int Orthop* 2009;33(6):1597-1601.
5. Sisto DJ, Sarin VK: Custom patellofemoral arthroplasty of the knee. *J Bone Joint Surg Am* 2006;88(7): 1475-1480.
6. Ackroyd CE, Newman JH, Evans R, Eldridge JD, Joslin CC: The Avon patellofemoral arthroplasty: Five-year survivorship and functional results. *J Bone Joint Surg Br* 2007;89(3):310-315.
7. Seisler AR, Sheehan FT: Normative three-dimensional patellofemoral and tibiofemoral kinematics: A dynamic, in vivo study. *IEEE Trans Biomed Eng* 2007;54(7): 1333-1341.
8. Mont MA, Haas S, Mullick T, Hungerford DS: Total knee arthroplasty for patellofemoral arthritis. *J Bone Joint Surg Am* 2002; 84(11):1977-1981.
9. Parvizi J, Stuart MJ, Pagnano MW, Hanssen AD: Total knee arthroplasty in patients with isolated patellofemoral arthritis. *Clin Orthop Relat Res* 2001;392: 147-152.
10. Lonner JH: Patellofemoral arthroplasty: Pros, cons, and design considerations. *Clin Orthop Relat Res* 2004;428:158-165.
11. Lonner JH: Patellofemoral arthroplasty: The impact of design on outcomes. *Orthop Clin North Am* 2008;39(3):347-354, vi.
12. Krajca-Radcliffe JB, Coker TP: Patellofemoral arthroplasty: A 2- to 18-year followup study. *Clin Orthop Relat Res* 1996;330: 143-151.
13. Lonner JH, Mehta S, Booth RE Jr: Ipsilateral patellofemoral arthroplasty and autogenous osteo-

chondral femoral condylar transplantation. *J Arthroplasty* 2007; 22(8):1130-1136.

14. Argenson JN, Flecher X, Parratte S, Aubaniac JM: Patellofemoral arthroplasty: An update. *Clin Orthop Relat Res* 2005;440:50-53.
15. Leadbetter WB, Ragland PS, Mont MA: The appropriate use of patellofemoral arthroplasty: An analysis of reported indications, contraindications, and failures. *Clin Orthop Relat Res* 2005;436: 91-99.
16. Komistek RD, Kane TR, Mahfouz M, Ochoa JA, Dennis DA: Knee mechanics: A review of past and present techniques to determine in vivo loads. *J Biomech* 2005;38(2):215-228.
17. van Jonbergen HP, Werkman DM, Barnaart LF, van Kampen A: Long-term outcomes of patellofemoral arthroplasty. *J Arthroplasty* 2010;25(7):1066-1071.
18. Lonner JH: Patellofemoral arthroplasty. *J Am Acad Orthop Surg* 2007;15(8):495-506.
19. Burstein D: Tracking longitudinal changes in knee degeneration and repair. *J Bone Joint Surg Am* 2009; 91(suppl 1):51-53.
20. Wheaton AJ, Casey FL, Gougoutas AJ, et al: Correlation of T1rho with fixed charge density in cartilage. *J Magn Reson Imaging* 2004; 20(3):519-525.
21. Hollinghurst D, Stoney J, Ward T, Pandit H, Beard D, Murray DW: In vivo sagittal plane kinematics of the Avon patellofemoral arthroplasty. *J Arthroplasty* 2007; 22(1):117-123.
22. van Jonbergen HP, Werkman DM, van Kampen A: Conversion of patellofemoral arthroplasty to total knee arthroplasty: A matched case-control study of 13 patients. *Acta Orthop* 2009;80(1):62-66.
23. Fulkerson JP: Alternatives to patellofemoral arthroplasty. *Clin Orthop Relat Res* 2005;436:76-80.
24. van Jonbergen HP, Poolman RW, van Kampen A: Isolated patellofemoral osteoarthritis. *Acta Orthop* 2010;81(2):199-205.
25. Dahm DL, Al-Rayashi W, Dajani K, Shah JP, Levy BA, Stuart MJ: Patellofemoral arthroplasty versus total knee arthroplasty in patients with isolated patellofemoral osteoarthritis. *Am J Orthop (Belle Mead NJ)* 2010;39(10):487-491.
26. Lotke PA, Lonner JH, Nelson CL: Patellofemoral arthroplasty: The third compartment. *J Arthroplasty* 2005;20(4):4-6.
27. Delanois RE, McGrath MS, Ulrich SD, et al: Results of total knee replacement for isolated patellofemoral arthritis: When not to perform a patellofemoral arthroplasty. *Orthop Clin North Am* 2008;39(3):381-388, vii.
28. Leadbetter WB: Patellofemoral arthroplasty in the treatment of patellofemoral arthritis: Rationale and outcomes in younger patients. *Orthop Clin North Am* 2008; 39(3):363-380, vii.
29. Cartier P, Sanouiller JL, Grelsamer R: Patellofemoral arthroplasty: 2-12-year follow-up study. *J Arthroplasty* 1990;5(1):49-55.
30. Cartier P, Sanouiller JL, Khefacha A: Long-term results with the first patellofemoral prosthesis. *Clin Orthop Relat Res* 2005;436:47-54.
31. Kooijman HJ, Driessen AP, van Horn JR: Long-term results of patellofemoral arthroplasty: A report of 56 arthroplasties with 17 years of follow-up. *J Bone Joint Surg Br* 2003;85(6):836-840.
32. Paxton EW, Fithian DC: Outcome instruments for patellofemoral arthroplasty. *Clin Orthop Relat Res* 2005;436:66-70.
33. Utukuri MM, Khanduja V, Somayaji HS, Dowd GS: Patient-based outcomes in patellofemoral arthroplasty. *J Knee Surg* 2008; 21(4):269-274.
34. Hendrix MR, Ackroyd CE, Lonner JH: Revision patellofemoral arthroplasty: Three- to seven-year follow-up. *J Arthroplasty* 2008; 23(7):977-983.
35. Lonner JH, Jasko JG, Booth RE Jr: Revision of a failed patellofemoral arthroplasty to a total knee arthroplasty. *J Bone Joint Surg Am* 2006;88(11):2337-2342.

SECTION

6

Spine

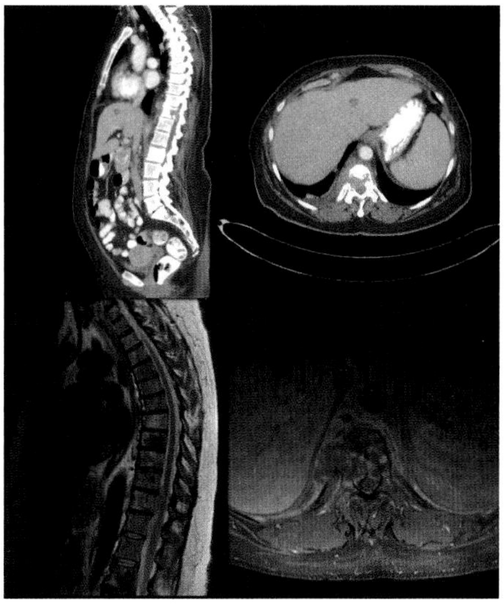

33 Modern Techniques in the Treatment of Patients With Metastatic Spine Disease

34 Lumbar Spinal Stenosis

33

Modern Techniques in the Treatment of Patients With Metastatic Spine Disease

Han Jo Kim, MD
Jacob M. Buchowski, MD
Charbel D. Moussallem, MD, FEBOT
Peter S. Rose, MD

Abstract

The treatment of metastatic disease to the spine involves a comprehensive evaluation of the patient and an individualized treatment plan based on the tumor type and location, the extent of the disease, and the general medical condition of the patient. Careful consideration of these factors dictates the treatment options, which include surgery, radiation, chemotherapy, and/or palliative options. Patients with a good overall prognosis may be considered candidates for more aggressive surgical resections, such as en bloc resections, whereas those with a poor prognosis may benefit from less invasive piecemeal resections to decompress the spine and restore neurologic function while minimizing the morbidity associated with more invasive procedures. The goals of surgery are tailored to the overall prognosis and should be aimed at optimizing the quality of the patient's life.

Instr Course Lect 2013;62:375-382.

The surgical management of metastatic disease of the spine continues to evolve. For most of the recent three decades, radiation therapy provided the mainstay of treatment for patients with symptomatic metastatic disease of the spine. Surgical treatment during this era often involved dorsal spinal cord decompression with no or limited spinal instrumentation.[1,2] These procedures generally provided only an indirect decompression of the spinal cord and often increased spinal instability. However, with advances in the understanding of metastatic processes in the spine and the evolution of surgical techniques and instrumentation, surgical treatment plays a prominent role in the care of patients with metastatic epidural spinal cord compression. Studies have now yielded level I evidence on the efficacy of surgery for metastatic disease of the spine for improving the quality of life and the outcomes in patients with spinal metastasis. Concurrently, advances in radiation oncology now allow high-precision targeting of tumors and increased efficacy when treating radioresistant lesions.[3] These advances together have led to important advances in the treatment of metastatic disease of the spine.

Research findings continue to identify appropriate candidates for surgical intervention for metastatic spinal disease as well as define optimal surgical and radiation therapy techniques. In considering treatment methods, it is essential to account for factors such as tumor type and/or biology, extent of disease, neurologic status, an individual patient's expectations, quality of life, and life expectancy. For example,

Dr. Buchowski or an immediate family member serves as a board member, owner, officer, or committee member of the American Academy of Orthopaedic Surgeons, the Cervical Spine Research Society, the North American Spine Society, the Orthopaedic Research and Education Foundation, the Scoliosis Research Society, and the Spine Arthroplasty Society; is a member of a speakers' bureau or has made paid presentations on behalf of Globus Medical and Stryker; serves as a paid consultant to or is an employee of CoreLink and Stryker; and has received research or institutional support from the Complex Spine Study Group and K2M. Dr. Rose or an immediate family member serves as a board member, owner, officer, or committee member of the American Academy of Orthopaedic Surgeons and the Minnesota Orthopedic Society. Neither of the following authors nor any immediate family member has received anything of value from or owns stock in a commercial company or institution related directly or indirectly to the subject of this chapter: Dr. Kim and Dr. Moussallem.

Table 1
Revised Evaluation System for the Prognosis of Metastatic Spine Tumors: Tokuhashi System[a]

Characteristic	Score
General condition (performance status)	
Poor (PS 10%-40%)	0
Moderate (PS 50%-70%)	1
Good (PS 80% to 100%)	2
Number of extraspinal bone metastases foci	
≥ 3	0
1-2	1
0	2
Number of metastases in the vertebral body	
≥ 3	0
2	1
1	2
Metastases to the major internal organs	
Unremovable	0
Removable	1
No metastases	2
Primary site of the cancer	
Lung, osteosarcoma, stomach, bladder, esophagus, pancreas	0
Liver, gallbladder, unidentified	1
Others	2
Kidney, uterus	3
Rectum	4
Thyroid, breast, prostate, carcinoid tumor	5
Palsy	
Complete (Frankel A, B)	0
Incomplete (Frankel C, D)	1
None (Frankel E)	2

PS = performance status.
[a]A higher score indicates a better prognosis. Criteria of predicted prognosis: Total score (TS) 0-8 = < 6 months; TS 9-11 = ≥ 6 months; TS 12-15 = ≥ 1 year.
Reproduced with permission from Tokuhashi Y, Matsuzaki H, Oda H, Oshima M, Ryu J: A revised scoring system for preoperative evaluation of metastatic spine tumor prognosis. *Spine (Phila Pa 1976)* 2005;30(19):2186-2191.

hematopoietic tumors reliably respond to radiation therapy and rarely require surgery for a compressive neurologic deficit alone. Aggressive surgical intervention may be futile in the face of an established neurologic deficit and/or rapidly advancing tumor refractory to treatments. However, many patients continue to present with symptomatic solid organ metastases and reasonable life expectancies and will benefit from a comprehensive evaluation by surgeons in concert with medical and radiation oncologists.

Surgical Staging and Assessing Prognosis

Although some patients clearly face a poorer prognosis than others, the prediction of life expectancy for any individual patient remains difficult and subject to error.[4] As new chemotherapeutic agents become available, older data may not apply to individual patients. For example, the treatment of metastatic renal cell carcinoma has changed dramatically since the approval of tyrosine kinase inhibitors in 2007; prognostic criteria from older cohorts of patients may not fully apply to contemporary clinical scenarios. Patients are generally considered candidates for aggressive surgical treatment of metastatic disease if their life expectancy exceeds 3 to 4 months, acknowledging the difficulties in accurately predicting this. Recent data have helped in understanding the role that a patient's age plays in predicting the benefit from surgical intervention.[5]

To aid in better estimating a prognosis, several scoring systems have been developed that take into consideration individual prognostic markers (such as primary tumor type and the presence of metastasis) and designate a score that provides an indication for the overall prognosis and/or life expectancy.[6-10] The Tomita scoring system was derived from a retrospective review of 67 patients and uses three main factors: grade of malignancy, visceral metastasis, and bone metastasis.[8] The revised Tokuhashi scoring system is different from the Tomita system in that it also considers performance status, types and locations of metastatic lesions, and paralysis with use of the Frankel classification to assign a score.[9] The initial Tokuhashi system was inconsistent in predicting prognosis and actual survival; however, the revised scoring system, developed after 1998 and reported subsequently in 2005, has an accuracy of up to 86% in prospective studies.[6,7,9,10] Both of the aforementioned scoring systems attempt to develop a score that will guide treatment algorithms and surgical options for managing metastatic spine disease. Generally speaking, the scores indicate an assessment on prognosis (in the Tokuhashi system, high scores indicate a good prognosis [**Table 1**]; in the Tomita system, lower scores indicate a good prognosis). This chapter's authors use these systems as a framework to guide the aggressiveness of treatment rather than as absolute cutoff points to define patient care.

Preoperative Optimization and Considerations

If aggressive surgical treatment is considered, the fitness of the patient for surgery is carefully assessed. This begins with a thorough history and physical examination to assess comorbidities and the overall condition of the patient. Preoperative medical optimization is an essential element in the management of patients with metastatic disease of the spine. Often enteral or parenteral supplemental nutrition is necessary in the perioperative period to optimize metabolic balance in the body toward an anabolic state to promote recovery and healing. Patient comorbidities must be managed in the postoperative period to anticipate complications and limit their manifestations. Complication rates after spine surgery for metastatic spine disease can be as high as 40%.[11,12] Recently, the Charlson Comorbidity Index has been used to predict the risk of 30-day postoperative complications in patients with metastatic spine disease.[12] In this study, a Charlson Comorbidity Index of 2 or more was associated with a five times higher likelihood of the development of a complication within 30 days after surgery. Efforts to anticipate and prevent complications in these patients will allow better selection of surgical candidates and likely improve patient outcomes.

Preoperative tumor embolization is used to minimize intraoperative blood loss for tumors that are prone to bleeding.[13] Although renal cell carcinoma is the most common hypervascular metastatic tumor, thyroid and hepatocellular carcinomas also benefit from embolization. Surgery is ideally performed within 24 to 48 hours after embolization to minimize revascularization of the tumor.

Patients are often treated with chemotherapy, so careful attention to the myelosuppressive effects of chemotherapy or potential wound-healing impairments is necessary in evaluating and managing patients perioperatively.

Surgical Planning Techniques

Surgical staging strategies are designed for planning surgical approaches for tumors of the spine; these should not be confused with overall oncologic staging to define the systemic extent of disease. Examples are the classification systems described by Tomita et al[8] (**Figure 1**) and the Weinstein, Boriani, and Biagini system[14,15] (**Figure 2**). The Weinstein, Boriani, and Biagini system provides an excellent template for planning en bloc resections of spinal tumors at a specific level, but it fails to take into consideration the possibility of multiple levels of involvement. In this respect, the classification system of Tomita et al[8] is more valuable; however, areas of resection are not noted in that classification system with the precision of the Weinstein, Boriani, and Biagini system.[8] Therefore, the Weinstein, Boriani, and Biagini classification system is an excellent tool for communicating the extent and location of a resection for tumors at a given level independent of the patient's prognosis.

Options and Considerations for Surgical Approach

Surgical management of spinal metastases is considered for four primary indications: compression of the neural elements; spinal instability, including pathologic fracture; unrelenting pain; and, rarely, when a histologic diagnosis must be established. Patients with metastatic spinal disease requiring surgical intervention may be treated with either an en bloc spondylectomy (considered in the rare patient with a solitary metastasis and favorable prognosis) or more commonly with an intralesional decompression and stabilization.

Traditionally, anterior approaches were used because they aided in achieving disease-free margins in en bloc spondylectomies. However, this chapter's authors routinely approach spondylectomies from an all-posterior approach to avoid the morbidity associated with an anterior approach. This applies to metastatic lesions in the thoracic as well as the lumbar spine, where a thoracotomy or laparotomy adds substantial morbidity and increases complications. Although disease-free margins are difficult to achieve without direct visualization of the anterior aspect of the spine, careful surgical planning with CT and MRI aids in guiding en bloc spondylectomies from an all-posterior approach. Stereotactic navigation may be useful in the surgical plan and execution of en bloc resections.[16] Although the Weinstein, Boriani, and Biagini system is still used to classify the location and exact position for resections, tomogram-based navigation systems may allow for more accurate resections with tumor-free margins from an all-posterior approach.[16] This is especially important for patients with the best prognosis and solitary spinal metastatic lesions for whom the goal is a curative resection and minimization of the tumor burden.

Frequently, clear margins and true en bloc spondylectomies cannot be performed because of the local extent of the tumor. This is especially true in patients in whom the metastatic lesion has spread to the posterior elements

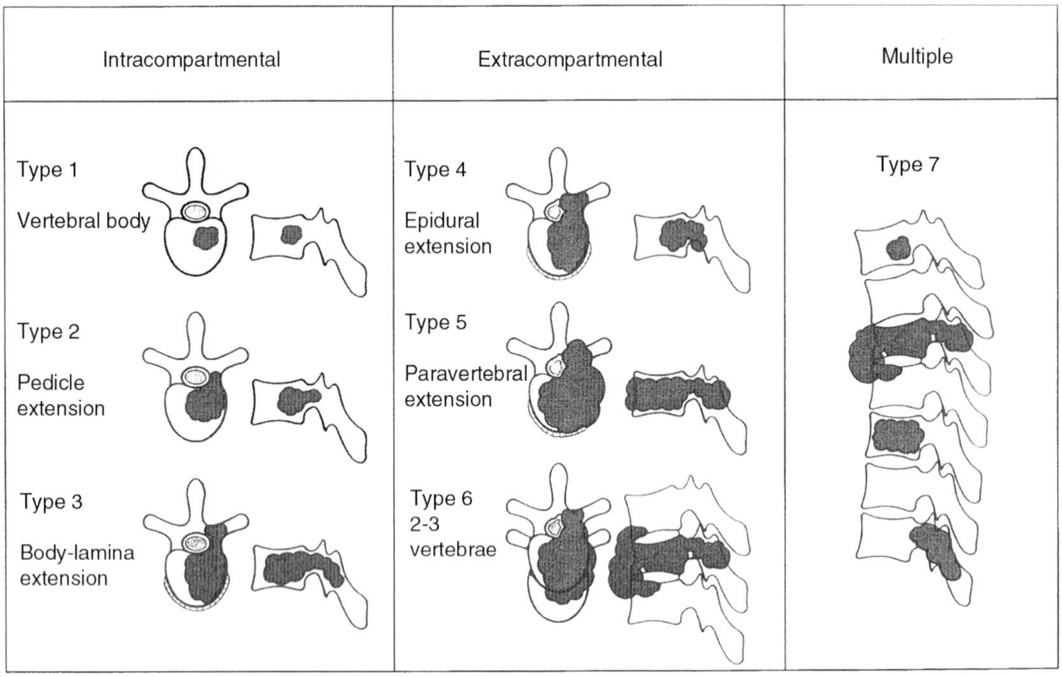

A

Scoring System

Point	Prognostic factors: Primary tumor	Prognostic factors: Visceral mets*	Prognostic factors: Bone mets**
1	Slow growth (breast, thyroid, etc)		solitary or isolated
2	Moderate growth (kidney, uterus, etc)	Treatable	Multiple
4	Rapid growth (lung, stomach, etc)	Un-treatable	

Prognostic score	Treatment goal	Surgical strategy
2 3	Long-term local control	Wide or marginal excision
4 5	Middle-term local control	Marginal or intralesional excision
6 7	Short-term palliation	Palliative surgery
8 9 10	Terminal care	Supportive care

*No visceral mets = 0 points
**Bone mets, including spinal mets

B

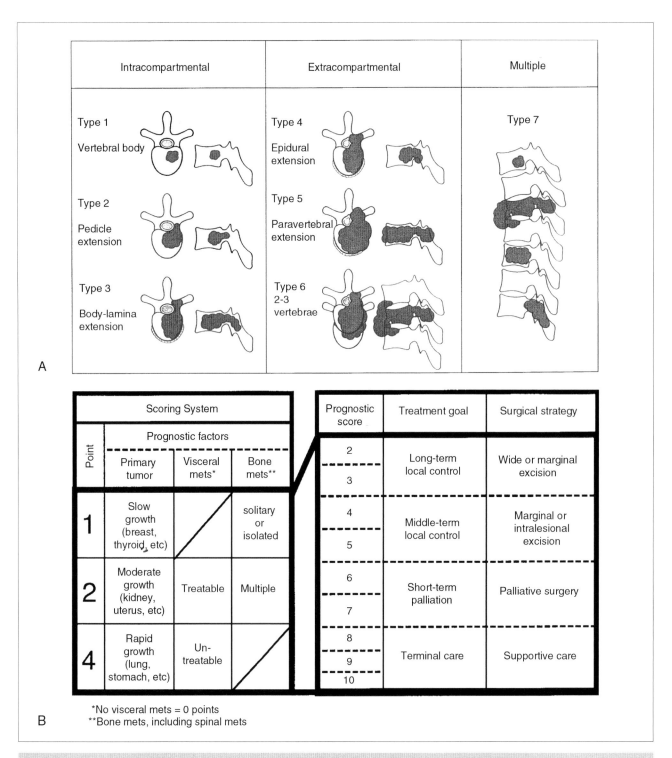

Figure 1 **A,** Illustration of the Tomita staging system showing the location and site of the lesion, which are used to produce a prognostic score. **B,** The score ultimately dictates the surgical strategy for the management of the metastatic lesion. A lower score indicates a good prognosis. Mets = metastasis. (Reproduced with permission from Tomita K, Kawahara N, Kobayashi T, Yoshida A, Murakami H, Akamaru T: Surgical strategy for spinal metastases. *Spine (Phila Pa 1976)* 2001;26(3):298-306.)

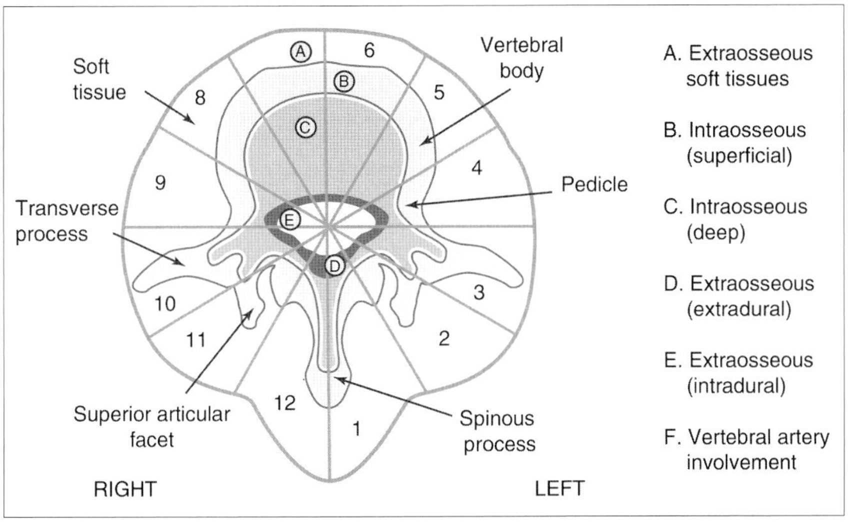

Figure 2 The modified staging system of Weinstein, Boriani, and Biagini from the Spine Oncology Study Group. The location of the lesion on the diagram, which is separated into radiating zones, dictates the type of surgical approach used for en bloc resection. For radiating zone 4-8 or 5-9, the procedure is vertebrectomy (double approach). For zone 2-5 or 7-11, the procedure is sagittal resection (double approach). For zone 10-3, the procedure is posterior arch resection (posterior approach). (Reproduced with permission from Boriani S, Weinstein JN, Biagini R: Primary bone tumors of the spine: Terminology and surgical staging. *Spine (Phila Pa 1976)* 1997;22(9): 1036-1044.)

through the lamina or vice versa from the lamina through the pedicle into the anterior vertebral body. In such situations, the most feasible approach is to achieve a marginal resection because a laminectomy and violation of the posterior elements are necessary to remove the anterior elements en bloc without injury to the spinal cord. In this respect, most vertebral en bloc resections are, at best, contaminated marginal resections. In such cases, postoperative radiation may aid in minimizing local disease recurrence.[3,17,18] Improved survival in patients treated with en bloc resection compared with those who have marginal resection for metastatic disease of the spine has not been documented. These procedures are technically demanding and are associated with a high rate of morbidity. For these reasons, this chapter's authors reserve these aggressive procedures for patients with a solitary metastasis following a long disease-free interval.

Most patients with metastatic spinal disease requiring surgical intervention are treated with an intralesional resection. The goals of surgery are to adequately decompress the neural elements, stabilize the spine, and achieve a gross total resection of the tumor. The offending tumor is most commonly located in the vertebral body; however, the surgical approach need not be anterior in all patients. In patients with multilevel disease or (nearly) circumferential dural compression, anterior approaches may not be suitable for decompression. Posterolateral transpedicular or costotransversectomy approaches have been increasingly used to provide safe and effective neural decompression and spinal stabilization while avoiding the morbidity (particularly pulmonary) associated with anterior approaches and providing the flexibility to extend the surgery over multiple symptomatic levels. Regardless of the approach used, adequate spinal fixation or instrumentation is necessary to provide immediate stability and avoid the use of spinal orthoses postoperatively. Usually, subsequent radiation therapy is used to minimize the risk of local tumor recurrence.

Reconstruction and Stabilization Considerations

Reconstruction of the anterior part of the spine after en bloc resections usually necessitates structural support. These options include metallic cages, cortical structural allografts, or methyl methacrylate bone cement (**Figure 3**). The selection of instrumentation used is based on patient-related factors and surgeon preference. Expandable cages can hold bone graft and allow for the possibility of a fusion; however, they are costly, require a greater exposure for insertion, and may compromise postoperative imaging studies.[19] Their use may be more beneficial for patients with a good long-term prognosis and those in whom a successful tumor-free margin was achieved intraoperatively so that postoperative radiation is not necessary. Cortical structural allografts may also provide benefits similar to those of an expandable cage at a fraction of the cost, but may lead to fatigue fracture and nonunion. Methyl methacrylate bone cement is an inexpensive and readily available option for immediate anterior column reconstruction. No comparative data exist to define the benefit of one method over the other in these circumstances.

Spinal instrumentation is used to restore stability after surgery for metastatic disease. For anterior procedures, plate-and-screw constructs are used; for posterior procedures, pedicle screw systems are used. As the healing potential of patients is uncertain in these cir-

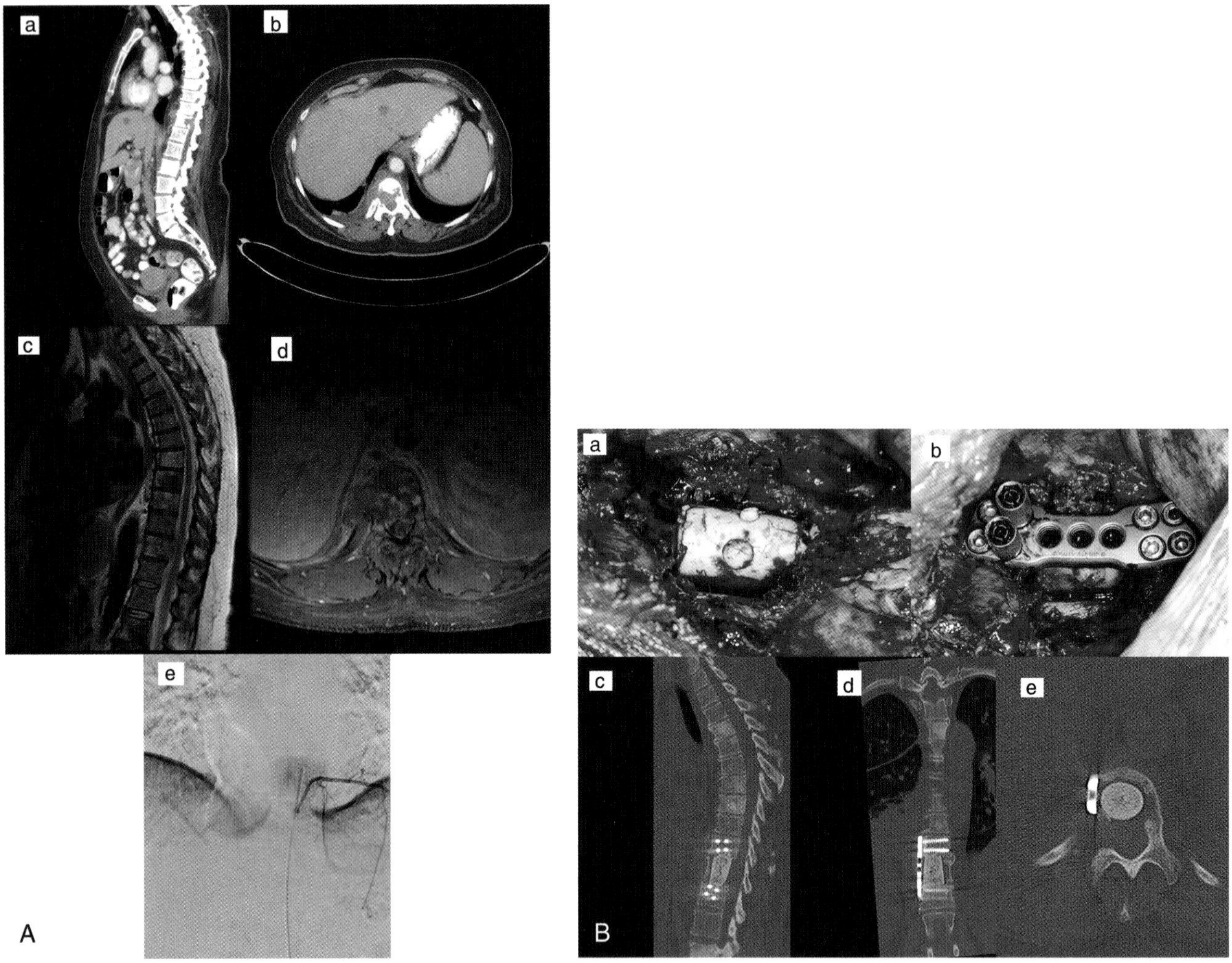

Figure 3 Imaging studies and intraoperative photographs of a 57-year-old woman in whom a T11 metastatic lesion from an adrenal cortical adenocarcinoma was diagnosed, with epidural cord compression and clinical signs of myelopathy. A right thoracotomy approach was used to visualize the anterolateral aspect of the vertebral column. A T11 corpectomy, including diskectomies at T10-T11 and T11-T12, was done. The reconstruction was performed with use of methyl methacrylate in a chest tube to minimize the risk of expansion and thermal injury to the spinal cord and surrounding structures. A locking plate was added to stabilize the construct. After the surgery, the patient was fully able to walk. **A,** Preoperative imaging included a sagittal CT scan showing a lytic lesion in the T11 vertebral body (a), an axial CT scan showing destruction of the posterior wall of the T11 vertebral body (b), a sagittal T2-weighted fast spin-echo MRI showing cord compression (c), an axial T1-weighted fat-saturated MRI showing epidural extension of the disease (d), and a spinal angiogram demonstrating that the anterior spinal artery arises from the left T9 vertebral artery (e). **B,** Intraoperative and postoperative images, include an intraoperative image showing the methyl methacrylate in a chest tube (a) and stabilization of the construct by a locked plate (b), a sagittal CT scan showing good sagittal balance of the spine (c), a coronal CT scan showing good alignment of the spine (d), and an axial CT scan showing adequate decompression of the spinal canal (e).

cumstances, robust fixation minimizes the likelihood of instrumentation failure during the patient's remaining life.

Less Invasive Options

When prognostic indicators are extremely poor, less invasive measures can be explored to relieve pain more than to decrease the tumor burden or achieve a decompression of the spinal cord.[20] Kyphoplasty and vertebroplasty are efficacious in addressing pain associated with vertebral compression fractures resulting from metastatic lesions from a solid organ tumor as well as multiple myeloma with minimal complications.[21-25] These procedures can be combined with radiation and chemotherapy with little concern for wound dehiscence and without much delay. Substantial pain control

Table 2
Radiosensitivity of a Tumor Based on Histologic Findings

Sensitivity	Tumor Histology
High	Leukemia, lymphoma, multiple myeloma, plasmocytoma, germ cell tumor
Intermediate	Breast, prostate, chondrosarcoma, nonmelanoma skin cancer, head and neck cancer, cervical, anal, nonsmall cell lung carcinoma
Low	Renal, thyroid, colon and small cell lung carcinoma, melanoma, sarcoma

can be achieved with this technique.[17,23,24,26] However, vertebroplasty and kyphoplasty do not allow for decompression of the spinal cord. Patients with a substantial loss of vertebral body height, posterior vertebral body cortex violation, or canal compromise are at increased risk during these percutaneous techniques. Preliminary data on percutaneous instrumentation coupled with limited open procedures for patients with metastatic disease have been favorably reported.[27]

Advances in Radiation Oncology

Radiation therapy is used in the treatment of patients with metastatic spinal disease to achieve local control of tumors. Traditionally, standard fractionated radiation therapy was used to achieve local control and minimize symptomatic local recurrence.[17] Standard radiation therapy provides excellent treatment of most patients with metastatic disease of the spine. Although the spinal cord and adjacent organs are exposed to radiation, the modest doses used and limited life expectancy of the patients makes the likelihood of radiation-associated complications less than 5%.

However, radioresistant tumors may not reliably respond to conventional radiation therapy techniques (**Table 2**). Repeat irradiation of recurrent tumor is problematic with conventional radiation therapy. Stereotactic delivery techniques that allow high-precision treatment of tumors have been developed.[3,17,18,28] The high-precision targeting of these techniques allows for hypofractionated treatment schemes to increase their effectiveness against radioresistant tumors. Further research continues to define the exact role of stereotactic radiation techniques in the treatment of patients with metastatic disease.[16]

If standard fractionated radiation therapy is used as an adjunct to surgery, postoperative use is recommended because preoperative radiation can increase the prevalence of surgical site infections and wound-healing complications. Although treatment is individualized, patients treated with anterior procedures can usually begin treatment in 2 to 3 weeks and those treated with posterior procedures in 3 to 4 weeks.

Summary

The treatment of metastatic disease remains a common clinical problem for spine surgeons. Patients with reasonable health and life expectancies are considered for surgical treatment when they present with compressive neurologic deficits from radioresistant tumors. Patient wishes, histologic findings, and the extent of spinal and extraspinal disease influence treatment decisions.

Many patients are managed without surgery. In those requiring surgical intervention, intralesional decompression and stabilization with postoperative radiation therapy is the mainstay of treatment. Patients are considered for aggressive en bloc resections if they present with a solitary metastasis after a long disease-free interval or have other unique clinical indications. Similarly, a subset of patients will benefit from high-precision and/or stereotactic radiation techniques. Surgery plays a powerful and increasing role in the treatment of these patients.

References

1. Young RF, Post EM, King GA: Treatment of spinal epidural metastases: Randomized prospective comparison of laminectomy and radiotherapy. *J Neurosurg* 1980; 53(6):741-748.
2. Patchell RA, Tibbs PA, Regine WF, et al: Direct decompressive surgical resection in the treatment of spinal cord compression caused by metastatic cancer: A randomised trial. *Lancet* 2005; 366(9486):643-648.
3. Shin JH, Chao ST, Angelov L: Stereotactic radiosurgery for spinal metastases: Update on treatment strategies. *J Neurosurg Sci* 2011; 55(3):197-209.
4. Nathan SS, Healey JH, Mellano D, et al: Survival in patients operated on for pathologic fracture: Implications for end-of-life orthopedic care. *J Clin Oncol* 2005; 23(25):6072-6082.
5. Chi JH, Gokaslan Z, McCormick P, Tibbs PA, Kryscio RJ, Patchell RA: Selecting treatment for patients with malignant epidural spinal cord compression-does age matter? Results from a randomized clinical trial. *Spine (Phila Pa 1976)* 2009;34(5):431-435.

6. Yamashita T, Siemionow KB, Mroz TE, Podichetty V, Lieberman IH: A prospective analysis of prognostic factors in patients with spinal metastases: Use of the revised Tokuhashi score. *Spine (Phila Pa 1976)* 2011;36(11): 910-917.
7. Tokuhashi Y, Matsuzaki H, Toriyama S, Kawano H, Ohsaka S: Scoring system for the preoperative evaluation of metastatic spine tumor prognosis. *Spine (Phila Pa 1976)* 1990;15(11):1110-1113.
8. Tomita K, Kawahara N, Kobayashi T, Yoshida A, Murakami H, Akamaru T: Surgical strategy for spinal metastases. *Spine (Phila Pa 1976)* 2001;26(3):298-306.
9. Tokuhashi Y, Matsuzaki H, Oda H, Oshima M, Ryu J: A revised scoring system for preoperative evaluation of metastatic spine tumor prognosis. *Spine (Phila Pa 1976)* 2005;30(19):2186-2191.
10. Tokuhashi Y, Ajiro Y, Umezawa N: Outcome of treatment for spinal metastases using scoring system for preoperative evaluation of prognosis. *Spine (Phila Pa 1976)* 2009;34(1):69-73.
11. Bauer H, Tomita K, Kawahara N, Abdel-Wanis ME, Murakami H: Surgical strategy for spinal metastases. *Spine (Phila Pa 1976)* 2002; 27(10):1124-1126.
12. Arrigo RT, Kalanithi P, Cheng I, et al : Charlson score is a robust predictor of 30-day complications following spinal metastasis surgery. *Spine (Phila Pa 1976)* 2011; 36(19):E1274-E1280.
13. Truumees E, Dodwad SN, Kazmierczak CD: Preoperative embolization in the treatment of spinal metastasis. *J Am Acad Orthop Surg* 2010;18(8):449-453.
14. Boriani S, Weinstein JN, Biagini R: Primary bone tumors of the spine: Terminology and surgical staging. *Spine (Phila Pa 1976)* 1997;22(9):1036-1044.
15. Chan P, Boriani S, Fourney DR, et al: An assessment of the reliability of the Enneking and Weinstein-Boriani-Biagini classifications for staging of primary spinal tumors by the Spine Oncology Study Group. *Spine (Phila Pa 1976)* 2009;34(4):384-391.
16. Smitherman SM, Tatsui CE, Rao G, Walsh G, Rhines LD: Image-guided multilevel vertebral osteotomies for en bloc resection of giant cell tumor of the thoracic spine: Case report and description of operative technique. *Eur Spine J* 2010;19(6):1021-1028.
17. Lanni TB Jr, Grills IS, Kestin LL, Robertson JM: Stereotactic radiotherapy reduces treatment cost while improving overall survival and local control over standard fractionated radiation therapy for medically inoperable non-small-cell lung cancer. *Am J Clin Oncol* 2011;34(5):494-498.
18. Haley ML, Gerszten PC, Heron DE, Chang YF, Atteberry DS, Burton SA: Efficacy and cost-effectiveness analysis of external beam and stereotactic body radiation therapy in the treatment of spine metastases: A matched-pair analysis. *J Neurosurg Spine* 2011; 14(4):537-542.
19. Alfieri A, Gazzeri R, Neroni M, Fiore C, Galarza M, Esposito S: Anterior expandable cylindrical cage reconstruction after cervical spinal metastasis resection. *Clin Neurol Neurosurg* 2011;113(10): 914-917.
20. Huang TJ, Hsu RW, Li YY, Cheng CC: Minimal access spinal surgery (MASS) in treating thoracic spine metastasis. *Spine (Phila Pa 1976)* 2006;31(16):1860-1863.
21. Bouza C, López-Cuadrado T, Cediel P, Saz-Parkinson Z, Amate JM: Balloon kyphoplasty in malignant spinal fractures: A systematic review and meta-analysis. *BMC Palliat Care* 2009;8:12.
22. Chew C, Craig L, Edwards R, Moss J, O'Dwyer PJ: Safety and efficacy of percutaneous vertebroplasty in malignancy: A systematic review. *Clin Radiol* 2011;66(1): 63-72.
23. Lane MD, Le HB, Lee S, et al: Combination radiofrequency ablation and cementoplasty for palliative treatment of painful neoplastic bone metastasis: Experience with 53 treated lesions in 36 patients. *Skeletal Radiol* 2011;40(1): 25-32.
24. Sandri A, Carbognin G, Regis D, et al: Combined radiofrequency and kyphoplasty in painful osteolytic metastases to vertebral bodies. *Radiol Med* 2010;115(2): 261-271.
25. Tancioni F, Lorenzetti M, Navarria P, et al : Vertebroplasty for pain relief and spinal stabilization in multiple myeloma. *Neurol Sci* 2010;31(2):151-157.
26. Lee B, Franklin I, Lewis JS, et al: The efficacy of percutaneous vertebroplasty for vertebral metastases associated with solid malignancies. *Eur J Cancer* 2009;45(9): 1597-1602.
27. Rose PS, Clarke MJ, Dekutoski MB: Minimally invasive treatment of spinal metastases: Techniques. *Int J Surg Oncol* 2011;2011: 494381.
28. Al-Mamgani A, Tans L, Teguh DN, van Rooij P, Zwijnenburg EM, Levendag PC: Stereotactic body radiotherapy: A promising treatment option for the boost of oropharyngeal cancers not suitable for brachytherapy. A single-institutional experience. *Int J Radiat Oncol Biol Phys* 2012;82(4): 1494-1500.

34

Lumbar Spinal Stenosis

Joe Y.B. Lee, MD
Peter G. Whang, MD
Joon Y. Lee, MD
Frank M. Phillips, MD
Alpesh A. Patel, MD, FACS

Abstract

Lumbar spinal stenosis affects many patients and is one of the most common reasons for spinal surgery in the elderly population. New research and surgical innovations have resulted in a better understanding of the disease and its diagnosis and treatment. To select the optimal treatment approach for each patient, it is helpful to review patient presentations, diagnostic workups, surgical and nonsurgical treatment options, evidence-based outcomes, and the pathophysiology of lumbar spinal stenosis.

Instr Course Lect 2013;62:383-396.

Lumbar spinal stenosis represents an important cause of pain and disability in the aging population.[1] The actual prevalence of symptomatic spinal stenosis is unknown because radiographic evidence of this condition does not always lead to clinical symptoms. Boden et al[2] performed a cross-sectional analysis of MRI findings in a population of asymptomatic individuals and found that between 30% and 90% of asymptomatic adults had a major spinal abnormality, including disk herniation, disk degeneration, and spinal stenosis. This study highlights the potential disconnection between MRI findings and patient symptoms, as well as the importance of accurately correlating clinical symptoms with radiographic findings.

The clinical presentation of lumbar spinal stenosis typically consists of back and leg pain, with the latter presenting as either neurogenic claudication or radicular leg pain. Neurogenic claudication arises from compression of the thecal sac, resulting in pain, numbness, heaviness, cramping, burning, or weakness in the lower extremities. These symptoms may not follow a dermatomal distribution and are characteristically worse with extension of the lumbar spine during walking or prolonged standing. Neurogenic claudication can be distinguished from vascular claudication in that neurogenic claudication is relieved by bending over, sitting, or leaning forward while walking (such as leaning against a shopping cart). Unlike neurogenic claudication, radicular leg pain arises from compression of particular nerve roots. Patients often describe pain in a specific dermatomal pattern corresponding to the compressed nerve root

Dr. Whang or an immediate family member is a member of a speakers' bureau or has made paid presentations on behalf of Baxter, Medtronic, and Stryker; serves as a paid consultant to or is an employee of Baxter, Cerapedics, Medtronic, Paradigm Spine, Smith & Nephew, and Stryker; serves as an unpaid consultant to DiFusion; and owns stock or stock options in DiFusion. Dr. Joon Lee or an immediate family member has received research or institutional support from Stryker. Dr. Phillips or an immediate family member has received royalties from Nuvasive and DePuy; serves as a paid consultant to or is an employee of DePuy, Kyphon, Stryker, and Nuvasive; and owns stock or stock options in Nuvasive, Baxano, Spinal Kinetics, Spinal Motion, Axiomed, Flexuspine, CrossTrees, Pearl Diver, BioAssets, Facet Solutions, and Pioneer. Dr. Patel or an immediate family member serves as a board member, owner, officer, or committee member of the American Academy of Orthopaedic Surgeons, the American College of Surgeons, the American Orthopaedic Association, AO Spine North America, the Cervical Spine Research Society, the Lumbar Spine Research Society, and the North American Spine Society; has received royalties from Amedica; serves as a paid consultant to or is an employee of Amedica, Biomet, GE Healthcare, Stryker, and Trinity Orthopaedics; and owns stock or stock options in Amedica, Cytonics, Nocimed, and Trinity Orthopaedics. Neither Dr. Joe Y.B. Lee nor any immediate family member has received anything of value from or owns stock in a commercial company or institution related directly or indirectly to the subject of this chapter.

and may have associated myotomal weakness. Severe disease leading to frank motor deficit or cauda equina syndrome is rare in patients with lumbar spinal stenosis. In patients with mild or moderate degenerative lumbar stenosis, rapid or catastrophic neurologic decline is rare.[3]

The physical examination is also an important component in diagnosing lumbar spinal stenosis. The patient may be observed in a flexed-forward seated position in the examination room. During standing and walking, these patients often continue to lean forward, with the hips and knees flexed; this expands the diameter of the spinal cord and thereby minimizes symptoms. Lumbar extension is frequently avoided and may reproduce the patient's symptoms. In the Spine Patient Outcomes Research Trial (SPORT) study, asymmetric reflexes were reported in 26% of the patients with symptomatic stenosis, 28% with motor weakness, and 29% with a sensory deficit.[4]

Pathophysiology

Compression of the neural elements occurs because of changes in the local anatomy, including the intervertebral disk, facet joint, and ligamentum flavum. Degeneration of the motion segment is believed to begin in the intervertebral disk.[5] Normally, the anulus fibrosus contains 60% type II collagen and 40% type I collagen, whereas the nucleus pulposus contains mostly type II collagen. With aging, the concentration of type I collagen increases as type II collagen decreases. This leads to increased desiccation of the disk because type I collagen is associated with less water content. Dehydration of the disk is worsened by the natural increase in the ratio of keratan sulfate to chondroitin sulfate that occurs with aging.[5]

The degenerative cascade, as described by Yong-Hing and Kirkaldy-Willis,[5] views the spine as a tripod, with the disk and the two facet joints comprising the three legs. Altered disk structure and loss in disk height are coupled with disruption of the anulus fibrosus, leading to bulging of the disk and the posterior longitudinal ligament. This may cause narrowing of the spinal canal and neural foramen. The shortened disk height also leads to buckling of the ligamentum flavum and increased stresses in the facet joints, potentiating facet degeneration and leading to hypertrophy and osteophyte formation. The changes in the ligamentum flavum and facet joints lead to further narrowing of the spinal canal, and the cycle of degeneration is propagated.

It has been theorized that facet joint osteoarthritis is associated with several factors. It is commonly believed that facet tropism (asymmetry between the facet joints) contributes to degenerative changes. Kalichman et al[6] reviewed CT scans of 188 individuals and found osteoarthritis was associated with more sagittally oriented facet joints. The abnormal kinematics of the posterior facets lead to joint hypertrophy, osteophyte formation, capsular thickening, subluxation, and synovial cyst formation.[7] These changes encroach into the spinal canal, causing central and/or lateral recess stenosis.

Another cause for clinical symptoms in patients with lumbar spinal stenosis may be directly related to instability or spondylolisthesis. Although instability is poorly described in the literature, it has been defined as greater than 3 mm of translation of one vertebral body on another or more than 10° of motion between adjacent end plates on flexion and extension radiographs.[8] Some investigators have differentiated dynamic versus static spondylolisthesis. Dynamic spondylolisthesis is defined as the presence of greater than 3 mm difference on flexion and extension radiographs, and static spondylolisthesis is defined as a slip that does not change with either flexion or extension.[9] Theoretically, in addition to the incremental stenosis associated with dynamic translation, shear forces applied at the motion segment cause added irritation to the exiting and traversing nerve roots.

Changes occur in the ligamentum flavum and further contribute to stenosis. Although the focus of discussion traditionally has been on buckling of the ligamentum flavum associated with a loss of disk height, there is growing evidence that identifies ligamentum flavum hypertrophy as a pathologic feature of spinal stenosis. Two major pathomechanisms have been proposed to account for ligamentum flavum hypertrophy: degenerative changes and mechanical stresses.[10] Degenerative changes have been attributed to the aging process, with a decrease in the elastin-to-collagen ratio contributing to fibrosis.[11] Mechanical stresses may also contribute to ligamentum flavum thickening through compensatory hypertrophy. Sairyo et al[12] reported on the pathomechanism of ligamentum flavum hypertrophy. The authors found transforming growth factor-β was related to the stimulation of fibrosis and summarized the process of ligamentum flavum hypertrophy as beginning with mechanical stress-inducing tissue damage that leads to inflammation, scarring, and fibrosis. Histologic studies have identified other inflammatory markers related to ligamentum flavum hypertrophy and fibrosis, including tissue inhibitors of matrix metalloproteinases.[13]

The combination of disk, facet, and ligamentum flavum degeneration leads to neurologic compression. However, because some individuals have neural compression without symptoms, it has been suggested that other factors in addition to mechanical neural compression are responsible for symptom generation.[14] Rydevik et al[15] described the pathophysiology of nerve root compression and showed capillary restriction and electrophysiologic alteration occurring with increased pressure on the thecal sac. Increasing pressure also leads to venous congestion of the intraneural microcirculation, arterial restriction, and decreased solute transportation across nerve root segments. Animal studies have shown that motor and sensory deficits occur when 50% compression of the cauda equina was reached.[16] Changes in the macroscopic and microscopic environment of the neural elements lead to a substantial inflammatory response. Multiple studies have identified the presence of matrix metalloproteinases, nitric oxide, interleukin-6, and prostaglandin E_2 with lumbar disk disease.[17,18] These inflammatory mediators and markers suggest that a biologic response, in addition to mechanical compression, plays an important role in the development of symptomatic stenosis. A genetic basis for the biologic response may, ultimately, differentiate symptomatic from asymptomatic patients.

Localization of Disease

Spinal stenosis can be localized to specific anatomic zones, including the central, lateral recess, foraminal, and extraforaminal regions.

Central Stenosis

Central stenosis refers to narrowing and compression within the lumbar spinal canal, medial to the facet joints and under the laminae. Central stenosis generally occurs because of the hypertrophied ligamentum flavum and lumbar disk prolapse and causes the dural sac to flatten in the anteroposterior dimension, resulting in a loss of normal cerebrospinal fluid space. Central stenosis generally causes bilateral leg symptoms (weakness and pain) and neurogenic claudication.

Lateral Recess Stenosis

Lateral recess stenosis refers to the area medial to the pedicle, under the superior articular process of the caudal vertebra. Lateral recess stenosis, also referred to as subarticular stenosis, is typically caused by degenerative changes in the facet joint and disk (hypertrophy, osteophytes), as well as hypertrophic subarticular ligamentum flavum. Stenosis in this region generally causes pain and weakness unilaterally in the distribution of the traversing nerve root. For example, lateral recess stenosis at the L4-5 level generally affects the traversing L5 nerve root.

Foraminal Stenosis

Foraminal stenosis refers to compression at the entrance and within the neural foramen formed by the superior and inferior pedicles, the facet joint dorsally, and the vertebral body and disks anteriorly. The most common reason for foraminal stenosis is disk protrusion into the foramina or osteophytic overgrowth of the superior articular facet into the neural foramina above.[5] A loss of cranial-caudal foraminal (pedicle-to-pedicle) height may be seen with progressive disk space narrowing, whereas a loss of normal foraminal width occurs with spondylolisthesis. Foraminal stenosis typically causes radicular pain in the dermatome of the exiting nerve root.

Diagnostic Imaging

Plain Radiography

If lumbar spinal stenosis is suspected, diagnostic testing often begins with plain radiography. Dynamic spondylolisthesis should be considered and is evaluated with flexion and extension lateral views in addition to AP and lateral views. Standard full-spine (36-inch cassette) standing radiographs should be obtained for any patient with scoliosis or sagittal malalignment. This allows assessment of the patient's global balance in both the coronal and sagittal planes. Bending and supine radiographs may also be considered if there is a kyphotic deformity. Plain radiographs may show narrowing of the neural foramina and spinal canal from spondylotic structures. Bone quality, ossification of ligamentous structures, ankylosis of the spine, erosion of the disk space, or pathologic bony changes should be assessed and correlated with clinical symptoms.

Magnetic Resonance Imaging

MRI provides detailed images of the bone, soft tissue, and neural structures. The degree of compression of the neural elements, the offending pathology, and the location of stenosis can be assessed with MRI. Characteristic pathologies to consider on MRI include facet arthropathy, ligamentum hypertrophy, disk bulges or herniations, and synovial cysts. MRI with contrast can be useful in patients who had prior surgeries and helps distinguish between disk herniation and scar tissue.[14] MRI also has been shown to be valuable in assessing dynamic stability in patients with degenerative lumbar disease. Rihn et al[19] found the presence of facet fluid on MRI to be associated with radiographic instability on flexion and extension views at L4-5, with a positive predictive value of 82%.

CT With Myelography

CT combined with myelography can be a useful diagnostic modality because it provides good contrast between the thecal sac, the surrounding soft tissue, and bony pathology. A CT myelogram is especially valuable in patients with unclear MRI findings, those who are unable to have an MRI, those with scoliosis, or those with previous spinal instrumentation. In patients with spinal stenosis, plain CT may not effectively identify areas of stenosis as well as myelography or MRI.

Nonsurgical Management

A systematic review of the literature by Watters et al[3] did not find sufficient evidence to support physical therapy as a stand-alone treatment of lumbar spinal stenosis, although some physicians believe that physical therapy may be an effective measure in controlling patient symptoms. In addition to traditional core strengthening programs, active aerobic exercises have been shown to improve symptoms.[20]

Nonsteroidal anti-inflammatory drugs (NSAIDs) are widely prescribed for the treatment of various spinal disorders. However, the exact role of inflammation in the pathogenesis of lumbar spinal stenosis remains uncertain, and the efficacy of NSAIDs has not been specifically investigated in patients with this condition. NSAIDs may also be associated with substantial costs and can be toxic in some patients. For these reasons, the American College of Rheumatology and the European League Against Rheumatism have both recommended acetaminophen as the initial therapy for spinal stenosis.[21]

Gabapentin is an anticonvulsant medication frequently used in the treatment of neuropathic pain syndromes. The addition of gabapentin to physical therapy and NSAID use in patients with lumbar spinal stenosis was found to increase walking distance and improve pain scores and the recovery of sensory deficits in a small clinical study.[22] Other drugs used to treat neuropathic pain include pregabalin, tricyclic antidepressants, and duloxetine; however, these drugs have not been studied in patients with lumbar spinal stenosis.

Calcitonin is a hormone secreted by the thyroid gland that has been reported to have analgesic and anti-inflammatory properties. Older, small trials have shown that intramuscular and subcutaneous administration of calcitonin improves walking distance and pain in some patients with lumbar spinal stenosis.[23-25] Because more recent studies reported no substantial benefit of nasally administered calcitonin compared with placebo, the efficacy of calcitonin for lumbar spinal stenosis remains uncertain.[26,27]

A trial epidural injection is reasonable if leg pain has not responded to simpler measures. Although Ng et al[28] found no difference in pain or walking distance in patients with lumbar spinal stenosis who received a single, transforaminal, epidural, steroid injection at 12-week follow-up, several other studies reported positive results.[29,30] Botwin et al[29] reported substantial improvement in pain and walking tolerance in patients treated with a multiple-injection protocol of transforaminal epidural steroid injections and followed for 12 months. In a retrospective review of 140 patients with lumbar spinal stenosis treated with either transforaminal or caudal epidural steroid injection, Delport et al[30] found that 32% of patients had pain relief at 2-month follow-up, and 53% of patients had improvement in their functional abilities. Based on a review of the literature, single injections may lead to short-term relief of symptoms from lumbar spinal stenosis, whereas a multiple-injection program may be more reliable in producing longer-term pain relief.[3]

Surgical Treatment

When conservative treatment fails in patients with lumbar spinal stenosis, surgical treatment may be indicated. The SPORT study examined the outcomes of patients who were randomized to surgical versus nonsurgical treatment of lumbar spinal stenosis.[31] Although a high crossover rate occurred, surgically treated patients maintained substantially greater improvements in pain and function through 4 years of follow-up compared with nonsurgically managed patients. A similar conclusion was reached by Kovacs et al[32] in a systematic review of five high-quality randomized controlled trials. The authors concluded that when 3 to 6 months of nonsurgical treatment is unsuccessful in patients with lumbar spinal stenosis, surgery was more effective than continued conservative treatment.

Decompressive Techniques

In patients in whom nonsurgical management has failed or who have progressive pain or neurologic deficits, surgical intervention may be the optimal treatment. Many surgical techniques can achieve the goals of decompressing the neural elements and preserving spinal stability. A wide laminectomy, with medial facetectomies and foraminotomies, is considered the traditional gold standard surgical treatment of symptomatic lumbar spinal stenosis. In a 10-year follow-up of patients treated with decompressive laminectomy for lumbar spinal stenosis, Iguchi et al[33] reported that more than 50% of the patients had good or excellent results. A prospective study of 101 elderly patients treated with decompressive laminectomy showed 87% satisfaction at 12-month follow-up.[34] During laminectomy, particular attention should be paid to preserving facet and pars integrity to prevent iatrogenic instability. Although effective in decompressing the neural elements, laminectomy is associated with risks, including infection, wound complications, postoperative pain, prolonged rehabilitation, and scar formation. Most importantly, laminectomy may lead to motion segment instability.[35] Multiple studies have reported between 4% and 31% recurrent stenosis or spondylolisthesis after facet-sparing laminectomy.[4,36-38]

Laminotomy may be considered to address the risks of iatrogenic instability associated with laminectomy. Laminotomy involves resection of the lamina, ligamentum flavum, and a partial area of the medial facet joint; it can be performed as a unilateral or bilateral procedure. The procedure retains the spinous process, interspinous ligament, and supraspinous ligament and may result in less interruption to the intrinsic stability of the spine. A cadaver study found substantially greater stability in spines treated with bilateral laminotomy versus facet-sparing laminectomy.[39] Multiple studies have shown that laminotomy is a clinically effective treatment for lumbar spinal stenosis.[36,40,41] In general, the location of the stenosis and the surgeon's experience and preference should guide the selection of the appropriate decompressive technique.

Minimally invasive surgery (MIS) has also been suggested as a possible means of reducing the risks associated with traditional surgical techniques for lumbar spinal stenosis. The rationale for MIS involves focal decompression specifically directed toward the compressive pathology. These techniques require precise localization of the stenotic pathology, with the greatest ability to treat compression typically occurring at the level of the interlaminar window. MIS decompression involves less soft-tissue dissection and resection of the posterior osteoligamentous arch and greater preservation of stabilizing structures.[42] The potential benefits of MIS may include avoidance of the morbidity inherent in open procedures and minimization of epidural scar formation and postoperative low back pain. In a prospective evaluation of patients treated with MIS decompression, Weiner et al[43] found that 87% of patients reported high satisfaction rates. Biomechanical studies also support the potential clinical benefits of MIS decompression, showing greater preservation of normal segmental motion, which may effectively minimize the risk of postoperative instability and the progression of adjacent-level degeneration.[44,45]

MIS decompressive procedures for lumbar spinal stenosis include interlaminar fenestration (laminotomy), partial/interspinous laminectomy, spinous process osteotomy, and laminoplasty.[46] In laminoplasty, the laminofacet junction is targeted with a guidewire under fluoroscopic guidance. Muscles and fascia are sequentially dilated to facilitate the placement of a tubular or expandable retractor. Decompression can be accomplished through an ipsilateral laminotomy (unilateral or bilateral). Undercutting of the medial facet joint and removal of hypertrophied ligamentum flavum can then be done to expose the thecal sac and nerve roots. The pars interarticularis and supraspinous/interspinous ligaments are preserved. Bilateral decompression can be accomplished through a unilateral laminotomy. Typically, the spinal canal is approached from the more symptomatic side. Once ipsilateral decompression is completed, the working channel may be angled medially to reach the contralateral side. The base of the spinous process and the contralateral lamina/facet is undercut to facilitate visualization, and decompression is continued laterally to the level of the contralateral pedicle[47] (**Figure 1**).

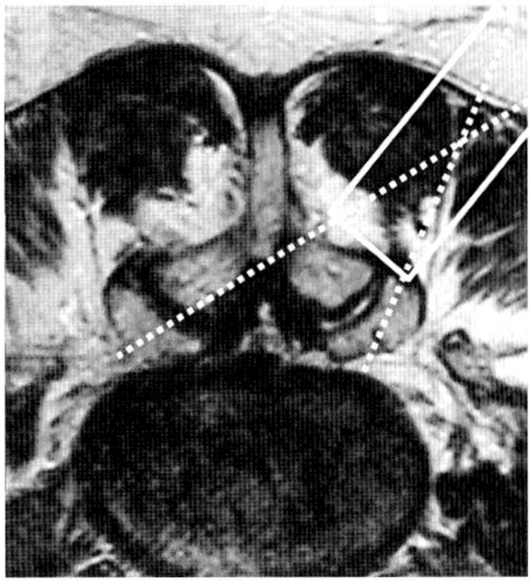

Figure 1 Cross-sectional MRI scan shows the path of access for minimally invasive decompression. A unilateral approach can be used to access both the ipsilateral (solid lines) and contralateral lateral recess as well as the central canal (dashed lines). (Reproduced with permission from Kim CW, Siemionow K, Anderson DG, Phillips FM: The current state of minimally invasive surgery. *J Bone Joint Surg Am* 2011;93(6):582-596).

The clinical outcomes of MIS decompression appear to be similar to those reported after laminectomy. Multiple series have reported success rates approaching 90%, with no increase in postoperative subluxation, even in patients with degenerative spondylolisthesis.[48,49] In a retrospective study of 374 patients treated with unilateral MIS decompression for lumbar spinal stenosis, Costa et al[41] found that 87.9% of patients reported clinical benefits, with a 0.8% incidence of postoperative instability. Khoo and Fessler[50] compared MIS laminotomy to laminectomy and found the short-term outcomes to be equivalent, but with less morbidity in the MIS group. In a randomized study comparing MIS laminotomy (unilateral and bilateral) to laminectomy, Thomé et al[47] found the greatest improvement and the lowest complication rate in patients treated with bilateral MIS laminotomy, with unilateral MIS laminotomy comparable to laminectomy. In a more recent study,

Rahman et al[40] compared MIS decompression to open laminectomy and observed less surgical blood loss, shorter surgical times and hospital stays, and fewer complications with the MIS technique.

Despite promising results, there remains a paucity of level I data establishing the safety and efficacy of MIS decompression, and the reported results have not been uniformally positive. Most studies have looked at small or heterogenous patient populations, lacked a control group, or had short follow-up periods. Kelleher et al[51] reviewed patients with lumbar spinal stenosis treated with MIS decompression and reported a substantially higher rate of revision surgery in patients with scoliotic deformity. Ikuta et al[52] compared minimally invasive and open laminotomy and found similar short-term outcomes, but with a higher complication rate in the MIS group. Pitfalls in MIS decompression arise from suboptimal visualization of pathology, which may compromise the extent of the neural decompression, be more technically challenging, and lengthen surgical times. Complications include inadequate decompression or residual stenosis, fracture or progressive instability, neurologic injuries, dural tears, epidural hematomas, and wound infections.[53]

Overall, MIS decompressive techniques can achieve similar clinical outcomes with the potential for less morbidity than open procedures. Preserving stabilizing structures may decrease the risk of iatrogenic instability and avoid the need for concomitant fusion. However, limited access procedures should not be performed at the expense of completing an adequate decompression. Additional long-term, prospective, randomized clinical trials are necessary to compare the safety and efficacy of MIS decompressive techniques.

Interspinous Process Spacers

Interspinous devices have been used in lumbar spinal stenosis with the rationale that they may indirectly decompress the neural elements, unload the spinal structures, and decrease segmental instability. The interspinous device is a central spacer placed between adjacent spinous processes to limit extension. The implant is maintained in the interspinous space with lateral wings or secured with attached cables. The decompressive role of interspinous devices was studied by Richards et al[54] using cadaver spines. The authors found that by applying an interspinous device, the canal area increased by 18%, the canal diameter increased by 10%, and the subarticular diameter increased by 50%. The foraminal area increased by 25%, and the foraminal width increased by 41%.[54] Interspinous devices are indicated in symptomatic neurogenic claudication with radiographic evidence of spinal stenosis with or without degenerative spondylolisthesis and provide considerable claudication relief with sitting and flexion. They are contraindicated in patients with substantial spinal instability or deformity, including isthmic spondylolisthesis, high-grade degenerative spondylolisthesis, and scoliosis greater than 25°. Interspinous devices are also contraindicated in patients with bony ankylosis, cauda equina syndrome, and severe osteoporosis.

Although the implant technique varies based on the device used, commonalities exist in the surgical approach. The lumbar spine is maintained in flexion for the procedure, which may be done with the patient in the lateral decubitus position or prone on a Wilson frame. Supraspinous ligaments must be preserved during the exposure. The interspinous space is distracted to facilitate implantation of the device. Interspinous device placement also has been combined with direct decompression of the spinal segment, but the rationale for its use in this setting is not supported by the literature.

Lindsey et al[55] studied the biomechanics of interspinous devices in cadavers and found flexion and extension substantially decreased at the level of the implant, with rotation and lateral bending not affected. Other biomechanical studies have found evidence that interspinous devices may minimize facet loading and reduce intradiscal pressures, while preserving the range of motion at adjacent segments.[56-58]

The X-Stop (Medtronic, Memphis, TN) interspinous device was studied by the product developers in a prospective, randomized clinical trial comparing the X-Stop to nonsurgical treatment of lumbar spinal stenosis. The study included 191 patients and had a minimum 2-year follow-up. Substantially greater clinical improvement occurred in the X-Stop group, with 73.1% of patients satisfied with the procedure compared with 35.9% in the control group.[59] The X-Stop is approved by the FDA to treat one- or two-level disease (based on the number of spinal segments).

A prospective case-controlled study by Richter et al[60] evaluated patients with lumbar spinal stenosis treated with decompression with and without implantation of the Coflex (Paradigm Spine, New York, NY) interspinous device. Both groups had substantial improvements in pain relief and functional outcomes, but the interspinous device did not appear superior to traditional decompression. Sobottke et al[61] reviewed 129 patients with lumbar spinal stenosis treated with an X-Stop, Wallis (Zimmer Spine, Bordeaux, France), or DIAM (Medtronic) interspinous device. Despite the finding that the X-Stop provided greater improvements in radiographic parameters, no substantial differences in symptom relief among the different interspinous devices were reported.

Despite the simplicity and potential benefit of interspinous devices, infrequent complications have occurred, including fracture, implant migration, neurologic sequelae, and persistent and/or recurrent symptoms. Barbagallo et al[62] reviewed 69 patients treated with X-Stop and found a 10.1% incidence of complications and a 7.2% reoperation rate. In a small series by Verhoof et al,[63] 4 of 12 patients reported no symptom relief, and recurrent symptoms developed within 2 years in an additional 3 patients. These seven patients required revision surgery for decompression and fusion. Similarly, Bowers et al[64] reported an overall complication rate of 38% and a reoperation rate of 85% in their series of 13 patients treated with X-Stop. Risk factors for complications included overdistraction, osteoporosis, and preexisting adjacent-level degeneration. Burnett et al[65] evaluated the cost effectiveness of nonsurgical management, laminectomy, or an interspinous device for lumbar spinal stenosis and concluded that laminectomy was the most cost-effective strategy for symptomatic patients.

Degenerative Spondylolisthesis

Surgical technique in treating spinal stenosis with degenerative spondylolisthesis is focused on a thorough neurologic decompression, including the central canal, lateral recess, and neural foramina. The necessity for a concomitant fusion with decompression remains controversial.

Herkowitz and Kurz[66] compared 50 patients treated with or without noninstrumented fusion, with autologous intertransverse bone grafting. At a minimum 2.4-year follow-up, good to excellent results were achieved in 96% of the patients with concomitant arthrodesis compared with 44% of the patients without arthrodesis. Subsequent radiographic evidence of fusion did not, however, predict outcomes.

In a multicenter comparison (SPORT study) between surgical and nonsurgical treatment of spinal stenosis with spondylolisthesis, 352 of 372 patients had decompression with a concomitant arthrodesis, with or without instrumentation.[67] At 2-year follow-up, the surgical group had statistically significant ($P < 0.05$) improvement of symptoms compared with the nonsurgical group. Those with degenerative spondylolisthesis and associated spinal stenosis were specifically reviewed at a 4-year follow-up. The authors reported substantially greater pain relief and improvement in function in the surgically treated patients compared with those treated nonsurgically. The SPORT study could not compare decompression only with decompression and fusion because of the small number of patients in the nonfused group.[68] Although these results suggest that arthrodesis should be performed with degenerative spondylolisthesis, there are conflicting findings in the literature regarding the benefit of an isolated decompression procedure.

Preservation of the facet joints, paraspinal muscle attachments, and posterior ligamentous structures (supraspinatus and infraspinatus ligaments) has been postulated to prevent postoperative instability. Hatta et al[69] reported on 105 consecutive patients, 30 with degenerative lumbar spondylolisthesis, treated with muscle- and ligament-sparing decompression. Although limited by the study's short-term follow-up (mean, 21.3 months; range, 8 to 44 months), the authors reported neurologic improvement in all patients and no neurologic complications. Sasai et al[48] reported the results of microdecompression (bilateral decompression through a unilateral approach) in a comparison of patients with and without spondylolisthesis. This approach protects the midline ligamentous structures and the contralateral paraspinal muscle attachments. The authors reported a higher percentage of slip in the patients with spondylolisthesis but no difference in clinical (back pain or Oswestry Disability Index scores) or neurologic outcomes at intermediate-term follow-up (mean, 46 months; range, 24 to 71 months). Additional factors, such as a loss of disk height, bridging osteophytes, and patient age, may influence the decision between fusion and nonfusion surgery; however, these factors have not yet been validated in the literature.

The use of instrumentation is also a variable in spinal fusion procedures. The addition of instrumentation has been shown to improve fusion rates, but its effect on the clinical outcome of patients is unclear.[70,71] Direct comparisons between instrumented and noninstrumented fusions have been done, with an early study finding no significant difference in global patient satisfaction but increased surgical time, blood loss, and revision rates with instrumentation.[72] In a randomized prospective study of 129 patients with 5-year follow-up, the authors reported no significant difference in functional results and pain surveys between patients who received instrumentation versus no instrumentation.[73] However, in a more recent study of 94 patients with a mean age of 70 years, instrumentation was shown to have superior clinical results and fusion rates compared with no instrumentation.[74] In a prospective study of 47 patients treated with decompression with posterior arthrodesis, Kornblum et al[70] reported substantially worse results in patients with pseudarthrosis compared with those with a solid fusion. Almost all of the patients in the SPORT study were treated with pedicle screw instrumentation, preventing a comparison between groups.[67] Based on the current literature, instrumentation has been shown to improve fusion results, and there is growing evidence that this improves clinical outcomes at long-term follow-up.

Degenerative Scoliosis

The surgical treatment of adult scoliosis that is refractory to nonsurgical management is challenging for surgeons. Several surgical options are available depending on the patient's symptoms and the degree and type of deformity. Decompression alone may be indicated for patients with stenotic or radicular symptoms and mild scoliosis. In patients with radiculopathy or neurogenic claudication, a relatively minor degree of scoliosis (less than 20°), and no anterolisthesis or rotatory listhesis, a limited decompressive procedure without concomitant fusion may be done.[75] Given the limited nature of the surgery, success is predicated on identifying the precise location of the neural compression responsible for the patient's symptoms. During decompression, meticulous care must be used to preserve the posterior stabilizing structures. Kelleher et al[51] reviewed the results of patients with and without deformity treated with minimally invasive decompression for lumbar spinal stenosis. The authors reported equivalent clinical results despite the presence of scoliosis; however, patients with lateral listhesis had a substantially higher rate of revision surgery.

Decompression and instrumented arthrodesis is usually required when treating patients with lumbar spinal stenosis with more advanced spinal deformity and coronal and sagittal plane imbalance. Arthrodesis may prevent progression of the deformity after the destabilizing effects of a laminectomy. Wide foraminal decompression may be needed, notably in the concavity of the curve, further destabilizing the deformity. Preoperative predictors of progression of scoliotic deformity include curves of greater magnitudes, rotatory listhesis (typically L3 or L4), abnormal motion in bending films, sagittal plane instabilities, and lumbar flatback.[76]

Decision making regarding the proper surgical technique for degenerative scoliosis is challenging. The surgeon should consider whether there is a need to include interbody fusions, fuse the entire scoliotic curve, or extend the fusion to the sacrum. The surgical goals should be to accomplish adequate decompression, maintain or restore spinal stability, and achieve spinal balance with adequate lordosis. The use of interbody fusion via either an anterior or a posterior approach may facilitate deformity correction and enhance fusion rates.[77] Tsai et al[78] retrospectively reviewed 58 patients treated with instrumented posterior lumbar interbody fusion for degenerative lumbar scoliosis and found a 72% patient satisfaction rate and good correction in coronal and sagittal balance.

Ideally, fusion should span the apex of any scoliosis. If the curve extends more proximally, or if there is advanced degeneration with kyphotic deformity in the upper lumbar spine, the fusion may need to be extended to the thoracic spine. Transfeldt et al[79] compared the outcomes of patients with scoliosis and lumbar spinal stenosis treated with decompression only, decompression with limited fusion, and decompression with full fusion. The authors found a 56% complication rate in the full fusion group versus 40% in the limited fusion group and 10% in the decompression-only group. Although significant Cobb angle correction (39° to 19°) and high patient satisfaction rates were achieved in the full fusion group, the Oswestry Disability Index score did not improve significantly. In the group treated with limited fusion, the Medical Outcomes 36-Item Short Form and the Oswestry Disability Index scores improved significantly. Revision surgeries were performed in 10% of the group treated with decompression only, with three repeat decompressions; 33% of the group was treated with limited fusion because of pseudarthrosis and wound-related issues; and 37% of the full fusion group was treated for pseudarthrosis, instrumentation revision, and wound-related issues. No adjacent segment degeneration was reported in any of the groups. Poor outcomes were related to sacrum-to-curve apex fusions and positive postoperative sagittal imbalance. Cho et al[80] also compared short fusions to long fusions in adult patients with scoliosis. Although significantly better Cobb angle correction was achieved in the long fusion group versus the short fusion group (22° to 6° versus 16° to 10°, respectively; P = 0.001), no difference in lordosis correction was reported between the groups. Adjacent-segment disease occurred in 36% of the group treated with short fusion compared with 23% of those treated with long fusion. Although a cutoff for the size of the Cobb angle was not clearly defined, the authors concluded that short fusion is sufficient for patients with a small Cobb angle and good spinal balance. Long fusion should be performed for patients with a severe Cobb angle and rotatory subluxation to minimize adjacent-segment disease.

Edwards et al[81] compared matched cohorts of adult scoliosis patients treated with fusion from the thoracic spine to either L5 or the sacrum. The authors concluded that long fusions to the sacrum improved sagittal balance but required more secondary surgical procedures and had a higher frequency of complications than fusions ending at L5. For fusions to L5, subsequent subadjacent disk degeneration was more common and associated with a forward shift in sagittal balance.

Instrumented arthrodesis procedures for the treatment of degenerative scoliosis have traditionally been associated with substantial complication risks, long surgical times, greater blood loss, and extended hospitalizations. Using the Scoliosis Research Society morbidity and mortality database, Sansur et al[82] retrospectively reviewed the complications of adult patients who had surgery for scoliosis; 4,980 cases were identified. The authors reported an overall complication rate of 13.4%, with no significant difference between patients with degenerative versus idiopathic scoliosis. Substantially higher complication rates were associated with osteotomies, revision surgery, and combined anterior-posterior approaches. In a retrospective review of 103 adult patients treated with long fusion from the thoracic spine to the pelvis for degenerative scoliosis, Howe et al[83] reported a 4% mortality rate, a 12% major complication rate, and a 35% rate of unplanned return to the operating room.

Minimally Invasive Lateral Interbody Fusion

Over the past decade, less invasive surgical approaches to neural decompression and fusion have been popularized and have recently been applied in the treatment of degenerative scoliosis. An example of this is the application of the less invasive lateral approach to the spine. The lateral interbody fusion procedure, using a minimally invasive retroperitoneal approach to the interbody space through the psoas muscle, has been reported in recent years. In general, the lumbar plexus and roots tend to reside in the posterior third of the psoas, so a transpsoas approach should ideally be within the anterior half of the psoas.[84] When traversing the psoas muscle, electromyographic monitoring is performed to assess the proximity of extraforaminal nerve roots and/or lumbar plexus traveling within the psoas muscle. After the dilator has traversed the psoas muscle to the interspace, sequential dilators are passed over the initial dilator, and the final retractor is placed (**Figure 2**). Electromyographic monitoring should be used throughout this approach to avoid nerve root injury. After placement of the retractor, the disk space is prepared and the interbody device is placed. Supplemental posterior fixation can then be performed.

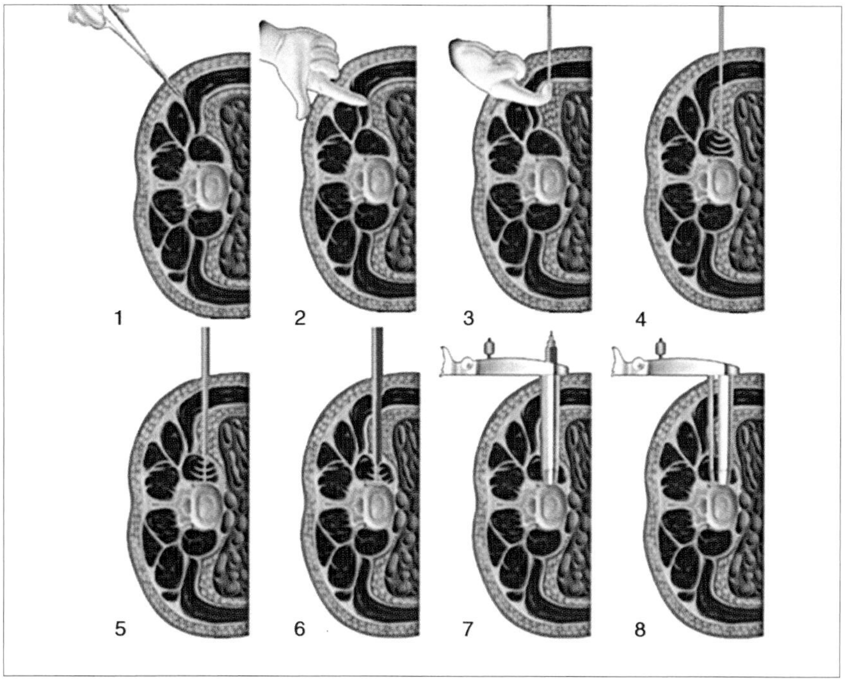

Figure 2 Diagrammatic representation of the sequential steps involved in the far lateral or transpsoas approach to the intervertebral disk space. (1) Incision in a lateral intermuscular space. (2) Blunt dissection into the retroperitoneal space. (3) Guidance of the far lateral approach (second skin incision) into the retroperitoneal space. (4 and 5) Diagrammatic representation of entry into the psoas muscle and electrophysiologic monitoring of the lumbar plexus during dilator placement and positioning. (6) Placement of a guidewire into the disk space. (7) Placement of the retractor around the dilators. (8) Expansion of the retractors and removal of the dilators to provide visualization of the disk space. (Courtesy of NuVasive, San Diego, CA.)

The lateral surgical approach for interbody fusion and deformity correction in the scoliotic spine can be more complicated than approaches used in degenerative spinal conditions. The anatomic variations, stiffness, rotary listhesis with aberrant position of the vasculature, and extensive osteophyte formation make attention to detail important. This approach relies on excellent intraoperative radiographic imaging to prevent neurologic or vascular injury. True lateral and AP radiographs are essential to guide the surgeon to the optimal trajectory to the interspace. Given the segmental deformities often seen in scoliosis, the operating table and fluoroscopy may need to be adjusted at each level to ensure optimal radiographic imaging. Using the widest interbody device possible that engages the stronger ring apophysis is recommended to avoid subsidence; lordotic cages are also recommended to restore or increase lordosis in patients with preoperative kyphosis.

Mundis et al[85] recommended approaching the spine from the concavity because this allows for soft-tissue release on the side of the spine that is contracted. Because the concavity is typically the site of foraminal narrowing, restoring the disk height from the concave side may improve foraminal height with indirect neural decompression. Access through the concavity decreases the number of incisions needed to treat the surgical levels (up to six levels through two small lateral incisions) and allows an easier approach to L4-5, where the iliac crest may otherwise obstruct access from the convexity. Positioning with the concavity up will also facilitate intraoperative reduction of the scoliotic curve through flexion of the operating table. Correction of the spinal deformity is enhanced by releasing the anulus fibrosus on the far side of the disk space; a Cobb elevator may be useful to facilitate this release and can be confirmed with fluoroscopy. Great care should be taken to avoid violation of the vertebral end plates to ensure that good disk space distraction is achieved by the interbody implant; this is particularly important in a patient with osteoporosis. Judicious use of fluoroscopy during diskectomy and end plate preparation may help reduce the risk of penetrating the end plates.

Anand et al[86] reported on 2-year follow-up of adult deformity correction with a MIS lateral interbody fusion technique and percutaneous screws posteriorly. The average blood loss was 241 mL for the anterior surgery and 231 mL for the posterior procedure. The coronal Cobb angle improved from 22° to 7° at final follow-up. The overall complication rate was 21%, which compared favorably with the rates of historic control subjects. Wang and Mummaneni[87] reported the results of their study of 23 patients with spinal deformity treated with a lateral MIS approach. The mean Cobb angle improved from 31.4° to 11.5° at the 13.5-month follow-up. The average blood loss was 477 mL. Complications occurred in 9 of 23 patients (39%), although the complications in 6 patients were transient, including thigh pain, dysesthesia, and paresthesias.

Dakwar et al[88] treated 25 patients for degenerative scoliosis with lateral interbody fusion. The overall complication rate was low, with rhabdomyolysis requiring hemodialysis in one patient, asymptomatic graft subsidence in one patient, and asymptomatic implant failure in one patient. Transient thigh numbness on the side of the approach developed in 3 of 25 patients (12%).

Isaacs et al[89] prospectively studied 107 patients treated with a lateral approach for degenerative scoliosis. Twenty-eight percent of the patients had at least one comorbidity. On average, 4.4 levels per patient (range, 1 to 9 levels) were treated. Supplemental pedicle screw fixation was used in 75.7% of the patients, 5.6% had lateral fixation, and 18.7% had standalone interbody fusion. The mean surgical time was 178 minutes, and blood loss was 50 to 100 mL. The mean hospital stay was 2.9 days for a single setting combined anterior-posterior surgery. Major complications occurred in 13 patients (12.1%); these included 2 (1.9%) medical and 12 (11.2%) surgical complications. Of the procedures that involved only less invasive techniques (lateral interbody stand-alone technique or percutaneous instrumentation), 9% of patients had one or more major complications, and 6.5% had transient leg pain and/or weakness. In those with supplemental open posterior instrumentation, 20.7% had one or more major complications.

Although initial data are promising, high-quality evidence for MIS treatment is lacking. Reports to date typically involve smaller curves. Additional comparative data, including larger curve magnitudes and sagittal inbalance, are needed before MIS treatments can be considered an equivalent alternative to standard procedures.

Summary

Lumbar spinal stenosis affects a large proportion of the aging population. A clearer understanding of the disease process has the potential to provide better preventive and medical treatment options and has led surgeons to more effective means of intervention. A broad spectrum of treatment options has been developed to address the wide range of disease severity and patient variables. Medical modalities, physical therapy, and injections are frequently used in the initial treatment of lumbar spinal stenosis, with varied results. When conservative measures fail, surgical treatment may be the best option in appropriately selected patients. In recent years, high-quality studies have supported the clinical and cost effectiveness of surgical intervention in this patient population. Recently, MIS techniques have been used in the treatment of patients with lumbar spinal stenosis, with and without associated spinal deformity. Long-term and comparative studies, however, are lacking. An understanding of a patient's comorbidities and expectations along with the surgeon's skills and experience should guide the selection of the optimal treatment choice.

References

1. Suri P, Rainville J, Kalichman L, Katz JN: Does this older adult

with lower extremity pain have the clinical syndrome of lumbar spinal stenosis? *JAMA* 2010; 304(23):2628-2636.

2. Boden SD, Davis DO, Dina TS, Patronas NJ, Wiesel SW: Abnormal magnetic-resonance scans of the lumbar spine in asymptomatic subjects: A prospective investigation. *J Bone Joint Surg Am* 1990; 72(3):403-408.
3. Watters WC III, Baisden J, Gilbert TJ, et al: Degenerative lumbar spinal stenosis: An evidence-based clinical guideline for the diagnosis and treatment of degenerative lumbar spinal stenosis. *Spine J* 2008;8(2):305-310.
4. Weinstein JN, Tosteson TD, Lurie JD, et al: Surgical versus nonsurgical therapy for lumbar spinal stenosis. *N Engl J Med* 2008; 358(8):794-810.
5. Yong-Hing K, Kirkaldy-Willis WH: The pathophysiology of degenerative disease of the lumbar spine. *Orthop Clin North Am* 1983;14(3):491-504.
6. Kalichman L, Suri P, Guermazi A, Li L, Hunter DJ: Facet orientation and tropism: Associations with facet joint osteoarthritis and degeneratives. *Spine (Phila Pa 1976)* 2009;34(16):E579-E585.
7. Wilby MJ, Fraser RD, Vernon-Roberts B, Moore RJ: The prevalence and pathogenesis of synovial cysts within the ligamentum flavum in patients with lumbar spinal stenosis and radiculopathy. *Spine (Phila Pa 1976)* 2009; 34(23):2518-2524.
8. Frymoyer JW, Selby DK: Segmental instability: Rationale for treatment. *Spine (Phila Pa 1976)* 1985;10(3):280-286.
9. Boden SD, Wiesel SW: Lumbosacral segmental motion in normal individuals: Have we been measuring instability properly? *Spine (Phila Pa 1976)* 1990;15(6): 571-576.
10. Fukuyama S, Nakamura T, Ikeda T, Takagi K: The effect of mechanical stress on hypertrophy of the lumbar ligamentum flavum. *J Spinal Disord* 1995;8(2): 126-130.
11. Kosaka H, Sairyo K, Biyani A, et al: Pathomechanism of loss of elasticity and hypertrophy of lumbar ligamentum flavum in elderly patients with lumbar spinal canal stenosis. *Spine (Phila Pa 1976)* 2007;32(25):2805-2811.
12. Sairyo K, Biyani A, Goel V, et al: Pathomechanism of ligamentum flavum hypertrophy: A multidisciplinary investigation based on clinical, biomechanical, histologic, and biologic assessments. *Spine (Phila Pa 1976)* 2005;30(23): 2649-2656.
13. Park JB, Lee JK, Park SJ, Riew KD: Hypertrophy of ligamentum flavum in lumbar spinal stenosis associated with increased proteinase inhibitor concentration. *J Bone Joint Surg Am* 2005;87(12):2750-2757.
14. Borenstein DG, O'Mara JW Jr, Boden SD, et al: The value of magnetic resonance imaging of the lumbar spine to predict low-back pain in asymptomatic subjects: A seven-year follow-up study. *J Bone Joint Surg Am* 2001; 83(9):1306-1311.
15. Rydevik BL, Pedowitz RA, Hargens AR, Swenson MR, Myers RR, Garfin SR: Effects of acute, graded compression on spinal nerve root function and structure: An experimental study of the pig cauda equina. *Spine (Phila Pa 1976)* 1991;16(5):487-493.
16. Delamarter RB, Bohlman HH, Dodge LD, Biro C: Experimental lumbar spinal stenosis: Analysis of the cortical evoked potentials, microvasculature, and histopathology. *J Bone Joint Surg Am* 1990;72(1):110-120.
17. Kang JD, Georgescu HI, McIntyre-Larkin L, Stefanovic-Racic M, Donaldson WF III, Evans CH: Herniated lumbar intervertebral discs spontaneously produce matrix metalloproteinases, nitric oxide, interleukin-6, and prostaglandin E2. *Spine (Phila Pa 1976)* 1996;21(3): 271-277.
18. O'Donnell JL, O'Donnell AL: Prostaglandin E2 content in herniated lumbar disc disease. *Spine (Phila Pa 1976)* 1996;21(14): 1653-1656.
19. Rihn JA, Lee JY, Khan M, et al: Does lumbar facet fluid detected on magnetic resonance imaging correlate with radiographic instability in patients with degenerative lumbar disease? *Spine (Phila Pa 1976)* 2007;32(14):1555-1560.
20. Whitman JM, Flynn TW, Childs JD, et al: A comparison between two physical therapy treatment programs for patients with lumbar spinal stenosis: A randomized clinical trial. *Spine (Phila Pa 1976)* 2006;31(22):2541-2549.
21. American College of Rheumatology Ad Hoc Group on Use of Selective and Nonselective Nonsteroidal Antiinflammatory Drugs: Recommendations for use of selective and nonselective nonsteroidal antiinflammatory drugs: An American College of Rheumatology white paper. *Arthritis Rheum* 2008;59(8):1058-1073.
22. Yaksi A, Ozgönenel L, Ozgönenel B: The efficiency of gabapentin therapy in patients with lumbar spinal stenosis. *Spine (Phila Pa 1976)* 2007;32(9):939-942.
23. Eskola A, Alaranta H, Pohjolainen T, Soini J, Tallroth K, Slätis P: Calcitonin treatment in lumbar spinal stenosis: Clinical observations. *Calcif Tissue Int* 1989; 45(6):372-374.
24. Eskola A, Pohjolainen T, Alaranta H, Soini J, Tallroth K, Slätis P: Calcitonin treatment in lumbar spinal stenosis: A randomized, placebo-controlled, double-blind, cross-over study with one-year

follow-up. *Calcif Tissue Int* 1992; 50(5):400-403.

25. Porter RW, Miller CG: Neurogenic claudication and root claudication treated with calcitonin: A double-blind trial. *Spine (Phila Pa 1976)* 1988;13(9):1061-1064.
26. Podichetty VK, Segal AM, Lieber M, Mazanec DJ: Effectiveness of salmon calcitonin nasal spray in the treatment of lumbar canal stenosis: A double-blind, randomized, placebo-controlled, parallel group trial. *Spine (Phila Pa 1976)* 2004;29(21):2343-2349.
27. Tafazal SI, Ng L, Sell P: Randomised placebo-controlled trial on the effectiveness of nasal salmon calcitonin in the treatment of lumbar spinal stenosis. *Eur Spine J* 2007;16(2):207-212.
28. Ng L, Chaudhary N, Sell P: The efficacy of corticosteroids in periradicular infiltration for chronic radicular pain: A randomized, double-blind, controlled trial. *Spine (Phila Pa 1976)* 2005; 30(8):857-862.
29. Botwin KP, Gruber RD, Bouchlas CG, et al: Fluoroscopically guided lumbar transformational epidural steroid injections in degenerative lumbar stenosis: An outcome study. *Am J Phys Med Rehabil* 2002;81(12):898-905.
30. Delport EG, Cucuzzella AR, Marley JK, Pruitt CM, Fisher JR: Treatment of lumbar spinal stenosis with epidural steroid injections: A retrospective outcome study. *Arch Phys Med Rehabil* 2004;85(3):479-484.
31. Weinstein JN, Tosteson TD, Lurie JD, et al: Surgical versus nonoperative treatment for lumbar spinal stenosis four-year results of the Spine Patient Outcomes Research Trial. *Spine (Phila Pa 1976)* 2010;35(14):1329-1338.
32. Kovacs FM, Urrútia G, Alarcón JD: Surgery versus conservative treatment for symptomatic lumbar spinal stenosis: A systematic review of randomized controlled trials. *Spine (Phila Pa 1976)* 2011; 36(20):E1335-E1351.
33. Iguchi T, Kurihara A, Nakayama J, Sato K, Kurosaka M, Yamasaki K: Minimum 10-year outcome of decompressive laminectomy for degenerative lumbar spinal stenosis. *Spine (Phila Pa 1976)* 2000; 25(14):1754-1759.
34. Jakola AS, Sørlie A, Gulati S, Nygaard OP, Lydersen S, Solberg T: Clinical outcomes and safety assessment in elderly patients undergoing decompressive laminectomy for lumbar spinal stenosis: A prospective study. *BMC Surg* 2010; 10:34.
35. Lee CK: Lumbar spinal instability (olisthesis) after extensive posterior spinal decompression. *Spine (Phila Pa 1976)* 1983;8(4): 429-433.
36. Fu YS, Zeng BF, Xu JG: Long-term outcomes of two different decompressive techniques for lumbar spinal stenosis. *Spine (Phila Pa 1976)* 2008;33(5): 514-518.
37. Fox MW, Onofrio BM, Onofrio BM, Hanssen AD: Clinical outcomes and radiological instability following decompressive lumbar laminectomy for degenerative spinal stenosis: A comparison of patients undergoing concomitant arthrodesis versus decompression alone. *J Neurosurg* 1996;85(5): 793-802.
38. Mullin BB, Rea GL, Irsik R, Catton M, Miner ME: The effect of postlaminectomy spinal instability on the outcome of lumbar spinal stenosis patients. *J Spinal Disord* 1996;9(2):107-116.
39. Lee MJ, Bransford RJ, Bellabarba C, et al: The effect of bilateral laminotomy versus laminectomy on the motion and stiffness of the human lumbar spine: A biomechanical comparison. *Spine (Phila Pa 1976)* 2010;35(19):1789-1793.
40. Rahman M, Summers LE, Richter B, Mimran RI, Jacob RP: Comparison of techniques for decompressive lumbar laminectomy: The minimally invasive versus the "classic" open approach. *Minim Invasive Neurosurg* 2008;51(2): 100-105.
41. Costa F, Sassi M, Cardia A, et al: Degenerative lumbar spinal stenosis: Analysis of results in a series of 374 patients treated with unilateral laminotomy for bilateral microdecompression. *J Neurosurg Spine* 2007;7(6):579-586.
42. Guiot BH, Khoo LT, Fessler RG: A minimally invasive technique for decompression of the lumbar spine. *Spine (Phila Pa 1976)* 2002;27(4):432-438.
43. Weiner BK, Walker M, Brower RS, McCulloch JA: Microdecompression for lumbar spinal canal stenosis. *Spine (Phila Pa 1976)* 1999;24(21):2268-2272.
44. Bresnahan L, Ogden AT, Natarajan RN, Fessler RG: A biomechanical evaluation of graded posterior element removal for treatment of lumbar stenosis: Comparison of a minimally invasive approach with two standard laminectomy techniques. *Spine (Phila Pa 1976)* 2009;34(1): 17-23.
45. Hamasaki T, Tanaka N, Kim J, Okada M, Ochi M, Hutton WC: Biomechanical assessment of minimally invasive decompression for lumbar spinal canal stenosis: A cadaver study. *J Spinal Disord Tech* 2009;22(7):486-491.
46. Yagi M, Okada E, Ninomiya K, Kihara M: Postoperative outcome after modified unilateral-approach microendoscopic midline decompression for degenerative spinal stenosis. *J Neurosurg Spine* 2009; 10(4):293-299.
47. Thomé C, Zevgaridis D, Leheta O, et al: Outcome after less-invasive decompression of lumbar spinal stenosis: A randomized comparison of unilateral lamin-

otomy, bilateral laminotomy, and laminectomy. *J Neurosurg Spine* 2005;3(2):129-141.

48. Sasai K, Umeda M, Maruyama T, Wakabayashi E, Iida H: Microsurgical bilateral decompression via a unilateral approach for lumbar spinal canal stenosis including degenerative spondylolisthesis. *J Neurosurg Spine* 2008;9(6): 554-559.
49. Pao JL, Chen WC, Chen PQ: Clinical outcomes of microendoscopic decompressive laminotomy for degenerative lumbar spinal stenosis. *Eur Spine J* 2009;18(5): 672-678.
50. Khoo LT, Fessler RG: Microendoscopic decompressive laminotomy for the treatment of lumbar stenosis. *Neurosurgery* 2002;51 (5, suppl):S146-S154.
51. Kelleher MO, Timlin M, Persaud O, Rampersaud YR: Success and failure of minimally invasive decompression for focal lumbar spinal stenosis in patients with and without deformity. *Spine (Phila Pa 1976)* 2010;35(19):E981-E987.
52. Ikuta K, Arima J, Tanaka T, et al: Short-term results of microendoscopic posterior decompression for lumbar spinal stenosis: Technical note. *J Neurosurg Spine* 2005; 2(5):624-633.
53. Ikuta K, Tono O, Tanaka T, et al: Surgical complications of microendoscopic procedures for lumbar spinal stenosis. *Minim Invasive Neurosurg* 2007;50(3): 145-149.
54. Richards JC, Majumdar S, Lindsey DP, Beaupré GS, Yerby SA: The treatment mechanism of an interspinous process implant for lumbar neurogenic intermittent claudication. *Spine (Phila Pa 1976)* 2005;30(7):744-749.
55. Lindsey DP, Swanson KE, Fuchs P, Hsu KY, Zucherman JF, Yerby SA: The effects of an interspinous implant on the kinematics of the instrumented and adjacent levels in the lumbar spine. *Spine (Phila Pa 1976)* 2003;28(19):2192-2197.
56. Swanson KE, Lindsey DP, Hsu KY, Zucherman JF, Yerby SA: The effects of an interspinous implant on intervertebral disc pressures. *Spine (Phila Pa 1976)* 2003;28(1):26-32.
57. Wilke HJ, Drumm J, Häussler K, Mack C, Steudel WI, Kettler A: Biomechanical effect of different lumbar interspinous implants on flexibility and intradiscal pressure. *Eur Spine J* 2008;17(8):1049-1056.
58. Wiseman CM, Lindsey DP, Fredrick AD, Yerby SA: The effect of an interspinous process implant on facet loading during extension. *Spine (Phila Pa 1976)* 2005;30(8): 903-907.
59. Zucherman JF, Hsu KY, Hartjen CA, et al: A multicenter, prospective, randomized trial evaluating the X STOP interspinous process decompression system for the treatment of neurogenic intermittent claudication: Two-year follow-up results. *Spine (Phila Pa 1976)* 2005;30(12):1351-1358.
60. Richter A, Schütz C, Hauck M, Halm H: Does an interspinous device (Coflex) improve the outcome of decompressive surgery in lumbar spinal stenosis? One-year follow up of a prospective case control study of 60 patients. *Eur Spine J* 2010;19(2):283-289.
61. Sobottke R, Schlüter-Brust K, Kaulhausen T, et al: Interspinous implants (X Stop, Wallis, Diam) for the treatment of LSS: Is there a correlation between radiological parameters and clinical outcome? *Eur Spine J* 2009;18(10):1494-1503.
62. Barbagallo GM, Olindo G, Corbino L, Albanese V: Analysis of complications in patients treated with the X-Stop Interspinous Process Decompression System: Proposal for a novel anatomic scoring system for patient selection and review of the literature. *Neurosurgery* 2009;65(1): 111-120.
63. Verhoof OJ, Bron JL, Wapstra FH, van Royen BJ: High failure rate of the interspinous distraction device (X-Stop) for the treatment of lumbar spinal stenosis caused by degenerative spondylolisthesis. *Eur Spine J* 2008;17(2):188-192.
64. Bowers C, Amini A, Dailey AT, Schmidt MH: Dynamic interspinous process stabilization: Review of complications associated with the X-Stop device. *Neurosurg Focus* 2010;28(6):E8.
65. Burnett MG, Stein SC, Bartels RH: Cost-effectiveness of current treatment strategies for lumbar spinal stenosis: Nonsurgical care, laminectomy, and X-STOP. *J Neurosurg Spine* 2010;13(1): 39-46.
66. Herkowitz HN, Kurz LT: Degenerative lumbar spondylolisthesis with spinal stenosis: A prospective study comparing decompression with decompression and intertransverse process arthrodesis. *J Bone Joint Surg Am* 1991;73(6): 802-808.
67. Weinstein JN, Lurie JD, Tosteson TD, et al: Surgical compared with nonoperative treatment for lumbar degenerative spondylolisthesis: Four-year results in the Spine Patient Outcomes Research Trial (SPORT) randomized and observational cohorts. *J Bone Joint Surg Am* 2009;91(6):1295-1304.
68. Weinstein JN, Lurie JD, Tosteson TD, et al: Surgical versus nonsurgical treatment for lumbar degenerative spondylolisthesis. *N Engl J Med* 2007;356(22):2257-2270.
69. Hatta Y, Shiraishi T, Sakamoto A, et al: Muscle-preserving interlaminar decompression for the lumbar spine: A minimally invasive new procedure for lumbar spinal canal stenosis. *Spine (Phila Pa 1976)* 2009;34(8):E276-E280.

70. Kornblum MB, Fischgrund JS, Herkowitz HN, Abraham DA, Berkower DL, Ditkoff JS: Degenerative lumbar spondylolisthesis with spinal stenosis: A prospective long-term study comparing fusion and pseudarthrosis. *Spine (Phila Pa 1976)* 2004;29(7):726-734.

71. Fischgrund JS, Mackay M, Herkowitz HN, Brower R, Montgomery DM, Kurz LT: Degenerative lumbar spondylolisthesis with spinal stenosis: A prospective, randomized study comparing decompressive laminectomy and arthrodesis with and without spinal instrumentation. *Spine (Phila Pa 1976)* 1997;22(24):2807-2812.

72. Thomsen K, Christensen FB, Eiskjaer SP, Hansen ES, Fruensgaard S, Bünger CE: The effect of pedicle screw instrumentation on functional outcome and fusion rates in posterolateral lumbar spinal fusion: A prospective, randomized clinical study. *Spine (Phila Pa 1976)* 1997;22(24): 2813-2822.

73. Christensen FB, Stender Hansen E, Laursen M, Thomsen K, Bünger CE: Long-term functional outcome of pedicle screw instrumentation as a support for posterolateral spinal fusion: Randomized clinical study with a 5-year follow-up. *Spine (Phila Pa 1976)* 2002;27(12):1269-1277.

74. Andersen T, Christensen FB, Niedermann B, et al: Impact of instrumentation in lumbar spinal fusion in elderly patients: 71 patients followed for 2-7 years. *Acta Orthop* 2009;80(4):445-450.

75. San Martino A, D'Andria FM, San Martino C: The surgical treatment of nerve root compression caused by scoliosis of the lumbar spine. *Spine (Phila Pa 1976)* 1983;8(3):261-265.

76. Korovessis P, Piperos G, Sidiropoulos P, Dimas A: Adult idiopathic lumbar scoliosis: A formula for prediction of progression and review of the literature. *Spine (Phila Pa 1976)* 1994;19(17): 1926-1932.

77. Jagannathan J, Sansur CA, Oskouian RJ Jr, Fu KM, Shaffrey CI: Radiographic restoration of lumbar alignment after transforaminal lumbar interbody fusion. *Neurosurgery* 2009;64(5):955-964.

78. Tsai TH, Huang TY, Lieu AS, et al: Functional outcome analysis: Instrumented posterior lumbar interbody fusion for degenerative lumbar scoliosis. *Acta Neurochir (Wien)* 2011;153(3):547-555.

79. Transfeldt EE, Topp R, Mehbod AA, Winter RB: Surgical outcomes of decompression, decompression with limited fusion, and decompression with full curve fusion for degenerative scoliosis with radiculopathy. *Spine (Phila Pa 1976)* 2010;35(20):1872-1875.

80. Cho KJ, Suk SI, Park SR, et al: Short fusion versus long fusion for degenerative lumbar scoliosis. *Eur Spine J* 2008;17(5):650-656.

81. Edwards CC II, Bridwell KH, Patel A, Rinella AS, Berra A, Lenke LG: Long adult deformity fusions to L5 and the sacrum: A matched cohort analysis. *Spine (Phila Pa 1976)* 2004;29(18): 1996-2005.

82. Sansur CA, Smith JS, Coe JD, et al: Scoliosis research society morbidity and mortality of adult scoliosis surgery. *Spine (Phila Pa 1976)* 2011;36(9):E593-E597.

83. Howe CR, Agel J, Lee MJ, et al: The morbidity and mortality of fusions from the thoracic spine to the pelvis in the adult population. *Spine (Phila Pa 1976)* 2011; 36(17):1397-1401.

84. Park DK, Lee MJ, Lin EL, Singh K, An HS, Phillips FM: The relationship of intrapsoas nerves during a transpsoas approach to the lumbar spine: Anatomic study. *J Spinal Disord Tech* 2010;23(4): 223-228.

85. Mundis GM, Akbarnia BA, Phillips FM: Adult deformity correction through minimally invasive lateral approach techniques. *Spine (Phila Pa 1976)* 2010; 35(26, suppl):S312-S321.

86. Anand N, Rosemann R, Khalsa B, Baron EM: Mid-term to long-term clinical and functional outcomes of minimally invasive correction and fusion for adults with scoliosis. *Neurosurg Focus* 2010; 28(3):E6.

87. Wang MY, Mummaneni PV: Minimally invasive surgery for thoracolumbar spinal deformity: Initial clinical experience with clinical and radiographic outcomes. *Neurosurg Focus* 2010; 28(3):E9.

88. Dakwar E, Cardona RF, Smith DA, Uribe JS: Early outcomes and safety of the minimally invasive, lateral retroperitoneal transpsoas approach for adult degenerative scoliosis. *Neurosurg Focus* 2010; 28(3):E8.

89. Isaacs RE, Hyde J, Goodrich JA, Rodgers WB, Phillips FM: A prospective, nonrandomized, multicenter evaluation of extreme lateral interbody fusion for the treatment of adult degenerative scoliosis: Perioperative outcomes and complications. *Spine (Phila Pa 1976)* 2010;35(26, suppl): S322-S330.

SECTION

7

Pediatrics

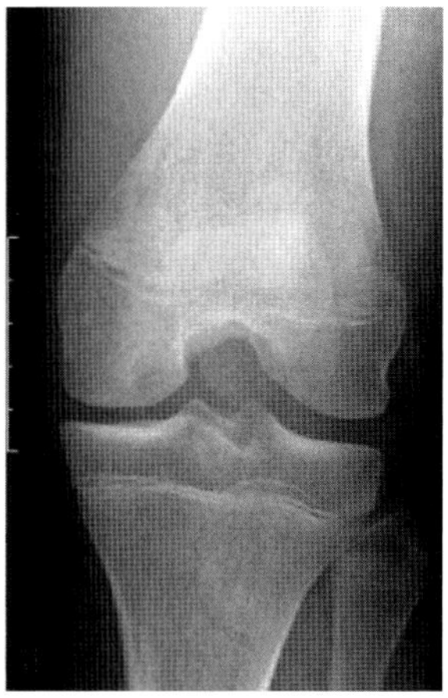

Symposium
35 Orthopaedic Aspects of Child Abuse

Symposium
36 Hip Septic Arthritis and Other Pediatric Musculoskeletal Infections in the Era of Methicillin-Resistant *Staphylococcus aureus*

Symposium
37 Advances in Hip Preservation After Slipped Capital Femoral Epiphysis

Symposium
38 Approach to the Pediatric Supracondylar Humeral Fracture With Neurovascular Compromise

39 Shoulder Instability in the Young Athlete

40 Patellofemoral Instability in Skeletally Immature Athletes

DVD **41** Juvenile Osteochondritis Dissecans of the Knee: Current Concepts in Diagnosis and Management

35

SYMPOSIUM

Orthopaedic Aspects of Child Abuse

Keith D. Baldwin, MD, MPH
Susan A. Scherl, MD

Abstract

Child abuse is one of the most serious problems encountered by on-call orthopaedic surgeons. There are adverse sequelae to both overdiagnosing and underdiagnosing this condition. Orthopaedic surgeons generally manage orthopaedic aspects of child abuse but should be aware of the associated injuries, diagnoses, prognoses, and natural history of abuse. Because fractures are the second most common presenting injury in children after skin lesions, orthopaedic surgeons are often on the front lines of treatment. No specific fracture is pathognomonic of child abuse, although some patterns, such as posterior rib fractures, metaphyseal corner fractures, and fractures in various stages of healing, are highly suggestive of abuse. Although metabolic bone disease is much rarer than child abuse, the child should be tested so treatment can be initiated, if needed, or for the purpose of demonstrating due diligence in the event of court proceedings. A diagnosis of child abuse is an understandably contentious issue; therefore, orthopaedic surgeons should be aware of injury patterns and differential diagnoses.

Instr Course Lect 2013;62:399-403.

Child abuse and neglect or nonaccidental injury in children is a common occurrence. The diagnosis is clinical and has implications for the medical, legal, and social management of the child. The diagnosis can be difficult to make for both clinical and interpersonal reasons. The literature can be confusing and may result in misperception and misdiagnosis by the clinician. There are serious consequences for the child in both overdiagnosing and underdiagnosing child abuse and neglect. As such, many centers are moving toward a multidisciplinary model to diagnose and treat this condition. Although many attempts have been made to identify fracture patterns common to abuse, no radiographic findings or fracture patterns are pathognomonic of child abuse and neglect. Although it is impossible to determine by radiographic findings alone if a child is the victim of abuse or neglect, some fractures and fracture patterns have high specificity for abuse.

Background

Battered child syndrome was first described by Kempe et al[1] in 1962. The authors based their description of the syndrome on fractures, skin bruising, and subdural hematomas. They estimated that 25% of fractures in children younger than 1 year and 10% to 15% of fractures in children younger than 3 years were the result of child abuse.[1] As a result of this report and others, since 1967, all 50 states have instituted mandatory reporting laws for suspected child abuse. Each year, 3.3 million cases of child abuse and neglect affecting 6 million children are reported, and 2 million of these cases (62%) are deemed to merit investigation.[2] Twenty-five percent of the reports are substantiated,[2] which translates to an abuse rate of 10/1,000 children in the United States. Overall, there are 702,000 unique victims per year. In 2009, there were 1,770 fatalities or 2.3 fatalities per 100,000 children. Almost one third (32%) of the victims are younger than 4 years; however, 81% of fatalities occur in children in this age group.[2] Eighty percent of the perpetrators are the victim's parents, 7% are relatives other than the

Dr. Baldwin or an immediate family member owns stock or stock options in Pfizer. Dr. Scherl or an immediate family member serves as a board member, owner, officer, or committee member of the American Academy of Orthopaedic Surgeons, the Orthopaedic Trauma Association, and the Pediatric Orthopaedic Society of North America and receives royalties from UptoDate and Lippincott.

parents, 54% are women, and 80% are 20 to 49 years old. A skeletal injury is sustained in 10% to 70% of abused children, and 30% to 50% of abused children are referred to an orthopaedic surgeon for consultation.[2]

Nonorthopaedic Injuries

Neglected and abused children may have several types of nonorthopaedic injuries. The most common physical injuries are skin lesions (bruises, scrapes, and burns), with fractures the second most common presenting injury.[3] Some nonorthopaedic injuries can cause more long-term damage than fractures. Emotional and sexual abuses are among the most sinister types of abuses. Sexual abuse is estimated to occur in 10% of neglected and abused children. Failure to thrive or malnutrition may be manifestations of child neglect. In addition to fractures, clinicians must be aware of soft-tissue injuries, burns, soft-tissue trauma, or subdural hemorrhages (such as shaken baby syndrome).[1]

Soft-tissue injuries, such as bruises, welts, laceration, and bites, are the most common manifestations of abuse.[3] These injuries will often be clustered and in the shape of the object that was used to strike the child. These injuries will be located in areas that would be atypical for accidental injury, such as the back, buttocks, or mucosal surfaces.[3] Burns can be in the form of cigarette burns, typically to the palms of the hands or the soles of the feet. Immersions or scalding burns may be present. When these injuries are identified, they are believed to represent severe abuse because of the premeditation involved. Internal injuries may be present, particularly in very young children with immature skeletons. These can be injuries to the abdominal viscera or wall and must be differentiated from injuries resulting from an automotive child restraint. One entity that bears special mention is shaken baby syndrome; this condition is characterized by subdural hematoma, retinal hemorrhage, and posterior rib fractures.[1,4] Shaken baby syndrome is important to identify because of the potential for catastrophic outcomes if the clinical triad is missed.

Fractures

Child abuse and neglect become increasingly likely as the etiology of a fracture in younger children. Although 50% of fractures secondary to abuse occur in children younger than 1 year, a fracture in a child in that age group does not necessarily indicate that abuse has occurred.[4] No particular fracture pattern, location, or morphology is pathognomonic of abuse. Fracture patterns (such as spiral, transverse, and buckle) can indicate the direction of mechanical force (bending, torsion, and compression) but not the etiology of that mechanical force.

However, some findings show a high propensity for an abusive etiology. Among these are posterior rib fractures, metaphyseal corner fractures, complex skull fractures, and long-bone fractures in children who have not yet learned to walk. Bilateral acute fractures and multiple fractures in various stages of healing are believed to represent suspicious injuries.[5] Isolated long-bone fractures, simple skull fractures, and clavicle fractures are believed to have less specificity for an abusive etiology.

A single transverse fracture is the most common long-bone fracture seen in abused children.[6] This pattern occurs in approximately 13% of victims. King et al[6] reported that the humerus is the most frequently fractured bone in abused children, followed by the tibia and then the femur. However, in a study of a group of patients who had accidental trauma, the tibia was more commonly injured in abuse than the femur or humerus.[7] Pierce et al[8] developed an injury plausibility model for femoral fractures resulting from falls on stairs. They found that transverse fractures were more suspicious than spiral fractures and believed the injury was more suspicious if the parent was unable to consistently describe the child's final position after the fall when relating the patient history.[8] Baldwin et al[9] produced a similar model, which found that a patient history suspicious for abuse, multiple injuries, and a patient younger than age 18 months were predictive of an abusive etiology 92.3% of the time. Schwend et al[10] studied 139 children younger than 4 years. They reported that 13 children (9%) were likely abused, and only 3 of those children were ambulatory. More than 50% of the referrals to child protective services in that study were deemed unnecessary. They concluded that, without substantiating evidence, a femoral fracture in a walking child is unlikely to be the result of abuse.[10]

Examinations

History and Physical Examination

The history and physical examination can provide important clues to the etiology of an injury, particularly in suspicious circumstances. It is important to ask or be aware of the answers to some vital questions. What is the caretaker's account of the injury? Was the injury witnessed? Does the story given to the physician differ from that given to emergency medical technicians or emergency room doctors? What is the caretaker's attitude toward the child and medical personnel? What is the child's demeanor? Are other social mitigating factors involved?[4,11,12]

The physical examination of the child can be challenging, particularly in situations involving an infant who cannot provide information. The child must be examined from head to toe, with particular attention to any deformities, evidence of burns, bruises, or other injuries, especially in locations where accidental trauma is unlikely. A careful neurovascular examination must be administered, as well as an eye examination if shaken baby syndrome is suspected. In certain circumstances, a genitourinary examination should be considered, although subspecialty consultation is appropriate in these situations.

Radiologic Examination

A thorough radiologic examination is critical if child abuse or neglect is suspected. The involved bone must be adequately imaged for both documentation and treatment purposes. AP and lateral views of the involved extremity are mandatory.[5] The clinician should also consider other radiologic modalities, both for diagnostic and potentially therapeutic reasons.

A skeletal survey is often recommended if child abuse or neglect is suspected. This survey consists of AP and lateral views of the skull and chest, lateral views of the spine, AP views of the pelvis and the long bones of the extremities and feet, PA oblique views of the hands, and additional views in at least two projections if there are abnormal findings.[5] A single AP radiograph of the entire infant is not acceptable because the detail is insufficient, and it does not provide standard interpretable views of the extremities.[5] A skeletal survey is mandatory in cases of suspected abuse when the child is younger than 2 years, and it is highly recommended in any child younger than 1 year with a fracture, a child with extensive fractures, a child with a history of one or more fractures, or a child with a personal or family history of fragile bones.[13] On skeletal survey, 50% of abused children will have a single fracture, 21% will have two fractures, 12% will have three fractures, and 17% will have more than three fractures.[6] It is important to be aware that a skeletal survey will not show some fractures. Rib fractures are often difficult to detect. It is estimated that only 36% of rib fractures are detected with a skeletal survey. Because rib fractures become apparent later when callus begins to form,[14] the skeletal survey should be repeated in 2 weeks if there is a high suspicion of child abuse. This later survey is also useful to date injuries. When evaluating a skeletal survey, the clinician must keep in mind that early in the healing process, between days 2 and 10, resolution of soft-tissue injuries generally occur. Starting at day 4 and peaking at days 10 to 14, periosteal new bone forms. This is followed by a loss of fracture definition, which peaks at 2 to 3 weeks after injury. Soft callus forms during this time frame as well, followed by hard callus, which peaks at 3 to 4 weeks after injury and is followed by remodeling, which occurs over a period of years.[15]

In certain circumstances, ultrasound can be useful to detect acute subperiosteal hemorrhages if radiographs are normal but the clinical examination suggests a fracture. Occult, long-bone fractures and costochondral injuries also can be detected with ultrasound.[5] Bone scans may be used in the acute setting if plain radiographs are negative. Difficulty arises when fractures are near growth plates because of the increased baseline blood flow in these areas.[5] Bone scans may be overly sensitive in patients with infection or nontraumatic increased blood flow to the bone.

Differential Diagnoses

Injuries resulting from metabolic bone disease and inherited conditions causing fragile bones can be mistaken for child abuse and neglect. Osteogenesis imperfecta (OI), rickets, renal disease, the adverse effects on bone from medications (such as corticosteroids or seizure medicines), or disuse osteopenia from a condition that limits or prevents ambulation (such as cerebral palsy) can be among the differential diagnoses for fragile bones.[16,17] Very young children may have birth trauma or Caffey disease, which is a painful, self-limiting condition in patients younger than 1 year. Mandibular involvement is characteristic of Caffey disease and is unusual in nonaccidental injuries.

Metabolic bone disease can be difficult to differentiate from child abuse and neglect because fractures in pathologic bone can mimic highly specific fractures resulting from abuse. However, child abuse and neglect is much more common (10/1,000 children) than a condition such as OI (1/20,000 children). A detailed workup for metabolic bone disease is useful because it potentially decreases the number of erroneous abuse reports, allows treatment if metabolic bone disease is diagnosed, and provides documentation if the case goes to trial and the possibility of the condition is raised in court.

A metabolic workup starts with a history and physical examination. Patients with OI can present with blue tinted sclera, dental abnormalities, or hearing problems. Babies with rickets tend to have poor muscle tone and are small and generally floppy. There is often noticeable genu varum in toddlers with rickets and exaggerated genu valgum in slightly older patients with rickets. Children with rickets may also have poor dentition. Other conditions, such as seizures or cerebral palsy, will be apparent from the history or physical examination. A suspicious history of injuries should always prompt an investigation because patients with metabolic bone disease may also be victims of abuse. It should be noted that a patient history and physical examination have a low predictive value for metabolic bone disease.[16] Most cases of OI are the result of de novo mutation.[16]

Laboratory, radiologic, and genetic studies can confirm or rule out the diagnosis of metabolic bone disease. Blood urea nitrogen and creatinine can be used to assess kidney function and determine whether brittle bones are secondary to renal disease. Alkaline phosphatase, serum calcium, and phosphate levels are useful to assess the metabolic state of the bone and may be altered in conditions such as uremia, hyperparathyroidism, and rickets. Vitamin D levels should be obtained if rickets are suspected.

Plain radiographs can provide clues regarding bone disorders causing severely brittle bones. Children with rickets characteristically have widened physes, and those with severe OI may have physes that appear disorganized. Patients taking bisphosphonate therapy for brittle bones may have zebra lines adjacent to bone physes. Dual-energy x-ray absorptiometry scans can be useful in diagnosing OI. The bones of children with this condition almost universally show decreased bone mineral density. The establishment of standards to reliably demonstrate this decreased bone density is being investigated. Current recommendations are to obtain two dual-energy x-ray absorptiometry studies 4 to 6 months apart. In that time frame, these studies will typically show an increase in bone density in children who do not have metabolic bone syndrome, whereas no increase in bone density will be shown in children with OI.

Genetic testing is useful but tends to have a high rate of false negative results. Fibroblast culturing has a 15% false-negative rate, and DNA testing has a 5% false-negative rate. These rates seem low; however, when it is considered that the incidence of child abuse and neglect is approximately 20 times the rate of OI, the value of a negative test is limited. As such, these tests are helpful if positive; but if negative, they do not effectively rule out OI.

Medicolegal Issues

Most fractures that result from child abuse can be managed nonsurgically. However, the nebulousness of the diagnosis of child abuse and neglect and the serious consequences for patients and families of overdiagnosing or underdiagnosing the condition presents difficulties for orthopaedic surgeons. Few studies address this conundrum.[17] Pandya et al[17] reported on studies that directly compared injuries that were mistaken for child abuse but were later discredited.[18,19] A recent study of 61 patients who were misdiagnosed as abused or neglected but who actually had OI showed that 88% had clinical or radiographic signs of OI, but the condition was confirmed by DNA or skin biopsy in only 50% of the patients.[16] Some major issues identified by this study were that confirmatory tests take weeks to months to be processed, and findings from the history and physical examination are soft and inconclusive. The mandate of the rule of law is to err on the side of protecting the child. Some experts believe that children with OI and other chronic illnesses are more likely to be abused than healthy children, although the literature does not support or refute this theory.

All physicians must report suspected child abuse and neglect. The physician has no liability for an erroneous report made in good faith; however, reports may not be retracted after they are made. Many tertiary centers have multidisciplinary teams to deal with suspected child abuse and neglect. These teams consist of social workers, pediatricians, radiologists, geneticists, and other specialists. These teams are tailored to identify and report child abuse if suspected.

It is important to remember there is a difference between testifying in court as an expert and as a treating physician. Experts provide opinions, whereas a treating physician may testify only regarding his or her examination observations and the care given. The opposing side will dwell on the issue of absolute versus reasonable certainty. For example, unless an instance of suspected nonaccidental injury has been directly witnessed by the person testifying, he or she cannot be absolutely certain that it did not occur from a fall or other injury mechanism. However, in a child who has an injury with a high specificity for abuse and an unconvincing explanation regarding how the injury occurred, the testifying witness can be reasonably certain of a nonaccidental injury mechanism. If a metabolic workup has been done with no diagnosis of metabolic bone disease, this line of questioning by the attorney is closed. Additional lines of questioning are usually related to falls. The defense will inquire about the possibility that the injury resulted from a fall. Data show that a fall from a household height results in a long-bone fracture in 1 in 750 occurrences.[20]

Summary

Child abuse is a clinical diagnosis based on the patient's history and physical examination and radiographic findings. No particular fracture is pathognomonic for abuse, although certain injury patterns are highly suggestive of abuse as the mechanism of injury. Transverse long-bone fractures are more common than spiral fractures in cases of abuse. An isolated radiograph will not confirm or refute whether a child was the victim of abuse. Long-bone fractures in nonambulatory children are always suspicious; therefore, the physician should consider a workup for the presence of metabolic bone disease.

A multidisciplinary team is best equipped to manage and diagnose child abuse. Orthopaedic surgeons and other physicians involved in the care of the child should work as the child's advocate and rule out other potential conditions if a diagnosis of child abuse is being considered. Institutional resources are invaluable in the triage of this socially complex condition.

References

1. Kempe CH, Silverman FN, Steele BF, Droegemueller W, Silver HK: The battered-child syndrome. *JAMA* 1962;181(1):17-24.
2. US Department of Health & Human Services, Administration for Children and Families: *Child Maltreatment* 2009. http://www.acf.hhs.gov/programs/cb/pubs/cm09/cm09.pdf. Accessed March 15, 2012.
3. McMahon P, Grossman W, Gaffney M, Stanitski C: Soft-tissue injury as an indication of child abuse. *J Bone Joint Surg Am* 1995; 77(8):1179-1183.
4. Kocher MS, Kasser JR: Orthopaedic aspects of child abuse. *J Am Acad Orthop Surg* 2000;8(1): 10-20.
5. Diagnostic imaging of child abuse. *Pediatrics* 2000;105(6): 1345-1348.
6. King J, Diefendorf D, Apthorp J, Negrete VF, Carlson M: Analysis of 429 fractures in 189 battered children. *J Pediatr Orthop* 1988; 8(5):585-589.
7. Pandya NK, Baldwin K, Wolfgruber H, Christian CW, Drummond DS, Hosalkar HS: Analysis at a level I pediatric trauma center. *J Pediatric Orthop* 2009;29(6): 618-625.
8. Pierce MC, Bertocci GE, Janosky JE, et al: Femur fractures resulting from stair falls among children: An injury plausibility model. *Pediatrics* 2005;115(6):1712-1722.
9. Baldwin K, Pandya N, Wolfgruber H, Drummond D, Hosalkar H: Femur fractures in the pediatric population: Abuse or accidental trauma? *Clin Orthop Relat Res* 2011;469(3):798-804.
10. Schwend RM, Werth C, Johnston A: Femur shaft fractures in toddlers and young children: Rarely from child abuse. *J Pediatr Orthop* 2000;20(4):475-481.
11. Akbarnia BA, Akbarnia NO: The role of orthopedist in child abuse and neglect. *Orthop Clin North Am* 1976;7(3):733-742.
12. Lane WG, Dubowitz H: What factors affect the identification and reporting of child abuse-related fractures? *Clin Orthop Relat Res* 2007;461:219-225.
13. Ludwig S: *Pediatric Emergency Medicine*, ed 5. Philadelphia, PA, Lippincott Williams & Wilkins, 2006, p 1761.
14. Kleinman PK, Schlesinger AE: Mechanical factors associated with posterior rib fractures: Laboratory and case studies. *Pediatr Radiol* 1997;27(1):87-91.
15. Kleinman P, : *Diagnostic Imaging of Child Abuse*. Baltimore, MD, Williams & Wilkins, 1987, p 112.
16. Singh K M, Dichtel L: Osteogenesis imperfecta misdiagnosed as child abuse. *J Pediatr Orthop B* 2011;20(6):440-443.
17. Pandya NK, Baldwin K, Kamath AF, Wenger DR, Hosalkar HS: Unexplained fractures: Child abuse or bone disease? A systematic review. *Clin Orthop Relat Res* 2011;469(3):805-812.
18. Lang C: Unexplained fractures: Child abuse or bone disease. A systematic review. *Clin Orthop Relat Res* 2011;469(11):3253-3254.
19. Karst WA: Letter to the editor: Unexplained fractures. Child abuse or bone disease: A systematic review. *Clin Orthop Relat Res* 2011;469(9):2654-2655.
20. Helfer RE, Slovis TL, Black M: Injuries resulting when small children fall out of bed. *Pediatrics* 1977;60(4):533-535.

36

SYMPOSIUM

Hip Septic Arthritis and Other Pediatric Musculoskeletal Infections in the Era of Methicillin-Resistant *Staphylococcus aureus*

Martin J. Morrison III, MD
Martin J. Herman, MD

Abstract

Pediatric musculoskeletal infections can cause devastating complications (including death) in this era of methicillin-resistant Staphylococcus aureus *and other virulent bacterial strains. The complexity and severity of these infections require timely diagnosis and treatment. A thorough emergency department evaluation, diagnostic workup, and early surgical intervention can influence outcomes. Septic arthritis of the hip is best treated with open drainage and antibiotic therapy to avoid osteonecrosis of the hip and joint damage. Because of genetic changes and inducible resistance, methicillin-resistant* Staphylococcus aureus *causes more complex infections than in the past. Deep, soft-tissue abscesses; pyomyositis; osteomyelitis; and septic arthritis often occur concurrently, causing destruction of musculoskeletal tissue. Severe and life-threatening complications, such as septic emboli, deep venous thrombosis, and multiorgan system failure may result from these infections.*

Instr Course Lect 2013;62:405-414.

Musculoskeletal infections in children pose treatment challenges to caregivers and are associated with potentially serious complications. A variety of pathologies and presentations within different age groups, from neonates to adolescents, can cause difficulties in making an accurate and timely diagnosis. Sequelae of a delayed or missed diagnosis may have a great effect on the child.[1] Specialists from many fields, including primary care, pediatric emergency medicine, orthopaedic surgery, infectious diseases, radiology, and critical care, play a vital role in the diagnosis and treatment of musculoskeletal infections and in preventing associated morbidity and mortality. This chapter discusses the modern concepts of hip septic arthritis in children and the emerging trends surrounding soft-tissue infections caused by methicillin-resistant *Staphylococcus aureus* (MRSA). Emphasis is placed on patient evaluation in the emergency department, an efficient diagnosis, and the practical management of children presenting with potentially serious musculoskeletal infections in the era of drug-resistant bacteria that are more invasive and destructive than pathogens of the past.

Hip Septic Arthritis

Hip septic arthritis is a potentially devastating musculoskeletal infection of childhood that most commonly affects children younger than 5 years.[2] Hip septic arthritis usually results from hematogenous bacteria that infiltrate and infect the hip joint, but it may be caused by the spread of contiguous bacterial infections of soft tissue, muscle, and bone. Bacterial enzymes and the child's inflammatory response to the infection directly damage hip cartilage and potentially result in chondrolysis within as few as 6 to 12 hours of

Dr. Herman or an immediate family member serves as a board member, owner, officer, or committee member of the American Academy of Orthopaedic Surgeons and the Pediatric Orthopaedic Society of North America. Neither Dr. Morrison nor any immediate family member has received anything of value from or owns stock in a commercial company or institution related directly or indirectly to the subject of this chapter.

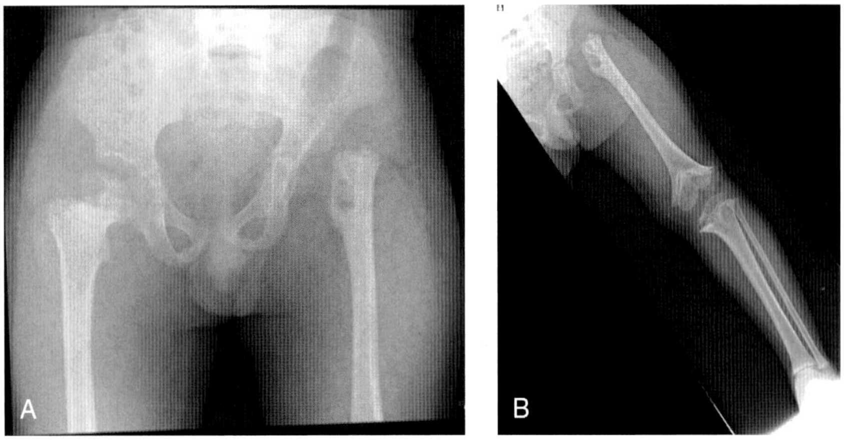

Figure 1 AP radiographic images of the pelvis (**A**) and left lower extremity (**B**) of a 5-year-old boy showing sequelae of a delay in the diagnosis of multifocal methicillin-sensitive *S aureus* (MSSA) osteomyelitis and septic arthritis. Note the extensive deformity of the hip and knee joints secondary to sepsis.

Table 1
Top Differential Diagnoses for Hip Septic Arthritis Based on Etiology

Etiology	Differential Diagnosis
Trauma	Fracture (consider child abuse)
	Slipped capital femoral epiphysis
Other infections	Toxic synovitis
	Myositis
	Osteomyelitis
Malignancy	Soft-tissue sarcoma
	Leukemia
Inflammatory	Juvenile idiopathic arthritis
	Lyme disease
Osteonecrosis	Legg-Calvé-Perthes disease
	Sickle cell anemia

exposure to pus. The hip, unlike other joints, is also affected by the increase in intracapsular pressure that occurs in association with hip septic arthritis. This increase in pressure may lead to osteonecrosis of the proximal femur and damage to the hip chondroepiphysis, resulting in abnormalities of hip development or joint destruction. A prolonged increase in intracapsular pressure can lead to capsular distension, which can cause hip joint instability over time. In extreme cases, systemic illness and even death can result from septic arthritis of the hip, especially in neonates, immunocompromised children, and patients who are diagnosed late. Early diagnosis, open surgical hip drainage, and antibiotic therapy lead to successful outcomes for most children with septic arthritis.[3]

Clinical Presentation

A child with a septic hip may present to the emergency department with a wide range of clinical symptoms. The list of potential diagnoses is extensive. A systematic and efficient diagnostic approach is needed because a long delay in diagnosing a septic hip can have serious consequences (**Figure 1**).The workup of a child presenting to the emergency department with hip irritability, refusal to bear weight, or limp starts with a thorough and focused history. Although a history of antecedent trauma may lead the clinical examination toward a traumatic etiology of the pain, septic arthritis must still be included in the differential diagnoses. Respiratory or other recent infections should alert the practitioner to other possible infectious causes, particularly viral illnesses. Other worrisome clinical findings include the presence of a fever greater than 38.5°C for more than 24 hours, a more prolonged complaint of pain, and systemic findings such as lethargy or a lack of eating or drinking. Clues to MRSA colonization may be elicited by a history of skin lesions, boils, or "bug or spider" bites.

A careful physical examination is mandatory; positive findings may vary based on the child's age. General irritability; pseudoparalysis of the lower extremity; or holding the hip in flexion, abduction, and external rotation may be the only signs of a septic hip in a newborn. Fever, tenderness, and limited hip range of motion are not always seen in children in this age range. Toddlers and school-age children typically present with a fever and either a limp or a refusal to bear weight on the affected limb. Guarded hip range of motion, particularly with passive internal rotation and extension, are common findings. For children of all ages, palpation of the entire extremity; the pelvis, including the sacroiliac joints; and the lumbar spine is crucial for detecting areas of swelling or tenderness. The most important differential diagnoses to consider are fractures and musculoskeletal infections, such as toxic synovitis of the hip (**Table 1**).

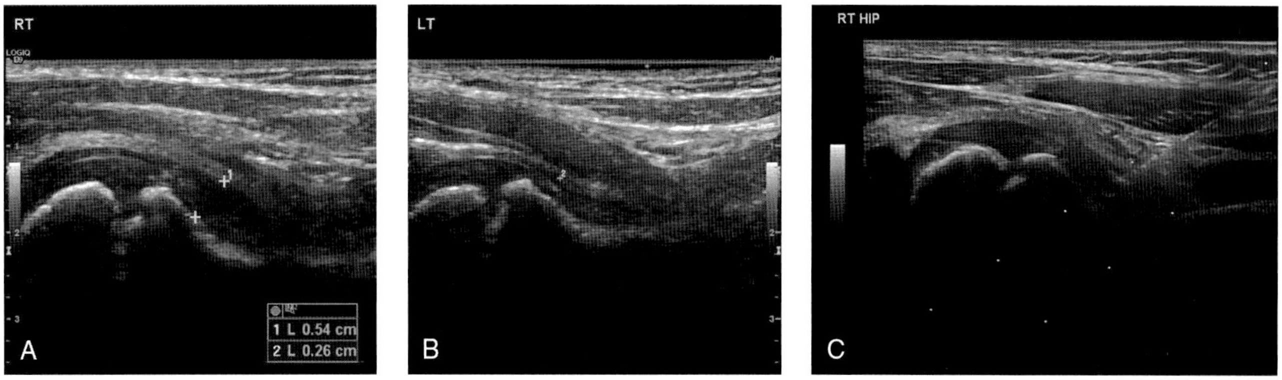

Figure 2 Sagittal ultrasound images of septic right hip (**A**), with comparison image of the uninvolved left hip (**B**). Note effusion quantified by on-image markers determining the distance between the hip capsule and femoral metaphysis, a measure of the amount of fluid in the hip joint. **C,** Sagittal ultrasound image of the septic right hip during ultrasound-guided aspiration. The hyperechoic area on the right side of the image shows the oblique path of entry of the aspiration needle.

Diagnostic Tests

Imaging

At the time of the initial evaluation of any child with a suspected septic hip, radiographs should be obtained of the entire affected limb and pelvis. Fractures, bone tumors, signs of infection, and other abnormalities can be ascertained from a careful examination of high-quality radiographs. Findings suggestive of septic arthritis include blurring of the periarticular fat pad and an increase in hip joint space greater than 2 mm compared with the contralateral side.[4] Normal radiographic findings, however, are common in children with septic arthritis.

Ultrasound plays the most important role in imaging septic arthritis of the hip, with a sensitivity as high as 95% for detecting excessive fluid in the hip joint.[5] Ultrasound evaluation of the child's hip is somewhat user-dependent, can be misleading if bilateral hips are involved because frequently the "well" hip is imaged first to determine the "normal" appearance of the hip, and is sometimes unable to detect small fluid accumulations seen early in the course of the disease. Ultrasound-guided aspiration of the joint may be done at the time of the initial diagnostic evaluation; only local anesthetic or limited sedation of the child is usually needed[6] (**Figure 2**).

MRI with contrast is the best imaging modality for evaluating children when the diagnosis is not clear from radiographic and ultrasound findings or if there is a high suspicion for contiguous musculoskeletal infections or infections that do not involve the hip joint directly but cannot be clinically differentiated from septic arthritis.[7] This chapter's authors believe that the rise of increasingly more virulent infections requires that almost all children diagnosed with hip septic arthritis be evaluated with MRI to rule out associated infections of bone or muscle that may alter the surgical management or the duration of antibiotic therapy after hip drainage.[8]

Laboratory Tests

A complete blood count, erythrocyte sedimentation rate (ESR), C-reactive protein (CRP) level, and blood cultures are needed for any child with suspected septic arthritis of the hip. An elevation of the white blood cell (WBC) count, elevation of the ESR greater than approximately 30 mm/h, and elevation of the CRP level of 2 mg/dL are findings that, at St. Christopher's Hospital for Children in Philadelphia, signal concern for septic arthritis of the hip in a child with fever, hip pain, and an effusion diagnosed on ultrasound. Care must be taken to note the units used by individual laboratories when reporting CRP levels because some levels are reported in mg/L. The criteria of Kocher et al,[9] however, are the best method for differentiating a child with a septic hip from one with toxic synovitis. An analysis of the fluid aspirated from the affected hip is helpful in the diagnosis. Cloudy fluid and a positive Gram stain (seen in 50% of the patients), and more than 50,000 to 75,000 WBCs/mm³ are important indicators of a septic hip. Blood and hip aspirate cultures are positive in approximately 50% of patients with septic arthritis of the hip. This information is useful for selecting antibiotics but does not aid in the initial diagnosis because laboratory analysis of the cultures takes approximately 24 hours.

Toxic Synovitis Versus Septic Arthritis

Kocher et al[9] developed an algorithm to aid in the diagnosis of septic arthritis of the hip. The algorithm predicts the likelihood of septic arthritis versus transient synovitis based on several independent clinical factors: the inability

Table 2
Differentiating Septic Arthritis From Toxic Synovitis: Factors to Consider

Factor	Parameter
Temperature	> 38.6°C
WBC count	> 12,000 cells/mL
ESR	> 40 mm/h
Weight-bearing status	Inability to bear weight
CRP level	> 2.0 mg/dL

to bear weight, a temperature greater than 38.5°C, a WBC count greater than 12,000 cells/mm³, and an ESR greater than 40 mm/h. These factors have become known as the Kocher criteria. When all four criteria are present, septic arthritis was diagnosed in 99.6% of patients versus 93.1% in whom three of four factors were present, 40.0% in whom two of four were present, 3.0% in whom one of four was present, and 0.2% with no predictors present. Some authors have disputed the use of these criteria,[10,11] but subsequent studies have corroborated the findings.[12,13]

The CRP level, not considered in Kocher's original work, was subsequently introduced into the diagnostic algorithm. Levine et al[14] used the CRP level as a screening tool to rule out septic arthritis in patients. The CRP level was found to have a high negative predictive value when it was less than 1.0 mg/dL. In their study, Caird et al[13] applied the Kocher criteria with the addition of CRP. Although the authors confirmed that CRP level and ESR were both important independent predictors of septic arthritis, they deemed the CRP level to be a stronger independent predictor. When a CRP level greater than 2.0 mg/dL was added as a factor to the Kocher criteria, findings were similar to those established in Kocher's 1999 study. The presence of all five factors resulted in a 97.5% chance of septic arthritis, four of five factors indicated a 93.1% chance, three of five an 82.6% chance, two of five a 62.4% chance, and one of five a 36.7% chance (**Table 2**).

Treatment

Antibiotics

After blood cultures have been drawn and the hip has been aspirated, antibiotic administration can begin. If the diagnosis is equivocal and the child is not systemically ill with signs of sepsis, antibiotics may be withheld while the child is observed for 6 to 12 hours in the hospital if other tests, such MRI or bone scans, will be obtained. Parenteral antibiotics that provide a broad spectrum of coverage for the most common organism that causes septic arthritis in that patient's age group are given (**Table 3**).[15] *S aureus* is the most common causative organism in septic arthritis.[16] The next most common bacteria include group A β-hemolytic Streptococcus, *Streptococcus pneumoniae*, and *Enterobacter*.[2,16] Septic arthritis caused by *Haemophilus influenzae* has been almost eliminated since the introduction of the *H influenzae* type b vaccine.[2,16] There has been a recent increase in infections cause by MRSA and *Kingella kingae* (likely because of improved culture techniques and media).[2,16] The ideal empiric antibiotic regimen takes into account past positive regional and institutional cultures and sensitivities and is adjusted based on bacterial culture results from serum, aspirate, and surgical samples.

Open Drainage of Septic Arthritis

The treatment for all children with presumed hip septic arthritis is open drainage.[2] An anterior Smith-Peterson approach is most commonly used. After making a slightly oblique incision approximately 2 to 4 cm parallel to the inguinal ligament and approximately 1 to 2 cm distal to it over the hip joint, the interval between the tensor fascia lata and sartorius is divided, and the lateral border of the rectus femoris is identified. The rectus femoris is then dissected laterally, exposing the hip capsule. An incision is made in the capsule (ideally over the femoral neck), and a small window of capsular tissue is removed to ensure that the drainage portal remains open. The joint fluid is cultured, and the joint is then vigorously irrigated. Closure over a drain, which is sewn in for later removal, is performed, and a sterile dressing is applied.

The drain may be removed after drainage has slowed substantially or has ceased, typically 1 to 2 days after surgery. The child's temperature, comfort level, joint range of motion, and serum CRP level should be carefully monitored while parenteral antibiotics are administered. Most children show clinical improvement and diminution of the CRP level within 2 to 4 days of open drainage. Repeat ultrasound or MRI and repeat surgical interventions may be warranted if there is minimal clinical improvement. The duration of antibiotic administration varies based on many factors, including the infecting organism, the extent of the infection, and the postoperative clinical course; however, it is typically administered for 7 to 14 days, first parenterally, then orally.

Table 3
Empiric Antibiotic Recommendations for Pediatric Musculoskeletal Infections

Age Group	Antibiotic	Dose (mg/kg)	Route	Frequency
Pediatric and adolescent patients	Clindamycin	10	IV	Every 6 hours
	Clindamycin	8	PO	Every 8 hours
	Vancomycin[a]	15	IV	Every 6 hours, initially[b,c]
	Rifampin[d]	10	IV or PO	Every 24 hours
Neonatal (younger than 1 month)	Ampicillin/sulbactam	150	IV	Every 6 hours
	Gentamicin[e]	2	IV	Every 8 hours[b]
Neonatal (to 3 months)	Vancomycin[e]	15	IV	Every 6 hours, initially[b,c]
	Ceftriaxone[e]	100	IV	Every 24 hours

IV = intravenous, PO = oral
[a]Recommended for suspected sepsis or severe infection.
[b]Peak and trough measured after third dose.
[c]Target peak, 45 µg/mL; target trough, 15 µg/mL.
[d]Used in conjunction with vancomycin in cases of osteomyelitis.
[e]Recommended in combination.

Serial Aspiration

Serial aspiration has been used as an alternative to open drainage for septic arthritis of the hip. No studies have directly compared the benefits of serial aspirations with open irrigation and débridement. Proponents of less invasive methods have argued that morbidity and hospital stays are reduced with serial aspiration, which still provides the benefits of joint decontamination and decompression.

Givon et al[17] performed serial, ultrasound-guided aspirations on 34 children with hip septic arthritis. In the 34 children with septic hips, 6 required surgery because of a clogged or dislodged needle. The remaining 28 children were managed with serial aspirations, and 24 were successfully treated with serial aspirations alone. Four hips were subsequently treated with open arthrotomy because of a failure to improve. Overall, no complications were reported. In the children treated with surgical débridement, none had poor outcomes despite the delay before open treatment.

Pääkkönen et al[18] reported on 62 consecutive patients with septic hip arthritis who were treated initially with serial hip aspiration. After analysis of the clinical and laboratory responses, only 12 patients required a formal arthrotomy; many of those patients had contiguous osteomyelitis. This chapter's authors believe that this method requires more careful study before it is considered an option equivalent to open drainage for children with hip septic arthritis. Serial aspiration is not recommended at this time.

Recent Trends

In a 2011 study, Griffet et al[19] described a technique using percutaneous aspiration, irrigation, and débridement to treat septic arthritis in children. Nineteen of 52 patients (36%) with septic arthritis had septic hips. All were treated with fluoroscopically assisted aspiration with an indwelling catheter and subsequent irrigation. All of the children were immobilized during the irrigation and drainage period. The authors reported that their technique resulted in successful outcomes with complete resolution of symptoms in all but one patient. One patient had intermittent pain and no associated decreased range of motion.

Harel et al[20] reported on a randomized, double-blinded, placebo-controlled study in which dexamethasone (0.15 mg/kg every 6 hours for 4 days) was administered to children with septic arthritis of the hip. Although the authors do not recommend the administration of steroids in the face of fulminant infection, it should be emphasized that in this study all of the septic hips were treated with antibiotics and open surgical drainage and/or serial aspirations in addition to steroid administration. When compared with placebo, the treatment group had a shorter duration of fever, fewer local inflammatory signs, a quicker return to a normal ESR, a shorter period of parenteral antibiotic administration, and a shorter hospital stay.

Arthroscopic Drainage

As early as 1993, Chung et al[21] reported excellent outcomes in older children and adolescents treated with arthroscopic lavage for hip septic arthritis. More recently, El-Sayed[22] compared arthroscopic débridement with open surgery. All of the patients had excellent outcomes, and those treated

Table 4
The Rise of Community-Acquired MRSA: Studies From the Pediatric Orthopaedic Literature

Study (Year)	Findings
Arnold et al[26] (2006)	10-fold increase in MRSA infections; 91% of MRSA infections required surgery.
Gafur et al[23] (2008)	2.8-fold increase in osteomyelitis, 30% of all infections cultured MRSA, and high incidence of contiguous infection.
Vander Have et al[25] (2009)	26% of MRSA patients had deep venous thrombosis or septic emboli, 15% of patients with MRSA had multiorgan failure, and 100% of patients with MRSA infections required surgery.

with arthroscopic débridement had a shorter hospital stay. This chapter's authors believe that arthroscopic lavage of the hip for children with hip septic arthritis is a reasonable option for surgeons who are skilled in hip arthroscopy and have appropriately sized equipment to perform this procedure effectively and safely in children. However, it may be difficult to organize appropriate equipment and personnel to perform hip arthroscopy emergently in some institutions.

Emerging Concepts

In a large study of musculoskeletal infections at one institution, which repeated a similar study from 25 years prior, Gafur et al[23] reported two important emerging concepts about septic arthritis in children. Although the incidence of septic arthritis has not changed over a 20-year period, the causative organisms are different. Culture-proven MRSA septic arthritis, which was not reported in the prior era, is now commonplace and accounts for a substantial percentage of staphylococcal-related septic arthritis. More importantly, septic arthritis now often occurs with contiguous infections, including osteomyelitis, pyomyositis, and soft-tissue abscesses. These contiguous infections result from MRSA and virulent methicillin-sensitive *Staphylococcus* species. Modern era infections from these organisms have also resulted in more frequent and serious complications.[23]

Methicillin-Resistant *S aureus*

In the 1990s, hospital-acquired MRSA became an important pathogen. Musculoskeletal infections caused by hospital-acquired MRSA were problematic because of the bacteria's resistance to common drugs, such as penicillin and cephalosporin. The virulence and complications of these infections, however, were not substantially different from methicillin-sensitive *S aureus* (MSSA) infections identified and treated during the same time period. At the turn of the 21st century, however, new strains of these resistant pathogens were identified that were primarily acquired in the community rather than in the hospital.[24,25] These new strains of community-acquired MRSA, like hospital-acquired MRSA, possess the *mecA* gene cassette, which conveys the organism's resistance to β-lactam antibiotics.[24,25] More importantly, community-acquired MRSA, unlike hospital-acquired MRSA, is also capable of producing powerful tissue cytotoxins, the end product of Panton-Valentine leukocidin (*pvl*) genes,[24,25] among others, which cause musculoskeletal infections capable of tissue invasion, destruction, and complications that had not been previously seen. The advent of these so-called superbugs has changed the approach to musculoskeletal infections in children.

Several US centers have reported a rise in the number of infections, an increase in the extent of tissue damage, a greater need for surgical management, and more severe complications associated with the increase in community-acquired MRSA isolates in these centers[23,25,26] (**Table 4**). Extensive, concurrent infections of joints, bones, muscles, and soft tissues are more common and may require multiple surgical débridements (**Figure 3**). Previously, uncommon complications, such as deep venous thrombosis (DVT), septic pulmonary emboli, and multiorgan system failure, were reported with an unexpectedly high frequency at all of these centers (**Figure 4**).

Vander Have et al[25] called community-acquired MRSA a game changer. Because of community-acquired MRSA, this chapter's authors have revised several aspects of care for children with musculoskeletal infections. Four important changes have evolved, including the need for a thorough emergency department evaluation, a more important role for surgical management, the implementation of more complex antibiotic regimens, and increased active surveillance of complications secondary to MRSA infections.

Emergency Department Evaluation

A thorough emergency department evaluation is now more crucial because the initial presentation of musculoskeletal infections varies from child to child and from organism to organism. Subtle signs of systemic illness other

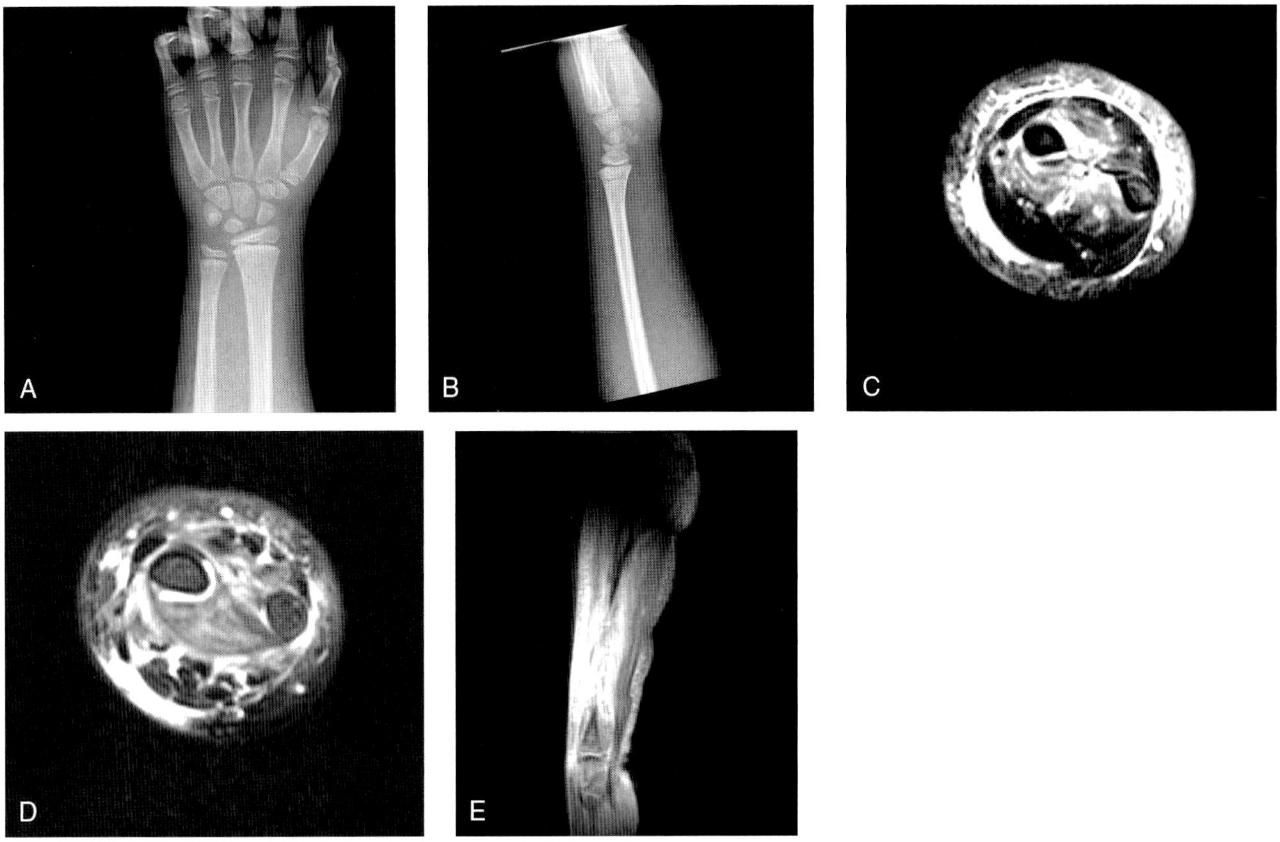

Figure 3 AP (**A**) and lateral (**B**) radiographs of the left wrist of a 7-year-old girl transferred to St. Christopher's Hospital for Children in Philadelphia with a 2-day history of left wrist pain and fever up to 103.1°F. Examination revealed severe swelling and erythema of her entire left forearm, with diffuse tenderness of the entire forearm and upper arm. The radiographs are significant for soft-tissue swelling without signs of bony involvement or periosteal reaction. Subsequent T2-weighted axial MRI (**C** and **D**) and sagittal (**E**) images of the left forearm show extensive cellulitis, myositis, and subperiosteal abscess about the radius. The patient required emergent surgery to treat distal radius community-acquired MRSA osteomyelitis with contiguous pyomyositis. Multiple surgical débridements and skin grafting were needed.

than an elevated temperature, such as sustained tachycardia or mild hypotension, must be considered potential signs of serious illness even if the initial clinical findings are minimal. A history of an insect bite or pustules on the skin combined with painful cellulitis and limb tenderness that extends beyond the area of cellulitis is a scenario that is concerning for an MRSA infection. At St. Christopher's Hospital for Children in Philadelphia, children who present with any of these emergency department findings are admitted to the hospital (some to the intensive care unit) for observation, the administration of antibiotics, and further imaging studies.

Ju et al[27] attempted to differentiate MRSA from MSSA osteomyelitis using parameters at the time of the patient's hospital admission. A temperature greater than 38°C, a hematocrit level less than 34%, a WBC count greater than 12,000 cells/mm³, and a CRP level greater than 1.3 mg/dL were parameters that were correlated with a predictive value. MRSA osteomyelitis was diagnosed in 92% of children with all four findings. A 45% predictive value was reported with three of four findings, 10% with two of four findings, 1% with one of four findings, and 0% when no criterion was present. It is important to note, however, that regardless of the predictive values determined by any algorithm, the diagnosis of serious musculoskeletal infections must be made with a high index of suspicion based on a careful and thorough patient evaluation, a review of imaging findings, and analysis of laboratory studies.

The Role of Surgery

Surgical treatment now has a more important role because the virulence of the infecting organisms causes tissue damage that often can be treated only with débridement. Gafur et al[23] reported that there is a hierarchy of severity of tissue involvement, with severity in the following decreasing order: osteomyelitis, septic arthritis,

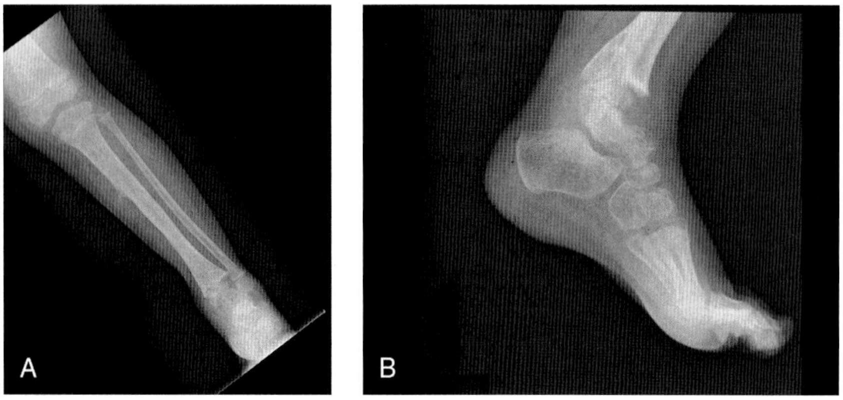

Figure 4 AP radiograph (**A**) of the left tibia and lateral radiograph (**B**) of the left ankle of a 4-year-old girl 2 years after treatment for extensive MRSA myositis and osteomyelitis of the left leg and septic arthritis of the left ankle. These images show extensive changes to the distal tibia and avascular changes of the talus. During treatment, septic emboli were found, and the patient required care in the intensive care unit for 3 weeks and ventilatory support for 1 week. Seven surgical débridements were performed during the patient's hospitalization.

pyomyositis, and abscess. More importantly, modern infections are often complicated by contiguous tissue involvement in addition to the primary sites of infection. An MRI with contrast is important for surgical planning because it can determine the full extent of the infection. Serial débridements are increasingly needed to drain pus and remove devitalized tissue.

Complex Antibiotic Regimens

More complex antibiotic regimens are necessary for empiric coverage on admission because of the rise of bacterial resistance. Reasonable recommendations for antibiotic coverage are shown in **Table 3**.[23] Antibiotic regimens, however, are best established locally from isolates previously identified in other patients in the community or ideally from cultures and sensitivities of the patient being treated. Although *Staphylococcus* and *Streptococcus* species remain the most common pathogens, community-acquired MRSA and MSSA, in particular, require drug combinations to ensure broad coverage. Vancomycin remains the most effective drug to treat MRSA. At St. Christopher's Hospital for Children in Philadelphia, vancomycin is used as empiric treatment only in children who have systemic sepsis or severe infections on admission; these limitations on use are an attempt to prevent overuse of the drug and the development of resistance over time. Clindamycin, in combination with another agent, is the primary choice for empiric treatment of most musculoskeletal infections based on the 2010 antibiogram of this chapter's authors. Because some *Staphylococcus* species may develop an inducible resistance to clindamycin, the D-test must be performed on all isolates to ensure that, despite an initial sensitivity to clindamycin, the organism does not become resistant to it with exposure.[28] The D-test entails plating the *Staphylococcus* isolate on Mueller-Hinton agar. Antibiotic disks (clindamycin and erythromycin) are used for disk diffusion testing. Each is placed 15 mm from the center of the plate and analyzed after incubation for 18 hours at 35°C. A negative D-test is illustrated by two circular zones of inhibition for 13 mm or greater around the erythromycin and 21 mm or greater for the clindamycin. If a circular zone of 13 mm or less is apparent around the erythromycin, but a D-shaped zone 21 mm or greater around the clindamycin appears, then the D-test is positive for inducible clindamycin resistance. Antibiotic choices should be made in consultation with a pediatric infectious disease service in nearly all cases.

Active Surveillance for Complications

Active surveillance for complications secondary to MRSA infections is required to improve outcomes for the child. Limb swelling or focal cord-like tenderness, either near the site of intravenous catheters or away from them, may be signs of DVT. In one study, DVT developed in one third of patients with osteomyelitis and another contiguous infection.[23] Doppler ultrasound studies are best for diagnosing DVT; treatment with anticoagulants may be appropriate for some patients.

Shortness of breath, chest pains, or decreasing oxygen saturation as determined by pulse oximetry or the analysis of blood gases may indicate the development of septic emboli. Although many children are managed only with supplemental oxygen, in some extreme situations, ventilator support is necessary. This chapter's authors recommend the use of a multidisciplinary care team in an intensive care setting for any child who has or is at risk for the development of these complications.

Multiorgan system failure, limb amputation, and death are also known complications of serious MRSA infections.[29] Patients and families must be informed of the potential for devastating outcomes in children with severe MRSA infections.

Summary

Published studies and the experiences of this chapter's authors have confirmed an increase in the severity of many pediatric musculoskeletal infections over the past decade. Community-acquired MRSA, with drug resistance and increased virulence from *pvl* genes, has radically changed the treatment of these infections. A careful clinical evaluation to establish a diagnosis and effective early treatment provides the best chance for successful outcomes. Surgical treatment now plays a vital role in managing all pediatric musculoskeletal infections. An understanding of the bacteriology of these infections allows the surgeon, in consultation with an infectious disease specialist, to choose the most effective antibiotic regimens. Multidisciplinary care of the child with a severe infection provides the best opportunity for identifying and treating complications such as DVT and septic emboli. Patients, families, and caregivers must be made aware of the potential for devastating outcomes from modern pediatric infections despite appropriate management.

References

1. Forlin E, Milani C: Sequelae of septic arthritis of the hip in children: A new classification and a review of 41 hips. *J Pediatr Orthop* 2008;28(5):524-528.
2. McCarthy JJ, Dormans JP, Kozin SH, Pizzutillo PD: Musculoskeletal infections in children: Basic treatment principles and recent advancements. *Inst Course Lect* 2005;54:515-528.
3. Choi IH, Pizzutillo PD, Bowen JR, Dragann R, Malhis T: Sequelae and reconstruction after septic arthritis of the hip in infants. *J Bone Joint Surg Am* 1990; 72(8):1150-1165.
4. Jung ST, Rowe SM, Moon ES, Song EK, Yoon TR, Seo HY: Significance of laboratory and radiologic findings for differentiating between septic arthritis and transient synovitis of the hip. *J Pediatr Orthop* 2003;23(3):368-372.
5. Zamzam MM: The role of ultrasound in differentiating septic arthritis from transient synovitis of the hip in children. *J Pediatr Orthop B* 2006;15(6):418-422.
6. Cavalier R, Herman MJ, Pizzutillo PD, Geller E: Ultrasound-guided aspiration of the hip in children: A new technique. *Clin Orthop Relat Res* 2003;415: 244-247.
7. Browne LP, Mason EO, Kaplan SL, Cassady CI, Krishnamurthy R, Guillerman RP: Optimal imaging strategy for community-acquired Staphylococcus aureus musculoskeletal infections in children. *Pediatr Radiol* 2008;38(8): 841-847.
8. Jaramillo D: Infection: Musculoskeletal. *Pediatr Radiol* 2011; 41(suppl 1):S127-S134.
9. Kocher MS, Zurakowski D, Kasser JR: Differentiating between septic arthritis and transient synovitis of the hip in children: An evidence-based clinical prediction algorithm. *J Bone Joint Surg Am* 1999;81(12):1662-1670.
10. Luhmann SJ, Jones A, Schootman M, Gordon JE, Schoenecker PL, Luhmann JD: Differentiation between septic arthritis and transient synovitis of the hip in children with clinical prediction algorithms. *J Bone Joint Surg Am* 2004;86(5):956-962.
11. Sultan J, Hughes PJ: Septic arthritis or transient synovitis of the hip in children: The value of clinical prediction algorithms. *J Bone Joint Surg Br* 2010;92(9):1289-1293.
12. Kocher MS, Mandiga R, Zurakowski D, Barnewolt C, Kasser JR: Validation of a clinical prediction rule for the differentiation between septic arthritis and transient synovitis of the hip in children. *J Bone Joint Surg Am* 2004; 86(8):1629-1635.
13. Caird MS, Flynn JM, Leung YL, Millman JE, D'Italia JG, Dormans JP: Factors distinguishing septic arthritis from transient synovitis of the hip in children: A prospective study. *J Bone Joint Surg Am* 2006;88(6):1251-1257.
14. Levine MJ, McGuire KJ, McGowan KL, Flynn JM: Assessment of the test characteristics of C-reactive protein for septic arthritis in children. *J Pediatr Orthop* 2003;23(3):373-377.
15. Copley LA: Pediatric musculoskeletal infection: Trends and antibiotic recommendations. *J Am Acad Orthop Surg* 2009;17(10): 618-626.
16. Kang S-N, Sanghera T, Mangwani J, Paterson JM, Ramachandran M: The management of septic arthritis in children: Systematic review of the English language literature. *J Bone Joint Surg Br* 2009;91(9):1127-1133.
17. Givon U, Liberman B, Schindler A, Blankstein A, Ganel A: Treatment of septic arthritis of the hip joint by repeated ultrasound-guided aspirations. *J Pediatr Orthop* 2004;24(3):266-270.
18. Pääkkönen M, Kallio MJ, Peltola H, Kallio PE: Pediatric septic hip with or without arthrotomy: Retrospective analysis of 62 consecutive nonneonatal culture-positive cases. *J Pediatr Orthop B* 2010; 19(3):264-269.
19. Griffet J, Oborocianu I, Rubio A, Leroux J, Lauron J, Hayek T: Percutaneous aspiration irrigation drainage technique in the management of septic arthritis in children. *J Trauma* 2011;70(2): 377-383.
20. Harel L, Prais D, Bar-On E, et al: Dexamethasone therapy for septic arthritis in children: Results of a randomized double-blind placebo-controlled study. *J Pediatr Orthop* 2011;31(2):211-215.
21. Chung WK, Slater GL, Bates EH: Treatment of septic arthritis of the

hip by arthroscopic lavage. *J Pediatr Orthop* 1993;13(4):444-446.

22. El-Sayed AM: Treatment of early septic arthritis of the hip in children: Comparison of results of open arthrotomy versus arthroscopic drainage. *J Child Orthop* 2008;2(3):229-237.
23. Gafur OA, Copley LA, Hollmig ST, Browne RH, Thornton LA, Crawford SE: The impact of the current epidemiology of pediatric musculoskeletal infection on evaluation and treatment guidelines. *J Pediatr Orthop* 2008;28(7):777-785.
24. Martínez-Aguilar G, Avalos-Mishaan A, Hulten K, Hammerman W, Mason EO Jr, Kaplan SL: Community-acquired, methicillin-resistant and methicillin-susceptible Staphylococcus aureus musculoskeletal infections in children. *Pediatr Infect Dis J* 2004;23(8):701-706.
25. Vander Have KL, Karmazyn B, Verma M, et al: Community-associated methicillin-resistant Staphylococcus aureus in acute musculoskeletal infection in children: A game changer. *J Pediatr Orthop* 2009;29(8):927-931.
26. Arnold SR, Elias D, Buckingham SC, et al: Changing patterns of acute hematogenous osteomyelitis and septic arthritis: Emergence of community-associated methicillin-resistant Staphylococcus aureus. *J Pediatr Orthop* 2006;26(6):703-708.
27. Ju KL, Zurakowski D, Kocher MS: Differentiating between methicillin-resistant and methicillin-sensitive Staphylococcus aureus osteomyelitis in children: An evidence-based clinical prediction algorithm. *J Bone Joint Surg Am* 2011;93(18):1693-1701.
28. Yilmaz G, Aydin K, Iskender S, Caylan R, Koksal I: Detection and prevalence of inducible clindamycin resistance in staphylococci. *J Med Microbiol* 2007;56(pt 3):342-345.
29. Gwynne-Jones DP, Stott NS: Community-acquired methicillin-resistant Staphylococcus aureus: A cause of musculoskeletal sepsis in children. *J Pediatr Orthop* 1999;19(3):413-416.

37

SYMPOSIUM

Advances in Hip Preservation After Slipped Capital Femoral Epiphysis

Emmanouil Morakis, MD
Ernest L. Sink, MD

Abstract

The metaphyseal deformity, in even a mild slipped capital femoral epiphysis (SCFE), results in acetabular labral and cartilage injury. SCFE is the most extreme form of femoroacetabular impingement, and the mechanism of cartilage and labral injuries is similar. Recent surgical advances for treating femoroacetabular impingement have made it possible to consider applying these techniques to the surgical treatment of SCFE deformities to lessen the risk of secondary osteoarthritis. The goals of treatment are to arrest slip progression and restore normal proximal femoral anatomy, thereby decreasing damage to the hip joint secondary to impingement. In situ pinning is the most effective treatment to halt short-term slip progression; outcomes are favorable in many hips. In medical centers with substantial experience with hip preservation techniques, open or arthroscopic osteochondroplasty can be used to treat mild SCFE, and a modified Dunn epiphyseal reorientation can be used for more severe deformities to decrease the potential for secondary osteoarthritis.

Instr Course Lect 2013;62:415-428.

Slipped capital femoral epiphysis (SCFE) is one of the more common hip disorders in pediatric and adolescent populations. The annual incidence in the United States has been reported as 8.8 to 10.80 cases per 100,000 children.[1,2] The usual age at the initial diagnosis is 13 to 15 years for boys and 11 to 13 years for girls, which corresponds to the ages of peak skeletal growth in each group.[3,4] Younger age at the time of diagnosis is typical for patients with an underlying endocrinopathy or other pathology.[5] Risk factors for SCFE include obesity, acetabular retroversion, proximal femoral retroversion, hypothyroidism, growth hormone therapy, and Down syndrome. A higher incidence of SCFE also has been reported in blacks and people from the Pacific Islands. Although the etiology of SCFE has not been fully elucidated, physeal abnormalities and biochemical factors have been attributed to a weakened physis. The frequency of bilaterality varies depending on the study but ranges from 19% to 60%.[6-8]

Clinical Presentation and Classification

The clinical presentation of SCFE is characterized by groin pain, knee pain, and/or a limp. The hip should be examined in patients with known risk factors who present with knee pain. Physical examination will show an externally rotated gait and a positive Drennan sign (obligatory external rotation with hip flexion). Signs of SCFE on AP radiographs may be subtle and include epiphyseal widening and/or a Klein line (a line drawn up the lateral surface of the femoral neck that does not touch the femoral head). Lateral views may show a posteriorly directed epiphysis. MRI is occasionally needed to confirm the presence of SCFE. Because there is significant morbidity associated with SCFE, a prompt, accurate diagnosis and treatment are critical.

Dr. Sink or an immediate family member serves as a board member, owner, officer, or committee member of the Pediatric Orthopaedic Society of North America and serves as a paid consultant to or is an employee of Pivot. Neither Dr. Morakis nor any immediate family member has received anything of value from or owns stock in a commercial company or institution related directly or indirectly to the subject of this chapter.

SCFE is classified according to the duration of symptoms, the severity of the physeal fracture on radiographs, and the ability of the patient to bear weight. Historically, SCFE was classified temporally as acute (duration of symptoms less than 3 weeks), chronic (symptoms lasting more than 3 weeks), or acute-on-chronic (duration of symptoms more than 3 weeks with a sudden increase in pain and disability).[9-11] Southwick[12] classified SCFE according to the severity of the slip: mild (< 30°), moderate (30° to 60°), or severe (> 60°). The degree of slip is calculated by subtracting the epiphyseal shaft angle of the unaffected side (angle of the epiphysis to the femoral shaft measured on a frog-lateral radiograph) from the corresponding angle on the affected side. A value of 12° is used in children with bilateral disease.

In an attempt to provide a system with better prognostic value, Loder et al[13] classified SCFE as stable or unstable. Patients with stable SCFE have the ability to ambulate with or without crutches, whereas those with unstable SCFE are prevented by pain from bearing weight, even when using crutches. The association of SCFE and osteonecrosis of the femoral head has been documented, with reported frequencies of 1.4% for a stable slip and from 14.8% to 21.4% for an unstable slip.[14,15]

The natural history of untreated SCFE includes eventual closure of the physis and fusion of the epiphysis with the femoral metaphysis at skeletal maturity.[16,17] However, an untreated SCFE may progress into a severe chronic or an acute-on-chronic slip before closure of the physis. Carney et al[18] reported progression of the slip soon after diagnosis in 6 of 36 hips (17%), with a chronic slip that initially had been treated only symptomatically. In a report from southern Sweden, Ordeberg et al[19] reported on a cohort with untreated or symptomatically treated SCFE. At a mean of 47 years, 19 of 33 hips (57.5%) had increased displacement; however, the deterioration from the standpoint of pain, limp, and decreased hip mobility was slight. Patients with a pronounced slip had a higher incidence of arthrosis.

The risk for the development of degenerative osteoarthritis in SCFE correlates with the severity of the femoral head slip and osteonecrosis secondary to treatment.[16,18] Because slip progression cannot be predicted, stabilization of the slip is advisable.[20] A variety of treatment methods have been described to stabilize the epiphyseal slip. Some of these methods are solely of historic interest (hip spica cast and bone graft epiphysiodesis), and some are rarely used in North America (in situ fixation with multiple pins, modified Dunn technique, and intertrochanteric osteotomy with internal fixation).[21-27]

The most common and preferred treatment for a stable SCFE is in situ fixation with a single, centrally located screw.[28,29] Study results show that in situ fixation is an effective treatment method for all SCFE deformities, has the lowest complication rates (osteonecrosis and chondrolysis), and achieves excellent short- and long-term outcomes.[30] Most patients remain asymptomatic for many years after in situ fixation. For the patients who remain symptomatic after in situ fixation, various proximal femoral osteotomies have been described.[12,31-33]

The description of femoroacetabular impingement (FAI) by Ganz et al[34] and the study of the proximal femoral geometry of SCFE by Rab[35] provided new insights into the pathomechanics of SCFE and its potentially causative relationship with degenerative osteoarthritis. Intra-articular approaches in the surgical treatment of SCFE, such as arthroscopy and surgical hip dislocation, have provided evidence of early cartilage damage, even in mildly displaced slips.[36-39] Because there is growing clinical evidence that FAI after SCFE leads to early degenerative osteoarthritis,[40] treatment goals are changing. The slipped epiphysis should be stabilized, and treatment complications should be avoided; however, there is a growing trend of addressing FAI to avoid degenerative osteoarthritis and improve long-term outcomes. **Table 1** summarizes current treatment options for SCFE.

In Situ Pinning

In situ fixation of SCFE remains the gold standard of treatment.[28,41] The goals of in situ fixation are to prevent slip progression and avoid complications, specifically osteonecrosis and chondrolysis. This technique is the most reproducible, with minimal complications reported for most patients.

Diverse techniques are available for in situ fixation. Consideration has been given to the type (smooth pins, threaded pins, or threaded screws) and number (one screw, two screws, or multiple pins) of implants, as well as the use of fixation with or without compression across the physis.[42]

Most orthopaedic surgeons favor in situ fixation using a single, central screw placed under fluoroscopic guidance, with the option of a second screw for additional stability and rotational control in an unstable SCFE.[28] This technique provides reliable results with a high rate of successful outcomes and a low incidence of slip progression, osteonecrosis, and chondrolysis.[29] In a prospective study, Aronson and Carlson[43] reported on 44 children (58 hips) followed for a mean of 3 years (range, 2 to 6 years) after in situ fixation with a single screw. They reported good to excellent results in 54 of 58 hips (93%), with one case of os-

Table 1
Current Treatment Options for SCFE

	No Prior Treatment	Prior In Situ Pinning
Mild slip angle (0° to 30°), minimal translation	In situ pinning In situ pinning with osteochondroplasty Open Arthroscopic	Osteochondroplasty only Arthroscopic Open anterior approach Surgical hip dislocation
Moderate to severe slip angle (> 30°)	In situ pinning with delayed osteotomy if painful with limited function In situ pinning with concurrent osteotomy (intertrochanteric) Modified Dunn reduction	Surgical hip dislocation ± osteotomy Femoral neck osteotomy

teonecrosis, no cases of chondrolysis, and three other complications (one fracture, one loss of fixation, and one slip progression). Subsequent studies document similar successful results and low complication rates in patients with SCFE treated with single-screw, in situ fixation.[44-46]

In a study with a mean follow-up of 41 years, Carney et al[18] reported good outcomes (mean Iowa hip score of 85) in 11 patients treated with in situ pinning. The authors reported one case of osteonecrosis and no cases of chondrolysis. In a study of 140 patients with SCFE treated with pinning or nailing in situ (mean follow-up, 28 years), Hägglund et al[47] observed radiographic signs of osteoarthritis in 24% of the patients; however, 72% of all hips were pain free at follow-up. In a Swedish study of 59 hips treated for SCFE (mean follow-up, 31 years), the authors reported excellent clinical outcomes (Harris hip score 90 or higher on a scale of 100) in 52 hips (88%) and radiographic evidence of reduced joint space in 18 hips (30.5%).[30] Wensaas et al[48] retrospectively studied 76 hips treated for SCFE with either screw fixation in situ, bone-peg epiphysiodesis, or bone-peg epiphysiodesis combined with a corrective femoral osteotomy. The authors reported 71% good clinical outcomes (Harris hip score of 85 or higher on a scale of 100). Twenty percent of the hips had radiographic evidence of hip osteoarthritis in the 28 hips treated with in situ screw fixation after a mean follow-up of 33 years.

For a stable SCFE, the preferred technique of most surgeons is percutaneous insertion of a single, long-threaded or fully threaded stainless steel screw on a radiolucent table or fracture table. A technique using two C-arms can facilitate screw placement when using the fracture table. The benefits of a radiolucent table include easier and faster setup, particularly for bilateral pinning; better visualization of the hip joint in obese patients; the ability to take the hip joint through a range of motion during the surgery; and less radiation exposure compared with surgery using a fracture table.[49-51] One technical consideration is the tendency to bend the guidewire when flexing and abducting the hip to obtain a lateral view. This can be overcome with careful partial abduction of the hip and concomitant tilting of the fluoroscopy machine.

The screw diameter should be at least 6.5 mm or larger, depending on the size of the child. Fully threaded or long-threaded stainless steel screws with reverse cutting threads are preferred over titanium or short, partially threaded screws because they are easier to remove.[52-54] Fully threaded screws provide higher biomechanical strength to the femoral neck compared with 16-mm partially threaded screws.[55-57] In situ fixation requires that the screw be advanced through the physis into the epiphysis, with an attempt to engage at least five threads into the epiphysis to prevent slip progression.[58] The safest position for the tip of the screw is in the center of the epiphysis in both planes. In this position, injury to the lateral epiphyseal vessels supplying the femoral epiphysis is avoided, and there is a lower risk of unrecognized joint penetration.[59,60] The tip of the screw should be more than 4 mm from the subchondral bone on the frog-lateral view or 6 mm on the AP view to avoid joint penetration.[61]

After inserting the screw and before removing the guidewire, fluoroscopy is used to confirm that the tip of the screw does not penetrate into the hip joint. Using live imaging, the hip is rotated from full extension and internal rotation to maximal flexion and external rotation. During this maneuver, the tip of the screw appears to approach and then withdraw from the subchondral bone (approach-withdraw phenomenon). The instant of change from approach to withdrawal represents the true position of the tip of the screw.[62,63] If the SCFE is stable, partial weight bearing with crutches can begin and will continue for 4 to 6 weeks.

A second screw can be used in unstable SCFEs to increase stability and rotational control.[64,65] In an animal model, Segal et al[64] reported 312% increased torsional stiffness for a two-screw construct of a nonreduced SCFE compared with the single-screw construct. When the SCFE was reduced, the torsional stiffness was still increased by 137% on the two-screw construct. In another animal study, two screws provided twice the relative torsional stiffness and strength compared with fixation with a single screw.[66]

Two-screw fixation is not recommended for a stable SCFE. Clinical studies have reported favorable outcomes for single-screw fixation.[43,45,46,67] The increase in the number of implants (screws or pins) has been shown to correlate with higher complication rates, mainly hip joint perforation.[68,69]

The disadvantage of in situ SCFE fixation is the presence of residual metaphyseal deformity, which is proportionate to the slip severity. The prominent metaphysis impinges on the acetabulum, causing labral and cartilage injuries, potentially leading to hip pain and degenerative arthritis.[36,38] Gait abnormalities observed in patients with SCFE treated with in situ pinning have been attributed to the femoral head and metaphyseal deformities. Abnormal gait patterns may contribute to uneven stresses on the joint, leading to degenerative osteoarthritis.[70,71]

Screw head impingement has been recognized as a possible cause of hip pain, restricted hip range of motion, and decreased hip function in patients with SCFE treated with in situ fixation.[72] Goodwin et al[72] reported impingement of the screw head on the anterior acetabular rim of cadaver specimens, which simulated in situ fixation in moderate and severe SCFEs. Pinning with a starting point lateral to the intertrochanteric line on the AP radiographic view minimized the risk of screw head impingement.

Despite the early favorable outcomes of this treatment approach, recent studies are unclear about its long-term effectiveness. Larson et al[73] presented the results of a retrospective study of 146 patients (176 hips) treated with in situ fixation for SCFE at a mean follow-up of 16 years. The authors reported that approximately 33% of the patients had residual pain, 12% needed subsequent reconstructive surgery, and degenerative osteoarthritis severe enough to warrant total hip arthroplasty was likely to develop in 5% of the patients 20 years after in situ fixation.

Mild and Stable SCFE

Most orthopaedic surgeons recommend in situ pinning to treat a mild SCFE (Southwick angle < 30°).[29,74] Follow-up studies have reported favorable outcomes with this treatment method for mild deformities.[10,18]

Recent studies have provided evidence that questions the benign natural history of mild SCFE treated with in situ pinning. Leunig et al[38] reported on 13 patients with SCFE who were treated with surgical hip dislocation. Intraoperative acetabular cartilage damage ranging from chondromalacia to full-thickness cartilage loss and labral injuries (such as contusions, erosions, and tears) was observed. These injuries were also noted in the three patients with mild SCFE. The authors observed impingement of the prominent metaphysis of the femoral neck on the anteromedial acetabulum and labrum with hip flexion and internal rotation. It was concluded that mechanical damage of the labrum and cartilage, even in patients with a mild SCFE, may lead to cartilage degeneration and osteoarthritis.

The observations of Leunig et al[38] were confirmed in a study of 36 patients with SCFE who were treated with surgical hip dislocation for chronic symptoms. The authors reported cartilage damage and/or labral injuries in seven of eight patients with a mild slip.

Rab[35] proposed using a three-dimensional computer model to distinguish two types of mechanical damage (impaction and inclusion) to the cartilage and labrum determined by the size of the metaphyseal prominence. In an impaction injury, the very prominent metaphyseal segment of a severe slip impinges on the acetabular rim and levers the femoral head out of the acetabulum. Clinical manifestations include limited hip range of motion, external rotation during gait, and difficulty sitting. This mechanism may cause a pattern of posterior acetabular and labral injury with global chondral thinning. In an inclusion injury, the metaphyseal segment is less prominent (mild SCFE or remodeled SCFE). The rough metaphysis can enter the hip joint and cause erosions to the smooth acetabular cartilage and injuries to the labrum with hip motion.

In a retrospective study of 36 patients with SCFE treated with in situ pinning of the femoral head using a single cannulated screw, 32% had clinical signs of impingement at a mean follow-up of 6.1 years.[75] Among the patients with a mild SCFE, 30% reported pain and had clinical signs of FAI.

These studies suggest that removing the metaphyseal prominence that results in impingement may have some benefit in the long-term sequelae of a mild SCFE deformity. Therefore, some surgeons now treat a mild SCFE with in situ pinning and concurrently perform an osteoplasty of the metaphysis via an arthroscopic or open approach to prevent labral and chondral injuries.[36,76,77] Despite the lack of long-term results, excellent early outcomes have been reported. Leunig et al[77] described the surgical technique and results of three patients with a mild SCFE treated with in situ pinning and arthroscopic osteoplasty. In situ pinning of the affected hip was followed by arthroscopic evaluation and the repair of chondral and labral injuries. An osteoplasty of the prominent metaphyseal segment was performed, and its adequacy was evaluated with fluoroscopy. At the postoperative follow-up (range, 6 to 23 months), all patients were asymptomatic, had returned to their previous activities, had negative impingement tests, and presented without obligate external rotation of the hip with flexion.

Current evidence indicates in situ pinning as the treatment of choice for mild SCFE. An anterior open or an arthroscopic approach can be used to restore the head-neck offset and provide a more functional range of hip motion (at least 90° of hip flexion and 20°of internal rotation). An osteoplasty may be considered based on the current understanding of the pathomechanics of FAI in patients with mild SCFE. Prospective studies with long-term follow-up are needed to evaluate the safety and effectiveness of new treatment approaches compared with in situ fixation alone.

Moderate and Severe Stable SCFE

The clinical outcomes of patients with SCFE have been shown to correlate with the severity of the slip; patients with moderate and severe SCFE have poorer functional results on long-term follow-up studies. In a retrospective study of 124 patients at mean follow-up of 41 years, Carney et al[18] reported worse outcomes for patients with moderate and severe slips compared with patients with mild slips.

Despite the poorer long-term prognosis, most orthopaedic surgeons prefer in situ fixation for moderate to severe slips.[41] Aggressive attempts at forced reduction have been related to increased rates of osteonecrosis. Published studies indicated that in situ fixation is safer in the short term, with reproducible good results and low complication rates.[43-46] This treatment option addresses the immediate goal, which is to prevent slip progression.[78] Many patients remain asymptomatic for many years after in situ pinning. Remodeling of the femoral head deformity occurs until the closure of the physis, which partially improves the head deformity.[79,80] However, the amount of remodeling is not enough to restore normal femoral head and neck shape.[80,81] The remodeling potential also decreases with increasing slip severity.[82]

Castañeda et al[83] evaluated 105 patients (129 hips) with severe slips treated with in situ pinning with a single screw at an average follow-up of 66 months (minimum 5 years). The mean Iowa hip score for these patients was 84.75; among these, those with adequate screw placement based on criteria described by Stambough et al[69] had excellent clinical results (mean Iowa hip score = 89.69). In patients with moderate or severe SCFE treated with in situ pinning, those who remain or become symptomatic can be treated later with some form of reorientation osteotomy of the proximal femur and/or osteoplasty of the head-neck prominence.[12,26,31,84]

Various methods have been proposed to address both epiphyseal instability and deformity in moderate and severe SCFE. The goal of treatment is to prevent early clinical dysfunction of the hip and the development of degenerative osteoarthritis. In a retrospective nonrandomized study, Diab et al[85] compared 10 children with chronic, severe SCFE treated with in situ fixation with 10 children treated with in situ fixation and concurrent flexion intertrochanteric osteotomy. The average follow-up interval was 6.8 years. An intertrochanteric osteotomy, as originally described by Imhäuser,[31] was used to correct the relatively posterior and inferior positions of the epiphysis with flexion and internal rotation of the distal fragment. The patients treated with a combination of in situ fixation and intertrochanteric osteotomy had improved flexion and internal rotation of the hip compared with the control group; however, there was no difference in functional outcomes between the groups as measured by the Harris hip score. The authors concluded that early outcomes of severe slips were not improved with this combined treatment. However, the effect of the osteotomy on preventing degenerative hip joint changes remains unknown because longer follow-up periods are needed.

A study by Witbreuk et al[27] presented the results of treating 28 patients with moderate or severe SCFE with in situ fixation combined with an Imhäuser intertrochanteric osteotomy. The average follow-up was 8.2 years. The patients showed improved flexion, adduction, and internal rotation. Functional outcomes based on the Harris hip score were good to excellent in 71% of the patients. Outcomes based on the Medical Outcomes 36-Item Short Form survey were not substantially different from those of the general population matched for age. No cases of osteonecrosis or chondrolysis were reported.

Schai and Exner[86,87] reported on 51 patients with moderate to severe chronic SCFE treated with in situ fixation and an Imhäuser intertrochanteric osteotomy. At an average follow-up of 24.1 years, 55% of the patients had good results (asymptomatic without activity limitations, hip range of motion within 10° compared with the

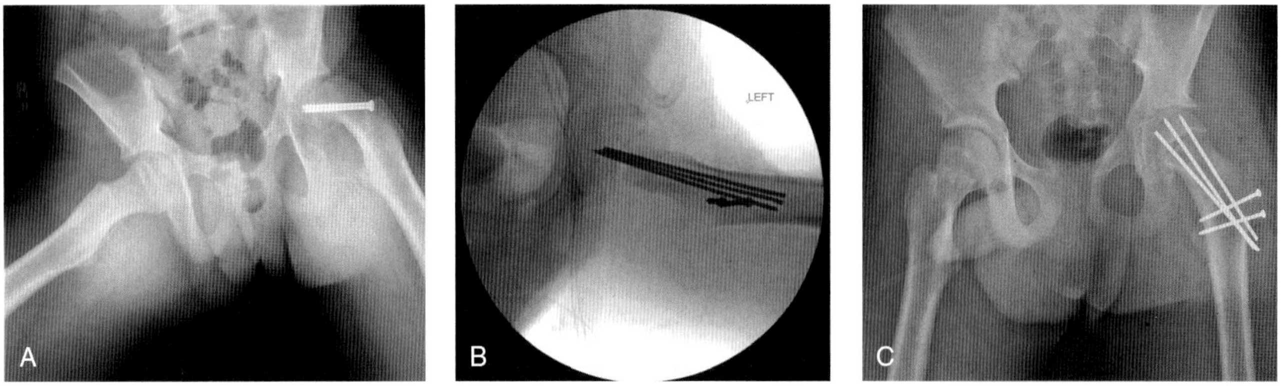

Figure 1 **A,** Preoperative lateral radiograph of the hip of a 13-year-old boy with a severe SCFE. **B,** Intraoperative lateral image of the hip during treatment with the modified Dunn technique after in situ pinning. **C,** Postoperative AP radiograph.

healthy contralateral hip, and no radiologic evidence of degenerative osteoarthritis). Early performance of an intertrochanteric osteotomy has the theoretic advantage of improving hip biomechanics, partially restoring hip joint incongruity, and minimizing the risk for the development of FAI and degenerative hip osteoarthritis.

The potential for restoring a normal femoral head shape and hip function will increase with increasing proximity of the corrective osteotomy to the physis, although the theoretic risk of osteonecrosis is greater. An extracapsular osteotomy at the base of the femoral neck was performed in 32 patients (36 hips) with moderate to severe slips.[88] At an average follow-up of 9 years, Abraham et al[88] reported good to excellent outcomes in 90% of the hips based on Southwick's criteria. The authors reported no cases of osteonecrosis, three cases of chondrolysis, and a limb-length discrepancy of more than 2 cm in six patients. Other approaches to correct the deformity with subcapital femoral osteotomies are less common because of higher complication rates, especially osteonecrosis.[89-91]

Ganz et al[92] described a safe technique to surgically dislocate the hip and treat intra-articular pathology. Using this surgical approach, a modified Dunn subcapital osteotomy can be performed to restore the normal proximal femoral anatomy by epiphyseal reduction on a long retinacular flap[39,93] (**Figure 1**). Through a lateral incision and using a trochanteric flip osteotomy, the hip is surgically dislocated. If the hip is unstable, the femoral epiphysis is provisionally stabilized in situ with threaded Kirschner wires to avoid stretching the retinacular vessels before dislocating the hip. A long retinacular flap is developed containing the periosteum of the femoral neck, the retinacular vessels, and short external rotators. This retinacular flap preserves the blood supply to the femoral epiphysis. The residual physeal cartilage is removed from the femoral epiphysis, and any callus formation from the femoral neck is resected. The femoral head is reduced in anatomic position on the femoral neck, taking care to avoid tension on the retinacular flap or entrapment of it between the head and neck. The reduced femoral head is then fixed with fully threaded Kirschner wires. Throughout the procedure, perfusion to the femoral epiphysis is evaluated with a laser Doppler flowmetry head probe by drilling a 2-mm hole that should bleed or with an intracerebral pressure probe.[26,38,39]

Excellent results have been reported with this technique.[76,94] Ziebarth et al[76] reported on 40 patients with SCFE treated with a modified Dunn technique at two medical centers. The clinical outcomes, measured with the Merle d'Aubigné-Postel scale and the Harris hip score, were almost normal. The authors reported three delayed unions, one heterotopic ossification, one patient with residual impingement, and three hardware failures. No osteonecrosis or chondrolysis were reported.

Huber et al[94] reported on 28 patients (30 hips) treated with the same technique. The mean postoperative slip angle was 5.2°, 26 of 28 patients had excellent clinical outcome (measured with the Harris hip score and the Western Ontario and McMaster Universities Osteoarthritis Index [WOMAC] questionnaire). The authors reported four implant failures and documented one patient with osteonecrosis who had shown no evidence of epiphyseal perfusion intraoperatively. Slongo et al[26] reported similar excellent outcomes in 23 patients using this treatment approach, with few complications (one patient with osteonecrosis, one with osteoarthritis, and one failure of fixation).

Currently, in situ pinning is the preferred treatment for moderate or severe SCFE in most patients. The modified Dunn technique or proximal femoral osteotomy can be considered a treatment option. Favorable medium-term outcomes (range, 1 to 8.4 years) with this approach have been reported from surgeons at medical centers with considerable experience with the technique of surgical hip dislocation and cannot be generalized to all orthopaedic surgeons. Longer follow-up studies will provide data for comparison with the current preferred treatment option of in situ pinning.

Unstable SCFE

Osteonecrosis is recognized as the most devastating complication after SCFE and is the most common indication for total hip arthroplasty in patients with a history of SCFE.[13,95-97] Patients with osteonecrosis required total hip arthroplasty earlier (7.6 years) than those with degenerative joint disease or impingement (23.6 years).[97]

The etiology of osteonecrosis is not completely understood. It has been attributed to a compromise of the femoral head blood supply, either by iatrogenic factors (pin or screw position, reduction of the slip, or femoral neck osteotomy), the acute injury itself, or compression of the hematoma or chronic metaphyseal callous on the retinacular vessels after the epiphysis is reduced to the anatomic position.[13,29,98-100]

Palocaren et al[101] retrospectively evaluated 27 patients with unstable or acute SCFE and determined the risk factors associated with osteonecrosis of the femoral head after in situ pinning. Overall, the prevalence of osteonecrosis was 22.2%. Risk factors for the development of osteonecrosis after in situ pinning were preoperative slip angle (for every 1° increase in the slip angle there was a 4% increase in the risk of osteonecrosis; adjusted risk ratio = 1.04) and female sex (risk ratio = 4.15). Sankar et al[102] reported younger age and longer duration of symptoms as risk factors for osteonecrosis in a cohort of 70 patients with unstable SCFE. The overall incidence of osteonecrosis was 20%. Similarly, Kennedy et al[14] recognized younger age as a risk factor for osteonecrosis after an unstable SCFE; they reported that the patient's sex or severity of the slip were not statistically important risk factors.

Despite the unequivocal agreement of the prognosis of an unstable SCFE, there is still debate concerning many treatment aspects, including the appropriate time to perform surgery, the necessity of reduction maneuvers, the degree of reduction, the type and number of implants for stabilization, the role of joint decompression, and the need for prophylactic treatment of the contralateral side.

In a survey of 794 members of the Pediatric Orthopaedic Society of North America, approximately 31% of 263 respondents considered an acute or unstable SCFE an emergency, 57% as a condition requiring urgent treatment (less than 8 hours), and 12% as a condition that can be treated electively.[28] Most surgeons (84%) would treat an acute or unstable SCFE with in situ pinning after simple positioning on the fracture table, 11.8% with in situ pinning after manipulation and reduction, and 3% of surgeons would perform open reduction. Fixation with a single threaded screw was the preferred treatment option for 57.4%, and 40.3% would use two threaded screws. Most of the respondents (64.6%) did not recommend capsular decompression, whereas 25.9% would perform decompression via hip aspiration, and only 9.5% would perform open capsular decompression of the hematoma.

In a similar survey conducted by the European Pediatric Orthopaedic Society, 287 members were surveyed and 72 responded. Comparable results were reported, with 46% of the surgeons recommending reduction by simple positioning of the hip on the fracture table, 35% by manipulation, and 11% advising open reduction. Single-screw fixation was favored by 44% of the respondents, and 36% recommended two-screw fixation for severe unstable SCFE.[41]

Timing is one of the most debated factors in the treatment of an acute or unstable SCFE. It has been theorized that an acute or unstable slip causes the posterior blood vessels to kink or twist, leading to epiphyseal ischemia. In that sense, urgent reduction and stabilization of the slip may restore blood flow.[103] In their initial study on unstable SCFE, Loder et al[13] did not find a statistically significant difference in the osteonecrosis rates of patients treated urgently (less than 24 hours) and those treated later. However, the authors reported a significantly higher rate ($P = 0.012$) of osteonecrosis in patients treated within the first 48 hours compared with those treated later. Because of the retrospective nature of the study, the authors could not determine a cause-effect relationship between the timing of treatment and osteonecrosis rates.

Several studies investigated the correlation between the timing of treatment of an acute or unstable SCFE and the incidence of osteonecrosis.[13,14,103-105] Lowndes et al[106] reported on a meta-analysis of retrospective case-controlled studies assessing the relationship between the timing of treatment of an acute or unstable SCFE and the incidence of osteonecrosis. Analysis of these studies resulted in an odds ratio of 0.50 ($P = 0.441$), indicating that the odds for the development of osteonecrosis if the patient is treated within 24 hours were 50% compared with patients treated after 24 hours. In a retrospective study of 70 patients treated for an unstable SCFE, Sankar et al[102] did not find an association between surgical delay and the incidence of osteonecrosis.[102] Although the current literature does not provide conclusive evidence on the effect of timing and the development of osteonecrosis, most orthopaedic surgeons recommend treating an unstable SCFE as an urgent condition.[29,74,102,106-108]

Some authors have recommended decompression of the intra-articular hematoma to prevent osteonecrosis after an unstable SCFE.[103,105,107,109,110] An intracapsular hematoma after an acute or unstable SCFE may compromise the femoral head blood supply through a tamponade effect.[111,112] Increased intracapsular hip pressure, compared with the contralateral hip, has been reported in patients with an unstable SCFE.[110] Urgent treatment of an unstable SCFE with capsulotomy for decompression of the hip joint (especially following gentle reduction) has been strongly recommended.

Intracapsular decompression of the hip can be performed either with percutaneous aspiration or arthrotomy. Gordon et al[105] reported no osteonecrosis in 10 patients with an unstable SCFE who were treated within 24 hours with reduction of the slip, decompression, and fixation. In a study of 15 patients treated with urgent reduction arthrotomy and fixation for an unstable SCFE, Chen at al[107] reported osteonecrosis in 1 patient.

Another controversial aspect of unstable SCFE management is the safety of reducing the slipped epiphysis to attempt restoration of the normal anatomy. Most surgeons advocate in situ fixation or incidental reduction with positioning on the operating table for an unstable SCFE.[18,28,78] Recent studies have reported favorable results with gentle reduction within 24 hours of the onset of symptoms combined with capsular hematoma decompression.[103,107]

Parsch et al[113] reported on 64 children with an unstable SCFE, defined by sonographic presence of hip effusion, who were treated with hip joint capsulotomy with open reduction and fixation. Most patients (76%) were treated within 24 hours from the onset of symptoms. The hip capsule was exposed through an anterior Watson-Jones approach, and an anterior capsulotomy was done to decompress the joint from the effusion or hematoma. A gentle reduction maneuver was performed while the surgeon's index finger was used to control the reduction of the epiphysis on the metaphysis. Using fluoroscopy, the reduced epiphysis was fixed in place with three Kirschner wires. After a minimum follow-up of 12 months, the patients had an average slip angle of 10.6°, good clinical outcomes (mean Iowa hip score 94.5 of 100), and a 4.7% rate of osteonecrosis. In the 55 children who could not bear weight preoperatively, a 5.4% rate of osteonecrosis was reported.

Another reduction approach for an acute or unstable SCFE is the modified Dunn technique after surgical dislocation of the hip.[38,114] An almost anatomic reduction of the slipped epiphysis on the femoral neck has been reported along with protection of the epiphyseal blood supply and avoidance of leg shortening. The few medical centers that have experience with this approach have achieved excellent results.[26,39,76,94]

Authors have recommended that patients with an unstable SCFE should, at the least, be treated urgently, with hip joint decompression and fixation with one or two screws; the surgeon should not reduce the epiphysis further than the tidemark (the location of the epiphysis relative to the metaphysis before the destabilizing event). Other treatment options that may be considered depending on the surgeon's familiarity with the procedure are gentle open reduction (to the tidemark) through an anterior Watson-Jones approach and fixation with one or two screws or an open reduction with the modified Dunn technique through a surgical hip dislocation.

Painful Healed SCFE

After stabilization of the slipped epiphysis, patients with SCFE gradually regain function as symptoms resolve. The physis of the femoral head closes with time, but the deformity of the residual slip remains. The proximal femur acquires a typical radiographic appearance, which has been called a tilt deformity or pistol-grip deformity.[115,116]

Depending on the severity of the slip and the activities of the patient, symptomatic FAI can develop. The restrictions of hip motion and the point at which FAI occurs depend not only on the severity of the slip but also the shape of the remaining head deformity and the anatomic characteristics of the specific hip joint (coxa profunda; femoral or acetabular retroversion).[117]

The indications for restoring the residual head deformity after closure of the physis in asymptomatic patients with a history of SCFE pinning are not defined. Growing evidence from patients treated with surgical hip dislocation and advanced imaging show early cartilage wear and varying degrees of labral injuries in most patients with SCFE.[36,114,118,119] Generally, hips with less than 90° of flexion, no internal rotation at 90° of flexion, or a slip angle of more than 30° have a higher risk of future symptomatic FAI.[120]

The current indication for surgical correction of the residual deformity is a symptomatic patient with a limited arc of motion of the hip (flexion and internal rotation) that impedes activities. Various surgical approaches have been proposed. Intertrochanteric osteotomies can partially correct the deformity by creating a secondary deformity distally. The most popular intertrochanteric osteotomies were initially described by Southwick[12] and Imhäuser.[31] The Imhäuser intertrochanteric osteotomy corrects the deformity at the intertrochanteric level using mainly flexion and some internal rotation of the segment distal to the osteotomy.[87] This procedure can adequately correct deformities up to 60°, with minimal risk of osteonecrosis. Midterm and long-term follow-up studies (range, 7.5 to 24 years) of patients treated with an intertrochanteric osteotomy have reported favorable results.[121-125] The rates of osteonecrosis ranged from 0% to 6.67%, the radiographic evidence of degenerative osteoarthritis was 3.7% to 77%, and clinical outcomes were good or excellent in 71% to 85% of patients. The disadvantages of an intertrochanteric osteotomy are the creation of a second deformity distally and the limited amount of correction that it can provide (up to 60° of correction), which may not be enough for impingement-free hip range of motion because of the deformity of the metaphysis.[126]

An intra-articular approach through a surgical hip dislocation is an alternative option, which allows complete access to the head-neck deformity, accurate assessment of impingement, and the possibility of evaluating and repairing any intra-articular pathology. This approach allows for osteoplasty of the metaphyseal prominence, which is the greatest impediment to range of motion. Osteoplasty will decrease the degree of flexion required if an intertrochanteric osteotomy is still necessary.

An open approach through a surgical hip dislocation and osteoplasty is ideal for only mild and moderate deformities. The goal is to achieve at least 90° of hip flexion and 20° of internal rotation intraoperatively to provide functional hip range of motion. For more severe deformities, surgical hip dislocation and osteoplasty can be combined with an Imhäuser-type intertrochanteric osteotomy. This combination may be the best treatment for the most severe deformities because it addresses the metaphyseal component and decreases the degree of the osteotomy.[127] Spencer et al[128] evaluated the results of surgical hip dislocation and femoral neck osteoplasty, with and without concomitant intertrochanteric osteotomy, on 19 patients with FAI (12 had a history of SCFE). The average follow-up was 12 months. Among the 12 patients who had a history of SCFE, 6 were treated with an osteoplasty and 6 with combined osteoplasty and intertrochanteric osteotomy. The authors reported improved range of motion (flexion and internal rotation) and function and decreased pain (WOMAC score) in 9 of the 12 patients. Osteonecrosis did not develop in any of the patients. The patients who did not benefit from the surgical approach had existing extensive chondral injuries.[129]

Arthroscopic and mini-open approaches also have been used to successfully treat cam-type FAI after healing of SCFE.[130,131] With the arthroscopic approach, intra-articular pathology can be evaluated and repaired easily by experienced surgeons, and the femoral neck deformity can be restored with osteochondroplasty. Moderate and severe deformities can be technically difficult to treat arthroscopically, especially the superior and lateral portions of the prominence.

Summary

In situ fixation is still the preferred treatment option for SCFE. Long-term results are favorable for most patients, and it has a low complication rate and can prevent slip progression. An unstable SCFE should be treated urgently with at least gentle reduction and joint decompression or open reduction. A better understanding of the pathomechanics of FAI and recent evidence of chondral and labral injuries on even mild SCFE deformities dictates a redirection of treatment strategies for SCFE. The goals of treatment should be to arrest slip progression and restore normal proximal femoral anatomy to decrease the damage to the hip joint secondary to impingement. Symptomatic patients with a healed SCFE and mild residual deformity can be treated with arthroscopic or mini-open osteochondroplasty. Moderate and severe deformities can be corrected with an intertrochanteric osteotomy or with a surgical hip dislocation and osteoplasty. A combination of an intertrochanteric osteotomy with a surgical hip dislocation with osteoplasty may be the best treatment for the most severe deformities. Subcapital realignment of a slipped epiphysis with a surgical hip dislocation may be the ideal surgical option to restore the normal femoral head anatomy and stop slip progression. Early results from the few medical centers using this approach are promising. This is a technically demanding procedure with a steep learning curve and important complications if it is not performed correctly. Long-term patient outcomes will provide evidence of its effectiveness and safety by comparing it to the current gold standard of in situ fixation.

References

1. Larson AN, Yu EM, Melton LJ III, Peterson HA, Stans AA: Incidence of slipped capital femoral epiphysis: A population-based study. *J Pediatr Orthop B* 2010; 19(1):9-12.

2. Lehmann CL, Arons RR, Loder RT, Vitale MG: The epidemiology of slipped capital femoral epiphysis: An update. *J Pediatr Orthop* 2006;26(3):286-290.
3. Loder RT: The demographics of slipped capital femoral epiphysis: An international multicenter study. *Clin Orthop Relat Res* 1996;322:8-27.
4. Hägglund G, Hansson LI, Ordeberg G: Epidemiology of slipped capital femoral epiphysis in southern Sweden. *Clin Orthop Relat Res* 1984;191:82-94.
5. Loder RT, Wittenberg B, DeSilva G: Slipped capital femoral epiphysis associated with endocrine disorders. *J Pediatr Orthop* 1995;15(3):349-356.
6. Jerre R, Billing L, Hansson G, Karlsson J, Wallin J: Bilaterality in slipped capital femoral epiphysis: Importance of reliable radiographic method. *J Pediatr Orthop B* 1996;5(2):80-84.
7. Raid J, Bajelidze G, Gabbos PG: Bilateral slipped capital femoral epiphysis: Predictive factors for contralateral slip. *J Pediatr Orthop* 2007;27(4):411-414.
8. Hurley JM, Betz RR, Loder RT, Davidson RS, Alburger PD, Steel HH: Slipped capital femoral epiphysis: The prevalence of late contralateral slip. *J Bone Joint Surg Am* 1996;78(2):226-230.
9. Fahey JJ, O'Brien ET: Acute slipped capital femoral epiphysis: Review of the literature and report of ten cases. *J Bone Joint Surg Am* 1965;47:1105-1127.
10. Boyer DW, Mickelson MR, Ponseti IV: Slipped capital femoral epiphysis: Long-term follow-up study of one hundred and twenty-one patients. *J Bone Joint Surg Am* 1981;63(1):85-95.
11. Loder RT, Aronson DD, Greenfield ML: The epidemiology of bilateral slipped capital femoral epiphysis: A study of children in Michigan. *J Bone Joint Surg Am* 1993;75(8):1141-1147.
12. Southwick WO: Osteotomy through the lesser trochanter for slipped capital femoral epiphysis. *J Bone Joint Surg Am* 1967;49(5):807-835.
13. Loder RT, Richards BS, Shapiro PS, Reznick LR, Aronson DD: Acute slipped capital femoral epiphysis: The importance of physeal stability. *J Bone Joint Surg Am* 1993;75(8):1134-1140.
14. Kennedy JG, Hresko MT, Kasser JR, et al: Osteonecrosis of the femoral head associated with slipped capital femoral epiphysis. *J Pediatr Orthop* 2001;21(2):189-193.
15. Fallath S, Letts M: Slipped capital femoral epiphysis: An analysis of treatment outcome according to physeal stability. *Can J Surg* 2004;47(4):284-289.
16. Engelhardt P: Natural course of epiphysiolysis of the femur head. *Orthopade* 1994;23(3):195-199.
17. Aronsson DD, Loder RT: Treatment of the unstable (acute) slipped capital femoral epiphysis. *Clin Orthop Relat Res* 1996;322:99-110.
18. Carney BT, Weinstein SL, Noble J: Long-term follow-up of slipped capital femoral epiphysis. *J Bone Joint Surg Am* 1991;73(5):667-674.
19. Ordeberg G, Hansson LI, Sandström S: Slipped capital femoral epiphysis in southern Sweden: Long-term result with no treatment or symptomatic primary treatment. *Clin Orthop Relat Res* 1984;191:95-104.
20. Weinstein SL: Natural history and treatment outcomes of childhood hip disorders. *Clin Orthop Relat Res* 1997;344:227-242.
21. Betz RR, Steel HH, Emper WD, Huss GK, Clancy M: Treatment of slipped capital femoral epiphysis: Spica-cast immobilization. *J Bone Joint Surg Am* 1990;72(4):587-600.
22. Meier MC, Meyer LC, Ferguson RL: Treatment of slipped capital femoral epiphysis with a spica cast. *J Bone Joint Surg Am* 1992;74(10):1522-1529.
23. Adamczyk MJ, Weiner DS, Hawk D: A 50-year experience with bone graft epiphysiodesis in the treatment of slipped capital femoral epiphysis. *J Pediatr Orthop* 2003;23(5):578-583.
24. Rao SB, Crawford AH, Burger RR, Roy DR: Open bone peg epiphysiodesis for slipped capital femoral epiphysis. *J Pediatr Orthop* 1996;16(1):37-48.
25. Reize P, Rudert M: Kirschner wire transfixation of the femoral head in slipped capital femoral epiphysis in children. *Oper Orthop Traumatol* 2007;19(4):345-357.
26. Slongo T, Kakaty D, Krause F, Ziebarth K: Treatment of slipped capital femoral epiphysis with a modified Dunn procedure. *J Bone Joint Surg Am* 2010;92(18):2898-2908.
27. Witbreuk MM, Bolkenbaas M, Mullender MG, Sierevelt IN, Besselaar PP: The results of downgrading moderate and severe slipped capital femoral epiphysis by an early Imhauser femur osteotomy. *J Child Orthop* 2009;3(5):405-410.
28. Mooney JF III, Sanders JO, Browne RH, et al: Management of unstable/acute slipped capital femoral epiphysis: Results of a survey of the POSNA membership. *J Pediatr Orthop* 2005;25(2):162-166.
29. Aronsson DD, Loder RT, Breur GJ, Weinstein SL: Slipped capital femoral epiphysis: Current concepts. *J Am Acad Orthop Surg* 2006;14(12):666-679.
30. Hansson G, Billing L, Högstedt B, Jerre R, Wallin J: Long-term results after nailing in situ of slipped upper femoral epiphysis: A

30-year follow-up of 59 hips. *J Bone Joint Surg Br* 1998;80(1): 70-77.

31. Imhäuser G: Late results of Imhäuser's osteotomy for slipped capital femoral epiphysis. *Z Orthop Ihre Grenzgeb* 1977;115(5): 716-725.
32. Kramer WG, Craig WA, Noel S: Compensating osteotomy at the base of the femoral neck for slipped capital femoral epiphysis. *J Bone Joint Surg Am* 1976;58(6): 796-800.
33. Dunn DM, Angel JC: Replacement of the femoral head by open operation in severe adolescent slipping of the upper femoral epiphysis. *J Bone Joint Surg Br* 1978;60(3):394-403.
34. Ganz R, Parvizi J, Beck M, Leunig M, Nötzli H, Siebenrock KA: Femoroacetabular impingement: A cause for osteoarthritis of the hip. *Clin Orthop Relat Res* 2003; 417:112-120.
35. Rab GT: The geometry of slipped capital femoral epiphysis: Implications for movement, impingement, and corrective osteotomy. *J Pediatr Orthop* 1999;19(4): 419-424.
36. Sink EL, Zaltz I, Heare T, Dayton M: Acetabular cartilage and labral damage observed during surgical hip dislocation for stable slipped capital femoral epiphysis. *J Pediatr Orthop* 2010;30(1):26-30.
37. Futami T, Kasahara Y, Suzuki S, Seto Y, Ushikubo S: Arthroscopy for slipped capital femoral epiphysis. *J Pediatr Orthop* 1992;12(5): 592-597.
38. Leunig M, Casillas MM, Hamlet M, et al: Slipped capital femoral epiphysis: Early mechanical damage to the acetabular cartilage by a prominent femoral metaphysis. *Acta Orthop Scand* 2000;71(4): 370-375.
39. Leunig M, Slongo T, Kleinschmidt M, Ganz R: Subcapital correction osteotomy in slipped capital femoral epiphysis by means of surgical hip dislocation. *Oper Orthop Traumatol* 2007; 19(4):389-410.
40. Abraham E, Gonzalez MH, Pratap S, Amirouche F, Atluri P, Simon P: Clinical implications of anatomical wear characteristics in slipped capital femoral epiphysis and primary osteoarthritis. *J Pediatr Orthop* 2007;27(7):788-795.
41. Sonnega RJ, van der Sluijs JA, Wainwright AM, Roposch A, Hefti F: Management of slipped capital femoral epiphysis: Results of a survey of the members of the European Paediatric Orthopaedic Society. *J Child Orthop* 2011;5(6): 433-438.
42. Lehmann TG, Engesæter IO, Laborie LB, Rosendahl K, Lie SA, Engesæter LB: In situ fixation of slipped capital femoral epiphysis with Steinmann pins. *Acta Orthop* 2011;82(3):333-338.
43. Aronson DD, Carlson WE: Slipped capital femoral epiphysis: A prospective study of fixation with a single screw. *J Bone Joint Surg Am* 1992;74(6):810-819.
44. Ward WT, Stefko J, Wood KB, Stanitski CL: Fixation with a single screw for slipped capital femoral epiphysis. *J Bone Joint Surg Am* 1992;74(6):799-809.
45. Goodman WW, Johnson JT, Robertson WW Jr: Single screw fixation for acute and acute-on-chronic slipped capital femoral epiphysis. *Clin Orthop Relat Res* 1996;322:86-90.
46. de Sanctis N, Di Gennaro G, Pempinello C, Corte SD, Carannante G: Is gentle manipulative reduction and percutaneous fixation with a single screw the best management of acute and acute-on-chronic slipped capital femoral epiphysis? A report of 70 patients. *J Pediatr Orthop B* 1996;5(2): 90-95.
47. Hägglund G, Hansson LI, Sandström S: Slipped capital femoral epiphysis in southern Sweden: Long-term results after nailing/pinning. *Clin Orthop Relat Res* 1987;217:190-200.
48. Wensaas A, Svenningsen S, Terjesen T: Long-term outcome of slipped capital femoral epiphysis: A 38-year follow-up of 66 patients. *J Child Orthop* 2011;5(2):75-82.
49. Mohammed R, Johnson K, Bache E: Radiation exposure during in-situ pinning of slipped capital femoral epiphysis hips: Does the patient positioning matter? *J Pediatr Orthop B* 2010;19(4): 333-336.
50. Blasier RD, Ramsey JR, White RR: Comparison of radiolucent and fracture tables in the treatment of slipped capital femoral epiphysis. *J Pediatr Orthop* 2004; 24(6):642-644.
51. Lee FY, Chapman CB: In situ pinning of hip for stable slipped capital femoral epiphysis on a radiolucent operating table. *J Pediatr Orthop* 2003;23(1):27-29.
52. Ilchmann T, Parsch K: Complications at screw removal in slipped capital femoral epiphysis treated by cannulated titanium screws. *Arch Orthop Trauma Surg* 2006; 126(6):359-363.
53. Vresilovic EJ, Spindler KP, Robertson WW Jr, Davidson RS, Drummond DS: Failures of pin removal after in situ pinning of slipped capital femoral epiphyses: A comparison of different pin types. *J Pediatr Orthop* 1990; 10(6):764-768.
54. Lee TK, Haynes RJ, Longo JA, Chu JR: Pin removal in slipped capital femoral epiphysis: The unsuitability of titanium devices. *J Pediatr Orthop* 1996;16(1): 49-52.
55. Dragoni M, Heiner AD, Costa S, Gabrielli A, Weinstein SL: Biomechanical study of 16-mm threaded, 32-mm threaded, and

fully threaded SCFE screw fixation. *J Pediatr Orthop* 2012;32(1):70-74.

56. Miyanji F, Mahar A, Oka R, Pring M, Wenger D: Biomechanical comparison of fully and partially threaded screws for fixation of slipped capital femoral epiphysis. *J Pediatr Orthop* 2008;28(1):49-52.
57. Upasani V, Kishan S, Oka R, et al: Biomechanical analysis of single screw fixation for slipped capital femoral epiphysis: Are more threads across the physis necessary for stability? *J Pediatr Orthop* 2006;26(4):474-478.
58. Carney BT, Birnbaum P, Minter C: Slip progression after in situ single screw fixation for stable slipped capital femoral epiphysis. *J Pediatr Orthop* 2003;23(5):584-589.
59. Claffey TJ: Avascular necrosis of the femoral head: An anatomical study. *J Bone Joint Surg Br* 1960;42:802-809.
60. Nguyen D, Morrissy RT: Slipped capital femoral epiphysis: Rationale for the technique of percutaneous in situ fixation. *J Pediatr Orthop* 1990;10(3):341-346.
61. Senthi S, Blyth P, Metcalfe R, Stott NS: Screw placement after pinning of slipped capital femoral epiphysis: A postoperative CT scan study. *J Pediatr Orthop* 2011;31(4):388-392.
62. Moseley C: The approach-withdraw phenomenon in the pinning of slipped capital femoral epiphysis. *Orthop Trans* 1985;9:497.
63. Rooks MD, Schmitt EW, Drvaric DM: Unrecognized pin penetration in slipped capital femoral epiphysis. *Clin Orthop Relat Res* 1988;234:82-89.
64. Segal LS, Jacobson JA, Saunders MM: Biomechanical analysis of in situ single versus double screw fixation in a nonreduced slipped capital femoral epiphysis model. *J Pediatr Orthop* 2006;26(4):479-485.
65. Kishan S, Upasani V, Mahar A, et al: Biomechanical stability of single-screw versus two-screw fixation of an unstable slipped capital femoral epiphysis model: Effect of screw position in the femoral neck. *J Pediatr Orthop* 2006;26(5):601-605.
66. Snyder RR, Williams JL, Schmidt TL, Salsbury TL: Torsional strength of double- versus single-screw fixation in a pig model of unstable slipped capital femoral epiphysis. *J Pediatr Orthop* 2006;26(3):295-299.
67. Stevens DB, Short BA, Burch JM: In situ fixation of the slipped capital femoral epiphysis with a single screw. *J Pediatr Orthop B* 1996;5(2):85-89.
68. Blanco JS, Taylor B, Johnston CE II : Comparison of single pin versus multiple pin fixation in treatment of slipped capital femoral epiphysis. *J Pediatr Orthop* 1992;12(3):384-389.
69. Stambough JL, Davidson RS, Ellis RD, Gregg JR: Slipped capital femoral epiphysis: An analysis of 80 patients as to pin placement and number. *J Pediatr Orthop* 1986;6(3):265-273.
70. Siegel DB, Kasser JR, Sponseller P, Gelberman RH: Slipped capital femoral epiphysis: A quantitative analysis of motion, gait, and femoral remodeling after in situ fixation. *J Bone Joint Surg Am* 1991;73(5):659-666.
71. Song KM, Halliday S, Reilly C, Keezel W: Gait abnormalities following slipped capital femoral epiphysis. *J Pediatr Orthop* 2004;24(2):148-155.
72. Goodwin RC, Mahar AT, Oswald TS, Wenger DR: Screw head impingement after in situ fixation in moderate and severe slipped capital femoral epiphysis. *J Pediatr Orthop* 2007;27(3):319-325.
73. Larson AN, Sierra RJ, Yu EM, Trousdale RT, Stans AA: Outcomes of slipped capital femoral epiphysis treated with in situ pinning. *J Pediatr Orthop* 2012;32(2):125-130.
74. Uglow MG, Clarke NM: The management of slipped capital femoral epiphysis. *J Bone Joint Surg Br* 2004;86(5):631-635.
75. Dodds MK, McCormack D, Mulhall KJ: Femoroacetabular impingement after slipped capital femoral epiphysis: Does slip severity predict clinical symptoms? *J Pediatr Orthop* 2009;29(6):535-539.
76. Ziebarth K, Zilkens C, Spencer S, Leunig M, Ganz R, Kim YJ: Capital realignment for moderate and severe SCFE using a modified Dunn procedure. *Clin Orthop Relat Res* 2009;467(3):704-716.
77. Leunig M, Horowitz K, Manner H, Ganz R: In situ pinning with arthroscopic osteoplasty for mild SCFE: A preliminary technical report. *Clin Orthop Relat Res* 2010;468(12):3160-3167.
78. Weinstein SL, Carney BT: Slipped capital femoral epiphysis. *Curr Orthop* 1997;11(1):51-55.
79. O'Brien ET, Fahey JJ: Remodeling of the femoral neck after in situ pinning for slipped capital femoral epiphysis. *J Bone Joint Surg Am* 1977;59(1):62-68.
80. Bellemans J, Fabry G, Molenaers G, Lammens J, Moens P: Slipped capital femoral epiphysis: A long-term follow-up, with special emphasis on the capacities for remodeling. *J Pediatr Orthop B* 1996;5(3):151-157.
81. Wong-Chung J, Strong ML: Physeal remodeling after internal fixation of slipped capital femoral epiphyses. *J Pediatr Orthop* 1991;11(1):2-5.
82. Jones JR, Paterson DC, Hillier TM, Foster BK: Remodelling after pinning for slipped capital

femoral epiphysis. *J Bone Joint Surg Br* 1990;72(4):568-573.

83. Castañeda P, Macías C, Rocha A, Harfush A, Cassis N: Functional outcome of stable grade III slipped capital femoral epiphysis treated with in situ pinning. *J Pediatr Orthop* 2009;29(5):454-458.

84. Philippon MJ, Stubbs AJ, Schenker ML, Maxwell RB, Ganz R, Leunig M: Arthroscopic management of femoroacetabular impingement: Osteoplasty technique and literature review. *Am J Sports Med* 2007;35(9):1571-1580.

85. Diab M, Daluvoy S, Snyder BD, Kasser JR: Osteotomy does not improve early outcome after slipped capital femoral epiphysis. *J Pediatr Orthop B* 2006;15(2): 87-92.

86. Schai PA, Exner GU: Indication for and results of intertrochanteric osteotomy in slipped capital femoral epiphysis. *Orthopade* 2002; 31(9):900-907.

87. Schai PA, Exner GU: Corrective Imhäuser intertrochanteric osteotomy. *Oper Orthop Traumatol* 2007;19(4):368-388.

88. Abraham E, Garst J, Barmada R: Treatment of moderate to severe slipped capital femoral epiphysis with extracapsular base-of-neck osteotomy. *J Pediatr Orthop* 1993; 13(3):294-302.

89. Gage JR, Sundberg AB, Nolan DR, Sletten RG, Winter RB: Complications after cuneiform osteotomy for moderately or severely slipped capital femoral epiphysis. *J Bone Joint Surg Am* 1978;60(2):157-165.

90. Biring GS, Hashemi-Nejad A, Catterall A: Outcomes of subcapital cuneiform osteotomy for the treatment of severe slipped capital femoral epiphysis after skeletal maturity. *J Bone Joint Surg Br* 2006;88(10):1379-1384.

91. DeRosa GP, Mullins RC, Kling TF Jr: Cuneiform osteotomy of the femoral neck in severe slipped capital femoral epiphysis. *Clin Orthop Relat Res* 1996;322:48-60.

92. Ganz R, Gill TJ, Gautier E, Ganz K, Krügel N, Berlemann U: Surgical dislocation of the adult hip: A technique with full access to the femoral head and acetabulum without the risk of avascular necrosis. *J Bone Joint Surg Br* 2001; 83(8):1119-1124.

93. Leunig M, Slongo T, Ganz R: Subcapital realignment in slipped capital femoral epiphysis: Surgical hip dislocation and trimming of the stable trochanter to protect the perfusion of the epiphysis. *Instr Course Lect* 2008;57: 499-507.

94. Huber H, Dora C, Ramseier LE, Buck F, Dierauer S: Adolescent slipped capital femoral epiphysis treated by a modified Dunn osteotomy with surgical hip dislocation. *J Bone Joint Surg Br* 2011; 93(6):833-838.

95. Kallio PE, Paterson DC, Foster BK, Lequesne GW: Classification in slipped capital femoral epiphysis: Sonographic assessment of stability and remodeling. *Clin Orthop Relat Res* 1993;294: 196-203.

96. Kallio PE, Mah ET, Foster BK, Paterson DC, LeQuesne GW: Slipped capital femoral epiphysis: Incidence and clinical assessment of physeal instability. *J Bone Joint Surg Br* 1995;77(5):752-755.

97. Larson AN, McIntosh AL, Trousdale RT, Lewallen DG: Avascular necrosis most common indication for hip arthroplasty in patients with slipped capital femoral epiphysis. *J Pediatr Orthop* 2010; 30(8):767-773.

98. Tokmakova KP, Stanton RP, Mason DE: Factors influencing the development of osteonecrosis in patients treated for slipped capital femoral epiphysis. *J Bone Joint Surg Am* 2003;85-A(5):798-801.

99. Krahn TH, Canale ST, Beaty JH, Warner WC, Lourenço P: Long-term follow-up of patients with avascular necrosis after treatment of slipped capital femoral epiphysis. *J Pediatr Orthop* 1993;13(2): 154-158.

100. Maeda S, Kita A, Funayama K, Kokubun S: Vascular supply to slipped capital femoral epiphysis. *J Pediatr Orthop* 2001;21(5): 664-667.

101. Palocaren T, Holmes L, Rogers K, Kumar SJ: Outcome of in situ pinning in patients with unstable slipped capital femoral epiphysis: Assessment of risk factors associated with avascular necrosis. *J Pediatr Orthop* 2010;30(1):31-36.

102. Sankar WN, McPartland TG, Millis MB, Kim YJ: The unstable slipped capital femoral epiphysis: Risk factors for osteonecrosis. *J Pediatr Orthop* 2010;30(6): 544-548.

103. Peterson MD, Weiner DS, Green NE, Terry CL: Acute slipped capital femoral epiphysis: The value and safety of urgent manipulative reduction. *J Pediatr Orthop* 1997; 17(5):648-654.

104. Kalogrianitis S, Tan CK, Kemp GJ, Bass A, Bruce C: Does unstable slipped capital femoral epiphysis require urgent stabilization? *J Pediatr Orthop B* 2007; 16(1):6-9.

105. Gordon JE, Abrahams MS, Dobbs MB, Luhmann SJ, Schoenecker PL: Early reduction, arthrotomy, and cannulated screw fixation in unstable slipped capital femoral epiphysis treatment. *J Pediatr Orthop* 2002;22(3):352-358.

106. Lowndes S, Khanna A, Emery D, Sim J, Maffulli N: Management of unstable slipped upper femoral epiphysis: A meta-analysis. *Br Med Bull* 2009;90:133-146.

107. Chen RC, Schoenecker PL, Dobbs MB, Luhmann SJ, Szymanski DA, Gordon JE: Urgent reduction, fixation, and arthrotomy for unstable slipped

capital femoral epiphysis. *J Pediatr Orthop* 2009;29(7):687-694.

108. Wirth T: Slipped upper femoral epiphysis (SUFE). *Z Orthop Unfall* 2011;149(4):e21-e41, quiz e42-e43.

109. Heisel J: Acute slipped femur head epiphysis. Causes, surgical treatment, results. *Aktuelle Traumatol* 1987;17(2):48-54.

110. Herrera-Soto JA, Duffy MF, Birnbaum MA, Vander Have KL: Increased intracapsular pressures after unstable slipped capital femoral epiphysis. *J Pediatr Orthop* 2008;28(7):723-728.

111. Svalastoga E, Kiaer T, Jensen PE: The effect of intracapsular pressure and extension of the hip on oxygenation of the juvenile femoral epiphysis: A study in the goat. *J Bone Joint Surg Br* 1989;71(2):222-226.

112. Beck M, Siebenrock KA, Affolter B, Nötzli H, Parvizi J, Ganz R: Increased intraarticular pressure reduces blood flow to the femoral head. *Clin Orthop Relat Res* 2004;424:149-152.

113. Parsch K, Weller S, Parsch D: Open reduction and smooth Kirschner wire fixation for unstable slipped capital femoral epiphysis. *J Pediatr Orthop* 2009;29(1):1-8.

114. Leunig M, Fraitzl CR, Ganz R: Early damage to the acetabular cartilage in slipped capital femoral epiphysis: Therapeutic consequences. *Orthopade* 2002;31(9):894-899.

115. Murray RO: The aetiology of primary osteoarthritis of the hip. *Br J Radiol* 1965;38(455):810-824.

116. Stulberg SD, Cordell LD, Harris WH, Ramsey PL, MacEwen GD: *Unrecognized Childhood Hip Disease: A Major Cause of Idiopathic Osteoarthritis of the Hip*. St. Louis, MO, CV Mosby, 1975.

117. Mamisch TC, Kim YJ, Richolt JA, Millis MB, Kordelle J: Femoral morphology due to impingement influences the range of motion in slipped capital femoral epiphysis. *Clin Orthop Relat Res* 2009;467(3):692-698.

118. Miese FR, Zilkens C, Holstein A, et al: MRI morphometry, cartilage damage and impaired function in the follow-up after slipped capital femoral epiphysis. *Skeletal Radiol* 2010;39(6):533-541.

119. Zilkens C, Miese F, Bittersohl B, et al: Delayed gadolinium-enhanced magnetic resonance imaging of cartilage (dGEMRIC), after slipped capital femoral epiphysis. *Eur J Radiol* 2011;79(3):400-406.

120. Millis MB, Novais EN: In situ fixation for slipped capital femoral epiphysis: Perspectives in 2011. *J Bone Joint Surg Am* 2011;93(suppl 2):46-51.

121. Diab M, Hresko MT, Millis MB: Intertrochanteric versus subcapital osteotomy in slipped capital femoral epiphysis. *Clin Orthop Relat Res* 2004;427:204-212.

122. Maussen JP, Rozing PM, Obermann WR: Intertrochanteric corrective osteotomy in slipped capital femoral epiphysis: A long-term follow-up study of 26 patients. *Clin Orthop Relat Res* 1990;259:100-110.

123. Schai PA, Exner GU, Hänsch O: Prevention of secondary coxarthrosis in slipped capital femoral epiphysis: A long-term follow-up study after corrective intertrochanteric osteotomy. *J Pediatr Orthop B* 1996;5(3):135-143.

124. Kartenbender K, Cordier W, Katthagen BD: Long-term follow-up study after corrective Imhäuser osteotomy for severe slipped capital femoral epiphysis. *J Pediatr Orthop* 2000;20(6):749-756.

125. Rao JP, Francis AM, Siwek CW: The treatment of chronic slipped capital femoral epiphysis by biplane osteotomy. *J Bone Joint Surg Am* 1984;66(8):1169-1175.

126. Mamisch TC, Kim YJ, Richolt J, et al: Range of motion after computed tomography-based simulation of intertrochanteric corrective osteotomy in cases of slipped capital femoral epiphysis: Comparison of uniplanar flexion osteotomy and multiplanar flexion, valgisation, and rotational osteotomies. *J Pediatr Orthop* 2009;29(4):336-340.

127. Kuzyk PR, Kim YJ, Millis MB: Surgical management of healed slipped capital femoral epiphysis. *J Am Acad Orthop Surg* 2011;19(11):667-677.

128. Spencer S, Millis MB, Kim YJ: Early results of treatment of hip impingement syndrome in slipped capital femoral epiphysis and pistol grip deformity of the femoral head-neck junction using the surgical dislocation technique. *J Pediatr Orthop* 2006;26(3):281-285.

129. Rebello G, Spencer S, Millis MB, Kim YJ: Surgical dislocation in the management of pediatric and adolescent hip deformity. *Clin Orthop Relat Res* 2009;467(3):724-731.

130. Clohisy JC, McClure JT: Treatment of anterior femoroacetabular impingement with combined hip arthroscopy and limited anterior decompression. *Iowa Orthop J* 2005;25:164-171.

131. Byrd JW, Jones KS: Arthroscopic management of femoroacetabular impingement. *Instr Course Lect* 2009;58:231-239.

38

SYMPOSIUM

Approach to the Pediatric Supracondylar Humeral Fracture With Neurovascular Compromise

Corinna C. Franklin, MD
David L. Skaggs, MD

Abstract

Supracondylar fractures of the humerus are exceedingly common in pediatric patients but may present treatment challenges when complicated by neurovascular compromise. Patients presenting with poor perfusion should be treated with urgent reduction because this is a limb-threatening emergency. If perfusion does not improve, or if a previously perfused extremity loses perfusion after reduction, arterial exploration is warranted. Controversy exists over whether to observe or explore a reduced, perfused, but pulseless extremity with a supracondylar fracture. Minimal management requires that these injuries be carefully monitored for 48 hours for loss of perfusion or the development of compartment syndrome.

In general, nerve injuries accompanying supracondylar fractures of the humerus are neurapraxias and may be treated conservatively; however, nerve palsy with accompanying pulselessness warrants immediate exploration. Patients should be treated more urgently if excessive swelling, antecubital ecchymosis, skin puckering, an absent pulse, or fractures in the same limb are present. If a hand is not perfused or compartments are firm, emergent treatment should be considered.

Instr Course Lect 2013;62:429-433.

Supracondylar fractures of the humerus are exceedingly common pediatric fractures, accounting for 55% to 80% of elbow fractures in children.[1] Considerable controversy exists concerning the management of difficult supracondylar fractures, particularly regarding the treatment of fractures with vascular or nerve injury or compartment syndrome and the appropriate timing of fracture fixation. This chapter discusses approaches to treating supracondylar fractures with neurovascular compromise based on the available literature and the senior author's (DLS') experience in a level I pediatric trauma hospital (**Figure 1**).

Vascular Compromise

As many as 20% of pediatric patients with supracondylar fractures present with some form of vascular compromise.[1] Brachial artery injury in this setting affects approximately 60 children per year in the Unites States.[2] In a study of 1,255 consecutive pediatric patients with supracondylar fractures, Choi et al[1] found that 33 patients (2.6%) presented with a pulseless fracture. Other studies have cited vascular compromise rates of up to 20%, and brachial artery compromise has been reported in up to 11% of supracondylar fractures.[3,4] It is essential to determine whether the extremity is well perfused despite the lack of a pulse. The assessment of perfusion in the pulseless extremity can be difficult and is somewhat subjective; if there is doubt concerning adequate perfusion, it should be assumed that the extremity is not well perfused. A perfused but pulseless hand should be pink and warm, with capillary refill taking less than 2 sec-

Dr. Skaggs or an immediate family member serves as a board member, owner, officer, or committee member of the Pediatric Orthopaedic Society of North America, the Growing Spine Study Group, and the Scoliosis Research Society; has received royalties from Biomet; is a member of a speakers' bureau or has made paid presentations on behalf of Medtronic and Stryker; serves as a paid consultant to or is an employee of Medtronic, Stryker, and Biomet; and has received nonincome support (such as equipment or services), commercially derived honoraria, or other non–research-related funding (such as paid travel) from Medtronic (sold intellectual property of rod benders for $10,000). Neither Dr. Franklin nor any immediate family member has received anything of value from or owns stock in a commercial company or institution related directly or indirectly to the subject of this chapter.

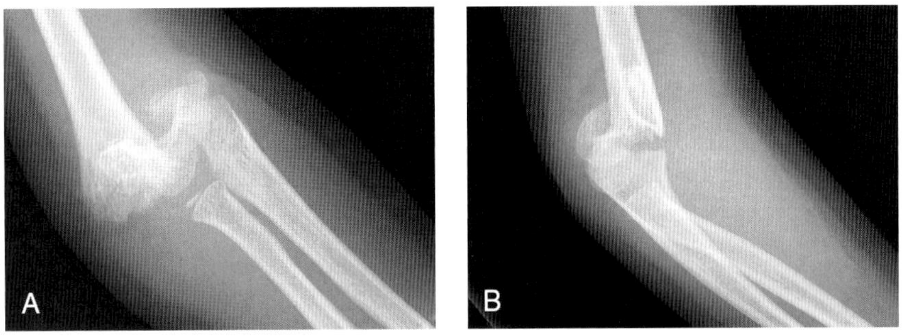

Figure 1 AP (**A**) and lateral (**B**) radiographic views of a displaced supracondylar fracture of the humerus.

onds. A cool, pale hand with sluggish capillary refill should be considered poorly perfused.

For a patient presenting with a supracondylar fracture with a pulseless and poorly perfused extremity, urgent reduction is indicated.[3] Gentle traction and 30° to 40° of flexion may be applied as soon as possible in the emergency department. A preoperative arteriogram is not indicated because no additional useful information can be ascertained. In an isolated supracondylar fracture of the humerus, if clinical signs clearly indicate vascular compromise, it can be assumed that the vascular injury is located at the fracture site.[1,5]

After reduction and fixation, the extremity should be reassessed. If the pulse returns and the extremity is well perfused, no further steps are needed. If the pulse is absent and the extremity remains poorly perfused, the artery should be explored. If a pulse was present before reduction and is absent after reduction, it should be assumed that the artery or adjacent tissue is trapped in the fracture site and is occluding the arterial flow. In this situation, it is usually necessary to open the fracture site for evaluation of the artery and fracture reduction.

Perfusion in a pulseless extremity can be difficult to assess, particularly if the coloring has been affected by the surgical preparation or the extremity is cool after being prepped and washed. Controversy exists over the appropriate treatment at this point—whether to explore the artery or admit the patient for 48 hours with elevation of the arm and close observation. Sabharwal et al[6] examined a small series of pulseless supracondylar fractures in which the artery was repaired and reported a high rate of residual stenosis and reocclusion. The authors recommended close observation rather than early surgical intervention. In contrast, a systematic review by White et al[3] recommended watchful waiting for a pulseless but perfused supracondylar fracture. The authors also suggested that if brachial artery revascularization is performed, it is likely to succeed, with high patency rates. In a series of 12 patients who had vascular reconstructions after supracondylar humeral fractures, Konstantiniuk et al[7] found that all the reconstructions were patent at a mean follow-up of 14 years.

Ramesh et al[8] reported on a series of seven pediatric patients with supracondylar humeral fractures who had a pulseless but perfused hand after reduction. Vascular exploration was not performed; the radial pulse returned in all the patients within 6 weeks, and no long-term complications were reported. Griffin et al[9] concluded that "a child with a pink pulseless hand post fracture reduction can be managed expectantly unless additional signs of vascular compromise develop" and indicated that neither angiography nor color duplex ultrasound add any valuable information in these cases.

Pulseless supracondylar fractures have a substantial risk for compartment syndrome and must be closely observed. Blakey et al[4] reported on a series of pediatric patients in whom contractures of the forearm and hand developed because of ischemia after a persistent, pink, pulseless supracondylar fracture. The authors recommended urgent exploration of the vessels and nerves if fracture reduction does not restore a pulse, and pain suggestive of a nerve lesion or ischemia persists.

If the patient has a pulseless but well-perfused hand after reduction, this chapter's authors recommend in-hospital observation for 48 hours. In two of our patients, perfusion was lost in the hand after reduction (at approximately 24 hours in one patient and 36 hours in the other patient). In both of these patients, the artery itself was not trapped in the fracture site, but adjacent tissue was trapped and caused a sharp kink in the artery. When the tissue was released, vascular perfusion was restored.

Perfusion in the presence of pulselessness at the time of presentation is predictive of the patient's outcome. Choi et al[1] reported that fracture reduction alone was sufficient treatment for all patients in their study who had a perfused but pulseless extremity, and additional vascular repair was not needed. Considerable controversy has existed over the urgency of reduction and fixation in a pulseless but perfused hand. Several recent studies suggest that undue delay in reducing a pink, pulseless supracondylar fracture may increase the risk of complications.[3,4]

The patient presenting with a pulseless and poorly perfused extremity has a much higher risk of a poorer

Table 1
Study Results: Supracondylar Humeral (SCH) Fractures With Neurovascular Compromise

Study	Patients and Fractures	Results	Recommendations/Conclusions
Blakey et al[4]	26 pink, pulseless SCH fractures	23 of 26: ischemic contracture	Urgent exploration of SCH fracture with pink, pulseless hand
Choi et al[1]	33 pulseless SCH fractures; 24 well-perfused, 9 poorly perfused	All well perfused did well; poorly perfused: 2 compartment syndromes, 4 vascular repairs	Patients with SCH fracture and poor perfusion are at risk for vascular repair and compartment syndrome
Gupta et al[15]	150 consecutive SCH fractures	50 patients had surgery ≤ 12 hours; 100 had surgery > 12 hours	No difference in complication rate or open reduction rate
Iyengar et al[12]	58 consecutive type 3 SCH fractures	23 had surgery ≤ 8 hours; 35 had surgery > 8 hours	No difference in need for open reduction or clinical outcome
Konstantiniuk et al[7]	12 SCH fractures with vascular reconstructions	All patent	Surgical reconstruction for SCH fracture with vascular lesion is effective
Leet et al[14]	153 type 3 SCH fractures	30 unsatisfactory results	No correlation between delay and unsatisfactory results or open reduction
Mangat et al[11]	19 pink, pulseless SCH fractures	11 treated conservatively, 4 of which required secondary intervention because of an entrapped artery	Anterior interosseous or median nerve palsy is strongly predictive of nerve or vessel entrapment
Mehlman et al[13]	198 displaced SCH fractures	52 treated ≤ 8 hours; 146 treated > 8 hours	No significant difference in complication rates between early and delayed surgery
Ramachandran et al[16]	11 SCH fractures with compartment syndrome	10 patients had severe swelling and a mean 22-hour delay until surgery	Significant swelling and delay in reduction may be warning signs for compartment syndrome
Ramesh et al[8]	7 pink pulseless SCH fractures	All patients managed expectantly; all pulses returned by 6 weeks	Watchful expectancy is appropriate for the pink, pulseless SCH fracture
Sabharwal et al[6]	13 pink pulseless SCH fractures	Early revascularization resulted in a high rate of reocclusion	Close observation of pink pulseless SCH fractures rather than early intervention is warranted
Shaw et al[5]	143 type 3 SCH fractures	17 had vascular compromise	Angiography not necessary

outcome. In the study by Choi et al,[1] nine patients presented with a pulseless and poorly perfused extremity. Four of those nine patients (44%) required vascular repair, and compartment syndrome developed in two of the patients (22%). This chapter's authors consider a pulseless and poorly perfused hand with a supracondylar fracture to be a limb-threatening condition that must be treated emergently. Consideration should be given to alerting the vascular surgery service when a patient presents with these injuries.

Patients with pulseless supracondylar humeral fractures are likely to have good outcomes with timely fracture reduction if the hand is well perfused. Fracture reduction should not be delayed for vascular studies or consultation. The goal of treatment is to maintain vascular perfusion, not necessarily return a pulse. Patients with pulseless but well-perfused hands should be closely observed for 24 to 48 hours postoperatively for loss of perfusion and/or the development of compartment syndrome.

Nerve Injury

Traumatic nerve injury associated with supracondylar humeral fractures has an incidence between 12% and 20%. Extension-type fractures most frequently lead to median or anterior interosseous nerve injuries. Flexion-type injuries more commonly affect the ulnar nerve and are usually neurapraxias that heal within 6 months. Isolated nerve injuries (those without vascular compromise) typically require observation only.[10]

In contradistinction, a pulseless hand with anterior interosseous or median nerve palsy warrants early exploration. Mangat et al[11] reported the presence of an entrapped or tethered artery in all the patients in their study (seven patients) who had a pulseless hand and nerve palsy at presentation, whereas only 20% of the patients without a nerve deficit had an entrapped or tethered artery. This chapter's authors believe that in patients with a supracondylar humeral fracture, nerve palsy, and pulselessness, early exploration of the fracture site to extricate a potentially entrapped artery is appropriate. Patients with supracondylar fractures who have either nerve

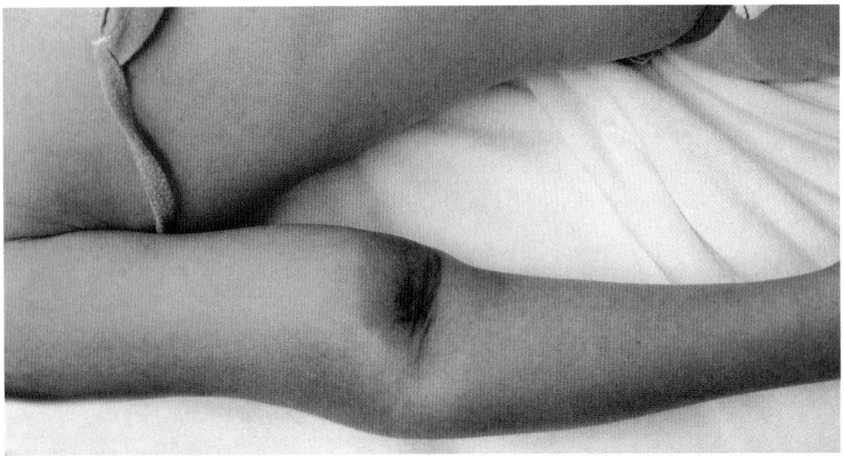

Figure 2 Antecubital ecchymosis should prompt urgent treatment of a supracondylar fracture of the humerus. (Courtesy of Children's Orthopaedic Center, Los Angeles, CA.)

palsy or a pulseless but perfused hand may be observed; in the presence of both conditions, exploration is indicated.

Surgical Timing

Considerable controversy exists concerning the appropriate timing for the fixation of supracondylar humeral fractures. It is debated whether these fractures should be fixed immediately (even in the middle of the night) or whether delay until the morning is acceptable. Based on several retrospective studies, the general finding is that some delay is acceptable and will not increase the risks of complications. Iyengar et al[12] and Mehlman et al[13] reported that a delay of more than 8 hours after injury was not associated with an increased risk of complications. Other authors found that delaying fracture fixation 12 hours to more than 21 hours after injury did not increase the risk of complications.[14,15] However, because these were retrospective studies, they may show only that the operating surgeons had good judgment in selecting the patients who required urgent treatment. It is imperative that a delay in treatment not be confused with a delay in the diagnosis; patients should be evaluated urgently, even if surgery is not to be performed immediately. The results of studies of pediatric patients with supracondylar humeral fractures with neurovascular compromise are summarized in **Table 1**.[1,4-8,11-16]

Compartment Syndrome

Despite improved knowledge and decision making, an analysis of data from the Healthcare Cost and Utilization Project shows that compartment syndrome occurs in an average of 32 children each year in the United States after a supracondylar humeral fracture.[2,16] Ramachandran et al[16] examined a series of low-risk pediatric patients with closed, low-energy, isolated fractures without vascular compromise for the occurrence of compartment syndrome. Ten patients with compartment syndrome were identified; the mean age of the children was 6 years. Associated factors were severe elbow swelling in 90%, sensory changes in 70%, and a mean delay to surgery of 23 hours. The authors suggested that patients with severe elbow swelling have an elevated risk for compartment syndrome if surgery is delayed. More urgent treatment is required in the presence of excessive swelling, antecubital ecchymosis or skin puckering, an absent pulse, or other fractures in the same limb (**Figure 2**). If a hand is not perfused or the compartments are firm, emergent treatment should be considered.

Summary

Pediatric supracondylar humeral fractures are common injuries; those with accompanying neurovascular compromise warrant particular attention. A patient who presents with a poorly perfused extremity should be treated with urgent reduction because this is a limb-threatening emergency. Arterial exploration is warranted if reduction does not restore perfusion to the limb or if a previously perfused extremity loses perfusion after reduction. Whether to explore or observe a reduced, perfused, but pulseless extremity with a supracondylar fracture remains a topic of debate. Minimal management mandates that these borderline cases be carefully monitored for at least 48 hours for loss of perfusion or the development of compartment syndrome. Isolated nerve injuries accompanying supracondylar fractures of the humerus are usually neurapraxias, which may be treated conservatively. However, the particular case of nerve palsy with accompanying pulselessness should be immediately explored. More urgent treatment is also important in the presence of excessive swelling, antecubital ecchymosis, skin puckering, an absent pulse, or other fractures in the same limb. If the hand is not perfused or the compartments are firm, emergent treatment should be considered.

References

1. Choi PD, Melikian R, Skaggs DL: Risk factors for vascular repair and compartment syndrome in the

pulseless supracondylar humerus fracture in children. *J Pediatr Orthop* 2010;30(1):50-56.

2. Roehrich J, Mehlman CT, Ying J: Paper No. 230. Epidemiology of vascular complications in supracondylar humerus fractures in the United States. *AAOS 2012 Annual Meeting Proceedings*. CD-ROM. Rosemont, IL, American Academy of Orthopaedic Surgeons, 2012, p 804.
3. White L, Mehlman CT, Crawford AH: Perfused, pulseless, and puzzling: A systematic review of vascular injuries in pediatric supracondylar humerus fractures and results of a POSNA questionnaire. *J Pediatr Orthop* 2010;30(4): 328-335.
4. Blakey CM, Biant LC, Birch R: Ischaemia and the pink, pulseless hand complicating supracondylar fractures of the humerus in childhood: Long-term follow-up. *J Bone Joint Surg Br* 2009;91(11): 1487-1492.
5. Shaw BA, Kasser JR, Emans JB, Rand FF: Management of vascular injuries in displaced supracondylar humerus fractures without arteriography. *J Orthop Trauma* 1990;4(1):25-29.
6. Sabharwal S, Tredwell SJ, Beauchamp RD, et al: Management of pulseless pink hand in pediatric supracondylar fractures of humerus. *J Pediatr Orthop* 1997; 17(3):303-310.
7. Konstantiniuk P, Fritz G, Ott T, Weiglhofer U, Schweiger S, Cohnert T: Long-term follow-up of vascular reconstructions after supracondylar humerus fracture with vascular lesion in childhood. *Eur J Vasc Endovasc Surg* 2011; 42(5):684-688.
8. Ramesh P, Avadhani A, Shetty AP, Dheenadhayalan J, Rajasekaran S: Management of acute "pink pulseless" hand in pediatric supracondylar fractures of the humerus. *J Pediatr Orthop B* 2011;20(3): 124-128.
9. Griffin KJ, Walsh SR, Markar S, Tang TY, Boyle JR, Hayes PD: The pink pulseless hand: A review of the literature regarding management of vascular complications of supracondylar humeral fractures in children. *Eur J Vasc Endovasc Surg* 2008;36(6):697-702.
10. Ramachandran M, Birch R, Eastwood DM: Clinical outcome of nerve injuries associated with supracondylar fractures of the humerus in children: The experience of a specialist referral centre. *J Bone Joint Surg Br* 2006;88(1): 90-94.
11. Mangat KS, Martin AG, Bache CE: The "pulseless pink" hand after supracondylar fracture of the humerus in children: The predictive value of nerve palsy. *J Bone Joint Surg Br* 2009;91(11):1521-1525.
12. Iyengar SR, Hoffinger SA, Townsend DR: Early versus delayed reduction and pinning of type III displaced supracondylar fractures of the humerus in children: A comparative study. *J Orthop Trauma* 1999;13(1):51-55.
13. Mehlman CT, Strub WM, Roy DR, Wall EJ, Crawford AH: The effect of surgical timing on the perioperative complications of treatment of supracondylar humeral fractures in children. *J Bone Joint Surg Am* 2001;83-A(3): 323-327.
14. Leet AI, Frisancho J, Ebramzadeh E: Delayed treatment of type 3 supracondylar humerus fractures in children. *J Pediatr Orthop* 2002;22(2):203-207.
15. Gupta N, Kay RM, Leitch K, Femino JD, Tolo VT, Skaggs DL: Effect of surgical delay on perioperative complications and need for open reduction in supracondylar humerus fractures in children. *J Pediatr Orthop* 2004;24(3): 245-248.
16. Ramachandran M, Skaggs DL, Crawford HA, et al: Delaying treatment of supracondylar fractures in children: Has the pendulum swung too far? *J Bone Joint Surg Br* 2008;90(9):1228-1233.

39

Shoulder Instability in the Young Athlete

Benton E. Heyworth, MD
Mininder S. Kocher, MD, MPH

Abstract

Shoulder instability is among the most common musculoskeletal injuries and overuse conditions in pediatric and adolescent athletes requiring orthopaedic care. Injury patterns in skeletally immature patients are unique to the developing musculoskeletal system and may be specific to the involved sport. It is helpful to have an outline of the basic diagnostic approaches and to review the literature that guides management principles in young athletes with shoulder instability.

Instr Course Lect 2013;62:435-444.

As participation in youth sports continues to increase in number and intensity, musculoskeletal injuries and overuse conditions in pediatric and adolescent athletes are becoming more common.[1-3] Although anterior cruciate ligament ruptures, meniscal tears, and osteochondritis dissecans lesions are often cited as evidence of these trends, upper extremity pathology in the young athlete is also occurring more frequently.[4] Shoulder instability is among the most common conditions requiring orthopaedic care, and familiarity with its different forms and treatment methods is critical for all physicians who care for pediatric and adolescent athletes. This chapter describes the various types of shoulder instability common in young patients, outlines a basic diagnostic approach, and reviews the literature guiding management principles in this specific population.

Shoulder Anatomy and Maturation

The proximal humeral physis contributes approximately 80% of the longitudinal growth of the upper extremity and typically fuses at ages 14 to 22 years. The hypertrophic zone of the physis is particularly vulnerable to the acute macrotraumatic and chronic microtraumatic forces that can occur in athletic activities.[5-9] Salter-Harris type I or II fractures of the proximal humerus should be ruled out for any suspected glenohumeral dislocation in a skeletally immature athlete.[10]

The capsuloligamentous and muscular structures of the shoulder serve as static and dynamic stabilizers. The dynamic stabilizers are the rotator cuff, deltoid, and scapulothoracic tendons and muscles, which exert a centralizing compressive force on the humeral head against the concavity of the glenoid during the midrange of motion. The static stabilizers (the glenohumeral ligaments, the capsule, the labrum, and the glenoid) function at the terminal range of motion to limit abnormal humeral head translation. Injury to these dynamic and static restraints creates a unique pattern of disability that can limit normal shoulder function in the young athlete.[11]

The young athlete's stage of maturation is a unique factor contributing to injury patterns. A skeletally immature athlete has less muscular development than an adult. During the period of rapid growth, there is a predisposition to repetitive overuse injury in the developing physis, as seen in proximal humeral epiphysiolysis or Little Leaguer's shoulder.[5,7,10,12-14] Changes in soft-tissue laxity may play an important role. For example, in a newborn,

Dr. Heyworth or an immediate family member serves as a board member, owner, officer, or committee member of the Pediatric Orthopaedic Society of North America Trauma Committee and Research in Osteochondritis Dissecans of the Knee. Dr. Kocher or an immediate family member serves as a board member, owner, officer, or committee member of the American Academy of Orthopaedic Surgeons, the American Orthopaedic Society for Sports Medicine, and the Pediatric Orthopaedic Society of North America; serves as a paid consultant to or is an employee of Biomet and OrthoPediatrics; and owns stock or stock options in Fixes 4 Kids and Pivot Medical.

the predominantly synthesized collagen is elastic type III; as the child grows, the ratio of type III to less elastic type I collagen decreases with each passing year. The role of abnormal collagen or connective tissues, as seen in Ehlers-Danlos syndrome, and the wide range of etiologies contributing to generalized ligamentous hyperlaxity should be considered in all young patients with shoulder instability. Individual variations in the ratio of type I to type III collagen may predispose a young athlete to multidirectional instability (MDI) of the shoulder secondary to laxity of the capsuloligamentous structures.[15-17]

Epidemiology

Injury patterns in the shoulder of the young athlete are often specific to the involved sport. Similar to other acute traumatic injuries of the shoulder, such as acromioclavicular separations and clavicle fractures, traumatic glenohumeral dislocation is more common in contact sports, such as football, rugby, and lacrosse.[18-20] Chronic overuse injuries of the shoulder are more common in overhead sports involving repetitive activity, including tennis, swimming, and baseball. Such injuries may include internal impingement and MDI, which generally should be considered more of a chronic condition than its traumatic anterior and posterior instability counterparts.[21-23] MDI is also associated with ligamentous hyperlaxity syndromes and collagen disorders, such as Ehlers-Danlos syndrome, in both athletic and nonathletic youth populations.

Although the glenohumeral joint allows a greater arc of motion than any other joint in the body, it is also the most commonly dislocated joint in adolescents and adults. Up to 40% of all primary dislocations occur in patients younger than 22 years.[24] Shoulder dislocations are relatively rare in skeletally immature patients; however, some studies have shown impressively high rates of injury in certain subpopulations of young athletes, such as hockey and football players.[25,26] Cleeman and Flatow[24] reported a 7% incidence of traumatic shoulder dislocations in a group of young hockey players.

Patterns of Instability

The three well-described anatomic patterns of glenohumeral instability are anterior, posterior, and multidirectional. Instability may also be classified according to the mechanism of injury, (specifically as traumatic or atraumatic), which has important treatment considerations. Inferior, superior, and intrathoracic dislocations are extremely rare, usually associated with severe trauma and high complication rates, and generally not relevant to the discussion of shoulder conditions in athletes.

The most common glenohumeral instability pattern in young athletes is anterior instability, which accounts for 85% to 95% of all instability cases.[8] Anterior instability is usually caused by a traumatic acute injury in contact sports or, less commonly, results from a microtraumatic repetitive overuse injury in pitchers or throwing athletes.[27,28] A large percentage of shoulder instability in some studied populations, such as young military personnel, involves subluxation or partial dislocation episodes rather than complete, frank dislocation.[20] Posterior labral injuries, also called reverse Bankart lesions, occur in approximately 2% to 10% of all patients with shoulder instability;[29,30] have been linked to a specific pattern of direct blows to the arm or repetitive athletic activities;[31,32] and can occur in association with seizures, electrocution injuries, and severe trauma. This injury pattern, in which macrotrauma or repetitive microtrauma usually occurs with the arm flexed, adducted, and internally rotated, can often be misdiagnosed or remain undiagnosed because of the complexity of symptoms and infrequency in presentation.[30] MDI, in which subluxation or dislocation occurs in more than one direction, is also rare and accounts for less than 5% of shoulder instability cases.[33] Understanding of the complex and varying pathophysiology of MDI continues to evolve, but it is seen more often in athletes who perform repetitive overhead activities such as throwers, swimmers, and gymnasts, and it is often bilateral. MDI also can be caused by congenital hyperlaxity, abnormalities of the glenoid, or weakness in the rotator cuff.[8,34]

Diagnosis

The diagnosis and basic understanding of a patient's shoulder instability can often be made based on a detailed history and physical examination. Patients with frank anterior dislocation of the glenohumeral joint will most often report having sustained a blow to the arm or hand, with the shoulder in a position of abduction and external rotation. The arm may have been outstretched to withstand a fall to the ground, or a player may have reached out to grab another player moving with speed. Posterior dislocation is much less common and initially may be missed. At the time of injury, the patient may report having withstood a direct blow with the arm in forward elevation, adduction, and internal rotation; that position is common in football lineman during play.[35,36] Rates of subluxation, relative to frank dislocation, are high in this pattern of instability.

Players who sustain frank anterior or posterior dislocations may present to the emergency department before or after the dislocation has been reduced. In many instances, a spontaneous reduction will have occurred; this is more common with chronic, recurrent anterior instability and MDI. More commonly, however, manual reduction is needed and can be facilitated by sedating the patient. A variety of reduction maneuvers can be performed.

The physical examination of a patient with a suspected acute dislocation is critical, particularly if there is a substantial delay in obtaining radiographs. In such instances, a sideline reduction may be considered. The first step in treating a traumatic shoulder injury is a meticulous neurovascular examination because an injury to the axillary nerve can occur in association with glenohumeral dislocation and should be understood and documented before any intervention.[18,37] A patient with an anterior dislocation will generally hold the arm at his or her side and will not tolerate attempted motion of the shoulder. A subacromial defect or concavity may be visible in the soft tissue, with the humeral head palpable anteriorly.

Although there is no consensus or guideline regarding the need for radiographic confirmation before reduction of a suspected glenohumeral dislocation, radiographs should be obtained whenever possible because of the possibility of a Salter-Harris fracture involving the growth plate. Radiographic assessment should include AP and Y-scapular lateral views and an axillary lateral view to clearly establish the location of the humeral head in relationship to the glenoid and assess for a possible fracture of the glenoid rim (a bony Bankart lesion) or the humeral head (a Hill-Sachs lesion). The West Point axillary view may be necessary if the patient cannot tolerate abduction, and the Stryker notch views may be helpful to assess for Hill-Sachs lesions.[38-40]

In the subacute setting or at an office visit after a dislocation, the physical examination should include a comprehensive shoulder assessment, with particular focus on instability maneuvers. Positive anterior apprehension and relocation tests are the classic findings associated with anterior instability, whereas a posterior jerk test is generally positive with posterior labral pathology.[41-43] An inferior sulcus sign is usually positive with MDI.[44-46] Load and shift testing in an appropriately relaxed patient, usually in the supine position, can detect the degree to which the humeral head can be subluxated or dislocated in the anterior or posterior directions.[47,48]

MRI or magnetic resonance arthrography should be obtained to confirm a suspected capsulolabral injury, such as a Bankart tear (a tear of the anteroinferior glenoid labrum), a posterior labral tear, or other associated injuries. Contrast material may not be needed to identify Bankart lesions and other shoulder conditions.[49] However, magnetic resonance arthrography remains the gold standard for advanced imaging of traumatic labral pathology. Although a high rate of rotator cuff tearing has been reported in adults in association with shoulder dislocations,[50] this finding has not been replicated in the pediatric or adolescent populations. However, in adolescents, superior labral anterior to posterior tears most commonly occur in association with shoulder instability patterns and concomitant anterior and posterior labral tears.[50-52] Radiographs and MRIs of patients with MDI are often normal, other than the presence of a patulous capsule with increased volume. If a bony Bankart lesion or large Hill-Sachs lesion is appreciated on radiographs, some physicians recommend CT to better understand and quantify the size of the bony defect because large defects may require alternative procedures or procedures in addition to simple labral repair or capsulorrhaphy.[53-55]

Management of Anterior Instability

The appropriate first-line treatment of a young athlete with a traumatic anterior dislocation remains controversial.[56,57] High rates of recurrent instability have been reported after a first dislocation in patients younger than 20 years.[12,58-60] Rowe[61] and Marans et al[62] reported 100% redislocation rates in small studies of skeletally immature patients treated nonsurgically. Robinson et al[63] prospectively assessed a series of 252 young patients (age range, 15 to 35 years) and reported that 56% of the patients had recurrent instability episodes at a mean follow-up of 13 months after nonsurgical management. Risk factors for redislocation included male sex and age younger than 20 years. The risk of dislocation recurrence continued to increase over a 5-year period (**Figure 1**). Although the causes of redislocation in young athletes are likely multifactorial, high-demand activities, collision sports, and ligamentous laxity have been proposed as contributors to the condition.[64] In a randomized study of first-time dislocations, patients treated with arthroscopic repair had a 76% lower risk of redislocation than patients treated with arthroscopic lavage and had better functional scores, higher return to previous activity level, and greater satisfaction, along with lower treatment costs.[65] In a prospective multicenter study, Hovelius et al[66] reported on a large cohort of patients with primary anterior shoulder dislocations who were followed for 25 years. More than 50% of the patients ages 12 to 25 years at the time of the primary dislocation had a recurrent dislocation, and redislocation was at least twice as common in this group as a comparable group of older patients. There was a clear trend in the younger subgroups toward a greater risk of

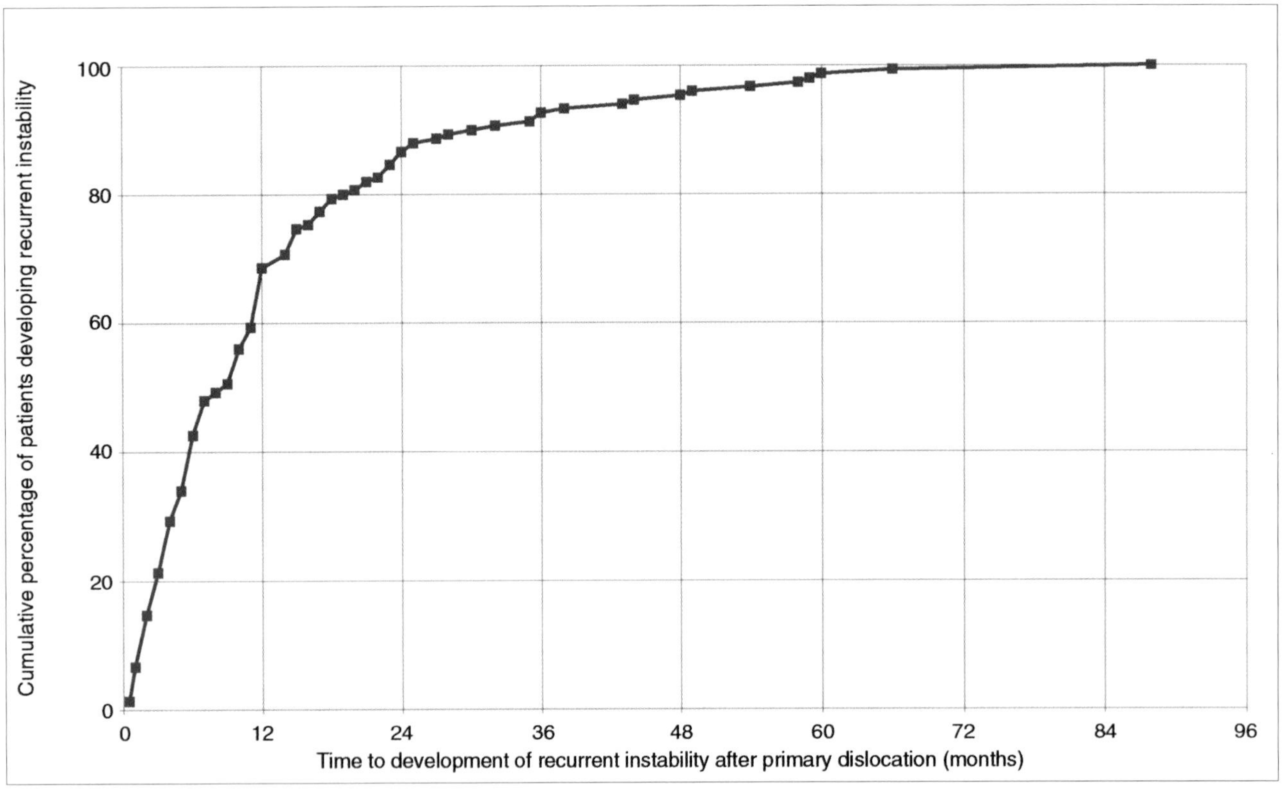

Figure 1 Graph showing the timing of the onset of instability in patients who had recurrent instability after a primary dislocation. (Reproduced with permission from Robinson CM, Howes J, Murdoch H, Will E, Graham CJ: Functional outcome and risk of recurrent instability after primary traumatic anterior shoulder dislocation in young patients. *J Bone Joint Surg Am* 2006;88(11):2326-2336.)

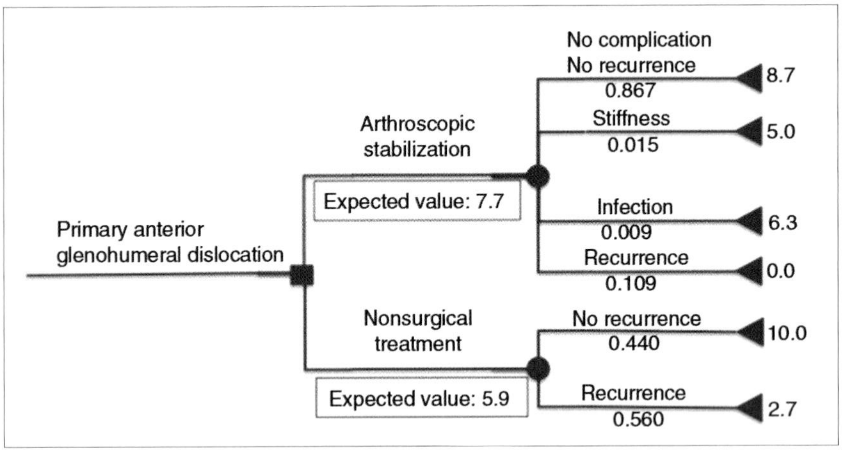

Figure 2 Decision tree reflecting decision analysis of surgical versus nonsurgical treatment of initial traumatic anterior glenohumeral dislocation. In this model, arthroscopic stabilization is the optimal management strategy. Per convention, utility data are placed to the right of the terminal nodes and probability data are placed under the terminal nodes. (Reproduced with permission from Bishop JA, Crall TS, Kocher MS: Operative versus nonoperative treatment after primary traumatic anterior glenohumeral dislocation: Expected-value decision analysis. *J Shoulder Elbow Surg* 2011;20(7):1087-1094.)

recurrence with younger age. Notably, the rate of recurrence reported by Robinson et al[63,65] for nonsurgically treated patients was 67% in all patients followed for 5 years, and the estimated probability for male teenagers ranged from 75% for a 19-year-old patient to 86% for a 15-year-old patient (**Table 1**).

In an attempt to reconcile the range of risk factors with subpopulations of dislocators, Bishop et al[67] used expected-value decision analysis to assess the optimal treatment strategy for patients with primary traumatic anterior glenohumeral dislocations (**Figure 2**). The authors concluded that arthroscopic stabilization was preferred over nonsurgical care by most patients. Sensitivity analysis was used to model the decision-making process for patients with different preferences or from different demographic groups. The model showed that patients who did not favor surgical treatment were those who had a low likelihood of recurrent instability with nonsurgical care; this group might include middle-aged or elderly patients. Others who would prefer nonsurgical treatment were those with an aversion to or reason to decline surgery, such as an in-season athlete who is willing to risk another dislocation rather than miss play.

Table 1
Age- and Sex-Specific Estimated Probability of Recurrent Instability in the First 2 Years After a Primary Glenohumeral Dislocation

Age (Years)	Males	Females
15	0.86	0.54
16	0.84	0.51
17	0.81	0.48
18	0.78	0.45
19	0.75	0.42
20	0.72	0.40
21	0.69	0.37
22	0.66	0.34
23	0.62	0.32
24	0.59	0.30
25	0.56	0.28
26	0.53	0.26
27	0.50	0.24
28	0.47	0.22
29	0.43	0.20
30	0.41	0.19
31	0.39	0.17
32	0.36	0.16
33	0.34	0.15
34	0.31	0.14
35	0.29	0.13

(Reproduced with permission from Robinson CM, Howes J, Murdoch H, Will E, Graham CJ: Functional outcome and risk of recurrent instability after primary traumatic anterior shoulder dislocation in young patients. *J Bone Joint Surg Am* 2006;88(11):2326-2336.)

Variations of Classic Anterior Instability

Certain subpopulations of dislocators or those with variations of classic anterior instability warrant additional discussion. Pathologic anterior instability should not be considered limited to frank dislocation events. Many patients may have labral tears with subluxation events alone; evidence suggests that such patients should be evaluated similarly to young athletes with true dislocations. Owens et al[68] prospectively analyzed the outcomes of 38 military cadets (mean age, 20 years) who had first-time subluxation events. Of those in whom MRI was obtained, 96% showed signs of a Bankart lesion, and 93% had signs of a Hill-Sachs lesion. More than 50% of the patients were treated surgically. Of those treated nonsurgically, 31% had recurrent subluxations or dislocations. Another variation of classic anterior instability is associated with a humeral avulsion of the glenohumeral ligament lesion, which is generally believed to be as or more debilitating than a Bankart tear. Cordischi et al[69] reported on 14 young patients (ages 10 to 13 years) with dislocations who were followed for 5.6 years. The three patients with a humeral avulsion of the glenohumeral ligament required surgery, whereas the other 11 patients had successful outcomes without surgery. Although debate continues regarding the optimal treatment in patients with first-time anterior dislocations, surgical treatment is generally recommended in young athletes with recurrent anterior instability episodes, despite adherence to a sound rehabilitation regimen.

Nonsurgical Treatment

Nonsurgical treatment of a primary anterior dislocation usually begins with a short 1- to 3-week period of sling immobilization of the shoulder. Because studies have not supported a benefit from postdislocation immobilization, it is generally prescribed for comfort only.[63,66] The optimal shoulder position for immobilization (internal or external rotation) is also controversial.[70-73] A randomized controlled study reported a 40% lower recurrence rate after 3 weeks of immobilization in external rotation compared with internal rotation.[72] These results have not yet been rigorously studied in multiple populations, and another randomized controlled study suggested that the two positions offer similar outcomes.[71] A course of physical therapy should be initiated early and should focus on periscapular and rotator cuff strengthening exercises. Following an appropriate rehabilitation program, patients should be reexamined to assess instability at a minimum of 4 to 6 weeks after the dislocation. Persistently positive apprehension and relocation signs increase the risks for recurrence.[74] A full range of motion, or at least fully functional range of motion for the specific sport, and strength symmetry should be present before clearance for return to play. There is no good evidence to support the effectiveness of protective shoulder braces, which are designed to control abduction and external rotation, in preventing recurrence. These braces are often poorly tolerated in the adolescent population; however, certain positional athletes, such as football lineman, may be reasonable candidates for a trial of bracing.[75]

Surgical Treatment

Surgical treatment includes repair of the capsulolabral injury, with or without additional capsulorrhaphy. Arthroscopic thermal capsulorrhaphy, which surged in popularity in the 1990s as an adjunctive and primary measure in shoulder instability surgery, has been more recently associated with concerning rates of chondrolysis, capsular tissue injury, recurrent instability, and revision surgery; its use is not recommended.[76] Both arthroscopic and open methods of anterior shoulder stabilization surgery have been described. Recurrence rates after arthroscopic repair with suture anchors have improved over time because of new methods, equipment, and implants and are now equal to those of a classic open Bankart procedure.[77-80] A meta-analysis that included studies of older arthroscopic techniques used in adults and children found that open procedures were more reliable for restoring stability and allowing the patient to return to work or sports. However, patients had better Rowe scores after arthroscopic repair, possibly because of lower rates of stiffness and better function.[81,82] There have been few studies of arthroscopic repair of shoulder instability in adolescents only. A retrospective study of 32 shoulders in patients ages 11 to 18 years reported 5 redislocations (16%) 2 years after arthroscopic repair, with 2 of the redislocations occurring in one patient with familial hyperlaxity.[83] Eleven of the patients returned to sports and had high scores on the Single Assessment Numeric Evaluation. Other studies, involving both adolescent and adult patients, have reported good results in adolescents.[47,83-85]

Management of Posterior Instability

Isolated posterior instability in contact athletes has become better understood and appreciated in recent decades.[86-88] Physical therapy is usually the first-line treatment, with a focus on strengthening of the posterior dynamic stabilizers, specifically the infraspinatus and teres minor muscles. When symptoms of persistent posterior pain or recurrent instability limit the activities of daily living, such as the ability to push a heavy door in nonathletic patients, or limit performance in young athletes, surgery may be considered. Generally, a posterior labral injury is seen on MRI but may appear intact in association with a reverse Hill-Sachs lesion or a suggestion of posterior capsular laxity.[19] Good to excellent results have been reported in multiple studies of both arthroscopic and open posterior stabilization procedures, although one retrospective comparative study in patients ages 15 to 35 years suggested the best results were achieved in a substratified cohort of arthroscopically treated patients.[17,87-90] When posterior instability recurs despite adequate arthroscopic treatment, an open approach should be considered. Good results have been reported in patients with a wide range of ages who had open treatment of recurrent posterior glenohumeral instability. A recurrence rate of 19%, no progressive articular degeneration seen at long-term follow-ups, and better results in younger patients and those without chondral defects have been reported.[35]

There are few published reports of outcomes for posterior instability in the pediatric and adolescent populations. A study by Kawam et al[91] assessed the outcomes of seven shoulders in six patients ages 9 to 17 years who were treated with shoulder stabilization using Putti-Platt-type capsulorrhaphy. One of the six patients required revision surgery, but all shoulders were stable at a mean follow-up of 9.4 years. One patient was limited in racquet sport participation because of shoulder apprehension. Validated outcome measures were not used in the study. The authors concluded that patient selection is critical, with the following requisite criteria for surgical consideration: history and physical examination findings specific for recurrent isolated posterior instability, failure of a minimum of 6 months of conservative therapy, significant disability, and the absence of psychologic factors (such as habitual dislocation for secondary gain) influencing the clinical picture. More research is needed to improve the understanding of posterior instability in the younger patient and its optimal management.

Management of MDI

Nonsurgical management is the mainstay of MDI treatment and generally achieves good results. A vigorous physical therapy program focusing on rotator cuff and periscapular strengthening is necessary to optimize the role of the dynamic stabilizers, the function of which are critical in patients with deficient static (ligamentous) stabilizers. Burkhead and Rockwood[92] reported an 80% rate of good or excellent results with an appropriate exercise program for a series of patients subject to recurrent atraumatic dislocations. Surgery is indicated for patients with symptoms that are debilitating or severely limit activities after at least 6 months of compliant rehabilitation. Arthroscopic or open capsulorrhaphy should focus on the symptomatic direction of the instability. Newer arthroscopic techniques have achieved encouraging results in adults and adolescents, including a return to sports in 89% and a satisfactory outcome in more than 90%.[93,94] Although MDI is commonly seen in the pediatric population, there are few reports focusing on younger patients. One study highlighted the association of MDI and the presence of Sprengel deformity, which should be assessed in all patients.[95]

Summary

The incidence of shoulder injuries in pediatric athletes is increasing, along with participation in high-demand sports by children at younger ages. Injury patterns in skeletally immature patients are unique to the developing musculoskeletal system and may be specific to the involved sport. A prompt and accurate diagnosis coupled with proper treatment can prevent long-term sequelae and expedite return to play. Although many injuries respond well to a nonsurgical regimen of rest and rehabilitation, surgical management is necessary in certain circumstances. Injury prevention strategies are also critical and should be encouraged in young athletes with risk factors for primary or recurrent injury.

References

1. Maffulli N, Longo UG, Spiezia F, Denaro V: Sports injuries in young athletes: Long-term outcome and prevention strategies. *Phys Sportsmed* 2010;38(2):29-34.
2. Bernhardt DT, Landry GL: Sports injuries in young athletes. *Adv Pediatr* 1995;42:465-500.
3. Injuries to young athletes: American Academy of Pediatrics. Committee on Pediatric Aspects of Physical Fitness, Recreation, and Sports. *Pediatrics* 1980;65(2): A53-A54.
4. Hill DE, Andrews JR: Stopping sports injuries in young athletes. *Clin Sports Med* 2011;30(4): 841-849.
5. Mariscalco MW, Saluan P: Upper extremity injuries in the adolescent athlete. *Sports Med Arthrosc* 2011;19(1):17-26.
6. Chen FS, Diaz VA, Loebenberg M, Rosen JE: Shoulder and elbow injuries in the skeletally immature athlete. *J Am Acad Orthop Surg* 2005;13(3):172-185.
7. Wasserlauf BL, Paletta GA Jr : Shoulder disorders in the skeletally immature throwing athlete. *Orthop Clin North Am* 2003; 34(3):427-437.
8. Mahaffey BL, Smith PA: Shoulder instability in young athletes. *Am Fam Physician* 1999;59(10): 2773-2782, 2787.
9. Ireland ML, Hutchinson MR: Upper extremity injuries in young athletes. *Clin Sports Med* 1995; 14(3):533-569.
10. Leonard J, Hutchinson MR: Shoulder injuries in skeletally immature throwers: Review and current thoughts. *Br J Sports Med* 2010;44(5):306-310.
11. Kvitne RS, Jobe FW: The diagnosis and treatment of anterior instability in the throwing athlete. *Clin Orthop Relat Res* 1993;291: 107-123.
12. Veltri DM: Shoulder instability in the young athlete. *Conn Med* 2010;74(8):465-468.
13. Hutchinson MR, Ireland ML: Overuse and throwing injuries in the skeletally immature athlete. *Instr Course Lect* 2003;52:25-36.
14. Adirim TA, Cheng TL: Overview of injuries in the young athlete. *Sports Med* 2003;33(1):75-81.
15. Debski RE, Sakone M, Woo SL, Wong EK, Fu FH, Warner JJ: Contribution of the passive properties of the rotator cuff to glenohumeral stability during anterior-posterior loading. *J Shoulder Elbow Surg* 1999;8(4):324-329.
16. Caprise PA Jr, Sekiya JK: Open and arthroscopic treatment of multidirectional instability of the shoulder. *Arthroscopy* 2006; 22(10):1126-1131.
17. Metcalf MH, Pon JD, Harryman DT II, Loutzenheiser T, Sidles JA: Capsulolabral augmentation increases glenohumeral stability in the cadaver shoulder. *J Shoulder Elbow Surg* 2001;10(6):532-538.
18. Robinson CM, Shur N, Sharpe T, Ray A, Murray IR: Injuries associated with traumatic anterior glenohumeral dislocations. *J Bone Joint Surg Am* 2012;94(1):18-26.
19. Robinson CM, Seah M, Akhtar MA: The epidemiology, risk of recurrence, and functional outcome after an acute traumatic posterior dislocation of the shoulder. *J Bone Joint Surg Am* 2011; 93(17):1605-1613.
20. Owens BD, Duffey ML, Nelson BJ, DeBerardino TM, Taylor DC, Mountcastle SB: The incidence and characteristics of shoulder instability at the United States Military Academy. *Am J Sports Med* 2007;35(7):1168-1173.
21. Heyworth BE, Williams RJ III: Internal impingement of the shoulder. *Am J Sports Med* 2009; 37(5):1024-1037.
22. Bae DS, Kocher MS, Waters PM, Micheli LM, Griffey M, Dichtel L: Chronic recurrent anterior sternoclavicular joint instability: Results of surgical management. *J Pediatr Orthop* 2006;26(1): 71-74.
23. Kocher MS, Waters PM, Micheli LJ: Upper extremity injuries in the

paediatric athlete. *Sports Med* 2000;30(2):117-135.

24. Cleeman E, Flatow EL: Shoulder dislocations in the young patient. *Orthop Clin North Am* 2000; 31(2):217-229.
25. Deitch J, Mehlman CT, Foad SL, Obbehat A, Mallory M: Traumatic anterior shoulder dislocation in adolescents. *Am J Sports Med* 2003;31(5):758-763.
26. Velin P, Four R, Matta T, Dupont D: Evaluation of sport injuries in children and adolescents. *Arch Pediatr* 1994;1(2):202-207.
27. Andrews JR, Sanders RA, Morin B: Surgical treatment of anterolateral rotatory instability: A follow-up study. *Am J Sports Med* 1985;13(2):112-119.
28. Cain EL Jr , Andrews JR, Dugas JR, et al: Outcome of ulnar collateral ligament reconstruction of the elbow in 1281 athletes: Results in 743 athletes with minimum 2-year follow-up. *Am J Sports Med* 2010;38(12):2426-2434.
29. Boyd HB, Sisk TD: Recurrent posterior dislocation of the shoulder. *J Bone Joint Surg Am* 1972; 54(4):779-786.
30. Provencher MT, LeClere LE, King S, et al: Posterior instability of the shoulder: Diagnosis and management. *Am J Sports Med* 2011;39(4):874-886.
31. Warren RF, Coleman SH, Dines JS: Instability after arthroplasty: The shoulder. *J Arthroplasty* 2002; 17(4, suppl 1):28-31.
32. Warren RF: Instability of shoulder in throwing sports. *Instr Course Lect* 1985;34:337-348.
33. Gerber C, Nyffeler RW: Classification of glenohumeral joint instability. *Clin Orthop Relat Res* 2002;400:65-76.
34. Hewitt M, Getelman MH, Snyder SJ: Arthroscopic management of multidirectional instability: Pancapsular plication. *Orthop Clin North Am* 2003;34(4):549-557.
35. Wolf BR, Strickland S, Williams RJ, Allen AA, Altchek DW, Warren RF: Open posterior stabilization for recurrent posterior glenohumeral instability. *J Shoulder Elbow Surg* 2005;14(2):157-164.
36. Schwartz E, Warren RF, O'Brien SJ, Fronek J: Posterior shoulder instability. *Orthop Clin North Am* 1987;18(3):409-419.
37. Tuckman GA, Devlin TC: Axillary nerve injury after anterior glenohumeral dislocation: MR findings in three patients. *AJR Am J Roentgenol* 1996;167(3): 695-697.
38. Kodali P, Jones MH, Polster J, Miniaci A, Fening SD: Accuracy of measurement of Hill-Sachs lesions with computed tomography. *J Shoulder Elbow Surg* 2011; 20(8):1328-1334.
39. Cho SH, Cho NS, Rhee YG: Preoperative analysis of the Hill-Sachs lesion in anterior shoulder instability: How to predict engagement of the lesion. *Am J Sports Med* 2011;39(11):2389-2395.
40. Farber JM, Buckwalter KA: Sports-related injuries of the shoulder: Instability. *Radiol Clin North Am* 2002;40(2):235-249.
41. Krueger D, Kraus N, Pauly S, Chen J, Scheibel M: Subjective and objective outcome after revision arthroscopic stabilization for recurrent anterior instability versus initial shoulder stabilization. *Am J Sports Med* 2011;39(1): 71-77.
42. Munro W, Healy R: The validity and accuracy of clinical tests used to detect labral pathology of the shoulder: A systematic review. *Man Ther* 2009;14(2):119-130.
43. Kim SH, Park JC, Park JS, Oh I: Painful jerk test: A predictor of success in nonoperative treatment of posteroinferior instability of the shoulder. *Am J Sports Med* 2004; 32(8):1849-1855.
44. Tzannes A, Paxinos A, Callanan M, Murrell GA: An assessment of the interexaminer reliability of tests for shoulder instability. *J Shoulder Elbow Surg* 2004; 13(1):18-23.
45. Tzannes A, Murrell GA: Clinical examination of the unstable shoulder. *Sports Med* 2002; 32(7):447-457.
46. McFarland EG, Campbell G, McDowell J: Posterior shoulder laxity in asymptomatic athletes. *Am J Sports Med* 1996;24(4):468-471.
47. Mazzocca AD, Cote MP, Solovyova O, Rizvi SH, Mostofi A, Arciero RA: Traumatic shoulder instability involving anterior, inferior, and posterior labral injury: A prospective clinical evaluation of arthroscopic repair of 270° labral tears. *Am J Sports Med* 2011; 39(8):1687-1696.
48. Deutsch A, Barber JE, Davy DT, Victoroff BN: Anterior-inferior capsular shift of the shoulder: A biomechanical comparison of glenoid-based versus humeral-based shift strategies. *J Shoulder Elbow Surg* 2001;10(4):340-352.
49. Potter HG, Jawetz ST, Foo LF: Imaging of the rotator cuff following repair: Human and animal models. *J Shoulder Elbow Surg* 2007;16(5, suppl):S134-S139.
50. Taylor DC, Arciero RA: Pathologic changes associated with shoulder dislocations: Arthroscopic and physical examination findings in first-time, traumatic anterior dislocations. *Am J Sports Med* 1997;25(3):306-311.
51. Eisner EA, Roocroft JH, Edmonds EW: Underestimation of labral pathology in adolescents with anterior shoulder instability. *J Pediatr Orthop* 2012;32(1): 42-47.
52. Cho HL, Lee CK, Hwang TH, Suh KT, Park JW: Arthroscopic repair of combined Bankart and SLAP lesions: Operative

techniques and clinical results. *Clin Orthop Surg* 2010;2(1):39-46.

53. Warner JJ, Kann S, Marks P: Arthroscopic repair of combined Bankart and superior labral detachment anterior and posterior lesions: Technique and preliminary results. *Arthroscopy* 1994; 10(4):383-391.
54. Latarjet M: Surgical technics in the treatment of recurrent dislocation of the shoulder (antero-internal). *Lyon Chir* 1965;61: 313-318.
55. Latarjet M: Treatment of recurrent dislocation of the shoulder. *Lyon Chir* 1954;49(8):994-997.
56. Good CR, MacGillivray JD: Traumatic shoulder dislocation in the adolescent athlete: Advances in surgical treatment. *Curr Opin Pediatr* 2005;17(1):25-29.
57. Walton J, Paxinos A, Tzannes A, Callanan M, Hayes K, Murrell GA: The unstable shoulder in the adolescent athlete. *Am J Sports Med* 2002;30(5):758-767.
58. Anakwenze OA, Huffman GR: Evaluation and treatment of shoulder instability. *Phys Sportsmed* 2011;39(2):149-157.
59. Meller R, Krettek C, Gösling T, Wähling K, Jagodzinski M, Zeichen J: Recurrent shoulder instability among athletes: Changes in quality of life, sports activity, and muscle function following open repair. *Knee Surg Sports Traumatol Arthrosc* 2007;15(3):295-304.
60. Uhorchak JM, Arciero RA, Huggard D, Taylor DC: Recurrent shoulder instability after open reconstruction in athletes involved in collision and contact sports. *Am J Sports Med* 2000;28(6): 794-799.
61. Rowe CR: Prognosis in dislocations of the shoulder. *J Bone Joint Surg Am* 1956;38(5):957-977.
62. Marans HJ, Angel KR, Schemitsch EH, Wedge JH: The fate of traumatic anterior dislocation of the shoulder in children. *J Bone Joint Surg Am* 1992; 74(8):1242-1244.
63. Robinson CM, Howes J, Murdoch H, Will E, Graham C: Functional outcome and risk of recurrent instability after primary traumatic anterior shoulder dislocation in young patients. *J Bone Joint Surg Am* 2006;88(11):2326-2336.
64. Johnson SM, Robinson CM: Shoulder instability in patients with joint hyperlaxity. *J Bone Joint Surg Am* 2010;92(6):1545-1557.
65. Robinson CM, Jenkins PJ, White TO, Ker A, Will E: Primary arthroscopic stabilization for a first-time anterior dislocation of the shoulder: A randomized, double-blind trial. *J Bone Joint Surg Am* 2008;90(4):708-721.
66. Hovelius L, Olofsson A, Sandström B, et al: Nonoperative treatment of primary anterior shoulder dislocation in patients forty years of age and younger: A prospective twenty-five-year follow-up. *J Bone Joint Surg Am* 2008;90(5):945-952.
67. Bishop JA, Crall TS, Kocher MS: Operative versus nonoperative treatment after primary traumatic anterior glenohumeral dislocation: Expected-value decision analysis. *J Shoulder Elbow Surg* 2011; 20(7):1087-1094.
68. Owens BD, Nelson BJ, Duffey ML, et al: Pathoanatomy of first-time, traumatic, anterior glenohumeral subluxation events. *J Bone Joint Surg Am* 2010;92(7):1605-1611.
69. Cordischi K, Li X, Busconi B: Intermediate outcomes after primary traumatic anterior shoulder dislocation in skeletally immature patients aged 10 to 13 years. *Orthopedics* 2009. http://www.healio.com/orthopedics/shoulder-elbow/journals/ORTHO/%7BA09E132F-99C2-41D1-9602-735976B1B597%7D. Accessed October 19, 2012.
70. Deyle GD, Nagel KL: Prolonged immobilization in abduction and neutral rotation for a first-episode anterior shoulder dislocation. *J Orthop Sports Phys Ther* 2007; 37(4):192-198.
71. Liavaag S, Brox JI, Pripp AH, Enger M, Soldal LA, Svenningsen S: Immobilization in external rotation after primary shoulder dislocation did not reduce the risk of recurrence: A randomized controlled trial. *J Bone Joint Surg Am* 2011;93(10):897-904.
72. Itoi E, Hatakeyama Y, Sato T, et al: Immobilization in external rotation after shoulder dislocation reduces the risk of recurrence: A randomized controlled trial. *J Bone Joint Surg Am* 2007; 89(10):2124-2131.
73. Handoll HH, Hanchard NC, Goodchild L, Feary J: Conservative management following closed reduction of traumatic anterior dislocation of the shoulder. *Cochrane Database Syst Rev* 2006; 1:CD004962.
74. Safran O, Milgrom C, Radeva-Petrova DR, Jaber S, Finestone A: Accuracy of the anterior apprehension test as a predictor of risk for redislocation after a traumatic shoulder dislocation. *Am J Sports Med* 2010;38(5):972-975.
75. Taylor DC, Krasinski KL: Adolescent shoulder injuries: Consensus and controversies. *J Bone Joint Surg Am* 2009;91(2):462-473.
76. Virk SS, Kocher MS: Adoption of new technology in sports medicine: Case studies of the Gore-Tex prosthetic ligament and of thermal capsulorrhaphy. *Arthroscopy* 2011;27(1):113-121.
77. Steinbeck J, Witt KA, Marquardt B: Arthroscopic versus open anterior shoulder stabilization: A systematic validation. *Orthopade* 2009;38(1):36-40.
78. Bottoni CR, Smith EL, Berkowitz MJ, Towle RB, Moore JH: Arthroscopic versus open shoulder

stabilization for recurrent anterior instability: A prospective randomized clinical trial. *Am J Sports Med* 2006;34(11):1730-1737.

79. Freedman KB, Smith AP, Romeo AA, Cole BJ, Bach BR Jr: Open Bankart repair versus arthroscopic repair with transglenoid sutures or bioabsorbable tacks for recurrent anterior instability of the shoulder: A meta-analysis. *Am J Sports Med* 2004;32(6):1520-1527.
80. Geiger DF, Hurley JA, Tovey JA, Rao JP: Results of arthroscopic versus open Bankart suture repair. *Clin Orthop Relat Res* 1997;337: 111-117.
81. Castagna A, Rose GD, Borroni M, et al: Arthroscopic stabilization of the shoulder in adolescent athletes participating in overhead or contact sports. *Arthroscopy* 2012;28(3):309-315.
82. Arce G, Arcuri F, Ferro D, Pereira E: Is selective arthroscopic revision beneficial for treating recurrent anterior shoulder instability? *Clin Orthop Relat Res* 2012; 470(4):965-971.
83. Jones KJ, Wiesel B, Ganley TJ, Wells L: Functional outcomes of early arthroscopic bankart repair in adolescents aged 11 to 18 years. *J Pediatr Orthop* 2007;27(2): 209-213.
84. Barrios-Moyano A, Negrete-Corona J, Chávez-Hinojosa E: Clinical and functional course of patients after arthroscopic repair of a Bankart lesion. *Acta Ortop Mex* 2009;23(5):281-285.
85. Owens BD, DeBerardino TM, Nelson BJ, et al: Long-term follow-up of acute arthroscopic Bankart repair for initial anterior shoulder dislocations in young athletes. *Am J Sports Med* 2009; 37(4):669-673.
86. Mair SD, Zarzour RH, Speer KP: Posterior labral injury in contact athletes. *Am J Sports Med* 1998; 26(6):753-758.
87. Tibone J, Ting A: Capsulorrhaphy with a staple for recurrent posterior subluxation of the shoulder. *J Bone Joint Surg Am* 1990; 72(7):999-1002.
88. Williams RJ III , Strickland S, Cohen M, Altchek DW, Warren RF: Arthroscopic repair for traumatic posterior shoulder instability. *Am J Sports Med* 2003;31(2): 203-209.
89. Bottoni CR, Franks BR, Moore JH, DeBerardino TM, Taylor DC, Arciero RA: Operative stabilization of posterior shoulder instability. *Am J Sports Med* 2005; 33(7):996-1002.
90. McIntyre LF, Caspari RB, Savoie FH III : The arthroscopic treatment of posterior shoulder instability: Two-year results of a multiple suture technique. *Arthroscopy* 1997;13(4):426-432.
91. Kawam M, Sinclair J, Letts M: Recurrent posterior shoulder dislocation in children: The results of surgical management. *J Pediatr Orthop* 1997;17(4):533-538.
92. Burkhead WZ Jr , Rockwood CA Jr: Treatment of instability of the shoulder with an exercise program. *J Bone Joint Surg Am* 1992; 74(6):890-896.
93. Bradley JP, Baker CL III, Kline AJ, Armfield DR, Chhabra A: Arthroscopic capsulolabral reconstruction for posterior instability of the shoulder: A prospective study of 100 shoulders. *Am J Sports Med* 2006;34(7): 1061-1071.
94. Baker CL III, Mascarenhas R, Kline AJ, Chhabra A, Pombo MW, Bradley JP: Arthroscopic treatment of multidirectional shoulder instability in athletes: A retrospective analysis of 2- to 5-year clinical outcomes. *Am J Sports Med* 2009;37(9): 1712-1720.
95. Hamner DL, Hall JE: Sprengel's deformity associated with multidirectional shoulder instability. *J Pediatr Orthop* 1995;15(5): 641-643.

40

Patellofemoral Instability in Skeletally Immature Athletes

William Hennrikus, MD
Tamara Pylawka, MD

Abstract

Acute patellofemoral dislocation is the most common acute knee disorder in children and adolescents. The predisposing factors for acute patellar dislocation are multifactorial.

Unless associated with substantial articular cartilage damage, nonsurgical management is typically used to treat a first-time acute patellofemoral dislocation in a skeletally immature athlete. In the setting of recurrent instability, surgical reconstruction is usually recommended. Surgical treatment of patellofemoral instability in the skeletally immature athlete is evolving from nonanatomic extensor mechanism surgical procedures to anatomic restorative procedures based on reconstitution of the medial patellofemoral ligament. The current goal of surgery is to restore the normal anatomy of the patellofemoral joint. Proper patient selection and attention to technical details are important in achieving good outcomes.

Instr Course Lect 2013;62:445-453.

Treatment of the skeletally immature athlete with an acute patellofemoral dislocation remains controversial, with long-term outcomes not well understood. In children, the incidence of patellofemoral dislocation is approximately 43 per 100,000 individuals, with a peak incidence at age 15 years.[1-3] The risk of acute dislocation and recurrent instability is particularly high in females ages 10 to 17 years.[4,5] After a first-time dislocation, young athletes may feel a sense of giving way, pain, or anxiety. Recurrent patellar dislocations often substantially impair their athletic performance. In 1952, Macnab[6] reported a 15% redislocation rate after a first-time dislocation, with 33% of the patients reporting pain and weakness after a dislocation. Other studies have reported a redislocation rate ranging from 20% to 44%.[4,7,8] Treatment is complicated by the presence of open growth plates, which precludes the use of osteotomies.[9-11] This chapter summarizes the pathoanatomy and natural history of patellofemoral instability in the skeletally immature athlete and discusses both nonsurgical and surgical treatment options for this condition.

Anatomy and Biomechanics of the Medial Patellofemoral Ligament

The medial patellofemoral ligament is the primary restraint to patellofemoral instability at 0° to 30° of flexion and overall provides more than 50% of the medial restraint to the patella.[12,13] The medial patellofemoral ligament is most taut in full knee extension with the quadriceps muscle contracted. The medial patellofemoral ligament aids in guiding the patella into the trochlear groove during early flexion. After the patella is engaged in the trochlear groove, the slope of the lateral facet provides the primary resistance to lateral translation.[14,15] Patellofemoral joint compression increases as flexion increases because of the increasing force vectors of the quadriceps and patellar tendons.[14]

Anatomically, the origin of the medial patellofemoral ligament is at the adductor tubercle on the medial femoral epicondyle near the distal femoral physis (**Figure 1**). The medial patellofemoral ligament inserts on the upper two thirds of the medial aspect of the patella and is approximately 55 mm

Dr. Hennrikus or an immediate family member serves as a board member, owner, officer, or committee member of the Pediatric Orthopaedic Society of North America and the Society of Military Orthopaedic Surgeons. Neither Dr. Pylawka nor any immediate family member has received anything of value from or has stock or stock options in a commercial company or institution related directly or indirectly to the subject of this chapter.

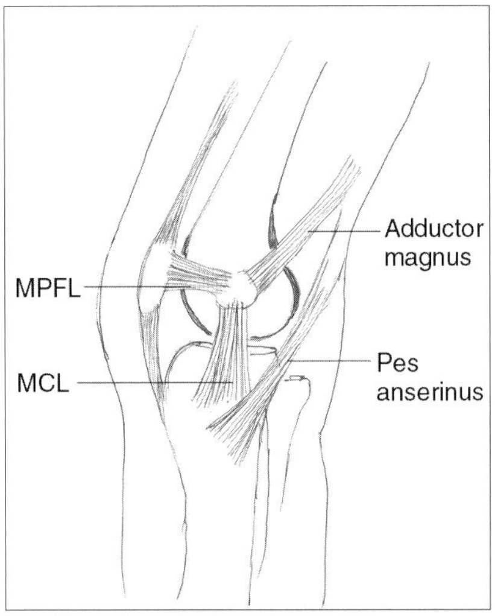

Figure 1 Illustration of the anatomy of the lateral aspect of the knee and the medial patellofemoral ligament (MPFL). MCL = medial collateral ligament.

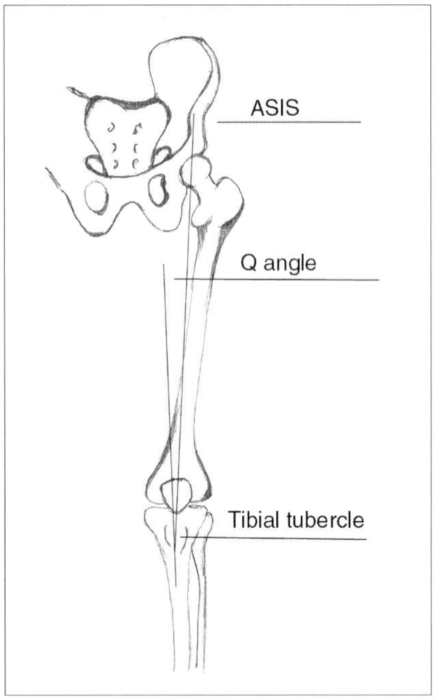

Figure 2 The Q angle. ASIS = anterior superior iliac spine.

long. The width of the patellar insertion is approximately 17 mm (range, 14 to 20 mm), and the width of the femoral origin is approximately 15 mm (range, 11 to 20 mm).[16] The medial patellofemoral ligament has two origins: a transverse origin from the osseous groove between the medial epicondyle and the adductor tubercle and an oblique origin from the leading edge of the medial collateral ligament.[17] The site of the femoral origin of the medial patellofemoral ligament is controversial. For example, in the skeletally immature athlete with open physes, Shea et al,[18] using radiographic analysis, suggested that the femoral origin of the medial patellofemoral ligament is 2 to 5 mm proximal to the distal femoral physis. However, in children, ligaments originate and insert into the epiphysis so that as the patient grows, the origin of the ligament does not migrate farther from the joint. In agreement with this principle, Nelitz et al,[19] also using radiographic analysis, suggested that the medial patellofemoral ligament origin is approximately 6 mm distal to the medial physis in the epiphysis. Similarly, Kepler et al,[20] using MRI analysis, demonstrated that the medial patellofemoral ligament origin was epiphyseal and approximately 5 mm distal to the medial femoral physis. Despite the debate about the exact location of the origin of the medial patellofemoral ligament, the three studies agree that the medial patellofemoral ligament origin is very near the physis; therefore, a drill hole in this area risks physeal injury.

Pathoanatomy of Patellar Instability

Clinical Findings

The pathoanatomy of patellofemoral instability is multifactorial. For example, patients who are at risk for patellofemoral instability often present with an increased quadriceps (Q) angle (**Figure 2**), ligamentous laxity, patella alta, trochlear dysplasia, external tibial torsion, and genu valgum. Patients also may demonstrate contractures of the iliotibial band, lateral retinaculum, and vastus lateralis muscle.[19-26] The gait may have a valgus thrust, valgus and internal rotation thrust, and excessive pronation of the foot.[24] The general core strength may be weaker, and vastus medialis oblique hypoplasia should be evaluated. Clinical examinations and/or signs that should be checked include the patellar glide test, the patellar apprehension sign, the tilt test, and the J sign.[24] Common additional injuries associated with a patellar dislocation on MRI include knee effusion, tears at the femoral insertion of the medial patellofemoral ligament, medial patellar bone bruises, and increased signal intensity in the vastus medialis muscle.[23]

Imaging

Radiographs of a patient with patellar instability should include AP, lateral, and Merchant views of the patella. Radiographs should be examined carefully for occult fractures. The presence of trochlear hypoplasia as well as patellar height, patellar tilt, and patellar subluxation should be noted.[21] If a large effusion exists, further investigation may warrant MRI examination. On the MRI examination, the tibial tuberosity–trochlear groove distance (**Figure 3**) and patellar tilt may be measured.[27] MRIs often can define where the medial patellofemoral ligament tear occurred. Sillanpää et al[28] reported medial patellofemoral ligament tears from the femur in 66% of patients, from the patella in 13%, and in the midsubstance in 21%. MRI nicely illustrates bone bruise patterns typical of patellar dislocation at the medial patellar facet and at the lateral femoral condyle.[29]

Epidemiology and Natural History of Acute Patellar Dislocation

Girls (ages 10 to 17 years) have the highest risk for patellar dislocation.[4] Of the patients sustaining a first-time dislocation, 61% were participating in a sporting activity at the time of dislocation. At the 5-year follow-up evaluation, both the patients with a first-time dislocation and those with subsequent subluxation-dislocation events did not present with substantial radiographic evidence of degenerative joint disease.[23] Overall, the reported redislocation rate after an initial patellar dislocation has ranged from 15% to 44%.[4,6-8]

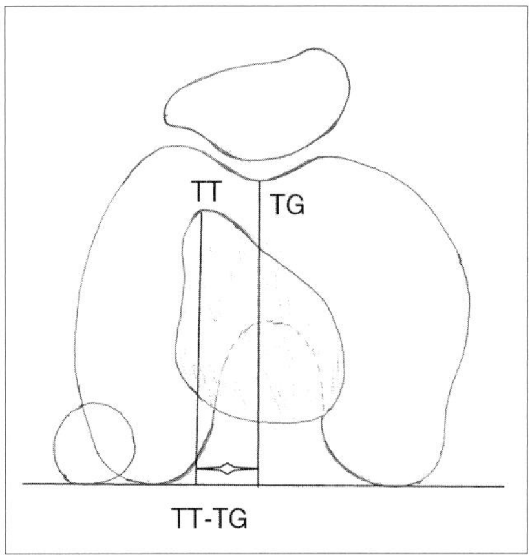

Figure 3 Measurement of the horizontal distance between the tibial tubercle (TT) and the center of the trochlear groove (TG).

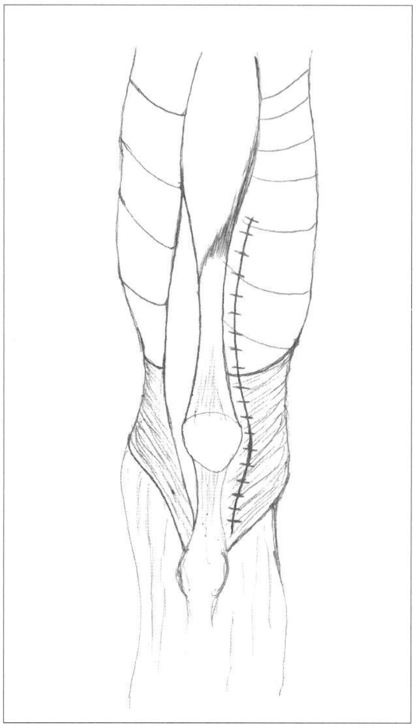

Figure 4 The Insall technique for proximal realignment includes an extensive open medial imbrication and lateral retinacular release.

Management of First-Time Patellar Dislocation

Nonsurgical management of a first-time traumatic patellar dislocation in a young athlete is recommended, except when there is an osteochondral fracture, an avulsion of the vastus medialis obliquus muscle, or additional intra-articular injuries such as a meniscal tear.[30-35] Nonsurgical management of patients with a first-time dislocation includes rehabilitation focused on vastus medialis obliquus and gluteal muscle strengthening, as well as core strengthening.[26,36] Taping and/or bracing with the goal to pull the patella away from the painful area may be considered.[37] Activity modification and proper sports training should be emphasized. An MRI examination may be warranted to evaluate the status of the cartilage if radiographic findings are normal and a large effusion is present. Palmu et al[38] reported on a randomized clinical trial of acute patellar dislocations in children and adolescents comparing surgical and nonsurgical treatment. The authors demonstrated that primary repair of the medial patellofemoral ligament and/or medial retinacular structures did not improve long-term subjective or functional results, supporting nonsurgical treatment of acute first-time patellar dislocation in children and adolescents.

Management of Recurrent Patellar Instability

Failure to improve after nonsurgical treatment and repeat dislocations are the most common indications for surgical care of patellar instability in the skeletally immature athlete.[35,37,39] More than 100 different types of surgical procedures for treating recurrent patellar dislocations have been described.[40] The surgical approach that is chosen is individualized for each patient and should treat the existing pathoanatomy contributing to the repeat dislocations.[40] Often, no single procedure corrects all patellofemoral problems.[41] Surgical options for patellofemoral instability in the skeletally immature athlete include proximal realignment, distal realignment, lateral release, medial patellofemoral ligament reconstruction, guided growth with tension-band plates, and combinations of these procedures. Osteotomies of the proximal part of the tibia and distal end of the femur are not indicated in patients in this young age group because of the risk of injury to the growth plate.

Proximal Realignment

Traditional proximal realignment techniques alter the medial-lateral patellar position by releasing a tight retinaculum lateral to the patella and tensioning loose structures medial to the patella. The classic proximal realignment procedure described by Insall et al[42] include an extensive open medial imbrication and lateral retinacular release (**Figure 4**). The Insall procedure has a success rate for preventing additional episodes of patellar dislocation of approximately 90%.[42,43] However, some authors have described high rates of patellofemoral pain and arthritis after this nonanatomic reconstruction.[44] Nam and Karzel[45] reported a mini-incision open medial reefing and arthroscopically assisted lateral release as an alternative proximal realignment method with similar (90%) success in preventing subsequent patellar insta-

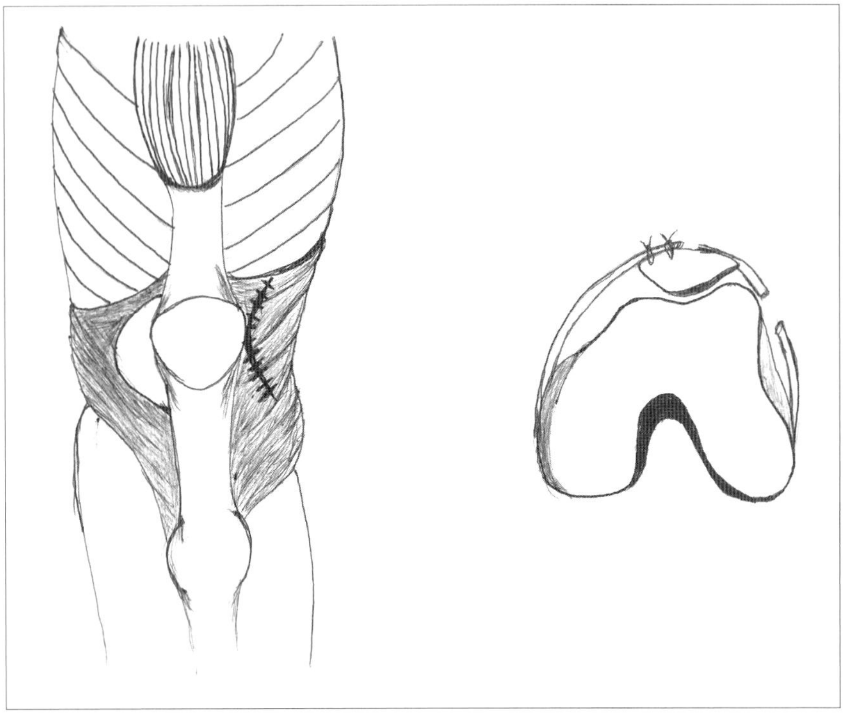

Figure 5 Arthroscopic lateral release with open medial reefing.

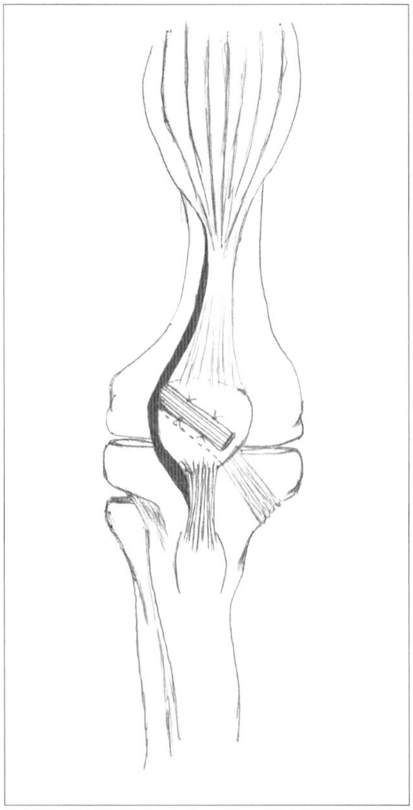

Figure 6 The Galeazzi semitendinosus tenodesis. See text for description.

bility with less potential morbidity and improved cosmesis (**Figure 5**).

Lateral Release

The role of lateral release in the treatment of patellofemoral instability has been reevaluated.[46-48] An isolated lateral release is not recommended for the treatment of patellar instability.[37,46,49] Lateral release alone does not align the patella more medially.[46,50] In cases of patellofemoral instability with normal alignment and no evidence of excessive patellar tilt, medial reefing without routine lateral release can be performed.[51] The current indications for performing a lateral release are abnormal patellar tilt by examination or imaging in the setting of anterior knee pain that has had unsuccessful conservative treatment or recurrent patellofemoral instability in combination with other surgical procedures.[46] Potential morbidity after lateral release includes hemarthrosis and medial instability.[47,49,52] For uncommon patients with anterolateral knee pain and symptoms of medial patellar instability after lateral release, open lateral retinacular closure surgery has been described.[53]

Distal Realignment

Distal realignment surgical procedures in skeletally immature patients aim to modify the proximal-distal and medial-lateral positions of the patella by soft-tissue transfer distal to the inferior pole of the patella.[54] Stanitski[55] recommended that a soft-tissue realignment procedure should include releasing the abnormal tethering vector, balancing the medial vector, and aligning the quadriceps-patellar-tibial mechanism. Distal realignment procedures include transfer of the semitendinosus tendon to the patella,[54,56,57] transfer of part or all of the patellar tendon medially to the periosteum or to the sartorius tendon,[58-60] and combination procedures including distal and proximal soft-tissue transfers.[58,61,62] The Galeazzi procedure includes a lateral release combined with transfer of the semitendinosus tendon to the medial patellar retinaculum or directly to the patella via an oblique drill hole through the patella[56,57,63] (**Figure 6**). Success rates greater than 80% for preventing subsequent patellar instability have been reported with the Galeazzi procedure.[56,57] The modified Roux-Goldthwait procedure is a combination distal and proximal soft-tissue transfer that includes a lateral release, plication of the medial retinaculum, advancement of the vastus medialis muscle, and medial transfer of the lateral half of the patellar tendon beneath the intact medial half to the sartorius insertion[58,62] (**Figure 7**). Success rates for preventing subsequent patellar instability of greater than 80% have been reported with the modified Roux-Goldthwait procedure.[62] Most recently, Joo et al[61] re-

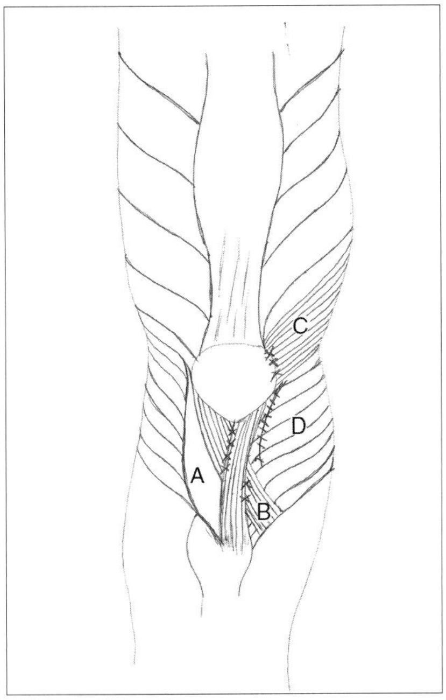

Figure 7 The modified Roux-Goldthwait procedure. A = lateral retinacular release, B = medial transfer of the lateral patellar tendon, C = advancement of the vastus medialis, and D = plication of the medial retinaculum.

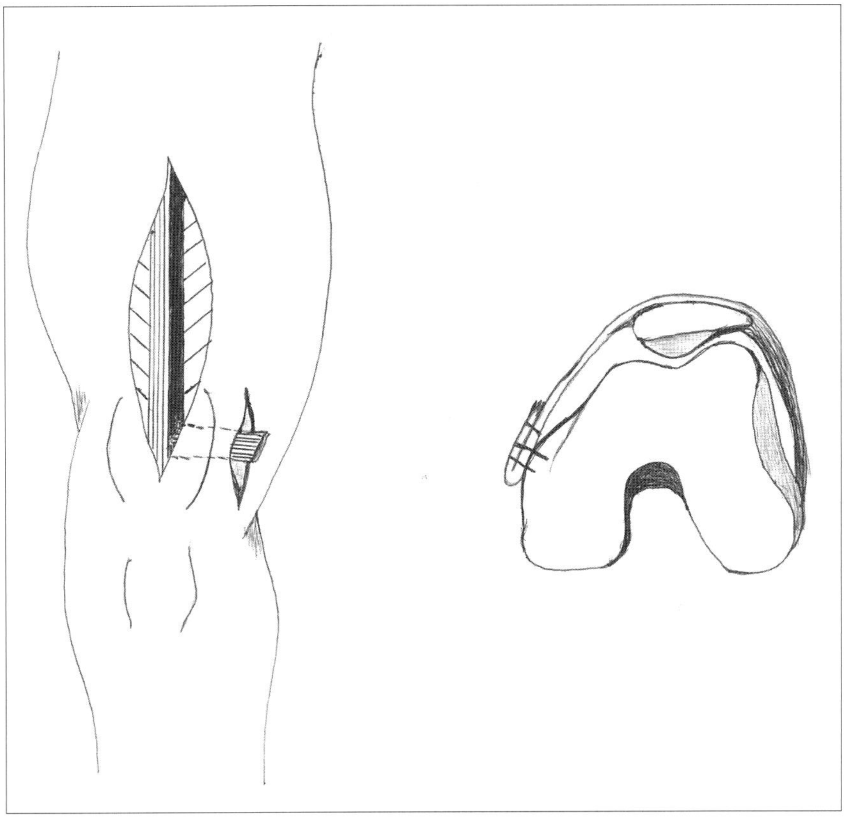

Figure 8 Medial patellofemoral ligament reconstruction with use of the medial third of the quadriceps tendon.

ported excellent results in a small case series of patients treated with the four-in-one procedure. The four-in-one procedure includes a lateral release, a vastus medialis muscle advancement, transfer of the semitendinosus tendon to the patella, and transfer of the lateral half of the patellar tendon to the medial tibial periosteum.[61] These proximal and distal realignment procedures involve shifting extensor mechanism tissue in various nonanatomic directions. Recently, the primary stabilizing role of the medial patellofemoral ligament has been emphasized as the key factor for patellar stability. The current trend in the treatment of patellofemoral instability in young athletes has evolved from nonanatomic extensor mechanism realignments to more anatomic procedures centered on reconstruction of the medial patellofemoral ligament.[12,13,39,64,65]

Medial Patellofemoral Ligament Reconstruction

The goal of soft-tissue reconstruction of the medial patellofemoral ligament is to reestablish the normal checkrein against lateral motion and create a tether to help restore normal passive motion of the patella, including allowing the patella to glide laterally approximately 9 mm. Medial patellofemoral ligament reconstruction is recommended for patients with repeat dislocation, whereas medial patellofemoral ligament repair is used more often for patients with a first-time dislocation in whom concomitant injuries are also being treated. Reconstruction is advocated over repair in patients with repeat dislocation because the chronically injured medial retinacular tissues are insufficient to establish a checkrein against lateral dislocation. Various graft choices have been used for medial patellofemoral ligament reconstruction, including hamstrings, patellar tendon, quadriceps, and adductor magnus.[66-70] Allograft can be considered if the patient has hyperlaxity.

Techniques that avoid injury to the growth plate should be used in the skeletally immature athlete. Two techniques in particular are safe and effective in this young, athletic population. Noyes and Albright[68] reported using an 8 × 70–mm strip of the medial part of the quadriceps tendon to reconstruct the medial patellofemoral ligament (**Figure 8**). The quadriceps graft is left attached to the superomedial border of the patella. The free end of the graft is passed between the synovium and the retinaculum to the medial femoral epicondyle and is sutured to the medial intermuscular septum. The remaining medial retinaculum is imbricated when the quadriceps tendon harvest site is closed. The graft is tensioned at 30° to 45° of knee flexion to allow for lateral patellar movement of up to 25% of the patellar width. A lateral release is added if tightness of the tissues prevents normal medial patellar translation with or without abnormal patellar tilting. Femoral or patellar drill holes are not used in this technique, so the risk of patellar fracture or injury to the distal femoral physis is reduced.[68]

Sillanpää et al[70] reported a technique using the adductor magnus tendon autograft that can also be of value when treating skeletally immature athletes with patellofemoral instability. The medial two thirds of the adductor tendon are harvested while leaving the distal insertion intact. A 12-cm strip of the medial aspect of the adductor magnus tendon is transferred via a tunnel between the capsule and the retinaculum and is fixed to the medial patellar margin with two suture anchors. The graft is tensioned at 30° of knee flexion with care to avoid overtightening by allowing lateral patellar glide similar to the contralateral knee.[70] Lateral release is not added to the procedure except in cases in which the patella cannot be medialized to the neutral position in the trochlear groove. The adductor magnus tendon reconstruction also avoids drill holes and minimizes the risk of a fracture or injury to the distal femoral physis.

Guided Growth

In young athletes, genu valgum of greater than 10° has been associated with patellofemoral instability and anterior knee pain.[71-73] Extraphyseal tension-band plating can be performed as a safe and minimally invasive technique to correct abnormal valgus in skeletally immature patients.[71-75] So-called guided growth to correct the genu valgum with the use of a tension-band plate across the distal femoral medial physis can gradually correct the angular deformity to neutral. Guided growth is considered for patients with greater than 10° of valgus and at least 12 months of growth remaining. Guided growth is typically not recommended before 8 years of age because until this age spontaneous correction of idiopathic genu valgum may occur.[71,76] The tension-band plates are removed when alignment is corrected. If rebound growth causes recurrent deformity, guided growth can be repeated safely.[71] The speed of correction decreases with increasing age because the physis grows at a slower rate as the patient approaches skeletal maturity.[71,73] Correction of approximately 0.7° per month in the femur and 0.3° per month in the tibia can be expected.[71,74]

Rehabilitation

The goal of the rehabilitation phase is to protect the patellar reconstruction while knee motion and strength are regained. Rehabilitation protocols vary by surgeon. Most surgeons use a brace for 3 to 6 weeks and allow a gradual increase in motion during this time. The use of ice packs and ice massage may be helpful. Partial weight bearing is allowed postoperatively and is progressed to full weight bearing over 4 to 6 weeks. Initial isometric exercises are supplemented with proprioceptive exercises, closed kinetic chain exercises, and, lastly, open chain exercises. Most patients can be expected to be able to jog by 3 to 4 months and return to full sporting activities by approximately 4 to 6 months.

Complications

Potential complications of the treatment of patellofemoral instability in the skeletally immature athlete include recurrent instability, patellofemoral pain, osteoarthritis, knee stiffness, wound infection, patellar fracture, medial instability, neuroma, and growth plate injury.[10,60,77,78] Patients should be adequately counseled preoperatively regarding potential complications.

References

1. Cash JD, Hughston JC: Treatment of acute patellar dislocation. *Am J Sports Med* 1988;16(3): 244-249.
2. Rünow A: The dislocating patella: Etiology and prognosis in relation to generalized joint laxity and anatomy of the patellar articulation. *Acta Orthop Scand Suppl* 1983;201:1-53.
3. Nietosvaara Y, Aalto K, Kallio PE: Acute patellar dislocation in children: Incidence and associated osteochondral fractures. *J Pediatr Orthop* 1994;14(4):513-515.
4. Fithian DC, Paxton EW, Stone ML, et al: Epidemiology and natural history of acute patellar dislocation. *Am J Sports Med* 2004; 32(5):1114-1121.
5. Nikku R, Nietosvaara Y, Aalto K, Kallio PE: Operative treatment of primary patellar dislocation does not improve medium-term outcome: A 7-year follow-up report and risk analysis of 127 randomized patients. *Acta Orthop* 2005; 76(5):699-704.
6. Macnab I: Recurrent dislocation of the patella. *J Bone Joint Surg Am* 1952;34(4):957-967.
7. Hawkins RJ, Bell RH, Anisette G: Acute patellar dislocations: The natural history. *Am J Sports Med* 1986;14(2):117-120.
8. Cofield RH, Bryan RS: Acute dislocation of the patella: Results of conservative treatment. *J Trauma* 1977;17(7):526-531.
9. Bollier M, Fulkerson JP: The role of trochlear dysplasia in patellofemoral instability. *J Am Acad Orthop Surg* 2011;19(1):8-16.

10. Tjoumakaris FP, Forsythe B, Bradley JP: Patellofemoral instability in athletes: Treatment via modified Fulkerson osteotomy and lateral release. *Am J Sports Med* 2010;38(5):992-999.
11. Utting MR, Mulford JS, Eldridge JD: A prospective evaluation of trochleoplasty for the treatment of patellofemoral dislocation and instability. *J Bone Joint Surg Br* 2008;90(2):180-185.
12. Bicos J, Fulkerson JP, Amis A: Current concepts review: The medial patellofemoral ligament. *Am J Sports Med* 2007;35(3):484-492.
13. Philippot R, Chouteau J, Wegrzyn J, Testa R, Fessy MH, Moyen B: Medial patellofemoral ligament anatomy: Implications for its surgical reconstruction. *Knee Surg Sports Traumatol Arthrosc* 2009;17(5):475-479.
14. Farahmand F, Tahmasbi MN, Amis AA: Lateral force-displacement behaviour of the human patella and its variation with knee flexion: A biomechanical study in vitro. *J Biomech* 1998;31(12):1147-1152.
15. Heegaard J, Leyvraz PF, Van Kampen A, Rakotomanana L, Rubin PJ, Blankevoort L: Influence of soft structures on patellar three-dimensional tracking. *Clin Orthop Relat Res* 1994;299:235-243.
16. Steensen RN, Dopirak RM, McDonald WG III: The anatomy and isometry of the medial patellofemoral ligament: Implications for reconstruction. *Am J Sports Med* 2004;32(6):1509-1513.
17. Baldwin JL: The anatomy of the medial patellofemoral ligament. *Am J Sports Med* 2009;37(12):2355-2361.
18. Shea KG, Grimm NL, Belzer J, Burks RT, Pfeiffer R: The relation of the femoral physis and the medial patellofemoral ligament. *Arthroscopy* 2010;26(8):1083-1087.
19. Nelitz M, Dornacher D, Dreyhaupt J, Reichel H, Lippacher S: The relation of the distal femoral physis and the medial patellofemoral ligament. *Knee Surg Sports Traumatol Arthrosc* 2011;19(12):2067-2071.
20. Kepler CK, Bogner EA, Hammoud S, Malcolmson G, Potter HG, Green DW: Zone of injury of the medial patellofemoral ligament after acute patellar dislocation in children and adolescents. *Am J Sports Med* 2011;39(7):1444-1449.
21. Dejour H, Walch G, Nove-Josserand L, Guier C: Factors of patellar instability: An anatomic radiographic study. *Knee Surg Sports Traumatol Arthrosc* 1994;2(1):19-26.
22. Monk AP, Doll HA, Gibbons CL, et al: The patho-anatomy of patellofemoral subluxation. *J Bone Joint Surg Br* 2011;93(10):1341-1347.
23. Redziniak DE, Diduch DR, Mihalko WM, et al: Patellar instability. *J Bone Joint Surg Am* 2009;91(9):2264-2275.
24. Reider B, Marshall JL, Warren RF: Clinical characteristics of patellar disorders in young athletes. *Am J Sports Med* 1981;9(4):270-274.
25. Sallay PI, Poggi J, Speer KP, Garrett WE: Acute dislocation of the patella: A correlative pathoanatomic study. *Am J Sports Med* 1996;24(1):52-60.
26. Powers CM: Rehabilitation of patellofemoral joint disorders: A critical review. *J Orthop Sports Phys Ther* 1998;28(5):345-354.
27. Balcarek P, Jung K, Frosch KH, Stürmer KM: Value of the tibial tuberosity-trochlear groove distance in patellar instability in the young athlete. *Am J Sports Med* 2011;39(8):1756-1761.
28. Sillanpää PJ, Peltola E, Mattila VM, Kiuru M, Visuri T, Pihlajamäki H: Femoral avulsion of the medial patellofemoral ligament after primary traumatic patellar dislocation predicts subsequent instability in men: A mean 7-year nonoperative follow-up study. *Am J Sports Med* 2009;37(8):1513-1521.
29. Paakkala A, Sillanpää P, Huhtala H, Paakkala T, Mäenpää H: Bone bruise in acute traumatic patellar dislocation: Volumetric magnetic resonance imaging analysis with follow-up mean of 12 months. *Skeletal Radiol* 2010;39(7):675-682.
30. Ahmad CS, Stein BE, Matuz D, Henry JH: Immediate surgical repair of the medial patellar stabilizers for acute patellar dislocation: A review of eight cases. *Am J Sports Med* 2000;28(6):804-810.
31. Christiansen SE, Jakobsen BW, Lund B, Lind M: Isolated repair of the medial patellofemoral ligament in primary dislocation of the patella: A prospective randomized study. *Arthroscopy* 2008;24(8):881-887.
32. Larsen E, Lauridsen F: Conservative treatment of patellar dislocations: Influence of evident factors on the tendency to redislocation and the therapeutic result. *Clin Orthop Relat Res* 1982;171:131-136.
33. Nikku R, Nietosvaara Y, Kallio PE, Aalto K, Michelsson JE: Operative versus closed treatment of primary dislocation of the patella: Similar 2-year results in 125 randomized patients. *Acta Orthop Scand* 1997;68(5):419-423.
34. Sillanpää PJ, Mäenpää HM, Mattila VM, Visuri T, Pihlajamäki H: Arthroscopic surgery for primary traumatic patellar dislocation: A prospective, nonrandomized study comparing patients treated with and without acute arthroscopic stabilization with a median 7-year follow-up. *Am J Sports Med* 2008;36(12):2301-2309.
35. Stefancin JJ, Parker RD: First-time traumatic patellar

dislocation: A systematic review. *Clin Orthop Relat Res* 2007;455: 93-101.

36. Beasley LS, Vidal AF: Traumatic patellar dislocation in children and adolescents: Treatment update and literature review. *Curr Opin Pediatr* 2004;16(1):29-36.
37. Colvin AC, West RV: Patellar instability. *J Bone Joint Surg Am* 2008;90(12):2751-2762.
38. Palmu S, Kallio PE, Donell ST, Helenius I, Nietosvaara Y: Acute patellar dislocation in children and adolescents: A randomized clinical trial. *J Bone Joint Surg Am* 2008;90(3):463-470.
39. Arendt EA, Fithian DC, Cohen E: Current concepts of lateral patella dislocation. *Clin Sports Med* 2002; 21(3):499-519.
40. Andrish J: The management of recurrent patellar dislocation. *Orthop Clin North Am* 2008;39(3): 313-327, vi.
41. Scuderi GR: Surgical treatment for patellar instability. *Orthop Clin North Am* 1992;23(4):619-630.
42. Insall J, Bullough PG, Burstein AH: Proximal "tube" realignment of the patella for chondromalacia patellae. *Clin Orthop Relat Res* 1979;144:63-69.
43. Abraham E, Washington E, Huang TL: Insall proximal realignment for disorders of the patella. *Clin Orthop Relat Res* 1989;248:61-65.
44. Panagopoulos A, van Niekerk L, Triantafillopoulos IK: MPFL reconstruction for recurrent patella dislocation: A new surgical technique and review of the literature. *Int J Sports Med* 2008;29(5): 359-365.
45. Nam EK, Karzel RP: Mini-open medial reefing and arthroscopic lateral release for the treatment of recurrent patellar dislocation: A medium-term follow-up. *Am J Sports Med* 2005;33(2):220-230.
46. Clifton R, Ng CY, Nutton RW: What is the role of lateral retinacular release? *J Bone Joint Surg Br* 2010;92(1):1-6.
47. Fithian DC, Paxton EW, Post WR, Panni AS; International Patellofemoral Study Group: Lateral retinacular release: A survey of the International Patellofemoral Study Group. *Arthroscopy* 2004;20(5): 463-468.
48. Gerbino PG, Zurakowski D, Soto R, Griffin E, Reig TS, Micheli LJ: Long-term functional outcome after lateral patellar retinacular release in adolescents: An observational cohort study with minimum 5-year follow-up. *J Pediatr Orthop* 2008;28(1):118-123.
49. Kolowich PA, Paulos LE, Rosenberg TD, Farnsworth S: Lateral release of the patella: Indications and contraindications. *Am J Sports Med* 1990;18(4):359-365.
50. Fulkerson JP: Diagnosis and treatment of patients with patellofemoral pain. *Am J Sports Med* 2002; 30(3):447-456.
51. Miller JR, Adamson GJ, Pink MM, Fraipont MJ, Durand P Jr: Arthroscopically assisted medial reefing without routine lateral release for patellar instability. *Am J Sports Med* 2007;35(4):622-629.
52. Hughston JC, Deese M: Medial subluxation of the patella as a complication of lateral retinacular release. *Am J Sports Med* 1988; 16(4):383-388.
53. Heyworth BE, Carroll KM, Dawson CK, Gill TJ: Open lateral retinacular closure surgery for treatment of anterolateral knee pain and disability after arthroscopic lateral retinacular release. *Am J Sports Med* 2012;40(2): 376-382.
54. Grelsamer RP: Patellar malalignment. *J Bone Joint Surg Am* 2000; 82(11):1639-1650.
55. Stanitski CL: Management of patellar instability. *J Pediatr Orthop* 1995;15(3):279-280.
56. Baker RH, Carroll N, Dewar FP, Hall JE: The semitendinosus tenodesis for recurrent dislocation of the patella. *J Bone Joint Surg Br* 1972;54(1):103-109.
57. Galeazzi R: New tendonous and muscular transplant applications. *Arch Ortop* 1922;38:315-325.
58. Fondren FB, Goldner JL, Bassett FH III: Recurrent dislocation of the patella treated by the modified Roux-Goldthwait procedure: A prospective study of forty-seven knees. *J Bone Joint Surg Am* 1985; 67(7):993-1005.
59. Gordon JE, Schoenecker PL: Surgical treatment of congenital dislocation of the patella. *J Pediatr Orthop* 1999;19(2):260-264.
60. Luhmann SJ, O'Donnell JC, Fuhrhop S: Outcomes after patellar realignment surgery for recurrent patellar instability dislocations: A minimum 3-year follow-up study of children and adolescents. *J Pediatr Orthop* 2011;31(1):65-71.
61. Joo SY, Park KB, Kim BR, Park HW, Kim HW: The "four-in-one" procedure for habitual dislocation of the patella in children: Early results in patients with severe generalised ligamentous laxity and aplasis of the trochlear groove. *J Bone Joint Surg Br* 2007; 89(12):1645-1649.
62. Marsh JS, Daigneault JP, Sethi P, Polzhofer GK: Treatment of recurrent patellar instability with a modification of the Roux-Goldthwait technique. *J Pediatr Orthop* 2006;26(4):461-465.
63. Moyad TF, Blakemore L: Modified Galeazzi technique for recurrent patellar dislocation in children. *Orthopedics* 2006;29(4): 302-304.
64. Schepsis AA, Rogers AJ: Medial patellofemoral ligament reconstruction: Indications and technique. *Sports Med Arthrosc* 2012; 20(3):162-170.

65. Hinton RY, Sharma KM: Acute and recurrent patellar instability in the young athlete. *Orthop Clin North Am* 2003;34(3):385-396.
66. LeGrand AB, Greis PE, Dobbs RE, Burks RT: MPFL reconstruction. *Sports Med Arthrosc* 2007; 15(2):72-77.
67. Camanho GL, Bitar AC, Hernandez AJ, Olivi R: Medial patellofemoral ligament reconstruction: A novel technique using the patellar ligament. *Arthroscopy* 2007; 23(1):e1-e4, 4.
68. Noyes FR, Albright JC: Reconstruction of the medial patellofemoral ligament with autologous quadriceps tendon. *Arthroscopy* 2006;22(8):e1-e7.
69. Steensen RN, Dopirak RM, Maurus PB: A simple technique for reconstruction of the medial patellofemoral ligament using a quadriceps tendon graft. *Arthroscopy* 2005;21(3):365-370.
70. Sillanpää PJ, Mäenpää HM, Mattila VM, Visuri T, Pihlajamäki H: A mini-invasive adductor magnus tendon transfer technique for medial patellofemoral ligament reconstruction: A technical note. *Knee Surg Sports Traumatol Arthrosc* 2009;17(5):508-512.
71. Boero S, Michelis MB, Riganti S: Use of the eight-plate for angular correction of knee deformities due to idiopathic and pathologic physis: Initiating treatment according to etiology. *J Child Orthop* 2011; 5(3):209-216.
72. Fabry G, MacEwen GD, Shands AR Jr: Torsion of the femur: A follow-up study in normal and abnormal conditions. *J Bone Joint Surg Am* 1973;55(8):1726-1738.
73. Guzman H, Yaszay B, Scott VP, Bastrom TP, Mubarak SJ: Early experience with medial femoral tension band plating in idiopathic genu valgum. *J Child Orthop* 2011;5(1):11-17.
74. Ballal MS, Bruce CE, Nayagam S: Correcting genu varum and genu valgum in children by guided growth: Temporary hemiepiphysiodesis using tension band plates. *J Bone Joint Surg Br* 2010;92(2): 273-276.
75. Stevens PM: Guided growth for angular correction: A preliminary series using a tension band plate. *J Pediatr Orthop* 2007;27(3): 253-259.
76. Salenius P, Vankka E: The development of the tibiofemoral angle in children. *J Bone Joint Surg Am* 1975;57(2):259-261.
77. Nomura E, Inoue M, Kobayashi S: Long-term follow-up and knee osteoarthritis change after medial patellofemoral ligament reconstruction for recurrent patellar dislocation. *Am J Sports Med* 2007;35(11):1851-1858.
78. Parikh SN, Wall EJ: Patellar fracture after medial patellofemoral ligament surgery: A report of five cases. *J Bone Joint Surg Am* 2011; 93(17):e97, 1-8.

41

Juvenile Osteochondritis Dissecans of the Knee: Current Concepts in Diagnosis and Management

Jacob F. Schulz, MD
Henry G. Chambers, MD

Abstract

Osteochondritis dissecans of the knee is a diagnosis that encompasses a wide spectrum of pathologies that can result in irreversible damage to articular cartilage and subchondral bone. Osteochondritis dissecans was first described more than 100 years ago, and despite substantial research on the topic, large gaps remain in the understanding of its etiology and optimal treatment.

An underlying vascular insult, resulting in separation of the progeny lesion from the parent subchondral bone, is a suspected cause but remains unproven. No single standardized classification exists to accurately predict long-term risk. Nonsurgical treatment with activity modification remains an option for stable lesions in young patients. Surgical treatment to encourage vascular ingrowth and healing is gaining popularity and represents a shift in thinking regarding the risk of disease progression. Unstable and displaced lesions remain a difficult treatment challenge. Various salvage procedures have shown promise, but the potential for long-term morbidity remains.

Instr Course Lect 2013;62:455-467.

Osteochondritis dissecans (OCD) is a common cause of knee pain and dysfunction in children and young adults. OCD is an acquired condition of unclear etiology, resulting in delamination and sequestration of subchondral bone, with or without damage to the overlying articular cartilage. OCD of the knee is variously classified according to its anatomic location, its appearance on radiographic studies, the chronologic age of the patient, and the extent of articular cartilage changes. The age and skeletal maturity of the patient is used to further subclassify the lesion into juvenile and adult forms and correlates highly with healing potential. The adult form of OCD is usually believed to be an unresolved juvenile lesion, but de novo adult lesions have been described.

Adult OCD lesions have a greater propensity for instability and typically follow a progressive and symptomatic clinical course. Juvenile lesions, by comparison, often present with an intact cartilaginous surface and have a higher potential for healing with activity modification. The long-term sequela of an unstable OCD lesion is an unremitting trend toward premature degenerative joint disease.[1]

The management of juvenile OCD depends on many factors related to both the lesion and the patient's characteristics. Nonsurgical treatment plays an important role for stable lesions in skeletally immature patients. Surgical management may be necessary in skeletally mature or maturing patients, particularly in those with unstable lesions. The goal of treatment is to avoid progression to the adult form and ultimately limit the likelihood of early arthrosis.

Epidemiology

Although the exact prevalence of OCD is unknown, the estimated

Dr. Chambers or an immediate family member serves as a board member, owner, officer, or committee member of the American Academy of Orthopaedic Surgeons, the American Academy for Cerebral Palsy and Developmental Medicine, and the Pediatric Orthopaedic Society of North America and serves as a paid consultant to or is an employee of Allergan Corporation, Merz Pharmaceuticals, and Orthopediatrics. Neither Dr. Schulz nor any immediate family member has received anything of value from or owns stock in a commercial company or institution related directly or indirectly to the subject of this chapter.

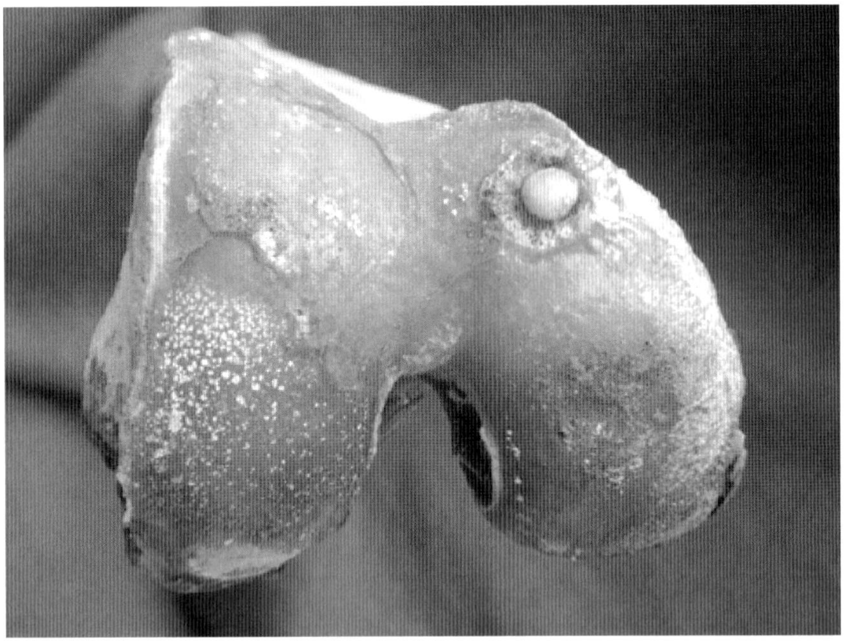

Figure 1 Photograph of the right distal femur from a naturally mummified female skeleton discovered in northern Chile and dated to approximately 2,000 BCE. The loose body has been repositioned in the condylar defect. (Reproduced with permission from Kothari A, Ponce P, Arriaza B, O'Connor-Read L: Osteochondritis dissecans of the knee in a mummy from northern Chile. *Knee* 2009;16(2):159-160.)

incidence ranges from 15 to 29 cases per 100,000 individuals.[2,3] Sex differences have been relatively consistent, with a male preponderance of 5:3 in most series. The mean age at OCD diagnosis appears to be decreasing, especially among girls. The reason for these trends has been linked to the increasing number of children, particularly girls, participating in competitive sports at a younger age, as well as the recognition of and vigilance for the condition on the part of caregivers.[4] Increased rates of serious knee injury and widespread use of MRI and arthroscopy have likely resulted in greater recognition of OCD lesions. Other contributing factors include early sport specialization, intensive single-sport training leading to overuse, and the loss of free play among this vulnerable population.

Most juvenile OCD lesions of the knee are located on the femoral side, with more than 70% located in the lateral aspect of the medial femoral condyle. Lateral condyle lesions, which are typically posterior and central lesions, account for 10% to 15% of lesions, whereas trochlear lesions account for less than 1%. Only 5% to 10% of OCD lesions are found in the patella but usually occur in the inferomedial area when present.

Etiology

OCD was first described by Paget in 1870; he called it "quiet necrosis." The name osteochondritis dissecans was coined by Konig in 1887 to describe an inflammatory process resulting in a dissection of the cartilage from the underlying subchondral bone.[5] The disease, however, predates both of these descriptions, as was shown in a 2009 report describing what appears to be bilateral OCD lesions of the knee in a 4,000-year-old naturally mummified skeleton of a middle-aged woman from northern Chile.[6] The rounded and smooth loose bodies in the bone suggest that the disease process had been present for a substantial period of time before death (**Figure 1**).

Several causes of OCD have been proposed, including inflammation, genetics, ischemia, ossification, and repetitive trauma; however, there is insufficient evidence to support a single etiology. The overlapping spectrum of osteochondral lesions and the lack of distinction between the adult and juvenile forms, together with the interchangeable and sometimes inappropriate use of terminology, contribute to the inconsistency regarding the diagnosis, management, and prognosis of OCD. Idiopathic OCD must also be differentiated from the similar-appearing osteochondral lesions resulting from osteonecrosis associated with chemotherapy, hemoglobinopathy, or steroid use.

Although the name osteochondritis suggests an inflammatory pathology, histologic evidence does not support this theory. Recent histopathologic studies have failed to identify either osteonecrosis of the OCD fragment or a relative ischemic watershed of the lateral aspect of the medial femoral condyle.[7,8] Yonetani et al[9] obtained cylindric osteochondral samples from eight patients with OCD who were arthroscopically evaluated. The authors identified two histologic patterns: (1) thick homogeneous hyaline cartilage alone with little fibrous tissue surrounding areas of separation and (2) nearly normal, thin hyaline cartilage above a mixed layer of hyaline cartilage and subchondral trabeculae and fibrous/fibrocartilaginous tissue at the areas of separation, indicating delayed union or nonunion. Early marrow stimulation or stabilization of even relatively stable lesions to promote healing was recommended.

Mubarak and Carroll[10] proposed a genetic predisposition to OCD when they identified lesions in 12 family members over four generations. A 13% to 30% incidence of bilateral OCD lesions, coupled with multiple case reports of patients with concomitant OCD lesions in several joints, also support some genetic etiology for the disease. Petrie,[11] however, identified only 1 relative with the disease in an examination of 86 first-degree relatives of 34 patients with OCD lesions. No other skeletal abnormalities were seen in Petrie's cohort, although OCD has been associated with dwarfism. To date, no specific genetic causative factor has been identified.

A traumatic etiology, either from acute macrotrauma or repetitive microtrauma, also has been proposed as the cause of OCD, particularly because of the increasing prevalence of this condition among athletes. In 1933, Fairbanks[12] suggested that OCD was the result of "violent rotation of the tibia, driving the tibial spine against the inner condyle." Although this theory may not account for all cases of OCD, especially those occurring on the patella or at other nontypical sites, the role of repetitive trauma has been supported by several experimental studies using animal models.[4] Repetitive trauma may induce a stress reaction resulting in a stress fracture of the underlying subchondral bone. Persistent loading may exceed the healing capabilities of that bone, resulting in necrosis of the fragment, separation from the underlying cartilage, and subsequent nonunion. Traumatic osteochondral fractures may result in lesions that appear identical to those of OCD; however, only one in five patients with this condition reports an inciting injury.[2]

In 1950, Rehbein[13] produced experimental lesions similar to those of OCD by repeated forced hyperextension of the knee combined with force placed on the femoral condyles through the patella. The role of altered mechanics in the development of OCD is further supported by the observation of lesions in patients with meniscal pathology, both in traumatic or congenital conditions. A 2007 report from Hashimoto et al[14] describes bilateral lateral femoral condyle OCD lesions arising after total meniscectomy for bilateral discoid lateral menisci. In a recent cohort study of 103 knees with OCD lesions, Jacobi et al[15] reported an association with the mechanical axis. Knees with medial femoral condylar lesions were more likely to have a varus mechanical alignment, whereas those in the lateral femoral condyle had a valgus moment. It is unclear whether the alignment causes a predisposition to the development of the lesion or the lesion causes the malalignment.

Healing of the avascular bone in OCD occurs by revascularization, and repair occurs by creeping substitution. When healing is incomplete, the interzone between the osteocartilaginous fragment and the surrounding cartilage is filled by dense fibrous tissue. These findings indicate delayed union or nonunion of the fracture.[16]

The relationship between adult and juvenile forms of OCD has not been fully elucidated. Although de novo cases have been reported, many physicians believe that adult lesions represent either an acute injury or a persistence of juvenile OCD.[17] For this reason, it has been argued that aggressive treatment of even asymptomatic lesions in skeletally immature patients may alter the natural history of the disease.

Clinical Presentation and Examination

Patients with juvenile OCD lesions typically present with poorly localized knee pain, which is exacerbated by exercise. Pain is commonly reported with deep flexion (climbing hills or stairs) or when rising from a prolonged seated position. Mechanical symptoms, such as locking or catching, or visible swelling may indicate the presence of a more advanced or unstable lesion, a loose body, or a concomitant meniscal injury.

The patient history should focus on the duration of symptoms, activities that exacerbate or relieve symptoms, and previous treatments. In athletes, the type of sport and the extent of participation should be fully investigated. Participation in nontraditional sports should not be dismissed as a possible exacerbating factor. Symptoms in the contralateral knee should be investigated, and underlying rheumatologic or vascular etiologies should be considered in the differential diagnoses. As with any report of vague knee pain in a skeletally immature child, the clinician should consider hip pathology that, if undiagnosed, could lead to substantial morbidity.

On physical examination, hip motion should be checked to investigate the possibility of referred pain. Visual inspection of the knee may reveal mild swelling, but substantial effusion is more likely related to an acute intra-articular pathology, such as an anterior cruciate ligament tear, a meniscal tear, patellar dislocation, or an acute osteochondral fracture. Maximal tenderness may be elicited over the anterior aspect of the medial femoral condyle with varying degrees of flexion, corresponding to the most common anatomic site of the lesion. The Wilson sign was first described in 1967 and is elicited by flexing the knee to 90°, fully rotating the tibia medially, and then gradually extending the knee.[18] The test is positive if there is pain at 30° of flexion; the pain is located over the medial femoral condyle anteriorly. Although

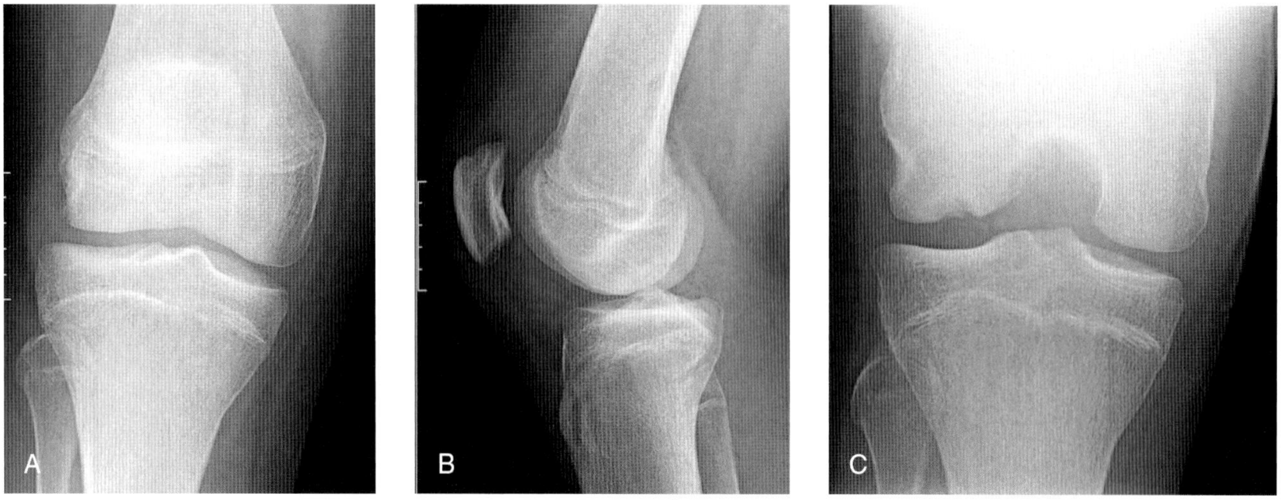

Figure 2 AP (**A**), lateral (**B**), and tunnel (**C**) views of the right knee of a 16-year-old boy show a large OCD lesion on the posterolateral femoral condyle. The lesion is nearly invisible on the AP view but is shown clearly on the tunnel view.

Table 1
Radiographic OCD Grading System According to Rodegerdts and Gleissner

Grade	Radiographic Appearance
I	Potentially depressed osteochondral fragment
II	Demarcation without sclerotic rim
III	Demarcation with sclerotic rim
IV	Nondisplaced partially detached fragment
V	Displaced fragment (loose body)

the Wilson sign is often negative in patients with an existing lesion, when pain is reported with the maneuver, it may be monitored to follow healing of the lesion.[19] An antalgic or external rotation gait may be observed, and atrophy of the quadriceps muscle may indicate a longer-standing lesion. Unstable lesions may produce crepitus or pain with motion. Bilateral involvement has been reported in 13% to 30% of patients, and, if present, is typically asymmetric in terms of size and symptoms.

Diagnostic Studies

Radiologic imaging is used to characterize OCD lesions and guide treatment. The ideal imaging study would distinguish lesions capable of healing spontaneously from those requiring surgical treatment. Although bone scintigraphy, MRI, and magnetic resonance arthrography allow better prediction of outcomes, no single imaging modality reliably predicts nonsurgical success. Multiple classification systems, based on plain radiography, bone scintigraphy, and MRI have been proposed. Because interpreting the stability of OCD lesions has proved elusive, no single system has gained wide acceptance. Skeletal maturity, the size of the lesion, and articular continuity remain the most predictive factors for assessing risks.

Plain Radiography

Plain radiography is the initial imaging modality of choice. AP and lateral radiographs are needed to rule out other bony injuries, evaluate skeletal maturity, and indicate the age of the lesion. They are necessary studies but not totally sufficient because posterior lesions may be clearly seen only on a flexed (tunnel or notch) view, and patellar lesions require a sunrise or Merchant view. Early lesions appear as a small radiolucency at the articular surface, whereas more advanced lesions have a well-demarcated segment of subchondral bone, the progeny lesion, with a lucent line separating it from the condyle or the parent bone[20] (**Figures 2** and **3**). The bone may appear radiodense compared with the surrounding bone. After the formation of a loose body, a crater remains on the surface of the affected condyle (**Table 1**) (**Figure 4**). Caution must be taken in evaluating plain radiographs in children younger than 7 years because asymptomatic irregularities of the distal femoral ossification center, usually in the posterior lateral condyle, are anatomic variations that may simu-

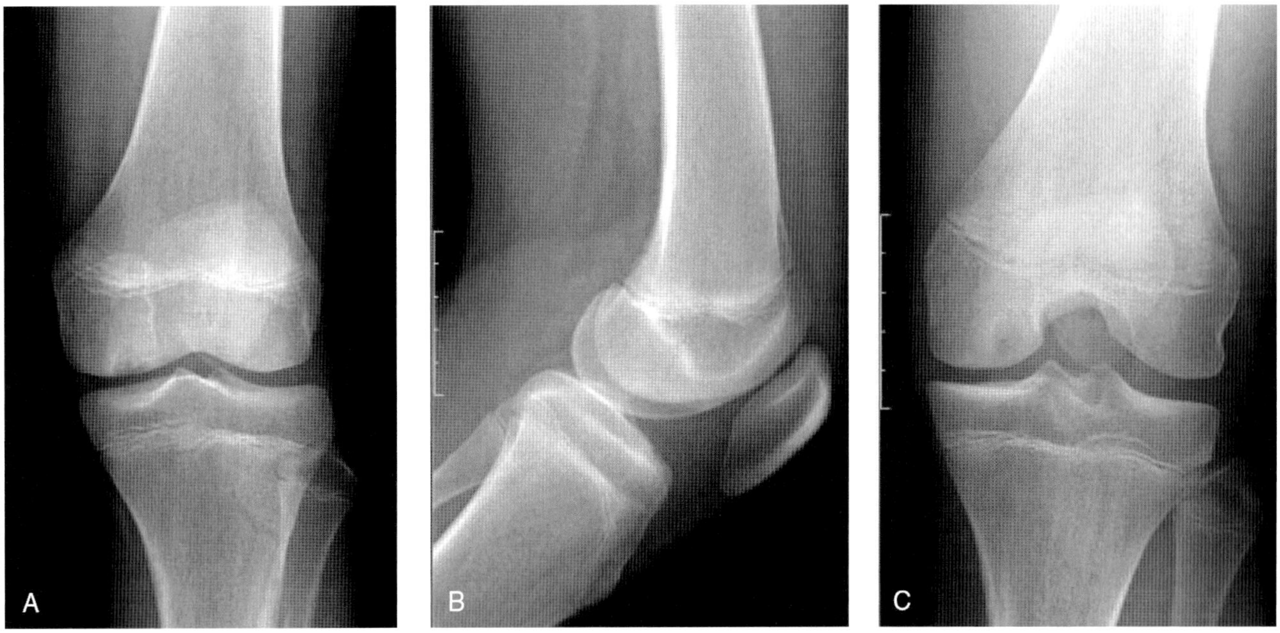

Figure 3 AP (**A**), lateral (**B**), and tunnel (**C**) radiographs of the left knee of a 13-year-old girl show an OCD lesion in its classic location on the lateral aspect of the medial femoral condyle.

late the appearance of OCD.[21] Given these irregularities, comparison views of the contralateral knee may be beneficial if the findings are questionable.

Bone Scintigraphy

Prior to the widespread use of MRI, technetium bone scans were used to assess the healing potential of OCD lesions. Cahill and Berg[22] developed a classification system for juvenile OCD based on the correlation of scintigraphic activity to blood flow and osteoblastic activity. Other investigators have pursued this imaging modality with moderate success. However, the need for repeat studies, time requirements, the perceived risk of the radioactive isotope, and the growth of MRI technology have rendered bone scintigraphy largely obsolete.

Magnetic Resonance Imaging

MRI is routinely used in the diagnostic evaluation of OCD to estimate the size of the lesion and the status of cartilage and subchondral bone[23] (**Figure 5**). MRI can identify the extent of bony edema, the appearance of high signal zones beneath the fragment, and the presence of loose bodies. After treatment has begun, MRI is a tool to assess interval healing (**Table 2**).

De Smet et al[24] described four MRI criteria on T2-weighted images that could be used to predict unstable OCD lesions: (1) a line of high signal intensity at least 5 mm in length between the OCD lesion and the underlying bone, (2) an area of increased homogeneous signal at least 5 mm in diameter beneath the lesion, (3) a focal defect of 5 mm or more in the articular surface, and (4) a high signal line traversing the subchondral plate into the lesion. The authors reported that a high signal line was found behind 74% of unstable lesions (**Figure 6**). Pill et al[25] applied and verified these findings to predict the success of nonsurgical treatment using MRI and clinical criteria. Lesion size and patient maturity also played an important role in predicting the success of nonsurgical treatment. A study by O'Conner et al[26] reported that MRI staging of an OCD lesion was improved from 45% to 85% by interpreting the high signal T2 line as a predictor of instability

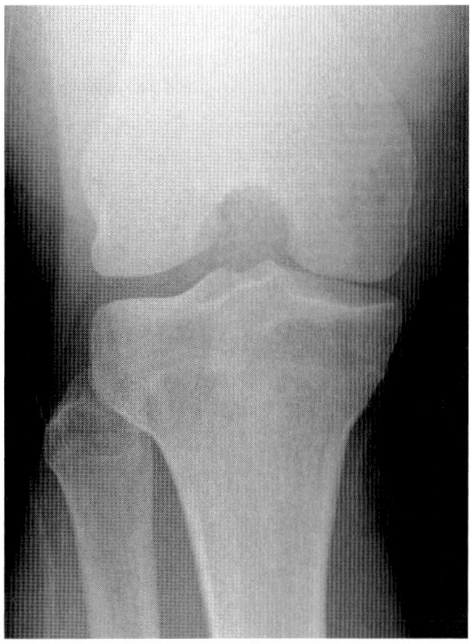

Figure 4 Tunnel radiograph of the right knee of a 17-year-old boy showing a loose body and osteochondral defect on the medial femoral condyle.

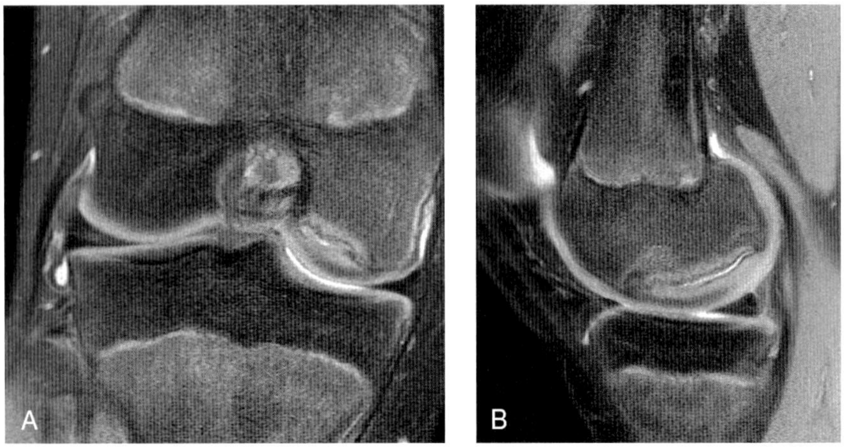

Figure 5 Coronal (**A**) and sagittal (**B**) proton density-weighted MRIs of an OCD lesion on the posterolateral aspect of the medial femoral condyle in a 10-year-old girl.

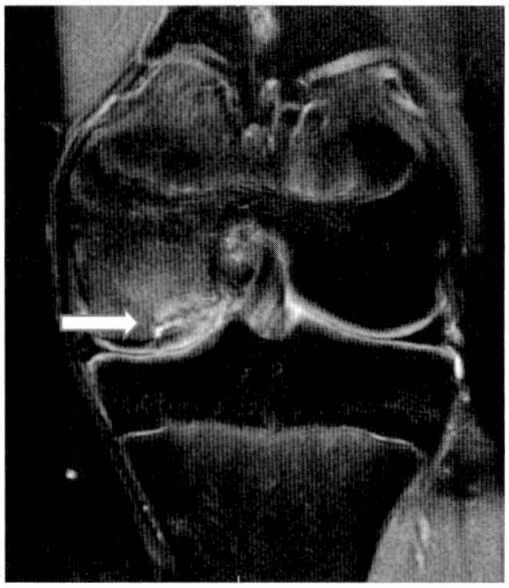

Figure 6 Coronal short tau inversion recovery image of an OCD lesion on the medial femoral condyle showing a high T2-weighted signal line (arrow) behind the lesion. The intensity is the same as that of the nearby synovial fluid, indicating instability of the lesion.

Table 2
MRI Classification of Juvenile OCD Lesions

Stage	Description
I	Small change of signal is present without clear margins of the fragment.
II	Osteochondral fragment with clear margins is present, but without fluid between the fragment and underlying bone.
III	Fluid is visible partially between the fragment and the underlying bone.
IV	Fluid is completely surrounding the fragment, but the fragment is still in situ.
V	The fragment is completely detached (loose body).

only when it is accompanied by a breach in the cartilage on the T1-weighted image.

Kijowski et al[27] reviewed the MRIs of 65 adult and juvenile patients treated with knee arthroscopy. Applying the four De Smet criteria resulted in 100% sensitivity but only 11% specificity for stable and unstable lesions in juvenile OCD. Similarly, Heywood et al[28] reported that MRI findings correlate poorly with fragment stability in juvenile OCD as determined at arthroscopy. The concordance between MRI and arthroscopic findings was 30%, indicating that MRI should not be used in isolation to determine the stability of juvenile OCD lesions.

The effectiveness of gadolinium-enhanced magnetic resonance arthrography also has been studied in predicting outcomes for patients with juvenile OCD. Although this imaging modality can reliably show the loss of continuity of the articular cartilage mantle, enhancement has not been shown to correlate with healing. Multiple studies have shown that smaller lesions are often associated with better clinical outcomes.[29,30]

Arthroscopic Evaluation

Arthroscopic probing of OCD lesions is the gold standard to which every imaging modality has been compared. The classification system of Guhl[31] remains the most widely used and is based on the examiner's ability to either define or displace the OCD lesion (**Table 3**). A more nuanced system, partially based on the quality of the articular surface, is currently being developed.

Current Evidence

The American Academy of Orthopaedic Surgeons has recently published a guideline for the diagnosis and treatment of OCD.[32] A complete review of the available literature produced only 16 articles of sufficient methodologic rigor to be included in formulating the guideline. Based on their review, the work group published a series of 16 recommendations. Of these, no recommendation was graded as strong, 2 were graded as weak, 4 were consensus statements, and 10 were inconclusive. These results underscore the limitations of the available literature and the paucity of high-level comparative studies to guide the treating surgeon. However, this guideline may allow surgeons to make reasonable recommendations to patients, help shape pro-

Table 3
Arthroscopic Staging System of Osteochondral Lesions

Stage	Arthroscopic Findings
I	Irregularity and softening of articular cartilage; no definable fragment
II	Articular cartilage breached; definable fragment not displaceable
III	Articular cartilage breached; definable fragment displaceable but attached by some overlying cartilage
IV	Loose body

spective research, and suggest the most appropriate course of treatment in a given set of circumstances.[33]

Nonsurgical Management

In the child with open physes and a stable lesion, nonsurgical management has historically been the first line of treatment. Cahill[4] reported that 50% of juvenile OCD lesions will heal within a 10- to 18-month period, provided the physis remains open and patient compliance is maintained. Controversy exists, however, regarding the best form of immobilization and activity modification in this group. Physicians who believe that OCD represents a form of subchondral fracture have argued for the use of a cast or knee immobilizer. Other physicians believe that strategies to maximize cartilage health should be used, and cartilage preservation should be the ultimate goal of treatment. Smillie[34] suggested that immobilization should not exceed 4 months in patients younger than 15 years, whereas Hughston et al[2] reported on the detrimental effects of prolonged immobilization, including stiffness, atrophy of the quadriceps, and, potentially, cartilage degeneration.

No consensus has been reached on the optimal type of immobilization for young patients with OCD. A cast allows rigid immobilization but cannot be removed for bathing; this makes it an unpopular choice for many families. A knee immobilizer may be removed for skin care but makes noncompliance, which can undermine treatment, much easier than discontinuing the use of a cast. Unloader braces have been used to allow range of motion but limit forces on the lesion. Difficulties with cost and compliance limit the effectiveness of all casts and braces.

A recent study of nonsurgical management of stable juvenile OCD lesions by Wall et al[35] reported that after 6 months of casting and unloader bracing, only 7 of 47 knees had completely reossified, whereas 16 of 47 had no progression toward healing. The size of the lesion at presentation was predictive of the healing potential, with larger lesions being less likely to heal. Although the authors continued to recommend an initial course of nonsurgical management, they cautioned that family expectations should be carefully managed.

In adolescents with closed or closing physes, low rates of spontaneous healing have been reported with conservative management.[36] In this population, surgery should be considered for patients with stable and smaller lesions to prevent the devastating long-term consequences of gonarthrosis.

Surgical Management

In skeletally immature patients with detached or unstable lesions (Guhl stage III or IV), or if a thorough course of conservative management has failed, surgical treatment is appropriate. Because of reduced healing potential, mature or maturing knees with OCD lesions should be treated surgically to achieve optimal outcomes.

The primary goals of surgical management are maintenance of joint congruity, stable fixation of unstable fragments, and repair of osteochondral defects.[37] Penetration of the subchondral bone is believed to promote vascular ingrowth to the lesion, allowing for healing of these nonunions. Multiple methods to achieve these goals have been studied in the literature, with good short- and medium-term results. Although arthroscopic techniques have replaced open surgery for all but the largest and most difficult lesions, the principles of OCD management must be respected to achieve optimal outcomes.

Accurately interpreting the results of the OCD treatments has proven controversial. Although clinical improvement is important, many patients (even those with large lesions) may be minimally symptomatic at the time of the baseline procedure. It has been proposed that the ultimate goal of treatment should be full and complete healing because the recurrence of lesions has not been reported, whereas the progression of lesions into adulthood has been proven. The true determinant of healing has not been established. Clinical examination, plain radiography, MRI, and second-look arthroscopy have been proposed as potential tools to verify healing; however, each modality presents a unique set of strengths and limitations.

For lesions that are stable to probing in the operating room, the promotion of vascular channels has been well described using transarticular or retroarticular techniques. Transarticular methods allow for direct visualization during drilling but create holes in the articular surface that must be filled with fibrocartilage over time (**Figure 7**). Retroarticular techniques avoid this potential complication but are

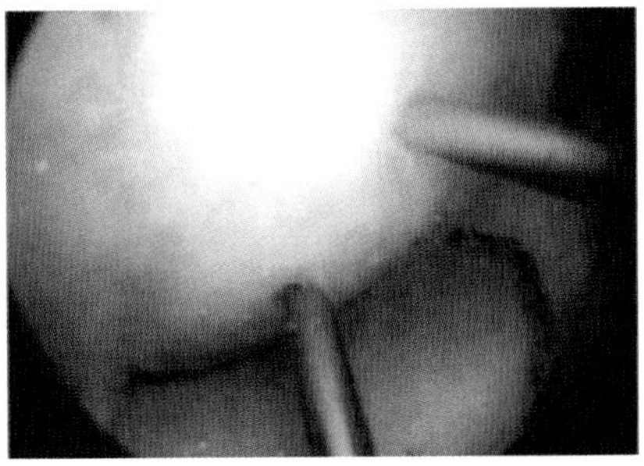

Figure 7 Arthroscopic image of transarticular drilling of a stable OCD lesion on the medial femoral condyle. (Reproduced with permission from Kocher MS, Tucker R, Ganley T, Flynn J: Management of osteochondritis dissecans of the knee: Current concepts review. *Am J Sports Med* 2006;34(7):1181-1191.)

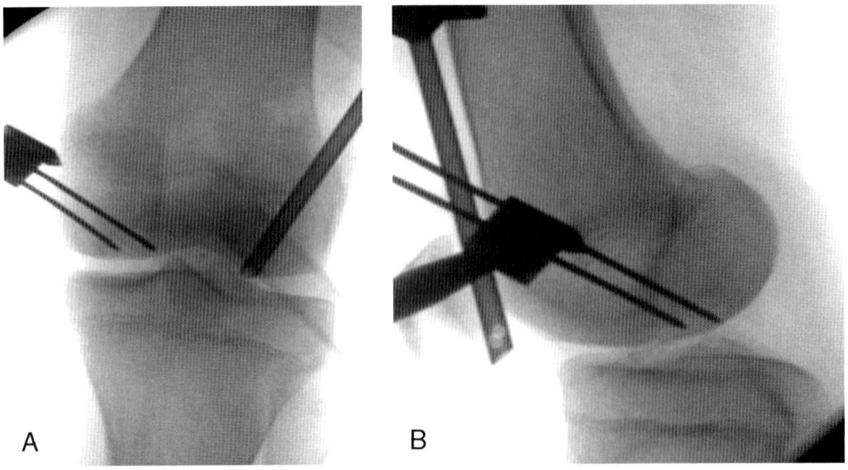

Figure 8 Intraoperative AP (**A**) and lateral (**B**) radiographs of the patient in Figure 3 showing retroarticular drilling of the OCD lesion.

considered a more technically demanding technique (**Figure 8**).

Open drilling, combined with reduction and internal fixation of osteochondral fragments, was first described by Smillie.[34] Arthroscopic techniques of transarticular drilling have been reported to result in predictably good outcomes. Aglietti et al[38] reported radiographic evidence of healing after arthroscopic transarticular drilling in 16 knees in 14 patients, all of whom were asymptomatic at 4 years after surgery.[38] Kocher et al[23] performed transarticular drilling in 30 knees (23 patients) and reported substantial healing and improvement in the Lysholm score at an average follow-up of 3.9 years. Younger age was predictive of better outcomes. Hayan et al[39] treated 40 consecutive patients with transarticular drilling and reported good to excellent clinical and radiographic outcomes in 97.5% and 95% of patients, respectively. Closed physes predicted a worse outcome, but healing rates were still high in skeletally mature patients.

Retroarticular drilling also has been shown to be an effective technique. Donaldson and Wojyts[40] reported on a series of patients treated with extra-articular drilling. Although 3 of 15 patients were lost to follow-up, the remaining 12 patients (13 knees) had excellent functional outcomes, with the exception of 1 patient with bilateral lesions who had a fair outcome in the contralateral knee.

In 2010, this chapter's senior author (HGC) reported on 59 children treated with a transepiphyseal method that allowed the placement of more drill holes in the lesion without violating the articular surface.[41] The mean time to return to activities was 2.8 months, and the mean percentage of radiographic healing was 98.2% at final follow-up. Forty-four of the 59 OCD lesions (75%) were successfully treated and showed 100% radiographic healing with an average time for healing of 11.9 months (range, 1.3 to 47.3 months). Large lesions took significantly longer to heal than small lesions, 15.3 months versus 8.8 months ($P = 0.032$). The percentage of radiographic healing at final follow-up approached significance, with large lesions (> 3.2 cm²) attaining a mean of 96.9% (SD = 6.4%) versus small lesions (< 3.2 cm²) with a mean of 99.4% (SD = 2.1%, $P = 0.083$). No surgical complications were observed.

Video 41.1: Retroarticular Drilling of Osteochondritis Dissecans. Henry G. Chambers, MD; Jacob F. Schulz, MD (3 min)

Boughanem et al[42] reported on the results of retroarticular drilling of 34 OCD lesions in 31 skeletally immature patients; 33 of 34 knees had improvement in the Lysholm score at an average follow-up of 4 years. Radiographic evidence of healing was found in 32 of 34 knees, although the two patients who did not have radiographic healing still reported symptomatic improvement. Ninety-two percent of the patients in the study were satisfied or very satisfied with their outcomes and would repeat the surgery again if needed.

In an attempt to reconcile these two techniques, Gunton et al[43] performed a systematic literature review comparing transarticular and retroarticular drilling of juvenile OCD lesions. Although the quality of the available literature limited their conclusions, the authors found no substantial difference in the healing rates or functional outcomes in either group at short-term follow-up. Longer-term studies are needed to determine if the transarticular method results in important changes in articular cartilage.

For lesions that are unstable based on MRI or arthroscopy, various fixation methods have been proposed. Complete débridement of the subchondral bed before refixation and the congruency of the articular surface afterward are key factors in successful treatment. If there is subchondral bone loss, autogenous bone graft should be packed into the defect before fixation. Recessed cannulated screws, headless screws, bioabsorbable screws and pins, as well as bone and osteochondral plugs, have all been used as fixation devices (**Figure 9**). Several studies have shown that bioabsorbable screws provide better fixation than smooth pins, although multiple sources have reported on the negative consequences related to biodegradation of the synthetic polymers and host response.[44,45] A recent animal study, however, suggests that poly-L-lactide implants may be no more reactive than metallic screws in cancellous bone.[46] More concerning are the reports of implants that have loosened and backed out, resulting in damage to adjacent articular surfaces[47,48] (**Figure 10**).

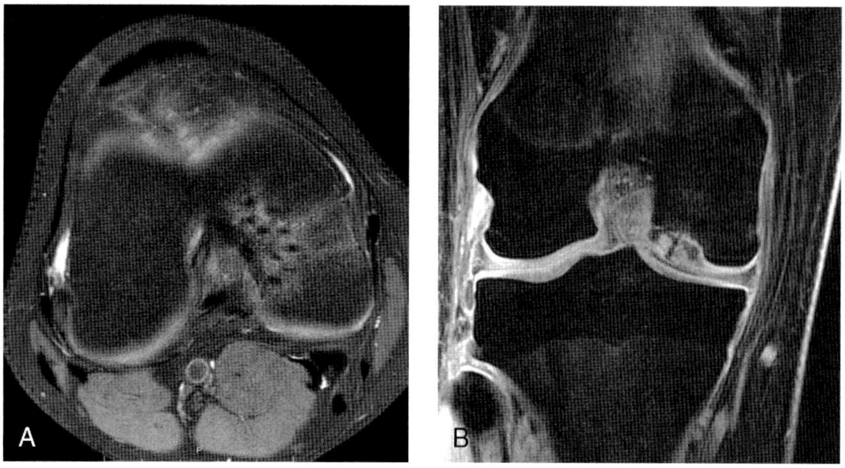

Figure 9 Postoperative axial (**A**) and coronal (**B**) MRIs of an OCD lesion on the medial femoral condyle of a 17-year-old boy. The lesions were fixed arthroscopically with absorbable nails.

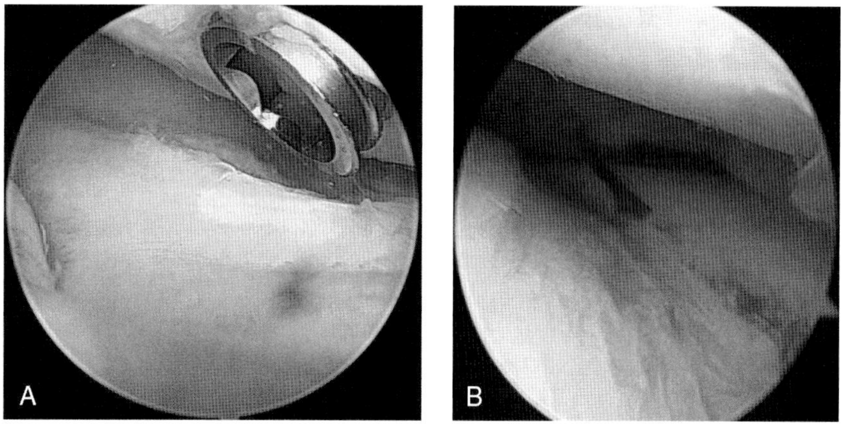

Figure 10 **A,** Arthroscopic view of a headless screw that has backed out of an OCD lesion on the medial femoral condyle. **B,** Arthroscopic view of the resultant defect from that screw on the medial tibial plateau.

Despite these concerns, a 2007 study by Kocher et al[49] evaluated healing rates in 26 patients with unstable lesions that were treated with various fixation devices. The authors reported an approximate 85% healing rate, including healing of all fully detached lesions. No differences were found based on the location, fixation method, or grade of the lesion. In 2010, Tabaddor et al[50] reported on 24 lesions treated with poly 96L/4D-lactide copolymer bioabsorbable implants and found a low rate of complications and a high rate of healing, with good to excellent outcomes in 22 of 24 patients.

Weckström et al[51] compared the outcomes of larger OCD lesions fixed with bioabsorbable nails or pins in skeletally mature patients. Compared with smooth pins, the nails have small barbs and a head to improve compressive hold in cancellous bone. Seventy percent of the lesions were greater than 300 mm² in size. With an average follow-up of 5.3 years, the authors reported that 75% of the nail group had good or excellent outcomes compared with 35% of the pin group. Radiographic evidence of healing supported these clinical results.

Salvage Procedures

If the OCD lesion has become fragmented or lacks sufficient bony backing (< 2 mm) for refixation, removal may be the only option. Various salvage procedures have been described in an attempt to replace the lost native hyaline cartilage. Drilling, abrasion arthroplasty, or microfracture attempt to promote the development of fibrocartilaginous substitute by recruiting pluripotent cells from the marrow elements by transgressing the subchondral bone. Multiple studies of adults

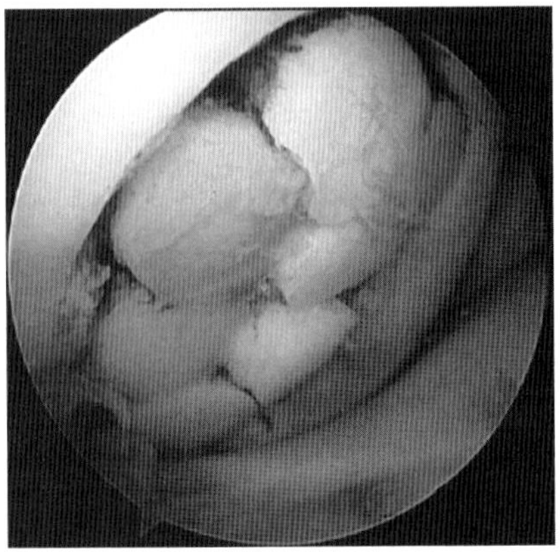

Figure 11 Osteochondral allograft transplantation for a 2.5 cm² OCD defect in the medial femoral condyle. (Reproduced with permission from Rimtautas G, Rasa S, Emilis C, Ramunas T: A prospective, randomized clinical study of osteochondral autologous transplantation versus microfracture for the treatment of osteochondritis dissecans in the knee joint in children. *J Pediatr Orthop* 2009; 29(7):741-748.)

support this method for small lesions (typically < 2 cm) but note progressively worsening arthrosis when used on larger lesions or at long-term follow-up.[37,52-54]

Harvesting hyaline cartilage from non–weight-bearing portions of a patient's own knee (osteochondral autograft transplant surgery) or a donor knee (osteochondral allograft surgery) and shaping the grafts to fit the area of cartilage loss is another salvage option. These are technically demanding procedures. Correctly reshaping the contour of the femoral condyle may be difficult.

In a study of 48 lesions in 46 patients, Pascual-Garrido et al[52] concluded that patients with adult OCD of the knee treated with surgical cartilage procedures, such as débridement, drilling, loose-body removal, arthroscopic reduction and internal fixation, microfracture, and osteochondral allograft or autologous chondrocyte implantation (ACI) showed durable function and symptomatic improvement at a mean follow-up of 4 years. Patients treated with arthroscopic reduction and internal fixation and loose-body removal had greater improvement in outcome scores than those treated with osteochondral allograft.

Gudas et al[53] compared the result of osteochondral autologous transplantation with microfracture in patients younger than 18 years with juvenile OCD. They found that both groups initially responded well to treatment, but at a mean follow-up of 4.2 years, more than 90% of the group treated with osteochondral autologous transplantation compared with 63% of the patients treated with microfracture maintained a good to excellent response. Both groups compared favorably with their preinjury level of pain and function (**Figure 11**).

Among the newest treatments of large cartilage defects in the knee is ACI, in which chondrocytes harvested from the patient's body are grown in a laboratory and then replanted in the defect with a matrix covering. This technique has been used in Europe for some time and is gaining new support in the United States. The role of ACI in the treatment of defects caused by juvenile OCD has not been fully elucidated but has shown promise in the adult population. Peterson et al[55] reported on 58 patients with OCD lesions of the knee, 7 of whom were younger than 18 years (mean age, 26 years). With an average lesion size of 5.8 cm², the authors concluded that using ACI to treat OCD lesions of the knee produces integrated repaired tissue and a successful clinical result in more than 90% of patients. They recommended the wider use of ACI for OCD lesions of the knee.

Although clinical success has been shown with ACI, the histologic quality of the reparative cartilage has proven less than ideal. Moriya et al[56] studied six patients ages 13 to 35 years who had been treated with ACI for an OCD lesion. At 1 year follow-up, a second-look arthroscopy was done for each patient, and the reparative cartilage was clinically assessed and biopsied. Compared with native cartilage, there was a substantial decrease in type I cartilage and an increase in type II cartilage. The concentration of glycosaminoglycans was also substantially decreased; this indicated lower quality cartilage, although functional improvements were still excellent.

No single surgical technique has yet been proven superior in the treatment of irreparable OCD lesions of the knee. The size and quality of the lesion, along with patient- and surgeon-specific factors, should guide the selection of the salvage technique.

Summary

OCD of the knee remains a difficult disease to treat more than a century after it was first described. Controversy exists regarding the underlying etiology, optimal diagnostic workup, and ultimate treatment. There is a need for high-quality studies to support current practices, along with standardization of nomenclature to allow accurate study comparisons. Predicting healing potential and lesion stability are major challenges for the treating surgeon. Although the juvenile form of OCD carries a more favorable prognosis, nonsurgical management will be unsuccessful in a subset of patients. The recent literature suggests that early surgical treatment can positively affect the medium-term prognosis; however, long-term studies are lacking. The results for various salvage procedures are promising and should improve with a better understanding of cartilage pathology.

References

1. Kocher MS, Tucker R, Ganley TJ, Flynn JM: Management of osteochondritis dissecans of the knee: Current concepts review. *Am J Sports Med* 2006;34(7):1181-1191.
2. Hughston JC, Hergenroeder PT, Courtenay BG: Osteochondritis dissecans of the femoral condyles. *J Bone Joint Surg Am* 1984;66(9):1340-1348.
3. Lindén B: The incidence of osteochondritis dissecans in the condyles of the femur. *Acta Orthop Scand* 1976;47(6):664-667.
4. Cahill BR: Osteochondritis dissecans of the knee: Treatment of juvenile and adult forms. *J Am Acad Orthop Surg* 1995;3(4):237-247.
5. Barrie HJ: Osteochondritis dissecans 1887-1987: A centennial look at König's memorable phrase. *J Bone Joint Surg Br* 1987;69(5):693-695.
6. Kothari A, Ponce P, Arriaza B, O'Connor-Read L: Osteochondritis dissecans of the knee in a mummy from northern Chile. *Knee* 2009;16(2):159-160.
7. Koch S, Kampen WU, Laprell H: Cartilage and bone morphology in osteochondritis dissecans. *Knee Surg Sports Traumatol Arthrosc* 1997;5(1):42-45.
8. Chiroff RT, Cooke CP III: Osteochondritis dissecans: A histologic and microradiographic analysis of surgically excised lesions. *J Trauma* 1975;15(8):689-696.
9. Yonetani Y, Nakamura N, Natsuume T, Shiozaki Y, Tanaka Y, Horibe S: Histological evaluation of juvenile osteochondritis dissecans of the knee: A case series. *Knee Surg Sports Traumatol Arthrosc* 2010;18(6):723-730.
10. Mubarak SJ, Carroll NC: Familial osteochondritis dissecans of the knee. *Clin Orthop Relat Res* 1979;140:131-136.
11. Petrie PW: Aetiology of osteochondritis dissecans: Failure to establish a familial background. *J Bone Joint Surg Br* 1977;59(3):366-367.
12. Fairbanks H: Osteo-chondritis dissecans. *Br J Surg* 1933;21:67-82.
13. Rehbein F: The origin of osteochondritis dissecans. *Langenbecks Arch Klin Chir Ver Dtsch Z Chir* 1950;265(1):69-114.
14. Hashimoto Y, Yoshida G, Tomihara T, et al: Bilateral osteochondritis dissecans of the lateral femoral condyle following bilateral total removal of lateral discoid meniscus: A case report. *Arch Orthop Trauma Surg* 2008;128(11):1265-1268.
15. Jacobi M, Wahl P, Bouaicha S, Jakob RP, Gautier E: Association between mechanical axis of the leg and osteochondritis dissecans of the knee: Radiographic study on 103 knees. *Am J Sports Med* 2010;38(7):1425-1428.
16. Herring JA, ed: *Tachdjian's Pediatric Orthopaedics*, ed 3. Philadelphia, PA, Saunders, 2002.
17. Garrett JC: Osteochondritis dissecans. *Clin Sports Med* 1991;10(3):569-593.
18. Wilson JN: A diagnostic sign in osteochondritis dissecans of the knee. *J Bone Joint Surg Am* 1967;49(3):477-480.
19. Conrad JM, Stanitski CL: Osteochondritis dissecans: Wilson's sign revisited. *Am J Sports Med* 2003;31(5):777-778.
20. Polousky JD: Juvenile osteochondritis dissecans. *Sports Med Arthrosc* 2011;19(1):56-63.
21. Milgram JW: Radiological and pathological manifestations of osteochondritis dissecans of the distal femur: A study of 50 cases. *Radiology* 1978;126(2):305-311.
22. Cahill BR, Berg BC: 99m-Technetium phosphate compound joint scintigraphy in the management of juvenile osteochondritis dissecans of the femoral condyles. *Am J Sports Med* 1983;11(5):329-335.
23. Kocher MS, Micheli LJ, Yaniv M, Zurakowski D, Ames A, Adrignolo AA: Functional and radiographic outcome of juvenile osteochondritis dissecans of the knee treated with transarticular arthroscopic drilling. *Am J Sports Med* 2001;29(5):562-566.
24. De Smet AA, Ilahi OA, Graf BK: Reassessment of the MR criteria for stability of osteochondritis dissecans in the knee and ankle. *Skeletal Radiol* 1996;25(2):159-163.
25. Pill SG, Ganley TJ, Milam RA, Lou JE, Meyer JS, Flynn JM: Role of magnetic resonance imaging and clinical criteria in predicting successful nonoperative treatment of osteochondritis dissecans in children. *J Pediatr Orthop* 2003;23(1):102-108.
26. O'Connor MA, Palaniappan M, Khan N, Bruce CE: Osteochondritis dissecans of the knee in children: A comparison of MRI and arthroscopic findings. *J Bone Joint Surg Br* 2002;84(2):258-262.
27. Kijowski R, Blankenbaker DG, Shinki K, Fine JP, Graf BK, De Smet AA: Juvenile versus adult osteochondritis dissecans of the knee: Appropriate MR imaging criteria for instability. *Radiology* 2008;248(2):571-578.
28. Heywood CS, Benke MT, Brindle K, Fine KM: Correlation of magnetic resonance imaging to arthroscopic findings of stability in juvenile osteochondritis dissecans. *Arthroscopy* 2011;27(2):194-199.
29. Bohndorf K: Osteochondritis (osteochondrosis) dissecans: A review and new MRI classification. *Eur Radiol* 1998;8(1):103-112.
30. De Smet AA, Ilahi OA, Graf BK: Untreated osteochondritis dissecans of the femoral condyles:

Prediction of patient outcome using radiographic and MR findings. *Skeletal Radiol* 1997;26(8): 463-467.

31. Guhl JF: Arthroscopic treatment of osteochondritis dissecans. *Clin Orthop Relat Res* 1982;167:65-74.
32. American Academy of Orthopaedic Surgeons: *Clinical Practice Guideline on the Diagnosis and Treatment of Osteochondritis Dissecans.* Rosemont, IL, American Academy of Orthopaedic Surgeons, December 2010. http://www.aaos.org/research/guidelines/OCD_guideline.pdf.
33. Chambers HG, Shea KG, Anderson AF, et al: Diagnosis and treatment of osteochondritis dissecans. *J Am Acad Orthop Surg* 2011; 19(5):297-306.
34. Smillie IS: Treatment of osteochondritis dissecans. *J Bone Joint Surg Br* 1957;39(2):248-260.
35. Wall EJ, Vourazeris J, Myer GD, et al: The healing potential of stable juvenile osteochondritis dissecans knee lesions. *J Bone Joint Surg Am* 2008;90(12):2655-2664.
36. Linden B: Osteochondritis dissecans of the femoral condyles: A long-term follow-up study. *J Bone Joint Surg Am* 1977;59(6): 769-776.
37. Steadman JR, Briggs KK, Rodrigo JJ, Kocher MS, Gill TJ, Rodkey WG: Outcomes of microfracture for traumatic chondral defects of the knee: Average 11-year follow-up. *Arthroscopy* 2003;19(5): 477-484.
38. Aglietti P, Buzzi R, Bassi PB, Fioriti M: Arthroscopic drilling in juvenile osteochondritis dissecans of the medial femoral condyle. *Arthroscopy* 1994;10(3):286-291.
39. Hayan R, Phillipe G, Ludovic S, Claude K, Jean-Michel C: Juvenile osteochondritis of femoral condyles: Treatment with transchondral drilling. Analysis of 40 cases. *J Child Orthop* 2010; 4(1):39-44.
40. Donaldson LD, Wojtys EM: Extraarticular drilling for stable osteochondritis dissecans in the skeletally immature knee. *J Pediatr Orthop* 2008;28(8):831-835.
41. Edmonds EW, Albright J, Bastrom T, Chambers HG: Outcomes of extra-articular, intra-epiphyseal drilling for osteochondritis dissecans of the knee. *J Pediatr Orthop* 2010;30(8): 870-878.
42. Boughanem J, Riaz R, Patel RM, Sarwark JF: Functional and radiographic outcomes of juvenile osteochondritis dissecans of the knee treated with extra-articular retrograde drilling. *Am J Sports Med* 2011;39(10):2212-2217.
43. Gunton MJ, Carey JL, Shaw CR, Murnaghan ML: Drilling juvenile osteochondritis dissecans: Retro- or transarticular? [published online ahead of print January 25, 2012] *Clin Orthop Relat Res.* PMID:20016956
44. Barfod G, Svendsen RN: Synovitis of the knee after intra-articular fracture fixation with Biofix: Report of two cases. *Acta Orthop Scand* 1992;63:680-681.
45. Fridén T, Rydholm U: Severe aseptic synovitis of the knee after biodegradable internal fixation: A case report. *Acta Orthop Scand* 1992;63:94-97.
46. Pihlajamäki H, Salminen S, Laitinen O, Tynninen O, Böstman O: Tissue response to polyglycolide, polydioxanone, polylevolactide, and metallic pins in cancellous bone: An experimental study on rabbits. *J Orthop Res* 2006;24:1597-1606.
47. Friederichs MG, Greis PE, Burks RT: Pitfalls associated with fixation of osteochondritis dissecans fragments using bioabsorbable screws. *Arthroscopy* 2001;17(5): 542-545.
48. Scioscia TN, Giffin JR, Allen CR, Harner CD: Potential complication of bioabsorbable screw fixation for osteochondritis dissecans of the knee. *Arthroscopy* 2001; 17(2):E7.
49. Kocher MS, Czarnecki JJ, Andersen JS, Micheli LJ: Internal fixation of juvenile osteochondritis dissecans lesions of the knee. *Am J Sports Med* 2007;35(5): 712-718.
50. Tabaddor RR, Banffy MB, Andersen JS, et al: Fixation of juvenile osteochondritis dissecans lesions of the knee using poly 96L/4D-lactide copolymer bioabsorbable implants. *J Pediatr Orthop* 2010;30(1):14-20.
51. Weckström M, Parviainen M, Kiuru MJ, Mattila VM, Pihlajamäki HK: Comparison of bioabsorbable pins and nails in the fixation of adult osteochondritis dissecans fragments of the knee: An outcome of 30 knees. *Am J Sports Med* 2007;35(9):1467-1476.
52. Pascual-Garrido C, Friel NA, Kirk SS, et al: Midterm results of surgical treatment for adult osteochondritis dissecans of the knee. *Am J Sports Med* 2009;37(suppl 1): 125S-130S.
53. Gudas R, Simonaityte R, Cekanauskas E, Tamosinas R: A prospective, randomized clinical study of osteochondral autologous transplantation versus microfracture for the treatment of osteochondritis dissecans in the knee joint in children. *J Pediatr Orthop* 2009;29(7):741-748.
54. Wright RW, McLean M, Matava MJ, Shively RA: Osteochondritis dissecans of the knee: Long-term results of excision of the fragment. *Clin Orthop Relat Res* 2004;424: 239-243.
55. Peterson L, Minas T, Brittberg M, Lindahl A: Treatment of osteochondritis dissecans of the knee with autologous chondrocyte transplantation: Results at two to ten years. *J Bone Joint Surg Am* 2003;85(suppl 2):17-24.

56. Moriya T, Wada Y, Watanabe A, et al: Evaluation of reparative cartilage after autologous chondrocyte implantation for osteochondritis dissecans: Histology, biochemistry, and MR imaging. *J Orthop Sci* 2007;12(3):265-273.

Video Reference

41.1: Chambers HG, Schulz JF: Video. *Retroarcticular Drilling of Osteochondritis Dissecans.* Philadelphia, PA, 2012.

SECTION

8

Sports Medicine

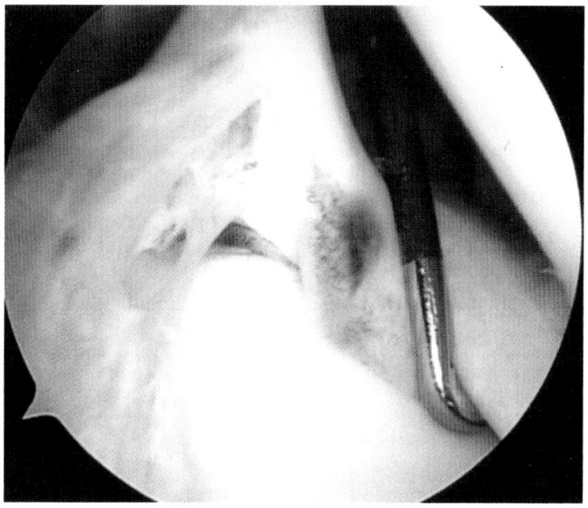

42 Superior Labrum Anterior to Posterior Injuries and Impingement

DVD 43 What Is a Clinically Important Superior Labrum Anterior to Posterior Tear?

44 Superior Labrum Anterior to Posterior Tears in Throwing Athletes

45 Superior Labrum Anterior to Posterior Tears and Glenohumeral Instability

DVD 46 Sports Hip Injuries: Assessment and Management

42

Superior Labrum Anterior to Posterior Injuries and Impingement

Michael G. Ciccotti, MD

Abstract

Superior labrum anterior to posterior (SLAP) tears and subacromial impingement are discrete shoulder pathologies that most often occur separately; however, in some patients the conditions occur simultaneously. Each pathology has specific clinical and radiographic characteristics, but some aspects are shared. Nonsurgical treatment is an important initial option for both SLAP tears and subacromial impingement. Surgical treatment options for SLAP tears include débridement or repair, whereas subacromial impingement is managed with decompression. When these pathologies occur together, it is essential to determine the primary cause of disability for a particular patient and treat it accordingly. In some patients, SLAP tears and subacromial impingement may be equally involved and will require combined treatment.

Instr Course Lect 2013;62:471-481.

The shoulder is exposed to many types of forces during the full spectrum of sport and occupational activities. Normally, a precise balance between the hard and soft tissues allows the performance of this wide range of activities. In some instances, however, that balance is lost and injury can occur. Imbalance can affect any or all of the shoulder structures; frequently, the superior labrum and/or the subacromial space are involved. Although superior labrum anterior to posterior (SLAP) tears and subacromial impingement can occur in relative isolation, these conditions can present simultaneously in some patients. This chapter will review SLAP injuries and subacromial impingement, focusing on the available epidemiologic data, the unique and shared characteristics of diagnosis, and the specific treatment options and outcomes. An algorithm for surgical treatment is provided for cases of simultaneous presentation.

Epidemiology

There is substantial information in the literature on SLAP injuries and subacromial impingement,[1-50] but less information has been published on the simultaneous occurrence of these two shoulder pathologies.[1-4] Several clinical studies have suggested that SLAP tears in patients younger than 40 years are most often seen with a concomitant anterior and/or posterior labral injury,[5] whereas SLAP tears in patients older than 40 years most often occur with rotator cuff or degenerative joint disease.[5,6] Imaging studies have suggested that asymptomatic changes can occur in both the superior labrum and the rotator cuff or subacromial space as patients age.[7-9] A recent review by Gorantla et al[13] suggested the occurrence of an increased number of superior labral injuries in youth and high-school overhead athletes. Data collected on elite level throwers have shown an increased number of superior labral tears occurring with time.[14] This information raises the question of whether SLAP injuries are occurring more frequently (perhaps because of the increased numbers of overhead athletes playing for longer periods of time) or if the increase is a reflection of enhanced awareness by physicians for this particular shoulder pathology.

Subacromial impingement occurs in patients participating in a variety of overhead sports or occupational

Dr. Ciccotti or an immediate family member serves as a board member, owner, officer, or committee member of the American Orthopaedic Society for Sports Medicine; serves as a paid consultant to or is an employee of Stryker; and has received research or institutional support from Arthrex.

activities.[9-12] In overhead throwing athletes particularly, it is believed to occur secondary to overuse or subtle shoulder instability. Radiographic studies have shown that alterations may occur in the rotator cuff, subacromial bursa, and acromial morphology with repetitive activity and/or advancing age.[7-9]

Although many studies have reported on SLAP injuries and subacromial impingement as separate entities, few epidemiologic data exist on these entities as a combined pathology.[6,10,11,13,15,17,20] Superior labral injuries have been associated with overhead or throwing sports in younger patients, whereas subacromial impingement has been associated with repetitive overhead work-related activities in older patients. Superior labral injuries have been reported to occur with other intra-articular pathologies (most commonly anterior or posterior labral tears), whereas subacromial impingement has been associated with other subacromial pathologies such as rotator cuff disease. Evidence suggests that asymptomatic changes can occur in the labrum, rotator cuff, and osseous structures of the shoulder.[7-9] These limited epidemiologic and review data do not clearly define these two shoulder pathologies and how they relate to each other.

Diagnosis

Although SLAP injuries and subacromial impingement have been previously defined from a clinical perspective, there are several important aspects of the history, examination, and imaging studies that help differentiate these two shoulder pathologies.

History

SLAP injuries are most often symptomatic in athletes younger than 40 years; superior labral changes seen on imaging studies or at arthroscopy in patients older than 40 years may not be the cause of symptoms.[15-19] In contrast, subacromial impingement has been most commonly identified in patients older than 40 years who are involved in repetitive, overhead, work-related activities.[1,9] Changes in the subacromial bursa and/or the rotator cuff in younger patients are believed to occur secondary to overuse and/or shoulder instability.[20] However, physiologic age does not always correlate with chronologic age; primary subacromial impingement may develop in younger patients, including overhead athletes, and primary superior labral pathology may develop in older patients and become a source of disability. In general, however, patients younger than 40 years are more likely to incur a SLAP injury, and those older than 40 years are more likely to have subacromial impingement.

SLAP tears and subacromial impingement are commonly associated with repetitive overhead activities. SLAP tears are commonly seen in the overhead throwing athlete, particularly those involved in baseball, javelin, basketball, and volleyball, but may occur in any athlete who has a traumatic injury that loads the superior labrum. Subacromial impingement is associated with repetitive overhead lifting and most often occurs in occupations that require such activities.

The type or quality of pain may help differentiate superior labral injuries from subacromial impingement. SLAP tears most often produce a sharp pain, which is felt deep or in the posterior aspect of the shoulder. The pain often is intermittent and associated with mechanical symptoms such as clicking, catching, and popping. With subacromial impingement, the pain is usually described as a dull ache localized to the anterior and lateral aspects of the shoulder. This pain may be progressive and persistent.

An identifiable traumatic event is often associated with a SLAP tear. A slow, progressive, insidious onset is often seen with subacromial impingement, although both of these entities can occur from a single event or with a slower onset.

Examination

Both SLAP tears and subacromial impingement may lead to decreased shoulder range of motion. SLAP tears often cause pain with maximum abduction and external rotation, as seen in the late cocking or early acceleration phases of throwing. On examination, progressive loss of internal rotation may be noted. Patients with subacromial impingement usually present with a painful arc of motion from approximately 80° to 140° in both forward flexion and abduction and often feel less discomfort either below or above that arc of motion. Strength may be diminished in both SLAP tears and subacromial impingement secondary to pain and shoulder deconditioning. Over time, an altered arc of motion compared with the contralateral shoulder may develop in the shoulder of the overhead throwing athlete. These athletes may have increased external rotation and decreased internal rotation in the dominant arm; however, the total arc of motion is usually symmetric with the nondominant shoulder. Decreases in internal rotation occur with time. If internal rotation deficits in the scapular plane are greater than 20° to 25° or the total arc of motion is 20° to 25° less than the contralateral shoulder, glenohumeral internal rotation deficit may be present.[21]

Specific tests have been suggested to help in diagnosing SLAP tears and subacromial impingement.[1,9] Many tests have been proposed for detecting SLAP pathology, including the commonly used O'Brien active compression test and the Mayo shear test.[22-26] The O'Brien active compression test is performed with the patient either sitting or supine to stabilize the scapula.[22] The shoulder is placed in 90° of forward flexion, with the elbow extended and the arm in 15° to 20° of adduction. Superior labral pathology may be indicated when resisted forward elevation with the thumb pointing caudally causes pain deep or along the posterior shoulder; this pain is relieved with the thumb pointing cephalad. The Mayo shear test is performed by circumducting the forward flexed shoulder; if a painful click or pop deep or along the posterior joint line occurs, a SLAP tear may be present.[25] Many studies, however, have shown that SLAP tears are clinically ambiguous.[27,28,29] Burkhart et al[30] correlated clinical testing with arthroscopically identified type II SLAP lesions in throwing athletes in an effort to more precisely determine which clinical tests are diagnostically helpful. In patients with an arthroscopically identified type II SLAP tear extending from the base of the biceps anteriorly, preoperative symptoms included anterior bicipital groove tenderness and positive Speed and O'Brien active compression tests. In patients with an arthroscopically identified type II SLAP tear extending from the base of the biceps posteriorly, the apprehension relocation test of Jobe was positive for posterior shoulder pain, which was relieved with reduction of the shoulder by a posteriorly directed force. The authors noted that in patients with a type II superior labral tear extending across the entire superior labrum from anterior to posterior, the anterior signs (bicipital groove tenderness and positive Speed and O'Brien active compression tests) and the posterior sign (apprehension and relocation test of Jobe for posterior shoulder pain) were present. However, no single positive test or combination of positive tests can reliably predict the presence of a SLAP tear. It has been suggested that a series of negative SLAP tests may help rule out a SLAP tear.[27-29]

Commonly performed tests for impingement include the Neer sign, the Hawkins sign, and the impingement injection test. The Neer sign is elicited by internally rotating the maximally forward-flexed arm. The Hawkins sign is elicited by abducting the arm to 90° in the scapular plane and internally rotating the upper arm. Positive Neer and Hawkins impingement signs are indicated by the generation of pain in patients with subacromial impingement and result from the thickened, inflamed bursa and/or rotator cuff impinging on the abnormal acromial morphology. The impingement injection test is performed by injecting approximately 5 to 6 mL of local anesthetic in the subacromial space of a patient with positive Neer and Hawkins signs. If the pain from the Neer and Hawkins signs is relieved or diminished after the injection, the impingement injection test is considered positive for subacromial impingement.

In addition to a focused shoulder examination, the scapula, spine, trunk, pelvis, and legs should be thoroughly examined. The kinetic chain theory suggests that the force necessary for throwing is initiated in the lower extremities, transmitted through the pelvis, and continued by trunk rotation to the upper extremity through the shoulder joint.[31-33] Weakness or deconditioning at any point along the kinetic chain may lead to increased forces in the shoulder and can result in a variety of pathologies, including SLAP injuries and/or rotator cuff and subacromial pathology. A thorough evaluation of the scapula and periscapular muscles; the cervical, thoracic and lumbar spine; the paraspinal muscles; and the core, pelvic, abdominal, hip, and leg musculature is needed to rule out a distant source of biomechanical malfunction that could lead to shoulder pain and disability.

Imaging

Plain AP radiographs in internal and external rotation along with axillary and outlet views are helpful in identifying bony sources of shoulder pain. Plain radiographs are usually normal in younger patients and patients with superior labral pathology. An altered acromial contour may be seen in patients with subacromial impingement.[9] Assessment of acromial morphology, as described by Bigliani et al,[9] may help diagnose subacromial impingement; however, asymptomatic patients have been identified with the full spectrum of acromial shapes.

MRI is one of the most commonly performed imaging studies for shoulder pathology, although there is some controversy on whether it is necessary for diagnostic purposes and if gadolinium enhancement is needed. Because studies have shown alterations in the superior labrum and the rotator cuff/ subacromial space in asymptomatic patients,[7,8,34] caution is needed when basing diagnostic and therapeutic decisions on imaging findings alone. Both superior labral and subacromial changes can exist on MRI in asymptomatic patients; therefore, imaging does not consistently differentiate these two shoulder pathologies as a possible source of shoulder disability in a specific patient.

Treatment Options

Both nonsurgical and surgical treatments have been proposed for SLAP injuries and subacromial impingement.

Nonsurgical Treatment

The initial treatment, especially when the clinical findings are ambiguous, should include nonsurgical measures such as rest from the offending sport or activity for 3 to 6 weeks depending on the severity of pain; heat and ice contrast to ease pain, improve flexibility, and diminish swelling; and nonsteroidal anti-inflammatory drugs to decrease the inflammatory process, if allowed by the patient's medical history. No particular anti-inflammatory drug has been identified as the optimal medication for either SLAP injuries or subacromial impingement.

An injection of local anesthetic combined with a corticosteroid can be diagnostic and therapeutic. Sequential injections in the subacromial and intra-articular spaces may more precisely identify the location of the pain. A subacromial injection that provides substantial symptom relief would indicate subacromial impingement as the primary source of pain, whereas an intra-articular injection providing pain relief would suggest intra-articular injury as the primary source of pain. Debate continues on the optimal combination of local anesthetic and corticosteroid and the number and frequency of injections. One possible combination is 2 mL of bupivacaine and 2 mL of Celestone (Schering-Plough, Whitehouse Station, NJ). If a patient has substantial but incomplete pain relief with a subacromial injection, a second injection may be given approximately 6 weeks later. After pain begins to diminish, a gentle progressive shoulder range-of-motion and stretching program is initiated. When the range of motion approaches normal, a rotator cuff and scapular strengthening program is begun and progresses from isometric through resistance exercises. All other nonshoulder issues are also addressed, including core, hip, and leg stability and strengthening. When the kinetic chain is normal, including a stable and strong core, hips, and legs along with good scapular control and a normal glenohumeral shoulder examination, sport-specific or work simulation exercises are instituted. Nonsurgical treatment for primary SLAP pathology may help to relieve symptoms, but true healing of the SLAP tear is debatable. A recent retrospective review of clinically documented SLAP tears by Edwards et al[35] reported a 49% success rate with nonsurgical treatment. All of the patients in the nonsurgical group had improvements in pain, function, and quality of life, and 71% of the athletes returned to their preinjury level of sports participation. Nonsurgical treatment is also successful for primary subacromial impingement, with studies reporting 90% to 95% good or excellent outcomes.[10-12,36]

Surgical Treatment

Surgical indications for both SLAP tears and subacromial impingement include persistent symptoms that are unresponsive to a structured nonsurgical treatment program of approximately 12 weeks' duration, inability to work, and difficulty sleeping and performing daily activities. In the elite or professional athlete, surgical treatment may be proposed more quickly to return the athlete to play in a more timely fashion.

Arthroscopic Evaluation

When surgical treatment is elected, arthroscopic evaluation may help to further differentiate SLAP tears from subacromial impingement. Arthroscopy is initiated in the glenohumeral joint, and all structures are thoroughly evaluated, including the rotator cuff, the intra-articular portion of the biceps, the glenoid and humeral articular surfaces, and the labrum (specifically the superior labrum). A variety of possible normal variations in the superior labrum can exist that may not indicate pathology.[18,19,37] Snyder et al[38] suggested that the superior labrum may be meniscoid-like and extend over the articular margin of the glenoid without being detached or torn. Huber and Putz[39] reported that a close evaluation of the labral articular cartilage interface is essential in determining a superior labral tear; the fibers of the undersurface of the superior labrum should be in close proximity to the articular margin of the superior glenoid rim. Burkhart and Morgan[40] and Wilk et al[41] suggested that throwing athletes may incur a peel-back phenomenon with repetitive throwing. The forces of throwing may cause the superior labrum to roll or peel off the superior glenoid rim with maximum abduction in external rotation. This hypermobility of the superior labrum may be a pain generator in throwing athletes and subsequently can lead to true SLAP tears. The peel-back phenomenon, if identified arthroscopically in a nonthrowing athlete or nonathlete, may not indicate true pathology. Arthroscopic evaluation is then continued in the subacromial space. It is essential to evaluate the thickness and brawniness of the bursal tissue as well as the smoothness of the superior aspect of the rotator cuff and the bony morphology of both the acromion and the distal clavicle.

There are specific clues that may help identify either a SLAP tear or subacromial impingement as the primary source of pain. Several features may be present in a true, symptomatic SLAP tear, including visible disruption of the superior labral fibers with fraying of the superior labral margin and hemorrhagic fibrous granulation-type tissue (**Figure 1**). Probing is essential to identify SLAP pathology. Lifting off of the superior labrum greater than 4 to 5 mm may suggest an unstable superior labrum, and exposed nonarticular glenoid beneath the superior labrum may indicate a SLAP tear (**Figure 2**). In the

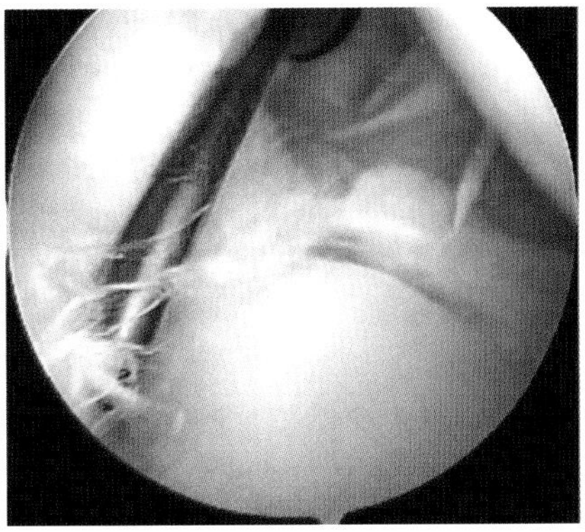

Figure 1 Arthroscopic view of superior labral fraying and fiber disruption at the site of a tear.

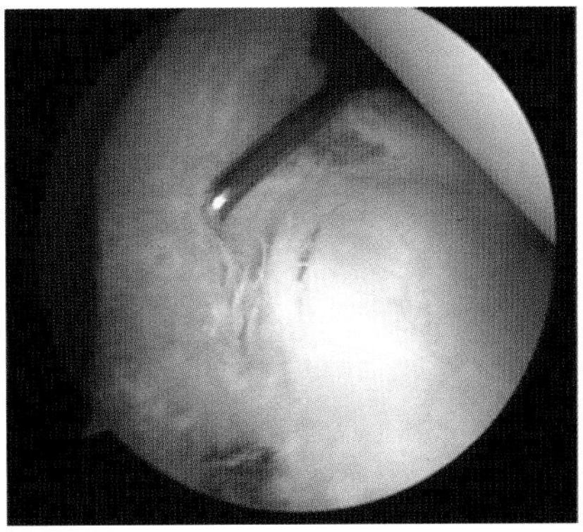

Figure 2 Arthroscopic view of exposed, nonarticular bone of the superior glenoid beneath a SLAP tear.

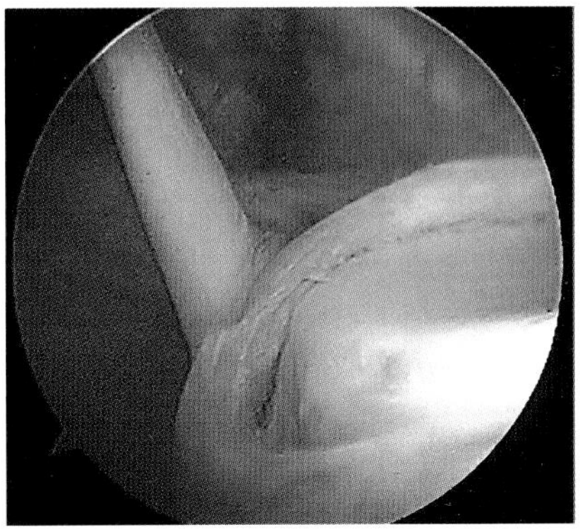

Figure 3 Arthroscopic view of superior labral instability as evidenced by peeling back of the superior labrum off the superior glenoid rim.

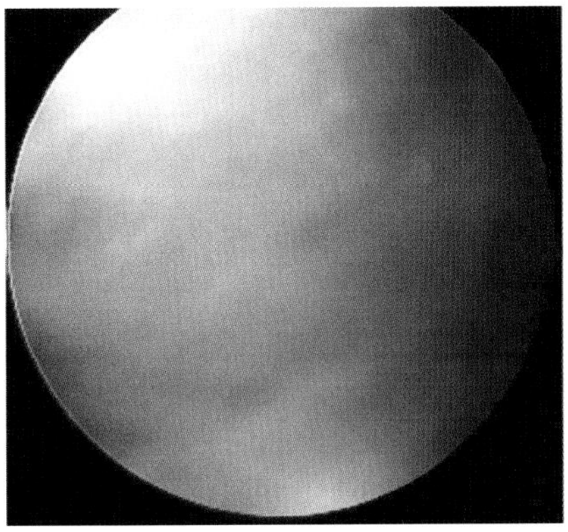

Figure 4 Arthroscopic view of thickened, hemorrhagic subacromial bursa.

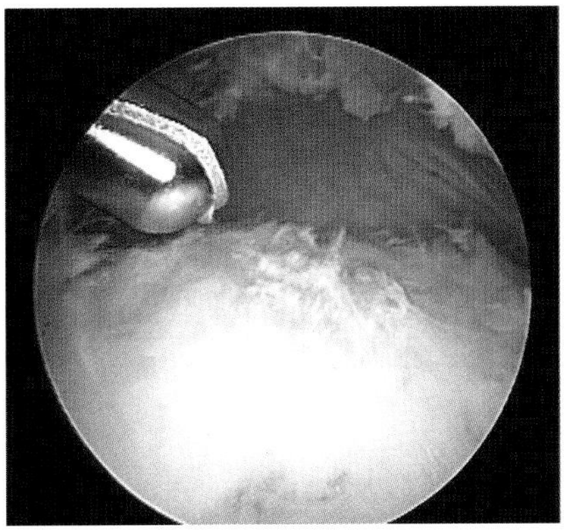

Figure 5 Arthroscopic view of rotator cuff fraying on the subacromial surface.

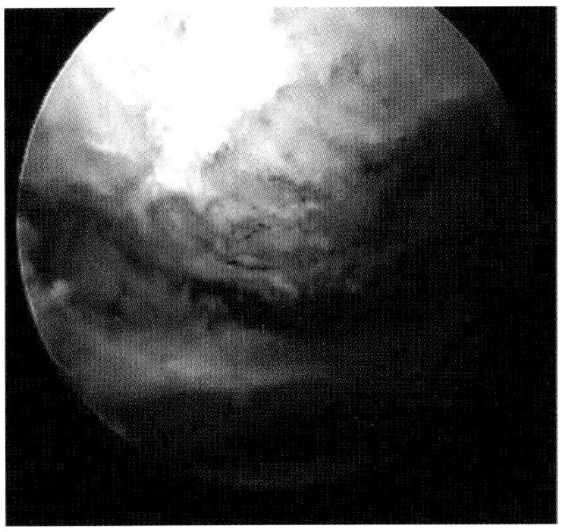

Figure 6 Subacromial spurring as viewed from a posterior portal.

overhead throwing athlete, instability of the superior labrum with abduction and external rotation in the operating room, as evidenced by peeling back of the superior labrum off the superior glenoid rim, is suggestive of a symptomatic SLAP tear (**Figure 3**). Examination of the subacromial space offers specific clues for subacromial impingement. Extremely thickened, hemorrhagic bursa with inflammation that makes visualization challenging indicates subacromial pathology (**Figure 4**). Fraying of the superior subacromial surface of the rotator cuff indicates a mechanical type of irritation from subacromial pathology (**Figure 5**). Anterior, lateral, and/or medial acromial bony spurring suggests mechanical subacromial impingement (**Figure 6**). Erythema of the coracoacromial ligament suggests that the ligament is generating mechanical irritation of the rotator cuff through the coracoacromial arch. Prominence and compression of the muscular or musculotendinous junction of the rotator cuff by the distal clavicle is also evidence of subacromial impingement. These clues may help identify either a SLAP tear or subacromial impingement as the primary pathologic process. The presence of these types of abnormalities in the superior labrum and subacromial space may indicate the presence of both pathologies in a particular patient.

SLAP Repair

Outcomes

Studies have identified reliable results with SLAP repair in young, overhead throwing athletes;[42-47] however, some authors caution against performing SLAP repairs in patients older than 40 years.[2,48-50] These authors believe that superior labral pathology may be an asymptomatic finding on advanced imaging or arthroscopic studies and often is not the true source of pain in this older patient population. Some studies suggest that SLAP repair in older patients can lead to substantial postoperative stiffness and altered shoulder function.[2,48-50]

More recently, two studies reported consistently good to excellent results in both older and younger patients treated with SLAP repair.[6,47] Alpert et al[47] evaluated the effect of age on the outcomes of arthroscopic repair of type II SLAP lesions in 52 patients treated with isolated arthroscopic repair. The patients were divided into two groups, those younger than 40 years (group I, 21 patients) and those older than 40 years (group II, 31 patients). The study population was followed for a minimum of 2 years and evaluated with postoperative validated outcome scores (American Shoulder and Elbow Surgeons [ASES] score and Medical Outcomes Study 12-Item Short Form score) and the visual analog scale for pain, range of motion, and ability to return to sports. The authors reported no statistically significant differences with respect to each parameter. Patients in group I (younger than 40 years) considered their shoulders to be 89% of normal, whereas patients in group II (older than 40 years) considered their shoulders to be 87% of normal. The satisfaction rates were statistically similar, with 95% of the patients in group I and 84% of the patients in group II satisfied with their outcomes. A nonstatistically significant increased length of time to regain full motion in the group of older patients was reported. The authors suggest that good to excellent results can be reliably obtained with arthroscopic repair of clinically symptomatic type II SLAP tears in both older and younger patients.

Neri et al[6] evaluated isolated type II SLAP lesions with respect to age-related outcomes of arthroscopic fixation in 50 patients. Twenty-five patients were younger than 40 years (group I) and 25 were 40 years or older (group II). All of the patients were followed for a minimum of 1 year and evaluated with postoperative validated shoulder scores (ASES scores), range of motion, and ability to return to sports. There were no statistically significant differences in any of the parameters between the two groups. Good to excellent results were obtained in 88% of the group I patients and 84% of the group II patients. Both groups showed equal ability to return to their preinjury level of sports after labral repair, although it took the older patients (group II) more time to return to their preinjury level. The authors concluded that most patients who are proper candidates for type II SLAP repair have good or excellent results regardless of age.

Technique

The literature suggests that SLAP repair is appropriate and reliable in consistent overhead athletes (particularly throwers) who experience decreased velocity and control and have examination findings consistent with a superior labral injury and no impingement signs.[2,3,6] MRI and arthroscopy should show identifiable SLAP abnormalities; an intact, viable biceps tendon; and no or minimal subacromial and rotator cuff abnormalities. The preferred technique of this chapter's author includes suture repair with the patient in a lateral decubitus position; an anterior suture shuttle portal and lateral transmuscular suture placement and a knot-tying portal are used.[51] The presence and full extent of the SLAP tear is confirmed with arthroscopy. The biceps tendon is thoroughly evaluated to confirm its integrity. If substantial biceps tendon pathology is present, biceps tenotomy or tenodesis may better relieve symptoms.[2,36,49,50]

This chapter's author believes that in the overhead athlete, and also perhaps in the overhead laborer, SLAP repair should be performed as well. The fibrous tissue between the superior labrum and the superior glenoid rim is débrided with an arthroscopic shaver. The superior glenoid rim is prepared with an arthroscopic shaver, a burr, and a rasp to create an optimal biologic healing bed without altering the contour of the superior glenoid. Bleeding of the superior glenoid rim is confirmed with direct arthroscopic visualization. Implants are placed in the superior glenoid rim posterior to the biceps, and their fixation is tested. The suture limbs are then shuttled through the superior labrum, posterior to the biceps in either a vertical or horizontal mattress fashion depending on the specific tear pattern. The number and location of implants is dependent on the extent of the tear and quality of the labral tissue. Two-point implant fixation is generally recommended. Debate continues regarding the precise location and type of implant as well as the optimal stitch configuration. Care is taken to maintain the knots on the nonarticular, capsular side of the labrum and not capture or tether the biceps at either its root or the capsule (**Figure** 7). The arm is then maneuvered in an abducted externally rotated position to ensure that the superior labrum is stable without tethering the biceps.

Subacromial Decompression

Several studies have suggested that subacromial decompression is a reliable procedure in older patients with isolated subacromial impingement.[9,10,12,36] In other studies, however, poor outcomes have been reported in younger patients treated with this procedure, and the authors have suggested that when treating the younger patient population (particularly throwing athletes), care must be taken to determine if subacromial impingement is the primary pathology or if it is secondary to an intra-articular labral tear or instability.[11,20] In the middle-aged patient, subacromial decompression is an appropriate procedure if there is limited participation in recreational overhead sports; a history of prolonged work-related overuse; examination findings consistent with impingement, including a positive injection test; no SLAP signs; and irregularities in the subacromial space and rotator cuff are identified on MRI and arthroscopy, with no superior labral changes.

The glenohumeral joint is thoroughly assessed through a posterior viewing portal and an anterior instrumentation portal. All of the intra-articular structures are evaluated. The arthroscope is then placed in the subacromial space, and the thickened inflamed bursa is carefully excised anterolaterally to posteromedially. Hemostasis is ensured with an electrothermal device. The rotator cuff is thoroughly evaluated, and any fraying is débrided. If substantial rotator cuff partial-thickness tearing is present, a repair is made depending on the depth, location, and extent of the rotator cuff injury. The coracoacromial arch is then evaluated with internal and external rotation of the humerus to identify mechanical impingement. An electrothermal device may be used to elevate the coracoacromial ligament off the anterior bony spur, with care taken to prevent transection or resection of the ligament. The acromion is thoroughly evaluated, including its anterior, lateral, and medial bony contours. The undersurface of the distal clavicle is also assessed. At this point in the procedure, a careful subacromial bony resection is performed by placing a pilot hole in the abnormal part of the spur with a 5-0 pineapple-shaped burr. The resection then proceeds from anterior to posterior and from lateral to medial; the spur is removed so that it is consistent with the depth of the previously placed pilot hole. This ensures 5 to 6 mm of bone resection, depending on the size of the spur. The subacromial space is evaluated from the lateral portal, and the burr is placed through the posterior portal (**Figure 8**). Additional resection is carried out if the burr sheath is not parallel to the undersurface of the acromion. The arm is then brought through a full range of motion to confirm that there is no mechanical impingement of the rotator cuff on the decompressed undersurface of the acromion and distal clavicle.

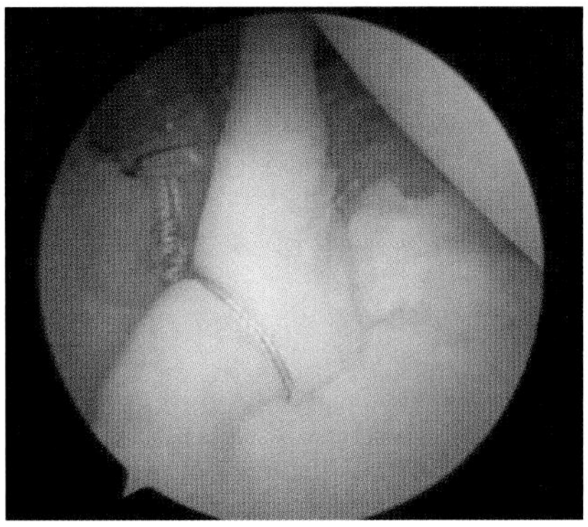

Figure 7 View of an arthroscopically repaired SLAP tear using suture implants.

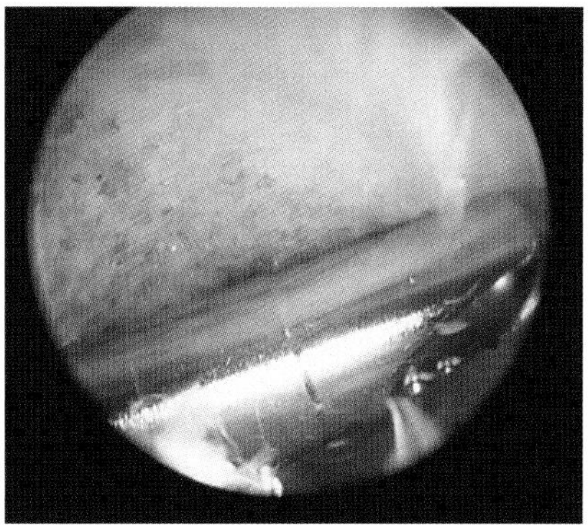

Figure 8 Arthroscopic visualization of the subacromial space from a lateral portal. A burr is placed through the posterior portal to assess the adequacy of decompression.

Combined SLAP Repair and Subacromial Decompression

In some patients, the history, physical examination, and imaging findings may suggest that both a SLAP tear and subacromial impingement are important contributors to shoulder disability. These patients may have a history of repetitive overhead activity and participation in overhead sports such as baseball or softball. The examination findings may indicate an intra-articular superior labral injury with an intact biceps tendon and subacromial impingement. Imaging studies and arthroscopy may show abnormalities in the superior labrum and the subacromial space. Despite the clinical logic of using a combined treatment approach, concern remains for the occurrence of postoperative stiffness and poor outcomes if both SLAP repair and subacromial decompression are performed.[2] Coleman et al[1] evaluated the outcomes of arthroscopic repair of type II SLAP lesions with and without acromioplasty in 50 patients. A structured, nonsurgical treatment program of at least 3 months' duration had been unsuccessful in all of the patients. The patients' preoperative examinations and MRI findings were consistent with the diagnosis of both a type II SLAP tear and subacromial impingement. Thirty-four patients were treated with isolated SLAP repair (group I), and 16 patients had SLAP repair and subacromial decompression (group II). All of the patients were evaluated with ASES and L'Insalata scores at a minimum follow-up of 2 years. There were no statistically significant ($P > 0.05$) differences in L'Insalata and ASES scores between the two groups. Sixty-five percent of the patients in group I were satisfied with their outcomes, whereas 81% in group II were satisfied ($P < 0.05$). The authors concluded that the combination of type II SLAP repair and subacromial decompression is a clinically acceptable and reproducible

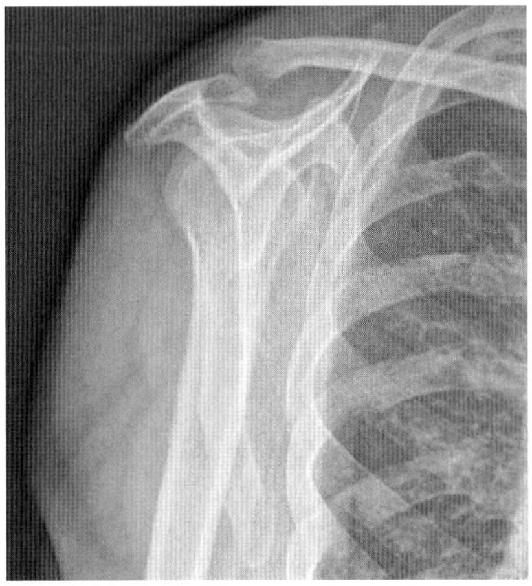

Figure 9 Plain radiograph of the shoulder (Y-view) showing a type II acromion.

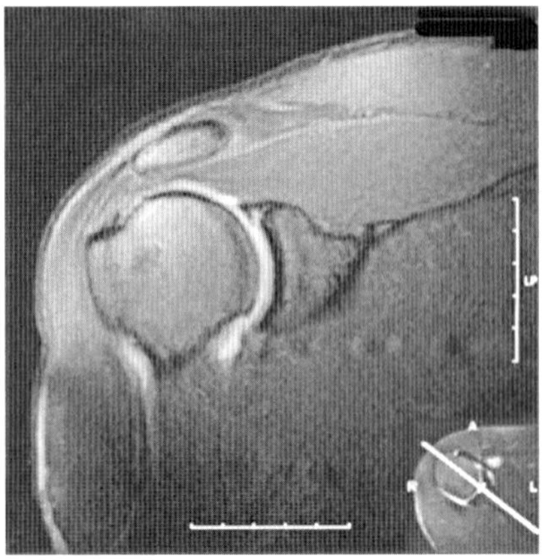

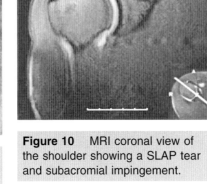

Figure 10 MRI coronal view of the shoulder showing a SLAP tear and subacromial impingement.

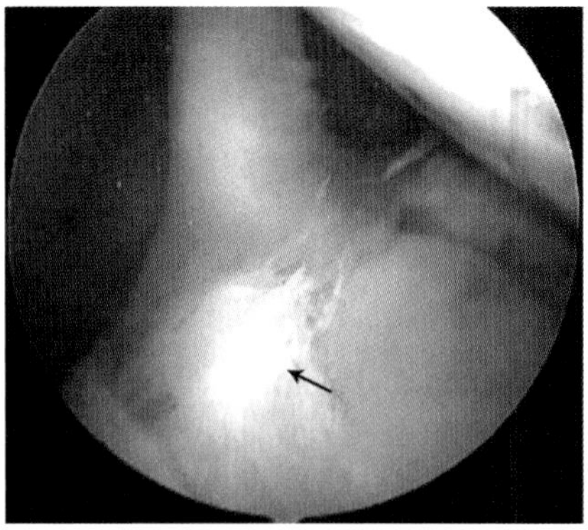

Figure 11 Arthroscopic view of the glenohumeral joint with evidence of a SLAP tear (arrow).

procedure with good clinical outcome scores in patients with preoperative evidence of both a symptomatic SLAP tear and subacromial impingement.

Postoperative Rehabilitation

Postoperative rehabilitation is essential to achieve optimal outcomes for patients treated with isolated or combined surgical treatments for SLAP injuries or subacromial impingement.[3,4,9,10,32,34,36,41,49,50] Range of shoulder motion should be closely monitored by the physician and the therapist. Alpert et al[47] reported that patients older than 40 years may take more than 3 months longer to achieve full range of motion than younger patients, but both groups reliably achieved full motion by final follow-up at a minimum of 2 years after surgery. A gentle progression of strengthening exercise for the rotator cuff and periscapular muscles follows range-of-motion exercises. All nonshoulder abnormalities should be addressed, including spine, core, hip, and leg deficiencies. After normal shoulder examination results, which are determined by comparison with the contralateral side, are achieved in terms of glenohumeral motion, rotator cuff strength, and specific labral and impingement tests along with a stable and strong core, hips, and legs, work simulation and/or sports-specific training is started. For patients treated with a SLAP repair and subacromial decompression, full return to overhead activities, particularly throwing sports, may take from 8 to 12 months.

Case Example

A 40-year-old man who worked at an automobile plant and played recreational baseball presented with 6 months of shoulder pain and difficulty with overhead activities. The patient recalled being injured while playing baseball but continued playing on a regular basis. His symptoms persisted after participation in a structured, nonsurgical treatment program. On examination, the patient had a painful arc of motion in both forward flexion and abduction between 80° and 145°. The Hawkins and Neer signs were positive. The O'Brien active compression test and the Mayo shear test were also positive. The scapula was well positioned, and there was no substantial glenohumeral internal rotation deficit. The patient's core, hips, and legs were strong and stable on examination. Plain radiographs (AP, internal and external rotation, Y, and axillary views) showed a type II acromion with no glenohumeral or acromioclavicular joint arthritis (**Figure 9**). Magnetic resonance arthrography identified a SLAP tear, rotator cuff tendinosis, and subacromial inflammation (**Figure 10**). An impingement injection test was performed by injecting local anesthetic into the subacromial space; substantial but incomplete improvement was obtained. Subsequently, additional local anesthetic was injected into the joint; nearly complete symptom resolution occurred. A SLAP tear and subacromial impingement were diagnosed. Nonsurgical treatment measures failed, and symptoms recurred. Because of the persistent symptoms, which interfered with work, sleep, and recreational activities, surgery was recommended. Shoulder arthroscopy identified a SLAP tear (**Figure 11**) and subacromial impingement (**Figure 12**). SLAP repair and subacromial decompression were performed, followed by a progressive postoperative rehabilitation program. The patient returned to work 4 months after surgery and to baseball 8 months after surgery.

Summary

SLAP injuries and subacromial impingement are two discrete shoulder

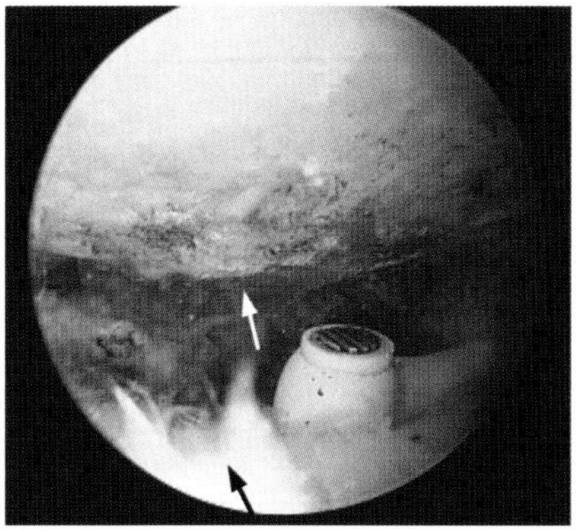

Figure 12 Arthroscopic view of the subacromial space with evidence of subacromial impingement (arrows).

pathologies that most often occur separately. These disorders, however, can occur simultaneously in some patients. Each condition has specific clinical and radiographic characteristics along with shared characteristics. If a structured nonsurgical treatment program is unsuccessful, surgical treatment of each condition in isolation can achieve reliable results in the patient with that isolated pathology. In patients with both pathologic conditions, the combination of SLAP repair and subacromial decompression is clinically acceptable. The combined procedure is reliable and achieves good clinical outcome scores in patients with a preoperative history and physical examination and imaging findings consistent with a symptomatic SLAP tear and subacromial impingement. A careful, structured postoperative rehabilitation program is essential to a successful outcome, especially in patients treated with a combined procedure.

References

1. Coleman SH, Cohen DB, Drakos MC, et al: Arthroscopic repair of type II superior labral anterior posterior lesions with and without acromioplasty: A clinical analysis of 50 patients. *Am J Sports Med* 2007;35(5):749-753.
2. Franceschi F, Longo UG, Ruzzini L, Rizzello G, Maffulli N, Denaro V: No advantages in repairing a type II superior labrum anterior and posterior (SLAP) lesion when associated with rotator cuff repair in patients over age 50: A randomized controlled trial. *Am J Sports Med* 2008;36(2):247-253.
3. Voos JE, Pearle AD, Mattern CJ, Cordasco FA, Allen AA, Warren RF: Outcomes of combined arthroscopic rotator cuff and labral repair. *Am J Sports Med* 2007; 35(7):1174-1179.
4. Forsythe B, Guss D, Anthony SG, Martin SD: Concomitant arthroscopic SLAP and rotator cuff repair. *J Bone Joint Surg Am* 2010; 92(6):1362-1369.
5. Kim TK, Queale WS, Cosgarea AJ, McFarland EG: Clinical features of the different types of SLAP lesions: An analysis of one hundred and thirty-nine cases. *J Bone Joint Surg Am* 2003; 85(1):66-71.
6. Neri BR, Vollmer EA, Kvitne RS: Isolated type II superior labral anterior posterior lesions: Age-related outcome of arthroscopic fixation. *Am J Sports Med* 2009; 37(5):937-942.
7. Reuss BL, Schwartzberg R, Zlatkin MB, Cooperman A, Dixon JR: Magnetic resonance imaging accuracy for the diagnosis of superior labrum anterior-posterior lesions in the community setting: Eighty-three arthroscopically confirmed cases. *J Shoulder Elbow Surg* 2006;15(5):580-585.
8. Waldt S, Burkart A, Lange P, Imhoff AB, Rummeny EJ, Woertler K: Diagnostic performance of MR arthrography in the assessment of superior labral anteroposterior lesions of the shoulder. *AJR Am J Roentgenol* 2004;182(5):1271-1278.
9. Bigliani LU, Morrison DS, April EW: The morphology of the acromion and its relationship to rotator cuff tears. *Orthop Trans* 1986; 10:228-232.
10. Williams GR, Kelley M: Management of rotator cuff and impingement injuries in the athlete. *J Athl Train* 2000;35(3):300-315.
11. Tibone JE, Jobe FW, Kerlan RK, et al: Shoulder impingement syndrome in athletes treated by an anterior acromioplasty. *Clin Orthop Relat Res* 1985;198:134-140.
12. Tibone JE, Elrod B, Jobe FW, et al: Surgical treatment of tears of the rotator cuff in athletes. *J Bone Joint Surg Am* 1986;68(6): 887-891.
13. Gorantla K, Gill C, Wright RW: The outcome of type II SLAP repair: Asystematic review. *Arthroscopy* 2010;26(4):537-545.
14. Eshelman T, Pfefferkorn M, eds: *Redbook: Major League Disability Analysis, 2010 Edition*. American Specialty Companies, Roanoke, IN, 2010.
15. Snyder SJ, Banas MP, Karzel RP: An analysis of 140 injuries to the superior glenoid labrum. *J Shoulder Elbow Surg* 1995;4(4): 243-248.
16. Ilahi OA, Labbe MR, Cosculluela P: Variants of the anterosuperior glenoid labrum and associated pathology. *Arthroscopy* 2002; 18(8):882-886.
17. Nam EK, Snyder SJ: The diagnosis and treatment of superior labrum, anterior and posterior (SLAP) lesions. *Am J Sports Med* 2003;31(5):798-810.
18. Bents RT, Skeete KD: The correlation of the Buford complex and SLAP lesions. *J Shoulder Elbow Surg* 2005;14(6):565-569.
19. Tischer T, Vogt S, Kreuz PC, Imhoff AB: Arthroscopic anatomy, variants, and pathologic findings in shoulder instability. *Arthroscopy* 2011;27(10):1434-1443.

20. Jobe FW, Kvitne RS, Giangarra CE: Shoulder pain in the overhand or throwing athlete: The relationship of anterior instability and rotator cuff impingement. *Orthop Rev* 1989;18(9):963-975.
21. Kibler WB: The role of the scapula in athletic shoulder function. *Am J Sports Med* 1998;26(2):325-337.
22. O'Brien SJ, Pagnani MJ, Fealy S, McGlynn SR, Wilson JB: The active compression test: A new and effective test for diagnosing labral tears and acromioclavicular joint abnormality. *Am J Sports Med* 1998;26(5):610-613.
23. Rhee YG, Lee DH, Lim CT: Unstable isolated SLAP lesion: Clinical presentation and outcome of arthroscopic fixation. *Arthroscopy* 2005;21(9):1099.
24. Guanche CA, Jones DC: Clinical testing for tears of the glenoid labrum. *Arthroscopy* 2003;19(5):517-523.
25. Cook C, Beaty S, Kissenberth MJ, Siffri P, Pill SG, Hawkins RJ: Diagnostic accuracy of five orthopedic clinical tests for diagnosis of superior labrum anterior posterior (SLAP) lesions. *J Shoulder Elbow Surg* 2012;21(1):13-22.
26. Ben Kibler W, Sciascia AD, Hester P, Dome D, Jacobs C: Clinical utility of traditional and new tests in the diagnosis of biceps tendon injuries and superior labrum anterior and posterior lesions in the shoulder. *Am J Sports Med* 2009;37(9):1840-1847.
27. McFarland EG, Kim TK, Savino RM: Clinical assessment of three common tests for superior labral anterior-posterior lesions. *Am J Sports Med* 2002;30(6):810-815.
28. Stetson WB, Templin K: The crank test, the O'Brien test, and routine magnetic resonance imaging scans in the diagnosis of labral tears. *Am J Sports Med* 2002;30(6):806-809.
29. Parentis MA, Glousman RE, Mohr KS, Yocum LA: An evaluation of the provocative tests for superior labral anterior posterior lesions. *Am J Sports Med* 2006;34(2):265-268.
30. Burkhart SS, Morgan CD, Kibler WB: The disabled throwing shoulder: Spectrum of pathology. Part II: Evaluation and treatment of SLAP lesions in throwers. *Arthroscopy* 2003;19(5):531-539.
31. Kibler WB: Biomechanical analysis of the shoulder during tennis activities. *Clin Sports Med* 1995;14(1):79-85.
32. Kibler WB, Livingston B, Chandler TJ: Shoulder rehabilitation: Clinical application, evaluation, and rehabilitation protocols. *Instr Course Lect* 1997;46:43-51.
33. Hirashima M, Yamane K, Nakamura Y, Ohtsuki T: Kinetic chain of overarm throwing in terms of joint rotations revealed by induced acceleration analysis. *J Biomech* 2008;41(13):2874-2883.
34. Applegate GR, Hewitt M, Snyder SJ, Watson E, Kwak S, Resnick D: Chronic labral tears: Value of magnetic resonance arthrography in evaluating the glenoid labrum and labral-bicipital complex. *Arthroscopy* 2004;20(9):959-963.
35. Edwards SL, Lee JA, Bell JE, et al: Nonoperative treatment of superior labrum anterior posterior tears: Improvements in pain, function, and quality of life. *Am J Sports Med* 2010;38(7):1456-1461.
36. Hawkins RJ, Abrams JS: Impingement syndrome in the absence of rotator cuff tear (stages 1 and 2). *Orthop Clin North Am* 1987;18(3):373-382.
37. Davidson PA, Rivenburgh DW: Mobile superior glenoid labrum: A normal variant or pathologic condition? *Am J Sports Med* 2004;32(4):962-966.
38. Snyder SJ, Karzel RP, Del Pizzo W, Ferkel RD, Friedman MJ: SLAP lesions of the shoulder. *Arthroscopy* 1990;6(4):274-279.
39. Huber WP, Putz RV: Periarticular fiber system of the shoulder joint. *Arthroscopy* 1997;13(6):680-691.
40. Burkhart SS, Morgan CD: The peel-back mechanism: Its role in producing and extending posterior type II SLAP lesions and its effect on SLAP repair rehabilitation. *Arthroscopy* 1998;14(6):637-640.
41. Wilk KE, Reinold MM, Dugas JR, Arrigo CA, Moser MW, Andrews JR: Current concepts in the recognition and treatment of superior labral (SLAP) lesions. *J Orthop Sports Phys Ther* 2005;35(5):273-291.
42. Neuman BJ, Boisvert CB, Reiter B, Lawson K, Ciccotti MG, Cohen SB: Results of arthroscopic repair of type II superior labral anterior posterior lesions in overhead athletes: Assessment of return to preinjury playing level and satisfaction. *Am J Sports Med* 2011;39(9):1883-1888.
43. Garofalo R, Mocci A, Moretti B, et al: Arthroscopic treatment of anterior shoulder instability using knotless suture anchors. *Arthroscopy* 2005;21(11):1283-1289.
44. Yian E, Wang C, Millett PJ, Warner JJ: Arthroscopic repair of SLAP lesions with a bioknotless suture anchor. *Arthroscopy* 2004;20(5):547-551.
45. Paxinos A, Walton J, Rütten S, Müller M, Murrell GA: Arthroscopic stabilization of superior labral (SLAP) tears with biodegradable tack: Outcomes to 2 years. *Arthroscopy* 2006;22(6):627-634.
46. Cohen DB, Coleman S, Drakos MC, et al: Outcomes of isolated type II SLAP lesions treated with arthroscopic fixation using a bioabsorbable tack. *Arthroscopy* 2006;22(2):136-142.
47. Alpert JM, Wuerz TH, O'Donnell TF, Carroll KM,

Brucker NN, Gill TJ: The effect of age on the outcomes of arthroscopic repair of type II superior labral anterior and posterior lesions. *Am J Sports Med* 2010; 38(11):2299-2303.

48. Weber SC: Surgical management of the failed SLAP repair. *Sports Med Arthrosc* 2010;18(3): 162-166.

49. Denard PJ, Ladermann A, Burkhart SS: Results according to age and workers' compensation status. *Arthroscopy* 2012;28(4):451-457.

50. Katz LM, Hsu S, Miller SL, et al: Poor outcomes after SLAP repair: Descriptive analysis and prognosis. *Arthroscopy* 2009;25(8): 849-855.

51. Ciccotti MG, Kuri JA II, Leland JM, Schwartz M, Becker C: A cadaveric analysis of the arthroscopic fixation of anterior and posterior SLAP lesions through a novel lateral transmuscular portal. *Arthroscopy* 2010;26(1):12-18.

43

What Is a Clinically Important Superior Labrum Anterior to Posterior Tear?

W. Ben Kibler, MD

Abstract

Knowledge is evolving regarding the importance of the superior labrum in shoulder function and dysfunction. Biomechanical and clinical studies are defining the role of the labrum in shoulder joint function and instability, and guidelines for the diagnosis and the treatment of disorders are emerging. There is a positive association between clinically important, symptomatic labral tears requiring treatment and alterations in labral anatomy. The diagnosis is based on the patient's history and clinical examination findings that indicate a loss of labral function. Labral injury can be confirmed with imaging studies and characterized by arthroscopic studies if surgery is necessary. Emerging data suggest that guided rehabilitation can achieve asymptomatic shoulder function in up to 50% of patients with clinically important labral injuries. Surgical treatment, if necessary, should address all aspects of the labral anatomy so that all the roles of the labrum in shoulder stability are restored.

Instr Course Lect 2013;62:483-489.

The exact role of the superior labrum in shoulder dysfunction remains unclear. Little emphasis was placed on the importance of the superior labrum until arthroscopic techniques and MRI allowed more detailed evaluations. Andrews et al[1] reported the presence of superior labrum anterior to posterior (SLAP) lesions in throwing athletes, and Snyder et al[2] developed a widely adopted (and sometimes modified) classification system. This classification system is observational and is based on arthroscopic visualization and criteria. As experience with the SLAP lesion increased, its importance as a key factor in the disabled throwing athlete was identified, and surgical techniques to treat this lesion were developed.[3-7] SLAP lesions are also being diagnosed and treated more frequently in nonthrowing patients. Current data from the American Board of Orthopaedic Surgery indicate a large increase in the number of SLAP surgeries in the past 10 years (Stephen Weber, MD, unpublished data presented at the American Shoulder and Elbow Surgeons specialty day presentation, San Francisco, CA, 2012). Surgeries for SLAP lesions have increased from 4% to 11% of all shoulder procedures and have become the second most common arthroscopic shoulder procedure.

Some experienced shoulder surgeons believe that SLAP lesions are being overdiagnosed or misdiagnosed as an aspect of shoulder pathology; consequently, shoulder dysfunction is sometimes inadequately treated, and the labral lesion may be overtreated. Published reports have found that physical examination testing, diagnostic imaging, and arthroscopic evaluation are imprecise in determining the role of SLAP tears in shoulder pathology and may contribute to the variable results from surgical repair of SLAP lesions.[8-13] To correct this problem, it is necessary to gain a better understanding of when a SLAP injury is contributing to shoulder dysfunction (a clinically important SLAP injury) and how it should be treated to restore the labrum's role in shoulder function.

Dr. Kibler or an immediate family member serves as a board member, owner, officer, or committee member of the International Society of Arthroscopy, Knee Surgery, and Orthopaedic Sports Medicine, and the American Orthopaedic Society for Sports Medicine; serves as an unpaid consultant to Alignmed; and owns stock or stock options in Alignmed.

Roles of the Labrum in Shoulder Function

Labral roles have been traditionally identified to include an attachment site for the biceps and a bumper to deepen the glenohumeral socket, minimize glenohumeral translation, and help increase capsular tension.[14,15] The actual role of the labrum as a mechanical bumper is controversial. The amount of increased mechanical glenohumeral translation after labral resection is only 10%, meaning that the labrum likely has other functional roles other than its role in mechanical stability.[16,17] Recent biomechanical studies have highlighted three other important functions of the labrum:(1) It acts as a deformable structure interposed between two surfaces, more evenly distributing contact pressures between the surfaces, increasing boundary lubrication, and maximizing concavity/compression characteristics, thus acting much like a washer between two surfaces. (2) The labrum acts as a pressure sensor to maximize proprioceptive feedback. (3) The labrum acts as an attachment site for muscles and ligaments and optimizes their tension.[15,17]

All of these roles allow the labrum to be the most precise of the elements that interact in controlling functional glenohumeral stability at high speeds of rotation, extreme changes in bony positions, and high applied loads. The other elements play more general roles. The bony components create some inherent stability and can be dynamically aligned similar to a "ball on a sea lion's nose" to confer general stability.[18] Muscular activations in co-contraction and agonist/antagonist and coordinated multisegmental activation patterns exert compressive forces that are maximally effective within ± 29.3° of glenohumeral angulation. Ligamentous components are effective passively at extremes of motion.[19-22] Clinically, an intact labrum will result in smooth shoulder motion in rotation, stable ball-and-socket kinematics, and maximal force transfer from the core and the legs through a stable linkage to the hand.

The Clinically Important SLAP Injury

The clinically important SLAP injury is one in which an anatomic alteration in the labrum results in findings of shoulder dysfunction that can be attributed to the loss of specific labral roles, which can be highlighted by certain physical examination tests for the injured labrum. It is a positive diagnosis, not a catch-all term in the presence of shoulder pain of unknown etiology.

Patient History

The patient's history will include findings suggestive of the loss of specific labral roles, including pain with external rotation/cocking, which indicates increased posterior superior translation;[4,16,17] weakness in clinical or functional arm strength, indicating pain and/or increased translation; symptoms of internal derangement (clicking, popping, catching, sliding), indicating loss of the bumper effect or washer effect; or decreased capsular tension and a feeling of a dead arm,[4] which indicates a loss of proprioceptive feedback, decreased capsular tension, and increased translation. Individually, these finding are not exclusive to labral injury; however, they point toward the loss of labral roles.

Examination

No single clinical test will conclusively demonstrate a clinically important SLAP tear. A comprehensive examination will show local and distant physiologic and biomechanical deficits that are commonly associated with a SLAP injury.

Kinetic chain deficits are present in most patients with SLAP injuries. Deficits in hip abductor or extensor strength, hip rotation flexibility, or core strength weakness have been identified in 50% of SLAP injuries.[23,24] These deficits can be identified in a screening examination using the one-leg stability series (a one-leg stance/one-leg half squat maneuver that correlates with hip and core strength).[24-26] Scapular dyskinesis (alteration of resting scapular position and dynamic scapular motion) is frequently seen in patients with labral injuries.[4,27,28] A clinical evaluation method based on the observation of the asymmetric medial border prominence in scapulohumeral rhythm with arm elevation and recording prominence as present or not present has been found to be clinically reliable.[29-31] The dynamic labral shear test has been shown to be clinically useful in evaluating labral injuries.[32] It is performed by abducting the arm and flexing the elbow to 90°. The arm is then abducted in the scapular plane to more than 120° and externally rotated to tightness. A shear load is applied to the joint by maintaining external rotation and horizontal abduction and lowering the arm from 120° to 60° of abduction (**Figure 1**). A positive test is indicated by reproducing pain and/or a painful click or catch in the joint line along the posterior joint line between 120° and 90° of abduction. The test has a sensitivity of 0.72, a specificity of 0.98, a positive predictive value of 0.97, and a positive likelihood ratio of 31.6.[32]

Glenohumeral internal rotation deficit is seen in virtually all patients with a SLAP injury and is predictive of future injury in asymptomatic patients.[33] Precise, reproducible measurements are possible with specific protocols that stabilize the scapula and measure glenohumeral motion using either a goniometer or an inclinometer[34,35] (**Figure 2**). Based on the experience of this

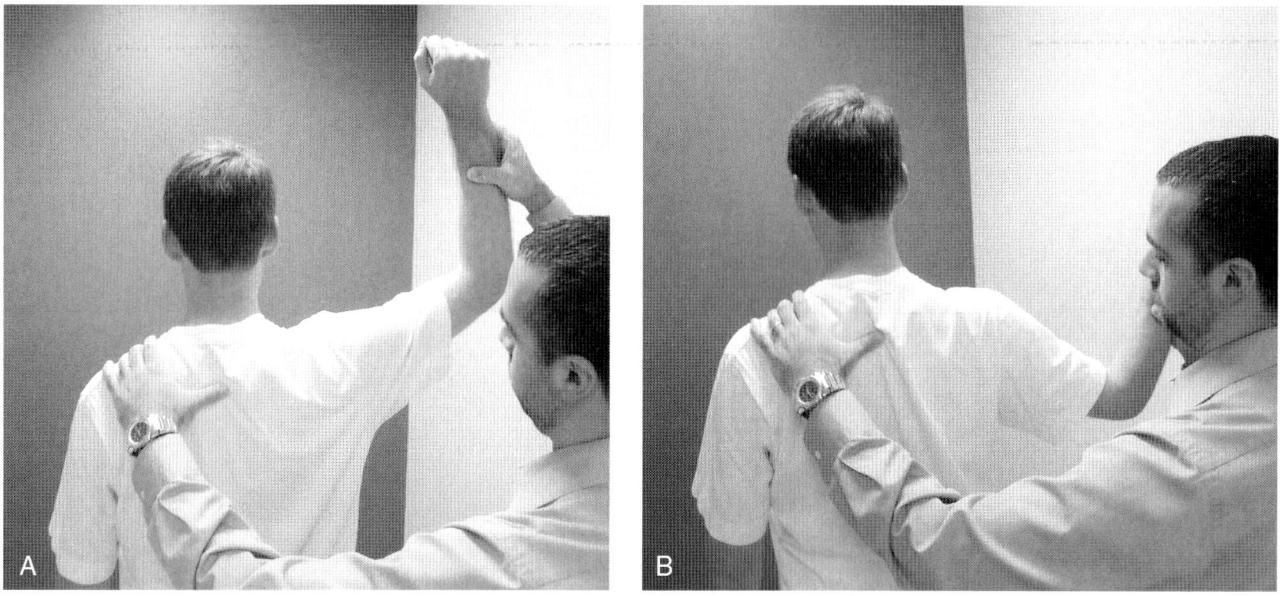

Figure 1 The dynamic labral shear test. **A,** The arm is placed in 130° of abduction in the scapular plane and is then moved into external rotation. **B,** The arm is moved down from 130° to 60° of abduction, which shears the humerus on the glenoid. A positive test is indicated by pain, a click, or a pop on the posterior joint line as the arm moves from 130° to 60°. (Reproduced with permission from Burkhart SS, Lo IK, Brady PC: *Burkhart's View of the Shoulder: A Cowboy's Guide to Advanced Shoulder Arthroscopy.* Philadelphia, PA, Lippincott Williams and Wilkins, 2006.)

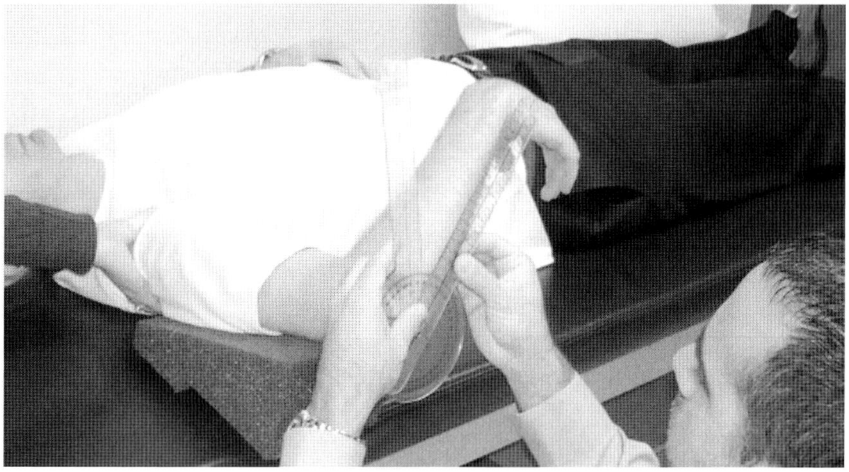

Figure 2 Clinical photograph of the standardized objective measurement of glenohumeral internal rotation.

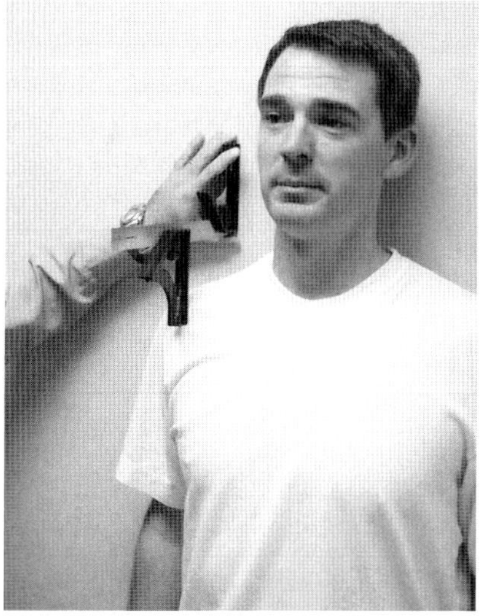

Figure 3 The double square measurement is used for assessing scapular forward posture. The patient stands against a wall in a relaxed posture. One arm of the double square is placed on the wall and the other is placed at the anterior edge of the acromion. A measurement in centimeters is taken from the wall. A bilateral measurement is taken for comparison.

chapter's author, scapular forward posture has been implicated as a negative factor for the successful nonsurgical treatment of patients with SLAP injuries. This posture results from weaker posterior scapular muscles and tight pectoralis minor muscles.[36] Clinical assessment by observation and palpation of the tight structures can be done and has been shown to be clinically reliable[37,38] (**Figure 3**).

Several specific intra-articular tests can provide clues to the loss of labral roles. A positive painful arc of motion test with Hawkins-type motion, with no pain relief with scapular posterior

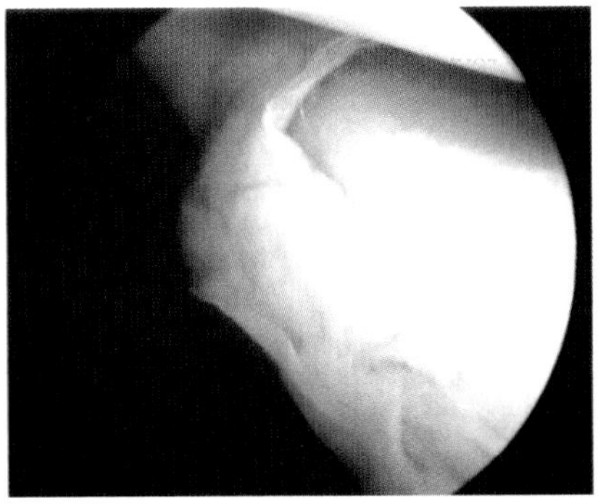

Figure 4 Arthroscopic image of a patient's right shoulder showing peel back of the glenoid labrum as it lifts off the glenoid from the 10-o'clock to the 12-o'clock position.

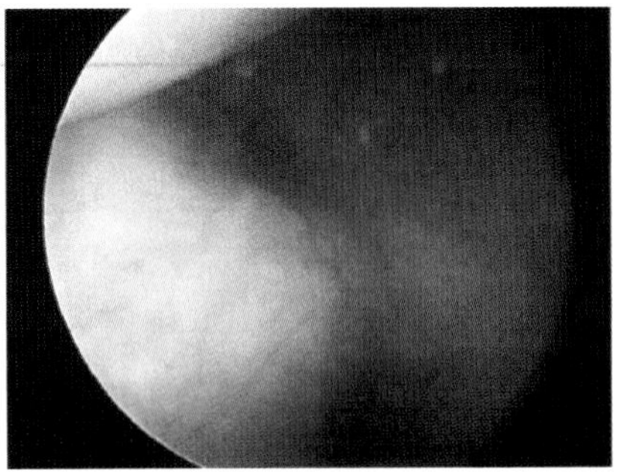

Figure 5 Arthroscopic image of a patient's right shoulder showing a loss of tension in the posterior band of the inferior glenohumeral ligament from the 7-o'clock to the 8-o'clock positions.

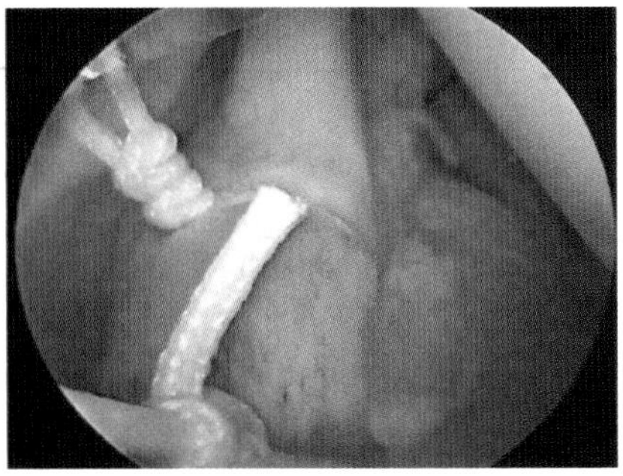

Figure 6 Arthroscopic image of a patient's right shoulder showing placement of sutures at the 10:30 and 11:30 clock positions to stabilize the peel-back lesion and reattach the labrum to the glenoid.

tilt in the scapula assistance test,[39] indicates increased translation. A positive O'Brien maneuver indicates loss of the washer effect, increased biceps tension, and increased translation. The dynamic labral shear test is clinically useful because it specifically replicates the peel-back phenomenon, in which the posterior superior labrum slides or peels off the glenoid as the arm moves into abduction and external rotation (**Figure 4**). A positive test indicates loss of biceps stability, loss of the washer effect, and increased translation.

The physical examination can provide findings that help construct a comprehensive picture of the deficits that cause or exacerbate the effects of the SLAP injury. These deficits should be addressed and restored as part of the treatment process—either nonsurgically or surgically.

The labral injury should be confirmed with MRI, magnetic resonance arthrography, or CT arthrography. Specific criteria have been developed to distinguish a labral alteration, but MRI is best viewed as a static estimation of the labral status and does not provide information about its dynamic roles. A percentage of patients will demonstrate labral tears on MRI without clinical symptoms related to loss of the labral roles.

Treatment

A clinically important SLAP injury should be treated, but surgical treatment is rarely the first option. Preliminary studies on the effect of structured rehabilitation on SLAP injuries in professional athletes (David Lintner, MD, personal communication, Lexington, KY, 2012) and this chapter's author's experience with active but nonprofessional athletes show that approximately 50% of SLAP injuries become functionally asymptomatic with guided rehabilitation. The rehabilitation programs have been designed to specifically address kinetic chain and scapular deficits, as well as muscle flexibility, strength, and strength balance deficits identified on the physical examination.[23,40]

If the rehabilitation program does not result in improvement in function, arthroscopy is recommended. The arthroscopic evaluation of the suspected labral injury must be specific. Arthroscopic findings most frequently associated with a clinically important labral injury that results in a loss of labral roles include (1) a type II or higher lesion denoting loss of attachment;[2] (2) a peel-back phenomenon, indicating increased compliance, a loss of the washer effect, and loss of the bumper effect;[4,16,17] (3) glenoid articular cartilage damage or chondromalacia, indicating increased translation and shear;[41] (4) loss of capsular tension indicated by a drive-through sign or loss of tension in the posterior band of the inferior glenohumeral ligament (**Figure 5**); and/or (5) excessive posterior inferior capsular thickness and scar indicating end-stage capsular damage that helps create a glenohumeral internal rotation deficit.[42] Care must be taken to differentiate labral detachment from anatomic variants, such as sublabral foramina, a Buford complex attachment of the middle glenohumeral ligament, or a meniscoid-like labral attachment that does not peel back.[43]

Video 43.1: Identification of the Labral Lesion. W. Ben Kibler, MD (2 min)

Based on these principles, a framework for arthroscopic treatment of a labral injury includes seven factors:

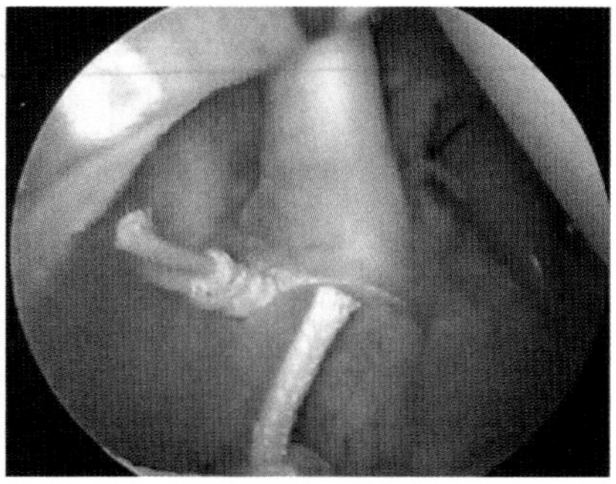

Figure 7 Arthroscopic image of a patient's right shoulder showing no tethering of the biceps as the arm goes into external rotation.

(1) Evaluation of the peel-back phenomenon, the labral injury, mobility, the glenoid surface, and capsular tension using direct visualization. (2) The placement of multiple anchors to secure at least two-point fixation of the labrum on the posterior superior glenoid (10:30 and 11:30 clock positions on the right shoulder). A double-loaded single anchor represents only one-point fixation (**Figure 6**). (3) The placement of enough posterior superior anchors to eliminate peel back. (4) An evaluation of biceps mobility to ensure adequate motion of the biceps in shoulder external rotation (**Figure 7**). (5) The rare placement of anchors and sutures in the anterior superior glenoid (12-o'clock to 2:30 clock positions on the right shoulder) to reduce the chance of biceps tethering. (6) An evaluation of the effect of the labral repair on the tension of the posterior band of the inferior glenohumeral ligament tension to ensure discernible tautness (**Figure 8**). (7) Assessment of total glenohumeral rotation to ensure that no external rotation has been lost.

DVD **Video 43.2:** Fixation of the Labral Lesion. W. Ben. Kibler, MD (5 min)

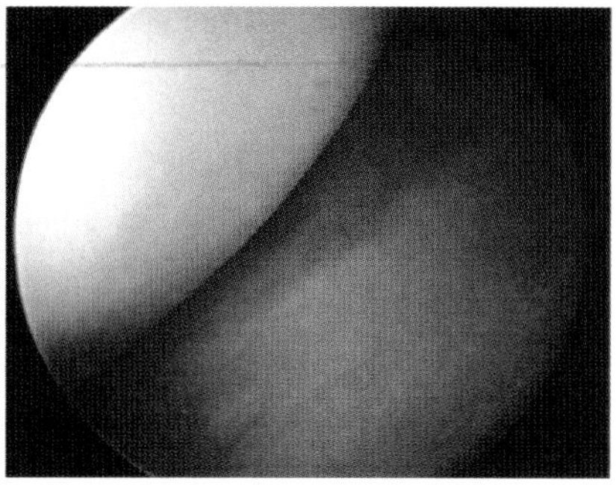

Figure 8 Arthroscopic image of a patient's right shoulder showing reconstitution of tension in the posterior band of the inferior glenohumeral ligament after suture anchor placement.

Summary

Clinically important SLAP tears exist. The optimum integration of clinical history, physical examination findings, imaging findings, and arthroscopic criteria has not been established. Diagnostic guidelines to determine a clinically important SLAP injury and the labral alteration that is associated with the dysfunction should be related to a demonstration of the loss of specific labral roles. Treatment guidelines should emphasize a structured rehabilitation program because approximately 50% of all lesions can be symptomatically resolved through rehabilitation. Surgical guidelines should also emphasize delineation of the loss of labral roles and their surgical restoration.

References

1. Andrews JR, Carson WG Jr, McLeod WD: Glenoid labrum tears related to the long head of the biceps. *Am J Sports Med* 1985; 13(5):337-341.
2. Snyder SJ, Karzel RP, Del Pizzo W, Ferkel RD, Friedman MJ: SLAP lesions of the shoulder. *Arthroscopy* 1990;6(4):274-279.
3. Burkhart SS, Morgan CD, Kibler WB: Shoulder injuries in overhead athletes: The "dead arm" revisited. *Clin Sports Med* 2000; 19(1):125-158.
4. Burkhart SS, Morgan CD, Kibler WB: The disabled throwing shoulder: Spectrum of pathology. Part I: Pathoanatomy and biomechanics. *Arthroscopy* 2003;19(4): 404-420.
5. Jazrawi LM, McCluskey GM III, Andrews JR: Superior labral anterior and posterior lesions and internal impingement in the overhead athlete. *Instr Course Lect* 2003;52:43-63.
6. Grossman MG, Tibone JE, McGarry MH, Schneider DJ, Veneziani S, Lee TQ: A cadaveric model of the throwing shoulder: A possible etiology of superior labrum anterior-to-posterior lesions. *J Bone Joint Surg Am* 2005;87(4): 824-831.
7. Trantalis JN, Lo IK: Superior labral anterior-posterior (SLAP) tears: Recent advances and outcomes. *Curr Orthop Pract* 2008; 19(5):530-534.
8. McFarland EG, Kim TK, Savino RM: Clinical assessment of three common tests for superior labral anterior-posterior lesions. *Am J Sports Med* 2002;30(6):810-815.
9. Jost B, Zumstein M, Pfirrmann CW, Zanetti M, Gerber C: MRI findings in throwing shoulders: Abnormalities in professional handball players. *Clin Orthop Relat Res* 2005;434:130-137.
10. Gobezie R, Zurakowski D, Lavery K, Millett PJ, Cole BJ, Warner JJ: Analysis of interobserver and intraobserver variability in the diagnosis and treatment of SLAP tears using the Snyder classification. *Am J Sports Med* 2008; 36(7): 1373-1379.
11. Morgan CD, Burkhart SS, Palmeri M, Gillespie M: Type II SLAP lesions: Three subtypes and their relationships to superior instability and rotator cuff tears. *Arthroscopy* 1998;14(6):553-565.

12. Radkowski CA, Chhabra A, Baker CL III, Tejwani SG, Bradley JP: Arthroscopic capsulolabral repair for posterior shoulder instability in throwing athletes compared with nonthrowing athletes. *Am J Sports Med* 2008;36(4):693-699.

13. Rhee YG, Lee DH, Lim CT: Unstable isolated SLAP lesion: Clinical presentation and outcome of arthroscopic fixation. *Arthroscopy* 2005;21(9):1099-1104.

14. Harryman DT II, Sidles JA, Harris SL, Matsen FA III: Laxity of the normal glenohumeral joint: A quantitative in vivo assessment. *J Shoulder Elbow Surg* 1992; 1(2):66-76.

15. Pagnani MJ, Warren RF: *The Upper Extremity in Sports Medicine*, ed 2. St Louis, MO, Mosby, 1995, pp 173-208.

16. Bankart AS, Cantab MC: Recurrent or habitual dislocation of the shoulder-joint, 1923. *Clin Orthop Relat Res* 1993;291:3-6.

17. Veeger HE, van der Helm FC: Shoulder function: The perfect compromise between mobility and stability. *J Biomech* 2007; 40(10):2119-2129.

18. Matsen FA III, Fu FH, Hawkins R, eds: *The Shoulder: A Balance of Mobility and Stability: Workshop, Vail, Colorado, September, 1992.* Park Ridge, IL, American Academy of Orthopaedic Surgeons, 1993.

19. Speer KP, Garrett WE: Muscular control of motion and stability about the pectoral girdle, in Matsen FA III, Fu F, Hawkins RJ, eds: *The Shoulder: A Balance of Mobility and Stability.* Rosemont, IL, American Academy of Orthopaedic Surgeons, 1994, pp 159-173.

20. Davids K, Glazier PS, Araújo D, Bartlett R: Movement systems as dynamical systems: The functional role of variability and its implications for sports medicine. *Sports Med* 2003;33(4):245-260.

21. Nichols TR: A biomechanical perspective on spinal mechanisms of coordinated muscular action. *Acta Anat (Basel)* 1994;151:1-13.

22. Nieminen H, Niemi J, Takala EP, Viikari-Juntura E: Load-sharing patterns in the shoulder during isometric flexion tasks. *J Biomech* 1995;28(5):555-566.

23. Burkhart SS, Morgan CD, Kibler WB: The disabled throwing shoulder: Spectrum of pathology. Part III: The SICK scapula, scapular dyskinesis, the kinetic chain, and rehabilitation. *Arthroscopy* 2003;19(6):641-661.

24. Kibler WB, Press J, Sciascia AD: The role of core stability in athletic function. *Sports Med* 2006; 36(3):189-198.

25. Crossley KM, Zhang WJ, Schache AG, Bryant A, Cowan SM: Performance on the single-leg squat task indicates hip abductor muscle function. *Am J Sports Med* 2011; 39(4):866-873.

26. Leetun DT, Ireland ML, Willson JD, Ballantyne BT, Davis IM: Core stability measures as risk factors for lower extremity injury in athletes. *Med Sci Sports Exerc* 2004;36(6):926-934.

27. Warner JJ, Micheli LJ, Arslanian LE, Kennedy J, Kennedy R: Scapulothoracic motion in normal shoulders and shoulders with glenohumeral instability and impingement syndrome: A study using Moiré topographic analysis. *Clin Orthop Relat Res* 1992;285: 191-199.

28. Laudner KG, Myers JB, Pasquale MR, Bradley JP, Lephart SM: Scapular dysfunction in throwers with pathologic internal impingement. *J Orthop Sports Phys Ther* 2006;36(7):485-494.

29. McClure PW, Tate AR, Kareha S, Irwin D, Zlupko E: A clinical method for identifying scapular dyskinesis: Part 1. Reliability. *J Athl Train* 2009;44(2):160-164.

30. Tate AR, McClure PW, Kareha S, Irwin D, Barbe MF: A clinical method for identifying scapular dyskinesis: Part 2. Validity. *J Athl Train* 2009;44(2):165-173.

31. Uhl TL, Kibler WB, Gecewich B, Tripp BL: Evaluation of clinical assessment methods for scapular dyskinesis. *Arthroscopy* 2009; 25(11):1240-1248.

32. Kibler WB, Sciascia AD, Dome DC, Hester PW, Jacobs C: Clinical utility of new and traditional exam tests for biceps and superior glenoid labral injuries and superior labrum anterior and posterior lesions in the shoulder. *Am J Sports Med* 2009;37(9):1840-1847.

33. Wilk KE, Macrina LC, Fleisig GS, et al: Correlation of glenohumeral internal rotation deficit and total rotational motion to shoulder injuries in professional baseball pitchers. *Am J Sports Med* 2011; 39(2):329-335.

34. Wilk KE, Reinhold MM, Macrina LC, et al: Glenohumeral internal rotation measurements differ depending on stabilization techniques. *Sports Health* 2009;1(2): 131-136.

35. Kibler WB, Sciascia A, Thomas SJ: Glenohumeral internal rotation deficit: Pathogenesis and response to acute throwing. *Sports Med Arthrosc* 2012;20(1):34-38.

36. Borstad JD, Ludewig PM: The effect of long versus short pectoralis minor resting length on scapular kinematics in healthy individuals. *J Orthop Sports Phys Ther* 2005;35(4):227-238.

37. Kluemper M, Uhl TL, Hazelrigg H: Effects of stretching and strengthening shoulder muscles on forward shoulder posture in competitive swimmers. *J Sport Rehabil* 2006;15(1):58-70.

38. Kibler WB, Sciascia AD: Current concepts: Scapular dyskinesis. *Br J Sports Med* 2010;44(5):300-305.

39. Kibler WB, McMullen J: Scapular dyskinesis and its relation to shoulder pain. *J Am Acad Orthop Surg* 2003;11(2):142-151.

40. Kibler WB, McMullen J, Uhl TL: Shoulder rehabilitation strategies, guidelines, and practice. *Oper Tech Sports Med* 2001;32(3): 527-538.

41. Savoie FH III, Field LD, Atchinson S: Anterior superior instability with rotator cuff tearing: SLAC lesion. *Orthop Clin North Am* 2001;32(3):457-461, ix.

42. Burkhart SS, Morgan CD, Kibler WB: The disabled throwing shoulder: Spectrum of pathology. Part II: Evaluation and treatment of SLAP lesions in throwers. *Arthroscopy* 2003;19(5):531-539.

43. Burkhart SS, Lo IK, Brady PC: *Burkhart's View of the Shoulder: A Cowboy's Guide to Advanced Shoulder Arthroscopy.* Philadelphia, PA, Lippincott Williams and Wilkins; 2006.

Video References

43.1: Kibler WB: Video. *Identification of the Labral Lesion.* Lexington, KY, 2012.

43.2: Kibler WB: Video. *Fixation of the Labral Lesion.* Lexington, KY, 2012.

44

Superior Labrum Anterior to Posterior Tears in Throwing Athletes

David M. Lintner, MD

Abstract

Superior labrum anterior to posterior (SLAP) tears and partial undersurface tears of the rotator cuff are common in experienced throwers, may be adaptive, and are only occasionally symptomatic. Pain in the shoulder of a throwing athlete with an MRI-documented SLAP tear or partial undersurface tear of the rotator cuff can be managed nonsurgically, with attention to posterior capsular contracture, scapular dyskinesia, and rotator cuff strength. The results of the surgical repair of SLAP lesions in the throwing athlete, with or without rotator cuff repair, are inferior to those of nonsurgical treatment. The cause of pain in the throwing athlete must be accurately diagnosed without reliance on MRI findings.

Instr Course Lect 2013;62:491-500.

Initially described by Andrews et al,[1] lesions of the superior labrum are a common cause of shoulder pain, particularly in overhead throwing athletes. Superior labrum anterior to posterior (SLAP) tears have been classified by Snyder et al[2] into types I, II, III, and IV; Maffet et al[3] further classified additional variations. All SLAP tears involve detachment of the superior quadrant of the labrum, including at least a portion of the biceps anchor. SLAP tears can occur as traumatic or attritional injuries; the presentation is different with each etiology. Traumatic injuries occur as a one-time event, typically with a traction injury in an anteroinferior direction or with forceful abduction of the arm. Notable is the acute onset of deep shoulder pain, which is often associated with mechanical symptoms such as catching, popping, or grinding; pain when attempting to lift heavy objects from below the waist; or pain when reaching in front of the body or overhead against resistance.

Attritional injuries occur because of repetitive stress and are more common in overhead athletes than are traumatic injuries. There are many proposed mechanisms of injury, some of which may occur in combination. One mechanism is the repeated alternating anterior and posterior traction from the biceps combined with twisting during repeated rotational movements of the arm in the overhead position.[4] Another involves the so-called peel-back mechanism. As the arm abducts and externally rotates, the force on the biceps coupled with the posterior glide of the humerus results in the peeling off of the posterosuperior quadrant of the glenoid in the posterior labrum.[4] Another injury mechanism is posteroinferior capsular tightness, which causes a posterosuperior shift of the humeral head during overhead activities and subsequent intrasubstance tearing or detachment of the posterosuperior labrum.[4-6]

Variability in the anatomy of the biceps origin can affect the level of strain in the superior labrum.[7] There is disagreement on whether the late cocking or the deceleration phase of throwing is most responsible for SLAP tears.[1,4,7-10] The peel-back mechanism implicates late cocking, whereas the proposed traction mechanism supports deceleration as the primary cause of tearing. Regardless of the origin,

Dr. Lintner or an immediate family member is a member of a speakers' bureau or has made paid presentations on behalf of Mitek; serves as a paid consultant to or is an employee of Mitek; and has received nonincome support (such as equipment or services), commercially derived honoraria, or other non–research-related funding (such as paid travel) from Breg and Mitek.

attritional SLAP tears in overhead athletes typically act in a different manner than traumatic lesions.[11] The high frequency of these lesions in asymptomatic throwing athletes has been confirmed.[12,13] When a lesion becomes symptomatic, the physician must determine the reason for the change in shoulder pain, whether it is attributable to the presence of a long-time tear of the superior labrum or another cause. This determination is more complicated than identifying a SLAP tear on an MRI scan. Most type II SLAP tears in competitive throwers are asymptomatic. The goal of treatment is to return the injured athlete to asymptomatic status with a minimum of morbidity and time lost from competition.

Accurate determination of the pain generator is necessary. There are many interacting factors in addition to the labral abnormality. Posteroinferior capsular contracture, anterior capsular laxity often seen in throwers, and partial-thickness undersurface tears of the rotator cuff resulting from traction overload and internal impingement may all play a role in pain generation. However, these findings are often present in asymptomatic throwing athletes. Scapulothoracic dyskinesia may cause otherwise asymptomatic structural abnormalities to become painful.[14-16] Each of these factors has an effect on the glenohumeral joint.

Issues Unique to Throwing Athletes

Competitive overhand throwing requires extreme motion of the shoulder that is repeated at high velocity tens of thousands of times per year over many years. The angular velocity of the shoulder is the fastest recorded human motion (7,000° per second).[17,18] The lack of bony stability allows tremendous motion of the shoulder but at the cost of little inherent stability. This combination of extremely high forces repeated tens of thousands of times results in adaptive and pathologic changes in the shoulder joint and surrounding tissues. A centered humeral head is imperative for providing a stable point to generate leverage for applying force to the baseball. However, the lack of inherent mechanical stability forces the soft tissues of the shoulder to work near their mechanical limits to provide static and dynamic stability in the presence of high compression, shear, and distraction forces during the various throwing phases. A confluence of circumstances increases the likelihood of injuries to the shoulder.

Upper extremity injuries in baseball are most closely correlated with the volume of throwing performed by the athlete.[19,20] It has been shown that increased external rotation and horizontal extension correlate with performance and velocity.[21,22] As year-round baseball play, pitching lessons, and backyard sessions with friends and family have become the norm, the number of throws that a typical baseball player performs in a year has steadily increased. More accomplished players (those who have increased throwing velocity) generally play on more teams and in more leagues; therefore, better pitchers usually pitch more frequently and put the most stress on their shoulders.

Increased external rotation and horizontal extension are imperative for high-level throwing performance. The structures that restrict these motions are the anteroinferior capsule and the mechanical abutment of the posterosuperior rotator cuff/greater tuberosity on the posterosuperior labrum (internal impingement). Gaining external rotation in the abducted and extended position requires increased laxity of the anterior and anteroinferior capsule as well as increased clearance in the posterosuperior quadrant of the shoulder. The peel-back of the superior labrum and undersurface detachment of the rotator cuff seen in internal impingement may facilitate this gain in external rotation. Peel-back of the posterosuperior labrum allows the labrum to move medially off the posterosuperior glenoid rim and can decrease mechanical impingement of the rotator cuff on the greater tuberosity, thus diminishing internal impingement and allowing greater external rotation and extension in the horizontal plane. At least in theory, labral peel-back and rotator cuff peel-off can be an adaptive change rather than a pathologic change, are not necessarily painful, and facilitate the hyperangulation needed for high-velocity throwing.

Competitive throwing is a highly repetitious unilateral activity that results in bony and soft-tissue adaptive changes in the shoulder. A shift in the arc of shoulder rotation, with a gain in external rotation and a commensurate loss in internal rotation, develops in experienced throwers. If this shift is symmetric (the gain in external rotation equals the loss of internal rotation) with the total arc of motion remaining equal to the opposite side, this shift is primarily caused by bony changes (such as humeral retroversion).[23-26] Stress-related bony and soft-tissue changes occur primarily during adolescence and progress with time in the overhead throwing athlete.[25-29] These changes, which allow increased external rotation, are considered normal and adaptive; however, a greater loss of internal rotation than the gain in external rotation indicates contracture of the posterior soft tissues.[4,14,15,27,30-32] In a throwing athlete with such a contracture, there is a decrease in the total arc of motion compared with the nondominant side, with a gain in external rotation and a relative loss of internal rotation. This condition is called glenohumeral internal rotation deficit (GIRD). This capsular asymmetry with posterior capsular contracture pushes the humeral head off-center in a posterosuperior direction and results in increased stress on the posterosuperior labrum and loss of humeral head centering on the glenoid.[5,6]

In patients with anterior capsular laxity, the ability of the rotator cuff to dynamically center the humerus on the glenoid is crucial for pain-free performance. Posterior capsular contracture, anterior capsular laxity, and posterosuperior labral detachment contribute to shoulder instability. Internal impingement is worsened by capsular contracture and scapulothoracic dyskinesia.[4,14,32,33] As the amount of scapular forward rotation and protraction increase, the mechanical impingement of the posterosuperior portion of the rotator cuff into the labrum increases, resulting in increased damage to the rotator cuff. With the changes in the passive stabilizers, the function of the shoulder is dependent on the ability of the rotator cuff to maintain stability of the humerus on the glenoid. If the rotator cuff is weak and/or inflamed, it is less able to maintain stability, and dynamic microinstability occurs. This results in diminished performance, with a progression toward pain with throwing.

The presence of posterior capsular tightness and scapular dyskinesia worsen the situation. Decreasing capsular tightness will decrease pain in the throwing shoulder in most athletes.[4,32] Programs for stretching the posterior capsule are successful in decreasing GIRD.[4,14,15,30,31,34] Improving scapular rhythm can result in short- and long-term improvements in pain and performance.[4,15,30,35,36] Edwards et al[37] reported a return to the same or a higher level of sports participation in 66% of the overhead athletes with SLAP tears who were treated nonsurgically.

The surgical repair of SLAP tears has mixed results in overhead athletes, with few studies reporting only on throwing populations. In an evaluation of the arthroscopic treatment of high-school, college, and professional throwers with type II SLAP tears, an 87% rate of return to the same level of competition at 1 year and 78% at 2 years was reported (GP Paletta, MD, San Diego, CA, unpublished data, 2011). Failed treatment was associated with a loss of external rotation. In a study of elite overhead athletes (most of whom were professional baseball players) treated with arthroscopic repair of type II SLAP lesions, Neri et al[38] reported that 57% returned to their pain-free preinjury levels of competition at final follow-up. Poorer success rates were reported in patients with a partial-thickness rotator cuff tear.[38,39] A substantially lower success rate has been reported with arthroscopic treatment of superior labral lesions in overhead athletes compared with nonoverhead athletes.[37,40,41] In a recent study of overhead athletes (including participants in baseball, softball, javelin, and tennis) Neuman et al[42] reported that throwers treated with arthroscopic repair perceived that they recovered 83% of their preinjury level of performance at midterm follow-up (mean, 3.5 years); however, it was not reported if the patients returned to their preinjury level of competition. The authors concluded that SLAP repairs resulted in improved shoulder function during routine daily activities, but consistent return to participation in elite throwing sports could be problematic. No current published studies have evaluated field performance data after SLAP repair or return to specific levels of play (such as Division 1 or Major League Baseball).

In an ongoing study, this chapter's author has collected data from 2000 to 2011 on a single Major League Baseball franchise and its minor league affiliate teams for all players with shoulder pain that required a secondary in-office evaluation. The treatment algorithm begins with an evaluation of the player done in the team's city by the athletic trainer and the local team physician. Initial treatment begins with modalities (ice, ultrasound, and electrical stimulation), exercise (rotator cuff strengthening and scapular posterior capsular stretches), and the administration of nonsteroidal anti-inflammatory drugs. Shoulder pain decreases in most players. However, if satisfactory progress is not achieved, the player is sent for a secondary evaluation by the head team physician. This evaluation includes a repeat history, reexamination, and, typically, MRI arthrography. This group of players makes up the study population and includes Major League (40-man roster players at the time of injury) and Minor League players (all others). The treatment proceeds as previously described, typically with increased attention to cross-body posterior capsular stretching and eccentric rotator cuff strengthening. Success is defined as return to play in professional competition at a minimum 1-year follow-up. SLAP lesions were documented on MRI in 79 players; 47 were pitchers. Of those pitchers completing the nonsurgical algorithm, 89% returned to professional competition. For those who underwent surgery, the success rate was 46% for pitchers and 71% for position players. The criterion for surgery was persistent pain that prohibited satisfactory performance despite documented improvement in GIRD and scapular kinetics after 6 weeks or more of the second rehabilitation trial. In those treated with suture repairs of deeply penetrating partial-thickness

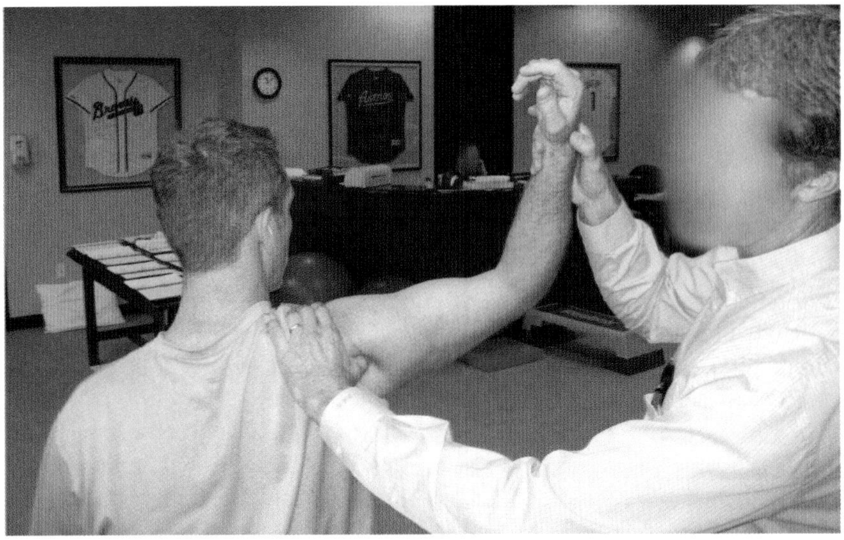

Figure 1 In the internal impingement test, the arm is exaggerated in external rotation and horizontal extension. The location of pain along the posterior joint line indicates entrapment of labral tissue or rotator cuff tissue in the posterior glenohumeral joint.

rotator cuff tears (high-grade internal impingement lesions), the success rate was much lower.

Presentation

The loss of centering of the humeral head (microinstability during throwing) is most commonly associated with loss of velocity and control, trouble getting loose (warming up sufficiently that the shoulder feels flexible and relaxed), and difficulty finishing pitches (getting the arm fully extended toward home plate to apply the last amount of spin to the baseball). Symptoms eventually progress to pain. This pain is most often located at the posterosuperior portion of the joint line during the cocking phase of throwing. The second most common site of pain is located more posterolaterally and occurs during the deceleration phase of throwing.

The physical examination typically shows positive labral signs (the O'Brien sign; the Kibler sign; a modified Jobe relocation sign, which is positive for pain rather than apprehension in the posterior shoulder and is relieved by posteriorly directed pressure; and the internal impingement sign). On testing, pain is elicited in the rotator cuff with resisted abduction in the scapular plane and resisted external rotation at 90° of forward flexion; posterior pain occurs with resisted flexion in the follow-through position. Scapulothoracic dyskinesia and GIRD also are common. Stretching the posterior capsule in the cross-body position can often duplicate the patient's pain.

Internal Impingement Sign

With the arm at the 90°-90° cocked position, the examiner stands behind the patient, places one hand on the thrower's shoulder with the thumb at the posterior joint line, and the other hand grasps the thrower's wrist. The arm is then pulled into horizontal extension and increased external rotation, imitating the maximum cocked position. It may be helpful to have the athlete stride forward with his or her opposite foot and initiate a throwing maneuver while the examiner provides resistance, pulling the arm into further abduction and external rotation. The thrower naturally allows the arm to go into further external rotation when instructed to throw the examiner's hand. During this maneuver, the examiner attempts to entrap the posterior labrum between the undersurface of the patient's posterosuperior rotator cuff/greater tuberosity, mimicking mechanical internal impingement, with the examiner's thumb on the posterior joint line searching for tenderness. Posterior pain is a positive finding; anterior pain is not (**Figure 1**).

The Deceleration Sign

With the arm in the cross-body position, below horizontal and approaching waist level, the humerus is internally rotated and the scapula is protracted. The patient should be instructed to resist downward pressure from the examiner's hand. This puts an eccentric load on the thrower's posterior rotator cuff and attempts to mimic deceleration during the follow-through phase of throwing (**Figure 2**). The difference between this position and that used in the O'Brien test is that the arm is placed at a lower level, at an increased level of cross-body adduction, and the scapula is protracted. A positive finding is posterior pain in the region of the posterior rotator cuff, which results from incompetence of the posterior rotator cuff. Anterior pain indicates an anterior disorder, such as biceps tendinitis, coracoid impingement, or a superoanterior labral tear with entrapment.

Posterior Capsular Tightness in the Supine Position

With the patient supine, the examiner stabilizes the lateral border of the scapula with the heel of the hand. This requires substantial pressure. While holding the shoulder in neutral rotation, with the forearm parallel to the shoulders, the examiner pushes the humerus across the chest into cross-body

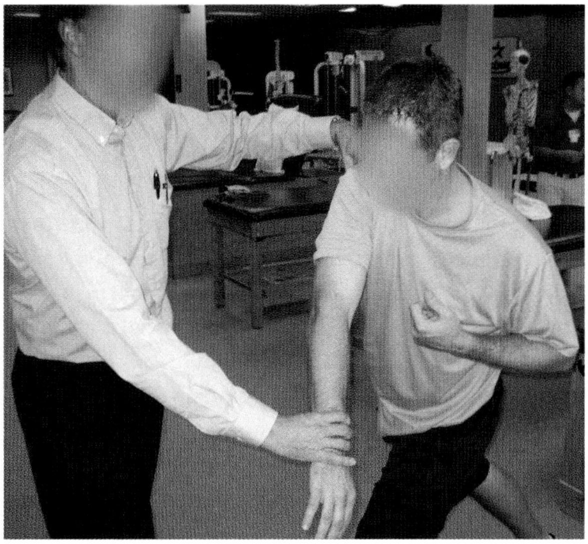

Figure 2 In the deceleration test, the patient's arm is placed in the follow-through position. The patient resists a downward force to the distal forearm. The location of pain indicates the probable location of pathology.

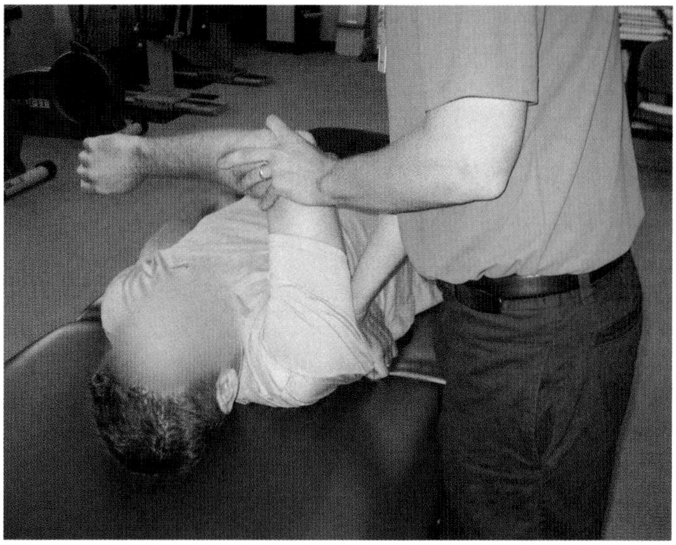

Figure 3 The cross-body stretch is identical to the maneuver used to measure posterior capsular tightness during the physical examination. The therapist's hand stabilizes the scapula. Significant force is required to hold the scapula while applying force to the humerus. The humerus should be held in neutral or internal rotation throughout the stretch.

adduction while preventing the scapula from moving (**Figure 3**). The arm should not be allowed to externally rotate (the hand should not be allowed to come above the opposite shoulder). The patient will feel a stretch in the posterior shoulder. If painful, the patient should be asked if the pain replicates the pain felt when throwing. A positive response indicates that the posterior capsular tightness is the source of pain, which is typically most prominent during the deceleration phase of throwing. Often, the humerus cannot move past vertical with the scapula stabilized on the dominant side, whereas the humerus on the contralateral side can easily be moved past the player's chin.

Imaging

AP, Stryker, and axillary radiographic views are helpful. The Stryker and axillary views allow assessment of the posteroinferior and posterior aspects of the glenoid, respectively, and can help detect a thrower's exostosis, calcification of the posterior labrum, or glenoid erosion. Because of the high rate of false-positive findings, MRI is only occasionally warranted. When performed, MRI should be done with a high-strength, closed magnet with intra-articular contrast and abduction external rotation positioning. This scanning is performed after completing the standard scan, with the athlete's arm placed in the abducted and overhead position; it provides a reasonable approximation of the position of the arm during the cocked phase of throwing. Although type II SLAP tears are usually obvious, more subtle findings include posterosuperior rotator cuff tearing, particularly delamination in the region of the posterior portion of the supraspinatus and the superior portion of the infraspinatus. In the standard sequences with the arm at the side, the rotator cuff is under tension, which often reduces the displacement of the layers of the rotator cuff. With the arm in the abducted and externally rotated positions, the tension is taken off the rotator cuff, and it will crumple or fold, resulting in differential tension on the various layers of the rotator cuff. This allows delamination planes to separate and become visible and is also helpful for visualizing the abutment of the rotator cuff on the posterior labrum. Tears of the posterosuperior labrum are more evident. The examiner should look for other subtle findings, such as a bulbous posterior labrum and early calcification in the posterior labrum. Because there may not be a frank tear in the labrum, these areas may be read as "normal" by the radiologist.

Before performing MRI, the patient and family should be informed that the scan will most likely show abnormalities such as a SLAP tear and a partial rotator cuff tear. It should be made clear that these findings are ubiquitous in throwers and are present in a high percentage of asymptomatic throwing athletes. The patient and family should understand that these lesions are typically benign. MRI should not be routinely used because the findings may cause unnecessary anxiety and do not affect the initial treatment of the thrower's shoulder.

Treatment Options and Decision Making

Timing Considerations

When evaluating the competitive thrower, there are often many parties involved in the decision-making process. The athlete, parents, coaches, and others will have concerns about how the treatment and recovery process will affect the recruiting and scouting process for a young baseball player. When considering treatment options, it is important for the physician to be aware of and sensitive to these timing issues, along with the emotional investment each party has in the treatment decisions. Fear and anxiety often permeate the decision-making process, and the physician's understanding and discussion of timing of college recruitment cycles and other career-affecting concerns can provide reassurance to the patient and his or her family.

For example, a high-school junior with shoulder pain that limits pitching ability in the fall of the athlete's junior year faces a dilemma. The prime recruiting and scouting season for colleges is the spring of the junior year and the summer after; therefore, the athlete must be capable of performing well at these times. Recovery time will be an important factor in the athlete's decision regarding surgical treatment. Because many players and their families expect a quick recovery after surgery, it is important to inform the concerned parties about the surgical procedure and provide a realistic timeline when throwing can be resumed and when the athlete can return to competitive play. For example, although many surgeons allow pitchers with SLAP repairs to begin throwing at approximately 4 months postoperatively, it can take an additional 3 to 6 months for the athlete to be capable of effective competitive throwing. Many pitchers describe the need for a full competitive season to reach their expected level of performance after SLAP surgery. In the example of the high-school junior with a documented SLAP lesion and symptoms in midfall, there is no urgency to consider surgery because surgery would likely prevent competition during the athlete's junior spring season and compromise performance the following summer. If an attempt at rehabilitation should fail and surgery is performed a few months after presentation, the patient should lose no additional important playing time compared with the choice of immediate surgery.

Nonsurgical Treatment

Nonsurgical management is the mainstay of treatment for the symptomatic thrower with a documented SLAP lesion. The presence of a SLAP lesion on MRI does not correlate with symptoms and should not be the focus of decision making. Rather, the function of the shoulder must be considered in the context of the kinetic chain, including the hips and trunk, the thoracic spine, and especially the scapula thoracic joint and posterior capsule. The SLAP lesion can be presumed to have been present chronically long before the onset of symptoms. Treatment should focus on restoring the shoulder to its presymptomatic status by addressing the proximate causes that provoked the symptoms. Most commonly, these causes include an alteration in the kinetic chain that produces shoulder decompensation and symptoms. A progressive tightening of the posterior capsule caused by acute[43] or sustained overuse;[4,27,28,30,44] a slight change in scapulothoracic posturing resulting in increased shear or internal impingement;[4,32,44] or weakness of the rotator cuff caused by fatigue, inflammation, or structural damage can cause symptoms.[16,35] Treatment should be tailored to these issues, with directed rotator cuff strengthening, training of scapular rhythm and posture, and assisted manual stretching and self-stretching of the posterior capsule.

The importance of correcting scapular dyskinesia can be easily demonstrated for the patient. Most patients will have a rounded posture while seated on the examination table. With the examiner's hand holding the scapula in that position while pulling the arm into the cocked position, the patient will feel a significant stretch on the anterior shoulder and posterior pain. With the patient sitting up straight, the examiner should again retract the scapula. Repeating the cocking maneuver in this position results in an obvious decrease in tension and pain in the shoulder and the elbow. This series of maneuvers usually helps to educate the patient on the importance of scapulothoracic posture in restoring healthy shoulder function and may instill confidence in the potential success of the rehabilitation program.

Surgical Treatment

Surgical decision making has evolved because of the mixed results of SLAP repair and the treatment of internal impingement lesions in throwers. Successful treatment should be defined as the return of the player to his or her prior level of performance rather than healing of a repaired labrum or rotator cuff or return to play. Loss of motion, particularly external rotation, correlates with impaired performance and is poorly tolerated in high-level throwers (GP Paletta, MD, San Diego, CA, unpublished data, 2011); therefore, the trend has been away from placing anchors anterior to the biceps root because of the possibility of tethering the

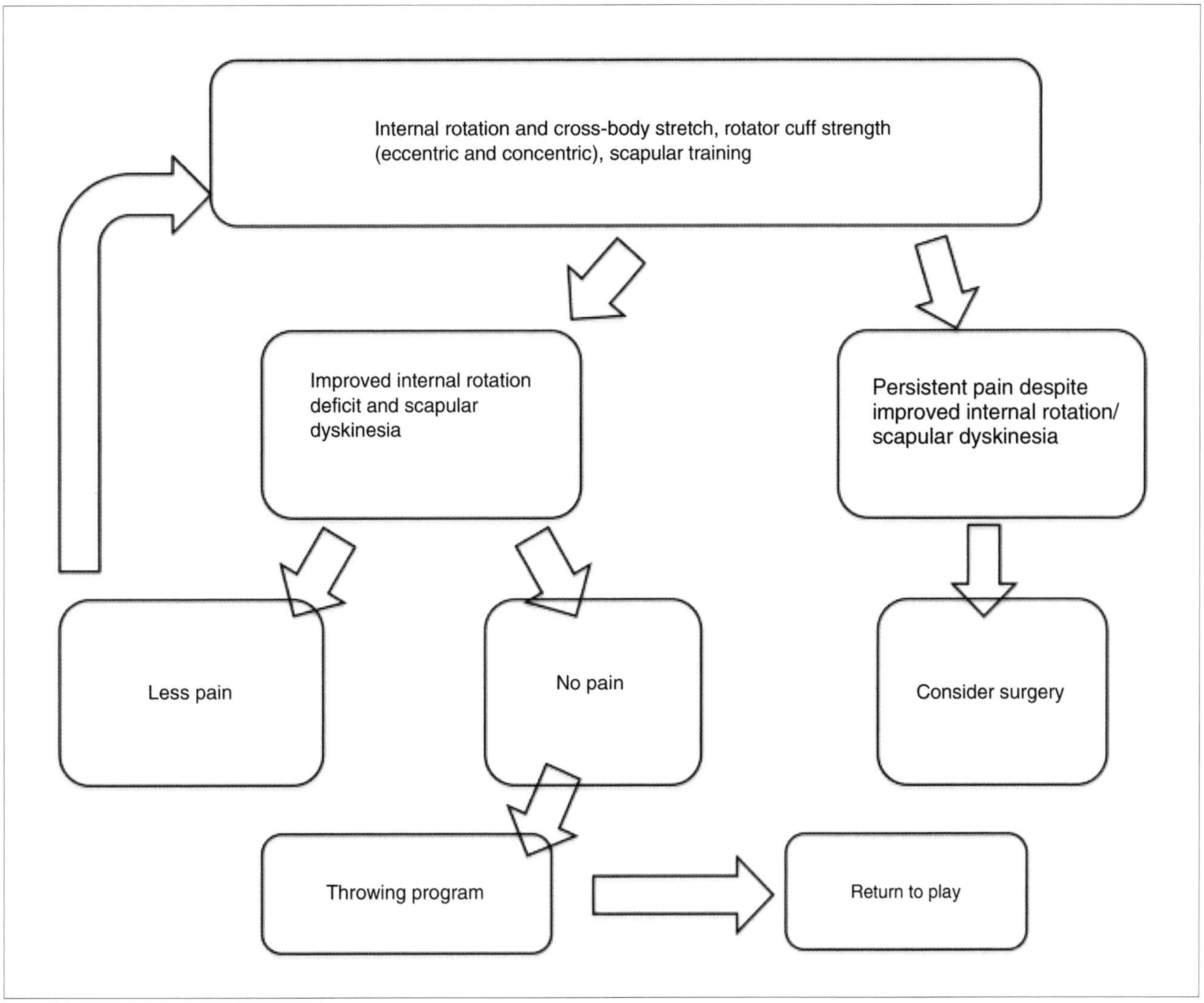

Figure 4 Algorithm for nonsurgical treatment. The time to completion is variable and dependent on the absence of pain and improvement in scapular dyskinesia and GIRD.

biceps and decreasing external rotation in the cocked position. Anatomic restoration of the footprint of the internal impingement lesion on the rotator cuff is no longer performed because of similar concerns. In a shoulder that can no longer compensate for the loss of dynamic stability caused by a type II SLAP lesion and impairment of the rotator cuff function, suture anchor repair of the posterosuperior labrum with débridement of the entrapped flaps of the rotator cuff is performed. For a deeply penetrating cuff tear, a top-to-bottom repair may be performed with no attempt to advance the tissue to the footprint. This procedure stabilizes the flaps and prevents propagation but does not effect an anatomic repair.

Treatment Algorithm

Based on the experience of this chapter's author with local scholastic, collegiate, and professional baseball organizations, a treatment algorithm for pain in the thrower's shoulder has been developed (**Figure 4**).

The algorithm should be used to evaluate the patient, along with the patient's history, physical, and, if appropriate, MRI findings. Observations from the team's athletic trainer or pitching coach and a discussion of changes in the player's workload, delivery, and type of pitches may also be helpful. The pain generator can usually be determined based on the examination findings.

As previously described, the patient is informed about the importance of proper scapulothoracic posture in decreasing shoulder pain and the perceived force across the shoulder and elbow joints. Rehabilitation should begin or resume, focusing on gaining posterior capsular flexibility and improving scapulothoracic movement patterns. Core and hip weakness, restricted movements, posterior capsular tightness, and scapulothoracic dyskinesia should be documented goniometrically or with digital photographs. The patient should be involved in improving these metrics. Initial rehabilitation requires a therapist who is skilled in the management of throwers' injuries. Manual stretching exercises are extremely helpful, particularly the cross-body stretch. This exercise is difficult to perform independently. Internal rotation stretches, such as sleeper stretches, are easier to perform independently but are less effective than the cross-body stretch. A subset of patients, however, will increase internal rotation with the performance of sleeper stretches but will not show improvement in the performance of cross-body stretching.

A skilled therapist should supervise scapulothoracic posture rehabilitation. All strengthening exercises should be done with the scapulae in the proper position, and all dynamic patterns should also be done while maintaining appropriate scapular posture. The cocking phase of throwing must be rehearsed repeatedly to capture the muscle memory necessary for the pitcher to maintain proper form without having to think about it when under pressure during competition. This requires the supervision of a skilled therapist who observes the scapula while the athlete performs the strengthening exercises, mock throwing drills, and actual throwing. The therapist provides immediate input and continuous feedback. Video analysis can be helpful but is not a substitute for real-time observation.

After the athlete begins to make progress with scapulothoracic rhythm and posterior capsular flexibility, work is initiated on "posing." The throwing motion is broken down into its component phases while the athlete focuses on the position of the legs and trunk and the appropriate scapular posture during each of these phases. Initially, the athlete will use single-leg balance on his or her stance leg and will practice maintaining a level pelvis, an erect spine, and set scapulae. The athlete will perform the motions with a ball and glove as would be used during normal pitching. This is believed to help trigger subliminal and subconscious pathways that are familiar to the athlete and improves the muscle-memory training. Each step is repeated dozens of times daily without actually throwing the ball. The athlete will progress to bringing the arm up to the cocked position while maintaining scapular posture, but instead of throwing the ball will return the arm back down to the side and return to the set position. Training often begins with the athlete standing with his or her back against a wall to ensure that the spine is erect and the scapula is held in the proper position while the arm is brought up to the cocked position. The athlete will initially note that the scapula in the retracted position feels highly abnormal and uncomfortable and will fatigue easily when trying to hold this position. The athlete must learn to feel comfortable with the scapula in the correct position to prevent reversion to the forward rotated/protracted position during the pressure of actual competition.

As the athlete learns how to clear the posterior glenoid rim from the greater tuberosity with correct scapular mechanics, he or she will progress toward actual throwing. Light throwing begins only when the posterior capsular contracture and scapulothoracic positioning have improved, although neither may have normalized. The progressive throwing program is halted if pain recurs, and the athlete returns to earlier phases of the rehabilitation program.

The graduated throwing program is best performed with the supervision of a therapist or coach who can recognize scapular posture and pelvic, arm, and elbow angles during the throw. The athlete should not return to his or her normal throwing motion because this would likely result in a relapse.

If the athlete still feels pain despite the improvement in posterior capsular flexibility and scapular posture, this indicates that the remaining structural abnormalities (such as a SLAP tear and/or a partial-thickness rotator cuff tear) are responsible for the symptoms. Surgery may be considered. If SLAP repair is performed, anchors are placed only behind the biceps anchor to avoid tethering the bicep. Flaps of the rotator cuff are débrided. Occasionally for a deeply (> 75% thickness) penetrating rotator cuff tear, side-to-side sutures are placed percutaneously.[45] Suture anchors are not used, and no attempt is made to reconstitute the anatomic footprint.

Summary

SLAP lesions and partial-thickness rotator cuff tears are common shoulder disorders (internal impingement) in overhead throwing athletes and are often asymptomatic. The development of pain is associated with contracture of the posterior soft-tissues causing GIRD and scapular dyskinesia. These conditions combine with impaired function of the rotator cuff to create a dynamic microinstability or loss of the ability to center the humeral head; this results in pain and impaired performance. Superior results are obtained with nonsurgical correction of GIRD and scapular dyskinesia compared with surgical repair. If nonsurgical care is not successful, repair of the posterosuperior labrum and débridement of the impinging flaps of soft tissue (labral or rotator cuff) should be performed. After surgical treatment, the prognosis for return to preinjury performance remains guarded.

References

1. Andrews JR, Carson WG Jr, McLeod WD: Glenoid labrum tears related to the long head of the biceps. *Am J Sports Med* 1985; 13(5):337-341.
2. Snyder SJ, Karzel RP, Del Pizzo W, Ferkel RD, Friedman MJ: SLAP lesions of the shoulder. *Arthroscopy* 1990;6(4):274-279.
3. Maffet MW, Gartsman GM, Moseley B: Superior labrum-biceps tendon complex lesions of the shoulder. *Am J Sports Med* 1995; 23(1):93-98.
4. Burkhart SS, Morgan CD, Kibler WB: The disabled throwing shoulder: Spectrum of pathology. Part III: The SICK scapula, scapular dyskinesis, the kinetic chain, and rehabilitation. *Arthroscopy* 2003;19(6):641-661.
5. Grossman MG, Tibone JE, McGarry MH, Schneider DJ, Veneziani S, Lee TQ: A cadaveric model of the throwing shoulder: A possible etiology of superior labrum anterior-to-posterior lesions. *J Bone Joint Surg Am* 2005;87(4): 824-831.
6. Clabbers KM, Kelly JD, Bader D, et al: Effect of posterior capsule tightness on glenohumeral translation in the late-cocking phase of pitching. *J Sport Rehabil* 2007; 16(1):41-49.
7. Yeh ML, Lintner D, Luo ZP: Stress distribution in the superior labrum during throwing motion. *Am J Sports Med* 2005;33(3): 395-401.
8. Kuhn JE, Lindholm SR, Huston LJ, Soslowsky LJ, Blasier RB: Failure of the biceps superior labral complex: A cadaveric biomechanical investigation comparing the late cocking and early deceleration positions of throwing. *Arthroscopy* 2003;19(4):373-379.
9. Pradhan RL, Itoi E, Hatakeyama Y, Urayama M, Sato K: Superior labral strain during the throwing motion: A cadaveric study. *Am J Sports Med* 2001;29(4):488-492.
10. Jobe FW, Moynes DR, Tibone JE, Perry J: An EMG analysis of the shoulder in pitching: A second report. *Am J Sports Med* 1984; 12(3):218-220.
11. Ide J, Maeda S, Takagi K: Sports activity after arthroscopic superior labral repair using suture anchors in overhead-throwing athletes. *Am J Sports Med* 2005;33(4):507-514.
12. Miniaci A, Mascia AT, Salonen DC, Becker EJ: Magnetic resonance imaging of the shoulder in asymptomatic professional baseball pitchers. *Am J Sports Med* 2002;30(1):66-73.
13. Connor PM, Banks DM, Tyson AB, Coumas JS, D'Alessandro DF: Magnetic resonance imaging of the asymptomatic shoulder of overhead athletes: A 5-year follow-up study. *Am J Sports Med* 2003;31(5):724-727.
14. Laudner KG, Myers JB, Pasquale MR, Bradley JP, Lephart SM: Scapular dysfunction in throwers with pathologic internal impingement. *J Orthop Sports Phys Ther* 2006;36(7):485-494.
15. Cools AM, Declercq G, Cagnie B, Cambier D, Witvrouw E: Internal impingement in the tennis player: Rehabilitation guidelines. *Br J Sports Med* 2008;42(3):165-171.
16. Burkhart SS: Internal impingement of the shoulder. *Instr Course Lect* 2006;55:29-34.
17. Fleisig GS, Andrews JR, Dillman CJ, Escamilla RF: Kinetics of baseball pitching with implications about injury mechanisms. *Am J Sports Med* 1995;23(2): 233-239.
18. Fleisig GS, Barrentine SW, Escamilla RF, Andrews JR: Biomechanics of overhand throwing with implications for injuries. *Sports Med* 1996;21(6):421-437.
19. Fleisig GS, Andrews JR, Cutter GR, et al: Risk of serious injury for young baseball pitchers: A 10-year prospective study. *Am J Sports Med* 2011;39(2):253-257.
20. Lyman S, Fleisig GS, Andrews JR, Osinski ED: Effect of pitch type, pitch count, and pitching mechanics on risk of elbow and shoulder pain in youth baseball pitchers. *Am J Sports Med* 2002; 30(4):463-468.
21. Atwater AE: Biomechanics of overarm throwing movements and of throwing injuries. *Exerc Sport Sci Rev* 1979;7:43-85.
22. Matsuo T, Escamilla RF, Fleisig G, et al: Comparison of kinematic and temporal parameters between different pitch velocity groups. *J Appl Biomech* 2001;17:1-13.
23. Crockett HC, Gross LB, Wilk KE, et al: Osseous adaptation and range of motion at the glenohumeral joint in professional baseball pitchers. *Am J Sports Med* 2002;30(1):20-26.
24. Reagan KM, Meister K, Horodyski MB, Werner DW, Carruthers C, Wilk K: Humeral retroversion and its relationship to glenohumeral rotation in the shoulder of college baseball players. *Am J Sports Med* 2002;30(3): 354-360.
25. Chant CB, Litchfield R, Griffin S, Thain LM: Humeral head retroversion in competitive baseball players and its relationship to glenohumeral rotation range of motion. *J Orthop Sports Phys Ther* 2007;37(9):514-520.
26. Drakos MC, Barker JU, Osbahr DC, et al: Effective glenoid version in professional baseball play-

ers. *Am J Orthop (Belle Mead NJ)* 2010;39(7):340-344.

27. Thomas SJ, Swanik KA, Swanik CB, Kelly JD: Internal rotation and scapular position differences: A comparison of collegiate and high school baseball players. *J Athl Train* 2010;45(1):44-50.

28. Kibler WB, Chandler TJ, Livingston BP, Roetert EP: Shoulder range of motion in elite tennis players: Effect of age and years of tournament play. *Am J Sports Med* 1996;24(3):279-285.

29. Sabick MB, Kim YK, Torry MR, Keirns MA, Hawkins RJ: Biomechanics of the shoulder in youth baseball pitchers: Implications for the development of proximal humeral epiphysiolysis and humeral retrotorsion. *Am J Sports Med* 2005;33(11):1716-1722.

30. Bach HG, Goldberg BA: Posterior capsular contracture of the shoulder. *J Am Acad Orthop Surg* 2006; 14(5):265-277.

31. Lintner D, Mayol M, Uzodinma O, Jones R, Labossiere D: Glenohumeral internal rotation deficits in professional pitchers enrolled in an internal rotation stretching program. *Am J Sports Med* 2007; 35(4):617-621.

32. Burkhart SS, Morgan CD, Kibler WB: The disabled throwing shoulder: A spectrum of pathology. Part I: Pathoanatomy and biomechanics. *Arthroscopy* 2003; 19(4):404-420.

33. Davidson PA, Elattrache NS, Jobe CM, Jobe FW: Rotator cuff and posterior-superior glenoid labrum injury associated with increased glenohumeral motion: A new site of impingement. *J Shoulder Elbow Surg* 1995;4(5):384-390.

34. McClure P, Balaicuis J, Heiland D, Broersma ME, Thorndike CK, Wood A: A randomized controlled comparison of stretching procedures for posterior shoulder tightness. *J Orthop Sports Phys Ther* 2007;37(3):108-114.

35. Burkhart SS, Morgan C: SLAP lesions in the overhead athlete. *Op Tech Sports Med* 2000;8(3): 213-220.

36. Kibler WB, Sciascia A: Current concepts: scapular dyskinesis. *Br J Sports Med* 2010;44(5):300-305.

37. Edwards SL, Lee JA, Bell JE, et al: Nonoperative treatment of superior labrum anterior posterior tears: Improvements in pain, function, and quality of life. *Am J Sports Med* 2010;38(7):1456-1461.

38. Neri BR, ElAttrache NS, Owsley KC, Mohr K, Yocum LA: Outcome of type II superior labral anterior posterior repairs in elite overhead athletes: Effect of concomitant partial-thickness rotator cuff tears. *Am J Sports Med* 2011; 39(1):114-120.

39. Van Kleunen JP, Field LD, Savoie FH: Return to high level throwing after combination infraspinatus repair, SLAP repair, and release of glenohumeral internal rotation deficit. *Arthroscopy* 2011;27(5): e32-e33.

40. Kim SH, Ha KI, Kim SH, Choi HJ: Results of arthroscopic treatment of superior labral lesions. *J Bone Joint Surg Am* 2002;84(6): 981-985.

41. Cohen DB, Coleman S, Drakos MC, et al: Outcomes of isolated type II SLAP lesions treated with arthroscopic fixation using a bioabsorbable tack. *Arthroscopy* 2006; 22(2):136-142.

42. Neuman D, Ciccotti MG, Bolsvert CB, Reiter B, Lawson K, Cohen SB: Results of arthroscopic repair of type II superior labral anterior posterior lesions in overhead athletes: Assessment of return to preinjury playing level and satisfaction. *Am J Sports Med* 2011;39(9):1883-1888.

43. Reinold MM, Wilk KE, Macrina LC, et al: Changes in shoulder and elbow passive range of motion after pitching in professional baseball players. *Am J Sports Med* 2008;36(3):523-527.

44. Myers JB, Laudner KG, Pasquale MR, Bradley JP, Lephart SM: Glenohumeral range of motion deficits and posterior shoulder tightness in throwers with pathologic internal impingement. *Am J Sports Med* 2006;34(3):385-391.

45. Brockmeier SF, Dodson CC, Gamradt SC, Coleman SH, Altchek DW: Arthroscopic intratendinous repair of the delaminated partial-thickness rotator cuff tear in overhead athletes. *Arthroscopy* 2008;24(8):961-965.

45

Superior Labrum Anterior to Posterior Tears and Glenohumeral Instability

Mandeep S. Virk, MD
Robert A. Arciero, MD

Abstract

Cadaver experiments and clinical studies suggest that the superior labrum–biceps complex plays a role in glenohumeral stability. Superior labrum anterior to posterior (SLAP) tears can be present in acute and recurrent glenohumeral dislocations and contribute to glenohumeral instability. Isolated SLAP tears can cause instability, especially in throwing athletes. Diagnosing a SLAP tear on the basis of the clinical examination alone is difficult because of nonspecific history and physical examination findings and the presence of coexisting intra-articular lesions. Magnetic resonance arthrography is the imaging study of choice for diagnosing SLAP tears; however, arthroscopy remains the gold standard for diagnosis. Arthroscopy is the preferred technique for the repair of a type II SLAP tear and its variant types (V through X) in acute glenohumeral dislocations and instability in younger populations. Clinical outcome studies report a low recurrence of glenohumeral instability after the arthroscopic repair of a SLAP tear in addition to a Bankart repair. Long-term follow-up studies and further advances in arthroscopic fixation techniques will allow a better understanding and improvement in outcomes in patients with SLAP tears associated with glenohumeral instability.

Instr Course Lect 2013;62:501-514.

A superior labrum anterior to posterior (SLAP) lesion is characterized by detachment of the superior labrum in the anteroposterior direction, with or without involvement of the biceps tendon. First described by Andrews et al[1] in 1985, these lesions can cause shoulder pain and disability. SLAP tears can occur in isolation, but they are commonly seen in association with other shoulder lesions, including rotator cuff tears, Bankart lesions, glenohumeral arthritis, acromioclavicular joint pathology, and subacromial impingement.[2] SLAP tears are a known pathologic entity in glenohumeral dislocations and contribute to glenohumeral instability. This chapter reviews the role of the superior labrum–bicep complex in the stability of the glenohumeral joint and discusses the management and clinical outcomes of SLAP tears in the presence of glenohumeral instability.

Biomechanical Role of the Superior Labrum–Biceps Complex

Glenohumeral stability is determined by a complex interplay of static and dynamic anatomic structures. The glenoid labrum provides stability to the glenohumeral joint by increasing the concavity of the glenoid and therefore increasing the contact surface of glenohumeral articulation. The labrum provides attachment to various glenohumeral ligaments that confer static stability to the shoulder joint. The superior labrum also confers glenohumeral stability, but its specific role is not well understood. The superior labrum provides attachment to the long head of the biceps and capsule and capsular ligaments, which all confer stability to the glenohumeral joint.

Dr. Arciero or an immediate family member is a member of a speakers' bureau or has made paid presentations on behalf of Arthrex; has received research or institutional support from Arthrex; and owns stock or stock options in Soft Tissue Regeneration. Neither Dr. Virk nor any immediate family member has received anything of value from or owns stock in a commercial company or institution related directly or indirectly to the subject of this chapter.

The long head of the biceps attaches partly to the supraglenoid tubercle and partly to the superior glenoid labrum. The attachment to the superior labrum can be posterior (type I), predominantly posterior with some anterior attachment (type II), equally anterior and posterior (type III), or predominantly anterior with some posterior attachment (type IV).[3] The middle glenohumeral ligament may insert onto the superior labrum instead of the glenoid.

The contribution of the superior labrum–biceps complex to shoulder stability is controversial and not well understood. Electromyographic analysis of volunteers with normal shoulders has demonstrated conflicting results with respect to the activity of the biceps during active shoulder motion.[4] Simulated experiments in cadavers, despite the inherent limitations of such studies, have resulted in an improved understanding of the pathophysiology of the superior labrum–biceps complex in glenohumeral instability.[5-10] In a dynamic cadaver shoulder model, Rodosky et al[5] showed that the long head of the biceps muscle contributes to the anterior stability of the glenohumeral joint and decreases the stress placed on the inferior glenohumeral ligament. McMahan et al[6] and Patzer et al[11] demonstrated that creating a simulated type II SLAP lesion increases anteroposterior and anteroinferior translation of the glenohumeral joint. Increased anteroposterior translation of the glenohumeral joint in simulated SLAP lesions in cadavers occurred only if the anterosuperior labral tear extended into the long head of the biceps.[7] Panossian et al[8] reported that repairing SLAP lesions can restore the increased glenohumeral translation seen in experimental SLAP tears in cadavers. However, other cadaver studies reported that repair of simulated SLAP tears alone does not completely restore normal glenohumeral translation, and a failure to address capsular deformation and laxity probably contributes to the residual instability.[9,10]

The blood supply to the labrum is derived from the suprascapular artery, the anterior humeral circumflex artery, and the posterior humeral circumflex artery.[12] The superior and the anterosuperior parts of the labrum are less well vascularized compared with the remaining labrum. Labral tears in areas of poorer vascularity are predisposed to compromised healing because of the precarious blood supply.

Pathogenesis

Cadaver experiments and studies in throwing athletes have lent credence to the commonly proposed mechanisms of injury to the superior labrum-biceps complex. Common mechanisms of injury leading to SLAP tears include traction insult or compressive injury to the superior labrum–biceps complex caused by heavy lifting, falls onto an outstretched hand, and chronic overhead throwing activities. Using a cadaver model, Clavert et al[13] reported on the role of shearing forces during a traumatic fall. When tested with a shoulder apparatus, simulated forward falls created SLAP tears in five of the five shoulders tested, whereas backward falls resulted in two SLAP tears in the five tested shoulders.

Throwing athletes are predisposed to SLAP tears by the increased external rotation in shoulder abduction and a tight posterior capsule. Increased external rotation of the shoulder in the late cocking phase generates increased torsional forces at the biceps anchor, resulting in a peel-back injury to the posterosuperior labrum.[14,15] The predisposition to injury is further compounded by the presence of increased tightness or contracture of the posteroinferior capsule. In the absence of posterior capsular tightness, the humeral head shifts posteroinferiorly in the late cocking position. However, after a simulated posterior capsular contracture and an anterior capsular stretch injury, the humeral head shifts posterosuperiorly with maximum external rotation. This leads to shear stress on the superior labrum.[16]

A SLAP tear is one of the pathologic lesions that can be present in acute and recurrent glenohumeral dislocations.[17-20] In a glenohumeral dislocation, a SLAP tear usually contributes to instability rather than being the essential lesion causing instability. In a cohort of patients with chronic anterior glenohumeral instability, Hantes et al[21] reported that the number of preoperative dislocations were higher in patients with a combined SLAP tear and Bankart lesion compared with those with a Bankart lesion alone. Some physicians believe that SLAP tears in recurrent glenohumeral instability are an end result of chronic instability rather than a reason for the initial instability.[18] Type I SLAP tears do not contribute to instability, and type III tears usually cause mechanical symptoms.[22] Type II and types IV through X SLAP tears can contribute to instability by disrupting the superior labrum–biceps complex and compromising the function of the entire capsular-labral complex[23-25] (**Table 1**).

Epidemiology and Classification of SLAP Lesions

There is a high incidence of associated labral injuries, including SLAP tears, in acute and recurrent glenohumeral dislocations.[17,19,20] However, no long-term clinical studies are available to accurately determine the true incidence of SLAP tears in association with glenohumeral instability. Arthroscopic and MRI examinations in patients with first-time or recurrent glenohumeral dislocations have shown wide variations in the prevalence of SLAP tears.[2,17-19,21,26-29] In 1990, Snyder et al[22] described four classic types of SLAP tears. Six additional types, which are extensions of type II tears, have since been added to the original classification system[23-25] (**Table 1**).

Table 1
Classification of SLAP Tears

SLAP Lesion	Tear Morphology
Type I	Fraying of the superior labrum
Type II	Detachment of the superior labrum–biceps anchor Predominantly anterior (type IIa) Predominantly posterior (type IIb) Combined anterior and posterior (type IIc)
Type III	Bucket-handle tear of the superior labrum with intact biceps anchor
Type IV	Bucket-handle tear of the superior labrum with extension into the biceps tendon
Type V	Anteroinferior Bankart-type labral disruption in continuity with type II lesion
Type VI	Type II lesion with an unstable labral flap tear
Type VII	Type II lesion with capsular extension anteriorly beneath the middle glenohumeral ligament
Type VIII	Type II lesion with extension into the posterior labrum
Type IX	Type II lesion with circumferential disruption of the labrum
Type X	Type II lesion combined with posteroinferior labral disruption (reverse Bankart lesion)

History and Physical Examination

Diagnosing a SLAP tear with a clinical examination alone is difficult, especially in patients with coexisting intra-articular pathologies. Pain is the most frequently reported symptom. The onset of pain is insidious in patients with chronic overuse injuries, and symptoms are usually acute after a traumatic injury. The locations and characteristics of pain are variable and nonspecific. Typically, symptoms are worsened with pushing, lifting, and overhead activities. A throwing athlete may report weakness, reduced performance in overhead activity, and pain.

Range of motion is usually preserved with isolated SLAP tears. Scapular mechanics may be altered as a result of pain, weakness, and mechanical symptoms. External rotation in the abducted position may reproduce mechanical symptoms. Although many provocative physical tests are available to assist in diagnosing SLAP tears[30-41] (**Table 2**), these tests vary in sensitivity and specificity, and there is no good evidence to support their validity.[42-44]

SLAP tears can be associated with glenohumeral instability. The instability pattern is usually anterior, but posterior instability can occur.[45] All SLAP tears do not result in instability; SLAP tear types II, IV, and V through X can cause instability.

Imaging

Plain radiographs, including AP, axillary, and outlet views of the shoulder, are usually the first diagnostic imaging studies performed. Magnetic resonance arthrography is the gold standard for diagnosing labral tears because it is highly sensitive and specific (> 95%) and is superior to conventional MRI.[46] Interestingly, magnetic resonance arthrography has not proved reliable in accurately differentiating various subtypes of labral tears,[46] but it is helpful in differentiating anatomic variants of superior labral tears (sublabral recess, sublabral foramen, Buford complex, and mobile glenoid labrum) from pathologic tears.[46-48] The labrum is typically a low-signal structure on all MRI sequences. Linear high signal within the labrum is an essential finding in labral tears. Other features indicative of a labral tear include irregular margins, abnormal morphology (bucket-handle or flap fragments), an increased degree of separation of the labrum from the glenoid surface, and extension of the contrast posterior to the biceps tendon.[46,47] The presence of a paralabral cyst is highly suggestive of a labral tear but not necessarily a SLAP lesion. Other associated lesions, including rotator cuff tears, Bankart lesions, and chondral lesions, also can be discerned with magnetic resonance arthrography. CT arthrography is an equally sensitive and specific alternative if magnetic resonance arthrography is contraindicated.[48,49]

Managing SLAP Tears and Instability

Historically, the surgical treatment of SLAP tears has included débridement, biceps tenotomy, biceps tenodesis, biceps repair, and labral reattachment.[50,51] Surgical management is indicated for persistent pain, mechanical symptoms, and instability. Relative contraindications for the repair of SLAP tears are the presence of glenohumeral arthritis, shoulder stiffness, and concomitant rotator cuff tears in elderly patients.[50,52]

Arthroscopic examination of the shoulder is the gold standard for diagnosing SLAP tears and is also a preferred technique for repairing the tears. A bare sublabral footprint, positive

Table 2
Common Provocative Physical Examination Tests for SLAP Tears

Test	Study (Year)	Description	Positive Test	Sensitivity[a]	Specificity[a]
Anterior slide test	Kibler et al[30] (1995)	In a sitting or standing position, the patient flexes his or her elbow and rests the hand's first web space on the ipsilateral hip with the thumb pointing posteriorly. The examiner then applies an axial load in an anterosuperior direction from the elbow up the shoulder.	Pain or click in the anterior or the posterior joint line.	~78%	~91%
Crank test	Liu et al[31] (1996)	The affected arm is elevated to 160° in the plane of the scapula, and the shoulder joint is loaded axially along the humeral shaft and rotated externally and internally.	Maneuver produces pain or mechanical symptoms.	91%	93%
Active compression test	O'Brien et al[32] (1998)	The affected shoulder is flexed to 90°, adducted 10° to 15°, and internally rotated with the elbow in full extension. A downward force is applied with the palm facing down (pronation), and the maneuver is then repeated with the palm facing up (supination).	Pain is present with forearm in pronation and disappears or diminishes in supination.	100%	~98%
Biceps load test 1	Kim et al[33] (1999)	In the supine position, the affected shoulder is placed in 90° abduction and external rotation, and an anterior apprehension test is performed. The patient is asked to actively flex his or her elbow against resistance.	Pain and apprehension stay the same or worsen.	~91%	~97%
Pain provocation test	Mimori et al[34] (1999)	In the sitting position, the affected shoulder is abducted to 90° and externally rotated by the examiner. This maneuver is tested first in maximal forearm supination and then maximum pronation.	Pain is present only in the prone position of the forearm or pain is more severe in the prone position compared with the supine position	100%	90%
Biceps load test 2	Kim et al[35] (2001)	In the supine position, the affected arm is elevated to 120° and externally rotated with the elbow in 90° flexion. The patient is asked to actively flex his or her elbow against resistance.	Patient reports pain with resisted elbow flexion.	~90%	~97%
Modified Jobe relocation test	Hammer et al[36] (2000)	In the supine position with the affected shoulder in 90° of abduction, the arm is externally rotated until the patient feels pain in the posterosuperior part of the shoulder. The arm is brought back to the starting position, and the maneuver is repeated but with a posteriorly directed force to the proximal humerus.	Relief of pain.	NA	NA
Resisted supination external rotation test	Myers et al[37] (2005)	In the supine position, the affected shoulder is abducted to 90°, the elbow is flexed to 70°, and the forearm is in neutral or slight pronation. The patient actively supinates the hand against resistance while the examiner externally rotates the shoulder to maximal limit.	Anterior or deep shoulder pain; clicking or catching in the shoulder or reproduction of symptoms that occur during throwing.	~83%	~82%

Table 2 (continued)
Common Provocative Physical Examination Tests for SLAP Tears

Test	Study (Year)	Description	Positive Test	Sensitivity[a]	Specificity[a]
Forced abduction test	Nakagawa et al[38] (2005)	The arm is forced into maximal abduction, and the patient is asked about pain. At this position, if pain is felt by the patient in the posterosuperior aspect of the shoulder, the elbow is flexed and the pain response is reevaluated.	Pain occurs posterosuperiorly with maximal abduction and diminishes with elbow flexion.	67%	67%
Passive compression test	Kim et al[39] (2007)	With the arm in a lateral position, the examiner stabilizes the shoulder by holding the AC joint and externally rotates the shoulder in 30° of abduction. The examiner then pushes the arm proximally while extending the arm, which results in a passive compression of the superior labrum onto the glenoid.	Pain or a painful click is elicited in the glenohumeral joint.	~82%	~86%
Supine flexion resistance test	Ebinger et al[40] (2008)	In the supine position, the patient is asked to rest the arm above the head in full elevation and then perform a resisted throwing motion.	Pain is felt by the patient deep inside the shoulder joint or on the dorsal aspect of the shoulder along the joint line.	80%	69%
Passive distraction test	Schlechter et al[41] (2009)	In the supine position, the affected shoulder is elevated to 150° with the elbow extended and forearm supinated. The forearm is gently pronated from the supinated position while maintaining a steady position of the upper arm.	Pain is reported deep inside the joint either anteriorly or posteriorly.	53%	94%

[a]As described by the inventor of the test. NA = not available, AC = acromioclavicular.

peel-back sign, displaceable biceps root, and positive drive-through sign are important arthroscopic findings associated with type II SLAP tears. Instability or increased anterior translation may be present. SLAP tears may be associated with a labral tear of the anteroinferior labrum (Bankart lesion) or the posteroinferior labrum (reverse Bankart lesion), or a circumferential disruption of the labrum may be present.

The surgical treatment of SLAP tears with glenohumeral instability is determined by the type and severity of the tear, the age and functional demands of the patient, and the presence of coexisting intra-articular lesions. In a young patient, type II SLAP tears are surgically treated by reattaching the superior labrum–biceps complex to the glenoid[51,53-58] (**Table 3**). Various methods of fixation, including metallic suture anchors, absorbable suture anchors, knotless suture anchors, and biodegradable suture tack fixation, can be used to reattach the superior labrum–biceps complex to the glenoid.[53-55,59] Biceps tenodesis is an effective alternative to SLAP reattachment for type II SLAP tears. In a prospective study of patients with isolated type II SLAP tears, Boileau et al[51] reported that patients treated with biceps tenodesis were more satisfied and had higher rates of return to their presurgical level of activity and sports participation compared with patients treated with SLAP repair. However, there was a substantial difference in the mean ages of the two groups (37 years in the repair group versus 52 years in the tenodesis group), and the study was not adequately powered. For SLAP tear types V through X, repair of the anterior or posterior labrum and the middle glenohumeral ligament is performed in addition to the superior labrum–biceps anchor complex. For type IV SLAP tears, the bucket-handle component of the labrum can be débrided in elderly patients or repaired in young patients. Multiple options exist for treating the torn biceps tendon. If damage to the biceps tendon is not substantial (less than one third the width of the tendon), débridement of the biceps tendon tear can be performed. Repair of the biceps tendon, tenodesis (in younger patients and/or those with higher functional demands), or tenotomy (in older patients and/or those with low functional demands) can be performed if the biceps tendon tear is more than one third the width of the tendon.[52,60-62]

Table 3
Clinical Studies Assessing Outcomes of Isolated Type II SLAP Tears

Study (Year)	Study Design	Follow-up	Outcome Measures	Surgical Details	Results and Complications
Neuman et al[55] (2011)	Retrospective; 30 overhead athletes	3.5 years	KJOC and ASES scores	Lateral decubitus or beach-chair position; posterior and transrotator cuff portal used; bioabsorbable suture anchors (range, 1-4 anchors)	Significant improvement in the postoperative outcome scores; athletes returned to ~84% of their preinjury level; ~93% satisfaction rate; three revision surgeries
Kaisidis et al[54] (2011)	Retrospective; 20 consecutive patients, including 17 athletes	2 years	Modified Constant-Murley score	Beach-chair position; anterior and posterior portals but no transrotator cuff portal; knotless suture anchors (range, 1-2 anchors)	Significant improvement in postoperative outcome and pain scores; 80% good or excellent outcomes and 95% patient satisfaction rate, 45% return to play (significantly earlier return and higher rate in patients younger than 40 years compared to those older than 40 years)
Boileau et al[51] (2009)	Prospective cohort; 25 patients, including 15 overhead athletes	35 months	Constant score	Beach-chair position; posterior, anterosuperior rotator interval or transrotator cuff interval portal used; SLAP repair with resorbable suture anchors (n = 10) or biceps tenodesis (n = 15) with interference screw fixation	Significant improvement in the postoperative outcome scores; lower satisfaction rate and return to preinjury level in the repair group (40% and 20%, respectively) compared with the tenodesis group (93% and 87%, respectively); four revision surgeries in the repair group
Yung et al[56] (2008)	Prospective cohort; 16 patients, including 13 overhead athletes	27.6 months	UCLA shoulder score	Lateral decubitus position; posterior, anterosuperior rotator interval and/or transrotator cuff interval portal; bioabsorbable knotless suture anchors (range, 2-4 anchors)	Significant improvement in the postoperative outcome scores; 87.5% excellent and good results; time to return to play at preinjury level was 9.4 months; overhead athletes had longer rehabilitation period and took longer time to return to play
Cohen et al[57] (2006)	Retrospective; 29 athletes, including 8 throwing and 21 nonthrowing athletes	3.7 years	ASES and L'Insalata questionnaire	Beach-chair position; posterior, anterosuperior rotator interval or transrotator cuff interval portal used; bioabsorbable tack fixation (range, 1-4 tacks)	Significant improvement in postoperative outcome scores, 69% of patients reported excellent/good outcome; 48% of athletes returned to preinjury level; overall patient satisfaction ~71%
Ide et al[58] (2005)	Prospective cohort; 40 athletes involved in overhead sports	41 months	Modified Rowe score	Lateral decubitus position; posterior and lateral transrotator cuff portal used; suture anchors (average, 2 anchors)	Significant improvement in postoperative modified Rowe scores; 75% returned to preinjury level; 90% had satisfactory outcome
Kim et al[53] (2002)	Retrospective; 30 athletes, including 18 overhead and 12 nonoverhead athletes	33 months	UCLA shoulder score and ability to return to preinjury level	Lateral decubitus position; posterior, anterosuperior, and anteroinferior rotator interval portals used; single minirevo screw	85% good/excellent outcome; 94% had satisfactory shoulder scores; 91% return to preinjury level; lower shoulder scores and lower percentage of return to preinjury level in athletes participating in overhead sports

KJOC = Kerlan Jobe Orthopaedic Clinic, ASES = American Shoulder and Elbow Surgeons, UCLA = University of California Los Angeles.

There are few long-term outcome data on the treatment of SLAP tears and instability[21,26,28,63-65] (**Table 4**). Most studies are retrospective, and long-term results are not available. Clinical studies have shown an increased incidence of redislocation and instability in young patients treated nonsurgically for acute glenohumeral dislocations. The age of the patient is the single most important predictor of redislocation and future instability.[66] The redislocation rate can be significantly reduced by arthroscopic repair in young patients compared with nonsurgical management.[67,68] However, there is a concern that combined repair of Bankart and SLAP tears may restrict the range of shoulder motion, especially external rotation in older patients. In a prospective nonrandomized study, Hantes et al[21] reported no substantial differences in shoulder stability, range of motion, and functional outcome scores in the patients treated with arthroscopic Bankart repair compared with the patients treated with arthroscopic repair of type V SLAP tears. Cho et al[28] reported favorable clinical results in patients with recurrent shoulder dislocations and type V tears (mean age, 24.2 years) compared with those with an isolated Bankart lesion. There were no limitations in range of motion of more than 10° at final follow-up, although patients with type V tears had a slower postoperative recovery of shoulder motion. In contrast, Takase[26] examined a cohort of patients with chronic, traumatic anterior instability to compare type II and IV tears with and without extension into a Bankart lesion. The SLAP tears that extended into a Bankart lesion were treated with débridement alone because those tears were believed to be secondary to recurrent episodes of dislocations and/or subluxations. The superior labrum was reattached in SLAP tears that did not communicate with a Bankart lesion. All of the Bankart lesions were repaired. Patients treated with SLAP tear débridement had similar redislocation rates and functional outcomes and substantially more external rotation compared with patients treated with SLAP lesion reattachment.

No association has been reported between the preoperative number of dislocations and the recurrence rate after labral repair in patients with traumatic glenohumeral instability in association with SLAP tears. Kim et al[63] reported good outcomes with arthroscopic repair of type V SLAP lesions in patients with primary as well as recurrent anterior glenohumeral dislocations. There were no substantial differences between the primary and recurrent dislocation groups with respect to the redislocation rate, shoulder range of motion, and outcome scores. In a prospective, nonrandomized study of 53 patients with anterior glenohumeral instability, Gartsman et al[27] reported no substantial differences between the number of preoperative dislocations and the recurrence rate after arthroscopic repair in the patients with associated SLAP tears. However, the authors found more severe labral tears in the patients with a higher number of preoperative dislocations. Habermeyer et al[69] reported similar findings in a prospective study of an observational cohort of patients with traumatic glenohumeral instability.

There is no universal consensus on whether SLAP repair should precede Bankart lesion repair or Bankart lesion repair should precede SLAP repair, although more surgeons favor the latter approach. Fixing a SLAP lesion first limits access to the Bankart lesion;[21,27,64] however, fixing a SLAP lesion first helps to anatomically reduce the Bankart lesion because of the bowstring effect of the superior labrum and could potentially result in decreased surgical time compared with repairing the Bankart lesion first.[28] Repair of a type IV SLAP tear represents a more unique situation. Baker and Romeo[61] reported that reducing a bucket-handle tear of the superior labrum provides a template for more anatomic repair of the Bankart lesion. However, even in this situation, the Bankart repair still precedes the final repair of the superior labrum.

Senior Author's Preferred Technique for Repairing SLAP Tears

This chapter's senior author (RAA) prefers that the patient be placed in a lateral decubitus position for all arthroscopic shoulder stabilization procedures. This position enhances exposure of the inferior portion of the glenohumeral joint and facilitates a modest amount of distraction when combined with a bump placed in the axilla (**Figure 1**). The increased exposure of the inferior aspect, and especially the inferior glenohumeral ligament–labral complex, improves drilling and instrumentation inferiorly and is necessary for proper repair. With slight distal traction of approximately 7 lb, the superior aspect of the joint can be adequately exposed for repair of the SLAP tear if indicated. The senior author does not perform a rotator interval closure as part of the SLAP tear repair in these combined lesions because of the risk of a loss of shoulder motion.

There are several more common presentations of SLAP tears with Bankart lesions. In the senior author's experience, combined SLAP tears and Bankart lesions occur with higher energy trauma (such as falls from a height, motor vehicle crashes, and downhill skiing injuries). The SLAP lesions occur primarily as a direct continuation of the Bankart lesion superiorly and often posteriorly and appear as type II lesions. The Bankart lesion

Table 4
Clinical Studies Assessing Outcomes of Combined Repair of a SLAP Tear and a Bankart Lesion

Study (Year)	Study Design	Follow-up	Outcome Measures	Surgical Details	Results and Complications
Kim et al[63] (2011)	Retrospective study; outcomes of arthroscopic repair of type V SLAP lesion in patients with primary dislocations (n = 42) was compared with patients with recurrent dislocations (n = 68)	2 years (minimum)	Constant and Rowe scores	Lateral position; posterior, anterosuperior, and anteroinferior portals used; absorbable suture anchors for repair; SLAP repair preceded Bankart repair in 52 patients and vice versa in 58 patients	No significant differences between two groups with respect to outcome measures, ROM testing, and revision surgery; shorter duration of surgery if Bankart repair preceded SLAP repair, but the differences in the duration of surgery were not significant
Takase[26] (2009)	Case series; outcomes of Bankart repair alone (n = 55) was compared with combined Bankart and SLAP repairs (15 type II and 5 type IV SLAP tears)	2.25 years	JOA and JSS shoulder instability scores	Beach-chair position; anterior, posterior, and anterosuperior portals used; SLAP repair was performed only if the SLAP lesion did not communicate with the Bankart lesion, otherwise débridement was performed; metallic and absorbable suture anchors	Significant improvement in the postoperative outcome scores in all groups; significant restriction of external rotation in the group with combined SLAP repair and Bankart repair compared with the group treated with débridement of SLAP tear and Bankart repair alone
Cho et al[28] (2010)	Retrospective study; outcomes of arthroscopic Bankart repairs (n = 15) compared with type V SLAP repairs (n = 15)	15 months	ASES and Rowe shoulder scores	Beach-chair position; posterior, anterior, anterosuperior, and Wilmington portals used; absorbable suture anchors used; mean number of suture anchors was 5.2; SLAP repair preceded Bankart repair	Significant improvement in the postoperative outcome scores; no significant difference between the two groups with respect to ROM and outcome scores at final follow-up, but ROM recovery was slower in the SLAP type V repair group
Hantes et al[21] (2009)	Retrospective study; failure rates of arthroscopic Bankart repair (n = 38) were compared to type V SLAP repair (n = 25)	2 years (minimum)	Constant and Rowe scores	Lateral position; posterior, anterosuperior, anteroinferior, and Wilmington portals used; absorbable suture anchors for repair; mean number of suture anchors for SLAP repair was 5.5; Bankart repair preceded SLAP repair	No significant differences between the two groups with respect to failure rate, outcome scores, and ROM
Warner et al[65] (1994)	Retrospective study; 7 athletes treated with arthroscopic repair of the anterior-inferior-superior-posterior labral detachment	> 1 year	ASES scores and L'Insalata questionnaire	Beach-chair position; posterior, anterosuperior rotator interval, or transrotator cuff interval portal used; absorbable suture anchors; SLAP repair preceded Bankart repair	Significant improvement in the postoperative outcome scores, one recurrent dislocation and one stiff shoulder; no significant difference in the side-to-side comparison of external rotation of the shoulder
Lo et al[64] (2005)	Retrospective study; 7 patients with combined type II SLAP and anterior and posterior labral lesions	41 months	Modified Rowe score	Lateral decubitus position; posterior, posterolateral, anterosuperior, low anterior, and Wilmington portals used; absorbable suture anchors used; mean number of suture anchors was 7.1; Bankart repair preceded SLAP repair	Significant improvement in postoperative modified Rowe scores; 75% returned to preinjury level; six patients were satisfied with the surgery

JOA = Japanese Orthopaedic Association, JSS = Japanese Shoulder Society, ASES = American Shoulder and Elbow Surgeons, ROM = range of motion.

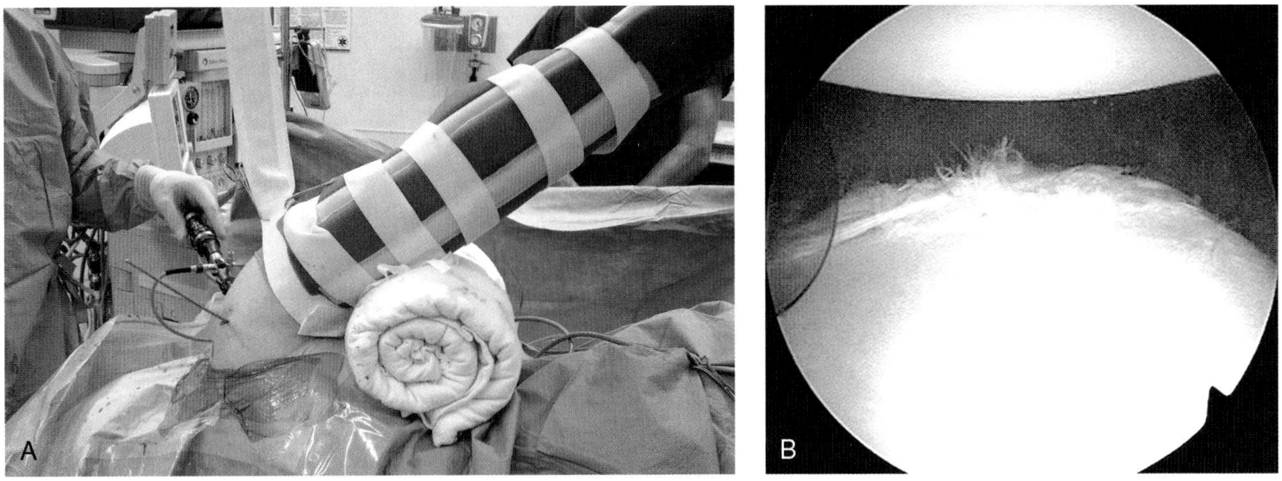

Figure 1 The lateral decubitus position with lateral and overhead traction and a bump under the axilla (**A**) is preferred for arthroscopic shoulder procedures to improve the superior and inferior arthroscopic exposure (**B**).

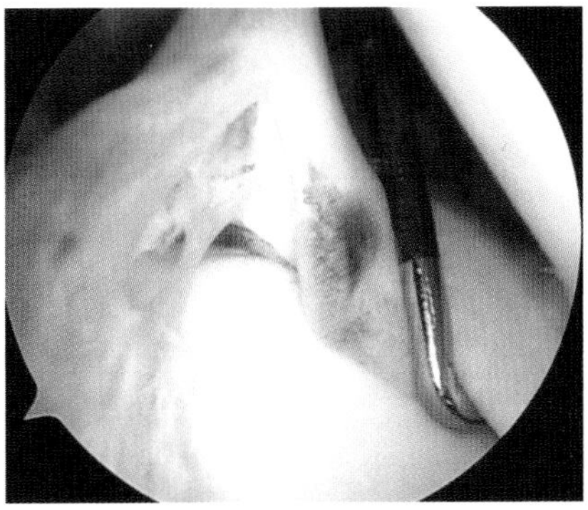

Figure 2 Arthroscopic view of a SLAP tear extending into the insertion of the long head of the biceps.

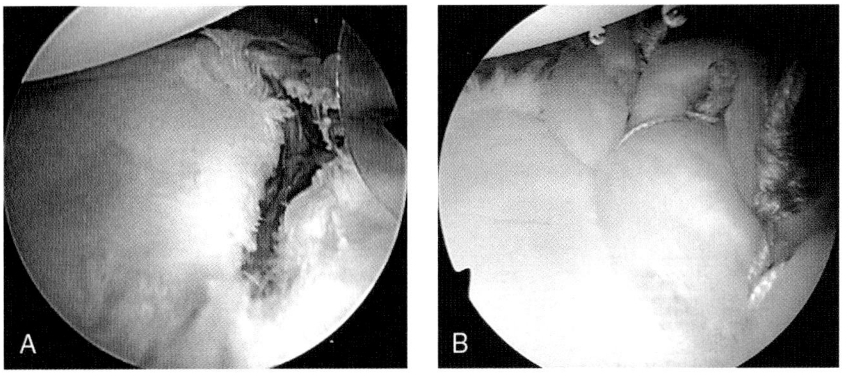

Figure 3 Type V SLAP tear showing the Bankart component before (**A**) and after repair (**B**).

may also present with a SLAP lesion that appears as a type IV lesion. This condition involves a substantial split in the labrum from the biceps anchor, with extension into the proximal biceps tendon. If the extension into the biceps tendon is substantial, the lesion is treated with a superior labral repair, Bankart repair, and subpectoral biceps tenodesis (**Figure 2**).

Technique 1: Continuous Type II SLAP Lesion With a Bankart Lesion

The lateral decubitus position is selected, and distal and overhead traction is generally used to treat a continuous type II SLAP lesion with a Bankart lesion. After performing diagnostic arthroscopy through a posterior portal, the arthroscope is moved to the anterosuperior portal, with 8.5-mm cannulas placed in the posterior and anterior midglenoid portals. The Bankart lesion is repaired first, typically with three to four double-loaded anchors, using a passing hook and suture shuttling technique (**Figure 3**).

The arthroscope is then moved back posteriorly. The anterosuperior portal, which was previously used for viewing, is enlarged, and another 8.5-mm cannula is placed. A suture anchor is then placed anterior to the biceps anchor, typically from the anterosuperior portal. The sutures are then passed using a suture hook loaded with a monofilament suture that serves as a passing suture to shuttle the nonabsorbable suture housed within the anchor (**Figure 4**). Sutures are passed in a mattress configuration to avoid suture knot prominence on the superior articular surface of the glenoid.

A second anchor is placed posterior to the biceps anchor, and the steps are repeated to complete the repair. Occasionally, if it is not possible to easily place the second anchor from the anterosuperior portal, a lateral portal (the so-called port of Wilmington portal) is used.

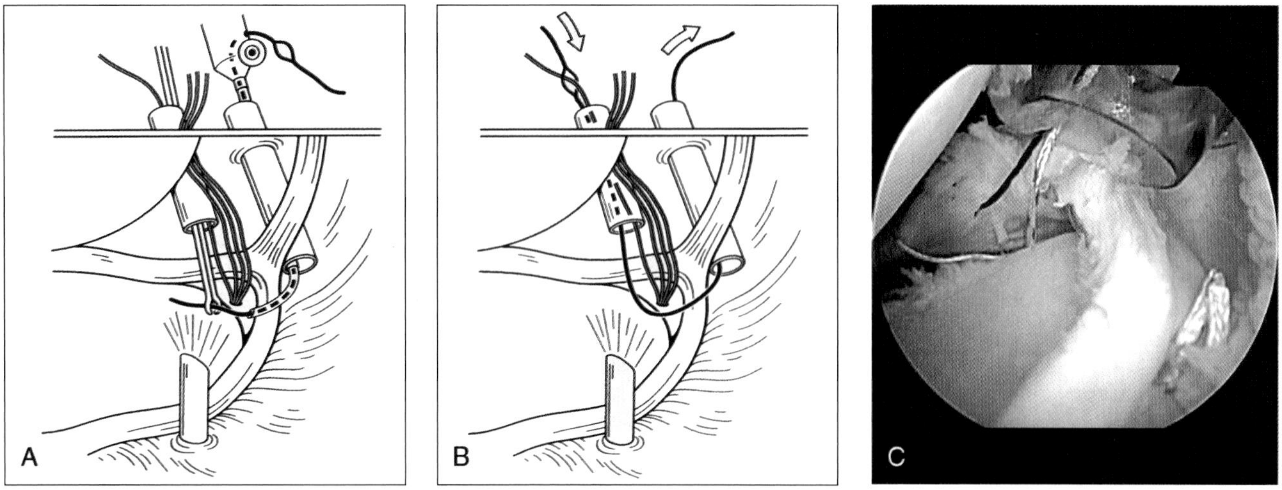

Figure 4 Illustrations and arthroscopic view of the repair of the superior labrum and biceps anchor using suture anchor. **A,** A suture anchor is placed anterior to the biceps anchor and sutures are then passed using a suture hook loaded with a monofilament suture. **B,** The monofilament suture serves as a passing suture to shuttle the nonabsorbable suture housed within the anchor. **C,** Arthroscopic view of the procedure described in B.

Technique 2: Separated Type II SLAP Lesion With a Bankart Lesion

Technique 2 is used when there is discontinuity between the type II SLAP and Bankart lesions. Because the SLAP tear is not in continuity with the mid and inferior labrum, this segment is unstable and can often be displaced into the upper 25% of the glenoid fossa, which impedes exposure. It is preferable to repair the SLAP lesion first to stabilize the superior labrum. The arthroscope is maintained posteriorly, and an anterosuperior portal and anterior midglenoid portal are instrumented with 8.5-mm cannulas as described previously. The arthroscope is then moved to the anterosuperior portal to complete the Bankart repair.

Technique 3: Type IV SLAP Lesion With a Bankart Lesion

The bucket-handle tear of the superior labrum is the unique feature of a combined type IV SLAP lesion with a Bankart lesion (**Figure 5**). If the labral split is thin, it is simply excised, the Bankart tear is repaired, and the superior labrum is repaired as described previously. If the labral split is large and comprises essentially the entire superior labrum, then it is incorporated into the superior labral repair with the use of suture anchors. Another option is to repair the labral split with simple sutures before the entire superior labrum–biceps anchor complex is repaired back to bone with suture anchors (**Figure 6**).

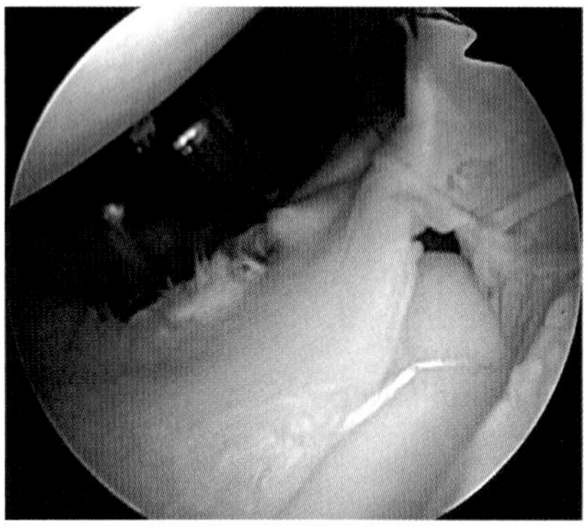

Figure 5 Arthroscopic view of a type IV SLAP tear with a bucket-handle fragment and a bald superior glenoid.

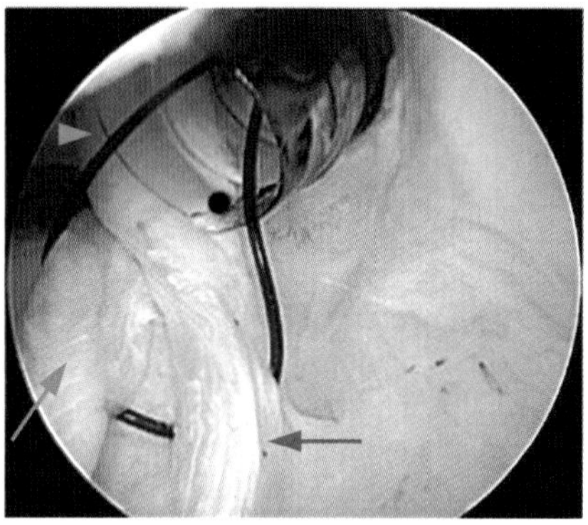

Figure 6 Arthroscopic view of the repair of a type IV SLAP tear with a large bucket-handle fragment (blue arrow). The bucket-handle fragment can be repaired with simple sutures before the entire superior labrum–biceps anchor complex is repaired back to bone with suture anchors. Biceps tendon = arrowhead. Superior labrum = red arrow.

In these situations, the superior exposure is often compromised, so repair of the type IV SLAP lesion before repair of the Bankart lesion is preferred as described in technique 2. This repair is more challenging and is typically reserved for young, high-demand patients with a displaced superior labral fragment. In older patients with a superior labral tear extending into the proximal biceps tendon, the fragment is excised, the superior labrum and

Bankart lesion are repaired, and a subpectoral biceps tenodesis is performed to complete the procedure. In patients who are candidates for surgical repair, this chapter's senior author prefers to perform the arthroscopic primary repair within 2 weeks of injury when the condition of the tissue is optimal. In addition to the Bankart repair, the inferior glenohumeral ligament is retensioned to treat any capsular stretching that occurred with the dislocation.

Postoperative Rehabilitation

The labrum heals over a period of 6 to 8 weeks. During this time, the labrum is protected from activities that can stress and disrupt the healing process. A shoulder sling is used for the first 4 to 6 weeks. The initial emphasis of the rehabilitation protocol is regaining and preserving shoulder range of motion. The rehabilitation regimen includes active-assisted motion consisting of forward elevation in the plane of the scapula and external rotation preformed at the side or at 45° of abduction in the plane of the scapula for the first 6 weeks. The next phase involves strengthening the muscles around the shoulder. Closed-chain exercises emphasizing scapular stability and deltoid function are initiated early and are followed by isometric and scapular strengthening exercises, which are gradually introduced between 3 and 4 months after surgery. The final phase of recovery involves a gradual return to the patient's previous activity level. In a competitive athlete, sports-specific training is started after 3 months, and return to competitive sports can be allowed at 6 months or longer.

Summary

An understanding of the role of the superior labrum–biceps complex in glenohumeral stability continues to evolve. SLAP tears have been shown to contribute to increased glenohumeral instability in both cadaver and clinical studies. Clinical studies suggest that repair of SLAP tears in young patients with acute or chronic glenohumeral instability favors optimal outcomes with lower redislocation and instability episodes. Prospective randomized studies and long-term follow-up will contribute to a better understanding of the role of SLAP tears in glenohumeral instability and the effect of SLAP repair on glenohumeral stability in patients with acute and recurrent glenohumeral dislocations.

References

1. Andrews JR, Carson WG Jr, McLeod WD: Glenoid labrum tears related to the long head of the biceps. *Am J Sports Med* 1985; 13(5):337-341.
2. Kim TK, Queale WS, Cosgarea AJ, McFarland EG: Clinical features of the different types of SLAP lesions: An analysis of one hundred and thirty-nine cases. *J Bone Joint Surg Am* 2003;85(1): 66-71.
3. Vangsness CT Jr, Jorgenson SS, Watson T, Johnson DL: The origin of the long head of the biceps from the scapula and glenoid labrum: An anatomical study of 100 shoulders. *J Bone Joint Surg Br* 1994;76(6):951-954.
4. Sakurai G, Ozaki J, Tomita Y, Nishimoto K, Tamai S: Electromyographic analysis of shoulder joint function of the biceps brachii muscle during isometric contraction. *Clin Orthop Relat Res* 1998;354:123-131.
5. Rodosky MW, Harner CD, Fu FH: The role of the long head of the biceps muscle and superior glenoid labrum in anterior stability of the shoulder. *Am J Sports Med* 1994;22(1):121-130.
6. McMahon PJ, Burkart A, Musahl V, Debski RE: Glenohumeral translations are increased after a type II superior labrum anterior-posterior lesion: A cadaveric study of severity of passive stabilizer injury. *J Shoulder Elbow Surg* 2004;13(1):39-44.
7. Pagnani MJ, Deng XH, Warren RF, Torzilli PA, Altchek DW: Effect of lesions of the superior portion of the glenoid labrum on glenohumeral translation. *J Bone Joint Surg Am* 1995;77(7):1003-1010.
8. Panossian VR, Mihata T, Tibone JE, Fitzpatrick MJ, McGarry MH, Lee TQ: Biomechanical analysis of isolated type II SLAP lesions and repair. *J Shoulder Elbow Surg* 2005;14(5):529-534.
9. Burkart A, Debski R, Musahl V, McMahon P, Woo SL: Biomechanical tests for type II SLAP lesions of the shoulder joint before and after arthroscopic repair. *Orthopade* 2003;32(7):600-607.
10. Mihata T, McGarry MH, Tibone JE, Fitzpatrick MJ, Kinoshita M, Lee TQ: Biomechanical assessment of type II superior labral anterior-posterior (SLAP) lesions associated with anterior shoulder capsular laxity as seen in throwers: A cadaveric study. *Am J Sports Med* 2008;36(8):1604-1610.
11. Patzer T, Habermeyer P, Hurschler C, et al: Increased glenohumeral translation and biceps load after SLAP lesions with potential influence on glenohumeral chondral lesions: A biomechanical study on human cadavers. *Knee Surg Sports Traumatol Arthrosc* 2011;19(10):1780-1787.
12. Cooper DE, Arnoczky SP, O'Brien SJ, Warren RF, DiCarlo E, Allen AA: Anatomy, histology, and vascularity of the glenoid labrum: An anatomical study. *J Bone Joint Surg Am* 1992;74(1): 46-52.
13. Clavert P, Bonnomet F, Kempf JF, Boutemy P, Braun M, Kahn JL: Contributions to the study of pathogenesis of type II superior labrum anterior-posterior lesions:

A cadaveric model of a fall on an outstretched hand. *J Shoulder Elbow Surg* 2004;13:45-50.

14. Burkhart SS, Morgan CD: The peel-back mechanism: Its role in producing and extending posterior type II SLAP lesions and its effect on SLAP repair rehabilitation. *Arthroscopy* 1998;14(6): 637-640.
15. Kuhn JE, Lindholm SR, Huston LJ, Soslowsky LJ, Blasier RB: Failure of the biceps superior labral complex: A cadaveric biomechanical investigation comparing the late cocking and early deceleration positions of throwing. *Arthroscopy* 2003;19(4):373-379.
16. Burkhart SS, Morgan CD, Kibler WB: The disabled throwing shoulder: Spectrum of pathology: Part I. Pathoanatomy and biomechanics. *Arthroscopy* 2003;19(4): 404-420.
17. Taylor DC, Arciero RA: Pathologic changes associated with shoulder dislocations: Arthroscopic and physical examination findings in first-time, traumatic anterior dislocations. *Am J Sports Med* 1997;25(3):306-311.
18. Yiannakopoulos CK, Mataragas E, Antonogiannakis E: A comparison of the spectrum of intra-articular lesions in acute and chronic anterior shoulder instability. *Arthroscopy* 2007;23(9):985-990.
19. Antonio GE, Griffith JF, Yu AB, Yung PS, Chan KM, Ahuja AT: First-time shoulder dislocation: High prevalence of labral injury and age-related differences revealed by MR arthrography. *J Magn Reson Imaging* 2007;26(4): 983-991.
20. te Slaa RL, Brand R, Marti RK: A prospective arthroscopic study of acute first-time anterior shoulder dislocation in the young: A five-year follow-up study. *J Shoulder Elbow Surg* 2003;12(6):529-534.
21. Hantes ME, Venouziou AI, Liantsis AK, Dailiana ZH, Malizos KN: Arthroscopic repair for chronic anterior shoulder instability: A comparative study between patients with Bankart lesions and patients with combined Bankart and superior labral anterior posterior lesions. *Am J Sports Med* 2009;37(6):1093-1098.
22. Snyder SJ, Karzel RP, Del Pizzo W, Ferkel RD, Friedman MJ: SLAP lesions of the shoulder. *Arthroscopy* 1990;6(4):274-279.
23. Morgan CD, Burkhart SS, Palmeri M, Gillespie M: Type II SLAP lesions: Three subtypes and their relationships to superior instability and rotator cuff tears. *Arthroscopy* 1998;14(6):553-565.
24. Powell SE: The diagnosis, classification, and treatment of SLAP lesions. *Oper Tech Sports Med* 2004;12:99-110.
25. Maffet MW, Gartsman GM, Moseley B: Superior labrum-biceps tendon complex lesions of the shoulder. *Am J Sports Med* 1995; 23(1):93-98.
26. Takase K: Risk of motion loss with combined Bankart and SLAP repairs. *Orthopedics* 2009;32(8).
27. Gartsman GM, Roddey TS, Hammerman SM: Arthroscopic treatment of anterior-inferior glenohumeral instability: Two to five-year follow-up. *J Bone Joint Surg Am* 2000;82(7):991-1003.
28. Cho HL, Lee CK, Hwang TH, Suh KT, Park JW: Arthroscopic repair of combined Bankart and SLAP lesions: Operative techniques and clinical results. *Clin Orthop Surg* 2010;2(1):39-46.
29. Segmüller HE, Hayes MG, Saies AD: Arthroscopic repair of glenolabral injuries with an absorbable fixation device. *J Shoulder Elbow Surg* 1997;6(4):383-392.
30. Kibler WB: Specificity and sensitivity of the anterior slide test in throwing athletes with superior glenoid labral tears. *Arthroscopy* 1995;11(3):296-300.
31. Liu SH, Henry MH, Nuccion SL: A prospective evaluation of a new physical examination in predicting glenoid labral tears. *Am J Sports Med* 1996;24(6):721-725.
32. O'Brien SJ, Pagnani MJ, Fealy S, McGlynn SR, Wilson JB: The active compression test: A new and effective test for diagnosing labral tears and acromioclavicular joint abnormality. *Am J Sports Med* 1998;26(5):610-613.
33. Kim SH, Ha KI, Han KY: Biceps load test: A clinical test for superior labrum anterior and posterior lesions in shoulders with recurrent anterior dislocations. *Am J Sports Med* 1999;27(3):300-303.
34. Mimori K, Muneta T, Nakagawa T, Shinomiya K: A new pain provocation test for superior labral tears of the shoulder. *Am J Sports Med* 1999;27(2):137-142.
35. Kim SH, Ha KI, Ahn JH, Kim SH, Choi HJ: Biceps load test II: A clinical test for SLAP lesions of the shoulder. *Arthroscopy* 2001; 17(2):160-164.
36. Hamner DL, Pink MM, Jobe FW: A modification of the relocation test: Arthroscopic findings associated with a positive test. *J Shoulder Elbow Surg* 2000;9(4): 263-267.
37. Myers TH, Zemanovic JR, Andrews JR: The resisted supination external rotation test: A new test for the diagnosis of superior labral anterior posterior lesions. *Am J Sports Med* 2005;33(9):1315-1320.
38. Nakagawa S, Yoneda M, Hayashida K, Obata M, Fukushima S, Miyazaki Y: Forced shoulder abduction and elbow flexion test: A new simple clinical test to detect superior labral injury in the throwing shoulder. *Arthroscopy* 2005;21(11):1290-1295.
39. Kim YS, Kim JM, Ha KY, Choy S, Joo MW, Chung YG: The passive compression test: A new clinical test for superior labral tears of the shoulder. *Am J Sports Med* 2007;35(9):1489-1494.
40. Ebinger N, Magosch P, Lichtenberg S, Habermeyer P: A new

SLAP test: The supine flexion resistance test. *Arthroscopy* 2008; 24(5):500-505.

41. Schlechter JA, Summa S, Rubin BD: The passive distraction test: A new diagnostic aid for clinically significant superior labral pathology. *Arthroscopy* 2009;25(12): 1374-1379.
42. Jones GL, Galluch DB: Clinical assessment of superior glenoid labral lesions: A systematic review. *Clin Orthop Relat Res* 2007;455: 45-51.
43. Dessaur WA, Magarey ME: Diagnostic accuracy of clinical tests for superior labral anterior posterior lesions: A systematic review. *J Orthop Sports Phys Ther* 2008;38(6): 341-352.
44. McFarland EG, Tanaka MJ, Garzon-Muvdi J, Jia X, Petersen SA: Clinical and imaging assessment for superior labrum anterior and posterior lesions. *Curr Sports Med Rep* 2009;8(5):234-239.
45. Savoie FH III, Holt MS, Field LD, Ramsey JR: Arthroscopic management of posterior instability: Evolution of technique and results. *Arthroscopy* 2008;24(4): 389-396.
46. Chang D, Mohana-Borges A, Borso M, Chung CB: SLAP lesions: Anatomy, clinical presentation, MR imaging diagnosis and characterization. *Eur J Radiol* 2008;68(1):72-87.
47. Lin E: Magnetic resonance arthrography of superior labrum anterior-posterior lesions: A practical approach to interpretation. *Curr Probl Diagn Radiol* 2009; 38(2):91-97.
48. Waldt S, Metz S, Burkart A, et al: Variants of the superior labrum and labro-bicipital complex: A comparative study of shoulder specimens using MR arthrography, multi-slice CT arthrography and anatomical dissection. *Eur Radiol* 2006;16(2):451-458.
49. Kim YJ, Choi JA, Oh JH, Hwang SI, Hong SH, Kang HS: Superior labral anteroposterior tears: Accuracy and interobserver reliability of multidetector CT arthrography for diagnosis. *Radiology* 2011; 260(1):207-215.
50. Gartsman GM, Hammerman SM: Superior labrum, anterior and posterior lesions: When and how to treat them. *Clin Sports Med* 2000;19(1):115-124.
51. Boileau P, Parratte S, Chuinard C, Roussanne Y, Shia D, Bicknell R: Arthroscopic treatment of isolated type II SLAP lesions: Biceps tenodesis as an alternative to reinsertion. *Am J Sports Med* 2009; 37(5):929-936.
52. DaSilva MA, Cole BJ: Arthroscopic superior labrum anterior to posterior repair. *Oper Tech Orthop* 2008;18:53-61.
53. Kim SH, Ha KI, Kim SH, Choi HJ: Results of arthroscopic treatment of superior labral lesions. *J Bone Joint Surg Am* 2002;84(6): 981-985.
54. Kaisidis A, Pantos P, Heger H, Bochlos D: Arthroscopic fixation of isolated type II SLAP lesions using a two-portal technique. *Acta Orthop Belg* 2011;77(2):160-166.
55. Neuman BJ, Boisvert CB, Reiter B, Lawson K, Ciccotti MG, Cohen SB: Results of arthroscopic repair of type II superior labral anterior posterior lesions in overhead athletes: Assessment of return to preinjury playing level and satisfaction. *Am J Sports Med* 2011;39(9):1883-1888.
56. Yung PS, Fong DT, Kong MF, et al: Arthroscopic repair of isolated type II superior labrum anterior-posterior lesion. *Knee Surg Sports Traumatol Arthrosc* 2008;16(12): 1151-1157.
57. Cohen DB, Coleman S, Drakos MC, et al: Outcomes of isolated type II SLAP lesions treated with arthroscopic fixation using a bioabsorbable tack. *Arthroscopy* 2006; 22(2):136-142.
58. Ide J, Maeda S, Takagi K: Sports activity after arthroscopic superior labral repair using suture anchors in overhead-throwing athletes. *Am J Sports Med* 2005;33(4):507-514.
59. Samani JE, Marston SB, Buss DD: Arthroscopic stabilization of type II SLAP lesions using an absorbable tack. *Arthroscopy* 2001; 17(1):19-24.
60. Duthcheshen NT: Superior labrum anterior posterior lesions in the overhead athlete: Current options for treatment. *Oper Tech Sports Med* 2007;15:96-104.
61. Baker CL III, Romeo AA: Combined arthroscopic repair of a type IV SLAP tear and Bankart lesion. *Arthroscopy* 2009;25(9): 1045-1050.
62. Gregush RV, Snyder SJ: Superior labral repair. *Sports Med Arthrosc* 2007;15(4):222-229.
63. Kim DS, Yi CH, Yoon YS: Arthroscopic repair for combined Bankart and superior labral anterior posterior lesions: A comparative study between primary and recurrent anterior dislocation in the shoulder. *Int Orthop* 2011; 35(8):1187-1195.
64. Lo IK, Burkhart SS: Triple labral lesions: Pathology and surgical repair technique-report of seven cases. *Arthroscopy* 2005;21(2): 186-193.
65. Warner JJ, Kann S, Marks P: Arthroscopic repair of combined Bankart and superior labral detachment anterior and posterior lesions: Technique and preliminary results. *Arthroscopy* 1994; 10(4):383-391.
66. Arciero RA, Taylor DC: Primary anterior dislocation of the shoulder in young patients: A ten-year prospective study. *J Bone Joint Surg Am* 1998;80(2):299-300.
67. DeBerardino TM, Arciero RA, Taylor DC, Uhorchak JM: Prospective evaluation of arthroscopic

stabilization of acute, initial anterior shoulder dislocations in young athletes: Two- to five-year follow-up. *Am J Sports Med* 2001; 29(5):586-592.

68. Arciero RA, Wheeler JH, Ryan JB, McBride JT: Arthroscopic Bankart repair versus nonoperative treatment for acute, initial anterior shoulder dislocations. *Am J Sports Med* 1994;22(5):589-594.
69. Habermeyer P, Gleyze P, Rickert M: Evolution of lesions of the labrum-ligament complex in posttraumatic anterior shoulder instability: A prospective study. *J Shoulder Elbow Surg* 1999;8(1): 66-74.

46

Sports Hip Injuries: Assessment and Management

Bryan T. Kelly, MD
Travis G. Maak, MD
Christopher M. Larson, MD
Asheesh Bedi, MD
Ira Zaltz, MD

Abstract

Over the past 10 years, the understanding, assessment, and management of hip pain and injuries in the athlete have improved. Traditionally, the evaluation of hip pain and injuries was limited to obvious disorders, such as hip arthritis and fractures, or disorders that were previously considered to be simply soft-tissue strains and contusions, such as groin pulls, hip pointers, and bursitis. Two parallel tracks of progress have improved understanding of the complexities of hip joint athletic injuries and the biomechanical basis of early hip disease. In the field of sports medicine, improved diagnostic skills now allow better interpretation of debilitating intra-articular hip disorders and their effects on core performance. In the field of hip preservation, there has been an evolution in understanding the effects of biomechanical mismatches between the femoral head and the acetabulum on the development of early hip damage, injury, and arthritis. The integration of these two parallel fields has accelerated the understanding of the importance of hip biomechanics and early hip injury in human performance and function.

Instr Course Lect 2013;62:515-531.

This chapter reviews contemporary concepts for assessing and managing athletic hip injuries within a sport-specific framework. Common injury patterns in contact sports, throwing and swinging sports, running and cutting sports, dance and gymnastics, as well as developmental hip injuries in pediatric athletes, are discussed. Assessment and treatment guidelines are provided for athletes with symptomatic labral pathology and impingement, traumatic subluxations and dislocations, chondral injuries to the hip joint, muscular contusions and strains, stress fractures, abductor injuries, snapping hip syndromes, dysplasia, the hypermobile hip, and apophyseal avulsion injuries in pediatric athletes.

Hip Injuries in the Contact Athlete

Femoroacetabular Impingement

Basic Principles

Femoroacetabular impingement (FAI) of the hip joint is a well-documented disorder caused by cam impingement (abnormal sphericity of the femoral head), rim impingement (an excessive anterolateral acetabular bony prominence), or a combination of these pathologies.[1] FAI has been associated with injuries such as labral tears, chondral delamination, and osteoarthrosis.[1-4] Cam-type impingement is most often seen in the young male athlete.[5,6] This impingement occurs with flexion and

Dr. Kelly or an immediate family member serves as a paid consultant to or is an employee of Smith & Nephew; serves as an unpaid consultant to Pivot Medical and A2 Surgical; has received research or institutional support from Pivot Medical; and owns stock or stock options in Pivot Medical and A3 Surgical. Dr. Larson or an immediate family member serves as a paid consultant to or is an employee of Smith & Nephew and A2 Surgical and owns stock or stock options in A3 Surgical. Dr. Bedi or an immediate family member serves as a board member, owner, officer, or committee member of the American Orthopaedic Society for Sports Medicine and the American Academy of Orthopaedic Surgeons; serves as a paid consultant to or is an employee of Biomimetics Therapeutics and Smith & Nephew; and owns stock or stock options in A3 Surgical. Dr. Zaltz or an immediate family member has received research or institutional support from DePuy. Neither Dr. Maak nor any immediate family member has received anything of value from or owns stock in a commercial company or institution related directly or indirectly to the subject of this chapter.

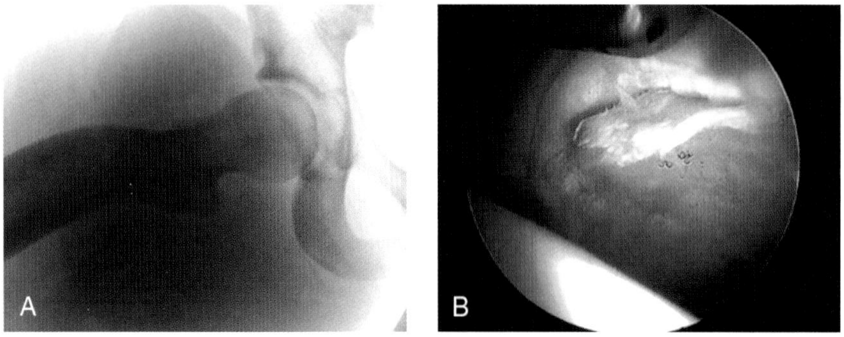

Figure 1 **A,** Dunn lateral radiographic view of an aspheric femoral head consistent with a cam lesion. **B,** Intra-articular arthroscopic image of a chondrolabral separation and a transition zone with cartilage delamination.

internal rotation of the hip joint, which forces the prominent femoral head-neck junction into contact with the anterolateral aspect of the acetabular chondrolabral junction. Repeated impingement results in increased shear and direct impact forces, with subsequent intrasubstance labral tears, chondrolabral separation, chondral delamination, and intrasubstance labral ossification[7] (**Figure 1**).

In contrast to cam impingement, rim impingement more commonly occurs in middle-aged female athletes.[5,6] Rim impingement results from increased anterolateral acetabular overcoverage that leads to a similar reduction in the functional hip flexion arc and subsequent impingement on the anterolateral femoral head-neck junction. Excessive global acetabular retroversion, coxa profunda, and protrusio have also been identified as contributors to this impingement mechanism.[5,6] Resultant trauma to the anterior labrum and direct trauma from the femoral head contrecoup impact on the posteroinferior acetabular cartilage may occur.[5,6] Because a combination of mixed cam- and rim-type impingements can occur, both types should be considered when impingement is suspected as the etiology of hip pain in an athlete.[5]

Assessment

The patient's history, physical examination findings, and a focused diagnostic evaluation are used to guide management decisions and optimize treatment outcomes. The typical patient with FAI reports groin pain, specifically with hip hyperflexion.[5] Functional activities of the hip, including standing from a sitting position, climbing stairs, extensive ambulation, or athletic participation, may exacerbate or precipitate groin pain.[5,6,8,9] Mechanical symptoms, including clicking, popping, and catching with hip motion, may also occur.

A focused physical examination should assess range of motion, strength, and stability of the involved hip and the contralateral asymptomatic extremity. A finding of limited internal rotation with the hip flexed to 90° is particularly important. An impingement test should be conducted using passive hip hyperflexion, adduction, and internal rotation, which re-create the most common pathologic position of FAI. The test is positive if the maneuver elicits pain that is identical to that experienced with FAI. Other provocative tests also have been described to assess areas of atypical bony impingement.[10,11]

The diagnostic evaluation for FAI should include an AP pelvic radiograph and an elongated neck or modified Dunn lateral view of the affected hip.[12] A false profile view should be obtained if there is suspicion for concomitant underlying dysplasia. These radiographs allow evaluation of acetabular version and identification of the crossover sign, in which the superolateral border of the anterior wall of the acetabulum can be seen intersecting or crossing over the inferomedial border of the posterior wall.[13] The Dunn view allows improved evaluation of the femoral head-neck geometry, identification of the cam-type lesion, and calculation of an alpha angle, which estimates the severity of the impingement.

MRI with or without gadolinium contrast of the affected hip will allow accurate delineation of the periarticular soft-tissue structures, including the femoral and acetabular chondral surface, labrum, capsule, and surrounding extra-articular tendinous insertions. CT with three-dimensional reconstruction and femoral version analysis provides a more detailed analysis of the proximal femoral and acetabular geometry. A fluoroscopically guided, intra-articular, analgesic and steroid injection can be used as a diagnostic and therapeutic tool along with the patient's history and physical examination. This diagnostic tool can be extremely effective in differentiating between intra-articular and extra-articular hip pathology.

Treatment Guidelines

Nonsurgical management of FAI includes oral nonsteroidal anti-inflammatory drugs (NSAIDs), physical therapy, and intra-articular analgesic/steroidal injections. Nonsurgical management is often ineffective in patients with an identifiable pathology because patients with FAI are typically young, active, and have a mechanical pathology.[6]

Surgical treatment includes acetabuloplasty, femoral head osteoplasty, chondroplasty, labral resection, and repair through both open and arthroscopic approaches.[14] Arthroscopic treatment of FAI has become increasingly popular because it is a minimally invasive approach and provides good visualization (**Figure 2**). The indications for choosing an arthroscopic versus an open surgical approach depend on a thorough understanding of the size and location of the mechanical deformity and the expertise of the treating surgeon.

Several studies have documented excellent early results with open and arthroscopic management of FAI.[15-17] Early data suggested that labral and acetabular rim resection achieved better results compared with labral resection alone.[15] A more recent study has suggested that labral preservation with refixation and acetabular rim débridement may provide superior results.[16] This technique is the preferred method of this chapter's authors.

Video 46.1: Arthroscopic Management of Pincer- and Cam-Type Femoroacetabular Impingement. Christopher M. Larson, MD; Rebecca M. Stone, ATC (7 min)

Rehabilitation and Return to Play

Focused rehabilitation after open or arthroscopic treatment of FAI will improve postoperative range of motion and strength and reduce pain and the time needed to return to play. The rehabilitation regimen should begin immediately after surgery. The patient should maintain 20-lb, foot-flat weight-bearing status with crutch assistance for the first 2 postoperative weeks if a femoral head-neck osteoplasty is performed or 4 to 6 weeks if a chondral repair including microfracture is performed. Early rehabilitation should focus on maximizing passive range of motion, reducing any soft-tissue irritation, and allowing postoperative healing of the periarticular structures. Strength training typically begins after 4 weeks, but care is taken to avoid overly aggressive protocols to minimize the risk for soft-tissue inflammation and tendinitis. Strength, coordination, reaction time, and proprioception are assessed at regular intervals postoperatively. Return to athletic participation is recommended only after the affected hip approaches 90% of the condition of the contralateral extremity. Impact activities should not be permitted for a minimum of 3 to 4 months to allow completion of osseous remodeling, especially after femoral head-neck osteoplasty.

Subluxation and Dislocation

Basic Principles

Posterior hip instability ranges from subluxation to frank dislocation. The most common traumatic mechanism of injury during athletic competition is a fall with a posteriorly directed force onto a flexed and adducted hip.[18-20] Atraumatic and lower energy mechanisms of hip instability also have been described.[11,21,22] Hip dislocations have been reported in American football, skiing, rugby, gymnastics, jogging, basketball, biking, and soccer.[11,21,22]

In the athlete with FAI, the functional range of motion required in athletic competition is often greater than the limited physiologic motion allowed by the cam and/or pincer lesions. Attempts to increase flexion and internal rotation can result in anterior engagement between the cam lesion and the anterior acetabulum, which levers the femoral head posteriorly. This levering can lead to failure of the posterior soft-tissue and osseous structures, a posterior acetabular rim fracture, and/or a posterior capsulolabral tear in addition to a crush injury to the anterior labrum[18,23] (**Figure 3**). In certain instances, a posterior hip subluxation or dislocation may be the first manifestation of occult FAI in competitive athletes.[24] Increased levering forces during athletic competition could result in hip subluxation.

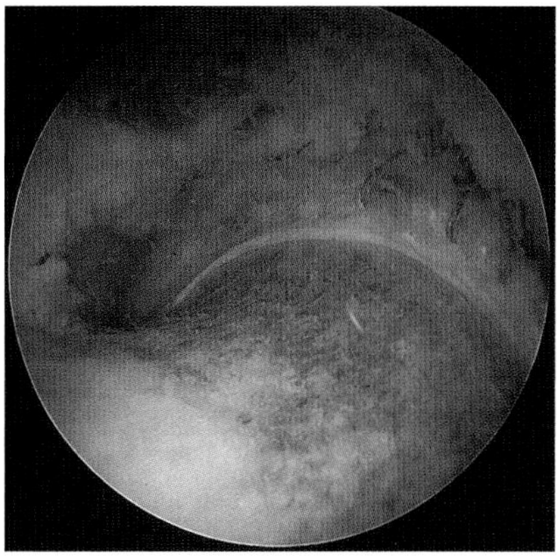

Figure 2 Arthroscopic image showing the spherical contour of the femoral head at the head-neck junction in a patient treated with cam lesion decompression.

Assessment

Patients present with painful limitation of hip motion and often report discomfort in the hip when at rest. A high index of suspicion is needed to avoid missing this injury, which is often misdiagnosed as a muscle strain.[11,18,19-22,25] Careful assessment of the injury mechanism is important. Although a fall on a flexed knee is the most commonly described mechanism, forceful impact on a hyperextended, internally rotated knee can result in posterior hip subluxation in the athlete with underlying limited internal rotation.

Unrecognized posterior subluxation of the hip with subsequent osteonecrosis can be a devastating injury.[26] The classic triad of findings after posterior hip subluxation as Moorman et al[19] described in eight American football

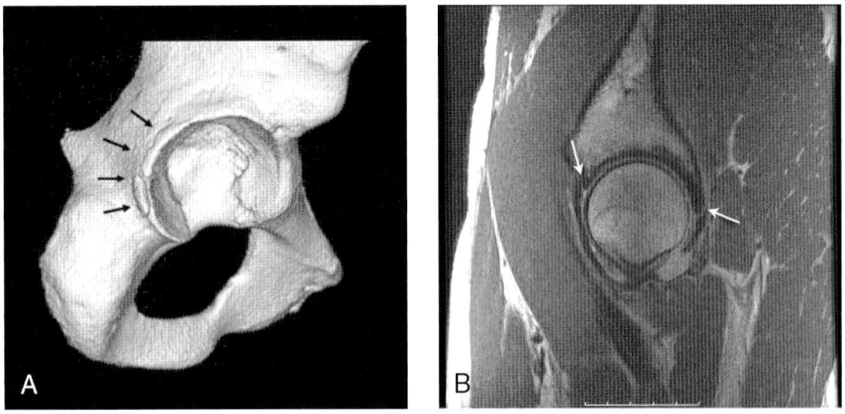

Figure 3 **A,** Three-dimensional CT scan of a patient who is a lacrosse player who sustained a posterior hip subluxation with a posterior rim fracture (arrows). **B,** MRI scan showing injury to the posterior labrum with concomitant crushing of the anterior labrum. Arrows indicate the posterior acetabular rim fracture.

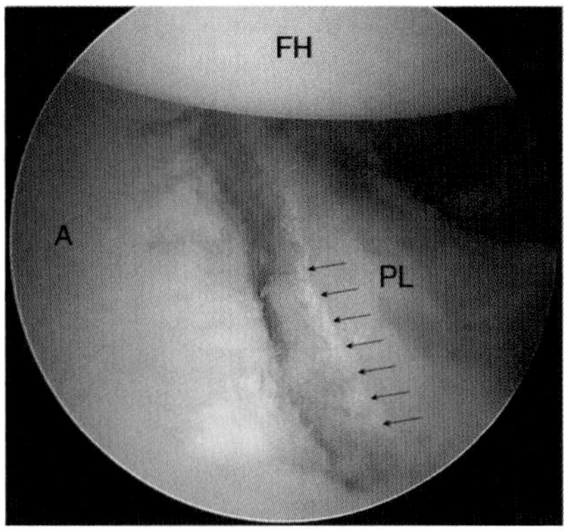

Figure 4 Arthroscopic image showing a posterior labral tear (arrows) with the associated bony avulsion attached to the labral fragment. FH = femoral head, A = anterior, PL = posterior labrum.

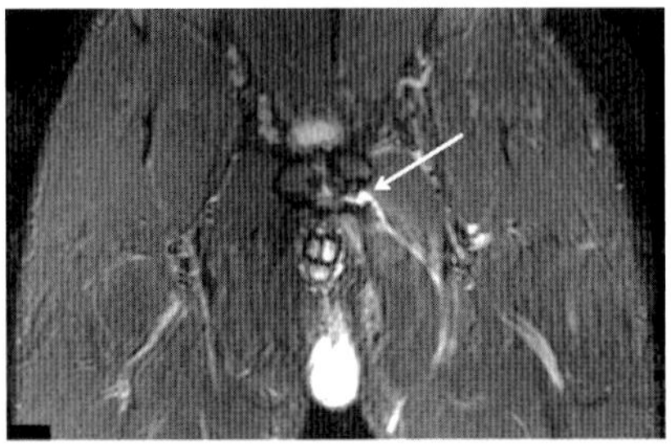

Figure 5 Coronal MRI scan of the thigh of a 23-year-old man who is a National Hockey League player shows an acute proximal adductor longus rupture (arrow). The injury was treated nonsurgically and resulted in return to play without restrictions.

players included hemarthrosis, iliofemoral ligament disruption, and posterior acetabular hip fractures (**Figure 4**). Supine AP pelvic, Dunn lateral, and Judet plain radiographs should be obtained for athletes with suspected hip subluxation. CT is helpful in identifying small, posterior, bony acetabular hip avulsions and is also helpful in assessing underlying impingement or dysplasia. MRI is important for evaluating injury to the capsule, ligamentum teres, and labrum and identifying loose bodies and translational sheer injuries to the articular cartilage.

Treatment Guidelines

In the presence of substantial hemarthrosis, fluoroscopically guided aspiration helps decompress the joint, reduces pain, and may reduce the risk for subsequent osteonecrosis. Protected weight bearing for 2 to 6 weeks is recommended depending on the size and location of the acetabular lip fracture. Early surgical intervention is required if the bony fragment renders the hip unstable, if there are loose fragments in the central compartment that may result in third-body wear injury to the articular cartilage, or if the labrum is incarcerated in the joint, resulting in nonconcentric joint reduction. If after a course of protected weight bearing followed by progressive strengthening and attempts at a functional return to sports there is persistent pain or a sense of instability, surgery should be delayed. If either early or delayed surgery is required, any underlying, predisposing structural abnormality should be treated concurrently.

Return to Play

Athletes are allowed to return to play after radiographic union of the acetabular lip fragment and after progression to asymptomatic full strength and range of motion. A progression to sport-specific activities in a supervised environment is advised to ensure that there is no residual instability or pain.

Myotendinous Injuries About the Hip and the Pelvis

Myotendinous injuries of the hip and the pelvis in athletes are increasingly being recognized. Optimal physical conditioning and full recovery from injury prior to game situations can reduce the risk of preseason hip and groin injuries. Risks are often elevated because of the reduced schedule of off-season training. Most myotendinous injuries are treated with activity modification, ice, analgesic agents, and a gradual resumption of athletic activity after the restoration of functional strength. The roles for physical therapy and platelet-rich plasma injections are evolving, but studies are lacking on their efficacy in treating acute and chronic myotendinous injuries. Some specific injuries deserve special attention.

Proximal Adductor Injuries

Adductor strains are common in athletes who participate in cutting and pivoting sports and ice hockey. Acute injuries involving the adductor longus (**Figure 5**) are typically self-limiting; however, chronic, athletic-related, proximal adductor pain has been associated with underlying FAI in up to 94% of athletes.[27] Chronic, recalcitrant, proximal adductor pain can be treated with surgical tenotomy, which provides pain relief and allows return to sports for most athletes. Complete proximal adductor ruptures have been reported in athletes. Although both surgical and nonsurgical treatments have been recommended, a National Football League study reported a quicker return to sports activity (6 weeks versus 3 months) after nonsurgical treatment, with all patients returning to play regardless of the treatment.[28]

Rectus Femoris Injuries

Rectus femoris strain typically results from sprinting or kicking. This injury can involve the central or the peripheral tendon. Greater disability is reported with central tendon involvement, which can lead to a painful proximal mass that in rare instances may require surgical excision. Heterotopic bone formation and chronic healed anterior inferior iliac spine (AIIS) avulsions can lead to subspine/AIIS impingement (**Figure 6**). This injury can result in pain and limited hip flexion that may require decompression of the AIIS. Complete proximal rectus femoris avulsions also occur. A study by Gamradt el al[29] reported on the nonsurgical treatment of 11 professional athletes with proximal avulsions of the rectus femoris. All the athletes returned to play within 6 to 12 weeks.

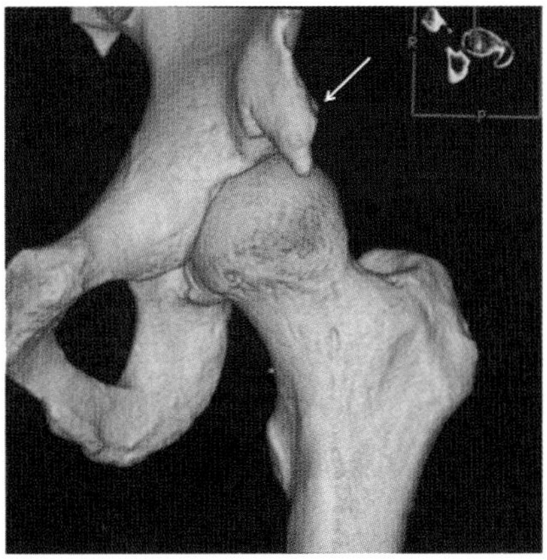

Figure 6 Three-dimensional CT scan of a man who is a National Football League player who previously sustained a proximal rectus femoris rupture. The scan shows ossification of the rectus origin (arrow), which resulted in subspine AIIS impingement, associated hip flexion limitations, and pain. The inset shows a two-dimensional axial view of the involved hip. After arthroscopic decompression of the AIIS, the athlete returned to play without limitations or pain.

Proximal Hamstring Injuries

Proximal hamstring strains can lead to prolonged periods of disability compared with middle and distal myotendinous injuries. Chronic proximal hamstring tendinopathy is commonly seen in distance runners. For the rare recalcitrant injury, semimembranosus tenotomy or proximal hamstring débridement and repair can be considered.[30] Acute, complete, proximal hamstring ruptures occur infrequently but require a high index of suspicion for diagnosis (**Figure 7**). Patients with MRI evidence of a complete two- or three-tendon proximal rupture with greater than 2 cm retraction may benefit from early surgical repair to avoid long-term deficits in strength and athletic disability.[31,32] Distal fractional lengthening and repair and, more recently, proximal hamstring reconstruction with allograft have resulted in improved strength and function for patients with symptomatic chronic proximal hamstring ruptures.[31]

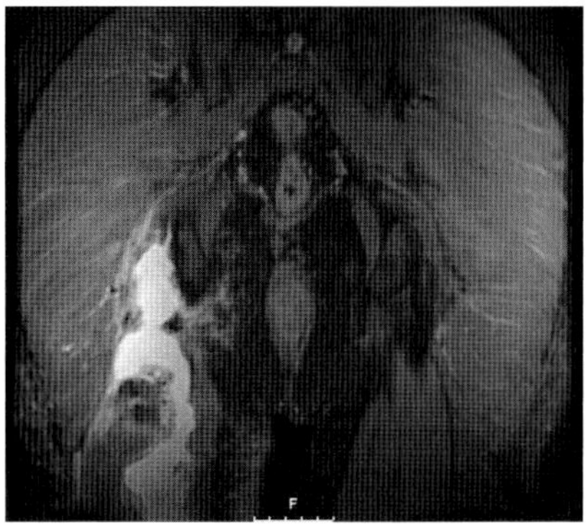

Figure 7 Coronal MRI scan of a 36-year-old patient who sustained an injury while water skiing shows a complete proximal hamstring avulsion. The avulsion was surgically repaired 2 weeks after injury.

Other Muscle Strain Injuries

Although injuries can involve virtually any muscle about the hip and pelvis, some injury patterns identified on physical examination or MRI should alert the clinician to seek a secondary cause of the athlete's pain. Signal change in the psoas adjacent to the hip capsule may indicate prior anterior hip subluxation. Signal change in the posterior hip musculature adjacent to the capsule may be indicative of a posterior hip subluxation. It should be recognized that recurrent or chronic myotendinous injuries about the hip and pelvis may be associated with athletic pubalgia (also called sports hernia) or other compensatory injuries secondary to underlying intra-articular hip disorders.

Contusions About the Hip and Pelvis

Quadriceps Contusions

Quadriceps contusions typically result from a direct blow to the quadriceps muscle that crushes the deep muscula-

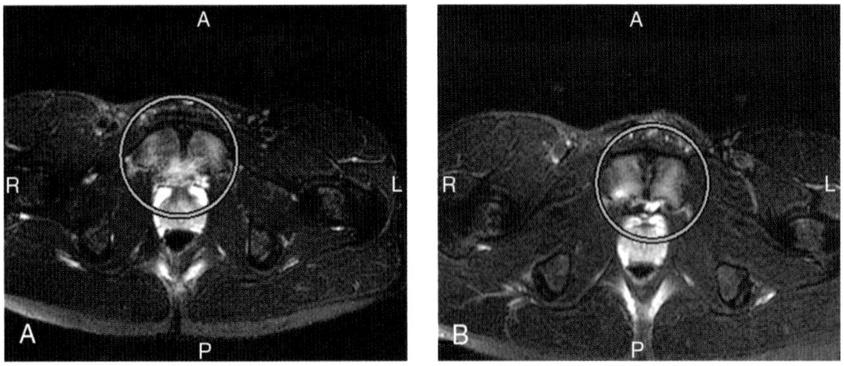

Figure 8 **A** and **B,** Axial MRI scans showing high signal intensity in the pubis secondary to stress overload of the pubic symphysis associated with osteitis pubis. Bone marrow edema in the pubic symphysis caused by osteitis pubis is shown in the circled areas.

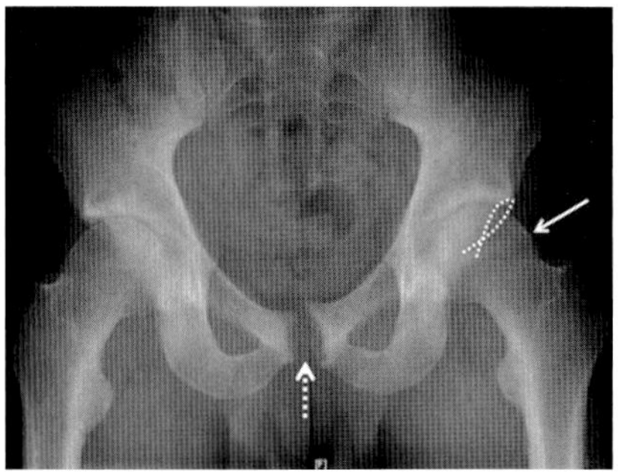

Figure 9 AP radiograph of the pelvis of a 23-year-old patient who is a collegiate soccer player shows osteitis pubis (dashed arrow), acetabular retroversion (dotted loop), and cam-type morphology of the proximal femur (solid arrow). The patient was treated with an arthroscopic procedure to correct FAI and concomitant athletic pubalgia/sports hernia repair.

ture against the femur. Studies have shown a decrease in disability time when patients are treated with a focused knee-flexion protocol.[33,34] A study of 47 naval midshipmen with quadriceps contusions showed that passively flexing the knee to 120° within 10 minutes of injury and holding that position for 24 hours resulted in a mean disability time of 3.5 days.[33] Aggressive stretching and heat producing modalities should be avoided. The area of injury should be padded to decrease the risk for further injury and myositis ossificans.

Hip Pointers

Hip pointers result from a contusion to the iliac crest, which is protected only by a layer of subcutaneous fat. Higher-level athletes may require acute management with an anesthetic injection to the iliac crest to continue sports participation in the same game or event. Padding the area until full recovery will minimize the risk of recurrent injury.

Morel-Lavallee Lesions

Morel-Lavallee lesions can occur in athletes as degloving of the skin and subcutaneous tissue from the neighboring fascia, with the peritrochanteric region at particular risk.[35] Initial treatment with compression and cryotherapy resolves up to 50% of these injuries. If this treatment fails, early aspiration, with or without doxycycline sclerodesis, can be curative.[35]

Athletic Pubalgia (Sports Hernia)

Definition and Presentation

Athletic pubalgia or sports hernia is defined as exertional lower abdominal pain with or without associated proximal adductor-related pain.[36,37] Athletes typically present with the insidious onset of increasing, exercise-induced, lower abdominal and/or adductor-related pain. The physical examination often reveals tenderness to palpation above the inguinal ligament over the abdominal obliques, transversus abdominis, and at the rectus abdominis/conjoined tendon. Pain also may be elicited over these structures with resisted sit-ups. Tenderness to palpation and with resisted adduction may be noted over the adductor, pectineus, and gracilis tendons.

Imaging Studies

Plain radiographs may be normal in patients with athletic pubalgia or may show evidence of osteitis pubis (**Figure 8**). Although MRI can be inconclusive, recent studies have noted that perisymphyseal edema, proximal adductor/gracilis/pectineus abnormalities, and disruptions of the rectus abdominis/adductor aponeurosis are consistent with athletic pubalgia[37] (**Figure 9**). In some instances, intra-articular hip pathology and athletic pubalgia can coexist. Imaging studies may show findings consistent with FAI, along with intra-articular labral and chondral abnormalities.[38]

Differential Diagnosis

The underlying pain generators associated with athletic-related hip and pelvic pain can be elusive; a multidisciplinary approach is often required to obtain a diagnosis. Athletic pubalgia and potential underlying intra-articular hip pathology are common findings. Other differential diagnoses include psoas disorders, pudendal neuralgia, sciatic nerve entrapment, upper lumbar discogenic pain, pelvic and proximal femoral stress fractures, and gastrointestinal and genitourinary disorders. Diagnostic anesthetic injections into the hip joint, pubic symphysis, psoas bursa, and proximal adductors/pubic cleft followed by athletic activity or physical examination can help determine the source of the disability.

Treatment

Initial activity modification and a well-balanced rehabilitation program focusing on core stability should be implemented. The patient should avoid lifting heavy objects and perform low repetition, deep hip flexion weight training augmented with occasional corticosteroid injections into the pubic symphysis, adductor/pubic cleft, and hip joint. If conservative measures are unsuccessful, various surgical approaches for managing athletic pubalgia can decrease the time needed to return to athletic activity.[36,37] These approaches include broad pelvic floor repairs and modified hernia repairs, with or without adductor releases.[36,37]

FAI and Athletic Pubalgia

There is increasing evidence that symptoms of athletic pubalgia can develop in a subset of athletes from hip joint motion limitations secondary to FAI. Studies have shown an increased incidence of chronic groin pain and osteitis pubis in athletes with limited hip internal rotation.[39,40] One study reported that 94% of the athletes with long-standing proximal adductor-related pain had radiographic evidence of FAI.[27] A recent biomechanical study reported increased symphyseal motion in the presence of cam-type FAI, which could contribute to the development of osteitis pubis and athletic pubalgia.[41] In a study of athletes with both FAI and athletic pubalgia-related findings, surgical management resulted in a return to sports without limitations in 50% and 25% of the athletes after isolated FAI and sports hernia surgery, respectively.[38] Surgical management of both pathologies produced an 89% rate of return to sports without limitations.[38] It appears that motion limitations from FAI can lead to extra-articular compensatory patterns that result in athletic pubalgia in some athletes. These studies support an association between FAI and athletic pubalgia and emphasize the importance of managing both disorders in select patients to minimize the time lost from athletics and maximize successful outcomes.

Hip Injuries in the Overhead Athlete

Hip pathology associated with acetabular labral tears in the overhead athlete is an area of growing interest in the field of sports medicine. The mechanics of overhead sports, particularly throwing a baseball or a football, shooting a lacrosse ball, and hitting a tennis ball, may increase the potential for labral tears associated with FAI and instability. Axial and torsional forces under loading may predispose overhead athletes to traumatic labral pathology. The positional requirements and movement patterns of the athlete involved in overhead sports incorporate movements that can cause the bony deformities associated with FAI to abut the labrum and produce injury. These movement patterns also require excessive rotation that can lead to rotational instability. The labrum and capsuloligamentous structures are at risk for injury during different phases of the overhead activity.

FAI and laxity can be linked to intra-articular hip disorders, and the abnormal mechanics caused by these deformities may lead to altered movement patterns in the torso and upper extremity. Although upper extremity injuries are more common than hip injuries, pathologic stress on the torso, shoulder, and elbow may be a result of poor hip mechanics in overhead activities. One study examining pitching mechanics found that shoulder and elbow forces were substantially linked to pelvic rotation.[42] The importance of the lower extremity in generating forward momentum in throwing has been documented.[43] If optimal stride distance and lead leg foot placement does not occur because of decreased strength, restricted range of motion, pain, and/or apprehension in the lead or back hip, an overhead athlete will not properly generate torque from the pelvis and lower extremity. In pitching, leg drive is correlated with wrist velocity and is responsible for approximately 50% of the throwing velocity.[43,44] Similarly, more than 50% of the energy produced in a tennis serve is generated from the trunk and legs.[45] If this leg drive does not occur, the upper extremity may be responsible for generating a greater proportion of forces required for the overhead activity. The link between hip pathology, changes in movement pattern, and injury risk in the torso, shoulder, and elbow requires further study.

The basic assessment, treatment, and return-to-play guidelines for the overhead athlete with underlying hip impingement follow the previously outlined recommendations. The recognition of the hip as a potential contributor to upper extremity dysfunction in the overhead athlete should be considered in the complete evaluation of these athletes.

Hip Injuries in the Endurance Athlete

Stress Fractures of the Femoral Neck and the Pelvic Ring

Basic Principles

Although insufficiency fractures occur in elderly patients with osteoporosis because of inadequate bone mineral density and compressive and tensile strength, stress fractures in athletes are the result of excessive, repetitive, submaximal stresses experienced by physiologically normal bone. Many factors can contribute to an athlete's risk of

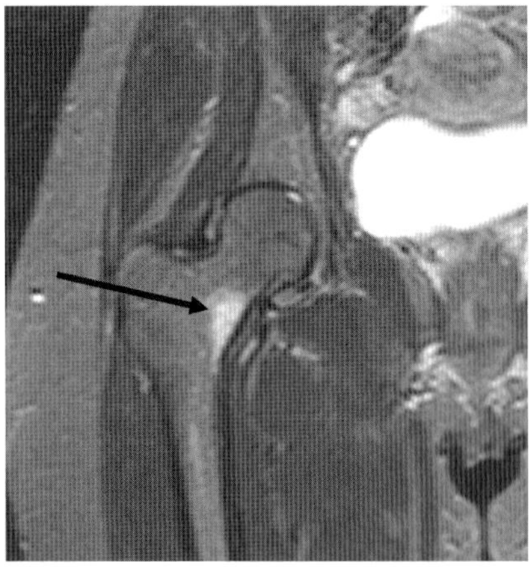

Figure 10 A coronal short tau inversion recovery image of the hip of a 45-year-old- woman with right hip pain 2 weeks after running a 5-km race shows increased signal intensity (arrow). This signal intensity pattern is consistent with an early-stage stress reaction fracture.

developing a stress fracture, including bone mineral density, bone vascularity, systemic factors (hormonal status, diet, collagen abnormalities, and metabolic bone disorders), and the type of sports activity. Muscular weakness or imbalance may also increase the risk for a stress fracture because excessive forces are concentrated on underlying bone.

Stress fractures can affect any endurance athlete but commonly occur in women.[46] Female endurance athletes attempt to minimize body fat to maintain a high level of athletic performance. With decreased body fat, estrogen levels decrease; this may lead to decreased bone mineral density and an increased risk of stress fractures. Male endurance athletes also are at risk for stress fractures because of a similar decrease in sex steroids (such as testosterone).[47] A decrease in testosterone results in increased activity in osteoclasts and subsequent bone resorption. The combination of paradoxical bone resorption and repetitive excessive loading greatly increases the risk of stress fractures.

Assessment

Patients with femoral neck or pelvic ring stress fractures typically report groin or pelvic pain that is exacerbated by weight bearing or intense activity and relieved by rest. This pain often occurs after an abrupt increase in the frequency, duration, or intensity of training, such as training for a marathon, a triathlon, or another endurance event. Patients may present with an antalgic gait. Although it is difficult to reproduce pain with palpation because of the overlying soft tissue, patients report pain with internal and external rotation at the extremes of hip range of motion. In patients with sacral insufficiency fractures, pain is elicited with flexion, abduction, and external rotation of the hip; there may be pelvic brim tenderness, but this finding is not sensitive because of the amount of soft tissue overlying the pelvis. If a sacral insufficiency fracture is suspected, careful neurologic examination is critical to detect nerve impingement from callus formation within and around neural foramina.

The radiographic location of the stress fracture guides treatment, especially with regard to the femoral neck. The location of a femoral neck stress fracture is classified as either tension sided (on the superior neck) or compression sided (on the inferior aspect of the femoral neck). Plain radiography is the first-line imaging modality, despite the fact that studies may be normal for 2 to 3 weeks after the onset of symptoms. Later radiographic studies may show periosteal reaction, cortical lucency, sclerosis, or a fracture line. Initial radiographs should include AP, AP pelvis, and lateral views of the affected hip.

Compression-type fractures show sclerotic thickening of the inferior cortex of the femoral neck, often with a hazy radiolucent center. Careful correlation with the patient history will differentiate this fracture from an osteoid osteoma, which may have a similar radiographic appearance. Tension-sided fractures appear as transverse and lucent and are perpendicular to the superior aspect of the femoral neck. The pelvis may be evaluated for contralateral hip pathology as well as stress fractures of the pelvic ring and sacrum. Inlet and outlet views of the pelvis may be used to evaluate the pelvic ring and sacrum.

Although nuclear imaging has been used in the past with success, axial imaging modalities are currently favored as the studies of choice after plain radiography.[48] With focal symptoms such as hip and groin pain, MRI can be used to directly evaluate the area of interest. MRI is advantageous because it can be used to rule out other differential diagnoses, including soft-tissue abnormalities. On MRI, stress fractures have decreased signal intensity on T1-weighted images and increased signal intensity on short tau inversion recovery and T2-weighted images (**Figure 10**).

Treatment Guidelines

Prior to treating the stress fracture locally, global abnormalities must be addressed. These include hormonal and nutritional deficiencies and the evaluation of connective tissue disease if clinically warranted. Activity modification is the mainstay of treatment for stress fractures of the femoral neck and the pelvis.

In compression-sided stress fractures of the inferior femoral neck, the bone is inherently stable and nonsurgical treatment is used. Displacement of compression-sided femoral neck stress fractures is extremely rare. Activity modification (with or without protected weight bearing) and expectant management are usually successful. Conversely, a tension-sided stress fracture should raise clinical concern because the biomechanical forces causing distraction at the fracture site increase the risk for the development of a displaced femoral neck fracture, with the possible complications of osteonecrosis, varus malunion, delayed union, and nonunion.[49] Initial management with internal fixation may avoid complications. Radiographic displacement is an indication for urgent percutaneous fixation with cannulated screws (**Figure 11**). Patients are typically managed with protected weight bearing for up to 12 weeks, which is guided by the resolution of symptoms and radiographic signs of healing.

Most patients with sacral and pelvic ring stress fractures are treated nonsurgically. Activity modification and close follow-up are the mainstays of treatment.

Rehabilitation and Return to Play

The patient's symptoms and radiographic signs of healing guide the full return to athletic activity. In patients with low-risk stress fractures about the hip and pelvic ring (compression-sided femoral neck, pelvic ring, and sacrum fractures), activity should be adjusted to attain a pain-free level for 4 to 8 weeks and is dependent on the severity of the symptoms and the injury. Crutches can be used for comfort, but weight bearing may be done as tolerated in uncomplicated injuries. As symptoms improve, patients can progress to light, low-impact physical activity and then to full activity if pain continues to decrease. This typically takes 3 to 6 weeks with low-grade lesions and up to 16 weeks with high-grade lesions.[50]

After patients with high-risk stress fractures (tension-sided fractures of the femoral neck) are stabilized surgically, they may return to play after symptoms have completely resolved and there is no pain with provocative examination maneuvers or with activities.[51] Follow-up radiography is typically helpful to assess hardware placement and radiographic healing.

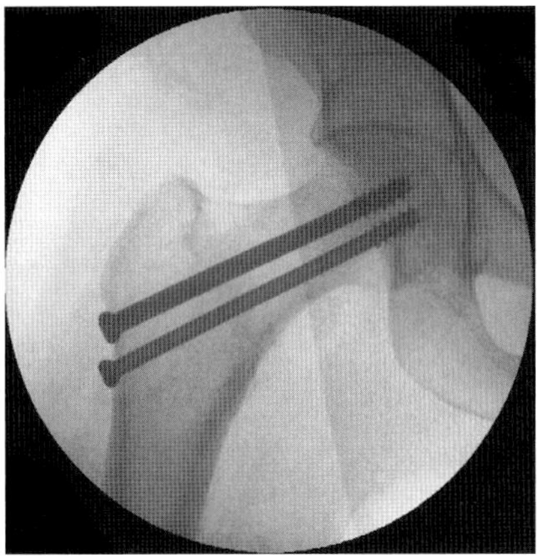

Figure 11 Fluoroscopic image of two percutaneous screws placed in the femoral neck of a 45-year-old patient who is a runner with a tension-sided stress fracture.

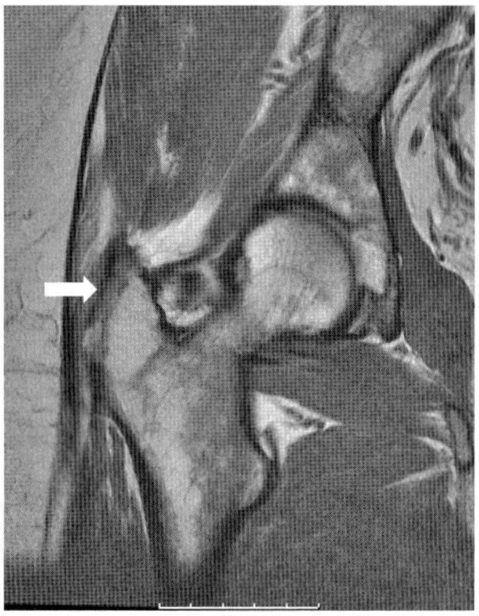

Figure 12 Coronal MRI scan of a high-grade tear of the anterolateral band insertion of the gluteus medius tendon (arrow) with adjacent soft-tissue edema. The gluteus minimus tendon is moderately degenerated.

Abductor Failure

Basic Principles

Hip abductor musculature is attached to the greater trochanter of the femur in a fashion analogous to the attachment of the rotator cuff to the shoulder. Acute and chronic injury to the gluteus medius and gluteus minimus can cause failure and tearing of the tendon insertions similar to that of a rotator cuff tear. These clinical entities, along with recalcitrant trochanteric bursitis, are referred to as greater trochanteric pain syndrome and have a peak occurrence between the fourth and sixth decades of life. This syndrome is four times more common in women than in men. Often, the initial pathology occurs in the tendinous insertions on the greater trochanter, with secondary involvement of the adjacent bursae because bursal distension is uncommon.[52-54]

Assessment

On presentation, patients report lateral hip pain centered over the greater trochanter. Occasionally, a patient may report a specific injury or a pop; however, this injury may also be chronic. Groin pain indicates a separate pathology that requires evaluation of the intra-articular pathology. On physical examination, patients typically report tenderness to palpation of the greater trochanter and either pain-limited or true weakness of the hip abductors depending on the size of the tear.

Although plain radiography is the initial study of choice to rule out osseus pathology, the diagnosis of abductor failure is largely based on MRI and ultrasound findings. In those with intractable greater trochanteric pain syndrome, 45% to 50% of patients have gluteus medius tendon tears demonstrated by MRI or ultrasound.[53,55] On MRI, these tears have high signal intensity on T2-weighted sequences and intermediate signal intensity on T1-weighted sequences (**Figure 12**).

Treatment Guidelines

Although most patients with greater trochanteric pain syndrome respond to

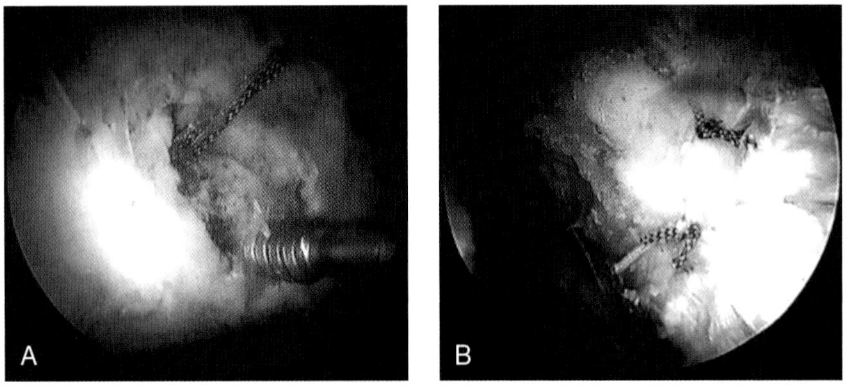

Figure 13 **A,** Arthroscopic image of a gluteus medius tear off the lateral facet with two suture anchors placed to restore the natural footprint. **B,** Arthroscopic image of the repair of the gluteus medius tendon with two double-loaded 5.5-mm peak anchors.

conservative management, recalcitrant pain is often caused by gluteus medius or minimus tendon tears. Surgical treatment may be considered if nonsurgical management (activity modification, physical therapy, and oral NSAIDs) for a minimum of 6 months is unsuccessful.

Both open and endoscopic surgical techniques have been described with good to excellent results in most patients.[56] Similar to rotator cuff repair in the shoulder, the tendon and footprint insertion may be débrided and repaired using suture anchors (**Figure 13**). In a prospective study of 10 patients treated with arthroscopic abductor repair with a minimum 2-year follow-up, all patients had complete resolution of pain in the lateral hip. Nine of the 10 patients (90%) had complete return of abductor strength based on manual muscle testing, 1 regained 80% abductor strength, and all of the patients maintained full hip range of motion. At 1-year follow-up, modified Harris hip scores and hip outcome scores normalized to 92 and 93 points, respectively.[57-59] All of the patients reported normal or nearly normal subjective hip function.[60]

Massive abductor tears with retraction are rare in this patient cohort and require open repair with tissue mobilization. Irreparable massive tears may be reconstructed with flap transfer of the gluteus maximus or allograft reconstruction.[61]

Rehabilitation and Return to Play

Postoperative rehabilitation after endoscopic repair consists of 6 weeks of crutch-protected weight bearing with 20 lb of pressure on the operative extremity. An abduction brace is used for 6 weeks to protect the repair from accidental trauma and stress. Gentle passive range of motion begins 1 week postoperatively, progressing to active range of motion and abductor strengthening at 6 weeks. Twelve weeks postoperatively, strengthening continues and sport-specific activities begin at 16 weeks. Running is allowed after abductor strength equals that of the unaffected side and is followed by full clearance for return to play.[60] A similar algorithm can be used for open repairs after surgical wound healing is stable. Return to play after nonsurgical management is guided by improvement in the patient's symptoms and begins with targeted physical therapy, strengthening, and progression of activities as tolerated.

Dysplasia and the Unstable Hip

Basic Principles

Understanding hip instability associated with dance and gymnastic sports illustrates the complex range of hip instability that may be related to specific maneuvers and exacerbated by acetabular and femoral malformations. Dance and gymnastic sports involve a complex combination of movements requiring extreme maximum, repetitive transverse, coronal, and sagittal plane range of motion. Passive range of motion data gathered from a large cohort of classic ballet dancers suggest that there is loss of hip motion with age that requires compensatory lumbar motion. This age-related motion loss may lead to increased stress on the hip in end motion.[62] Recent data suggest that certain motions, even in normal hip joints, produce leverage between various parts of the upper femur on either the acetabular rim or pelvis. Experiments with professional dancers using motion capture analysis showed femoroacetabular translation when the hip reached terminal motion.[63,64] Underlying acetabular malformations and variations in upper femoral morphology have an effect on the mechanical consequences of dance and gymnastic-like activities. Increased femoral anteversion or anterior acetabular hypoplasia can lead to increased strain within the acetabular labrum, especially when the hip is positioned repetitively in external rotation and abduction.[65] Increased strain is placed on the labra of dancers and gymnasts with mild underlying acetabular dysplasia who repetitively load the hip in extension.[66,67]

Assessment

Hip pain associated with activities similar to gymnastic sports or dance is challenging to diagnose and treat. The objective of the clinical and radiographic assessment is to establish the hip joint as the source of pain because soft-tissue injuries associated with repetitive activity are prevalent in this group of patients. It is important to obtain a careful history beginning with the onset of pain and the precipitating factors, the character of the discomfort, the location of the symptoms, the type of mechanical symptoms (such as locking, catching, crepitus, and instability), activity tolerance, and the transition of pain (such as flexion to extension, or pain with increased intra-abdominal pressure). It is also important to identify patients with atypical pain patterns, such as those with night pain, genital pain, or associated neurologic symptoms.

The objective of the physical examination is to characterize the mechanical characteristics of the hip joint and attempt to identify the anatomic structure that could be generating pain. Careful palpation of the hip region is used to identify inflamed structures. Passive motion testing and assessment of femoral torsion assists in understanding the motion limitations of the hip. Neurologic testing can identify specific patterns of weakness or spine-related problems that are associated with hip dysfunction.[68] Provocative tests are performed to identify specific patterns of activity-related instability.

Plain radiography, MRI, or CT is used to unify a suspected diagnosis and characterize the hip joint anatomy (**Figure 14**). Specific patterns of hip deformity are identifiable on radiographs by measuring the anterior and lateral center-edge angles, the acetabular depth-width ratio, the Tönnis angle, and the orientation of the acetabular walls. Less specific findings associated with hip instability include an increased neck-shaft angle, a high fovea, eversion of the epiphysis, and sclerosis of the lateral acetabular sourcil. CT can supplement plain radiographic information, whereas MRI is helpful in characterizing labral morphology and associated labral and articular cartilage damage that may be present inside the hip joint.

Treatment Guidelines

An incremental therapeutic approach should be used to treat patients engaged in repetitive athletic activities that produce hip instability with subtle anatomic deformity. The approach begins with a period of activity modification that ranges from complete rest to modified exercise and is combined with a course of anti-inflammatory medication and exercises to strengthen abdominal and pelvic muscles that may have weakened. The specific movements that precipitated the mechanical abnormality should then be identified, and efforts should be made to modify these mechanics to alleviate symptoms. The use of intra-articular cortisone may be considered for selected patients for diagnostic and therapeutic purposes. If nonsurgical therapy fails and the athlete continues to have athletic-related pain or daily discomfort, surgical treatment should be considered.

The goal of surgical treatment is to correct the underlying mechanical abnormality that is contributing to pain generation. Because the correction of hip instability most often involves acetabular reorientation, special care must be taken during surgery to limit motion loss after femoral head coverage is increased. Some surgeons have reported using capsulorrhaphy to stabilize subtly unstable hip joints, but there are few data on outcomes.[69] Patients who do not respond to nonsurgical treatment can elect acetabular reorientation. Athletes with borderline hip dysplasia present a challenging treatment dilemma with respect to simply managing intra-articular pathology versus corrective osteotomies.

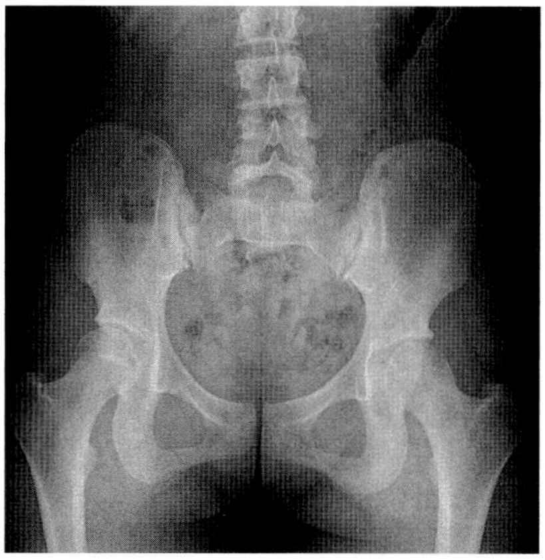

Figure 14 Radiograph showing a mildly dysplastic hip joint in a female patient who is a dancer. Impingement-related hip instability was seen when the hip was placed in maximum flexion and external rotation.

Return to Play

Patients usually can return to play if the pain resolves following a period of rest and education to correct the movements causing the mechanical abnormality or after successful surgical treatment. In either circumstance, return to play is not recommended until adequate hip abductor strength is achieved. The patient should return to play in a graduated fashion and in a structured, supervised environment.

The Hypermobile Hip Without Dysplasia

Basic Principles

There is no accurate definition of a hypermobile hip, although the term is used frequently, especially in female athletes with ligamentous laxity who present with hip pain. The term should be used diagnostically only when all other potential causes of pain are excluded. Anatomic entities that are often present in patients with ligamentous laxity include torsional abnormalities such as femoral antever-

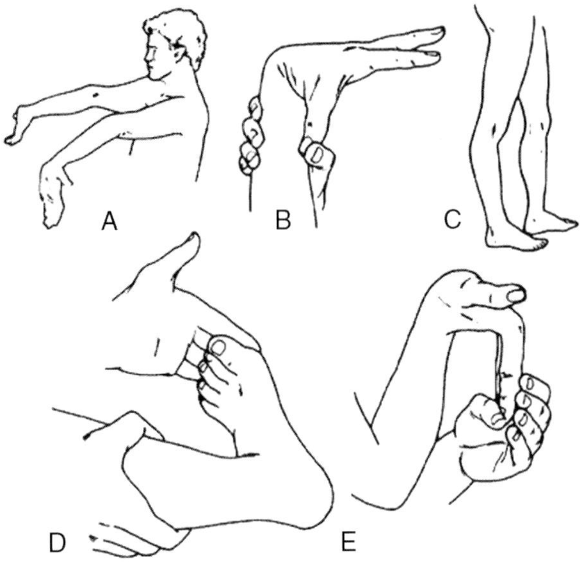

Figure 15 Illustrations of the five signs of ligamentous laxity described by Wynne-Davies. **A,** Elbow extension. **B,** Thumb touching forearm. **C,** Knee extension. **D,** Ankle dorsiflexion. **E,** Metacarpophalangeal joint extension. (Adapted with permission from Wynne-Davis R: Acetabular dysplasia and familial joint laxity: Two etiological factors in congenital dislocation of the hip. *J Bone Joint Surg Br* 1970;52(4):704-716)

sion, subtle acetabular dysplasia, psoas tendinitis, and central (core) muscle weakness.[70,71] Generalized ligamentous laxity, which is usually defined using the Wynne-Davies criteria, may relate to subtle activity-dependent instability[72] (**Figure 15**).

Assessment

The assessment of a patient with hip pain begins with a careful history, physical examination, and radiographic evaluation. Because hip pain associated with ligamentous laxity is diagnosed after excluding all other potential structural deformities that can produce pain, it is often necessary to use high-resolution MRI and CT to evaluate for labral and chondral damage and femoral and tibial torsion. Patients also should be evaluated for signs of connective tissue disorders, such as Marfan and Ehlers-Danlos syndromes. Diagnostic injections may be necessary to determine if intra-articular anesthesia can relieve the patient's symptoms.

Treatment Guidelines

It is challenging to treat patients with hip pain with ligamentous laxity if there is no identifiable structural deformity. Often, the patients have associated symptoms of bursitis that should be treated with a course of NSAIDs or that may respond to appropriate injections. Physical therapy to strengthen lower abdominal, paraspinal, and pelvic hip muscles can relieve some discomfort. There is a very limited role for surgical treatment in hip pain associated with ligamentous laxity. Occasionally, when a patient responds appropriately to an intra-articular injection, an arthroscopic examination is considered. When performing arthroscopy, it is essential to perform a minimal capsulotomy and repair or, in some instances, plicate the capsule when complete.[73]

Return to Play

It is safe for the athlete to return to play if there is satisfactory relief of symptoms following a period of rest, therapy, or surgery. Muscle strength should be satisfactory to help prevent future injuries, and return to play should be gradual, with an emphasis on modifying body mechanics to prevent reinjury.

Pediatric Hip Injuries in Sports

Apophyseal Avulsion Injuries

Basic Principles

The human hip and pelvis develop from a single mass of mesenchymal tissue that forms the upper femur and the entire pelvis. The ilium, ischium, and pubis comprise the pelvis and acetabulum. Toward the end of skeletal maturation, the femoral and pelvic apophyses become recognizable radiographically and include the lesser trochanter, the greater trochanter, the pubis, the ischial tuberosity, the iliac crest, the anterior superior iliac spine, and the AIIS. The apophyseal plate is composed of columnar-arranged chondrocytes located between primary and secondary sites of ossification where muscles either originate or insert. Pelvic and upper femoral avulsion injuries most commonly occur during adolescence;[74] however, they can occur until the mid-20s when the iliac apophyses fuse. These injuries often occur with an eccentric muscle contraction.[75] The ischial tuberosity and the AIIS are the two most commonly avulsed apophyses[76] (**Figure 16**). Severe complications after avulsion injuries are rare, with femoral head necrosis reported after greater trochanteric avulsion.[77]

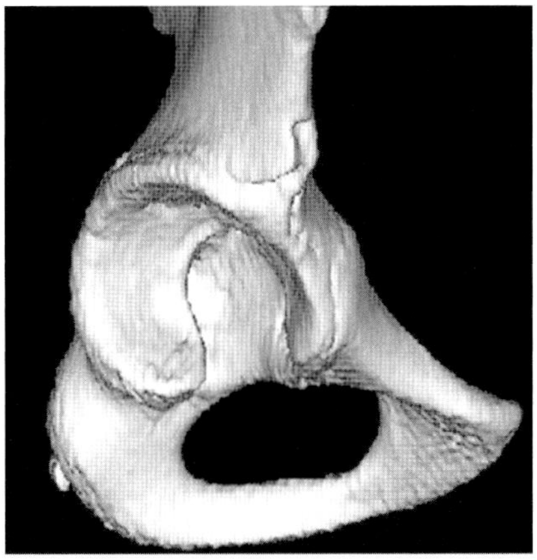

Figure 16 Three-dimensional CT scan showing the anatomy of ischial and AIIS apophyses, which are the two most common apophyseal avulsion fractures.

Assessment

The diagnosis of an avulsed apophysis is usually straightforward. Athletes experience a sudden injury, often accompanied by a popping sensation, which is accompanied by pain that can interfere with weight bearing. Physical findings include limitation of motion, swelling, and tenderness. Radiographic examination is necessary to confirm the diagnosis of an avulsion injury and exclude concomitant pathology. In rare instances, CT may be necessary to accurately gauge the degree of avulsion.

Treatment Guidelines

Pelvic avulsion injuries are usually self-limiting disorders that heal without specific orthopaedic intervention. If weight bearing is painful, crutches can be used. Acutely, ice and NSAIDs are useful at reducing pain and swelling. Rarely, a displaced ischial tuberosity or iliac crest avulsion injuries may require surgical fixation. The decision to repair an avulsion with surgery depends on the magnitude of the avulsion and the potential for the development of symptomatic weakness, nonunion, or a painful exostosis at the site of healing.

Return to Play

As with other minor avulsion fractures, patients can return to play after the injury has healed and the athlete has regained his or her preinjury level of flexibility and strength.

Slipped Capital Femoral Epiphysis and Developmental FAI

Basic Principles

Upper femoral deformity is associated with symptomatic FAI and labral disease. The pathogenesis of the deformity was considered akin to the development of a slipped capital femoral epiphysis (SCFE), with posterior translation of the epiphysis leading to prominence of the anterolateral femoral metaphysis and a pistol grip deformity. Anthropologic and radiographic evidence suggest distinct etiologies of SCFE and cam-type upper femoral morphologies. Despite a similar radiographic appearance at skeletal maturity, the pathoanatomy is different. The anatomy and mechanics of SCFE is well understood. Weakness of the upper femoral physis leads to anterior translation of the metaphysis relative to the neck of the femur. Although there is anatomic variability related to slip chronicity, the epiphysis remains normally shaped but abnormally aligned. In contrast, cam-type morphology will likely develop slowly depending on the morphology of the upper femoral chondroepiphysis. When the trochanteric apophysis and upper femoral epiphysis are coalesced, persistent epiphyseal tissue localized to the anterolateral and lateral femoral neck form an aspheric extension of the femoral head[78,79] (**Figure 17**).

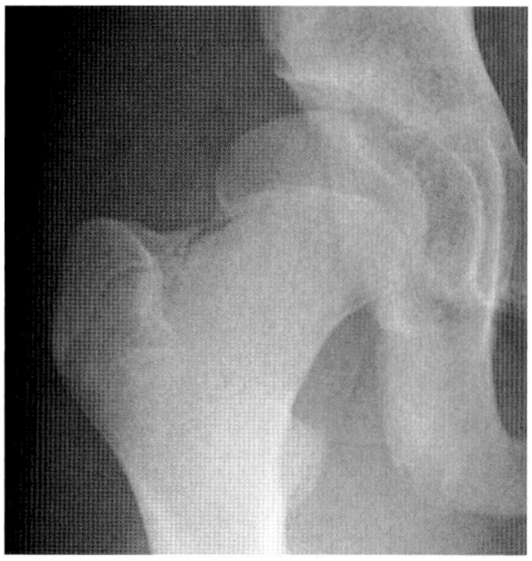

Figure 17 Radiograph showing coalescence of an adolescent trochanter and upper femoral epiphysis, which has been associated with the development of cam-type morphology.

Assessment

Hip pain that is caused by FAI or chronic SCFE is usually localized to the groin, the peritrochanteric area, the buttock, or the thigh and may be associated with mechanical symptoms. Usually, a patient with a slipped epiphysis has a history of SCFE treatment. Occasionally, there is no history of a childhood diagnosis of SCFE. Radiographically differentiating between cam-type morphology and mild, healed, chronic SCFE can be difficult using an AP radiograph; however, a lateral radiograph will show anterior metaphyseal translation that is not present with a cam-type femoral neck.

Treatment Guidelines

Treatment depends on the patient's history, degree of discomfort, and MRI appearance of the articular cartilage. Surgical decision making is dependent on the shape and orientation of the femoral neck as well as the extent of gait disturbance. Treatment options include arthroscopic osteoplasty or open femoral neck osteoplasty, which is usually performed through a surgical dislocation. Intertrochanteric osteotomy may be required to completely address the deformity.

Return to Play

Patients are permitted to return to play

after the hip pain resolves. For those with excessive arthrosis who are not surgical candidates, pain is managed conservatively, and sports participation is dependent on the patient's symptoms. After surgery, patients are permitted to return to sports participation after sufficient time has passed to permit healing, and muscle strength is normal. All patients are advised to avoid maximum hip flexion to prevent irritation to the acetabular rim.

Summary

The parallel developments in the assessment and treatment of hip injuries in the subspecialties of orthopaedic sports medicine and hip preservation have resulted in a more sophisticated understanding of the etiology of symptomatic hip pathology. The clear relationship between mechanical malalignment in the hip and the subsequent development of labral and chondral injury and extra-articular injury can be magnified in the setting of athletic activity because of the increased load on the joint during sports participation. In many instances, the earlier detection of hip injuries allows more timely and effective treatment. A thorough evaluation of the mechanism of injury, a detailed physical examination, and accurate interpretation of radiographic and advanced imaging studies are essential in the workup of an athlete with hip pain. Although surgical outcomes continue to improve with better techniques, continued emphasis on patient selection and the appropriate treatment of the underlying intra-articular pathology and structural malalignment are necessary for further advancements.

References

1. Ganz R, Parvizi J, Beck M, Leunig M, Nötzli H, Siebenrock KA: Femoroacetabular impingement: A cause for osteoarthritis of the hip. *Clin Orthop Relat Res* 2003; 417:112-120.
2. Byers PD, Contepomi CA, Farkas TA: A post mortem study of the hip joint: Including the prevalence of the features of the right side. *Ann Rheum Dis* 1970;29(1): 15-31.
3. Leunig M, Beck M, Woo A, Dora C, Kerboull M, Ganz R: Acetabular rim degeneration: A constant finding in the aged hip. *Clin Orthop Relat Res* 2003;413:201-207.
4. Seldes RM, Tan V, Hunt J, Katz M, Winiarsky R, Fitzgerald RH Jr: Anatomy, histologic features, and vascularity of the adult acetabular labrum. *Clin Orthop Relat Res* 2001;382:232-240.
5. Khanduja V, Villar RN: The arthroscopic management of femoroacetabular impingement. *Knee Surg Sports Traumatol Arthrosc* 2007;15(8):1035-1040.
6. Parvizi J, Leunig M, Ganz R: Femoroacetabular impingement. *J Am Acad Orthop Surg* 2007; 15(9):561-570.
7. Lavigne M, Parvizi J, Beck M, Siebenrock KA, Ganz R, Leunig M: Anterior femoroacetabular impingement: Part I. Techniques of joint preserving surgery. *Clin Orthop Relat Res* 2004;418:61-66.
8. Crawford JR, Villar RN: Current concepts in the management of femoroacetabular impingement. *J Bone Joint Surg Br* 2005;87(11): 1459-1462.
9. Philippon MJ, Stubbs AJ, Schenker ML, Maxwell RB, Ganz R, Leunig M: Arthroscopic management of femoroacetabular impingement: Osteoplasty technique and literature review. *Am J Sports Med* 2007;35(9):1571-1580.
10. Fitzgerald RH Jr: Acetabular labrum tears: Diagnosis and treatment. *Clin Orthop Relat Res* 1995; 311:60-68.
11. Anderson K, Strickland SM, Warren R: Hip and groin injuries in athletes. *Am J Sports Med* 2001; 29(4):521-533.
12. Meyer DC, Beck M, Ellis T, Ganz R, Leunig M: Comparison of six radiographic projections to assess femoral head/neck asphericity. *Clin Orthop Relat Res* 2006;445: 181-185.
13. Reynolds D, Lucas J, Klaue K: Retroversion of the acetabulum: A cause of hip pain. *J Bone Joint Surg Br* 1999;81(2):281-288.
14. Ganz R, Gill TJ, Gautier E, Ganz K, Krügel N, Berlemann U: Surgical dislocation of the adult hip a technique with full access to the femoral head and acetabulum without the risk of avascular necrosis. *J Bone Joint Surg Br* 2001; 83(8):1119-1124.
15. Larson CM, Giveans MR: Arthroscopic debridement versus refixation of the acetabular labrum associated with femoroacetabular impingement. *Arthroscopy* 2009; 25(4):369-376.
16. Philippon MJ, Briggs KK, Yen YM, Kuppersmith DA: Outcomes following hip arthroscopy for femoroacetabular impingement with associated chondrolabral dysfunction: Minimum two-year follow-up. *J Bone Joint Surg Br* 2009;91(1):16-23.
17. Sampson TG: Arthroscopic treatment of femoroacetabular impingement: A proposed technique with clinical experience. *Instr Course Lect* 2006;55:337-346.
18. Feeley BT, Powell JW, Muller MS, Barnes RP, Warren RF, Kelly BT: Hip injuries and labral tears in the national football league. *Am J Sports Med* 2008;36(11):2187-2195.
19. Moorman CT III, Warren RF, Hershman EB, et al: Traumatic posterior hip subluxation in American football. *J Bone Joint Surg Am* 2003;85(7):1190-1196.
20. Philippon MJ, Kuppersmith DA, Wolff AB, Briggs KK: Arthroscopic findings following trau-

matic hip dislocation in 14 professional athletes. *Arthroscopy* 2009; 25(2):169-174.

21. Pallia CS, Scott RE, Chao DJ: Traumatic hip dislocation in athletes. *Curr Sports Med Rep* 2002; 1(6):338-345.
22. Shindle MK, Ranawat AS, Kelly BT: Diagnosis and management of traumatic and atraumatic hip instability in the athletic patient. *Clin Sports Med* 2006;25(2):309-326, ix-x.
23. Bankart A: The pathology and treatment of recurrent dislocation of the shoulder joint. *J Bone Joint Surg Br* 1938;26:23-29.
24. Shindle MK, Voos JE, Heyworth BE, et al: Hip arthroscopy in the athletic patient: Current techniques and spectrum of disease. *J Bone Joint Surg Am* 2007; 89(suppl 3):29-43.
25. Weber M, Ganz R: Recurrent traumatic dislocation of the hip: Report of a case and review of the literature. *J Orthop Trauma* 1997; 11(5):382-385.
26. Cooper DE, Warren RF, Barnes R: Traumatic subluxation of the hip resulting in aseptic necrosis and chondrolysis in a professional football player. *Am J Sports Med* 1991;19(3):322-324.
27. Weir A, de Vos RJ, Moen M, Hölmich P, Tol JL: Prevalence of radiological signs of femoroacetabular impingement in patients presenting with long-standing adductor-related groin pain. *Br J Sports Med* 2011;45(1):6-9.
28. Schlegel TF, Bushnell BD, Godfrey J, Boublik M: Success of nonoperative management of adductor longus tendon ruptures in National Football League athletes. *Am J Sports Med* 2009;37(7): 1394-1399.
29. Gamradt SC, Brophy RH, Barnes R, Warren RF, Thomas Byrd JW, Kelly BT: Nonoperative treatment for proximal avulsion of the rectus femoris in professional American football. *Am J Sports Med* 2009; 37(7):1370-1374.
30. Lempainen L, Sarimo J, Mattila K, Vaittinen S, Orava S: Proximal hamstring tendinopathy: Results of surgical management and histopathologic findings. *Am J Sports Med* 2009;37(4):727-734.
31. Folsom GJ, Larson CM: Surgical treatment of acute versus chronic complete proximal hamstring ruptures: Results of a new allograft technique for chronic reconstructions. *Am J Sports Med* 2008;36(1):104-109.
32. Sallay PI, Friedman RL, Coogan PG, Garrett WE: Hamstring muscle injuries among water skiers: Functional outcome and prevention. *Am J Sports Med* 1996;24(2): 130-136.
33. Aronen JG, Garrick JG, Chronister RD, McDevitt ER: Quadriceps contusions: Clinical results of immediate immobilization in 120 degrees of knee flexion. *Clin J Sport Med* 2006;16(5):383-387.
34. Ryan JB, Wheeler JH, Hopkinson WJ, Arciero RA, Kolakowski KR: Quadriceps contusions: West Point update. *Am J Sports Med* 1991;19(3):299-304.
35. Matava MJ, Ellis E, Shah NR, Pogue D, Williams T: Morel-Lavallée lesion in a professional American football player. *Am J Orthop (Belle Mead NJ)* 2010; 39(3):144-147.
36. Brown RA, Mascia A, Kinnear DG, Lacroix V, Feldman L, Mulder DS: An 18-year review of sports groin injuries in the elite hockey player: Clinical presentation, new diagnostic imaging, treatment, and results. *Clin J Sport Med* 2008;18(3):221-226.
37. Meyers WC, McKechnie A, Philippon MJ, Horner MA, Zoga AC, Devon ON: Experience with "sports hernia" spanning two decades. *Ann Surg* 2008;248(4): 656-665.
38. Larson CM, Pierce BR, Giveans MR: Treatment of athletes with symptomatic intra-articular hip pathology and athletic pubalgia/sports hernia: A case series. *Arthroscopy* 2011;27(6):768-775.
39. Verrall GM, Hamilton IA, Slavotinek JP, et al: Hip joint range of motion reduction in sports-related chronic groin injury diagnosed as pubic bone stress injury. *J Sci Med Sport* 2005;8(1): 77-84.
40. Verrall GM, Slavotinek JP, Barnes PG, Esterman A, Oakeshott RD, Spriggins AJ: Hip joint range of motion restriction precedes athletic chronic groin injury. *J Sci Med Sport* 2007;10(6):463-466.
41. Birmingham P: The effect of dynamic femoroacetabular impingement on pubic symphysis motion: A cadaveric study. *Am J Sports Med* 2012;40(5):1113-1118.
42. Wight J, Richards J, Hall S: Influence of pelvis rotation styles on baseball pitching mechanics. *Sports Biomech* 2004;3(1):67-83.
43. MacWilliams BA, Choi T, Perezous MK, Chao EY, McFarland EG: Characteristic ground-reaction forces in baseball pitching. *Am J Sports Med* 1998;26(1): 66-71.
44. Stodden DF, Langendorfer SJ, Fleisig GS, Andrews JR: Kinematic constraints associated with the acquisition of overarm throwing: Part I. Step and trunk actions. *Res Q Exerc Sport* 2006; 77(4):417-427.
45. Kibler WB: The 400-watt tennis player: Power development for tennis. *Med Sci Tennis* 2009; 14:5-8.
46. Barrow GW, Saha S: Menstrual irregularity and stress fractures in collegiate female distance runners. *Am J Sports Med* 1988;16(3): 209-216.
47. Voss LA, Fadale PD, Hulstyn MJ: Exercise-induced loss of bone

density in athletes. *J Am Acad Orthop Surg* 1998;6(6):349-357.

48. Prather JL, Nusynowitz ML, Snowdy HA, Hughes AD, McCartney WH, Bagg RJ: Scintigraphic findings in stress fractures. *J Bone Joint Surg Am* 1977;59(7): 869-874.

49. Johansson C, Ekenman I, Törnkvist H, Eriksson E: Stress fractures of the femoral neck in athletes: The consequence of a delay in diagnosis. *Am J Sports Med* 1990; 18(5):524-528.

50. Arendt EA, Griffiths HJ: The use of MR imaging in the assessment and clinical management of stress reactions of bone in high-performance athletes. *Clin Sports Med* 1997;16(2):291-306.

51. Diehl JJ, Best TM, Kaeding CC: Classification and return-to-play considerations for stress fractures. *Clin Sports Med* 2006;25(1):17-28, vii.

52. Gordon EJ: Trochanteric bursitis and tendinitis. *Clin Orthop* 1961; 20:193-202.

53. Bird PA, Oakley SP, Shnier R, Kirkham BW: Prospective evaluation of magnetic resonance imaging and physical examination findings in patients with greater trochanteric pain syndrome. *Arthritis Rheum* 2001;44(9):2138-2145.

54. Kingzett-Taylor A, Tirman PF, Feller J, et al: Tendinosis and tears of gluteus medius and minimus muscles as a cause of hip pain: MR imaging findings. *AJR Am J Roentgenol* 1999;173(4):1123-1126.

55. Connell DA, Bass C, Sykes CA, Young D, Edwards E: Sonographic evaluation of gluteus medius and minimus tendinopathy. *Eur Radiol* 2003;13(6):1339-1347.

56. Kagan A II: Rotator cuff tears of the hip. *Clin Orthop Relat Res* 1999;368:135-140.

57. Byrd JW, Jones KS: Prospective analysis of hip arthroscopy with 2-year follow-up. *Arthroscopy* 2000;16(6):578-587.

58. Martin RL, Kelly BT, Philippon MJ: Evidence of validity for the hip outcome score. *Arthroscopy* 2006;22(12):1304-1311.

59. Martin RL, Philippon MJ: Evidence of reliability and responsiveness for the hip outcome score. *Arthroscopy* 2008;24(6):676-682.

60. Voos JE, Shindle MK, Pruett A, Asnis PD, Kelly BT: Endoscopic repair of gluteus medius tendon tears of the hip. *Am J Sports Med* 2009;37(4):743-747.

61. Whiteside LA: Surgical technique: Transfer of the anterior portion of the gluteus maximus muscle for abductor deficiency of the hip. *Clin Orthop Relat Res* 2012; 470(2):503-510.

62. Steinberg N, Hershkovitz I, Peleg S, et al: Range of joint movement in female dancers and nondancers aged 8 to 16 years: Anatomical and clinical implications. *Am J Sports Med* 2006;34(5):814-823.

63. Charbonnier C, Kolo FC, Duthon VB, et al: Assessment of congruence and impingement of the hip joint in professional ballet dancers: A motion capture study. *Am J Sports Med* 2011;39(3): 557-566.

64. Charbonnier C, Magnenat-Thalmann N, Becker CD, Hoffmeyer P, Menetrey J: An integrated platform for hip joint osteoarthritis analysis: Design, implementation and results. *Int J Comput Assist Radiol Surg* 2010; 5(4):351-358.

65. Safran MR, Giordano G, Lindsey DP, et al: Strains across the acetabular labrum during hip motion: A cadaveric model. *Am J Sports Med* 2011;39(suppl):92S-102S.

66. Daniel M, Iglic A, Kralj-Iglic V: Hip contact stress during normal and staircase walking: The influence of acetabular anteversion angle and lateral coverage of the acetabulum. *J Appl Biomech* 2008; 24(1):88-93.

67. Henak CR, Ellis BJ, Harris MD, Anderson AE, Peters CL, Weiss JA: Role of the acetabular labrum in load support across the hip joint. *J Biomech* 2011;44(12): 2201-2206.

68. Casartelli NC, Maffiuletti NA, Item-Glatthorn JF, et al: Hip muscle weakness in patients with symptomatic femoroacetabular impingement. *Osteoarthritis Cartilage* 2011;19(7):816-821.

69. Philippon MJ: The role of arthroscopic thermal capsulorrhaphy in the hip. *Clin Sports Med* 2001; 20(4):817-829.

70. Adib N, Davies K, Grahame R, Woo P, Murray KJ: Joint hypermobility syndrome in childhood: A not so benign multisystem disorder? *Rheumatology (Oxford)* 2005;44(6):744-750.

71. Roussel NA, Nijs J, Mottram S, Van Moorsel A, Truijen S, Stassijns G: Altered lumbopelvic movement control but not generalized joint hypermobility is associated with increased injury in dancers: A prospective study. *Man Ther* 2009;14(6):630-635.

72. Wynne-Davies R: Acetabular dysplasia and familial joint laxity: Two etiological factors in congenital dislocation of the hip. A review of 589 patients and their families. *J Bone Joint Surg Br* 1970;52(4): 704-716.

73. Martin HD, Savage A, Braly BA, Palmer IJ, Beall DP, Kelly B: The function of the hip capsular ligaments: A quantitative report. *Arthroscopy* 2008;24(2):188-195.

74. Orava S, Ala-Ketola L: Avulsion fractures in athletes. *Br J Sports Med* 1977;11(2):65-71.

75. Vandervliet EJ, Vanhoenacker FM, Snoeckx A, Gielen JL, Van Dyck P, Parizel PM: Sports-related acute and chronic avulsion

injuries in children and adolescents with special emphasis on tennis. *Br J Sports Med* 2007; 41(11):827-831.

76. Moeller JL: Pelvic and hip apophyseal avulsion injuries in young athletes. *Curr Sports Med Rep* 2003;2(2):110-115.

77. O'Rourke MR, Weinstein SL: Osteonecrosis following isolated avulsion fracture of the greater trochanter in children: A report of two cases. *J Bone Joint Surg Am* 2003;85(10):2000-2005.

78. Serrat MA, Reno PL, McCollum MA, Meindl RS, Lovejoy CO: Variation in mammalian proximal femoral development: Comparative analysis of two distinct ossification patterns. *J Anat* 2007; 210(3):249-258.

79. Siebenrock KA, Schoeniger R, Ganz R: Anterior femoroacetabular impingement due to acetabular retroversion: Treatment with periacetabular osteotomy. *J Bone Joint Surg Am* 2003;85(2): 278-286.

Video Reference

46.1: Larson CM, Stone RM: Video. *Arthroscopic Management of Pincer- and Cam-Type Femoroacetabular Impingement.* Edina, MN, 2011.

SECTION

9

Orthopaedic Medicine

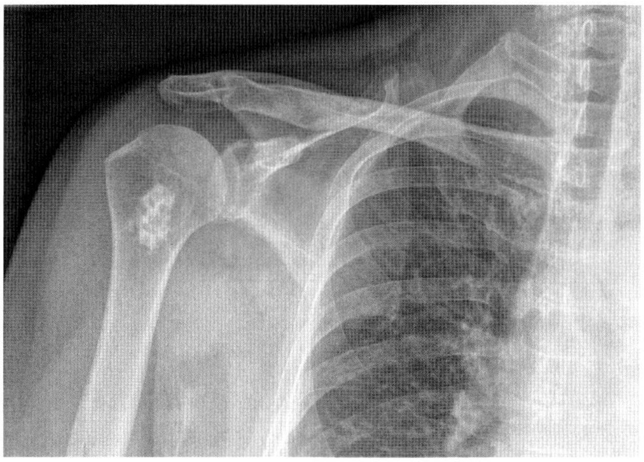

47 Malignant and Benign Bone Tumors That You Are Likely to See

47

Malignant and Benign Bone Tumors That You Are Likely to See

Valerae O. Lewis, MD
Carol D. Morris, MD
Theodore W. Parsons III, MD, FACS

Abstract

Although primary malignancies of bone are rare, thousands of benign bone tumors are diagnosed annually. It is important to be able to distinguish benign lesions from malignant lesions and differentiate those lesions that can be watched versus lesions that require further treatment and referral to an orthopaedic oncologist. Learning to distinguish these entities and their appropriate treatment or triage will positively affect the patient and the surgeon's practice.

Instr Course Lect 2013;62:535-549.

Although primary malignancies of bone are rare, thousands of benign bone tumors and reactive conditions are diagnosed annually. The treatment and prognosis of these tumors vary widely. It is important to be able to distinguish benign lesions from malignant lesions (those lesions that can be watched versus those lesions that require further treatment and referral to an orthopaedic oncologist). Early in the 20th century, Codman[1,2] recognized the rarity of bone tumor lesions and established a registry of bone tumor cases. It was from this registry that radiographic features were established to delineate benign from malignant bone tumors.[1-3] Combining information from Codman's registry with material from the Armed Forces Institute of Pathology, the features that distinguish slow-growing and aggressive lesions were further delineated. Radiographs should be reviewed as gross pathology, not as two-dimensional black-and-white pictures. Although the workup of bone tumors may require many imaging modalities, radiography should always be the first step in evaluating a bone lesion. The interpretation of other studies should never be attempted without clear biplanar radiographs.

Radiographic Evaluation

Enneking Criteria

Plain radiographs can delineate the location of the bone tumor, the growth characteristics, and the presence or absence of a matrix. Radiographs should be used to find the area of pathology, and four questions, as taught by the orthopaedic surgeon William D. Enneking, should be asked: (1) Where is the lesion? (2) What is the effect of the lesion on the bone? (3) What is the effect of the bone on the lesion? (4) What additional clues are present? The answers to these questions will help establish the differential diagnoses and determine whether the lesion is benign or malignant. It should then be determined if the lesion represents a bone tumor, a soft-tissue tumor, or joint disease.

Bone tumors often involve the bone more centrally rather than eccentrically and obey the Phemister law of lesion distribution, which states that

Dr. Lewis or an immediate family member serves as a board member, owner, officer, or committee member of the Western Orthopaedic Association, the American Academy of Orthopaedic Surgeons, the Musculoskeletal Tumor Society, and Orthopedics Today and has received research or institutional support from Stryker for the MD Anderson Musculoskeletal Oncology Course. Dr. Morris or an immediate family member serves as a board member, owner, officer, or committee member of the American Academy of Orthopaedic Surgeons. Dr. Parsons or an immediate family member serves as a board member, owner, officer, or committee member of the Society of Military Orthopaedic Surgeons, the Musculoskeletal Tumor Society, the Michigan Orthopaedic Society, the American Orthopaedic Association, and the American Academy of Orthopaedic Surgeons.

Table 1
Relationship of Biologic Activity to the Type of Tumor Margin and Periosteal Reaction

Growth Rate	Internal Margins	Periosteal Reaction
Slow	Geographic (I)	Solid
	IA IB IC	Continuous
Intermediate	Moth-eaten (II)	Shells Ridged Lobulated Smooth
Fast	Permeative (III)	Lamellated
Fastest	Nonvisible	Spiculated or none

malignant and benign bone tumors occur in regions of the most rapid growth.[4] Bone tumors usually do not invade a joint or cartilage and usually display some specific reaction that can be helpful in arriving at a diagnosis or narrowing the differential diagnoses.

The questions regarding the effect of the lesion on bone and the effect of the bone on the lesion address the margin around a bone lesion. The perception of a bone margin depends on the location of the tumor in the bone (cortical versus cancellous), the degree of bone loss, and the amount of adjacent bone available for contrast.[3] The epiphysis, metaphysis, and diaphysis of the bone have different internal characteristics and types of medullary bone. The epiphysis and metaphysis have compact cancellous medullary bone, and the diaphysis has scant fatty medullary bone. Lesions that may be evident in the metaphysis would not be as evident in the diaphysis. It is difficult to discern the ends of a diaphyseal lesion because there is little contrast provided by fatty medullary bone. Madewell et al[3] postulated that this lack of contrast explains why some metaphyseal lesions may seem to disappear with growth. Remodeling of the surrounding cancellous bone and bone growth "move" the lesion from the metaphysis, with structural cancellous bone, into the diaphysis, which contains only a scant amount of cancellous bone that makes the margins of the lesion less apparent.

Lesion Margins

Lodwick et al[5] developed a classification system that categorizes the transitional margin around a lesion and aids in diagnosing and determining the prognosis of the lesion (**Table 1**). In general, the prognosis for the patient is less favorable with the increasing grade of the lesion, and more aggressive lesions are higher-grade lesions.

Mankin Criteria

To determine the malignity or benignity of a lesion, Mankin developed four radiographic evaluation criteria that together are scored from 0 to 4.[6] In general, malignant lesions are all higher-grade lesions. Lesions are evaluated on the size of the lesion (big is bad; small is good), the presence or absence of a margin, the presence or absence of cortical destruction, and the presence or absence of a soft-tissue mass. Malignant lesions tend to have a score of 4, with a larger size, poor margination, cortical destruction, and a soft-tissue mass. However, infections and giant cell tumor of bone (a benign lesion) can have the score of 4, whereas some metastatic diseases may have a score of only 1 or 2.

Periosteal Reaction

The surface changes of the bone seen on radiographs also provide clues to a lesion's aggressiveness. A periosteal reaction is the formation of new bone in response to a stimulus. Changes in the underlying bone result in shifts in the periosteum (a periosteal reaction). The periosteal reaction must mineralize to become visible on a radiograph. Periosteal changes can be classified as continuous or interrupted, and the pattern of the periosteal reaction depends on the manner and the time it takes for it to be produced and ossify. Depending on the age of the patient, this process can take from 10 to 20 days. A periosteal reaction in response to a lesion may be amorphous (thick), laminated (layered), or spiculated (sunburst), and it depends on the type of stimulus and changes to the bone. The latter two periosteal reactions represent aggressive growth. Slow-growing lesions result in minimal periosteal stimuli and generate few periosteal changes. The configuration of the periosteal reaction reflects the biologic activity of the tumor.

Tumor Location and Multiplicity

Although the differential diagnosis can be established based on the appearance of the internal margin of the lesion and the periosteal reaction, the location of the tumor within the bone also aids in the development of a differential diagnosis (**Figure 1**). **Table 2** lists the differential diagnoses based on the location of the tumor within the skeleton. Because bone tumors have a site and age predilection, knowledge of the patient's age and tumor location will help narrow the differential diagnosis.

Knowledge of the multiplicity of the lesion will also aid in the differential diagnosis. If the lesions exist in multiple bones, with normal bone intervening, the range of the differential

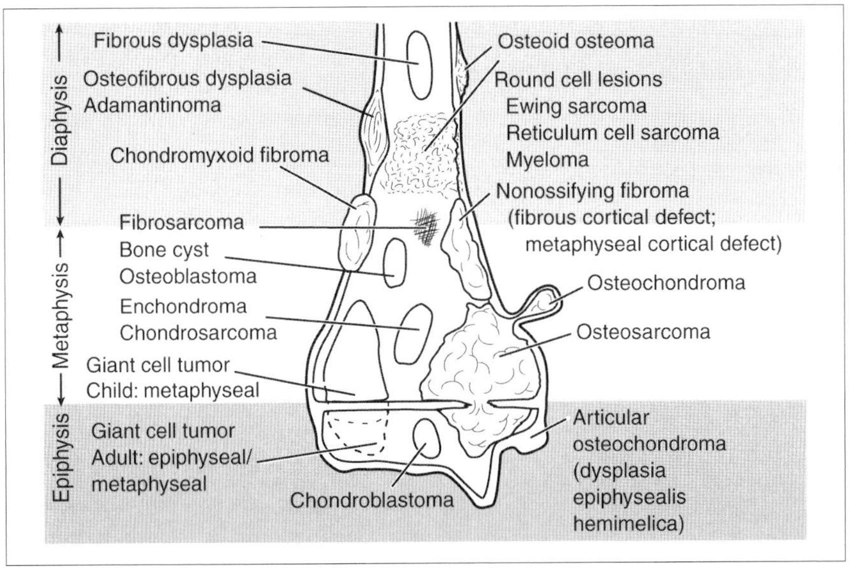

Figure 1 Illustration showing frequent sites of bone tumors.

Table 2
Differential Diagnosis Based on Tumor Site

Site	Tumor
Sacrum	Chordoma, giant cell tumor, and metastases
Tibia	Adamantinoma versus osteofibrous dysplasia
Posterior femur	Parosteal osteosarcoma
Aggressive bone-forming metaphyseal lesions in young patient	Osteosarcoma
Surface lesion: knob-like	Osteochondroma and parosteal osteosarcoma
Surface aggressive bone lesion	Periosteal osteosarcoma, high-grade surface osteosarcoma, and periosteal chondrosarcoma

diagnosis is sharply reduced. For the most part, multiple bones are involved in fibrous dysplasia, histiocytosis, sarcoidosis, infections, hereditary multiple exostosis syndrome, osteochondromas, Ollier disease, Maffucci syndrome, Paget disease, myeloma, and skeletal metastases. Joint disease can also mimic a bone tumor; however, it generally occurs in more than one bone and should, by definition, involve both sides of the joint (although both sides may not be equally affected). Signs of synovial inflammation are often present. The joint space is frequently narrowed, and juxtacortical osteopenia is common, can be severe, and can be out of proportion to the extent of the disease. This is particularly true when bone disease is associated with tuberculosis or rheumatoid arthritis and its variants. The most common etiologies that cause changes in the bone on both sides of the joint are hematoma, pus, pannus, pigmented villonodular synovitis, tuberculosis, and osteoarthritis.

Tumor Matrix

Radiographs also provide information regarding the status of the tumor matrix. Bone tumor and tumor-like conditions can be divided into those that produce a matrix and those that do not. There are three types of bone formations that can be seen on radiographs and are associated with bone tumors and tumor-like conditions:[7] direct formation of tumor osteoid, as in osteosarcoma; enchondral bone formation, described as rings or arcs and seen in chondrosarcoma; and reactive new bone, as described in periosteal reactions and reinforcing margins about benign lesions. Discussion of the specific patterns seen in different tumors is beyond the scope of this chapter; however, the matrix patterns associated with malignant osteoid-producing lesions (such as osteosarcoma) is dependent on the amount of mineralization present and can range from solid (sharp edges) to cloudy or ivory-like, hazy, ill-defined edges. The matrix pattern associated with tumor cartilage is stippled or flocculent, and the rings and arcs represent bony rims about the cartilage nodules. Most instances of calcifications of the medullary canal represent a cartilage tumor or a medullary infarct. The conditions can be hard to distinguish, but a cartilage tumor looks more like popcorn balls and a medullary infarct looks more like smoke up a chimney.

Characteristic Findings

Radiographs remain the first line in the diagnosis of a bone tumor. **Table 3** includes some key radiologic buzzwords to describe characteristic findings and their corresponding diagnoses. However, after a differential diagnosis is made, additional imaging modalities can be useful in establishing the final diagnosis.

Other Imaging Modalities

MRI is the imaging modality of choice for localization, characterization, and

Table 3
Key Radiologic Bone Tumor Buzzwords and Related Diagnoses

Radiologic Buzzwords	Diagnosis
Soap bubble	Aneurysmal bone cyst
Blow-out	Aneurysmal bone cyst
Nidus	Osteoid osteoma
Popcorn balls	Cartilage tumors
Smoke up a chimney	Bone infarct
Scallops from within	Fibrous dysplasia
Ground glass	Fibrous dysplasia
Sled runner tracks	Ollier disease and Maffucci syndrome
Sunburst pattern	Osteosarcoma
Bear bite	Fibrosarcoma or malignant fibrous histiocytoma
Permeative or moth-eaten	Round cell tumors

staging of bone tumors. MRI provides a three-dimensional anatomic delineation. It can be used to evaluate the intraosseous extent of the tumor and the bone marrow involvement and integrity. MRI can identify the presence of a soft-tissue mass and delineate its relationship to the neurovascular bundle and the surrounding soft tissues. In patients with malignant disease and those receiving systemic treatment, MRI can be used to evaluate the response to chemotherapy. When limb salvage is a treatment option, MRI is critically important in surgical planning and the determination of the resection margin. By emphasizing the various characteristics of the radiofrequency pulse (strength, frequency, or the time at which the signal is measured), different pulse sequences can be created. The different sequences assist in visualizing and highlighting different tissues and their characteristics.

Gadolinium contrast used with MRI is important when evaluating musculoskeletal tumors. Gadolinium can differentiate cystic from solid lesions by providing rim enhancement of the cystic lesions. It highlights enhanced viable tumor tissue from nonenhanced necrotic tissue and is useful in assessing treatment response or guiding the biopsy needle.

CT is helpful in delineating the osseous anatomy. It can be used to evaluate cortical integrity and mineralization by showing subtle mineralization within the bone. Although CT is not the primary imaging modality in the evaluation of bone tumors, it is a useful adjuvant to MRI.

Benign Bone Tumors

In general, patients with benign bone tumors have an excellent prognosis. Perhaps the single most important aspect of treating these patients is to be sure that the condition is benign. The orthopaedic surgeon should use a diagnostic strategy to reach the correct treatment plan. Some lesions have pathopneumonic features that allow great confidence in the benign diagnosis. Other lesions are questionable and warrant biopsy. It is best to use a multidisciplinary approach in which a complete history and physical examination are correlated with imaging findings in conjunction with consultations with a radiologist, a surgeon, or a pathologist with knowledge of musculoskeletal neoplasms. Most lesions, even when asymptomatic, deserve serial imaging to document maintenance of a benign clinical pattern.

The most common benign bone tumors are reviewed with regard to their presentation, characteristic imaging findings, and most likely treatment plan. The tumors can be classified by tissue type (osseous, cartilaginous, fibrous, cystic, or other) because this classification facilitates narrowing of the differential diagnosis (**Table 4**).

Osteoid Osteoma

Osteoid osteoma is a benign, bone-forming tumor that typically affects children and adolescents. It is characterized by small size (< 1.5 cm), limited growth potential, and a distinctive pain pattern of nocturnal exacerbation; pain is usually relieved with nonsteroidal anti-inflammatory drugs or aspirin. It has been reported in virtually every bone but most commonly occurs in the cortices of long bones, with the proximal femur being the most common site. On physical examination, there is often a focal area of point tenderness if the tumor is subcutaneous. Within the spine, osteoid osteoma occurs in the posterior elements, and patients may present with a painful scoliosis secondary to muscle spasm.

Characteristic imaging findings include dense cortical thickening on plain radiographs and a target-shaped central nidus on CT scans (**Figure 2**). The nidus can be more difficult to localize on MRI secondary to the substantial surrounding edema. The tumor is always hot on a technetium Tc-99m bone scan. The current standard of care for lesions in the long bones and pelvis is CT-guided percutaneous radiofrequency ablation, in which an electrode is inserted via a cannula in the center of the lesion and heated for a specified period of time to create a zone of necrosis.[8] This technique is associated with local recurrence rates of less than 10%. Surgical removal is usually reserved for tumors in which radiofrequency ablation is deemed unsafe, such as those near the

Table 4
Common Benign Bone Tumors According to Tissue Type

Tissue Type	Tumor
Osseous (bone forming)	Osteoid osteoma Osteoblastoma Osteoma/bone island Osteochondroma
Cartilaginous	Enchondroma Chondroblastoma Chondromyxoid fibroma Periosteal chondroma
Fibrous	Fibrous cortical defect Nonossifying fibroma Fibrous dysplasia Osteofibrous dysplasia
Cystic	Unicameral bone cyst Aneurysmal bone cyst
Other	Giant cell tumor Langerhans cell histiocytosis/eosinophilic granuloma Hemangioma

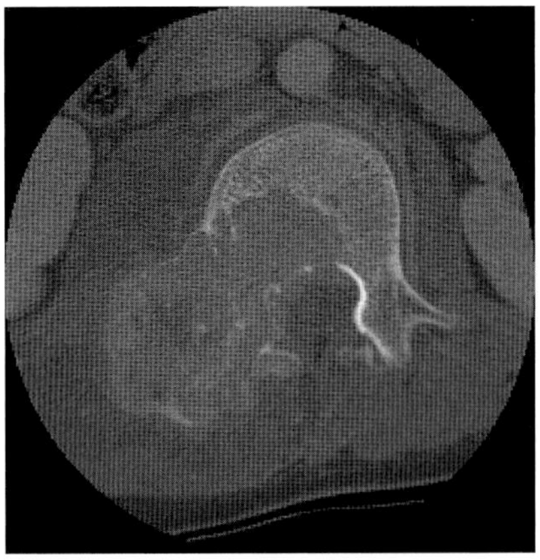

Figure 3 CT scan of a spinal osteoblastoma. The lesion is locally aggressive with substantial expansion of the bone and loss of mineralization. It is almost always confined by a thin periosteal shell of bone, which helps to differentiate it from osteosarcoma.

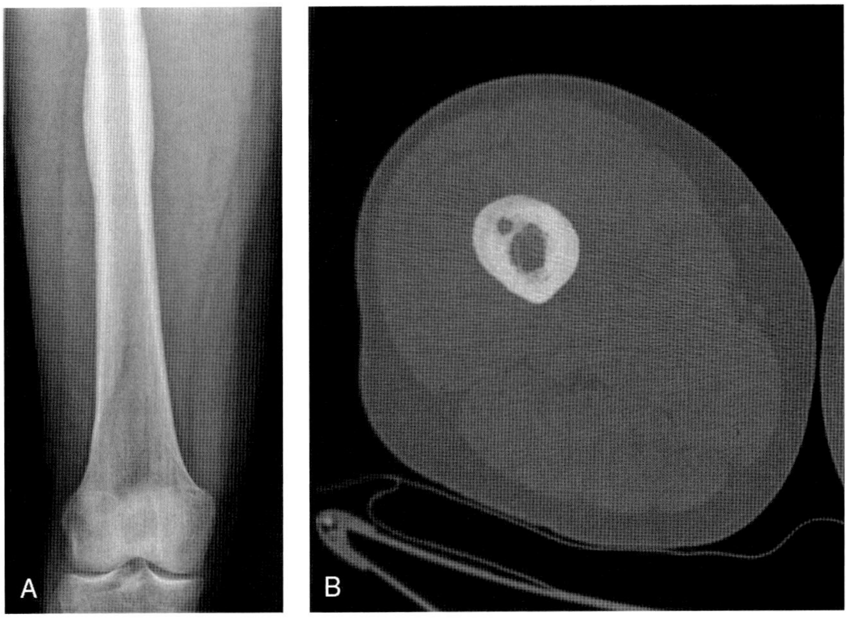

Figure 2 Classic radiographic and CT appearance of osteoid osteoma. **A,** Radiograph shows dense cortical sclerosis. The central nidus is often subtle and difficult to identify. **B,** Axial CT scan clearly shows a nidus within the cortex.

spinal cord or certain subchondral locations. Treatment with only nonsteroidal anti-inflammatory drugs, although not recommended, has been reported with resolution of symptoms at approximately 3 years.

Osteoblastoma

Osteoblastoma is histologically identical to osteoid osteoma but is larger in size (> 2 cm) and has a more aggressive clinical course. Whereas osteoid osteoma is a self-limiting condition, osteoblastoma typically progresses and recurs if not completely excised. Although these tumors may occur in any bone, most arise in the spine (usually within the posterior elements) and are equally distributed among the cervical, thoracic, and lumbar regions.[9] Pain is not typically relieved by nonsteroidal anti-inflammatory drugs. A wide range of radiographic appearances has been described, including radiolucency on radiographs and cortical expansion (**Figure 3**). Because of the aggressive local nature of osteoblastomas, the diagnosis can be challenging. The imaging and histology may be confused with osteosarcoma. Complete intralesional surgical excision is the treatment of choice. Local adjuvants, such as cryoablation or phenol, may be used to reduce the local recurrence rate, which has been reported as high as 20%.

Osteochondroma

Osteochondromas or exostoses are surface tumors consisting of a bony stalk covered with a cartilage cap. They represent the most common benign bone tumor, although their true incidence is

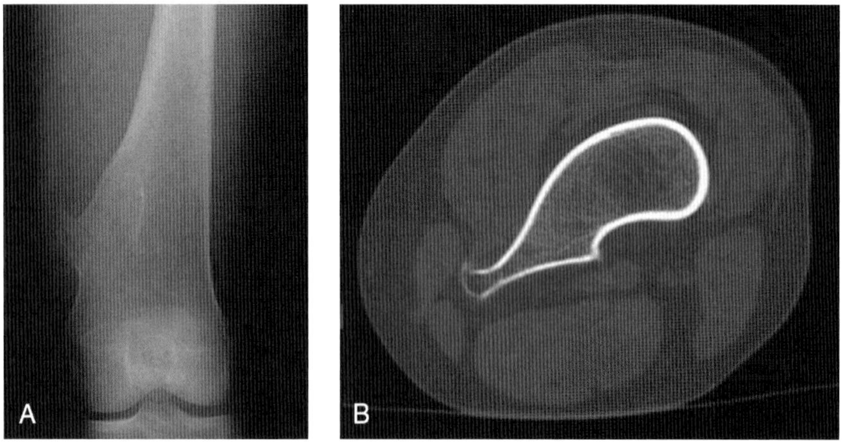

Figure 4 **A,** Typical radiographic appearance of a pedunculated osteochondroma on the metaphysis, with the stalk pointing away from the physis. **B,** CT scan confirms both the cortical and medullary continuity.

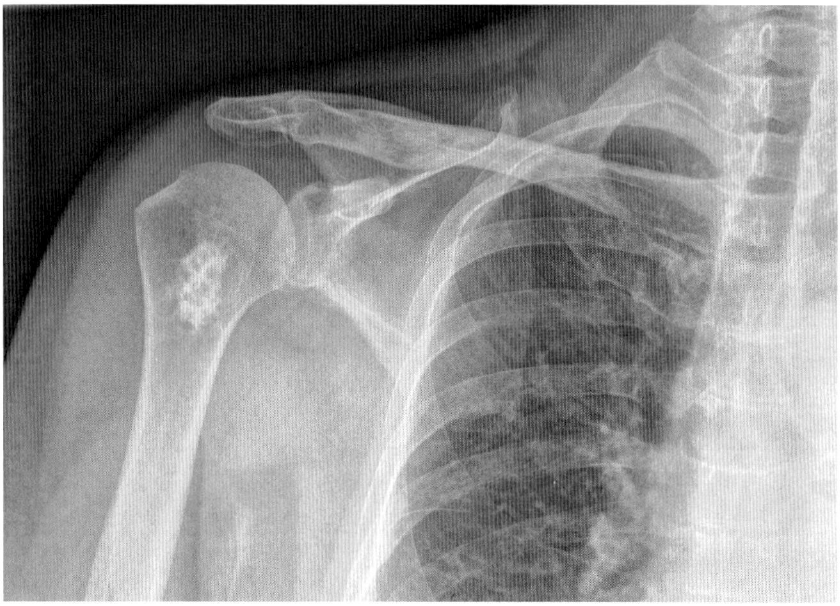

Figure 5 Typical radiographic appearance of an enchondroma in the proximal humerus. Note the ring-like pattern of calcification.

unknown. Technically, an osteochondroma is a developmental defect of bone that is believed to arise from aberrant physeal cartilage that grows independently of and at the same rate as the epiphysis, resulting in a bony prominence on the metaphyseal side of the growth plate. Recent investigations have suggested that inactivation of the *EXT1* gene may be necessary for the development of this condition, but the pathogenesis of the disorder is poorly understood.[10] Osteochondromas have a characteristic imaging appearance, showing a bony stalk with cortical and medullary continuity with the underlying bone (**Figure 4**). Growth of the lesion continues until the patient reaches skeletal maturity. Approximately 1% of solitary osteochondromas will undergo malignant transformation to chondrosarcoma, whereas a malignancy may develop during the lifetime in up to 10% of patients with multiple hereditary exostoses. Worrisome signs of malignancy include pain, continued growth of the lesion after skeletal maturity, and cartilage cap thickness greater than 2 cm. Asymptomatic osteochondromas do not require treatment. Lesions that appear at a younger age tend to become more symptomatic with time and may benefit from surgical excision.

Enchondroma

Enchondromas are benign, hyaline cartilage tumors located in medullary bone. They are the second most common benign bone tumor. Most enchondromas are solitary in nature but may involve more than one bone or more than one site in a single bone. They are most commonly diagnosed in patients ages 20 to 50 years and are most often found incidentally. The most common anatomic location for enchondromas is the small bones of the hand. Radiographic features are punctate rings and arcs of calcification (**Figure 5**).

It has been well documented that enchondromas can undergo malignant change to chondrosarcoma. Solitary enchondromas are likely associated with malignant transformation in less than 1% of cases, whereas multiple enchondromas are associated with Ollier disease and Maffucci syndrome and have a much higher rate of malignant change. High-grade or dedifferentiated chondrosarcomas are relatively easy to differentiate from their benign counterparts, whereas it is challenging to differentiate low-grade chondrosarcoma and enchondroma. Although attempts have been made to establish firm criteria, the diagnosis of low-grade chondrosarcoma relies heavily on many clinical factors (pain), radiographic findings (including size, amount of endosteal scalloping, uptake on bone scans), and the suspicion of the treating physician.[11] After removal, most enchondromas require continued follow-up but usually do not require surgical intervention. The type and frequency of monitoring is highly variable among physicians.

Chondroblastoma

Chondroblastoma is a rare cartilage-forming tumor found in the epiphysis or apophysis of skeletally immature patients. Although considered a benign tumor, 1% to 2% of chondroblastomas develop pulmonary metastases. They are typically discovered in the second decade of life and are most commonly located in the distal femur. Pain is the most common presenting symptom. These tumors have a lytic radiographic appearance, although the findings may be quite subtle. MRI usually confirms the diagnosis, showing a well-circumscribed lesion confined to the epiphysis, with substantial surrounding bony edema (**Figure 6**). Secondary aneurysmal bone cysts have been reported in up to 25% of patients and are believed to be associated with a higher rate of local recurrence. The standard of treatment of chondroblastoma is curettage of the lesion, which is usually followed with bone grafting.[12] Cement, not bone grafting, has been used in older patients. The local recurrence rate is approximately 15% and may be decreased with the use of local adjuvants, such as liquid nitrogen, phenol, or argon beam coagulation.

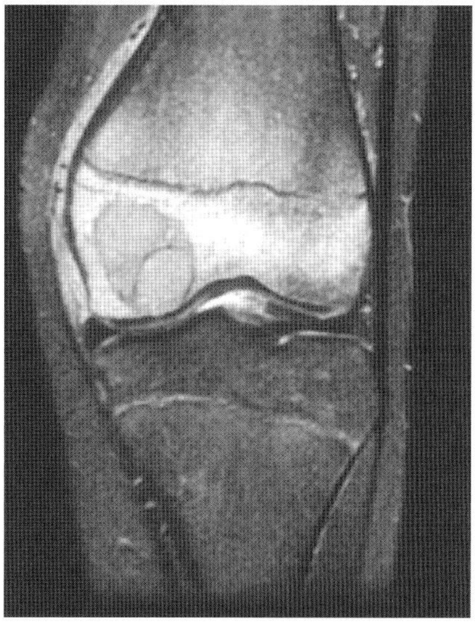

Figure 6 MRI of a chondroblastoma of the distal femur. The lesion is isolated to the epiphysis and associated with surrounding bony edema.

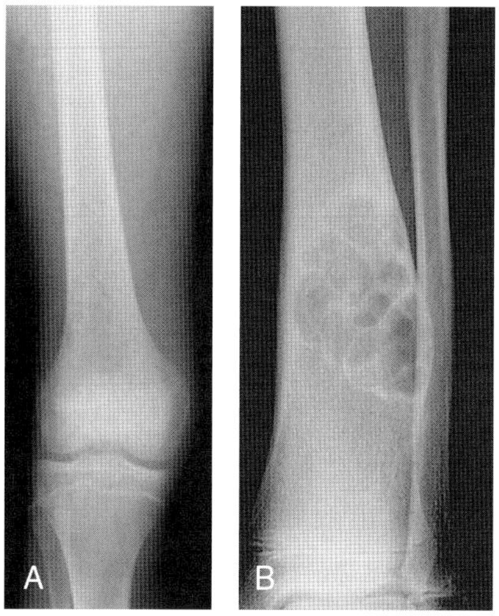

Figure 7 **A,** AP radiograph of a classic fibrous cortical defect involving the cortex of the lateral distal femoral metaphysis. **B,** Lateral radiograph of a nonossifying fibroma involving the medullary cavity of the distal tibia.

Fibrous Cortical Defects and Nonossifying Fibroma

Fibrous cortical defects and nonossifying fibromas are histologically identical lesions with different imaging characteristics. Fibrous cortical defects are confined to the cortex, whereas nonossifying fibromas involve the medullary cavity (**Figure 7**). A fibrous cortical defect is an incidentally found lesion that does not require further imaging. Most of these lesions are asymptomatic. Nonossifying fibromas can become symptomatic when they reach a critical size or from an injury resulting in a pathologic fracture. Under these circumstances, curettage and bone grafting, with or without internal fixation, may be necessary.[13,14] In the absence of fracture or impending fracture, biopsy and surgery are not needed. In general, both of these entities spontaneously regress with time.

Fibrous Dysplasia

Fibrous dysplasia is a developmental anomaly of bone in which a fibro-osseous proliferation replaces normal bone. This process is driven by a missense mutation in the *GNAS* gene. Most patients are younger than 30 years, and pain is the most common presenting symptom. On radiography, the lesions are centrally located in the medullary canal with a ground glass–appearing matrix and cortical thinning (**Figure 8**). Most lesions are monostotic. Multifocal disease exists as a polyostotic variant without an associated syndrome or in conjunction with McCune-Albright syndrome (endocrinopathies) or Mazabraud syndrome (soft-tissue myxomas). Polyostotic forms can involve the entire skeleton or be confined to single limb bud. Surgical treatment is reserved for painful lesions, pathologic fractures, or progressive deformity. Bone grafting of the lesion typically results in replacement of the graft material with additional fibro-osseous tissue. Bone graft substitutes have been used with some success.[15] Medical management of the disease with bisphosphonates is currently under investigation.[16]

Unicameral Bone Cyst

A unicameral bone cyst (UBC) is a benign, fluid-filled cyst; its etiology is largely unknown. A UBC is more likely a reactive or developmental lesion than a true neoplasm. These cysts are typically diagnosed in children but may present for the first time in adulthood. UBCs are most often discovered

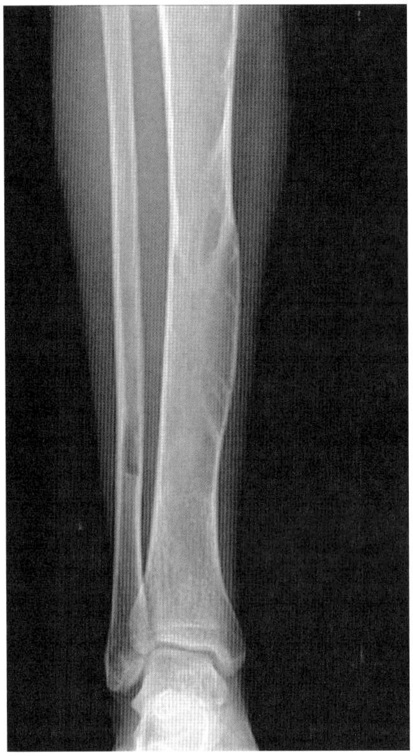

Figure 8 AP radiograph showing fibrous dysplasia involving most of the tibia and focally in the fibula. Note the hazy "ground glass" matrix and marked cortical thinning leading to scalloping in some areas.

because of pain from an associated fracture. Radiographs show unilocular or septated lucency, with thinning of the cortex most commonly in the proximal humerus followed by the proximal femur. In fractured cysts, cortical fracture fragments or the so-called fallen leaf sign may be present. UBCs are classified as active when they are within 1 cm of the physis and latent as they progress to a diaphyseal location. The term simple bone cyst should be avoided because the management of symptomatic refractory lesions is not a simple process. Observation is the treatment of choice for small or asymptomatic lesions and is often used after the first pathologic fracture. Active treatment options include steroid injection, open curettage, bone grafting, and percutaneous injection of marrow or graft substitutes.[17-19] The success of each method is variable, although nearly equivalent local recurrence rates have been reported.

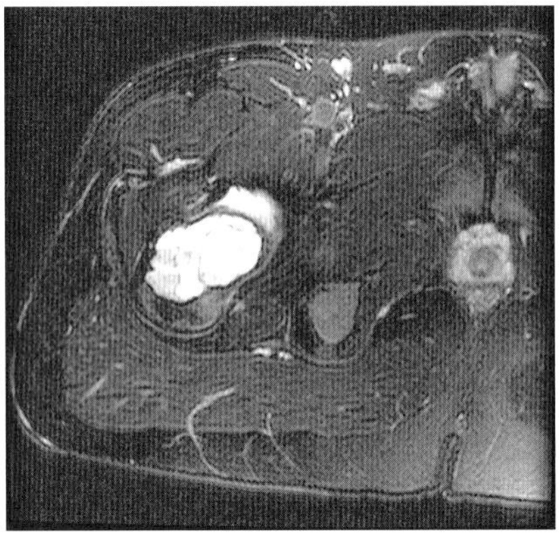

Figure 9 Axial fat-suppressed MRI scan of an ABC of the proximal femur. Fluid-fluid levels are seen in which the light color represents serum and the darker color represents blood.

Aneurysmal Bone Cyst

An aneurysmal bone cyst (ABC) is a benign bone tumor composed of blood-filled spaces separated by fibrous septae. A primary ABC is believed to be a neoplasm with a described translocation at chromosome 17, whereas a secondary ABC (associated with another primary bone tumor) is believed to be reactive. The most common tumors associated with secondary ABCs are giant cell tumors, UBCs, and chondroblastomas, although these lesions may possibly be associated with any tumor. Patients present with pain, swelling, and sometimes pathologic fracture. Radiographically, these lesions appear with expansion or an aneurysm of the bone, typically with an intact rim of cortex. Axial MRI shows the fluid-fluid levels seen in these tumors (**Figure 9**). Because fluid-fluid levels alone are not unique to ABCs, a broad differential diagnosis, including telangiectatic osteosarcoma, must be carefully considered. Some lesions may have an aggressive course and require biopsy to confirm the diagnosis. ABCs are typically treated with extended curettage, followed by bone grafting or local adjuvant and cement.[20,21] In large lesions, internal fixation may be required. Embolization has been described as an alternative treatment in lesions in difficult anatomic locations.[22] Local recurrence is reported as high as 30%. Local adjuvants have been shown to effectively lower the recurrence rate.

Giant Cell Tumor

Giant cell tumors are locally aggressive benign tumors that typically arise in the ends of the long bones, the pelvis, and the sacrum in adults ages 20 to 40 years. Typically, patients present with pain, swelling, and joint stiffness. Radiographically, giant cell tumors appear as lytic, eccentric lesions involving the epiphysis and metaphysis of long bones, with the distal femur and proximal tibia accounting for 50% of sites. Over time, the tumors can exhibit soft-tissue extension. Surgery is the treatment of choice. Because giant cell tumors tend to be locally aggressive and are associated with progressive bone destruction, observation is not recommended. Because of their aggressive appearance, biopsy is always indicated to rule out another process. After the histology is confirmed, the giant cell tumor is usually removed with extended curettage and a local adjuvant with or without internal fixation. Wide excision is reserved for expendable bones or tumors that have extensive local destruction. Local recurrence rates vary according to the treatment method: curettage without adjuvant (approximately 50%), curettage with adjuvant (5% to 25%), and wide excision (< 1%). Like chondroblastoma, giant cell tumor is associated with benign pulmonary metastases in approximately 2% of cases.[23-27]

Malignant Tumors of Bone

It has been estimated that 2,500 to 3,000 new bone sarcomas are diagnosed each year in the United States (soft-tissue sarcomas are approximately three times more common).[28] Recognizing these malignant bone lesions and understanding the appropriate evaluation and treatment is critical to providing quality patient care.

Patient Evaluation

A patient with an aggressive lesion of bone must be carefully evaluated.[29] The evaluation begins with a careful patient history, including attention to pain patterns, constitutional symptoms, family history, and rapidity of symptom onset. The involved bone/joint area is then examined to assess regional adenopathy, evidence of possible articular involvement, and the potential risk of fracture. Appropriate laboratory studies should be obtained, including a complete blood count, serum protein electrophoresis, urine protein electrophoresis, and chemistry panel, along with specific laboratory tests (such as thyroid function, prostate-specific antigen, and urine analysis) if metastatic carcinoma is being considered.

Appropriate plain radiographic studies should be obtained to analyze the lesion and its appearance. The behavior of the lesion (lytic or blastic, aggressive or nonaggressive, geographic or permeative) and the bony response should be identified. Other supporting studies, such as a whole-body bone scan, CT, and MRI of the affected bone, should be obtained as indicated. Radiography and CT of the lungs are necessary in the presence of a primary malignancy of bone, and a screening CT of the chest, abdomen, and pelvis is usually necessary if metastatic carcinoma is suspected.

Tissue diagnosis is necessary in an aggressive-appearing lesion or a lesion whose diagnosis is uncertain on imaging studies. Although the general orthopaedic surgeon may be comfortable dealing with metastatic carcinoma, most other biopsies of aggressive lesions should be done under the direction of a musculoskeletal oncologist.

Osteosarcoma

Osteosarcoma is the most common primary malignancy of bone (excluding myeloma) and is a lesion of malignant bone cells. This tumor has several subtypes, but high-grade intramedullary osteosarcoma is the most common type.[30] Most lesions present as high-grade, extracompartmental lesions of bone (Enneking stage IIB lesions).

Osteosarcoma is a disease of younger patients and generally occurs in the second decade of life, with males afflicted more commonly than females. A second peak occurs in the sixth decade and is usually associated with Paget sarcoma. There are approximately 1,000 cases per year in North America.

This lesion is generally a metaphyseal lesion of long bones and is predominantly found in the distal femur, proximal tibia, proximal humerus, and pelvis. As with most malignancies, pain is the most common presenting symptom. Generally progressive, the presence of pain when at rest and night pain should cause concern. Most patients eventually notice fullness near the associated joint, with impaired motion, swelling, and weakness. Fifteen percent of patients present with a pathologic fracture.

Radiographs usually show a mixed lytic or blastic lesion with cortical destruction, extension into the soft tissue, and periosteal reactions, including a Codman triangle, hair-on-end or sunburst pattern, or an onion-skin appearance. Occasionally these lesions are purely lytic or purely blastic (**Figure 10**). Bone scans show an extremely hot lesion that generally appears larger than its radiographic appearance. MRI should include the entire bone to look for the presence of skip lesions (discontiguous tumor in the same bone), which occur in approximately 10% of patients and portend a worse prognosis. MRI is excellent for delineating the extent of the bone and soft-tissue involvement and identifying the surrounding anatomy and at risk structures. MRI can help identify tumor spread in an adjacent joint and determine if limb salvage is possible. The lesion typically shows dark to intermediate signal on T1-weighted images, and bright signal on T2-weighted images. T1-weighted, gadolinium contrast images are generally bright and may overestimate the extent of the tumor because of the hyperemia that typically surrounds the lesion.[31]

Osteosarcoma is an aggressive lesion that tends to quickly progress. There is a clear association with the retinoblastoma tumor-suppressor gene, the *p53* gene mutations, and older patients with Paget disease. Several oncogenes have been identified in osteosarcoma. No known chromosomal translocation has been associated with this tumor. Histologically, the appearance of lacey (fine, delicate) osteoid in the midst of the malignant cells is the classic appearance. Cells generally exhibit substantial pleomorphism, with numerous mitotic figures. These malignant areas permeate through the existing trabeculae of the host bone and anneal onto the normal, lamellar host bone.

Osteosarcoma is usually treated with neoadjuvant multiagent chemotherapy, followed by local control of the lesion with wide resection (limb-salvage or amputation) and then additional adjuvant chemotherapy. Radiation is generally not used, al-

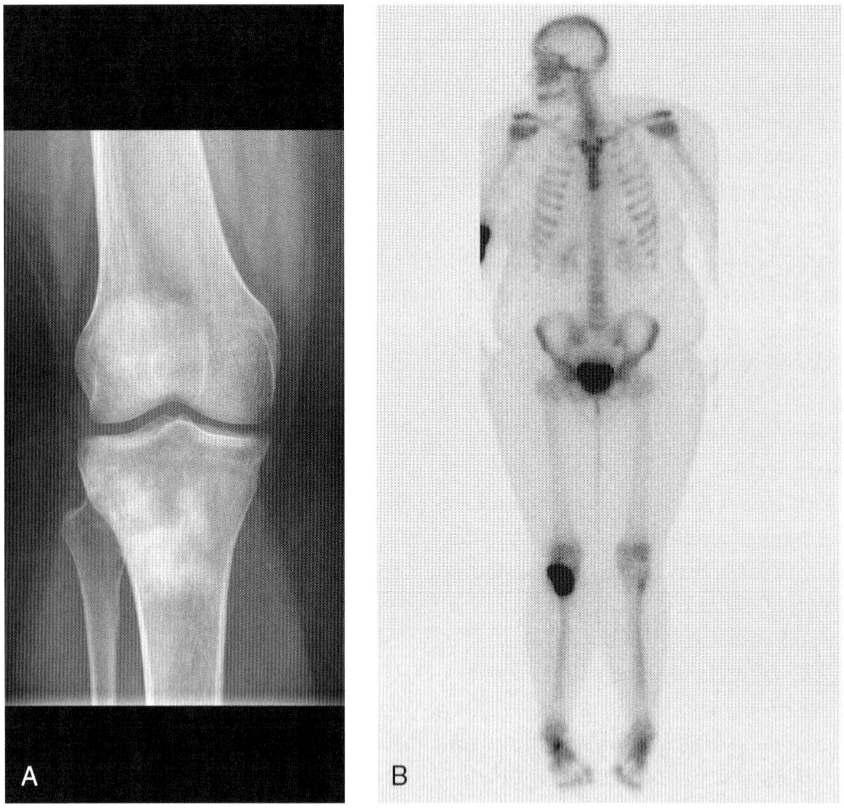

Figure 10 **A,** AP radiograph of the knee showing a blastic lesion in the proximal tibia, with early lateral cortical destruction and extension into the soft tissue, typical of osteosarcoma. **B,** The bone scan shows the typical intense uptake in these lesions.

though it may be added if positive margins are discovered after surgical treatment. Patients with lesions that demonstrate more than 90% necrosis after chemotherapy generally have an improved prognosis. Patients with tumors with a persistent elevation of lactic dehydrogenase and alkaline phosphatase tend to have a worse prognosis. The overall prognosis remains approximately 70% survival at 5 years. Patients with pelvic lesions or those that present with metastatic disease generally have a 5-year survival rate of 20% to 25%.[32]

Osteosarcoma may less frequently present as one of several specific subtypes. Parosteal osteosarcoma is a low-grade surface subtype lesion that presents in the second to third decades of life and is more common in women. These lesions present as an indolent, slowly progressing mass with swelling and loss of motion in the joint (generally knee). This lesion has the radiographic appearance of being stuck on the surface of the bone (the posterior distal femur is the classic presentation) and is densely ossified. These lesions tend to be fibrogenic on histologic section and can look fairly bland, almost like fibrous dysplasia. Treatment is wide resection, and the survival rate is approximately 90% at 5 years if complete resection is achieved. A dedifferentiated form can present (generally after multiple local recurrences), which has a much more aggressive course.

Periosteal osteosarcoma is a rare subtype that presents in young patients (second decade of life) and is almost always located in the diaphysis of the tibia or the femur. This is a painful lesion that generally has a sunburst or hair-on-end appearance in the middle of the lesion, with the lesion itself arising in the periosteum (often with some hazy density). The underlying cortex often has a saucerized appearance. Periosteal osteosarcoma tends to be chondroblastic on histologic section, with malignant osteoid present. Treatment is generally the same as for classic osteosarcoma (chemotherapy and wide surgical resection). Survival is approximately 75% to 80% at 5 years.

Telangiectatic osteosarcoma is a rare subtype that presents in a manner similar to conventional osteosarcoma (age group, symptoms, and location) but is purely lytic and has the radiographic appearance of a very aggressive ABC, which is in the radiographic differential diagnosis. On MRI, the presence of fluid-fluid levels is common. Nearly 25% of patients present with a pathologic fracture because of the aggressive lytic nature of the lesion. It is important not to misdiagnose these malignant lesions as ABCs. Histologically, large lakes of blood are present, occasionally with benign-appearing giant cells; however, the stromal cells appear malignant and often have mitotic figures. Malignant osteoid is not a major histologic feature in these tumors. Treatment and prognosis is essentially the same as that of classic osteosarcoma.

Ewing Sarcoma and Primitive Neuroectodermal Tumor

Ewing sarcoma is the third most common primary sarcoma of bone and is a malignant lesion of small round blue cells (round cell lesion). The cell of origin is unknown. Current thinking is that primitive neuroectodermal tumor is a differentiated neural lesion, and Ewing sarcoma is the more dedifferentiated lesion.[33] Bone marrow biopsy is required in the staging process.

This lesion presents in young individuals, with most patients in the second decade of life. Males are affected more commonly than females. This tumor is uncommon in African Americans. Common locations include the pelvis, femur (particularly the proximal and diaphyseal femur), humerus, and tibia; however, the tumor has been reported at virtually all locations. Pain is the most common clinical presentation. Swelling with loss of normal limb function is also common. Patients often present with fever, an elevated erythrocyte sedimentation rate and white blood cell count, which are suggestive of an infection. Care must be taken not to assume infection in young patients with these constitutional symptoms.

Radiographs show a lytic lesion that is permeative in appearance, often extensive, and has substantial periosteal reaction (classic onion-skin appearance) (**Figure 11**). The lesion often has a diaphyseal location. The general architecture of the bone remains, but it looks fuzzy because of subtle bone destruction. Plain radiographs generally suggest the presence of a soft-tissue mass. Radiographically, these lesions may look like osteosarcoma or any of the other aggressive round cell lesions of bone (such as infection, eosinophilic granuloma, or lymphoma).

Bone scans show a very hot lesion, often extending well beyond the expected area based on plain radiographs alone. MRI is helpful in defining the margins of the lesion, the extent of marrow involvement, and the often large soft-tissue mass that is associated with the tumor. The lesion shows intermediate signal on T1-weighted MRI and very bright signal on T2-weighted and gadolinium contrast images. Diffuse involvement of the surrounding musculature is common. Positron emission tomography shows intense uptake at the tumor site and is helpful in identifying occult disease and following the response of the lesion to chemotherapy.

The 11:22 chromosomal translocation (which produces the *EWS/FLI1* fusion gene) is nearly always present; if not present, the diagnosis is suspect. The tumor stains CD-99 positive. Histologically, the tumor is composed of "sheets" of small, round blue cells with poorly defined borders, minimal cytoplasm, and prominent nuclei. Grossly, the tumor looks like pus, which along with the presenting symptoms can result in a misdiagnosis. No real stroma exists, and necrosis can be a prominent feature. Pseudorosettes may be present. Mitotic figures are not typically a prominent feature of this tumor.

These aggressive lesions are treated with neoadjuvant chemotherapy followed by local control of the lesion, generally with wide resection; however, radiation is also effective. Controversy exists on whether surgery is a better treatment than radiation. In patients presenting with metastatic disease or with pelvic lesions, radiation may be more acceptable. However, radiation carries risks for fracture, growth disturbances, contractures, and secondary malignancy. After local control is achieved, patients receive several cycles of neoadjuvant chemotherapy. The 5-year survival rate in extremity lesions is approximately 70%, but in pelvic lesions or in patients with metastases, the 5-year survival rate is approximately 25%.[34] Metastasis generally presents in the lungs but may present in the bones.

Chondrosarcoma

Chondrosarcoma is the second most common primary sarcoma of bone. It may be a primary (de novo) lesion or a secondary lesion (arising from a preexisting chondroid lesion, such as osteochondroma). Chondrosarcoma is the result of malignant cartilage-forming cells.[35] Most of these lesions present as relatively low-grade lesions and slow-growing intracompartmental lesions of bone (Enneking stage IA).

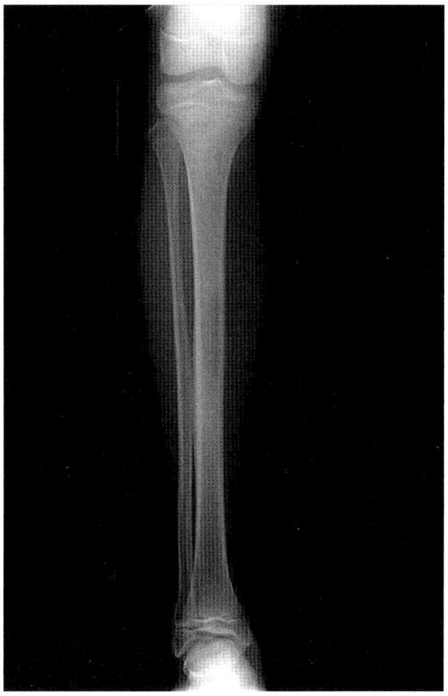

Figure 11 AP radiograph of the tibia shows a common diaphyseal presentation in Ewing sarcoma, with periosteal reaction and a "hazy" appearance to the bone secondary to destructive changes.

Chondrosarcoma usually presents in patients between 40 and 60 years of age. The most common locations include the pelvis, ribs, femur, and proximal humerus. Patients often present with a dull, achy pain, often of months' duration. The pain may be located over the involved bone or may be more diffuse. Night pain or dull pain when at rest is common. The presentation can be subtle and quite variable. This lesion, in particular, requires careful correlation of clinical, radiographic, and histologic findings to establish the proper diagnosis.

Radiographs generally show a destructive lesion with evidence of mineralization (approximately 75% of cases) and cortical changes (erosions, expansion of bone, and destructive areas). In patients with advanced

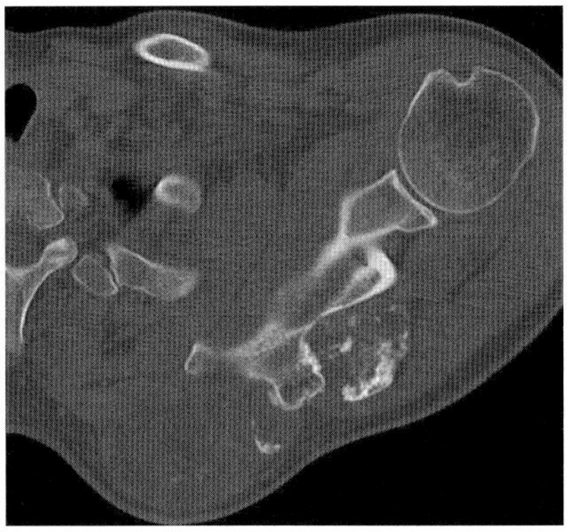

Figure 12 CT scan shows the typical punctate calcifications seen in this chondrosarcoma of the scapula. Extensive soft tissue involvement can be seen.

chondrosarcoma, a soft-tissue mass may be present. Progressive radiographic features (noted on serial radiographs) combined with clinical findings are the best method for determining malignant transformation or malignant behavior in a chondroid lesion. The bone scan is typically hot; the presence of a cold bone scan generally rules out chondrosarcoma. CT shows a destructive lesion that usually has punctate mineral density (well visualized on CT), occasionally with a soft-tissue mass. CT is particularly helpful in evaluating pelvic and scapular lesions (**Figure 12**). MRI shows a wet (high signal) lesion on T2-weighted images (low signal on T1-weighted images) that is inhomogeneous with areas of decreased signal and often demonstrates extension of the lesion beyond the expected margin seen on plain radiographs. Positron emission tomography is not typically used but can show increased metabolic activity in higher-grade lesions; however, it cannot reliably distinguish low-grade malignant lesions from enchondromas.

Younger patients tend to have lower-grade lesions than older patients. Axial lesions tend to have a worse prognosis and exhibit more aggressive behavior than appendicular lesions. Larger size lesions (> 5 to 7 cm) also portend a worse prognosis. Chondrosarcoma is typically slow growing and may be present for months or years before detection. The t(9;22) translocation is present in approximately 30% of myxoid chondrosarcomas. The ability of the tumor to degrade and migrate through tissue is believed to be caused, in part, by the collagenase production of the tumor cells. Chondrosarcomas are lobular chondroid lesions with increased cellularity and myxoid changes. Higher-grade lesions tend to have areas of multiple nuclei, greater cellularity, and tumor permeation around the host bone lamellae. Lower-grade lesions may be difficult to distinguish from benign cartilage tumors. The pathologist should be informed of the location of any biopsied lesion because benign cartilage tumors from the hand and feet or from a periosteal location also can be fairly cellular and may result in a misdiagnosis.

Wide resection is the treatment of choice in grade II or III lesions. Because these lesions do not respond to chemotherapy or radiation, appropriate resection of the tumor is key to a successful outcome.[36] In some instances, a low-grade lesion in a long bone may be treated with extended intralesional curettage with adjuvant treatment (such as phenol or argon beam therapy). The 5-year survival rate depends on the grade of the lesion: grade I, greater than 90%; grade II, approximately 75%; and grade III, less than 50%. The risk of late recurrence is approximately 20%. These lesions can be difficult to evaluate and stage and generally should be treated by a musculoskeletal oncologist.

Secondary chondrosarcomas arise from a preexisting chondroid lesion (such as an enchondroma or osteochondroma) and generally present in a similar fashion to an intramedullary lesion. In the preexisting osteochondroma, the tumor arises out of the cartilage cap that is thickened (historically reported as a cap thicker than 2 cm). These tumors are treated with wide resection in primary chondrosarcomas.

Dedifferentiated chondrosarcoma is the most malignant tumor of the chondrosarcoma family and is a very aggressive lesion with a poor prognosis. Approximately 10% of chondrosarcomas, especially long-standing lesions, transform into this high-grade lesion. This tumor histologically demonstrates a bimorphic pattern of malignant cartilage cells with superimposed high-grade spindle cells. The 5-year survival rates for patients with dedifferentiated chondrosarcoma are less than 20%. Patients are treated with resection. The use of chemotherapy is controversial; evidence of improved outcomes in these patients has not been clearly shown.

Multiple Myeloma

Myeloma is the most common primary malignancy of bone, although some physicians consider it a marrow tumor or systemic disease rather than a bone tumor. Myeloma produces immunoglobulins (Ig), generally IgG or IgA.[37] A myeloma spike is demonstrated in most patients on electrophoresis, either serum or urine (which identifies the light chain or Bence Jones protein).

Most patients presenting with myeloma are older than 40 years. Myeloma and metastatic carcinoma are the two primary considerations in patients with multiple bone lesions. Males are affected more frequently than females. Unlike Ewing sarcoma, this lesion is common in African Americans. The spine, ribs, pelvis, skull, and major long bones are the most common presenting locations, and pain is the most common symptom. Patients may present with weakness, weight loss, anemia, and a history of recurrent infections (because this tumor affects bone marrow). Pathologic fractures, particularly in the spine, are fairly common. Common laboratory findings include an elevated erythrocyte sedimentation rate, hypercalcemia, amyloidosis, and positive serum or urine protein electrophoresis.

Radiographs show purely lytic, punched-out lesions (particularly in flat bones) in multiple locations (**Figure 13**). There is rarely substantial periosteal reaction, and long bones may have the fuzzy or hazy appearance common to round cell lesions. Often the bones appear osteopenic. Bone scanning is not a reliable screening tool because the lesion frequently does not incite a substantial osteoblastic response in the underlying bone. Skeletal surveying remains the screening method of choice. MRI shows the typical dark-to-intermediate T1-weighted signal and the bright T2-weighted signal seen in other round cell lesions. MRI is helpful in identifying the extent of the tumor and the marrow involvement; it is particularly helpful in identifying spine lesions, which frequently can be occult.

The presence of one major and one minor criteria or three minor criteria are usually necessary to establish the diagnosis. Major criteria include positive histologic tissue analysis (plasmacytoma at biopsy), more than 30% plasma cells in bone marrow, and serum IgG levels greater than 3.5 g/dL. Minor criteria include 10% to 30% plasma cells in bone marrow, lytic bone lesions, and elevated serum or urine protein levels. Elevated β-2 microglobulin levels portend a worse prognosis. This tumor stains positive in the presence of CD38. Histologically, this lesion demonstrates sheets of plasma cells. These cells have the "clock face" chromatin in the eccentric nuclei, the "Hoffa bench" clear zone in the cytoplasm juxtaposed to the nuclei, and abundant eosinophilic cytoplasm. Mitotic figures are generally absent.

Patients are treated with chemotherapy and bisphosphonates (to help decrease the lytic bone lesions and the incidence of pathologic fractures). Radiation may be used for focal lesional control, and surgery is generally reserved for patients who require fixation and/or stabilization to maintain skeletal integrity (similar to the treatment of metastatic carcinoma).[38] The overall survival rate with this disease is poor, with approximately 10% survival at 10 years.

Lymphoma

Lymphoma is a clonal proliferation of mature B cells and is generally a non-Hodgkin lymphoma. Primary lymphoma of bone is rare. The typical orthopaedic presentation is extranodal disease to bone.

Patients with lymphoma generally present in the fifth decade of life, although individuals of any age can be affected, with males more commonly affected than females. Common locations include the femur, spine, and pelvis. Patients typically present with persistent pain, occasionally a soft-tissue mass, and may manifest neurologic symptoms if the lesion is located in the spine. Fever, night sweats, and weight loss (so-called B symptoms) may be present. Pathologic fractures are fairly common in patients with these lesions.

Radiographs typically show a lytic, permeative, classic round cell lesion that maintains the basic architecture of the bone, with subtle bone destruction (fuzzy appearance). At times, there may be little to no change apparent on plain radiographs; conversely, a focal lytic lesion may be seen (**Figure 14**). This tumor may occasionally have a blastic appearance if there is little bony reaction to the underlying lesion. A bone scan is generally very hot but may occasionally show little uptake. MRI appearance is similar to that of myeloma, with a dark-to-intermediate T1-weighted signal and a bright T2-weighted signal in the tumor. A large associated soft-tissue mass is very common. Positron emission tomography can be useful in evaluating the presence of multiple sites and the response to treatment.[39]

Lymphomas are delicate lesions that can be difficult to biopsy because it is

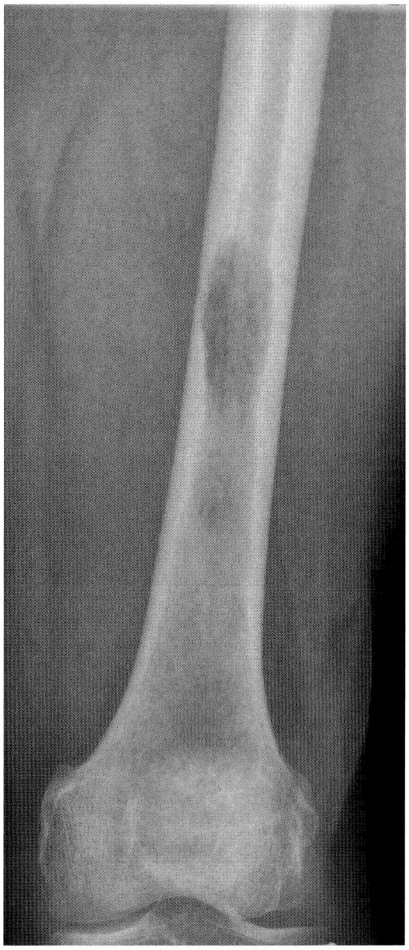

Figure 13 AP radiograph of the femur shows the typical lytic, punched-out appearance seen in myeloma. Often there are multiple lesions. (This patient had multiple bone involvement.)

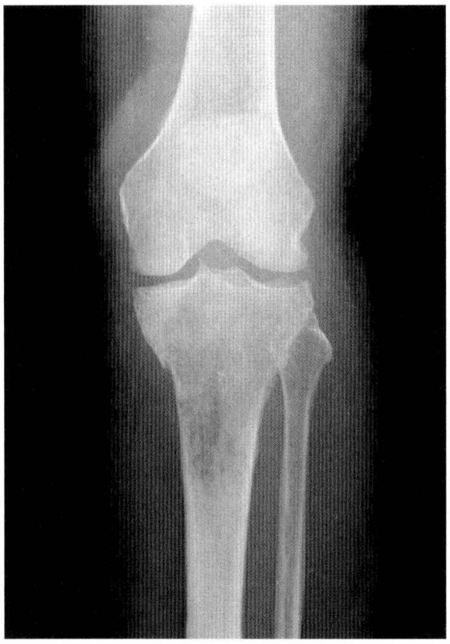

Figure 14 AP radiograph of the knee shows the lytic destructive changes common in lymphoma in the proximal tibia. Note that the bone has a washed out appearance, which is typical of round cell lesions.

easy to crush the tissue and impair histologic evaluation. Risk factors include immunodeficiency for any reason or the presence of persistent infection. Lymphoma cells stain positive for CD20 and CD45. Histologically, this is a round cell lesion that shows variable, enlarged lymphocytes (sizes vary considerably), which are clearly larger than most round cell lesions. There is little background stroma in these lesions, and mitotic figures are common. These lesions typically show a very infiltrative pattern into the underlying tissue.

Lymphomas are treated with chemotherapy, which is often quite effective. Occasionally, radiation is used for large focal lesions that otherwise do not respond to treatment. Surgical intervention is generally necessary only to maintain skeletal integrity, particularly in the presence of pathologic fractures. The overall prognosis is generally quite good, with 5-year survival rates of approximately 70%.

Summary

Malignant bone tumors are rare; however, improper treatment of these tumors can result in poor outcomes for patients. It is very important to distinguish benign bone lesions from malignant bone lesions. The ability to discern which lesion requires observation, surgical care, or referral to an orthopaedic oncologist will benefit both the orthopaedic surgeon and the patient.

References

1. Codman EA: The classic: The registry of bone sarcomas as an example of the end-result idea in hospital organization. 1924. *Clin Orthop Relat Res* 2009;467(11): 2766-2770.
2. Codman EA: The classic: Registry of bone sarcoma. Part I: Twenty-five criteria for establishing the diagnosis of osteogenic sarcoma. Part II: Thirteen registered cases of "five year cures" analyzed according to these criteria. 1926. *Clin Orthop Relat Res* 2009; 467(11):2771-2782.
3. Madewell JE, Ragsdale BD, Sweet DE: Radiologic and pathologic analysis of solitary bone lesions: Part I. Internal margins. *Radiol Clin North Am* 1981;19(4): 715-748.
4. Phemister DB: Cancer of the bone and joint. *J Am Med Assoc* 1948;136(8):545-554.
5. Lodwick GS, Wilson AJ, Farrell C, Virtama P, Dittrich F: Determining growth rates of focal lesions of bone from radiographs. *Radiology* 1980;134(3):577-583.
6. Parsons TW: Imaging interpretation of oncologic musculoskeletal conditions: Understanding what you see! Part III: Extremity bone tumors. http://www.aaosnotice.org/2011_Proceedings/tumor_metabolic_disease.html. Accessed October 5, 2012.
7. Sweet DE, Madewell JE, Ragsdale BD: Radiologic and pathologic analysis of solitary bone lesions: Part III. Matrix patterns. *Radiol Clin North Am* 1981;19(4): 785-814.
8. Rosenthal DI, Hornicek FJ, Torriani M, Gebhardt MC, Mankin HJ: Osteoid osteoma: Percutaneous treatment with radiofrequency energy. *Radiology* 2003;229(1): 171-175.
9. Ozaki T, Liljenqvist U, Hillmann A, et al: Osteoid osteoma and osteoblastoma of the spine: Experiences with 22 patients. *Clin Orthop Relat Res* 2002;397:394-402.
10. Porter DE, Simpson AH: The neoplastic pathogenesis of solitary and multiple osteochondromas. *J Pathol* 1999;188(2):119-125.
11. Marco RA, Gitelis S, Brebach GT, Healey JH: Cartilage tumors: Evaluation and treatment. *J Am Acad Orthop Surg* 2000;8(5): 292-304.
12. Springfield DS, Capanna R, Gherlinzoni F, Picci P, Campanacci M: Chondroblastoma: A review of seventy cases. *J Bone Joint Surg Am* 1985;67(5):748-755.
13. Moretti VM, Slotcavage RL, Crawford EA, Lackman RD, Ogilvie CM: Curettage and graft alleviates athletic-limiting pain in benign lytic bone lesions. *Clin Orthop Relat Res* 2011;469(1): 283-288.
14. Easley ME, Kneisl JS: Pathologic fractures through nonossifying fibromas: Is prophylactic treatment warranted? *J Pediatr Orthop* 1997;17(6):808-813.
15. Irwin RB, Bernhard M, Biddinger A: Coralline hydroxyapatite as bone substitute in orthopedic oncology. *Am J Orthop (Belle Mead NJ)* 2001;30(7):544-550.
16. Chapurlat RD: Medical therapy in adults with fibrous dysplasia of bone. *J Bone Miner Res* 2006; 21(suppl 2):114-119.

17. Rougraff BT, Kling TJ: Treatment of active unicameral bone cysts with percutaneous injection of demineralized bone matrix and autogenous bone marrow. *J Bone Joint Surg Am* 2002;84(6): 921-929.
18. Capanna R, Campanacci DA, Manfrini M: Unicameral and aneurysmal bone cysts. *Orthop Clin North Am* 1996;27(3):605-614.
19. Wright JG, Yandow S, Donaldson S, Marley L; Simple Bone Cyst Trial Group: A randomized clinical trial comparing intralesional bone marrow and steroid injections for simple bone cysts. *J Bone Joint Surg Am* 2008;90(4): 722-730.
20. Dormans JP, Hanna BG, Johnston DR, Khurana JS: Surgical treatment and recurrence rate of aneurysmal bone cysts in children. *Clin Orthop Relat Res* 2004;421: 205-211.
21. Marcove RC, Sheth DS, Takemoto S, Healey JH: The treatment of aneurysmal bone cyst. *Clin Orthop Relat Res* 1995;311: 157-163.
22. de Gauzy JS, Abid A, Accadbled F, Knorr G, Darodes P, Cahuzac JP: Percutaneous Ethibloc injection in the treatment of primary aneurysmal bone cysts. *J Pediatr Orthop B* 2005;14(5):367-370.
23. Malawer MM, Bickels J, Meller I, Buch RG, Henshaw RM, Kollender Y: Cryosurgery in the treatment of giant cell tumor: A long-term followup study. *Clin Orthop Relat Res* 1999;359:176-188.
24. Saiz P, Virkus W, Piasecki P, Templeton A, Shott S, Gitelis S: Results of giant cell tumor of bone treated with intralesional excision. *Clin Orthop Relat Res* 2004;424: 221-226.
25. Turcotte RE, Wunder JS, Isler MH, et al: Giant cell tumor of long bone: A Canadian Sarcoma Group study. *Clin Orthop Relat Res* 2002;397:248-258.
26. Algawahmed H, Turcotte R, Farrokhyar F, Ghert M: High-speed burring with and without the use of surgical adjuvants in the intralesional management of giant cell tumor of bone: A systematic review and meta-analysis. [Epub July 27, 2010]. *Sarcoma.*
27. Lewis VO, Wei A, Mendoza T, Primus F, Peabody T, Simon MA: Argon beam coagulation as an adjuvant for local control of giant cell tumor. *Clin Orthop Relat Res* 2007;454:192-197.
28. Siegel R, Ward E, Brawley O, Jemal A: Cancer statistics, 2011: The impact of eliminating socioeconomic and racial disparities on premature cancer deaths. *CA Cancer J Clin* 2011;61(4):212-236.
29. Parsons TW III, Filzen TW: Evaluation and staging of musculoskeletal neoplasia. *Hand Clin* 2004;20(2):v, 137-145.
30. Damron TA, Ward WG, Stewart A: Osteosarcoma, chondrosarcoma, and Ewing's sarcoma: National Cancer Data Base Report. *Clin Orthop Relat Res* 2007;459: 40-47.
31. Sanders TG, Parsons TW III: Radiographic imaging of musculoskeletal neoplasia. *Cancer Control* 2001;8(3):221-231.
32. Hornicek FJ: Osteosarcoma of bone, in Schwartz HS, ed: *Orthopaedic Knowledge Update: Musculoskeletal Tumors*, ed 2. Rosemont, IL, American Academy of Orthopaedic Surgeons, 2007, pp 163-174.
33. Dehner LP: Primitive neuroectodermal tumor and Ewing's sarcoma. *Am J Surg Pathol* 1993; 17(1):1-13.
34. Patterson FR, Basra SK: Ewing's sarcoma, in Schwartz HS, ed: *Orthopaedic Knowledge Update: Musculoskeletal Tumors*, ed 2. Rosemont, IL, American Academy of Orthopaedic Surgeons, 2007, pp 175-183.
35. Lee FY, Mankin HJ, Fondren G, et al: Chondrosarcoma of bone: An assessment of outcome. *J Bone Joint Surg Am* 1999;81(3): 326-338.
36. Seo SW, Remotti F, Lee FY: Chondrosarcoma of bone, in Schwartz HS, ed: *Orthopaedic Knowledge Update: Musculoskeletal Tumors*, ed 2. Rosemont, IL, American Academy of Orthopaedic Surgeons, 2007, pp 185-195.
37. Nau KC, Lewis WD: Multiple myeloma: Diagnosis and treatment. *Am Fam Physician* 2008; 78(7):853-859.
38. Epstein J, Walker R: Myeloma and bone disease: "The dangerous tango." *Clin Adv Hematol Oncol* 2006;4(4):300-306.
39. Schaefer NG, Strobel K, Taverna C, Hany TF: Bone involvement in patients with lymphoma: The role of FDG-PET/CT. *Eur J Nucl Med Mol Imaging* 2007;34(1): 60-67.

SECTION

10

The Practice of Orthopaedics

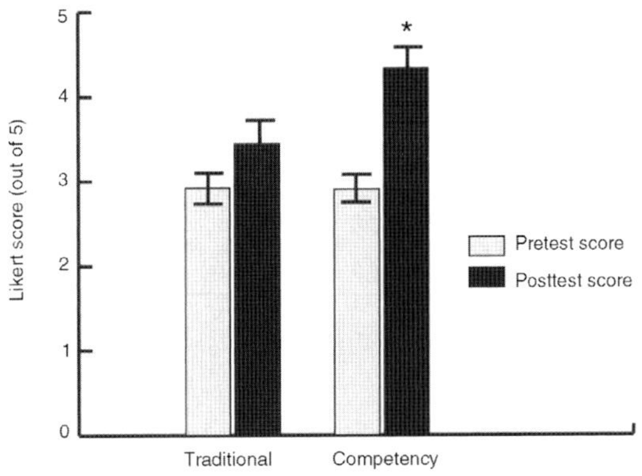

48 Orthopaedic Residency Education: A Practical Guide to Selection, Training, and Education

Symposium
49 Competency-Based Education: A New Model for Teaching Orthopaedics

Symposium
50 Resident Education in the Systems-Based Practice Competency

Symposium
51 I Feel Disconnected: Learning Technologies in Resident Education

52 The Emerging Case for Shared Decision Making in Orthopaedics

53 Surviving and Winning a Professional Negligence Lawsuit

48

Orthopaedic Residency Education: A Practical Guide to Selection, Training, and Education

Kenneth A. Egol, MD
Douglas R. Dirschl, MD
William N. Levine, MD
Joseph D. Zuckerman, MD

Abstract

The education of orthopaedic residents is an important responsibility shared by all those involved in residency training. The education of orthopaedic residents begins with the selection process, which recognizes the importance of choosing qualified individuals who can successfully complete the training program. Education during the 5 years of required training entails the acquisition of a body of knowledge, the development of surgical skills, and the exhibition of a level of professionalism consistent with being a physician and surgeon. Residency training also requires an evaluation of performance and, when necessary, measures to improve performance or correct inappropriate behaviors. The goal at the end of the 5-year training period is to have well-qualified, skilled, and knowledgeable orthopaedic surgeons who can enter practice and provide the highest level of patient care.

Instr Course Lect 2013;62:553-564.

The training of orthopaedic residents is a common thread shared by many orthopaedic surgeons regardless of subspecialty interest, location, or hospital affiliation. However, unlike the clinical areas of orthopaedic surgery for which there is extensive research and documented outcomes, there is a paucity of available research regarding residency training in orthopaedic surgery. Because applications for available positions as orthopaedic residents exceed the number of available positions, residency training programs have access to some of the best and brightest medical students. This chapter will focus on the selection, training, and education of orthopaedic residents.

Selection

Resident Attributes

Orthopaedic residency candidates should possess several attributes that may contribute to their success during residency training. More than 30 years ago, the Steering Committee on Resident Selection for the American Orthopaedic Association specified three specific areas that may predict resident performance: cognitive skills, noncognitive factors (affective domain), and motor abilities. Without evidence, committee members determined certain cognitive measures (such as the achievement of medical school honors and election to the Alpha Omega Alpha Honor Medical Society) that they believed correlated with success during residency training. A broader view of a candidate's cognitive skills by evaluating performance in the undergraduate setting, during medical school, and

Dr. Egol or an immediate family member serves as a board member, owner, officer, or committee member of the Orthopaedic Trauma Association Research Committee and the American Academy of Orthopaedic Surgeons Instructional Course Lecture Committee; has received royalties from Exactech; has received research or institutional support from Stryker, Synthes, and OREF; and owns stock or stock options in Johnson & Johnson. Dr. Dirschl or an immediate family member serves as a board member, owner, officer, or committee member of the American Orthopaedic Association; has received royalties from Biomet; and serves as a paid consultant to or is an employee of Stryker and Amgen. Dr. Levine or an immediate family member serves as a board member, owner, officer, or committee member of the American Orthopaedic Association and has received research or institutional support from Stryker. Dr. Zuckerman or an immediate family member has received royalties from Exactech and owns stock or stock options in Neostem and Joint Innovation Technology.

Table 1
Comparison of Perceived Importance of Residency Selection Criteria

Question	Program Director Ranking	Applicant Ranking	Significant Difference in Ranking[a]
Elective rotation performance	1	4	
USMLE step 1 score	2	2	
Class rank in medical school	3	3	
Formality and politeness at interview	4	5	
Personal appearance	5	9	*
Ethical question	6	10	*
Letter of recommendation from an orthopaedic surgeon	7	1	*
Alpha Omega Alpha Honor Medical Society membership	8	7	
Medical school reputation	9	11	
Dean's letter	10	6	
Thank you letter	24	24	
Skills testing	25	19	*
Psychological testing	26	22	

[a]The asterisk indicates a significant difference ($P < 0.05$) in the rank given by applicants versus program directors.
USMLE = United States Medical Licensing Examination.
(Adapted with permission from Bernstein AD, Jazrawi LM, Elbeshbeshy B, DellaValle CJ, Zuckerman JD: An analysis of orthopaedic residency selection criteria. *Bull Hosp Jt Dis* 2002;61(1-2):49-57.)

during interviews was also considered necessary.

The affective domain is defined as the personal and professional values of an applicant, including integrity, trustworthiness, responsibility, reliability, and accountability. The committee considered the evaluation of this domain to be important in gauging a future resident's performance.[1] To determine which personality traits were necessary for successful residency performance, the committee analyzed a survey completed by residents entering 33 different orthopaedic programs. Results showed that a poorly performing resident was less likely to describe himself or herself as well adjusted, competent, and thorough.[1,2] The components of affective domain are highly subjective and are, therefore, difficult to assess.[1,3-8] Predictors of success related to affective domain often require personal interaction and the direct observation of candidates, which may be time consuming and difficult to accomplish. Societal goals and responsibilities and the attributes necessary to achieve those goals are also important considerations in selecting future orthopaedic surgeons. The American Academy of Orthopaedic Surgeons (AAOS) promotes diversity in the field as the best method for treating a diverse patient population.[3]

The third domain recognized as a predictor of resident performance is the psychomotor domain, which encompasses the technical and motor skill set required to safely practice orthopaedic surgery. Almost no data are available regarding affective domain or motor abilities as factors in predicting a resident's likelihood of success or failure. Although these domains form the basis of evaluation of resident selection, they have not yet been incorporated into the Accreditation Council for Graduate Medical Education (ACGME) core competencies.

Survey Findings

In 2002, Bernstein et al[5] surveyed 91 orthopaedic residency applicants interviewing at a large university-based residency program and 109 orthopaedic program residency directors throughout the United States to determine their views on the most important criteria involved in the resident selection process (**Table 1**). The orthopaedic applicants believed that a letter of recommendation from an orthopaedic surgeon was the most important factor, followed by the score on the United States Medical Licensing Exam (USMLE) step 1 and then class rank in medical school. The three most important factors for the residency directors were performance of a rotation at the residency director's program, the USMLE step 1 score, and rank in medical school. The study also found an important difference in opinion between orthopaedic candidates and residency directors on 12 of the 26 criteria, which suggested a lack of communication between the two groups.[5,8]

A 2004 study by Bajaj and Carmichael[4] surveyed 46 orthopaedic residency applicants and 35 orthopaedic faculty members at programs throughout Texas. Each group ranked the importance of different attributes of orthopaedic residency candidates. Applicants believed that performance on a local rotation, USMLE step 1 scores, and letters of recommendation were the most important factors in obtaining a residency position. Faculty members reported that performances on local rotation, class rank, and at interview were the three most important selection criteria. Both groups reported that research participation, sex, and race were the three least important selection criteria.

Predictors of Success

One difficulty in selecting prediction criteria is establishing a universal measure of successful training. Most studies evaluating selection criteria have included successful promotion to the chief year, passing part 1 of the American Board of Orthopaedic Surgery (ABOS) certifying examination on the first attempt, and the absence of disciplinary issues during training as measures of successful training. It is also important to note that substandard performance during training may not predict failure as a practicing physician. In many instances, good doctors have failed the board examination before passing it. The cognitive domain has been extensively studied. Objective academic criteria have historically been emphasized in the orthopaedic residency selection process. Although the correlation between predictors of and successful performance during residency have not been clearly established,[4,7,9,10] many studies have stressed the growing importance of affective domain as a predictor of success.[1-15]

Cognitive Domain

Medical School Performance

Historically, medical school performance has been a selection criterion in orthopaedic residency programs. In 1989, Clark et al[6] attempted to determine the characteristics of applicants that were predictive of successfully matching into orthopaedic surgery training programs. Data were gathered from 288 applications of candidates applying in a single year to two different orthopaedic residency programs in Texas. Applicants who obtained a residency position were more often members of the Alpha Omega Alpha Honor Medical Society, had higher Medical College Admission Test scores, achieved higher National Board of Medical Examiners (NBME)-1 scores, and had a higher medical school grade point average compared with applicants who did not obtain a match. Applicants were less likely to successfully match if they were foreign citizens graduating from foreign medical schools or had previous residency experience in other fields.

Alpha Omega Alpha Honor Medical Society

Based on 2011 statistics, 27.1% of US seniors matching into orthopaedic training programs were members of the Alpha Omega Alpha Honor Medical Society.[16] A 2002 study by Dirschl[3] analyzed several applicant factors to determine which, if any, were predictive of a successful residency performance. The outcomes of success used in this study were the orthopaedic in-training examination (OITE) scores, ABOS part 1 scores, the amount of research involvement, and faculty evaluations. Higher third-year clinical grades specifically correlated with a better evaluation. Achieving Alpha Omega Alpha Honor Medical Society status was the second strongest predictor of a successful residency and correlated with better overall performance evaluations.

United States Medical Licensing Examination

Studies have reported that higher USMLE step 1 scores correlate with improved performance during residency and higher OITE scores.[9-11] In 2005, Carmichael et al[9] evaluated potential predictors of success during residency using OITE average percentile scores as the main outcome measure. Application information and OITE scores for 60 orthopaedic residents over an 8-year period in two participating Texas residency programs were analyzed. Residents who scored higher than 220 on the USMLE step 1 and residents who were married were more likely to have higher OITE scores. In 2008, Spitzer et al[11] performed a thorough analysis to determine which preselection factors correlated with success during residency. When residents were divided into two groups, good or poor performers, only performance on the OITE correlated with performance outcomes.

Because of timing issues, orthopaedic residency programs place less emphasis on USMLE step 2 scores than step 1 scores. Bajaj and Carmichael[4] reported that orthopaedic faculty place slightly more importance on USMLE step 2 results than do residents. Both applicants and faculty ranked the USMLE step 2 score lower in importance than the USMLE step 1 score.

Clark et al[6] reported that applicants with very high NBME-2 scores or very low NBME-2 scores (older terminology for the USMLE scores) were substantially more likely to match or not match, respectively, into a residency program. However, no pure cutoff values were determined between the two groups. No other study included USMLE step 2 scores as a possible predictor for residency success.

Medical School Rank

Residency program directors and applicants rank the reputation of the medical school attended as having moderate to high importance (ranked 9th and 11th, respectively, of 26 criteria) in the selection process.[5] In a study by Thordarson et al,[12] selection committee members ranked medical school affiliation as the fifth most important of nine criteria when ranking applicants for residency. Medical school reputation and ranking have been analyzed as a possible predictor of success during residency. Turner et al[10] used medical school reputation as a component of the quantitative composite scoring tool that was found to be predictive of OITE scores and ABOS oral examination passing rates. Spitzer et al[11] reported that a higher medical school ranking (based on *US News and World Report* rankings) was predictive of a higher average OITE score.

Dean's Letter

Although both orthopaedic applicants and residency program directors hold the value of a dean's letter of recommendation (also known as a medical school performance evaluation) in high regard, these letters have been described as unclear or unreliable predictors of a resident's success.[5] The dean's letter provides a summary of a candidate's performance in medical school and may provide insight into an applicant's level of involvement in other medical school–related activities. Code words (such as poor, fair, good, excellent, or outstanding) have been used to place students in certain tiers in comparison with classmates and former graduates. Many letters specifically state that they do not use code words or compare students, which make the evaluations a less reliable predictor of residency program success. Spitzer et al[11] attempted to correlate letters of recommendation from deans with performance during residency. The authors did not find any relationship between the code words used in the final line of the letter and performance outcomes.

Affective Domain

Bernstein et al[5] found the affective domain to be an especially important criterion for orthopaedic programs when considering applicants for residency. Four of the six highest ranked resident selection criteria cited by program directors involved the personal evaluation of a candidate and his or her level of professionalism. These criteria included performing a rotation at the director's program, formality and politeness during the interview, personal appearance at the interview, and performance on ethical questions at the interview. These four criteria were also ranked among the top 10 criteria for applicants surveyed; however, candidates ranked each criterion that incorporated affective domain slightly lower than the residency directors. Most residency directors believed that the most important part of an interview and personal statement was to learn more about the candidate as a person.[5] In a study by Gilbart et al,[13] orthopaedic faculty in 13 Canadian training programs ranked enthusiasm, work ethic, and interpersonal skills as the three criteria that most closely correlated with a high applicant ranking. As early as 1981, the American Orthopaedic Association Steering Committee on Resident Selection cited examples of academically qualified residents who dropped out or were dismissed from training programs because of a poor attitude. Character flaws were considered the main cause for dropouts and dismissals.[1]

Clark et al[6] reported that the most common reason for the discipline of residents or dismissal from orthopaedic training programs was shortcomings in affective domain. The study also concluded that noncognitive factors were the most important predictor of the future professionalism of orthopaedic surgeons. It has been suggested that the evaluation of a candidate's moral reasoning through testing may provide more valuable insight into his or her affective domain than interviews. The Defining Issues Test-2 is one such measure that has been used in evaluating the thinking strategies of medical students and orthopaedic residents. The use of such tests could also help minimize the time required to assess affective domain because some residency programs use professional personnel, such as human resource specialists, to evaluate the personal and professional values of applicants.[14]

Screening Tools

In 2006, Dirschl et al[15] used the results from a prior study to formulate an academic score, which was designed to screen applicants based on objective academic criteria. The study analyzed and compared applicant data from 1,006 completed orthopaedic residency applications to the University of North Carolina School of Medicine over a 2-year period with the applications and performance of 20 graduates of the affiliated residency program over a 5-year period. The study found that higher academic scores were fairly predictive of OITE and ABOS scores but not of faculty performance evaluations.

Turner et al[10] examined several possible predictors of success among 64 orthopaedic residents over a 5-year period at the Mayo Clinic. Predictors of success were the USMLE step 1 score, Alpha Omega Alpha Honor Medical Society membership, junior year clerkship honors grades, and the quantitative composite scoring tool score. Final residency year OITE scores, ABOS written and oral examination pass/fail status, and attainment of chief resident associate status were used as the outcome measures for successful residency performance. The study found that higher quantitative composite scoring tool scores correlated most strongly with higher OITE scores and an increased ABOS written and oral examination passing rate. Achieving honors grades during clinical clerkships was the strongest predictor of attainment of chief resident associate status.[10]

Interview Strategies

The interview is an essential component of the selection process. A candidate selected for an interview has already completed the initial evaluation based on the strength of his or her application and/or the evaluation of the applicant's clinical rotation performance. The most important goal of the interview is to evaluate the applicant, particularly with respect to presentation, appearance, and interpersonal skills. The interview also presents an opportunity to showcase the residency program; each applicant should be given as much information as possible about the strengths and weaknesses of the program. Although orthopaedic residency programs are very competitive, with more than 20% of applicants from US medical schools failing to find a match, the goal for each program director should be to select the most qualified applicants so that the 5 years of training are completed with a superlative performance. In this context, programs compete for the best and brightest residents.

In addition to the formal interview, applicants interact with program personnel in many settings, such as a social event the evening before the interview, informal exchanges during tours, and breakfast and lunch events. All of these interactions provide input into the selection process.

Approaches for Selecting Interviewees

Each residency program follows its own approach for selecting candidates to interview. Some programs use specific parameters, such as a minimum USMLE step 1 score or membership in the Alpha Omega Alpha Medical Honor Society, to pare down the large number of applications. Although this approach makes the review process easier, it arbitrarily removes talented applicants from the pool. The New York University Hospital for Joint Diseases residency program uses a scoring system for each applicant that includes consideration of the USMLE step 1 score, membership in the Alpha Omega Alpha Honor Medical Society, letters of recommendation, the dean's letter, research activities, extracurricular activities, and the applicant's personal statement (**Figure 1**). Each application is reviewed by two members of the selection committee, and the scores are combined. This allows stratification of the applicants from the highest score to the lowest score and identifies the top applicants to be considered for the 72 available interview positions. Regardless of the method used to select applicants for interviews, the most important goal is to offer interviews to the applicants who are most likely to successfully complete residency training with a superlative performance.

Structure of the Interview

The interview is a mandatory component of the selection process and should be structured to yield the optimal amount of information to assist each program director in compiling a list of applicants for the match. The first variable to consider is the number of interviews and the number of interviewers. In some programs, applicants have one or two lengthy interviews with members of the selection committee, whereas other programs prefer multiple interviews that include all committee members. At the New York University Hospital for Joint Diseases, each member of the selection committee interviews each candidate. This allows each member of the committee to compare and contrast the entire application pool; this method is believed essential for the ranking process. The interviews are 10 to 12 minutes in length. Each candidate has six interviews. In five interviews, the candidate meets with two members of the selection committee; in the sixth interview, he or she meets with the three executive chief residents, who are also members of the selection committee.

To optimize the information obtained during the interview process, the department of human resources at the New York University School of Medicine was asked to provide input. These experts advised on the structure and function of the interview and introduced the concept of the behavioral-based structured interview (BBSI). This type of interview focuses on the applicant's experiences, assesses past behavior as a predictor of future behavior, and allows a comparison among the applicants who respond to similar questions addressed at understanding their experiences and behaviors. Although the BBSI is the recognized standard interviewing method outside of medicine, its use in the residency selection process has been limited; however, residency programs are now embracing this approach, and some data suggest that it offers benefits compared with previous approaches.[17,18]

The BBSI can be used to evaluate patient-centered/compassionate care, being a team player, intellectual awareness and inquisitiveness, contributions to the community, a passion for teaching, amicability and resourcefulness, honesty and ethical behavior, and learning and professional growth. The

Overall Score: ☐

NYU Hospital for Joint Diseases Application Review Scoring Sheet

Applicant Name: ____________________ Reviewer: ______________

Medical School: ____________________

Rotation at NYU Hospital for Joint Diseases? Y N Score on Rotation? __________

Chief Resident on Rotation: ____________________

Faculty Preceptor: ____________________

****

1. USMLE Score: Step 1: ______________ ☐

Step 2: ______________

(Step 1 >250: 5; 240-249: 4; 230-239: 3; 220-229: 2; 200-219: 1; <200:0)

2. AOA ☐

(Yes: 1; No: 0 – Note: Case Western, UC Davis, Harvard, Stanford, UConn, Mayo, Yale Do Not Have AOA Chapters)

3. Medical School Class/Dean's Letter ☐

(Top 25%: 4; Top 50%: 3; Top 75%: 2; Bottom 25%: 1 Bonus Point for Top 25% for Schools Without AOA Chapter)

4. Letters of Recommendation ☐

(Superlative: 4; Good: 3; Fair: 2; Poor: 1)

5. Research Activity ☐

(Year of Dedicated Research or NIH Experience: 4; > 5 Published Papers/Presentations: 3; 2-5 Papers/Presentations: 2; Some Quality Research Activity: 1; Little to No Research Activity: 0)

6. Extracurricular Activities ☐

(Well Rounded/Leadership Activities: 3; Moderate Involvement: 2; Some Involvement: 1; Little Extracurricular Activities: 0)

7. Personal Statement ☐

(Well Written/Exceptional Story: 3; Adequate: 2; Fair: 1; Poorly Written: 0)

Total Score **(maximum = 24)** ☐

Figure 1 The New York University Hospital for Joint Diseases Application Review Scoring Sheet.

BBSI is based on the premise that past performance is the best indicator of future performance. Instead of asking a typical question such as, "What are your strengths and weaknesses?" the BBSI asks questions to gain insight into the candidate's decision-making skills, critical thinking, interpersonal communication skills, and the ability to handle difficult situations. The concept is to ask open-ended questions in a specific area that allows the applicant to describe a situation and discuss his or her behavior.

In evaluating patient-centered and compassionate care, the candidate may be requested to "Tell me about a time when you had to deal with an angry or an unhappy patient." In assessing the candidate as a team player, a possible request could be, "Tell me about a time in medical school when you felt like a team player, when your success was team based and not individually based." In the area of intellectual awareness and inquisitiveness, the request posed could be, "Tell me about a diagnostic dilemma and how you obtained the information needed to provide the patient's care." In the area of contributing to the overall good of the community, the question could be, "Tell me about a time you gave back to your community, why you did it and how it made you feel." To evaluate the applicant's commitment and passion for teaching, which is an essential role for each resident, a possible request could be, "Tell me about your most satisfying teaching experience and why it was so satisfying for you." To evaluate the applicant's amicability and ability to handle difficult situations, the request could be, "Tell me about a frustrating situation that made you angry, why it made you angry, and how you addressed the problem." To evaluate honesty and ethical behavior, two approaches can be used. First, the candidate can be asked, "Tell me about a time when you faced an ethical dilemma." This provides an open-ended opportunity for the applicant to describe a specific situation. Another approach is to provide a specific scenario for the applicant to address. This chapter's authors have used the scenario approach for many years and have learned that although there may clearly be some wrong answers, there is also a range of correct answers. An equally important component of the answer is the applicant's thought process and rationale for the approach selected. To evaluate the commitment to learning and professional growth, the applicant could be asked to "describe a situation in which you learned from a mistake."

In the interview process at the New York University Hospital for Joint Diseases, each of the five faculty interviews uses one of the eight areas of questioning, and the same question is posed to each applicant so a comparison can be made among all the applicants interviewed. In addition to the behavioral-based questions, the interviewers should also pose other appropriate questions suggested by the conversation and try to gain a general sense of what it would be like to work with the applicant for the 5 years of residency training. The interview with the chief residents is structured differently. Each chief resident is asked to specifically evaluate the candidate's fit into the residency program of the New York University Hospital for Joint Diseases.

Pitfalls of the Interview Process

All interviews have potential pitfalls for both the interviewees and the interviewers. Although an extensive discussion in this area is beyond the scope of this chapter, it is important to be aware of some common pitfalls, such as the central tendency effect, which is the tendency of the interviewer to view all applicants as centered around the mean with difficulty stratifying the candidates along a continuum. The "just like me" pitfall is the tendency for interviewers to more favorably view candidates who are similar to themselves. The "stereotype" pitfall is the tendency for an interviewer to view candidates similarly and with preconceived opinions based on specific characteristics (for example, older or younger candidates, holders of PhDs), rather than to evaluate each candidate individually. There is also the "leniency-strictness" pitfall, in which some interviewers inappropriately ignore red flags, whereas others may overweigh the importance of a specific incident or an element of the application, rather than evaluating each applicant based on every component of the process. Some interviewers may ignore relevant information and use irrelevant information. This is the tendency for the interviewer to either ignore important information or overemphasize unimportant findings, possibly in support of a preconceived impression. The "first impression" pitfall refers to the tendency for the interviewer to make up his or her mind based on the initial impression of the applicant with limited information (for example, a weak handshake that starts the interview). There is also the pitfall of overweighting isolated negative behavior. This pitfall is characterized by assigning undue and excessive importance to one specific negative incident. This pitfall is common because it makes it easier to come to a decision on the good and bad candidates.

Core Competencies: Origin and Measurement

Background

The first surgical residency training program was started at Johns Hopkins Hospital in the late 1890s and was based on the German model of regimen and discipline. Before that time, surgical training was haphazard, there often was no established end point, and medical education was quite uneven. Flexner[19] was commissioned to evaluate the 155 US medical schools in existence in the early 1900s. His report meticulously detailed the disparate quality and highlighted that "for twenty-five years past there has been an enormous over-production of uneducated and ill trained medical practitioners." Flexner also recommended reducing the number of medical schools in the United States from 155 to 31.[19]

In 1984, an 18-year-old woman named Libby Zion was admitted to New York Hospital with a fever of unknown origin and jerking body movements. Although the cause of her death on the day after admission remains unsolved (the presumptive diagnosis was malignant hyperthermia caused by an interaction of an monoamine oxidase inhibitor and meperidine), a grand jury investigation pushed by her father, Sidney Zion (a prominent journalist and former federal prosecutor), led to charges of 38 acts of gross negligence and incompetence against the intern and resident caring for her.[20] All charges were subsequently dropped; however, the New York State Health Commissioner empowered Dr. Bertrand Bell, chair of Internal Medicine at Albert Einstein College of Medicine, to further investigate the case. Bell's investigation took 17 months and resulted in changes to the state health code, which subsequently became known as New York State Hospital Code 405 (enacted on July 1, 1989).[21] The main conclusion of Bell's investigation was that attending supervision was seriously lacking. Recommendations for work-hour restrictions were made that limited the work week to no more than 80 hours and eliminated working for more than 24 consecutive hours (later amended to 24 plus 3 hours to allow handoffs).

Core Competencies

The ACGME initiated the Outcome Project and in 1999 mandated that all graduate medical education programs assess a resident's competencies in six areas: patient care, medical knowledge, practice-based learning and improvement, interpersonal skills, professionalism, and systems-based practice. The first phase of the project ended in 2002, with the goal that all programs would incorporate the core competencies in their teaching and evaluation programs. Phase 2 extended from 2002 to 2006. Programs were asked to show evidence of learning in all six domains and that competency-based evaluations tools were being implemented. Phase 3 of the project will end in 2016. Benchmark programs are to be identified by the completion of this final phase.[22]

Since the implementation of the core competency requirements 12 years ago, orthopaedic surgery residency programs have been working on methods of implementation, evaluation, and documentation. In a 2006 survey of residency directors and residents, both groups believed that patient care and medical knowledge were the most important core competencies, and practice-based learning and improvement and systems-based practice were the least important. The survey also reported that most orthopaedic residency programs used at most 4 tools (case logs, written examinations, 360° evaluations, and patient surveys) for resident evaluations, although the ACGME recommended the use of 12 evaluation tools.[23]

After the widespread implementation of the core competencies into residency programs, it became apparent that better documentation and evaluation of the competencies were needed. Some evaluation tools have been successfully used to document and evaluate the six core competencies in graduate medical education.

Patient Care

Residents must be capable of providing patient care that is compassionate, appropriate, and effective for the treatment of health disorders and the promotion of good health. Patient care can be divided into inpatient, operating room, and outpatient care. Tools for the inpatient evaluation include team rounds, with peer-to-peer evaluation; and 360° evaluations, including evaluations from nursing staff, social workers, physical and occupational therapists, and ward clerks. Tools used for the operating room assessment include faculty evaluations and 360° evaluations from senior and junior residents, fellows, and the operating room nursing staff. A surgical skills assessment form is used to assess what may be considered the seventh core competency—surgical skills. Outpatient clinic evaluation tools include a miniclinical evaluation in which an attending physician serves as an observer in a real-time patient evaluation by a resident.[24] Keys to the effectiveness of this tool are immediate constructive feedback, debriefing, and the implementation of corrective actions if deficiencies are identified.

Medical Knowledge

Residents must demonstrate knowledge of established and evolving biomedical, clinical, epidemiologic, and social behavioral sciences, as well as the application of this knowledge to patient care. Many physicians believe that medical knowledge is the easiest core competency to subjectively evaluate by rating a resident's performance in all facets of the residency program, including the resident's performance in the operating room, interactive conferences, the outpatient clinic, and when consulting with the attending physician.

Performance on the OITE can be used as an objective measure of medical knowledge. Public display of the examination results or decision making with respect to promotion and graduation are clearly prohibited, but it is often helpful for a resident to compare his or her scores with those of the in-training peer group and all residents in orthopaedic residency programs.

Practice-Based Learning and Improvement

Residents must demonstrate the ability to investigate and evaluate the care of their patients, appraise and assimilate scientific evidence, and continuously improve patient care based on constant self-evaluation and lifelong learning. Because self-evaluation is critical to this competency, this element has been incorporated into the residency program at the New York University Hospital for Joint Diseases. Residents are asked to complete a self-assessment evaluation at the beginning of each academic year and at 6 months thereafter. These self-evaluations are reviewed by the program director at biannual meetings with the residents to assess the goals achieved, the need for improvement, and the development of future objectives and goals.

Evidence-based medicine can be evaluated with a morbidity and mortality conference (a standardized form has been developed to document the resident's presentation), indications conferences, journal clubs, and through research projects. Quality improvement can be assessed by assigning quality improvement projects to residents and having them present these projects to the department or a resident quality council as used at the New York University Hospital for Joint Diseases. This council serves as a conduit for residents to present problems encountered at the hospital that affect patient care and develop plans of action to rectify the problems. Teaching skills, like medical knowledge, are assessed in all facets of the program, including the operating room, conferences, inpatient rounds, and the outpatient clinic.

Interpersonal Skills

Residents must demonstrate interpersonal and communication skills that result in the effective exchange of information and collaboration with patients, their families, and health professionals. This competency can be assessed with patient surveys and from 360° evaluations from attending staff, including fellows, peer residents (senior and junior), office coordinators, registered nurses, physician's assistants, medical assistants, and orthotists.

Professionalism

Residents must show a commitment to carrying out professional responsibilities and adhering to ethical principles. This competency is measured with 360° evaluations and assessments by faculty and department personnel as described in the preceding section.

Systems-Based Practice

Residents must be aware of and responsive to the healthcare system in the larger context and have the ability to effectively use other system resources to provide optimal care. This core competency can be evaluated with coding reviews (either local or national); AAOS modules on resident education and practice management; morbidity and mortality conferences; and working with nursing, social services, and the rest of the treatment team on discharge planning for inpatients after orthopaedic procedures. More information on the systems-based practice competency is available in chapter 50.

Coming Changes

The next step in completing the implementation of the core competencies into resident education will begin on July 1, 2013, when the Milestone Project begins. The Residency Review Committee, ABOS, and ACGME jointly sponsored the Milestone Project to assist in the implementation of phase 3 of the Outcome Project, which will develop patient-derived outcomes and assessment tools of the core competencies. This group has identified 17 commonly performed procedures for orthopaedic conditions, including anterior cruciate ligament injuries, ankle arthritis, ankle fractures, carpal tunnel syndrome, diabetic foot, femoral and tibial shaft fractures, distal radius fractures, elbow fractures, hip and knee osteoarthritis, hip fractures, lumbar disorders, meniscal tears, metastatic bone disease, neck pain, rotator cuff injuries, pediatric septic arthritis, and supracondylar humeral fractures. The adequacy of an orthopaedic resident's training will be assessed, in part, on achieving specific milestones for each procedure.

Residents Who Do Not Measure Up

The implementation of the six ACGME core competencies has, in some respects, changed how orthopaedic residents are trained and has totally changed methods of documenting the success of orthopaedic residency training. Success or failure in residency training is now categorized and documented in terms of the core competencies. The methods used to identify and correct a resident's difficulties with orthopaedic training are similar to remediation methods of the past.[25-28]

Traditionally, residency training was believed to occur in the cognitive, psychomotor, and affective realms. To ascertain the resident's area or areas of difficulty, it is helpful to know which of the core competencies are associated with each realm. The cognitive realm is clearly associated with the core competency of medical knowledge. The psychomotor realm maps to the realm of patient care; however, patient care also includes some of the cognitive realm because a surgeon cannot be an effective clinician without both cognitive and psychomotor excellence. The remaining four core competencies all map to the affective realm. This domain encompasses professional attitudes, beliefs, and behaviors and includes competencies in practice-based learning and improvement, interpersonal and communication skills, professionalism, and systems-based practice.

If a resident is having difficulties mastering the affective realm, it may be possible to sort out whether the issue is related to interpersonal skills or systems-based practice; however, the effort to make this distinction may not be worthwhile. It is more efficient to attribute resident difficulties to medical knowledge (the cognitive realm), patient care (the psychomotor and cognitive realms), or professional behaviors (the affective realm).

Difficulties Acquiring Medical Knowledge

Difficulties related to acquiring medical knowledge, although the simplest difficulties to diagnose and remedy, are also the least common. Most orthopaedic residents are among the highest scorers in their medical schools on standardized examinations, such as the USMLE series and shelf examinations for clinical rotations. Insufficient cognitive ability to acquire the knowledge necessary to complete orthopaedic training is unusual among orthopaedic residents. In rare instances, however, difficulties in acquiring knowledge may become known through questioning (the resident cannot answer appropriate questions posed in the course of clinical work), through conference participation (the resident does not participate or appears not to grasp the material during interactive conferences), and through scores obtained on the OITE. Residents with difficulties in this realm typically are encouraged to do more reading; however, these residents often do not know what to read. A structured reading program focusing on areas of weakness and specific texts and articles may assist them in building a knowledge base. A structured program for reading and preparing for conferences, surgical cases, and journal clubs will assist the resident in acquiring medical knowledge and in developing the habit of frequent and regimented reading to gain new knowledge and review existing knowledge.

Residents should begin with a base of knowledge acquired from textbooks and review articles and supplement those readings with specific journal articles for particular journal clubs, surgical cases, or teaching conferences. Review books and outlines should not be used as primary sources of learning because this may lead to a memorization of facts without a clear understanding of the underlying principles or an inability to assess the validity and applicability of the information. Review books and outlines should be used primarily in preparing for the ABOS part I examination.

The structured reading program should have specific goals, tasks, and deadlines. Scheduled periodic meetings (perhaps as often as weekly) with the resident and the faculty member responsible for the structured reading program should be conducted to discuss the assigned materials and ensure completion and comprehension. Such a program should be continued until there is evidence of substantial improvement; often, this will be when the next OITE examination scores are available and substantial improvement is indicated.

Although expectations and thresholds for cognitive performance may vary among training programs, residents scoring below the 20th percentile on the OITE should probably be placed on a structured reading plan. All residents should perform a literature search and write a paragraph about the correct answer to each incorrectly answered OITE question, but those scoring below the 20th percentile need further intervention because they are at substantial risk for failing the ABOS part I examination. A structured reading program with a faculty mentor can be a valuable technique to improve knowledge and performance.

Difficulties Regarding Patient Care

Residents experiencing difficulties in providing patient care are relatively simple to identify. Patients, hospital and clinic staff, fellow residents, and attending physicians can provide valuable information about performance in this area. Even when the problem is recognized, finding the root cause of the difficulty can be challenging. Patient care difficulties usually manifest as an inability to make a clinical decision, difficulty mastering surgical procedures and techniques, or as questionable and (rarely) dangerous patient-care decisions.

The inability to make a clinical decision usually stems from a lack of confidence or knowledge. It is important to understand which factor is involved because a lack of confidence requires support and reassurance, and a knowledge deficit requires a structured reading program. Lack of confidence in making the correct decision and fear of making an erroneous decision are normal and expected in residency training. Working in an environment where resident decisions are not permitted (care decisions are made entirely by the attending physician with no input or engagement with the resident) or where incorrect decisions result in harsh criticism can multiply the effects of low self-confidence and fear and can make it difficult for a resident to develop solid clinical decision-making skills. Each resident will respond differently in this regard, so it is important that attending physicians have the ability to vary their style and teaching approaches for different residents. It is appropriate to have the same expectation for all residents completing the residency program, but it is not appropriate to expect each resident to gain confidence at the same pace over the 5-year training period. Sensitivity to differences in self-confidence levels, engaging with residents to assure they can propose treatment decisions in a nonconfrontational environment, and having the flexibility and patience to explain the principles behind treatment decisions will assure the highest quality patient care and provide important skills for attending physicians.

Difficulty in mastering surgical procedures is common early in training because the natural pace of psychomotor learning varies among residents. With enough experience, most residents achieve adequate surgical skill by the end of training. Skills laboratories, simulators, courses, and other methodologies are helpful in shortening the learning curve for residents. Other methods of obtaining surgical experience will become even more important when further restrictions in the number of work hours decrease residents' exposure to surgical cases. Each training program should consider expanding its ability to provide surgery-specific psychomotor skills training outside the operating room in an effort to potentially improve the surgical competence of its residents. As with clinical decision making, attending physicians should take a calm and flexible approach to training individual residents in surgical skills. Clear communication and the setting of expectations are paramount. In advance of a surgical case, the attending surgeon and resident should discuss how the procedure will be done and which surgeon will perform each portion of the procedure. The resident must understand that performing only a portion of a surgical procedure is not a sign of a lack of confidence by the attending physician but is a means of ensuring that surgical learning occurs on a continuum, with mastery of certain skills before progression to more complex skills.

Difficulties Regarding Professional Behavior

Performance problems relating to professional behavior can masquerade as difficulties with knowledge or patient care, but a careful appraisal will properly identify the issue. For example, a resident with poor performance in teaching conferences and on the OITE may appear to have difficulties with cognitive performance; however, further inquiry may reveal that the resident spends hours each night playing video games rather than studying. This indicates that the true problem is a lack of dedication to medical training—an issue of professional behavior. Because poor professional behavior is related to the individual's values, beliefs, and personality traits, it is often the most difficult performance issue to remediate.

There is no single successful approach for correcting professional behavior problems. Institutions have different expectations, resources, and guidelines for assessing dedication, communication, and professionalism; however, several principles may make it easier to diagnose, manage, and prevent difficulties in this realm.

Observation Early in Training

Difficulties in professional behaviors are based on aspects of the individual's character that are present and reasonably well developed before entering the residency program. With observation, performance issues related to professional behavior are usually apparent at the outset of training. Program directors and attending physicians must be observant. Casual comments or other forms of feedback from nurses, other residents, operating room staff, and other hospital personnel should be sought and valued. Professional behavior issues are more easily remediated early in training.

Set Global and Local Expectations

It is important to set and clearly communicate behavioral standards. Many institutions have written standards of professionalism or a code of conduct that each physician and staff member must read and sign annually. Behavioral expectations should be established program wide (usually by the program director or chairman), with local expectations set by the faculty on each specific rotation. Expectations should be in written form for clarity, reference, and endurance.

Mentors as Appropriate Models

Behaviors tacitly modeled by faculty and fellows for the resident trainees have been referred to as the hidden curriculum. To ensure that a residency program has a minimum of behavioral problems, the faculty and fellows must be held to the same standards of behavior, conduct, and professionalism as the residents. Allowing faculty or fellows to behave badly sends a clear message to residents that such behavior is acceptable, and the program is not serious about maintaining professionalism. A disruptive faculty member must be disciplined. Because these matters are often beyond the authority of the residency program director, it is necessary to have the engagement and support of the chairman in setting and enforcing behavioral expectations for faculty and fellows.

Early and Frequent Communication

All feedback to residents should be timely, constructive, balanced, and depersonalized. It is much more difficult to discuss professional behavior than OITE scores, but attending physicians should not avoid giving feedback to residents about behavioral issues. Every faculty member should include feedback about professional behaviors in conversations with residents about performance. Program directors should include discussions about professional behaviors in meetings with residents about progress in the program.

Intervention

The few published studies on attempts to remediate behavioral problems indicate that complete remediation is almost never achieved, and partial remediation occurs less than 50% of the time.[1,2,4,5] Successful remediation efforts are usually initiated very early in training. When a resident has apparent behavioral issues, the program director should act quickly to set clear expectations, initiate counseling, and institute disciplinary procedures (up to and including dismissal) if progress is not achieved. The use of probation or other disciplinary tools will depend on the policies and procedures of the training institution. Program directors should be familiar with these policies and procedures.

Summary

In many ways, selecting, training, and evaluating orthopaedic surgery residents is a more complex task than treating the most complicated clinical disorders. Just as each patient needs to be evaluated individually to determine a treatment plan, the same concept applies to the training of orthopaedic residents. The goal of orthopaedic resident educators is to develop programs that successfully select and train residents who will graduate as knowledgeable, skilled, and caring orthopaedic surgeons who exhibit the highest level of professionalism. Achieving this goal requires commitment to each and every step of the training process.

References

1. Evarts CM: Resident selection: A key to the future of orthopaedics. *Clin Orthop Relat Res* 2006;449:39-43.
2. Evarts CM: On leadership. *J Bone Joint Surg Am* 1990;72(8):1119-1124.
3. Dirschl DR: Scoring of orthopaedic residency applicants: Is a scoring system reliable? *Clin Orthop Relat Res* 2002;399:260-264.
4. Bajaj G, Carmichael KD: What attributes are necessary to be selected for an orthopaedic surgery residency position: Perceptions of faculty and residents. *South Med J* 2004;97(12):1179-1185.
5. Bernstein AD, Jazrawi LM, Elbeshbeshy B, Della Valle CJ, Zuckerman JD: An analysis of orthopaedic residency selection criteria. *Bull Hosp Jt Dis* 2002-2003;61(1-2):49-57.
6. Clark R, Evans EB, Ivey FM, Calhoun JH, Hokanson JA: Characteristics of successful and unsuccessful applicants to orthopedic residency training programs. *Clin Orthop Relat Res* 1989;241:257-264.
7. Wagoner NE, Suriano JR, Stoner JA: Factors used by program directors to select residents. *J Med Educ* 1986;61(1):10-21.
8. Bernstein AD, Jazrawi LM, Elbeshbeshy B, Della Valle CJ, Zuckerman JD: Orthopaedic resident-selection criteria. *J Bone Joint Surg Am* 2002;84(11):2090-2096.
9. Carmichael KD, Westmoreland JB, Thomas JA, Patterson RM: Relation of residency selection factors to subsequent orthopaedic in-training examination performance. *South Med J* 2005;98(5):528-532.
10. Turner NS, Shaughnessy WJ, Berg EJ, Larson DR, Hanssen AD: A quantitative composite scoring tool for orthopaedic residency screening and selection. *Clin Orthop Relat Res* 2006;449:50-55.
11. Spitzer AB, Gage MJ, Looze CA, Walsh M, Zuckerman JD, Egol KA: Factors associated with successful performance in an orthopaedic surgery residency. *J Bone Joint Surg Am* 2009;91(11):2750-2755.
12. Thordarson DB, Ebramzadeh E, Sangiorgio SN, Schnall SB, Patzakis MJ: Resident selection: How we are doing and why? *Clin Orthop Relat Res* 2007;459:255-259.
13. Gilbart MK, Cusimano MD, Regehr G: Evaluating surgical resident selection procedures. *Am J Surg* 2001;181(3):221-225.
14. Self DJ, Baldwin DC Jr: Should moral reasoning serve as a criterion for student and resident selection? *Clin Orthop Relat Res* 2000;378:115-123.
15. Dirschl DR, Campion ER, Gilliam K: Resident selection and predictors of performance: Can we be evidence based? *Clin Orthop Relat Res* 2006;449:44-49.
16. Characteristics of applicants who matched to their preferred specialty in the 2011 main residency match. National Resident Matching Program website. Table ORS-1: Summary statistics for orthopaedic surgery, p 166. http://www.nrmp.org/data/chartingoutcomes2011.pdf. Accessed September 17, 2012.
17. Easdown L, Castro PL, Shinkle EP, Small L, Algren J: The behavioral interview, a method to evaluate ACGME competences in resident selection: A pilot project. *JEPM* 2005;7(1):1-10.
18. Strand EA, Moore E, Laube DW: Can a structured, behavior-based interview predict future resident success? *Am J Obstet Gynecol* 2011;204(5):446, e1-e446, e13.
19. Flexner A: Medical education in the United States and Canada: From the Carnegie Foundation for the Advancement of Teaching, Bulletin Number Four, 1910. *Bull World Health Organ* 2002;80(7):594-602.
20. Spritz N: Oversight of physicians' conduct by state licensing agencies: Lessons from New York's Libby Zion case. *Ann Intern Med* 1991;115(3):219-222.
21. Douglas RG Jr , Hayes JG, Roberts RB, Bardes CL: Bell Commission requirements: Doctors or factory workers? *Trans Am Clin Climatol Assoc* 1990;101:91-102.
22. Swing SR: The ACGME outcome project: Retrospective and prospective. *Med Teach* 2007;29(7):648-654.
23. Yaszay B, Kubiak E, Agel J, Hanel DP: ACGME core competencies: Where are we? *Orthopedics* 2009;32(3):171.
24. Norcini JJ, Blank LL, Duffy FD, Fortna GS: The mini-CEX: A method for assessing clinical skills. *Ann Intern Med* 2003;138(6):476-481.
25. Reamy BV, Harman JH: Residents in trouble: An in-depth assessment of the 25-year experience of a single family medicine residency. *Fam Med* 2006;38(4):252-257.
26. Adams KE, Emmons S, Romm J: How resident unprofessional behavior is identified and managed: A program director survey. *Am J Obstet Gynecol* 2008;198(6):692, e1-692, e5.
27. Veldenz HC, Scott KK, Dennis JW, Tepas JJ III , Schinco MS: Impaired residents: Identification and intervention. *Curr Surg* 2003;60(2):214-217.
28. Williams RG, Roberts NK, Schwind CJ, Dunnington GL: The nature of general surgery resident performance problems. *Surgery* 2009;145(6):651-658.

49

SYMPOSIUM

Competency-Based Education: A New Model for Teaching Orthopaedics

Benjamin A. Alman, MD
Peter Ferguson, MD, FRCSC
William Kraemer, MD, FRCSC
Markku T. Nousiainen, MD, FRCSC
Richard K. Reznick, MD

Abstract

The current methods used to train residents to become orthopaedic surgeons are based on tradition, not evidence-based models. Educators have only a limited ability to assess trainees for competency using validated tests in various domains. The reduction in resident work hours limits the time available for clinical training, which has resulted in some calls for lengthening the training process. Another approach to address limited training hours is to focus training in a program that allows residents to graduate from a rotation based on demonstrated competency rather than on time on a service. A pilot orthopaedic residency curriculum, which uses a competency-based framework of resident training and maximizes the use of available training hours, has been designed and is being implemented.

Instr Course Lect 2013;62:565-569.

The way medical students are trained to become competent orthopaedic surgeons is based on tradition, not evidence-based methods. The determination that resident trainees are competent to practice orthopaedic medicine is generally not based on validated assessment tools. In the past, the number of hours available each week for training in orthopaedic medicine was believed to be sufficient to ensure a resident's competency after 5 years of training. However, a reduction in resident work hours, in response to concerns for patient safety and reasonable working conditions, has limited the number of hours available for clinical training. Because fewer training hours are available, educators are rethinking methods to best train orthopaedic residents.[1-3] Some educators have recommended increasing the duration of the training period. An alternative approach is to maximize the educational use of the available training hours.[4]

To ensure that residents are appropriately trained in orthopaedic medicine, a program could allow residents to graduate from a rotation based on demonstrated competency rather than on time on a service. A pilot orthopaedic residency curriculum, which uses a competency-based framework of resident training and maximizes the use of the available training hours, was designed and implemented.[5] The rationale and organization of this novel, competency-based curriculum are described in this chapter. The steps to institute a pilot training program based on this curriculum and the early results of the first 3 years of the program are presented.

Dr. Alman or an immediate family member serves as a board member, owner, officer, or committee member of the Pediatric Orthopaedic Society of North America, the Shriners Research Advisory Board, and the Orthopaedic Research Society and has received research or institutional support from Infinity. Dr. Nousiainen or an immediate family member serves as a board member, owner, officer, or committee member of the Canadian Orthopaedic Association and the AOTK Computer Navigation North America committee. Dr. Reznick or an immediate family member serves as a board member, owner, officer, or committee member of Royal College Canada International. Neither of the following authors nor any immediate family member has received anything of value from or owns stock in a commercial company or institution related directly or indirectly to the subject of this chapter: Dr. Ferguson and Dr. Kraemer.

Methods

Rationale and Curriculum Design

The competency-based curriculum was designed on three main principles: (1) teach the appropriate level and spectrum of competencies required, (2) maximize the use of available training time, and (3) allow residents to progress through the program at their own rate.

A clinician can exhibit competency, proficiency, or expertise at a certain task.[6] Competency is having the necessary ability, knowledge, and/or skill to do something successfully. A competent orthopaedic surgeon would have the skills necessary to manage a clinical situation but may not have handled the particular problem or procedure in an independent manner. The objective of orthopaedic residency training is to achieve competency. Proficiency is the demonstrated ability to undertake a skill in an independent manner. For many tasks in orthopaedics, proficiency is expected of a clinical fellow. Expertise is demonstrated by extensive knowledge or ability beyond what is expected from the average clinician. Expertise is expected of the faculty teaching orthopaedic medicine.

The purpose of a residency program is not to create clinicians who are proficient at all subspecialty procedures, but it is important that they are proficient at skills (such as treating hip fractures) that a general orthopaedic surgeon would be expected to perform in his or her first months in practice. As such, the knowledge required for competency in each skill taught to residents was carefully considered so that education could be focused at the appropriate level.

The pilot orthopaedic residency curriculum was designed to cover all of the competencies necessary for training an orthopaedic surgeon, not only technical skills. The Canadian medical education directives for specialists (CanMEDS) competency framework of the Royal College of Physicians and Surgeons of Canada[7] was used to ensure that all areas are covered in the training curriculum. The CanMEDS framework categorizes competencies into seven domains: the medical expert, the collaborator, the manager, the health advocate, the scholar, the professional, and the communicator.

The program was structured so that residents could advance through training as quickly as possible. Trainees were assigned specific curricular objectives rather than being assigned to a particular service. Assessment tools were used to ensure that residents had reached certain performance benchmarks as they passed through a learning module. Procedural skill acquisition was incorporated into the early phases of the program to allow residents sufficient time to develop competency in all the CanMEDS competencies, such as collaborator, manager, health advocate, and communicator. Competency in basic arthroplasty was taught in the early phases of a resident's training, not when he or she became a midlevel or senior resident. Procedural skill acquisition included basic skills teaching that focused on the fundamental building blocks of becoming an orthopaedic surgeon. The first module was based in a simulation laboratory where trainees focused on learning how to use instruments, apply casts, use power tools, and manage routine patient interactions; frequent feedback was provided. This early curriculum was designed based on evidence that skills learned in a simulation laboratory can be transferred to the real world of the operating room.[8-11]

Curriculum Development and Implementation

The pilot curriculum was developed after an extensive process of communication, resulting in broad support from many orthopaedic surgeons on the faculty at the University of Toronto. The core curriculum of the Royal College of Physicians and Surgeons of Canada was used as a baseline. For each area in the curriculum, consensus was developed on what should be taught and the threshold for demonstrating competency. Based on this consultation, the curriculum was divided into 21 modules (**Table 1**), and an orthopaedic faculty member was recruited to lead each module. A working group evaluated the existing curricular objectives and reframed them in the context of 21 modules. The modules were grouped into three phases based on knowledge that could be a prerequisite for material taught in later modules. Trainees had to complete the phase one modules before starting the phase two modules, and so on.

Each module optimized the opportunity for both surgical and nonsurgical clinical experiences. An administrative assistant helped with scheduling the residents' training. In many of the modules, the residents rotated through more than one staff member and more than one hospital to optimize their clinical experiences.

In each module, the focus was on teaching the specific competencies, not the assignments that would traditionally be given to a resident on a particular clinical service. Providing service for patient care is an important competency for an orthopaedic surgeon and is a key component of professionalism in the CanMEDS framework. As such, the service components of a traditional residency, such as on-call service, were incorporated into the

Table 1
List of Modules in the Competency-Based Curriculum

Module	Phase 1
1	Introduction
2	Hip fracture
3	Basic fractures
4	Emergency surgery
5	Arthroscopy
6	Arthroplasty
7	Intensive care unit
8	Core training in surgery
9	CanMEDS core competencies
	Phase 2
10	Pediatric fractures
11	Spine
12	Foot and ankle
13	Basic science
14	Hand and upper extremity
15	Musculoskeletal medicine
	Phase 3
16	Oncology
17	Complex trauma
18	Complex arthroplasty/joint reconstruction
19	Pediatric orthopaedics
20	Sports
21	Research
Final	Integration

curriculum. Time expended performing redundant activities was removed from the curriculum. For example, a junior resident may make solo professional calls on hospital patients (prerounds) and then repeat those rounds with a senior level resident and then with a faculty member. These types of redundant activities were removed from the curriculum.

In the traditional training curriculum, there are several required off-service rotations. Discussions with current residents indicated that these rotations might not be the most efficient method of achieving the career-specific competencies required from off-service experiences. As such, the pilot curriculum was designed so that many core off-service objectives could be achieved as elements of the existing modules. This made the modules more relevant and reduced the time spent on rotations that provided more service than educational experience.

There are few standardized approaches to resident assessment that are rigorous and robust. A fundamental element of this pilot training model was to provide residents with real-time feedback on their progress. This allows an opportunity for self-improvement and helps the faculty determine when a particular resident has achieved a benchmark in a particular domain. Each of the 21 modules is associated with a multidimensional assessment algorithm, including multiple-choice questions, structured oral examinations, an objective structured assessment of technical skills,[12,13] multisource 360° feedback, patient assessments, management examinations,[14] observed history and physical examinations, and ward audits.

Early Results

Three residents were accepted into the pilot program each year starting in July 2009. Currently, the program is in its third year. Frequent internal and external evaluations of the program are performed. Residents in the new curriculum report an extremely high degree of satisfaction with this model of training. Competency-based residents, traditional-stream residents, and traditional-stream residents who had spent their initial rotations off service were asked to rate their confidence in their acquired skills. There was a main effect of the training stream ($P = 0.04$), with competency-based residents significantly more confident in their abilities.[15]

All the residents who entered the University of Toronto orthopaedic training program in 2009 and 2010 were tested on entry on their technical skills using the objective structured assessment of technical skills. They were subsequently retested to analyze whether there were differences in skill acquisition during the beginning part of their training. The tests involved the observation of casting techniques, preparation and draping of a limb, soft-tissue exposure, the use of power tools, wound closure, and communication in the operating room. The competency-based residents systematically showed better growth in their skill levels than the 10 traditional-stream residents[15] (**Figure 1**).

The surgical experiences of the trainees in the new and the conventional curriculums were compared. On average, each of the competency-based residents treated between two and three times the number of hip fractures

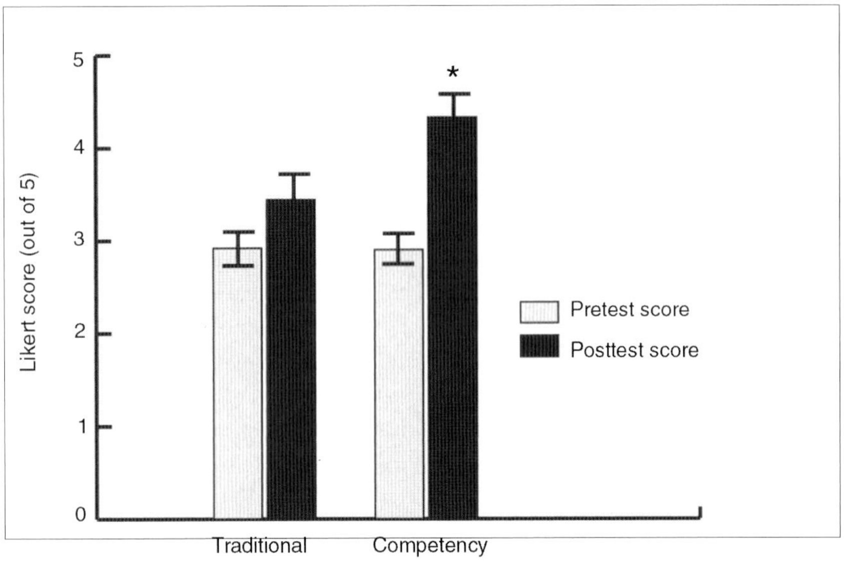

Figure 1 Bar graph of the mean scores of six basic technical skills from pretesting to posttesting after a 5-week intensive technical skills course for competency-based residents versus residents in a traditional training stream (mean and 95% CI (asterisk) indicating $P < 0.05$ compared with data from the traditional-stream residents). Residents in the competency-based curriculum had significantly higher scores compared with residents in the traditional-stream curriculum. Skills examined were aseptic technique, power tool usage, soft-tissue handling, casting, the AO bone fixation technique, and instrument identification.

than residents in the traditional stream in their first year in the training program.

Competency-based residents, their traditional-stream counterparts, and the faculty were extensively debriefed on the educational programs. The traditional-stream residents wanted to participate in the educational programs that were part of the competency-based curriculum, indicating that they believed the pilot program provided an educational advantage. The faculty generally believed that trainees in the competency-based stream were more prepared to perform surgery, which demonstrated the effectiveness of the skills lab in preparing trainees for real-life procedures. The intense evaluation process identified areas needing improvement early in the training process; this was believed to increase the flexibility of the curriculum and the assessment program's ability to identify deficiencies.

The initial cohort of trainees is in the third year of the pilot program. Of the three initial residents in the program, two are on track to complete all 21 modules in less than 4 years. As such, the curriculum appears to provide training in core competencies at an accelerated pace compared with the traditional 5-year residency training curriculum and still maintains the weekly working hour restrictions required to provide a safe working and learning environment.

Discussion

Because the competency-based curriculum is still in its initial phases, there has not been sufficient time to acquire definitive data comparing the new curriculum with traditional programs. The first vital evaluation of the program will be to determine if residents completing the new curriculum are at least equal in competency to those in the traditional steam at the completion of their training. The first cohort in the pilot program is still 1 year away from training completion. Although the new curriculum is still in an early stage, the accumulated information to date shows that the objectives of the new curriculum are being achieved.[15]

Because only 3 of the 12 residents accepted into the University of Toronto orthopaedic residency training program each year are trained using the new pilot curriculum, the scope of the pilot program is small in comparison with the entire training program. Training all orthopaedic residents using the pilot curriculum would increase the budget and the amount of time that faculty spend on residency education; however, the exact numbers of extra hours and increased costs have not been definitively calculated. Some aspects of the program can be easily applied to a larger residency cohort. For example, beginning in 2012, all orthopaedic residents at the University of Toronto participated in an orthopaedic boot camp, which was based on the first module of the new curriculum.[15]

It could be argued that the residents selected for the pilot program were extremely well motivated and did not represent average residents. Although that argument has validity, it is not possible to verify that the selected resident were better motivated or to determine the effect of their added motivation if it exists. However, on entry into the programs, there did not appear to be a substantial difference between residents selected for the competency-based stream versus those enrolled in the traditional stream. All residents accepted to the orthopaedic program were offered the opportunity to be part of the competency-based curriculum. Approximately 50% indicated their interest; from those, three were randomly selected for the pilot program.

Selected residents participated in an interview process suggested by the Royal College of Physicians and Surgeons of Canada to ensure that they were well informed about the implications of participation in the program.

One concern that has been raised is that the residents in the new curriculum will have good technical skills but will not perform as well in other domains. The program's faculty believe that the trainees are more mature, appear to be more confident, and have a richer sense of understanding of not only the basic elements of surgical procedures but also the nuances and complexities of the procedures compared with residents in the traditional stream. This may stem from the faculty allowing these residents to perform more tasks in the operating room and may also be related to the time these residents spent in the surgical skills laboratory acquiring a high level of capability in basic surgical procedures.

Summary

Although there are obvious logistic issues associated with implementing and administering a residency program based on such a competency-based curriculum, many of the lessons learned in the pilot program can be applied more broadly to the training of orthopaedic residents. The curriculum can focus on content that is appropriate to produce competency, provide flexibility in the time required on specific rotations, use simulation laboratories to enhance the rate of skills acquisition, and incorporate comprehensive evaluation tools to assess the resident's rate of learning. Using these principles, the time available for residency training may be used more effectively to give residents a greater degree of confidence and ensure that they are trained to the appropriate level of competency.

Acknowledgments

The authors would like to acknowledge the financial support for this project, which was provided from the Ministry of Health and Long Term Care of the Province of Ontario. The authors also want to acknowledge the support and cooperation for this project received form the Royal College of Physicians and Surgeons of Canada and the Office of Post-Medical Education, University of Toronto.

References

1. Baskies MA, Ruchelsman DE, Capeci CM, Zuckerman JD, Egol KA: Operative experience in an orthopaedic surgery residency program: The effect of work-hour restrictions. *J Bone Joint Surg Am* 2008;90(4):924-927.
2. Kusuma SK, Mehta S, Sirkin M, et al: Measuring the attitudes and impact of the eighty-hour work-week rules on orthopaedic surgery residents. *J Bone Joint Surg Am* 2007;89(3):679-685.
3. Friedlaender GE: The 80-hour duty week: Rationale, early attitudes, and future questions. *Clin Orthop Relat Res* 2006;449: 138-142.
4. Pellegrini VD Jr: Perspective: Ten thousand hours to patient safety, sooner or later. *Acad Med* 2012; 87(2):164-167.
5. Frank JR, Mungroo R, Ahmad Y, Wang M, De Rossi S, Horsley T: Toward a definition of competency-based education in medicine: A systematic review of published definitions. *Med Teach* 2010;32(8):631-637.
6. Dugger BH: Levels of performance for intravenous nursing practice. *J Intraven Nurs* 1993; 16(4):239-245.
7. Frank JR, Langer B: Collaboration, communication, management, and advocacy: Teaching surgeons new skills through the CanMEDS Project. *World J Surg* 2003;27(8):972-978, discussion 978.
8. Grantcharov TP, Kristiansen VB, Bendix J, Bardram L, Rosenberg J, Funch-Jensen P: Randomized clinical trial of virtual reality simulation for laparoscopic skills training. *Br J Surg* 2004;91(2): 146-150.
9. Seymour NE, Gallagher AG, Roman SA, et al: Virtual reality training improves operating room performance: Results of a randomized, double-blinded study. *Ann Surg* 2002;236(4):458-463, discussion 463-464.
10. Safir O, Dubrowski A, Williams C, Hui Y, Backstein D, Carnahan H: The benefits of fundamentals of laparoscopic surgery (FLS) training on simulated arthroscopy performance. *Stud Health Technol Inform* 2012;173:412-417.
11. Backstein D, Agnidis Z, Sadhu R, MacRae H: Effectiveness of repeated video feedback in the acquisition of a surgical technical skill. *Can J Surg* 2005;48(3): 195-200.
12. Martin JA, Regehr G, Reznick R, et al: Objective structured assessment of technical skill (OSATS) for surgical residents. *Br J Surg* 1997;84(2):273-278.
13. Faulkner H, Regehr G, Martin J, Reznick R: Validation of an objective structured assessment of technical skill for surgical residents. *Acad Med* 1996;71(12):1363-1365.
14. MacRae HM, Cohen R, Regehr G, Reznick R, Burnstein M: A new assessment tool: The patient assessment and management examination. *Surgery* 1997;122(2): 335-343, discussion 343-344.
15. Sonnadara RR, Van Vliet A, Safir O, et al: Orthopedic boot camp: Examining the effectiveness of an intensive surgical skills course. *Surgery* 2011;149(6):745-749.

50

SYMPOSIUM

Resident Education in the Systems-Based Practice Competency

Susanne M. Roberts, MD
Sandra Jarvis-Selinger, PhD
Daniel D. Pratt, PhD
Robert J. Lucking, MD
Kevin P. Black, MD

Abstract

More than 10 years after the establishment of the six core competencies by the Accreditation Council for Graduate Medical Education, systems-based practice remains an elusive subject to teach, measure, and document. A wide variety of methods have been reported that address teaching and assessing performance for the discrete parts of systems-based practice; however, no single approach has been described that encompasses the competency in its entirety. To better understand the current state of this competency, orthopaedic residents and educators from around the country were surveyed to determine which systems-based practice topics were being taught at their institutions, how these topics were being taught, and how resident performance was assessed. Seven focus group sessions were held with members involved in the care of musculoskeletal patients to determine what they believed were essential skills for residents to learn relative to the healthcare system. Using this information, a health systems rotation was created for first-year residents that incorporated several different teaching and assessment methods. This rotation has received positive feedback from residents, patients, and health professionals. Its effect on resident development will be tracked over the next 5 years.

Instr Course Lect 2013;62:571-576.

In 2001, the Accreditation Council for Graduate Medical Education (ACGME) Outcomes Project instituted a policy requiring graduating residents to demonstrate appropriate knowledge, skills, and behaviors in six core competencies and charged residency programs to measure and document resident accomplishments in these six areas.[1] The ACGME core competencies were chosen for their commonality across diverse medical specialties. The goals in establishing the competencies were to standardize specific expectations that would be applicable to all resident education and "enable conversations about the work of medicine."[2] However, perhaps nowhere in medicine is the conversation stalled more than in issues surrounding the core competency of systems-based practice (SBP). More than 10 years after the establishment of the core competencies, SBP remains an elusive subject to teach, measure, and document.[3-6] Few educators are comfortable enough with the complex, constantly shifting, and expanding healthcare system to serve as experts on SBP or assess resident knowledge and competency in this area.[7] Because residents are more focused on learning medical knowledge and patient care, competencies in other areas are perceived as less important.[8] In one study, only 10% of fourth-year medical students reported knowledge of SBP.[9] Because the ACGME has set SBP as a pillar of medical care, educators and residents must work to improve understanding, teaching methods, and assessment of this difficult core competency.

Expectations of SBP and Learning Approaches

Expectations

To allow the effectiveness of teaching to be measured, SBP competency must be deconstructed into more discrete parts. The ACGME has stated that res-

Dr. Black or an immediate family member serves as a board member, owner, officer, or committee member of the American Orthopaedic Association, the American Orthopaedic Society for Sports Medicine, and the Pennsylvania Orthopaedic Society. None of the following authors nor any immediate family member has received anything of value from or has stock or stock options held in a commercial company or institution related directly or indirectly to the subject of this chapter: Dr. Roberts, Dr. Jarvis-Selinger, Dr. Pratt, and Dr. Lucking.

idents must demonstrate competency in the following six expectations of SBP: (1) working effectively in various healthcare delivery settings and systems relevant to their clinical specialty; (2) coordinating patient care within the healthcare system relevant to their clinical activity; (3) incorporating considerations of cost awareness and risk-benefit analysis in patient and/or population-based care, as appropriate; (4) advocating for quality patient care and optimal patient care systems; (5) working on interprofessional teams to enhance patient safety and improve the quality of care; and (6) participating in identifying system errors and implementing potential systems solutions. Although a variety of approaches have been reported that address teaching and assessing performance for the discrete parts of SBP, no one method encompasses the SBP competency in its entirety.

Didactic Lectures

Didactic lecture series have been used by several programs across different specialties, and it has been reported that audience response systems support learner engagement and provide real-time feedback to the lecturer.[10,11] With or without audience response systems, morbidity and mortality conferences can be used as one method of tailoring established lectures within the residency curriculum to teach SBP.[12] David and Reich[8] developed an SBP/managed care curriculum in a monthly workshop lecture format for residents of internal medicine. The authors concluded that such lectures can increase the residents' understanding and comfort with various topics in managed care and SBP. Some didactic topics may lend themselves well to smaller groups, where information is provided by a facilitator who can encourage discussion. Small group sessions also lend themselves well to a case-based learning format to stimulate interest in the topic.[11]

Computer-Based Learning

Computer-based learning is a convenient method to organize SBP topics into learning modules, and residents' understanding can be easily assessed with web-based pretesting and posttesting.[13] At its core, however, the SBP competency is focused on the team aspect of the healthcare system and the ability of residents to effectively function within that team. In a paper on the use of web-based modules in SBP teaching and assessment, Eskildsen[14] stated, "Ideally, this product should be used in the context of a clinical rotation so that learners can expand their learning and acquire transferrable skills using this online tool as a starting point." A web-based system primarily encourages individualized learning in an isolated environment. Thus, computer-based learning is most appropriate and convenient for well-defined and individual learning experiences, such as basic patient safety information or healthcare system regulations. One notable exception was a web-based curriculum developed by Peters et al[15] that required interviews and consultations with members of the healthcare system and encouraged the kind of communication and mutual understanding that is an essential element of the SBP competency.

Group Projects

In direct contrast to the solitary learning experience of didactic and computer-based learning, participation in group projects can teach and assess residents' understanding of health systems and can strengthen residents' competency in teamwork with other healthcare providers and nonphysician members of the hospital staff.[16,17] In addition to enhancing collaboration skills, such programs can potentially identify inefficiencies in the system and may result in quality improvement projects. Evaluation may include assessment of the project's quality and effect as well as the quality of teamwork. One drawback of this approach was that residents were hesitant in giving less than good evaluations of their peers.[17] Although the strength of group projects lies in their collaborative nature, assessment of the individual resident may be difficult.

Simulation

Simulation as a method to teach SBP is a means of fostering collaboration and teamwork among residents and other healthcare providers. Wang and Vozenilek[18] described a simulation-based SBP curriculum for emergency medicine and noted that it allowed residents to interact with the healthcare team in a realistic way and within a controlled setting. The authors reported that residents could benefit from a debriefing session, even if they were not directly involved in the simulation. Larkin et al[19] reported that by developing and implementing a human factors curriculum, and focusing on interpersonal and communication skills, SBP, and professionalism, junior surgical residents experienced substantial improvement in empathic communication.

Experiential Learning

Through experiential SBP learning assignments, first-year medical residents reported having an increased appreciation of nonphysician members in the healthcare system and improved awareness of opportunities for efficiency in various patient-care tasks.[20] Such assignments provide valuable opportunities for building rapport with nonphysicians. Sutkin and Aronoff[21] reported improved resident appreciation for the training and responsibilities of office staff with a 2-day experiential learning assignment. Turley et al[22] reported a substantial increase in resident pretest-to-posttest knowledge after the implementation of a 5-day SBP rotation focusing on the interrelationships of patient care, clinical revenue, and the physician's role within the healthcare system.

Discussion

There may never be a more urgent time for emphasizing competency in SBP than the present. In addition to the challenges of teaching and assessing SBP, there is the reality that healthcare costs, quality, and safety have come under increased public scrutiny in the past decade. The healthcare system has become increasingly complex to understand and navigate. As legislation moves toward change, emphasis must be placed on the acquisition of SBP skills during residency training. The knowledge, judgment, and communication skills required for competency in SBP are essential to a resident's development as a health professional and to achieving success in the changing environment of health care in the coming decade. The essential commitment of a physician to lifelong learning must be applied to understanding interactions within the healthcare system to improve the safety, quality, and efficiency of patient care.

Authors have sought to develop a better understanding of the challenges associated with teaching, learning, and assessing SBP competency. This chapter describes knowledge gained from survey data from residents, educators, and a broad group of stakeholders in the healthcare system. Based on this information, an orthopaedic health systems rotation was created for postgraduate year 1 (PGY-1) residents at the Pennsylvania State University College of Medicine.

Data Collection

Survey of Orthopaedic Educators and Residents

To better understand how the SBP competency was being addressed, surveys were distributed to orthopaedic residents and educators attending a course on the effective educator, the resident leadership forum, and the meeting of the council of residency directors held at the 2010 conference of the American Orthopaedic Association. The response rate was 57%, with surveys collected from 69 orthopaedic residents and 62 orthopaedic faculty members.

The survey asked respondents which SBP topics were being taught at their institutions, how SBP was being taught, and how a resident's performance was assessed. Based on this chapter's authors review of the literature and experiences in resident education, 11 SBP areas were presented for consideration in the survey, including (1) practice management; (2) hospital finance; (3) professional finance; (4) scope of practice of midlevel providers and physician oversight responsibilities; (5) physician employment options; (6) the role of other nonphysician members of the healthcare team; (7) orthopaedic professional societies and infrastructure; (8) federal and state regulations; (9) quality measures, systems errors, and patient safety; (10) roles and relationships between different healthcare facilities and guidelines for admission; and (11) healthcare plans and access.

A respondent was asked if his or her residency program taught these topics (response options were yes, no, or do not know). In addition, the respondent was asked to describe how SBP was being taught. Possible responses included clinical observation, didactic case-based learning, online program, self-directed study, and quality improvement projects. A respondent was also asked how each competency area was assessed. Response choices included global evaluation form, written or web-based test, 360° evaluation, other, and not assessed.

Cross-Sectional Focus Groups

Seven semistructured focus group sessions were conducted with diverse stakeholders who participated in the care of musculoskeletal patients at the Pennsylvania State University College of Medicine. Focus group participants included five faculty members; six residents from the Department of Orthopaedics and Rehabilitation; four nursing leaders from the outpatient clinic, the inpatient orthopaedic floor, care coordination, and the operating room; five staff members from the areas of social work, inpatient physical therapy, and utilization review; five staff members from the areas of risk management, quality leadership (including the chief quality officer and the chief medical officer), and legal counsel; five senior hospital administrative leaders; and four community orthopaedic surgeons with whom residents had completed a rotation. Across the seven focus groups, a total of 34 individuals participated. Groups were selected to encourage participants to speak freely. Each session was led by three of this chapter's authors (KPB, DDP, and SJS), with the exception of the resident group (the department chairman [KPB] excused himself from those sessions). Discussions were recorded and transcribed verbatim.

A semistructured generic focus group protocol was used to support open conversation among the 34 participants regarding their understanding of the SBP competency, desired learning outcomes, gaps in residents' knowledge and behavior, current and proposed methods of teaching and assessment, and anticipated implementation barriers. The generic protocol was adapted to facilitate discussions with four major stakeholder categories: residents, orthopaedic faculty, community orthopaedic surgeons, and allied health professionals and hospital administrative staff. The semistructured nature of the focus groups meant that some questions were not directly asked, and some divergence from the protocol was permissible. Questions were intended to guide the facilitators. Procedures most closely associated with grounded theory were used to analyze focus group data by relying on a constant comparative method to develop salient themes arising from the discussions.[23]

Results

Survey of Orthopaedic Residents and Faculty

On average, faculty and residents reported that 56% of SBP topics were being taught. Wide variation was noticed among the individual topics, with 81% of faculty reporting that patient quality care, systems error, and patient safety were being taught, whereas only 47% of faculty reported that hospital finance and scope of practice of midlevel providers was being taught, and 40% reported that physician oversight was being taught. Most residents reported that professional finance; the role of nonphysician members of the healthcare team; and quality measures, systems error, and patient safety were not included in their curricula. Overall, the survey showed that formal teaching of the SBP competency is inconsistent across the United States with regard to curriculum content and representation of topics.

When queried about how SBP was being taught, 33% of the respondents reported that clinical observation was the most widely used method of teaching. Residents, in particular, reported that SBP topics were more likely to transpire through clinical observations and self-directed study, indicating that a more passive approach currently predominates in resident education on this competency. When taken together, both groups reported didactic case-based learning as the second most commonly used educational tool.

With regard to assessment methods, the most common response was that SBP was not assessed, as reported by 42% of residents and 29% of faculty. Of those who reported that assessment was occurring, the largest group (8%) stated that it occurred via global evaluation forms and written or web-based tests.

Cross-Sectional Focus Groups

Discussion with the seven focus groups complemented the disparities in resident education observed in the survey data and enriched the understanding of what various members of the health system believed were essential skills for residents to learn relative to the healthcare system. Those focus group members with direct responsibility for resident education admitted a lack of confidence in their understanding of the healthcare system and the SBP competency and questioned their ability to teach and assess it. Their perception of the SBP competency focused largely on efficiency in completing tasks. Discussions with residents revealed their inability to see the larger picture of the healthcare system because their education and personal goals primarily focused on acquisition of medical knowledge and technical skills and the efficient completion of discrete tasks.

Nonorthopaedic professionals focused their comments on SBP topics that were specific to their interactions with orthopaedic residents. For example, nurses, physician consultants, allied health members, and safety/quality leaders were passionate about the need for improved communication and collaboration skills as well as the need to reduce errors. Administrators emphasized the need to enhance residents' understanding of hospital operations, finance, law, and insurance.

Development of an Orthopaedic Health Systems Rotation

Through analyses of the survey and focus group data, it became apparent that SBP topics, such as finance, malpractice, and the medical-legal system, are extremely important to learn; however, the fundamental need for residents to learn how to effectively function as one part of a multidisciplinary team had been largely ignored. The knowledge on how to effectively function as a member of a team is not something that can be taught exclusively via didactic lecture or by reading journal articles; therefore, this chapter's authors developed a PGY-1 SBP rotation to address these shortcomings.

The goal of this initial learning opportunity is for interns to develop a better understanding of the healthcare system by observing care and the system through the eyes of the patient and other healthcare professionals. Interns are charged to consider what can be done, individually and collectively, to provide a safer, better, and more efficient experience for the patient.

During the first week, an intern is assigned two or three patients to follow from admission to discharge and is required to interview the patients and families and observe their interactions with healthcare providers as well as the interactions of providers with each other. The intern was expected to interview other healthcare providers to develop a better understanding of their roles in patient care and their views on what orthopaedic surgeons can do differently to improve communication and collaboration.

Required readings included two texts: *Understanding Patient Safety*[24] and *The Checklist Manifesto*.[25] Interns also participated in medical center patient safety and quality care review meetings and met with operating room medical and administrative leadership. Four months later, in the second week of the rotation, they attended lectures on the business of medicine and understanding diagnosis-related groups and were required to analyze a diagnosis-related group report for a four-physician joint arthroplasty service (for which they received a supplemental reading).

At the conclusion of each week, the interns provided a summary report and discussed their experiences with supervising faculty. In addition to sharing what they learned during each of these weeks, course faculty also sought to obtain feedback on what could be done to improve the learning experience for residents.

One class of interns has completed this health systems rotation and has been uniformly and enthusiastically positive about their experiences. The assigned readings were believed to provide invaluable background and perspectives which, when combined with their interactions with patients and other healthcare providers, resulted in essential new insights regarding their role in the healthcare system, threats to patient safety and quality of care, inefficiencies in the system, and opportunities for improvement. After attending patient safety and quality-of-care review meetings, interns reported that they were more interested in and better equipped to classify errors, perform a root cause analysis, and suggest solutions. During these meetings, interns enjoyed presenting their unique points of view regarding the larger picture of the care being delivered.

Patients and other healthcare providers also reported that they benefited from this health system rotation. Patients were receptive to sharing their experiences, and staff members were appreciative of the efforts made to provide orthopaedic residents with a better understanding of their roles in the healthcare system and opportunities to enhance communication and collaboration.

Summary

To provide patient care that is safe, efficient, and of the highest quality, it is essential to provide learning experiences for orthopaedic residents that prepare them to function as part of an effective healthcare team in a highly complex system. This chapter's authors believe that the described health systems rotation is a helpful first step in achieving these goals and are encouraged by feedback from the participating interns. The participants reported that the health system rotation prepared them for the pitfalls and dangers of the healthcare system and helped them suggest necessary and overdue improvements. The residents reported participating in discussions concerning avenues to effect change.

Much additional work is still needed. Resident education in this area needs to be continuous, developmental, and integrated into their 5-year curriculum and aligned with their level of experience. The current PGY-1 health systems rotation is being evaluated for possible improvements and expansion into years 2 through 5. Each class of residents will be tracked throughout the 5 years of their residency and into practice to see how their understanding and actions related to SBP develop over time and how the knowledge gained is implemented into orthopaedic practice after residency.

References

1. Bready LL: The graduate medical education community's responsibility for producing a fully trained physician. http://www.acgme.org/acgmeweb/Portals/0/PDFs/jgme-11-00-81-85%5B1%5D.pdf. Accessed October 15, 2012.
2. Batalden PB, Leach DC: Sharpening the focus on systems-based practice. *J Grad Med Educ* 2009; 1(1):1-3.
3. Didwania A, McGaghie WC, Cohen E, Wayne DB: Internal medicine residency graduates' perceptions of the systems-based practice and practice-based learning and improvement competencies. *Teach Learn Med* 2010;22(1):33-36.
4. Elwood D, Kirschner JS, Moroz A, Berliner J: Exploring systems-based practice in a sample of physical medicine and rehabilitation residency programs. *PM R* 2009;1(3):223-228.
5. Frenk J, Chen L, Bhutta ZA, et al: Health professionals for a new century: Transforming education to strengthen health systems in an interdependent world. *Lancet* 2010;376(9756):1923-1958.
6. Smith CS, Morris M, Langois-Winkle F, Hill W, Francovich C: A pilot study using cultural consensus analysis to measure systems-based practice performance. *Int J Med Ed* 2010; 1:15-18.
7. Harris EE, Abdel-Wahab M, Spangler AE, Lawton CA, Amdur RJ: Results of the Association of Directors of Radiation Oncology Programs (ADROP) survey of radiation oncology residency program directors. *Int J Radiat Oncol Biol Phys* 2009;74(2):327-337.
8. David RA, Reich LM: The creation and evaluation of a systems-based practice/managed care curriculum in a primary care internal medicine residency program. *Mt Sinai J Med* 2005;72(5):296-299.

9. Wasnick JD, Chang L, Russell C, Gadsden J: Do residency applicants know what the ACGME core competencies are? One program's experience. *Acad Med* 2010;85(5):791-793.
10. Mitchell JD, Parhar P, Narayana A: Teaching and assessing systems-based practice: A pilot course in health care policy, finance, and law for radiation oncology residents. *J Grad Med Educ* 2010; 2(3):384-388.
11. Davison SP, Cadavid JD, Spear SL: Systems-based practice: Education in plastic surgery. *Plast Reconstr Surg* 2007;119(1): 410-415.
12. Varkey P, Karlapudi S, Rose S, Nelson R, Warner M: A systems approach for implementing practice-based learning and improvement and systems-based practice in graduate medical education. *Acad Med* 2009;84(3): 335-339.
13. Kerfoot BP, Conlin PR, Travison T, McMahon GT: Web-based education in systems-based practice: A randomized trial. *Arch Intern Med* 2007;167(4):361-366.
14. Eskildsen MA: Review of Web-based module to train and assess competency in systems-based practice. *J Am Geriatr Soc* 2010; 58(12):2412-2413.
15. Peters AS, Kimura J, Ladden MD, March E, Moore GT: A self-instructional model to teach systems-based practice and practice-based learning and improvement. *J Gen Intern Med* 2008l;23(7):931-936.
16. Delphin E, Davidson M: Teaching and evaluating group competency in systems-based practice in anesthesiology. *Anesth Analg* 2008; 106(6):1837-1843.
17. Patterson BR, Kimball KJ, Walsh-Covarrubias JB, Kilgore LC: Effecting the sixth core competency: A project-based curriculum. *Am J Obstet Gynecol* 2008;199(5):561, e1-e6.
18. Wang EE, Vozenilek JA: Addressing the systems-based practice core competency: A simulation-based curriculum. *Acad Emerg Med* 2005;12(12):1191-1194.
19. Larkin AC, Cahan MA, Whalen G, et al: Human Emotion and Response in Surgery (HEARS): A simulation-based curriculum for communication skills, systems-based practice, and professionalism in surgical residency training. *J Am Coll Surg* 2010;211(2): 285-292.
20. Eiser AR, Connaughton-Storey J: Experiential learning of systems-based practice: A hands-on experience for first-year medical residents. *Acad Med* 2008;83(10): 916-923.
21. Sutkin G, Aronoff CK: Resident front office experience: A systems-based practice activity. *Med Educ Online* 2008;13:6.
22. Turley CB, Roach R, Marx M: Systems survivor: A program for house staff in systems-based practice. *Teach Learn Med* 2007; 19(2):128-138.
23. Charmaz K: *Inside Interviewing: New Lenses, New Concerns*. Thousand Oaks, CA, Sage Publications, 2003, pp 311-330.
24. Wachter W: *Understanding Patient Safety*. Columbus, OH, McGraw-Hill Companies, 2008.
25. Gawande A*: The Checklist Manifesto: How to Get Things Right*. New York, NY, Metropolitan Books, Henry Holt and Company, 2009.

51

SYMPOSIUM

I Feel Disconnected: Learning Technologies in Resident Education

April D. Armstrong, MD, FRCSC
Sandra Jarvis-Selinger, PhD

Abstract

With the rapid development of technology in medical education, orthopaedic educators are recognizing that the way residents learn and access information is profoundly changing. Residency programs are faced with the challenging problem that current educational methods are not designed to take full advantage of the information explosion and rapid technologic changes. This disconnection is often seen in the potentially separate approaches to education preferred by residents and orthopaedic educators. Becoming connected with residents requires understanding the possible learning technologies available and the learners' abilities, needs, and expectations. It is often assumed that approaches to strategic lifelong learning are developed by residents during their training; however, without the incorporation of technology into the learning environment, residents will not be taught the digital literacy and information management strategies that will be needed in the future. To improve learning, it is important to highlight and discuss current technologic trends in education, the possible technologic disconnection between educators and learners, the types of learning technologies available, and the potential opportunities for getting connected.

Instr Course Lect 2013;62:577-585.

More than four decades ago, Toffler's *Future Shock* prophetically described the need to manage the coming dramatic changes of the information age.[1] Those changes are here and are accelerating because of a multitude of technologic developments. The rapid development of learning technologies has and will continue to profoundly change the way residents learn and access information and will affect the way orthopaedic surgery is practiced now and in the future. As is the case with any academic training program, orthopaedic residency programs should educate residents for the current and future practice of orthopaedic medicine. The disconnection or gap exists because current educational methods are not designed to take full advantage of the information explosion and rapid technologic changes.[2] This disconnection is also seen in the disparate approaches to education used by residents and orthopaedic educators. For example, helping residents develop strategies to deal with information overload is becoming a critical element in their education. The faculty-resident relationship will fundamentally shift as new information resources are continually integrated into clinical activities. As Veillette and Harvey[2] write, "Orthopaedic education needs a fundamental change of focus from simply delivering content to developing the ability to manage these changes." Although managing the volume of information is one concern, residents must also learn to critically and scientifically navigate through new information to assign value to what they learn.

The Rise of the Machine

Many authors have noted the rapid

Dr. Armstrong or an immediate family member serves as a board member, owner, officer, or committee member of the American Shoulder and Elbow Surgeons and has received nonincome support (such as equipment or services), commercially derived honoraria, or other non–research-related funding (such as paid travel) from Zimmer. Neither Dr. Jarvis-Selinger nor any immediate family member has received anything of value from or owns stock in a commercial company or institution related directly or indirectly to the subject of this chapter.

rise of technology in medical education.[3-11] Several technologic trends are currently affecting and will continue to affect medical education.[5] Robin et al[5] reported five such trends, including the explosion of new information, the digitization of all information, the presence of new generations of learners, the emergence of new instructional technologies, and the accelerating pace of change.

The Explosion of Information

It has been estimated that knowledge has doubled every year since 1940, and it has been hypothesized that this rate is rapidly accelerating.[5,12,13] In a study conducted at the University of California–San Diego, the authors presented data on the information consumption of Americans in 2009.[12] According to this report, "Americans consumed information for about 1.3 trillion hours, an average of almost 12 hours per day. Consumption totaled 3.6 zettabytes and 10,845 trillion words, corresponding to 100,500 words and 34 gigabytes for an average person on an average day. A zettabyte is 10^{21} bytes, a million million gigabytes."

The Digitalization of Information

More information is being consumed in a digital format. The digitalization of information is supported by search engines such as Google Scholar and Google Books.[14,15] Jackson[16] reported that Google had estimated that there were more than 129 million books in the world, and Google had scanned 12 million books as of June 2010. Google plans to complete the scanning of all existing books by 2020, which will result in approximately 4 billion digitized pages and 2 trillion words.[16] Instant access to information is also facilitated by technology, which supports the ability of an individual to search, organize, filter, and synthesize millions of pieces of information quickly and efficiently. The search engine is a good example of the technology that allows locating, retrieving, reading, and digesting large amounts of information, which had not been possible in the past. (More senior readers will no doubt remember the days of card indexing, long library shelves, and the weight of seven or eight large reference texts).

A New Generation of Learners

The new generation of learners is correlated with the fact that the interaction with information has changed, and the current and upcoming generations are and will be immersed in this new technologic world. The new generation of learners, whom Prensky[17,18] calls digital natives, are individuals who have grown up in the digital world and use technology to communicate, record, and learn. As these digital natives reach medical school, important questions must be considered. What type of learners will they be (including how they are different than previous learners)? What changes are happening (and will happen) in medical education because of them? How will educators deal with the growing expectations to integrate technology into learning?

Educational changes will not only affect learners; educators will also be affected. Medical educators may belong to one of three groups: (1) digital immigrants, who learned technology after formal education and have adopted it but are not as immersed or natural with the digital world as the digital natives;[5,17] (2) digital settlers, who did not grow up immersed in technology but are very comfortable with technology and are similar to digital natives in their comfort and ease with using technology;[5,19] or (3) traditionalists, who did not grow up with technology and have not incorporated it into their teaching methods.[5]

New Instructional Technologies

The fourth trend outlined by Robin et al[5] is the emergence of new instructional technologies. This trend is not unique if technology is thought of as a modality for teaching. In many instances, new modalities for effectively presenting information have changed teaching methods. For example, many physicians may recall the change from blackboards (or whiteboards) to overhead projectors during their undergraduate education. Some may recall when the instant development of ideas in the classroom (such as writing on the blackboard) gave way to predesigned presentation tools such as PowerPoint (Microsoft, Redmond, WA) or even newer software options such as Prezi (Budapest, Hungary) or SlideRocket (San Francisco, CA). Both as students and teachers, physicians have seen how educational modalities and the introduction of technology into the teaching context have changed teaching, learning, and the practice of medicine.

Educational technology is not only creating better presentation methods; it is also changing the power structure of education itself. Christensen[20] wrote about the idea termed disruptive technologies in the world of business. Those technologies moved the power to the users and away from the traditional business organizations. For example, the introduction of digital photography combined with the increasing availability of photographic software, desktop computing, and color printers, gave users the ability to create, develop, and edit photographs at home and moved those activities away from photo-developing companies. In the realm of education and knowledge, Wikipedia (Wikipedia Foundation, San Francisco, CA) can be considered a disruptive technology in the field of creating and accessing information because it invades a realm typically owned and operated by companies such as Encyclopedia Britannica (Chicago, IL). Users can not only access information quickly and easily through sites such as Wikipedia but also create content.

The Rate of Change

The final trend to consider is the rate of change at which technology is being adopted into medical education. This rate of change is most directly related to the introduction of new instructional technologies, which are emerging at a mind-boggling rate. A consideration of the innovations in mobile telephone technology over the past 10 years provides a good idea of how quickly change is taking place. Another excellent example of the extraordinary rate of technologic change is the dramatic increase in the number of applications (known as apps) that have been created for mobile computing with smartphones. By December 2011, there were 522,857 active apps, developed by 122,478 active publishers, available for download.[21] This statistic also relates to the idea of disruptive technologies because individuals as well as corporations create apps. The top five categories of active apps are games (17%), books (11%), entertainment (10%), education (10%), and lifestyle (8%). Medical apps represent 2% or approximately 9,500 of the total number of active apps.

The rate at which apps are being produced is a good indication of how rapidly technology is changing and accelerating. In November 2008, an average of 97 apps became active each day of the month, with 25,303 total active apps available. In November 2010, an average of 714 apps became active each day of the month, with 519,831 active apps available. Such a rapid rate of change can contribute to the growing disconnection between residents and educators.

Disconnection

Prensky[17] describes the large discontinuity created as a result of the technologic trends that have rapidly changed the learning landscape over the past few decades. The educational context is not only changing, but Prensky[17] believes that students are thinking about and processing information in a fundamentally different manner than in past years. He describes two groups who he calls digital natives and digital immigrants. The digital native is the current student who is a native to the digital language of computers, video games, and the Internet. This group likes to receive information "really fast," likes to parallel process and multitask information, and functions best in a networking situation. Digital natives thrive on instant gratification and frequent rewards, prefer gaming to serious work, and have little patience for didactic lecture and step-by-step logic.

In contrast, digital immigrants are individuals not born into the digital world, but they have adapted more or less successfully to the new technologic environment. One important issue is that most digital natives are being taught by digital immigrants. Because the language of technology has been learned later in life by the digital immigrants, there may be a struggle for those educators to teach a population of residents (digital natives) that speaks an entirely new language. The educators (digital immigrants) may have little appreciation for the new cognitive and learning approaches of the residents (digital natives) and may be challenged by the pressure to change the learning landscape to accommodate ever-changing technologies. Educators may be resistant to technologic changes and may want to continue to teach in a slow, step-by-step fashion, not accepting the notion that learning can be fun. The educator may assume that his or her residents learn in the same way the educator learned and may not want to adopt new teaching methods. These factors contribute to the disconnection between learners and educators.

In the area of acceptance of technologic advancements, there is obviously a spectrum of comfort levels for both learners and educators. The digital native and the digital immigrant represent points along this spectrum, and there may or may not be a huge disparity in preferred learning approaches between these groups. In some cases, however, a huge disparity may exist, such as in the case of a senior faculty member and a postgraduate second-year resident. In others instances, such as those involving a new faculty member and a senior chief resident, there may be only a narrow gap or disconnection in learning and teaching approaches. The more important concept is that the rise of technologic advancements and the ever-increasing speed of adoption and adaptation to new methods will always create the possibility for a mismatch between the learner and the educator. The challenge is to acknowledge the possible disconnection and understand how educational technologies may be interfering with or enhancing the learning environment.

Educational Technologies

In addition to the technologic trends that continue to affect education and the disconnection with learners, educators are also continually faced with questions about learning modalities and their effectiveness. Educators must determine what kinds of technologies enhance learning. Because describing all the possible educational technologies is beyond the scope of this chapter, only three categories (online platforms, mobile computing, and social media) are discussed.

Online Platforms

Internet- or web-based technologies are the most common e-learning approaches in higher education, of which online courses are the most widely used. The course may be run exclusively online (with or without a facilitator) or may be a combination of online presentations and face-to-face interactions.[22] Popular web-based course software includes Blackboard (Blackboard Inc, Washington, DC), WebCT (Blackboard), and Moodle.

Course-based online learning is not the only use of web technologies. Shorter educational modules also have been created for surgical and orthopaedic residents.[23-25] Online resources available to orthopaedic residents include web-based textbooks, images, video clips, multimedia and case presentations, knowledge databases, e-mail, e-mail discussion lists, electronic forums, and technology-enabled conferences.[2] The American Academy of Orthopaedic Surgeons (AAOS) Orthopaedic Knowledge Online,[26] WorldOrtho,[27] and OrthoNet[28] are some websites that provide an extensive array of resources, including textbook-based notes, slide shows, practice examinations, and an overview of the history of orthopaedics.[2] For orthopaedic educators, websites such as MedEdPORTAL[29] provides teaching materials, assessment tools, and faculty development resources.

Mobile Computing

Mobile computing refers to any technology-enabled handheld devices, such as handheld computers, personal digital assistants, or smartphones. This sector of technologic hardware is rapidly expanding and is continually being redefined. Beyond what are traditionally considered smartphones, devices such as tablet computers (such as the iPad [Apple, Cupertino, CA], the BlackBerry Playbook [Research in Motion, Ontario, Canada], and the Galaxy Tab [Samsung, Ridgefield Park, NJ]) are also able to support mobile computing needs.

A 2009 study by Nielsen reported that 18% of mobile subscribers had smartphones, and more males than females used smartphones.[30] In the third quarter of 2011, 50% of mobile subscribers in the United States owned a smartphone, and 51% were female.[3,4,30-35] There has been a massive increase in the numbers of downloaded consumer apps for smartphones, with figures increasing from 300 million apps downloaded in 2009 to 5 billion in 2010.[36] In a recent national survey of the Accreditation Council for Graduate Medical Education orthopaedic surgery departments, Franko[4] found that 400 of 476 respondents (84%) had a smartphone, and 53% of the smartphone owners used apps in clinical practice.

There has been substantial research on the various ways mobile computing has been incorporated into medical education.[31,32,36] One of the most common methods of incorporating these devices into medical education is through the use of app- or program-based point-of-care information access. Residents now have instant access to apps and programs for medical calculators (such as MedMath, MedCalc, and Calculate), commercial databases (such as Epocrates [Epocrates Inc, San Mateo, CA]), and medical textbooks. The use of such apps represents a new learning experience. Although apps can digitize more traditional forms of education (such as video recordings of lectures and access to newsletters and articles), app-based education also provides access to novel ways of learning. Smartphone and iPad (Apple) apps that provide a spectrum of learning opportunities and useful clinical support systems are available to orthopaedic faculty members and residents.[4,33] These tools can be organized into six broad categories: (1) apps for surgical techniques and approaches, clinical examinations, and product guides (examples: Synthes [Synthes Inc, West Chester, PA], Stryker IVS [Stryker Interventional Spine, Kalamazoo, MI], and OpTech Live [Stryker]); (2) billing and coding apps (examples: Mobile Coder for Orthopedics and Mobile Coder for Foot and Ankle [Psygo, Redondo Beach, CA]); (3) tools for diagnoses (examples: CORE-Clinical Orthopaedic Exam [Clinically Relevant Technologies, Seattle, WA], SLIC [Digital Neurosurgeon, Maastricht, Netherlands], Scoligauge [Ockendon Partners, Shrewsbury, England], and iOrtho Lite [Amphetamobile, Upper Darby, PA]); (4) apps for three-dimensional interactive modeling (examples: iSpineCare [Anatomate-Apps, Mosman, Australia] and inMotion 3D [Stryker]); (5) reference and news apps (examples: AAOS Now [AAOS, Rosemont, IL], AO surgery reference [AO Foundation, Davos, Switzerland], OrthoAnatomy [Aesthete Software, St. Paul, MN], and Orthopaedics Hyperguide [Vindico Medical Education, Thorofare, NJ]); and (6) patient education apps (examples: FlipChart [Stryker] and Stryker IVS).

App-based learning can provide necessary repetition and reinforcement that is more difficult to achieve with traditional lecture-based approaches. Residents can access the app on demand and can replay, review, and rehearse areas they find challenging.

In addition to these informational tools, mobile computing can also support access to more traditional forms of education such as lectures and presentations. Similar to online platforms that support access to audio, video, and other interactive presentations, mobile computing can be used to access educational offerings. Mobile computing devices are commonly used to access podcasts of video or audio medical presentations. Podcasts of all types are available for download on iTunes (Apple). For example, the *Journal of Bone and Joint Surgery*, the *Journal of Medical Education*, the *British Medical Journal*, and many academic institutions have podcasts available for downloading. Podcasts allows physicians, residents, and medical students to view the latest research, review a clinical procedure or technique, or hear a lecture during a time convenient to the listener.[6,7,31] The asynchronous nature of podcasting allows users to access information anytime, anywhere, on any device. As Holzinger et al[32] comment, "the available mobile technology can enhance the shift from pure instructor-centered classroom teaching to constructivist learner-centered educational settings away from the classroom; for example in outside learning environments—medical education is a good example."

Social Media

Social media (also known as Web 2.0) is a new and emerging area within technology-enabled learning. Social media is a term given to web tools and applications designed to facilitate online interaction, discussion, and information sharing.[34,37] The development and use of these tools was originally created for entertainment and personal use; however, medical educators are recognizing that social media also has the potential to transform learning environments.[34] Some common examples are wikis (example, Wikipedia), blogs (example, kevinMD.com), electronic communities of practice (example, Orthopaedic Educators website),[38] social networks (examples, Facebook [Facebook Inc, Palo Alto, CA] and Twitter [Twitter Inc, San Francisco, CA]), videoconferencing (examples, Skype [Microsoft] and iChat [Apple]), and virtual worlds (example, Second Life [Linden Lab, San Francisco, CA]).

Wikis are interactive websites that allow users to add, modify, or delete content via web-based editing software.[6] Wikipedia is the most popular wiki, with more than 3.8 million content pages as of early 2012.[39] Many academic institutions have their own wiki platforms, where faculty and students can create their own wiki pages. Other wikis are specifically designed for medical educators, students, and residents. For example, one medical website (AskDrWiki) allows users with a medical background to publish review articles, clinical notes, pearls, and medical images.[40] Anyone with a medical background can contribute to or edit medical articles; however, the user must first create an account, which must include the individual's degree, training, and hospital or medical school affiliation. Ganfyd is a free medical wiki that allows registered medical practitioners to create and edit information.[41] It is a collaborative medical reference by medical professionals and invited nonmedical experts.

Another popular social media tool is the blog, a term coined by Peter Merholz, which is derived from a shortened version of weblog and is also used as a verb (blog) to describe the act of creating an online journal.[42] Blogs were one of the first social media tools and were built as interactive websites to track diary-like entries. Unlike static websites, blogs allow individuals to write articles and engage in one or more conversations with many readers.[42] Giustini[42] describes a blog known as Clinical Cases and Images.[43] This blog provides residents and clinicians with a collection of presurfed material; provides timely updates; and includes interactivity features, medical headlines, clinical images through Flickr [Yahoo, Sunnyvale, CA], and discussion areas for posting comments.

Virtual or electronic communities of practice are social networks of individuals who interact through technology-enabled platforms. Online communities can be used as a virtual coffee room, where physicians and residents can network with friends and colleagues.[31] These communities create opportunities to converse, get advice, share ideas and resources, and collaborate over a distance. One example is the website Orthopaedic Educators.[38] This electronic community of practice is an online learning environment that can be accessed by orthopaedic educators at any time or anywhere to positively affect orthopaedic education.[44] It creates an opportunity to build collaborative resources, share best practices, and discuss educational issues with other educators. Attributes of a successful electronic community of practice are voluntary involvement, self-organization, problem-focused material, distributed leadership, transparency, accountability, accessibility, shared identity, and sustainability.[44]

Boulos et al[45] described the potential of three-dimensional virtual worlds for medical education using the Second Life online platform and have compiled a resource page with information about such platforms (http://healthcybermap.org/sl.htm). The use of Second Life is illustrated with two case studies—HealthInfoIsland and the Virtual Neurologic Education Centre.[45] The authors conclude that there are financial and time-based learning and development costs and uptake barriers associated with the implementation of any technology; however, platforms such as Second Life have developed an "immersive, rich experience that combines many of the features of Web 2.0, such as group instant messaging, voice chat, profiles and real-time social networking, and a unique form of online social interaction that involves sharing various objects and creative collaboration on building and running places and services in the virtual world (user-generated content)."[45]

Discussion

Online platforms, mobile computing activities, and social media options are a few of many evolving educational technologies. A discussion of these types of technology (especially in the area of social media) must take into account the potential dangers and limitations of the technologies when applied in a clinical or educational setting. For example, educators must consider the issues of privacy and professionalism when deciding how technology will be integrated into residency programs.[46]

Getting Connected

Current students have been described as preferring digital literacy, experiential learning, interactivity, and immediacy.[47] It is also increasingly recognized that traditional teaching techniques may not be as effective for these students. With this in mind, educators are seeking methods to further enhance the teaching environment, adapt to the changing expectations of current learners, and get connected.

Training

The first step in getting connected is to educate and train the educator and the learner. Providing dedicated professional development time for members of the team will help in connecting the faculty educators (digital immigrants) and their students (digital natives). If the educator is trying to learn while teaching or is learning from the residents themselves, it detracts from the residents' learning opportunities and has less effect than dedicated, purposeful training. Using electronic medical records is a good example of a technologic development that may be more intuitive and have a shorter learning curve for residents than for faculty members. Using mobile devices or web interfaces to acquire patient information and results, chart and document findings to facilitate patient handovers,[48] or track a resident's performance[49] are innovative uses of technology but may be foreign to faculty members who were trained using a paper-based system. Such innovations save time, which is a premium commodity (especially given current resident work-hour restrictions).[48] Faculty educators should advocate and promote the development of innovative methods to care for patients but will need appropriate training and understanding of new technologies to optimize effectiveness.

Evaluating a Learner's Competency

Along with understanding technology, educators must also understand the needs and expectations of learners. Technology provides residents with instant access to knowledge; however, it still must be determined whether a specific resident is ready for the responsibilities inherent in caring for patients. Residents across all medical specialties value autonomy when dealing with patients as they gain experience, but this should not be confused with the mastery of autonomous self-directed learning and a comprehensive medical skills set. In an interview of 13 final-year, family-practice residents, Nothnagle et al[50] reported that the residents highlighted the need for more support and guidance in learning. With technology providing instant access to vast amounts of medical information, a resident may struggle with incorporating this information into practice and managing his or her own learning; however, in some instances, a resident may not recognize his or her personal limitations. A resident may believe that quickly accessing and reading information is the same as mastering the information. Faculty members may incorrectly assume that the resident has successfully mastered a topic if the educator does not probe to find the depth of the resident's knowledge. One method to ensure the mastery of knowledge is to go beyond simple recall questions and ask questions that require higher-order thinking or require the resident to apply the knowledge to a different situation. It is not uncommon to find a resident reading a web page on the diagnosis and treatment of the patient he or she is about to present in clinic. It can be difficult for the educator to know if the resident had the opportunity to consolidate and reflect on the material or if he or she is merely regurgitating information from short-term memory.

Faculty members must consider how resident competency is evaluated, even though the most technically savvy resident may appear to have all the correct answers. Recall aided by technology must not be confused with deep understanding. There is not enough evidence available to determine whether instant access to knowledge provided by technology is hurtful or helpful in gaining mastery of a subject.[51] The speed at which articles or textbooks can be accessed is helpful; however, it may be disadvantageous because digital natives spend less time on reflection, which is important for processing information. It would appear to be wise for educators to include reflection and critical thinking in the learning process. Surface learning (regardless of whether it is technologically enabled) will not provide the necessary knowledge and skill needed for clinical practice. A resident who quickly looks up an answer on the Internet often will spend little time reflecting on the newly gained information. Asking the same resident a question designed to apply this new knowledge to a different situation commonly results in the "deer in the headlights" look; he or she may know various facts but not yet appreciate how those facts relate in a larger context.

Carr[51] reports that people use a "form of skimming activity" when reading Internet material, which involves hopping from source to source, typically reading one or two pages, then jumping to the next article. This is known as the "power browse." It has been suggested that this weakens one's ability for deep reading and provides less time to make rich mental connections. It is vitally important for residents to take time to reflect on and process information because that practice promotes the ability to reason clinically, make sound judgments, and elicit appropriate information.[52] The role of faculty educators may shift from delivering content to becoming experts who provide structure and guidance for self-directed learning and training on how to reflect on that learning.[50]

Skill-Based Simulation Programs

The rise of technology has also contributed to the rise of skill-based simulation technologies. Time constraints related to resident work hours and the pressures of patient safety initiatives have clearly created a challenge to providing on-site surgical training. As a result, simulation teaching programs have been developed and will continue to become a common practice in residency programs. Simulation programs are already required in general surgery residency programs, and it is likely that they will soon be a mandated component of other procedural specialties. The topic of simulation programs is beyond the scope of this chapter, but the first step to "connecting" is accepting that these programs will likely become part of the orthopaedic educational environment.

Education issues relating to clinical simulation tools include the model's fidelity, transferability to real practice, and the ability to measure outcomes and provide feedback. A new concept evolving in this field is known as serious games, in which game-based knowledge technologies are being applied to teaching and learning.[53] Kapralos et al[53] suggest that a problem-based learning curriculum, using a game-based focus, can provide more predictable and timely content delivery and can be less dependent on the random flow of patient exposure. Simulation programs should be incorporated into residency training as a means of enhancing and amplifying, not replacing, the clinical teaching environment.

Improved Web-Based Resources

Other novel ways to improve connectivity with students and residents include increasing web-based links to course notes and resources, podcasting lectures so that they can be accessed again on handheld devices, using interactive response devices during lectures, and incorporating chat rooms or web-based collaborative learning centers into the teaching program.[47] The challenge to educators is to familiarize themselves with new technologic opportunities, become adept at using these technologies, determine the content that will be taught and how technology can be used to enhance the learning process, and reconsider the student evaluation process to make the educator a facilitator of reflective and critical thinking. As Coach George Allen has been credited with saying, "the future is now." Orthopaedic educators need to consider how best to train the new generation of surgeons, who will practice orthopaedics in the age of Google and Facebook.[54]

Summary

A disconnection between educators and learners exists because current educational methods are not designed to take full advantage of the information explosion and rapid technologic changes and because there is often a separate approach to education preferred by residents and orthopaedic educators. Getting connected with residents includes understanding new technologies and the needs and expectations of learners. It is often assumed that approaches to strategic lifelong learning are developed by residents during their training; therefore, incorporating technology into the learning environment will teach residents information management strategies to effectively and efficiently manage information overload now and in the future. Ultimately, the role of the orthopaedic educator is to bridge the disconnection and help residents to learn how to educate themselves.

References

1. Toffler A: *Future Shock*. New York, NY, Random House, 1970.
2. Veillette CJ, Harvey EJ: Implications for orthopaedic education. Canadian Orthopaedic Association, 2011. http://www.coa-aco.org/library/orthopaedic-informatics/the-information-age-implications-for-orthopaedic-education.html. Accessed March 5, 2012.
3. Lindquist AM, Johansson PE, Petersson GI, Saveman B-I, Nilsson GC: The use of the personal

digital assistant (PDA) among personnel and students in health care: A review. *J Med Internet Res* 2008;10(4):e31.

4. Franko OI: Smartphone apps for orthopaedic surgeons. *Clin Orthop Relat Res* 2011;469(7):2042-2048.
5. Robin BR, McNeil SG, Cook DA, Agarwal KL, Singhal GR: Preparing for the changing role of instructional technologies in medical education. *Acad Med* 2011; 86(4):435-439.
6. Boulos MN, Maramba I, Wheeler S: Wikis, blogs and podcasts: A new generation of Web-based tools for virtual collaborative clinical practice and education. *BMC Med Educ* 2006;6:41.
7. Masters K, Ellaway R: E-learning in medical education: Guide 32 part 2. Technology, management and design. *Med Teach* 2008; 30(5):474-489.
8. Wong G, Greenhalgh T, Pawson R: Internet-based medical education: A realist review of what works, for whom and in what circumstances. *BMC Med Educ* 2010;10:12.
9. Cook DA: Where are we with Web-based learning in medical education? *Med Teach* 2006; 28(7):594-598.
10. Ruiz JG, Mintzer MJ, Leipzig RM: The impact of e-learning in medical education. *Acad Med* 2006;81(3):207-212.
11. Lau F, Bates J: A review of e-learning practices for undergraduate medical education. *J Med Syst* 2004;28(1):71-87.
12. Bohn RE, Short JE: How much information? 2009 report on American consumers. San Diego, CA, 2009. Updated January, 2010. http://hmi.ucsd.edu/pdf/HMI_2009_ConsumerReport_Dec9_2009.pdf. Accessed March 5, 2012.
13. Lyman P, Varian HR: Reprint: How Much Information? *J Electron Publish* 2000;6(2).
14. Google Scholar. About Google Scholar. http://scholar.google.com/intl/en/scholar/about.html. Accessed March 5, 2012.
15. Google Books. http://books.google.com/. Accessed March 5, 2012.
16. Jackson J: Google: 129 million different books have been published. PC World. 2010. Available at http://www.pcworld.com/article/202803/google_129_million_different_books_have_been_published.html. Accessed March 5, 2012.
17. Prensky M: Digital natives, digital immigrants. *Horizon* 2001;9(5): 1-6. http://www.marcprensky.com/writing/prensky%20-%20digital%20natives,%20digital%20immigrants%20-%20part1.pdf. Accessed March 5, 2012.
18. Prensky M: Digital native, digital immigrants: Part II. Do they really think differently? *Horizon* 2001;9(5):7-13. http://www.marcprensky.com/writing/prensky%20-%20digital%20natives,%20digital%20immigrants%20-%20part2.pdf Accessed March 5, 2012.
19. Palfrey J, Gasser U: *Born Digital: Understanding the First Generation of Digital Natives.* New York, NY, Basic Books, 2008.
20. Christensen CM: *The Innovator's Dilemma: When New Technologies Cause Great Firms to Fail.* Boston, MA, Harvard Business Publishing, 1997.
21. Count of Active Applications in the App Store: 148Apps.biz website. http://148apps.biz/app-store-metrics/. Accessed March 5, 2012.
22. Ellaway R, Masters K: AMEE Guide 32: E-Learning in medical education. Part 1: Learning, teaching and assessment. *Med Teach* 2008;30(5):455-473.
23. Kalet AL, Coady SH, Hopkins MA, Hochberg MS, Riles TS: Preliminary evaluation of the Web Initiative for Surgical Education (WISE-MD). *Am J Surg* 2007; 194(1):89-93.
24. Shanedling J, Van Heest A, Rodriguez M, Putnam M, Agel J: Validation of an online assessment of orthopedic surgery residents' cognitive skills and preparedness for carpal tunnel release surgery. *J Grad Med Educ* 2010;2(3): 435-441.
25. Whitson BA, Hoang CD, Jie T, Maddaus MA: Technology-enhanced interactive surgical education. *J Surg Res* 2006;136(1): 13-18.
26. Orthopaedic Knowledge Online. American Academy of Orthopaedic Surgeons (AAOS) OrthoPortal. http://orthoportal.aaos.org/oko/default.aspx#tab1. Accessed March 5, 2012.
27. WorldOrtho website. http://www.worldortho.com/dev/index.php. Accessed March 5, 2012.
28. OrthoNet website. http://www.orthonet.on.ca. Accessed March 5, 2012.
29. MedEdPORTAL website. https://www.mededportal.org/. Accessed March 5, 2012.
30. State of the Media: Mobile Media Report Q3 2011. Nielsen website. 2011. http://nielsen.com/us/en/insights/reports-downloads/2011/state-of-the-media--mobile-media-report-q3-2011.html. Accessed March 5, 2012.
31. Ruskin KJ: Mobile technologies for teaching and learning. *Int Anesthesiol Clin* 2010;48(3):53-60.
32. Holzinger A, Nischelwitzer A, Meisenberger M: Examples for mobile interactive learning objects (MILOs). *Third International Conference on Pervasive Computing and Communications Workshop.* IEEE Computer Society, Washington, DC, 2005, pp 307-311.
33. Franko OI, Bhola S: iPad apps for orthopedic surgeons. *Orthopedics* 2011;34(12):978-981.

34. Chretien K, Arora V, Saarinen C, Ferguson B, Incorporating social media into medical education. *Academic Internal Medicine Insight* 2011;9(1):12-14.

35. Tamim RM, Bernard RM, Borokhovski E, Abrami PC, Schmid RF: What forty years of research says about the impact of technology on learning: A second-order meta-analysis and validation study. *Rev Educ Res* 2011;81(1):408-448.

36. Boulos MN, Wheeler S, Tavares C, Jones R: How smartphones are changing the face of mobile and participatory healthcare: An overview, with example from eCAALYX. *Biomed Eng Online* 2011;10(1):24.

37. Chou WY, Hunt YM, Beckjord EB, Moser RP, Hesse BW: Social media use in the United States: Implications for health communication. *J Med Internet Res* 2009; 11(4):e48.

38. Orthopaedic Educators website. http://ubc.communityzero.com/?org=orthopaedic. Accessed March 5, 2012.

39. Wikipedia. Statistics. http://en.wikipedia.org/wiki/Special:Statistics. Accessed March 5, 2012.

40. AskDrWiki website. http://askdrwiki.com/mediawiki/index.php?title=Physician_ Medical_ Wiki. Accessed March 5, 2012.

41. Ganfyd website. http://www.ganfyd.org/index.php?title=Main_Page. Accessed March 5, 2012.

42. Giustini D: How Web 2.0 is changing medicine. *BMJ* 2006; 333(7582):1283-1284.

43. Clinical Cases and Images website. http://clinicalcases.org/. Accessed March 5, 2012.

44. Jarvis-Selinger S, Armstrong A, Mehta S, Campion E, Black KP: Development of a supportive online learning environment for academic orthopaedic surgeons, in Ho K, Jarvis-Selinger S, Launcher HN, Cornelio J, Scott R, eds: *Technology Enabled Knowledge Translation for eHealth*. Berlin, Germany, Springer, 2012, pp 117-132.

45. Boulos MN, Hetherington L, Wheeler S: Second life: An overview of the potential of 3-D virtual worlds in medical and health education. *Health Info Libr J* 2007;24(4):233-245.

46. George DR, Dellasega C: Use of social media in graduate-level medical humanities education: Two pilot studies from Penn State College of Medicine. *Med Teach* 2011;33(8):e429-e434.

47. Skiba DJ, Barton AJ: Adapting your teaching to accommodate the net generation of learners. *Online J Issues Nurs* 2006;11(2):5.

48. Park J, Tymitz K, Engel AM, Welling RE: Computerized rounding in a community hospital surgery residency program. *J Surg Educ* 2007;64(6):357-360.

49. Wu BJ, Dietz PA, Bordley J IV, Borgstrom DC: A novel, web-based application for assessing and enhancing practice-based learning in surgery residency. *J Surg Educ* 2009;66(1):3-7.

50. Nothnagle M, Anandarajah G, Goldman RE, Reis S: Struggling to be self-directed: Residents' paradoxical beliefs about learning. *Acad Med* 2011;86(12):1539-1544.

51. Carr N: Is Google making us stupid? *Yearb Natl Soc Study Educ* 2008;107(2):89-94.

52. Wear D: Perspective: A perfect storm. The convergence of bullet points, competencies, and screen reading in medical education. *Acad Med* 2009;84(11):1500-1504.

53. Kapralos B, Cristancho S, Porte M, Backstein D, Monclou A, Dubrowski A: Serious games in the classroom: Gauging student perceptions. *Stud Health Technol Inform* 2011;163:254-260.

54. Jain SH: Practicing medicine in the age of Facebook. *N Engl J Med* 2009;361(7):649-651.

52

The Emerging Case for Shared Decision Making in Orthopaedics

Jiwon Youm, MS
Kate E. Chenok, MBA
Jeff Belkora, PhD
Vanessa Chiu, MPH
Kevin J. Bozic, MD, MBA

Abstract

The Institute of Medicine outlined a standard for patient-centered care, which has become the centerpiece of healthcare reform in the United States. Shared decision-making interventions, which include decision and communication aids, are formal embodiments of this philosophy. Although the concept of shared decision making has been shown to be an effective tool, and its relevance to orthopaedic medicine has been well documented, it has not been widely adopted by orthopaedic surgeons. It is helpful to examine the benefits of shared decision making, along with incentives to encourage adoption and implementation of this important philosophy.

Instr Course Lect 2013;62:587-594.

The Institute of Medicine outlined a standard for patient-centered care in its seminal publication *Crossing the Quality Chasm*.[1] Patient-centered care has since been the centerpiece of US healthcare reform in shared decision-making interventions, including decision and communication aids, which are formal embodiments of this philosophy. Although the concept of shared decision making and its relevance to orthopaedics have been well documented, and despite evidence that shows shared decision-making tools to be effective, shared decision making has not been widely adopted by orthopaedic surgeons. In this chapter, the benefits of shared decision making, barriers to adoption and implementation, and potential ways to encourage adoption are outlined from multiple perspectives: the patient, the provider, and the payer-purchaser. Resources for adopting shared decision making into clinical practice are provided, and opportunities and incentives to adopt shared decision making in orthopaedics are discussed.

Total joint arthroplasty of the hip and knee can be an effective procedure for reducing pain and improving function in patients with disabling osteoarthritis of the hip or knee.[2] Because the indications for total joint arthroplasty are heavily dependent on the quality of life and expectations of the patient, it is by definition a so-called preference-sensitive procedure. As with other preference-sensitive procedures, total joint arthroplasty utilization rates vary widely throughout different geographic regions of the United States.[3] A portion of this geographic variation may be attributed to patient characteristics such as sex, ethnicity, and age.[4-7] However, variations are not explained by differences in population characteristics alone.[8-10] Decisions are also affected by the calculations of patients

Dr. Bozic or an immediate family member serves as a board member, owner, officer, or committee member of the American Academy of Orthopaedic Surgeons, the Agency for Healthcare Research and Quality, the American Association of Hip and Knee Surgeons, the American Joint Replacement Registry, the American Orthopaedic Association, the California Joint Replacement Registry Project, the California Orthopaedic Association, and the Orthopaedic Research and Education Foundation. None of the following authors nor any immediate family member has received anything of value from or owns stock in a commercial company or institution related directly or indirectly to the subject of this chapter: Mr. Youm, Ms. Chenok, Dr. Belkora, and Ms. Chiu.

with regard to the trade-off among the perceived risks and benefits, their views on potential outcomes of surgery and the severity of their disease, their willingness to undergo surgery,[11] and their opinions about the role of their physician in medical decision making.[12,13] Studies have suggested that supply-induced demand (based on the density of specialist physicians in a particular geographic area), differences in physician practice patterns, or both may have a greater effect on the decision to use total joint arthroplasty than do patient or population characteristics.[14,15]

To address geographic variation in practice patterns, multiple healthcare stakeholders have suggested that an increased emphasis on informing patients, eliciting their preferences, and involving them in the choice of therapy are important tools.[10,14] The Institute of Medicine outlined a standard for patient-centered care in *Crossing the Quality Chasm*: "Providing care that is respectful of and responsive to individual patient preferences, needs, and values, and ensuring that patient values guide all clinical decisions."[1] Shared decision-making interventions are a formal embodiment of this philosophy.

What Is Shared Decision Making?

The term shared decision making was coined in 1982 in a report from the President's Commission for the Study of Ethical Problems in Medicine and Biomedical and Behavioral Research titled *Making Health Care Decisions: The Ethical and Legal Implications of Informed Consent in the Patient-Practitioner Relationship.*[16] At the time, Wennberg et al,[17] in a study from Dartmouth, had documented a wide variation in procedure rates and were conceptually isolating warranted from unwarranted variations. Other health services researchers noted that, in some conditions, physician recommendations often varied from care that had been proven effective.[18] These researchers defined effective care as care with known outcome rates, patient agreement on the ranking of outcomes, and a rate of good outcomes far outweighing the bad ones. Conversely, in preference-sensitive conditions, outcomes are uncertain and valued differently by different patients.[19] Examples of preference-sensitive conditions include hip osteoarthritis, knee osteoarthritis, prostate cancer, early-stage breast cancer, breast reconstruction, uterine fibroids, and coronary artery disease.

Shared decision making represented a movement to appeal to healthcare consumers to become informed and involved in their healthcare decision making so that they would obtain effective care when appropriate and negotiate preference-sensitive recommendations. By 1997, Charles et al[20] had expanded the concept of shared decision making to include active participation by all parties, the sharing of information about values as well as facts, and agreement on a course of action to be implemented.

The current model of shared decision making involves conversation between patients and physicians (or other providers) about the patients' options, needs, preferences, values, and possible outcomes. Frequently, but not exclusively, shared decision making can be facilitated by patient decision and communication aids. Decision aids are tools (print, video, or web-based resources) to inform patients about their choices and lead patients through critical reflection that will help them articulate their values and preferences. Decision aids are associated with increased patient knowledge and reduced decisional conflict or patient uncertainty about which choice best meets their needs.[21] Many groups have contributed to the development of decision aids, including the International Patient Decision Aid Standards Collaboration, Healthwise, Health Dialog, and the Informed Medical Decisions Foundation (**Table 1**). Tools developed for patients with hip and knee osteoarthritis include video testimony from patients with hip and knee osteoarthritis who have chosen and used different treatment options.[12]

Communication aids include question lists and consultation audio recordings and summaries. Question lists are associated with increased question asking,[22] whereas audio recordings and summaries are associated with increased information recall.[23] Often, a health coach will assist a patient in using communication aids, such as when a coach helps a patient develop a list of relevant questions and concerns to discuss with his or her physician and ensures that the patient can record visits and obtain after-visit summaries.[5,24,25] This approach has been used with breast cancer patients and has been tested in patients with hip and knee osteoarthritis.[12]

What Is the Evidence for Shared Decision Making?

Evidence has shown that shared decision-making tools, such as decision and communication aids, are effective in informing and involving patients in their treatment decisions, especially for preference-sensitive treatments such as total joint arthroplasty. Generally, informed and involved patients have better psychosocial and, in some cases, physical outcomes.[26]

The most comprehensive source of evidence for decision aids can be found in a Cochrane Review published in 2011.[21] This systematic review of 86 studies published through 2009

Table 1
Resources for Adoption of Shared Decision Making Into Clinical Practice

Organization	Resource Offered	Website Address
Informed Medical Decisions Foundation	Online video and print decision aids for a variety of conditions, including several related to orthopaedics (example, torn meniscus, early osteoarthritis, herniated disk, acute low back pain, chronic low back pain, knee osteoarthritis, hip osteoarthritis, spinal stenosis, and osteoporosis).	www.informedmedicaldecisions.org/
Health Dialog	Works with the Informed Medical Decisions Foundation to produce and distribute decision aids and has additional programs that incorporate health coaching.	www.healthdialog.com
CareCoach	Online and smartphone communication aids, which include audio recordings from real clinical encounters for different conditions; the ability to make a list of questions online and transfer them to a smartphone via apps; and the ability to record consultations using smartphone apps and store and share the recordings in an online "audio health record."	www.carecoach.com
National Health Service	Standardized online decision aid with a form that allows the user to print a summary to give to the provider.	www.nhsdirect.nhs.uk/DecisionAids/.aspx
Agency for Healthcare Research and Quality	Print and electronic resources for clinicians and patients, which includes an online interface for building and printing a list of questions for an upcoming visit.[a]	www.effectivehealthcare.ahrq.gov/index.cfm/tools-and-resources/patient-decision-aids/ for "Patient Decision Aids" and www.ahrq.gov/questions/ for "Questions Are the Answer"
Healthwise	Online decision aids for a wide variety of conditions, including those related to orthopaedics.	www.healthwise.org
Ottawa Hospital Research Institute	Links to freely available web-based decision aids and other commercially available decision aids for specific conditions.	http://decisionaid.ohri.ca/
Dartmouth-Hitchcock Center for Shared Decision Making	Guidelines on how to integrate decision aids and decision support into practice and training modules for decision support as a clinical skill.	www.med.dartmouth-hitchcock.org/csdm_toolkits.html
International Patient Decision Aid Standards Collaboration	Checklist for evaluating the quality of decision aids.	http://ipdas.ohri.ca/

[a]Decision aid only available for prostate cancer as of May 1, 2012.

provides substantial deployment of and evidence for the benefits provided by decision aids.

The Informed Medical Decisions Foundation and Health Dialog have implemented shared decision making for patients with hip and knee arthritis at a growing number of surgeon offices, health plans, and hospitals. One system-wide implementation has been at Group Health Cooperative in Seattle, where shared decision-making tools were implemented across 12 specialties, including orthopaedics. Study results have not yet been published, but the system has reported increased physician and patient satisfaction with decision quality.

What Are the Potential Benefits of Shared Decision Making?

Patient Perspective

The use of decision and communication aids increases patient knowledge and understanding of treatment options, risks, and benefits; creates more accurate expectations; increases active participation in decision making;[27] and reduces decisional conflict related to feeling uninformed.[21] The use of these aids also results in improvement in the match between patient values and subsequent treatment decisions,[14] higher patient satisfaction, and more informed decision making. Decision and communication aids may also reduce the overuse of certain elective surgical procedures (for example, those for a herniated disk) without apparent adverse effects on health outcomes.[28] They may also reduce disparities in access to care among ethnic groups.[29,30]

Provider Perspective

Time is one of the most valued commodities in modern medicine. Increasing clinical and administrative demands have resulted in decreased provider satisfaction.[31,32] The aforementioned Cochrane Review included nine studies that evaluated the effects of decision aids on consultation time (an 8-minute decrease to a 23-minute increase). However, results were not pooled, given the heterogeneity of the clinical setting (for example, atrial fibrillation, breast cancer genetic testing, and prostate cancer screening), the variability in the method used to record length of time, and the variability in distributing decision aids (before consultation or at the time of consultation). Perhaps most importantly, none of the nine aforementioned studies evaluated the effect of shared decision making on the length of a visit in orthopaedic practices. Thus, it remains unclear what effect shared decision-making tools will have on the length of an orthopaedic office visit.

There are many reasons why shared decision making could save time if decision aids are distributed before the appointment.[33] Patients may come with evidence-based information, not misconceptions (which often require time to clarify) that they picked up from the Internet and other sources.[34] A more informed patient may ask better questions that could also produce higher provider satisfaction.[24]

One recurring frustration for surgeons who treat patients with advanced arthritis of the hip or knee may be the amount of time spent discussing surgical techniques, implant options, and perioperative care protocols with patients who then opt for nonsurgical treatment. A major reason for this may be that physicians are not skilled at predicting patient preferences.[3] With decision aids, patients may advance in their stage of decision making before the office visit. Depending on the patient's preference toward surgical or nonsurgical treatment options, the orthopaedic surgeon can spend more time discussing the option already preferred by the patient. This may not necessarily reduce the length of the visit but would likely improve satisfaction for both patients and providers.

As the US population continues to age, demand for total joint arthroplasties is expected to increase. By 2030, the demand for total knee replacements in the United States is projected to increase by 673% to 3.48 million procedures.[35] This enormous increase in the number of patients with hip and knee arthritis will necessitate more efficient approaches to assessing patient preferences for managing these disabling conditions.

Shared decision-making tools can also decrease the risk of medical malpractice claims. Physicians who incorporate shared decision making are less likely to be sued for adverse outcomes because patients who participate in shared decision-making programs are more satisfied than those who do not.[36] Patients who are more satisfied with their treatment choices are less likely to pursue legal action in cases with adverse outcomes.[37]

Payer-Purchaser Perspective

Healthcare purchasers and health plans are also interested in using shared decision making. Costs for musculoskeletal care are one of the largest and most rapidly increasing components of medical costs.[38] Because patients themselves are increasingly responsible for sharing in the costs of their care, it is vital that patients be engaged in their treatment decisions and choose care that aligns with their preferences. Shared decision making results in higher-quality decisions, which may be associated with more appropriate and patient-centered use of surgical interventions.[11] Reduction in the overuse of elective surgery may be cost saving.[39,40] More importantly, as shared decision making reduces decisional conflict and time to treatment, patients may return to work earlier and be more productive.

Purchasers and health plans already offer a range of health education, second opinion, and wellness tools to their employees and members. Although many of these materials and services include the same evidence presented by shared decision-making tools, such as those developed by Health Dialog,[41] the information shared by the purchaser and payer cannot substitute for true shared decision making between the patient and his or her physician. Interviews with purchasers confirm the perceived importance of shared decision making and recognition that the tools they are providing are intended to be used by patients and their physicians. At the same time, purchasers believe that shared decision making is a vital component of high-quality care. Quality and process measures in use for patient-centered medical homes already include patient engagement measures, and it should be expected that measures for specialty care, such as those that will be used to evaluate accountable care organizations, may include similar measures.

What Are the Obstacles to Adopting and Implementing Shared Decision Making?

Patient Perspective

Patients often lack familiarity and experience with evaluating and expressing their values and preferences in conversations with physicians. In fact, more studies have shown that consumers have positive attitudes toward shared decision making rather than negative or passive attitudes; however, other studies have found lower rather than higher engagement in shared decision-making behavior.[42] Information overload may be a considerable barrier for patients whose health literacy is low. Decision-support intervention tools that are tailored to a patient's level of education may help to eliminate this barrier.

Provider Perspective

The initial barrier for most healthcare providers is limited familiarity with the concept of shared decision making and available tools.[43] Many providers also perceive that shared decision making creates an additional workflow burden and increases costs.

The greatest obstacle may be the fee-for-service payment system, which creates disincentives for physicians to spend substantial time emphasizing the potential benefits of nonsurgical treatment. If patients who use decision and communication aids are less likely to choose surgery,[21] physician concern about decreased procedure volumes and the resultant decrease in compensation is logical, expected, and understandable. Furthermore, physicians are not currently reimbursed for the additional time spent discussing treatment options.[44]

Health plans and purchasers are enthusiastic about the concept of patient engagement and providing information to patients on treatment alternatives for specific conditions that is culturally appropriate and tailored to the patient's literacy level. However, because approaches are frequently through third-party providers (such as Healthwise and Health Dialog), surgeons may not be aware of or prepared to take advantage of the patient's preparation through the use of these tools. Patients may be mistrustful of information regarding treatment options that is provided by their health plan or employer rather than their physician.

Collectively, these challenges necessitate the development of specialized systems and processes for widespread incorporation of shared decision-making tools into clinical practice.

Potential Ways to Encourage the Adoption of Shared Decision Making

Patient Perspective

To encourage the active participation of patients in shared decision making, they must first be educated in the benefits of actively engaging in their care, which can allow increased control over their health and treatment options. To facilitate engagement, access to decision and communication aids must be improved. Currently, decision and communication aids may be directly available to patients through their health plan (for example, Group Health Cooperative), or indirectly through a third party (for example, Health Dialog). The Agency for Healthcare Research and Quality Innovations Exchange also summarizes available decision aids and makes some of their own decision aids available. The Dartmouth-Hitchcock Medical Center has a library of decision aids available for its patients. However, patients outside these networks do not have ready access to decision and communication aids. Financial incentives must be created for patients. Payers and purchasers can incentivize patients through novel benefit designs (for example, a lower co-pay when engaging in shared decision making). Further research is needed to determine the role of providing culturally sensitive material and a level of detail appropriate for different levels of health literacy.

Provider Perspective

Despite several decades of research into the benefits of shared decision making, provider familiarity with shared decision making remains low.[7] This lack of familiarity likely stems from the absence of formal education in shared decision making during medical training. Thus, training in shared decision making should be incorporated into the medical school and postgraduate medical education curricula. For physicians who have completed their training, the range of tools in use by third parties should be widely publicized, patient decision aids should be made readily available, and physicians should be trained to take advantage of these tools.[45] Available resources and their web addresses are listed in **Table 1**. Shared decision-making training could be included as part of licensure or certification. Practice models must also be developed to facilitate implementation;[43] of note, shared decision making is currently being used at several demonstration sites for certain conditions.[46] It is likely that higher levels of evidence will be necessary to convince physicians who remain skeptical of the benefits of shared decision making.

Perhaps most importantly, both financial and medicolegal incentives must be created to facilitate widespread adoption of shared decision making. Financial incentives are especially important, given the concern of some primary providers that the adoption of shared decision-making tools may decrease the number of surgical procedures and provider compensation.

In general, practical protocols and incentives at the system level will be necessary to facilitate the widespread adoption of shared decision-making tools.

Opportunities for Orthopaedic Practices

Several federal and state mandates have been enacted to create both financial and medicolegal incentives for adopting shared decision making. The Patient Protection and Affordable Care Act (PPACA) of 2010 includes several demonstration projects that would provide additional reimbursement to clinicians who incorporate shared decision-making approaches into their practices. This could offset some of the costs associated with implementation and stimulate adoption of shared decision-making tools into clinical practices, especially if studies can demonstrate value in terms of improved patient satisfaction and more efficient use of resources. Sections 3506 and

3013 of PPACA specify funding for development, testing, and promotion of decision aids and for the development of quality measures that address patient-centered care and shared decision making. The PPACA established the Patient-Centered Outcomes Research Institute to focus on patient-reported outcomes measures, including shared decision making.

As the fundamental model of provider reimbursement shifts from fee-for-service to value-based payment, shared decision making will play a major role. For example, Medicare reimbursement will increasingly be tied to shared decision making.[47] The Hospital Value-Based Purchasing program, a provision of the PPACA that is funded by a 1% (and eventually 2%) withholding from participating hospitals' diagnosis-related group payments, will pay for better care based on clinical outcomes and patient experience. The latter is measured by the Hospital Consumer Assessment of Healthcare Providers and Systems hospital survey, which includes questions regarding provider assessment of patient preferences and values in medical decision making.

In the private sector as well as with Medicare, the move to new payment models (for example, bundled payments, accountable care organizations, and patient-centered medical homes) will eventually require orthopaedic surgeons to build shared decision making and other features of patient-focused care into their clinical workflow. In the final accountable care organizations ruling, patient engagement is one of the patient-centeredness criteria proposed by the Centers for Medicare and Medicaid Services.[48] According to that ruling, measures to promote patient engagement "may include, but are not limited to, the use of decision support tools and shared decision-making methods with which the patient can assess the merits of various treatment options in the context of his or her values and convictions." Patient activation increases adherence and improves outcomes.[49]

A parallel set of initiatives to improve informed consent is under way and will also encourage the use of shared decision making. Washington State passed legislation (Senate Bill 5930) in 2007 that provides for reduced professional liability for doctors who use shared decision-making interventions as part of an informed consent process. If a patient signs a written acknowledgment that he or she participated in shared decision making with the use of certified decision aids, the burden for establishing a legal claim against the physician for tort violation of informed consent changes from "a preponderance of evidence" to "clear and convincing evidence." A patient is also asked to identify the name of the decision aid and agree that questions were answered to his or her satisfaction. In effect, this legislation provides substantial legal protection to physicians and is an incentive to provide patients with certified decision aids proven to be effective in informing patients.

This is a critical time for orthopaedic surgeons to take a leading role in promoting shared decision making. A combination of legislative mandates, the creation of financial and medicolegal incentives for using shared decision making (and penalties for not using it), and growing interest among purchasers, health plans, and patients all create a time that is appropriate for action.

References

1. Institute of Medicine: *Crossing the Quality Chasm: A New Health System for the 21st Century*. Washington, DC, National Academies of Sciences; 2001.
2. Cushnaghan J, Bennett J, Reading I, et al: Long-term outcome following total knee arthroplasty: A controlled longitudinal study. *Ann Rheum Dis* 2009;68(5):642-647.
3. Fischer GS, Tulsky JA, Rose MR, Siminoff LA, Arnold RM: Patient knowledge and physician predictions of treatment preferences after discussion of advance directives. *J Gen Intern Med* 1998; 13(7):447-454.
4. Farley FA, Weinstein SL: The case for patient-centered care in orthopaedics. *J Am Acad Orthop Surg* 2006;14(8):447-451.
5. Leahy M: Viewing care through the eyes of patients and their families. *AAOS Now* 2010;4(10):16. http://www.aaos.org/news/aaosnow/oct10/clinical5.asp. Accessed November 9, 2012.
6. Weinstein JN: Partnership: Doctor and patient. Advocacy for informed choice vs. informed consent. *Spine (Phila Pa 1976)* 2005; 30(3):269-272.
7. Braddock C III, Hudak PL, Feldman JJ, Bereknyei S, Frankel RM, Levinson W: Surgery is certainly one good option: Quality and time-efficiency of informed decision-making in surgery. *J Bone Joint Surg Am* 2008;90(9):1830-1838.
8. Karlson EW, Daltroy LH, Liang MH, Eaton HE, Katz JN: Gender differences in patient preferences may underlie differential utilization of elective surgery. *Am J Med* 1997;102(6):524-530.
9. Byrne MM, Souchek J, Richardson M, Suarez-Almazor M: Racial/ethnic differences in preferences for total knee replacement surgery. *J Clin Epidemiol* 2006; 59(10):1078-1086.
10. Hudak PL, Clark JP, Hawker GA, et al: "You're perfect for the procedure! Why don't you want it?" Elderly arthritis patients' unwillingness to consider total joint arthroplasty surgery: A qualitative

study. *Med Decis Making* 2002; 22(3):272-278.

11. Weinstein JN, Clay K, Morgan TS: Informed patient choice: Patient-centered valuing of surgical risks and benefits. *Health Aff (Millwood)* 2007;26(3):726-730.
12. Bozic KJ, Chiu V: Emerging ideas: Shared decision making in patients with osteoarthritis of the hip and knee. *Clin Orthop Relat Res* 2011;469(7):2081-2085.
13. Katz JN, Wright EA, Guadagnoli E, Liang MH, Karlson EW, Cleary PD: Differences between men and women undergoing major orthopedic surgery for degenerative arthritis. *Arthritis Rheum* 1994;37(5):687-694.
14. Lurie JD, Weinstein JN: Shared decision-making and the orthopaedic workforce. *Clin Orthop Relat Res* 2001;385:68-75.
15. Ballantyne PJ, Gignac MA, Hawker GA: A patient-centered perspective on surgery avoidance for hip or knee arthritis: Lessons for the future. *Arthritis Rheum* 2007;57(1):27-34.
16. President's Commission for the Study of Ethical Problems in Medicine and Biomedical and Behavioral Research: *Making Health Care Decisions: The Ethical and Legal Implications of Informed Consent in the Patient-Practitioner Relationship*. Washington, DC, US Government Printing Office, 1982.
17. Wennberg JE, Barnes BA, Zubkoff M: Professional uncertainty and the problem of supplier-induced demand. *Soc Sci Med* 1982;16(7):811-824.
18. Center for the Evaluative Clinical Sciences: *A Dartmouth Atlas Project Topic Brief: Effective Care*. Lebanon, NH, Center for the Evaluative Clinical Sciences, 2007. http://www.dartmouthatlas.org/downloads/reports/effective_care.pdf. Accessed March 15, 2012.
19. Wennberg JE: *Tracking Medicine: A Researcher's Quest to Understand Health Care*. New York, NY, Oxford University Press, 2010.
20. Charles C, Gafni A, Whelan T: Shared decision-making in the medical encounter: What does it mean? (or it takes at least two to tango). *Soc Sci Med* 1997;44(5): 681-692.
21. Stacey D, Bennett CL, Barry MJ, et al: Decision aids for people facing health treatment or screening decisions. *Cochrane Database Syst Rev* 2011;10:CD001431.
22. Kinnersley P, Edwards A, Hood K, et al: Interventions before consultations for helping patients address their information needs. *Cochrane Database Syst Rev* 2007; 3:CD004565.
23. Pitkethly M, Macgillivray S, Ryan R: Recordings or summaries of consultations for people with cancer. *Cochrane Database Syst Rev* 2008;3:CD001539.
24. Belkora JK, Loth MK, Chen DF, Chen JY, Volz S, Esserman LJ: Monitoring the implementation of consultation planning, recording, and summarizing in a breast care center. *Patient Educ Couns* 2008;73(3):536-543.
25. Belkora JK, Teng A, Volz S, Loth MK, Esserman LJ: Expanding the reach of decision and communication aids in a breast care center: A quality improvement study. *Patient Educ Couns* 2011;83(2): 234-239.
26. Griffin SJ, Kinmonth AL, Veltman MW, Gillard S, Grant J, Stewart M: Effect on health-related outcomes of interventions to alter the interaction between patients and practitioners: A systematic review of trials. *Ann Fam Med* 2004;2(6):595-608.
27. Dartmouth-Hitchcock Medical Center: Patient resources: Center for Shared Decision Making. http://www.dhmc.org/shared_decision_making.cfm. Accessed November 9, 2012.
28. Deyo RA, Cherkin DC, Weinstein J, Howe J, Ciol M, Mulley AG Jr: Involving patients in clinical decisions: Impact of an interactive video program on use of back surgery. *Med Care* 2000; 38(9):959-969.
29. King JS, Eckman MH, Moulton BW: The potential of shared decision making to reduce health disparities. *J Law Med Ethics* 2011; 39(suppl 1):30-33.
30. Abellán Perpiñán JM, Sánchez Martínez FI, Martínez Pérez JE: How should patients' utilities be incorporated into clinical decisions? 2008 SESPAS Report. *Gac Sanit* 2008;22(suppl 1):179-185.
31. Dugdale DC, Epstein R, Pantilat SZ: Time and the patient-physician relationship. *J Gen Intern Med* 1999;14(suppl 1):S34-S40.
32. Saleh KJ, Quick JC, Sime WE, Novicoff WM, Einhorn TA: Recognizing and preventing burnout among orthopaedic leaders. *Clin Orthop Relat Res* 2009;467(2): 558-565.
33. Llewellyn-Thomas HA, Weinstein J, Mimnaugh D: Patients' decision aids for elective total joint replacement: A national survey to identify orthopaedic surgeons' preferences. *Med Decis Making* 2003; 23:551.
34. Bozic KJ, Smith AR, Hariri S, et al: The impact of direct-to-consumer advertising in orthopaedics. *Clin Orthop Relat Res* 2007; 458:202-219.
35. Kurtz S, Ong K, Lau E, Mowat F, Halpern M: Projections of primary and revision hip and knee arthroplasty in the United States from 2005 to 2030. *J Bone Joint Surg Am* 2007;89(4):780-785.
36. Frosch DL, Légaré F, Mangione CM: Using decision aids in

community-based primary care: A theory-driven evaluation with ethnically diverse patients. *Patient Educ Couns* 2008;73(3):490-496.

37. Fowler FJ Jr: Shared decision making and medical costs. Informed Medical Decisions Foundation. [updated September 2012]. http://informedmedicaldecisions.org/wp-content/uploads/2010/10/Perspectives_SDM-Cost_v2.pdf. Accessed November 9, 2012.
38. Haralson RH III, Zuckerman JD: Prevalence, health care expenditures, and orthopedic surgery workforce for musculoskeletal conditions. *JAMA* 2009;302(14):1586-1587.
39. Stacey D, Bennett C, Saarimamki A: *Shared Decision-Making in Health Care: Achieving Evidence-Based Patient Choice*, ed 2. New York, NY, Oxford University Press, 2009, pp 201-208.
40. Hawker GA, Wright JG, Coyte PC, et al: Determining the need for hip and knee arthroplasty: The role of clinical severity and patients' preferences. *Med Care* 2001;39(3):206-216.
41. The best medical decisions are those made together between doctor and patient. Health Dialog website. http://www.healthdialog.com/Main/Solutions/PopulationHealthSolutions/DECISIONDialog. Accessed November 9, 2012.
42. Williams N, Fleming C: *Issue Brief: Consumer and Provider Perspectives on Shared Decision Making: A Systematic Review of the Peer-Reviewed Literature*. Princeton, NJ, Mathematica, 2011.
43. Moulton B, King JS: Aligning ethics with medical decision-making: The quest for informed patient choice. *J Law Med Ethics* 2010;38(1):85-97.
44. Wennberg JE, Brownle S, Fisher ES, Skinner JS, Weinstein JN: Opportunities for the Congress and the Obama Administration. A Dartmouth Atlas White Paper. Lebanon, NH, The Dartmouth Institute for Health Policy & Clinical Practice, 2008. http://www.dartmouthatlas.org/downloads/reports/agenda_for_change.pdf. Accessed November 9, 2012.
45. Légaré F, Ratté S, Gravel K, Graham ID: Barriers and facilitators to implementing shared decision-making in clinical practice: Update of a systematic review of health professionals' perceptions. *Patient Educ Couns* 2008;73(3):526-535.
46. Frosch DL, Moulton BW, Wexler RM, Holmes-Rovner M, Volk RJ, Levin CA: Shared decision making in the United States: Policy and implementation activity on multiple fronts. *Z Evid Fortbild Qual Gesundhwes* 2011;105(4):305-312.
47. Wennberg JE, O'Connor AM, Collins ED, Weinstein JN: Extending the P4P agenda, part 1: How Medicare can improve patient decision making and reduce unnecessary care. *Health Aff (Millwood)* 2007;26(6):1564-1574.
48. Centers for Medicare and Medicaid Services: Shared Savings Program: Accountable Care Organizations. Updated May 29, 2012. https://www.cms.gov/Medicare/Medicare-Fee-for-Service-Payment/sharedsavingsprogram/index.html?redirect=/sharedsavingsprogram. Accessed May 5, 2012.
49. Skolasky RL, Mackenzie EJ, Wegener ST, Riley LH III: Patient activation and adherence to physical therapy in persons undergoing spine surgery. *Spine (Phila Pa 1976)* 2008;33(21):E784-E791.

53

Surviving and Winning a Professional Negligence Lawsuit

Douglas W. Lundy, MD, FACS
David D. Teuscher, MD

Abstract

Being served with a medical negligence lawsuit usually is a traumatic event for an orthopaedic surgeon. The course of litigation is long and tedious, and the defendant physician must be well prepared for the experience. It is imperative that the physician contact his or her insurance carrier immediately after being served with the complaint because many legal actions are time dependent. The insurance company will assign an attorney to defend the physician, and an effective team will be needed to mount a powerful defense. The defendant physician's deposition is among the most important aspects of the entire process. Extensive preparation for the deposition will strengthen the defense; but the physician must remember that the lawsuit will not be won during the deposition. Because the testimony of expert witnesses often decides the outcome of the case, it is important for the physician to help the attorney identify the best potential witnesses. A thorough knowledge of the tactics that the plaintiff's attorney may use during cross-examination can help ensure that the truth is clearly portrayed. The American Academy of Orthopaedic Surgeons Professional Compliance Program is designed to ensure that all testimony in medical liability cases is fair and factual.

Instr Course Lect 2013;62:595-601.

For most orthopaedic surgeons, a medical negligence lawsuit is among the worst experiences of their professional lives. Most physicians who have never been served with a lawsuit cannot comprehend the impact of learning that a patient is so angry and dissatisfied as to seek legal remediation. It is imperative that a physician in general and an orthopaedic surgeon in particular consider the probability of being sued during the course of their careers and prepare for the emotional impact. The initial reaction is likely to be an unpleasant visceral reaction as the sympathetic nervous system takes control of the body, leading to tachycardia, tachypnea, and xerostomia. The physician's mind might race on reading the negative, personally hurtful descriptions constructed by the patient's attorney. In addition to criticism of the patient's treatment, the physician is often portrayed as a careless monster with no compassion. At this moment, it is necessary to take a deep breath and remember that the document represents the plaintiff's best attempt to justify the lawsuit, every unfounded accusation can be rebutted, and the physician's professional reputation can be restored.

The Legal Process

The conduct of the legal system is foreign to most orthopaedic surgeons. Time is of the essence. Denial, in which the physician ignores the initial documents and hopes that the entire ordeal will disappear, is one of the worst reactions to being served with a lawsuit. It is imperative that the physician immediately contact his or her professional liability insurance carrier, preferably on the day that the lawsuit is served. A calm response can be expected because such lawsuits are an everyday occurrence for insurance com-

Dr. Lundy or an immediate family member serves as a board member, owner, officer, or committee member of the American Academy of Orthopaedic Surgeons, the American College of Surgeons, the Georgia Orthopaedic Society, and the Orthopaedic Trauma Association; is a member of a speakers' bureau or has made paid presentations on behalf of AO and Synthes; serves as an unpaid consultant to Synthes; and owns stock or stock options in Livengood Engineering. Dr. Teuscher or an immediate family member serves as a board member, owner, officer, or committee member of the American Academy of Orthopaedic Surgeons, the American Medical Association, the American Orthopaedic Foot and Ankle Society, the American Orthopaedic Society for Sports Medicine, TEXPAC, TMA, TOA, TPH, and WOA.

panies. Compare the situation to, for example, a fractured tibia, which represents a unique, catastrophic injury to the patient but is routine to an orthopaedic surgeon.

The complaint documents and the actions required are time sensitive. The insurance carrier should be provided with a copy of the complaint as soon as possible.[1] A delay in notifying advocates can negatively affect the physician's defense. The insurance provider will know the best medical liability defense attorneys in the area. The physician may inquire about specific attorneys but should carefully listen to the advice of his or her insurance representative. An experienced, focused, and effective team will be needed to help navigate the uncharted waters ahead.

One of the early advantages of the defense team is the right to immediately depose the plaintiff. If the physician's attorney believes the plaintiff and the plaintiff's attorney have not adequately prepared the case, including all of the elements critical to legally proving negligence, the physician's legal team may gain an early resolution of the case. However, some defense attorneys may prefer to delay the deposition until the facts are revealed because there may be only one opportunity to depose the plaintiff, and later discovery could strengthen the plaintiff's case at trial.[2]

It is important to understand the motives of the plaintiff's attorney. The attorney may consider the lawsuit to be an investment that will yield a substantial monetary sum relative to the required work and resources. In most lawsuits, the plaintiff does not pay the attorney unless the case is resolved in the plaintiff's favor. The plaintiff's attorney typically must fund the entire cost of pursuing the case. Attorneys decline many cases because the likelihood of prevailing at trial or the probable monetary damage award is insufficient to justify their investment. A more desirable case is one that is likely to settle before trial or has sensational details that may sway a jury to provide a large damage award with a minimal investment of resources.

As the lawsuit progresses, periods of frenzied activity are followed by long periods of relative inactivity. It is easy to become discouraged, but the defendant physician must pace himself or herself for a marathon ordeal. Maintaining a good attitude is critical to coping with the stress of the lawsuit. In some instances, the physician should lighten his or her clinical schedule for the purpose of spending time with family, who will be affected by the situation more than may be realized. With the attorney's permission and guidance, it is also wise to spend time with a faith leader, a close friend, or a trusted colleague.

Any statement made by the defendant physician can be admitted as evidence during the trial. Even a careless comment overheard by a staff member or another physician can be used against the defendant. Although it is important to receive emotional support from friends and family, the plaintiff and the specifics of the case should not be discussed. The physician-patient relationship is permanently severed when the physician is served with the lawsuit. Although a plaintiff may occasionally prefer to continue treatment with the defendant physician, the care of this patient should be transferred to another physician.

The stress of a lawsuit will often elicit specific reactions. Other patients may come to be regarded as potential litigants, and this negative reaction may change the verbal and nonverbal cues given to patients. The physician may start to practice defensive medicine in an attempt to avoid another lawsuit. This predictable, understandable response can increase the cost of providing health care and is one of the cited reasons why liability reform is integral to successful healthcare reform.[3]

Liability Insurance Survey

The American Academy of Orthopaedic Surgeons (AAOS) Professional Liability Insurance Survey Summary Report[4] is derived from a survey periodically sent to randomly selected AAOS fellows for the purpose of assessing current developments in medical liability. The 2011 survey was completed by 684 fellows and attained statistical significance. The respondents reported having been sued an average of 3.17 times during their careers. Because the respondents represented a cross section of orthopaedic surgeons at different stages of their professional lives, the average number of lawsuits over an entire career could not be calculated. However, an orthopaedic surgeon who becomes a defendant for the first time should be aware that many colleagues have undergone the same challenging experience.

The cases reported by the respondents most frequently were either dismissed or dropped; settlement was the third most frequent disposition. The orthopaedic surgeon was victorious in 92% of the cases that proceeded to trial. Seventy-six percent of the respondents reported that the threat of litigation to some extent affected their daily practice of orthopaedic surgery.

The Role of the Defense Attorney

The defense attorney is usually hired by the professional liability insurance company. It is important to recognize that although the attorney will represent the physician before the court, the attorney's responsibility to the insurance carrier is to minimize the payout. This inherent conflict of interest is likely to have nominal or nonexistent consequences because the goals of the defendant physician and the insurance carrier are usually the same.[5] Effective communication between the two parties and an understanding of state laws regarding settlement authority are important to ensure goodwill and a united front. Sometimes, however, one party prefers to settle the case, but the other party prefers a jury trial. In such instances, the defendant physician occasionally must retain an attorney at his or her own expense.

The attorney will expect the defendant physician to educate the legal team about the case and to honestly assess the quality of the care provided. The attorney will greatly benefit from the physician's thorough review of the medical literature, regardless of whether it supports the defendant's position. The physician can improve his or her chances of success in the case by taking an active, leading role in researching the literature. The plaintiff's attorney will be conducting the same type of research. It is critical that the defendant and the defense attorney have a trusting, collaborative relationship. The plaintiff's attorney and the jury may notice if the defendant physician does not listen to or respect his or her attorney. If necessary, the physician can request the insurance carrier to assign a different attorney.[2]

The defense attorney will rely on the defendant to identify experts who may be able to provide testimony to defend the care provided by the physician. The opinions of expert witnesses usually are important in determining the outcome of a case.[6] An orthopaedic surgeon who has written a definitive article on a relevant topic may be asked by both sides to appear as an expert witness. An experienced medical liability defense attorney will be able to identify successful expert witnesses based on the expert's reputation and experience. An excellent expert witness is able to testify without being distracted by cross-examination. However, the effectiveness of an expert witness sometimes is hindered if the expert has a reputation as a so-called hired gun. An expert from a distant city may be perceived as tailoring his or her testimony to suit the party being represented. On the other hand, the testimony of a local expert may be perceived as affected by a personal and professional relationship with the defendant physician. The 2011 AAOS Professional Liability Insurance Survey reported that the plaintiff's primary expert witness was from another state nearly twice as often as the defendant's primary expert witness (63.9% versus 38.7%, respectively).[4]

Medical Literature Review

The actual medical record is the most important body of information. A jury will expect the defendant physician to be well versed in the details of the medical record. The defendant also should be extremely knowledgeable about the medical literature related to the case. The defense attorney should be informed of any studies that tend to disagree with the treatment provided by the defendant physician. The defense team will need time to determine the best response if the plaintiff's attorney refers to those studies.[6,7]

The plaintiff's attorney will ask the defendant whether the literature was searched in preparing for the trial and what was found. The defendant physician and his or her attorney should discuss the answers to this line of questioning. The selection of expert witnesses can have a profound effect if the medical literature is adverse to the defendant physician. The defendant and his or her attorney should fully communicate before the court-imposed discovery deadline for naming expert witnesses. The defense attorney must have as much time as possible to locate expert witnesses who can support the care given to the patient.

Interrogatories

Interrogatories are a series of questions that each side sends to the other side. When first reading the interrogatories, the defendant may feel overwhelmed or angry. As is typical in liability lawsuits, the opposing attorney is provocatively seeking answers that can be exploited during the subsequent discovery and court proceedings. The defense attorney will limit the extent of answers or even object to specific questions.[1] The defendant physician should thoroughly review the case, the records, and the literature before assisting his or her attorney in completing the interrogatories.

The physician's attorney will provide advice concerning how much information is to be disclosed in the interrogatories. A good rule of thumb is to answer the plaintiff's attorney truthfully and succinctly, without elaboration. Physicians are used to being educators, but a well-intended explanation to an interrogatory or during the deposition or trial can inadvertently open a line of questioning that the plaintiff's attorney had not previously considered.

The defense attorney will send an equally exhaustive list of interrogatories to the plaintiff. The diversity of the questions may be surprising. The answers to the interrogatories will provide a starting point for the physician's attorney to question the plaintiff during the deposition. The defendant physician may be called on to assist his or her attorney in formulating questions for the plaintiff.

The curriculum vitae of the defendant physician will be carefully reviewed by the plaintiff's attorney. The document must be complete and accurate because any inconsistencies or gaps in the physician's training or practice will be probed. The plaintiff's attorney will request copies of any presentations given by the physician and will review any published material on subjects related to the case. The plaintiff's attorney will exploit the possibility of using the defendant's published words against him or her.[7,8]

The Deposition

The deposition is one of the most important events for the defendant physician. Like testimony at a trial, the deposition should be considered the equivalent of an extremely important oral board examination. Failure to prepare for the deposition or a poor deposition performance will badly damage the physician's defense. The importance of effective preparation cannot be overemphasized. The physician's attorney will help with preparation for the deposition, which should include a review of the entire medical record to avoid being "ambushed" by a fact recorded on the medical chart.[5]

Many physicians try to win the case during the deposition. It is reasoned that the patient's attorney will give up after hearing the truth about the care the patient received. This is not the correct way to approach the deposition. It should be concluded that the patient's attorney is convinced of the validity of the case. The defendant physician should be prepared to answer the deposition questions truthfully and succinctly.

It is highly advisable for the defendant physician and his or her attorney to review the physician's testimony before the deposition. Testimony should never appear to be rehearsed, but the attorney can offer advice on effectively and truthfully answering questions without harming the defendant's case.

The plaintiff's attorney commonly videotapes the defendant physician's deposition for review during trial preparation or plays selected portions during the trial. Videotaping also may be used as a means of intimidation. It is imperative for the defendant physician to be completely focused during the deposition; therefore, the location of the deposition can be important. The office of the defense attorney may be preferable to the physician's own office because it may offer fewer distractions.

The deposition is the dress rehearsal for the trial. The plaintiff's attorney is judging if the defendant physician is an effective witness and will be liked and respected by the jury. Because the deposition may be videotaped, the physician's dress, grooming, and humble professional demeanor are important to demonstrate expertise and gain empathy for the defendant physician.

There is disagreement regarding whether the defendant physician should attend the depositions of the plaintiff and the expert witnesses. The defendant physician's presence may unnerve the plaintiff and affect the deposition to the physician's benefit, but it also may anger the plaintiff or eventually increase a jury's sympathy for the plaintiff. The defense attorney may recommend that the physician not attend the plaintiff's deposition. It is extremely difficult to maintain silence and a professional demeanor while listening to several hours of testimony condemning one's character, judgement, and the treatment provided.

The defendant physician may be asked by his or her attorney to attend the depositions of the plaintiff's expert witnesses, with the hope that possible lines of cross-examination questioning will be detected. Many defendant physicians avoid attending these depositions because of concern about their own possible reactions to critical testimony.

The defendant physician should carefully review his or her own deposition and those of the plaintiff and the expert witnesses. The transcript of the defendant physician's deposition should be read as soon as it becomes available to assess its accuracy and identify any areas of concern. The deposition should be amended only with the advice of the physician's attorney; however, immediately amending the deposition is preferable to attempting to control damage after signing an incorrect deposition. During the trial, the plaintiff's attorney often asks the defendant physician to respond to specific points from an expert's deposition. It is advantageous to be knowledgeable about these depositions to avoid being surprised by their content. At trial, the defendant physician will undoubtedly be asked to read portions of his or her deposition aloud for the benefit of the jury, and there is no substitute for being extremely familiar with the contents of one's own deposition transcript.[5]

Trial Preparation

A good defense attorney will ensure that the defendant physician is well prepared before the trial. There is no substitute for knowing the entire medical record (especially important details from the patient's chart) and one's deposition transcript. It is important to be knowledgeable about the medical literature, especially as it pertains to the case. The defense attorney is likely to have an excellent idea of the tactics that the plaintiff's attorney may use to attack the testimony of the defendant and will aid the defendant in preparing for such attacks.

The defendant should practice testifying with the help of his or her attorney, just as the physician would prepare for an oral board examination with the help of a colleague. Practice can help to ease tension and enable the defendant to provide a truthful and accurate description of the events surrounding the case. The defendant physician should practice telling the story of the case to ensure that the relevant facts are explained so that the entire truth is made clear to the jury.

Settlement Talks

Medical negligence cases often are settled before trial. The reasons may include the limited potential for a damage award and questions concerning the defendant physician's responsibility. Settlement also may be in order if the opinions of the expert witnesses lead to concern that the case will be lost. However, many difficult cases should be vigorously defended through trial and, if necessary, the appellate courts. The decision should be made based on the facts of the individual case. If serious settlement discussion is indicated, it should begin as early as possible in the litigation process. Before settling a case, the defendant physician should be fully aware of how settlement will affect licensure, hospital privileges, medical liability insurance costs, and information in the National Practitioner Data Bank.

The Trial

The actual trial is both an intimidating and a welcome experience for the defendant physician. The courtroom and its proceedings are as uncomfortable a setting for most physicians as the operating room would be for most attorneys. Although the negative tone in which the plaintiff's attorney describes the case can be upsetting to a physician whose career has been dedicated to helping people, most defendant physicians are relieved that the trial date has finally arrived and are ready to see the case to conclusion. The trial may require that the physician take 1 week or more away from his or her practice. Scheduling the time away from the office can be difficult, especially considering the stigma associated with the reason for the absence. These factors can increase the stress associated with the trial. It is important for the physician to accept that he or she is undergoing an ordeal, block ample time from the schedule, and rely on colleagues to take care of patients.

Interaction with the plaintiff and his or her attorney during the trial is certain to be uncomfortable, and the two parties are likely to actively ignore one another. If contact is made, it is important to remember that the jury is watching and expects the physician to act professionally. Although the testimony of the plaintiff's expert witnesses can be difficult to listen to, the expert witnesses will not be encountered on a daily basis.

The defendant physician's courtroom testimony under oath is an opportunity to communicate directly with the jury. The defense attorney will ensure that all important points are communicated to the jury and will ask the physician specific questions during the direct examination. The defendant physician's attorney may want to discuss damaging points in the case during the direct examination to control how the information is delivered. It is important for the defendant to maintain eye contact with the jury during direct examination and show the jury that he or she is a caring and compassionate physician. The prepared answers should be given; the physician should not deviate from the defense strategy.

The cross-examination by the plaintiff's attorney is intended to show the jury that the physician is reckless and has no regard for patient safety or well-being. This offensive assault has the sole goal of damaging the defendant physician's reputation in the interest of winning the case. Through discovery and depositions, the plaintiff's attorney has come to know the defendant and will have a strategy for impeaching his or her testimony or provoking an inappropriate response. It is important to remember that controlling one's temper is mandatory, genuine humility is an asset, courtroom humor may backfire, the judge should be regarded as the smartest person in the courtroom, and a defendant who is liked and respected by the jury usually wins the case.

The courtroom is a theater in which the defendant is constantly being watched. The defendant's posture, appearance, and reactions will be observed by the jury. It is highly recommended that the defendant sit attentively with an upright bearing and avoid the use of electronic devices. The defendant should look at the person who is speaking. When the defendant is testifying, he or she should focus on the examining attorney and turn toward the judge only when the judge issues a ruling or instruction or asks a direct question. The defendant physician may occasionally turn toward the jury when providing a detailed explanation, especially when using a medical model, just as would be done when counseling a patient before surgery. Prolonged eye contact with the jury in general or individual jurors in particular should be avoided. Gestures such as a wink or a wave are not appropriate; jurors may react negatively if they believe the defendant is staring at them.

If the plaintiff's attorney asks inappropriate questions during the cross-examination, the defense attorney will protect the defendant by objecting to the judge. When there is an objection, the defendant should immediately cease answering the question until the judge has ruled on whether the answer must be completed. The defendant should always ask for the question to be repeated if there has been a delay or if the question cannot be remembered with certainty. In some states, the subject of medical liability reform cannot be discussed during direct or cross-examination, and a mention of this topic could result in a mistrial. Questions irrelevant to the case are not allowed during the cross-examination. The plaintiff's attorney may vigorously cross-examine the defendant to discredit his or her testimony, but harassment is not allowed. The defendant physician must rely on his or her attorney to object to the behavior of the opposing attorney, but he or she can be assured that juries often see through such tactics to the detriment of the plaintiff's case.

The plaintiff's attorney will often attempt to misrepresent the defendant's testimony to benefit the plaintiff's case; an innocent statement may be distorted into a damaging admission of guilt. Publications are available to help prepare the defendant physician to anticipate and counter such an attack.[9,10]

Any exaggerated or unsubstantiated aspects of the physician defendant's curriculum vitae will be questioned to make the physician appear untruthful. Any of the defendant's statements found on the Internet or in printed material will be compared with his or her curriculum vitae. The absence of membership in an appropriate organization may be used to question the physician's competence. Any self-promoting phrase, such as "nationally known," is prime ammunition for use during the cross-examination.[9]

Published articles and other writings of the defendant physician will be examined to determine whether the physician's own words can be used against him or her. The physician must be extremely familiar with his or her published works, especially if they are listed in the curriculum vitae. The defendant's presentations and handouts also can be used in rebuttal of his or her sworn testimony. The defense attorney must be advised ahead of time of any ethical, professional, financial, or personal problems to allow time for a prepared response if the plaintiff's attorney discloses such matters in court. If the defense attorney is prepared, the potential damage arising from a past mistake can be mitigated.

The defendant physician must be well prepared for the cross-examination. The plaintiff's attorney often will ask a question similar to the following: "In the interest of saving this busy court and the good men and women of the jury valuable time, I will agree to conduct this cross-examination as quickly as possible if you will agree to answer my questions with a 'yes' or 'no' if possible. Can we agree to this?" The defendant who agrees to such a "deal" has given away the right to explain the answers and control the testimony he or she is giving. It is important to remember that the plaintiff's attorney has devoted years honing his or her courtroom skills, just as the orthopaedic surgeon has honed his or her surgical skills. The plaintiff's attorney may attempt to force a defendant to quantify a variable that cannot be quantified, as in the following question: "If you are between 51% and 97% certain that you are right, could there be a 49% chance that you are wrong?" It is important that the defendant physician not accept such a supposition or be forced into quantifying something that is not quantifiable. If the defendant's testimony under cross-examination differs from his or her deposition, an appropriate explanation must be offered. The defendant must have complete knowledge of all statements made during his or her deposition.

Many medical liability cases are won or lost based on the testimony of expert witnesses. It is pleasant for a defendant to listen to a witness praising the care given to the patient, but professional composure must be maintained during all testimony. Good expert witnesses testify to the truth regardless of whom it will benefit, even though they commonly are referred to as plaintiff or defense witnesses. The expert witness who supports the defendant's treatment is extremely valuable to the defendant; however, the expression of appreciation must be controlled so that the jury does not misread the defendant's nonverbal cues.

Many cases are settled after the jury is seated or during the trial. An offer to settle may disrupt the rhythm and pace of the trial but may signal that the plaintiff has realized the limited chance of prevailing.

After all testimony is completed, the attorneys deliver their closing arguments. Negative comments from the plaintiff's attorney should be expected. The judge then gives instructions to the jury, and the stressful period of waiting for the jury's decision begins.

Most defendant physicians feel a tremendous sense of relief after the trial. Victory produces jubilation, but even a loss often leads to relief that the ordeal is over. The rules regarding appeal of the verdict vary between states, but inconsistencies during the trial may allow an appellate court to overturn a decision, resulting in a new trial. Many physicians are forever changed by the litigation experience. The joy associated with practicing medicine may be diminished, patients may be seen as potential litigants, and defensive medicine may become a more important consideration.

The AAOS Professional Compliance Program

The Professional Compliance Program of the AAOS is intended to ensure that expert testimony during legal proceedings is accurate and appropriate.[11] The AAOS program does not discourage AAOS fellows from serving as expert witnesses, but it requires them to behave in a professional manner and testify only to the truth of the case and the medical literature. These standards apply regardless of whether the statements of the expert witness are more favorable to the defendant or the plaintiff.

The AAOS has developed a fair method that ensures due process for all parties involved in the dispute. Filing a grievance under the AAOS program requires that the case must have reached its final disposition, and a grievance may be filed only against an AAOS fellow. The penalties available to the AAOS Board of Directors range from dismissal of the grievance to expulsion from fellowship in the Academy.

Summary

Medical negligence lawsuits are a source of considerable anxiety and stress for the defendant orthopaedic surgeon. Preparation for litigation is paramount for a successful defense, and the orthopaedic surgeon is strongly advised to heed the advice of his or her attorney. Education about the processes and tactics used during the depositions and trial will enable the orthopaedic surgeon to handle the events more wisely. Medical negligence lawsuits are inevitable in the modern tort system. Physicians can effectively assist in their defense and reduce the associated stress.

References

1. Dean M: *The Jurisprudent Physician*. Phoenix, AZ, Legis Press, 1999, pp 283-288.
2. Anderson RE: *Medical Malpractice: A Physician's Sourcebook*. Totowa, NJ, Humana Press, 2005, pp 30-39.
3. Sanbar SS, Firestone MH: *The Medical Malpractice Survival Handbook*. Philadelphia, PA, Mosby Press, 2007, pp 9-15.
4. American Academy of Orthopaedic Surgeons: *2011 Professional Liability Insurance Survey Summary Report*. Rosemont, IL, American Academy of Orthopaedic Surgeons, September 9, 2011.
5. Bal BS, Cowherd RR: The surgeon's role in assisting defense counsel. *AAOS Now* 2010;4(11): 30. http://www.aaos.org/news/aaosnow/nov10/managing5.asp. Accessed November 19, 2011.
6. Bal BS, Cowherd RR: Tips and pointers for depositions. *AAOS Now* 2010;4(11):35. http://www.aaos.org/news/aaosnow/nov10/managing6.asp. Accessed November 19, 2011.
7. Lundy DW: When you're on the "hot seat." *AAOS Now* 2008;2(5): 42. http://www.aaos.org/news/aaosnow/may08/managing7.asp. Accessed November 19, 2011.
8. Lundy DW, Weinstein SL: *Orthopaedic Knowledge Update 10*. Rosemont, IL American Academy of Orthopaedic Surgeons, 2011, pp 3-10.
9. Babitsky S, Mangraviti JJ: Defeating counsel's cross-examination tactics, in *Cross-Examination: The Comprehensive Guide for Experts*. Falmouth, MA, Seak, 2003, pp 303-342.
10. Babitsky S, Mangraviti JJ: *How to Become a Dangerous Expert Witness: Advanced Techniques and Strategies*. Falmouth, MA, Seak, 2005.
11. American Academy of Orthopaedic Surgeons: *Professional compliance program*. Rosemont, IL, American Academy of Orthopaedic Surgeons. http://www3.aaos.org/member/profcomp/profcomp.cfm. Accessed November 19, 2011.

Index

Page numbers with *f* indicate figures
Page numbers with *t* indicate tables

A

AAOS. *See* American Academy of Orthopaedic Surgeons
AAOS Professional Compliance Program, 600–601
AAOS Professional Liability Insurance Survey Summary Report, 596
ABC. *See* Aneurysmal bone cyst
Abductor failure, 523–524, 523*f*, 524*f*
Abductor weakness, 266
  rotational acetabular osteotomy and, 289
Abuse. *See* Child abuse
Accreditation Council for Graduate Medical Education (ACGME) core competencies
  background, 559
  changes coming to, 561
  interpersonal skills, 560–561
  medical knowledge, 560–562
  patient care, 560, 562–563
  practice-based learning and improvement, 560
  professionalism, 561, 563
  systems-based practice, 561, 571–575
Acetabular cartilage injury
  with acetabular retroversion, 307–308
  inspection during periacetabular osteotomy (PAO), 279–280
    management of, 281*f*, 282*f*, 282–284, 283*f*
    pathology of, 281*f*, 282*f*, 282–284, 283*f*
Acetabular dysplasia, 265
  anterior impingement test and, 267
  Chiari pelvic osteotomy for
    advantages and disadvantages of, 287, 288t, 290–292, 291*f*
    procedure for, 290
    results with, 292
  imaging of, 267–271
    CT, 269–270
    MRI, 270–271, 270*f*
    radiography, 267–269, 268*f*, 269*f*, 269*t*
  osteoarthritis and, 265
  patient evaluation with, 266–267
    history, 266
    patient consideration in rotational pelvic osteotomy (RPO), 271-273, 272t, 273f
    physical examination, 266–267, 267*t*
  rotational acetabular osteotomy for
    advantages and disadvantages of, 287, 288*t*, 289
    procedure for, 287–289, 288*f*
    results with, 289
  Tönnis angle, 267–268
  triple pelvic osteotomy for
    advantages and disadvantages of, 287, 288*t*, 289–290, 290*f*
    procedure for, 289
    results of, 290
Acetabular fractures, periprosthetic
  intraoperative, 321–322
  late, 322
  revision TKA for, 338, 338*f*
Acetabular labrum, 280
  Chiari pelvic osteotomy and, 292
  function of, 280
  during periacetabular osteotomy
    pathology, 280–281
    repair of, 281–282, 281*f*–282*f*
  tearing of, 280
Acetabular osteochondroplasty, 308
Acetabular osteolytic lesions, after THA, 208–209, 208*f*, 209*f*
Acetabular retroversion, 305, 306*f*
  patient with, 305–306
  after periacetabular osteotomy, 280
  radiographic assessment of, 306, 306*f*, 307*f*
  reverse periacetabular osteotomy for, 305, 308, 309*f*
    incision for, 309
    ischial osteotomy, 310, 310*f*
    planning for, 308–310
    positioning for, 308–309
    postoperative rehabilitation for, 312
    pubic bone osteotomy, 310
    research on, 312
    retroacetabular osteotomy, 311, 311*f*
    transverse iliac osteotomy, 310–311, 311*f*
  treatment of, 307–308
    acetabular osteochondroplasty for, 308
    decision-making tree for, 307–308, 308*f*, 309*f*
    options for, 308, 309*f*
    reasons for, 307, 307*f*
Acetabulum
  defect classification for, 217, 217*t*
  in mini-posterior approach to THA, 240–241, 241*f*
  in modified Watson-Jones approach to THA, 233, 233*f*, 234*f*
  osteolysis and THA revision for, 218–220, 219*t*, 220*f*, 221*f*
  in superior capsulotomy technique for THA, 248, 248*f*
ACGME core competencies. *See* Accreditation Council for Graduate Medical Education core competencies
Acromioclavicular (AC) joint exploration, for open rotator cuff repair, 107–108
Acromion, in open rotator cuff repair, 108–110, 108f, 109f, 110*f*, 111*f*, 112*f*
Adolescent athletes, shoulder instability in
  anterior instability, 436–440, 438*f*, 439*t*
  diagnosis, 436–437
  epidemiology, 436
  multidirectional instability, 436–437, 440–441
  posterior instability, 436–437, 440
  shoulder anatomy and maturation, 435–436
Affective domain attributes, 556
Alignment board, for proximal tibial fracture fixation, 70, 75*f*
Alpha Omega Alpha Honor Medical Society, 555

American Academy of Orthopaedic Surgeons (AAOS), bone defect classification system, 217, 217*t*
Amputation
on the battlefield, 8-10, 9*f*
for infection after TKA, 358
lower extremity
background, 35–36
battlefield and disaster relief efforts findings, 7–10, 8f, 9*f*
choice for, 38–39, 38*f*
choice for limb salvage, 39, 39*f*
decision for, 5
evaluation and initial treatment, 3–5, 4*f*, 5*f*
goals, 5–6
LEAP study findings, 6–7, 36–38
limb salvage compared with, 36–38, 37*t*
outcomes, 12–13
postoperative care, 10–12, 10*t*, 11*f*, 12*f*
prosthetic fitting, 10–12, 10*t*, 11*f*, 12*f*
Anatomic precontoured plates, for metadiaphyseal fractures, 43, 43*f*, 44*f*
Anatomic prosthesis, shoulder instability with, 138
Anderson Orthopaedic Research Institute (AORI) system for bone loss, 342
Aneurysmal bone cyst (ABC), 542, 542*f*
Ankle,
fusion, with pilon fractures, 30–31
posttraumatic arthritis in, 30
Anterior acetabular deficiency, 268, 268*f*
Anterior apprehension test maneuver, 267, 267*t*
Anterior capsulectomy, for anterior supine THA, 253–256, 254*f*, 255*f*, 256*f*
Anterior hip arthrotomy, with PAO, 281–282, 282*f*
Anterior iliofemoral approach
for Chiari pelvic osteotomy, 290
for rotational acetabular osteotomy, 288, 288*f*
for triple pelvic osteotomy, 289
Anterior impingement test
reverse periacetabular osteotomy and, 308
rotational pelvic osteotomy and, 266–267, 267*t*, 271
Anterior instability
after shoulder arthroplasty, 138
in young athletes, 436–440, 438*f*, 439*t*
Anterior supine THA, 251–252
acetabular component placement for, 255, 255*f*
anterior capsulectomy for, 253–256, 254*f*, 255*f*, 256*f*
complications with, 251–252, 259–260
discussion of, 259–260
experience with, 258–259, 259*t*
historical overview of, 251
hospitalization and rehabilitation protocol for, 256, 258
incisions for, 252–253, 254*f*
minimally invasive THA compared with, 238–239
perioperative factors, 258–259, 259*t*
prepping for, 252, 253*f*
recovery with, 259
revision surgery for, 251, 258–260, 259*t*
risks with, 252
Smith-Petersen interval for, 251–252
success rate of, 251
surgical technique for, 252–258, 253f, 254f, 255f, 256f, 257*f*, 258f
Antibiotics
for contaminated wounds, 4
for hip septic arthritis, 408, 409*t*
for MRSA infection, 409*t*, 412
for periprosthetic infection, 138
for shoulder arthroplasty, 121
after TKA, 353
Antigen-specific immune reactions, particle-induced, 204
Antiprotrusio cages, for acetabular defect repair, 219*t*, 220
Anulus fibrosus, 384
AO classification system
for proximal humeral fractures, 144
for proximal tibial fractures, 61, 62*f*
for wrist fractures, 183, 185*f*
Apophyseal avulsion injuries, 526–527, 527*f*
Arthritis. *See* Hip septic arthritis; Osteoarthritis; Patellofemoral arthritis; Rheumatoid arthritis
Arthrodesis
for infection after TKA, 358
with lumbar spinal stenosis, 389
Arthroplasty. *See specific arthroplasty surgeries*
Arthroscopic rotator cuff repair
acromioclavicular joint exploration, 107–108
acromion and coracoacromial ligament handling, 108–110, 108*f*, 109*f*, 110*f*, 111*f*, 112*f*
case example, 112–113, 112*f*, 113*f*
closure, 110–112
deltotrapezial approach, 106–107, 107*f*, 108*f*
postoperative immobilization and rehabilitation, 112
preoperative evaluation, 106
RAMPAGE procedure technique, 106
skin incision, 106, 107*f*
Arthroscopy. *See also* Dry arthroscopy
for thumb carpometacarpal (CMC) arthritis, 175, 175*f*
Athletes
hip injuries in, 515
athletic pubalgia, 520–521, 520*f*
contact, 515–518, 516*f*, 517*f*, 518*f*
contusions, 519–520
endurance, 521–526, 522*f*, 523*f*, 524*f*, 525*f*, 526*f*
myotendinous injuries, 518–519, 518*f*, 519*f*
overhead, 521
pediatric, 526–528, 527*f*
shoulder instability in young, 435–441
anterior instability, 436–440, 438*f*, 439*t*
diagnosis, 436–437
epidemiology, 436
multidirectional, 436–437, 440–441
patterns of instability, 436
posterior instability, 436–437, 440
shoulder anatomy and maturation, 435–436
SLAP injuries in throwing, 491–492
classification of, 502–503, 503*t*
epidemiology of, 502–503
history for, 503
imaging, 495–496, 503
managing, 503, 505, 506*t*, 507, 508*t*
pathogenesis of, 502, 503*t*

physical examination for, 503, 504t–505t
presentation of, 494–495
treatment, 496–498, 497f
Athletic pubalgia, 520–521, 520f
femoroacetabular impingement (FAI) and, 521
Autologous chondrocyte implantation (ACI), 464

B

Bankart lesions
continuous type II SLAP lesion with, 509, 509f, 510f
separated type II SLAP lesion with, 510
SLAP tears and, 505, 507, 509
type IV SLAP lesion with, 510–511, 510f
Battered child syndrome, 399
Battlefield amputations
casualty receiving facilities treatment, 8–10, 9f
complications, 10
initial treatment, 7–8, 8f
injury patterns, 7, 8f
Behavioral-based structured interview (BBSI), 557–559
Bicondylar tibial plateau fracture plating, 68, 71f
Bicycle test, 267, 267t
Bioabsorbable screws, 463, 463f
Bladder exstrophy, 305
Body mass index (BMI)
rotational pelvic osteotomy and, 271
THA considerations
anterior supine approach, 260
modified Watson-Jones approach, 230
Bone defect
classification of
acetabular, 217, 217t
femoral, 218, 218t
for revision TKA, 342
in revision TKA, 341
cement and screw reconstruction, 343
component shift for, 342–343
condyle-replacing hinged prosthesis, 346, 347f
increased resection for, 342–343
local autograft, 343, 344f
metaphyseal sleeves or cones, 345–346, 346f
particulate allograft, 343, 344f
preoperative assessment for, 341–342
prosthetic augments, 343–344
structural allografts, 344–345, 345f
treatment options for, 342–346
Bone grafting
for acetabular defect repair, 219–220, 220f
for femoral defect repair, 221–222
for knee defects, 343, 344f
for periprosthetic fractures around femoral component, 333
Bone healing, 41–43
Bone tumors
benign, 538, 539t
aneurysmal bone cyst (ABC), 542, 542f
chondroblastoma, 541, 541f
enchondroma, 540–541, 540f
fibrous cortical defects and nonossifying fibromas, 541, 541f
fibrous dysplasia, 541, 542f
giant cell tumor, 542–543
osteoblastoma, 539, 539f
osteochondroma, 539–540, 540f
osteoid osteoma, 538–539, 539f
unicameral bone cyst (UBC), 541–542
MRI and CT of, 537–538
malignant
chondrosarcoma, 545–546, 546f
Ewing sarcoma and primitive neuroectodermal tumor, 544–545, 545f
lymphoma, 547–548, 548f
multiple myeloma, 546–547, 547f
osteosarcoma, 543–544, 544f
patient evaluation for, 543
radiographic evaluation of
characteristic findings, 537, 538t
Enneking criteria, 535–536
lesion margins, 536, 536t
location and multiplicity, 536–537, 537f, 537t
Mankin criteria, 536
matrix, 537
periosteal reaction, 536

C

Caffey disease, 401
Calcaneus fractures, 31, 31f, 32f
Calcitonin, for lumbar spinal stenosis, 386
Callus, 41–43
Cam morphology, with acetabular retroversion, 307–308
Cam-type impingement, in hip, 282, 284
Cancellous grafting
for acetabular defect repair, 218–219
for femoral defect repair, 221–222
for knee defects, 343, 344f
Capsulorrhaphy arthropathy, 120
Capsulotomy. *See also* Superior capsulotomy technique for THA
for THA with modified Watson-Jones approach, 232, 232f
Carpal tunnel syndrome, 187
Central lumbar stenosis, 385
Ceramic heads, 222–223
Charcot arthropathy, 341
Charcot-Marie-Tooth disease, 266
Charlson Comorbidity Index, 377
Chiari pelvic osteotomy
advantages and disadvantages of, 287, 288t, 290–292, 291f
procedure for, 290
results with, 292
Child abuse
background, 399–400
differential diagnoses, 401–402
fractures, 399–400
medicolegal issues, 402
nonorthopaedic injuries, 400
patient history, 400–401
physical examination, 400–401
radiographic examination, 401

Childbirth
Chiari pelvic osteotomy and, 292
rotational acetabular osteotomy and, 289
triple pelvic osteotomy and, 290
Chondral injury. *See* Acetabular cartilage injury
Chondroblastoma, 541, 541*f*
Chondrolysis, slipped capital femoral epiphysis (SCFE) and, 416–417, 420
Chondromalacia
with acetabular retroversion, 307
with periacetabular osteotomy, 280
Chondrosarcoma, 545–546, 546*f*
Chopart injuries
biomechanics, 82, 82*f*
classification, 82–83, 83*f*
complications, 87
definitions, 79–80, 80*f*
diagnosis, 80*f*, 81*f*, 83–84, 84*f*
epidemiology, 79–80
injury mechanism, 82
osseous and soft-tissue anatomy, 80–82, 81*f*, 82*f*
outcomes, 87–88
cuboid and navicular fractures, 88–89, 89*f*
fusion or open reduction and internal fixation (ORIF) debate, 88
postoperative management, 86*f*, 87
preoperative planning/initial treatment, 84, 84*f*
treatment indications, 84
treatment technique, 85
definitive fixation of lateral column, 85*t*, 86
definitive fixation of medial column, 85*t*, 86–87, 86*f*
provisional fixation of medial column, 85–86, 85*t*, 86*f*
Clindamycin, for MRSA infection, 409*t*, 412
Coflex interspinous device, 388–389
Cognitive domain attributes
Alpha Omega Alpha Honor Medical Society, 555
dean's letter, 556
medical school performance, 555
medical school rank, 555–556
USMLE, 555
Combat application tourniquets, 8–9
Compartment syndrome
supracondylar humeral fracture with, 432, 432*f*
timing of surgical treatment of, 17–18
Competency-based orthopaedic residency curriculum
curriculum development and implementation, 566–567, 567*t*
discussion, 568–569
early results, 567–568, 568*f*
rationale and design, 566
Computer-based learning, 572
Cones. *See* Metaphyseal sleeves or cones
Congenital dysplasia, 258
Contact athlete, hip injuries in, 516*f*, 517*f*, 518*f*
Coracoacromial ligament, in open rotator cuff repair, 108–110, 108*f*, 109*f*, 110*f*, 111*f*, 112*f*
Core competencies
background, 559
changes coming to, 561
interpersonal skills, 560–561
medical knowledge, 560–562
patient care, 560, 562–563
practice-based learning and improvement, 560
professionalism, 561, 563
resident failure to measure up, 561–563
systems-based practice, 561, 571–575
Cortical defects, fibrous, 541, 541*f*
Cortical structural allografts, 379
Coxa valga, acetabular dysplasia with, 268
C-reactive protein (CRP)
in hip septic arthritis, 407–408
in MRSA infection, 411
in revision TKA, 341–342
in THA revision, 217
in TKA infection, 351–352
Crossover sign, 306, 306*f*
Cuboid fractures, 88–89, 89*f*
Cuff tear arthropathy (CTA), 118, 120
Cup-cage constructs, for acetabular defect repair, 219*t*, 220
Cysts
aneurysmal bone cyst, 542, 542*f*
unicameral bone cyst, 541–542

D

Damage control orthopaedics
for extremity, 24, 25*f*
history of, 22
inflammatory and resuscitation considerations in, 22–23, 23*t*
for patients with head injury, 23–24
Débridement
for infection after TKA, 353–354
arthroscopic, 353–354
open technique, 354, 355*t*, 356*t*
for mangled lower extremity, 4
for MRSA infection, 411–412, 412*f*
for open fractures, 19–20
for patellofemoral arthritis, 367
Deceleration sign, 494, 495*f*
Decompressive techniques
for degenerative scoliosis, 390–391
for lumbar spinal stenosis, 386–388, 387*f*
for slipped capital femoral epiphysis, 422
for subacromial impingement, 476–477, 477*f*
Deep venous thrombosis (DVT), MRSA infection with, 410, 412
Degenerative scoliosis, 390–391
Degenerative spondylolisthesis, 389–390
Deltoid-splitting approach, for proximal humeral fractures, 46–47, 47*f*
Deltopectoral approach, for proximal humeral fractures, 46–47, 149
Deltotrapezial approach, for open rotator cuff repair, 106–107, 107*f*, 108f
Deposition, for negligence lawsuits, 598
DIAM interspinous device, 388–389
Dislocation. *See specific dislocations*
Dislocation arthropathy, shoulder arthroplasty for, 120
Distal radius fracture. *See* Wrist fracture

Dorsal deltoid ligament, 169–170, 169*f*
Double innominate osteotomy of Sutherland and Greenfield, 289
Double square measurement, 485, 485*f*
Drive-through sign, 505
Dry arthroscopy, for acetabular chondral injury, 281*f*–282*f*, 283–284, 283*f*
Duloxetine, for lumbar spinal stenosis, 386
Dunn subcapital osteotomy, for SCFE, 420, 420*f*
Dunn technique, for SCFE treatment, 422
DVT. *See* Deep venous thrombosis
Dynamic labral shear test, 484, 485*f*
Dynamic spondylolisthesis, 384–385

E

Education. *See* Orthopaedic residency education
Ehlers-Danlos syndrome, rotational pelvic osteotomy and, 266
Emergency surgical treatment
  for compartment syndrome, 17–18
  for femoral neck fracture, 20–21, 20*t*, 21*t*
  for open fracture, 19–20
  for talar neck fracture, 21–22
  for vascular injury, 18–19
En bloc spondylectomy, 377, 379
Enchondroma, 540–541, 540*f*
Enneking criteria, 535–536
Epidural injection, for lumbar spinal stenosis, 386
Erythrocyte sedimentation rate (ESR)
  for hip septic arthritis, 407
  for revision TKA, 341–342
  for THA revision, 217
  for TKA infection, 351–352
Erythromycin, for MRSA infection, 409*t*, 412
EuroQol-5D, 266
Ewing sarcoma, 544–545, 545*f*
Exchange arthroplasty
  primary, 354
  two-stage, 354, 356–358, 356*f*, 356*t*, 357*f*, 357*t*
    antibiotics for, 354, 356
    outcomes for, 357*t*, 358
    readiness for reimplantation, 356–357
    static compared with articulating spacers, 356, 356*f*, 357*f*
Experiential learning, 572–573
Expert witnesses
  AAOS Professional Compliance Program for, 600–601
  in negligence lawsuits, 597, 600
Explosive blast injuries, lower extremity amputations after
  casualty receiving facilities treatment, 8–10, 9*f*
  complications, 10
  initial treatment, 7–8, 8*f*
  injury patterns, 7, 8*f*
Extension deformity, with intramedullary nailing of proximal tibial fractures, 64, 64*f*
External fixation
  for pilon fractures, 30
  for tibial plateau fractures, 30
  for wrist fracture, 192–193, 192*f*, 193*f*
Extra-articular proximal tibial fractures
  background, 61–62, 62*f*
  closed treatment, 62–63
  future directions, 74–75
  imaging, 62, 62*f*
  intramedullary nail treatment, 63–64, 63*f*, 63*t*, 64*f*
    blocking screws, 65–66, 68*f*
    mini-open reduction and internal fixation, 66, 69*f*
    nailing in relative extension, 64–65, 67*f*
    outcomes, 66–67, 69*t*
    portal placement, 64, 64*f*, 65*f*, 66*f*
    proximal fixation, 65
  plate treatment
    complications, 73
    fracture anatomy, 67–68, 70*f*, 71*f*
    locking plates, 69–70, 75*f*, 75*t*
    nonlocking plates, 70–72
    outcomes, 73–74
    percutaneous plating, 72–73
    surgical approaches, 68, 71*f*, 72*f*–73*f*, 74*f*

F

Facet joints
  with degenerative spondylolisthesis, 389
  in lateral recess stenosis, 385
  in lumbar spinal stenosis, 384
FAI. *See* Femoroacetabular impingement
Femoral anteversion, acetabular dysplasia with, 268
Femoral fracture
  anterior supine THA and, 258–259
  distal, locking plate fixation of, 49–51, 52*f*
  in endurance athletes, 521–523, 522*f*, 523*f*
    assessment of, 522, 522*f*
    basic principles of, 521–522
    rehabilitation, 523
    treatment guidelines for, 522–523, 523*f*
  periprosthetic, 324–325, 325*f*, 326*f*
    around femoral component, 333–337, 334*f*, 336*f*, 337*f*
  proximal, locking plate fixation of, 47–49, 49*f*, 50*f*, 51*f*
Femoral head deformity, acetabular dysplasia with, 268
Femoral neck fractures, timing of surgical treatment of, 20–21, 20*t*, 21*t*
Femoral osteolytic lesions, after THA, 209–210, 209*f*, 210*f*, 211*f*
Femoral retroversion, with acetabular retroversion, 307–308
Femoroacetabular impingement (FAI)
  athletic pubalgia and, 521
  chondral injury with, 282
  in contact sports, 515–517, 516*f*, 517*f*
    assessment of, 516
    basic principles of, 515–516, 515*f*
    rehabilitation, 517
    treatment for, 516–517, 517*f*
  femoral head-neck offset in, 284, 284*f*
  labrum in, 280
  periacetabular osteotomy and, 279–280
  reverse periacetabular osteotomy for, 308

slipped capital femoral epiphysis and, 416, 422–423, 527–528, 527*f*
Femur
in acetabular dysplasia, 268–269
in anterior supine THA, 255–256, 256*f*, 257*f*
in Chiari pelvic osteotomy, 291–292, 291*f*
defects in
bone grafting for, 343
classification for, 218, 218*t*, 342
component shift for, 342–343
increased resection for, 342–343
metaphyseal sleeves or cones for, 345–346, 346*f*
prosthetic augments for, 343–344
structural grafting for, 344–345, 345*f*
head-neck offset, 284, 284*f*
in mini-posterior approach to THA, 240–241, 240*f*
in modified Watson-Jones approach to THA, 233–234, 234*f*, 235*f*
osteolysis and THA revision for, 220–222
osteotomy of
in anterior supine THA, 255–256, 256*f*, 257*f*
in mini-posterior approach to THA, 240, 240*f*
in modified Watson-Jones approach to THA, 232–233, 233*f*
in superior capsulotomy technique for THA, 246–248, 247*f*, 248*f*
Fibromas, nonossifying, 541, 541*f*
Fibrous cortical defects, 541, 541*f*
Fibrous dysplasia, 541, 542*f*
Flexible intramedullary nails, 147
Fluoroscopic assistance
for anterior supine THA, 252, 254*f*
for transsartorial approach to PAO, 298–299, 299*f*
Foraminal stenosis, 385
Fractures. *See also specific fractures*
in child abuse, 399–400
Fragility fracture, of wrist, 186–187
Frankel classification, 376–377
Frykman classification, 183, 183*f*
Fusion
with calcaneus fractures, 31, 31*f*
with midfoot fractures, 88
with pilon fractures, 30–31

G

Gabapentin, for lumbar spinal stenosis, 386
Galeazzi procedure, 448, 448*f*
Gentamicin, for periprosthetic infection, 138
Giant cell tumor, 542–543
Glenohumeral internal rotation, 484–485, 485*f*
Glenohumeral stability
SLAP tears and, 501
classification of, 502–503, 503*t*
continuous type II SLAP lesion with Bankart lesion, 509, 509*f*, 510*f*
epidemiology of, 502–503
history for, 503
imaging for, 503
managing, 503, 505, 506*t*, 507, 508*t*
pathogenesis of, 502, 503*t*
physical examination for, 503, 504*t*–505*t*
postoperative rehabilitation, 511
preferred technique for repair of, 507, 509, 509*f*
separated type II SLAP lesion with Bankart lesion, 510
type IV SLAP lesion with Bankart lesion, 510–511, 510*f*
superior labrum–biceps complex and, 501–502
Glenoid
component loosening after shoulder arthroplasty, 139–140
preoperative morphology assessment, 115–116, 116*f*, 117*f*
shoulder arthroplasty surgical technique for
implant, 124–125
positioning, 126
preparation, 124, 126*f*
Graduated throwing program, 498
Grafting. *See* Bone grafting
Gram staining, for TKA infection, 352

H

Hannover Fracture Scale-98, 6, 36
Hawkins sign, 472, 485–486
Head injury, damage control orthopaedics and, 23–24
Hemiarthroplasty
for capsulorrhaphy arthropathy/dislocation arthropathy, 120
cuff tear arthropathy (CTA) outcomes, 120
osteonecrosis outcomes, 120
for proximal humeral fractures
indications, 155–156, 156*f*
rehabilitation, 158
results, 158–159, 159*f*
reverse shoulder arthroplasty, compared with, 160, 160*f*, 160*t*
surgical technique, 156–158, 156*f*, 157*f*, 158*f*
total shoulder arthroplasty (TSA) compared with
indications for hemiarthroplasty, 116*t*–117*t*, 117–118
in patients with OA, 118–119, 118*t*, 119*t*
Hemostatic dressing, 8, 8*f*
Hip disability and osteoarthritis outcomes score (HOOS), 266
Hip dislocation
in contact athlete, 517–518, 518*f*
after mini-posterior approach to THA, 238–239
Hip dysplasia
acetabular retroversion in, 305
chondral injury with, 282
in endurance athletes, 524–525, 525*f*
labrum in, 280
periacetabular osteotomy with, 279
Hip fracture, rotational acetabular osteotomy and, 289
Hip injuries in athletes, 515
athletic pubalgia, 520–521, 520*f*
contact athletes, 515–518, 516*f*, 517*f*, 518*f*
femoroacetabular impingement, 515–517, 516*f*, 517*f*

subluxation and dislocation, 517–518, 518*f*
contusions, 519–520
endurance athletes, 521–526
abductor failure, 523–524, 523*f*, 524*f*
dysplasia and unstable hip, 524–525, 525*f*
hypermobile hip, 525–526, 526*f*
stress fractures of femoral neck and pelvic ring, 521–523, 522*f*, 523*f*
myotendinous injuries, 518–519, 518*f*, 519*f*
overhead, 521
pediatric, 526–528, 527*f*
apophyseal avulsion injuries, 526–527, 527*f*
slipped capital femoral epiphysis and developmental FAI, 527–528, 527*f*
Hip pointers, 520
Hip resurfacings, 223
Hip septic arthritis, 405–406
clinical presentation of, 406, 406*f*, 406*t*
diagnostic tests for, 407–408
imaging, 407, 407*f*
laboratory tests, 407
toxic synovitis compared with, 407–408, 408*t*
emerging concepts in, 410
treatment for, 408–410
antibiotics, 408, 409*t*
arthroscopic drainage, 409–410
open drainage of, 408
recent trends in, 409
serial aspiration, 409
Hip subluxation, 517–518, 518*f*
Hormones, osteoarthritis correlation with, 171
Hueter approach. *See* Anterior supine THA
Humeral component, for shoulder arthroplasty, 126–127, 127*f*
periprosthetic fracture management and, 136–137
for proximal humeral fractures, 156, 156*f*
Humeral fractures. *See* Proximal humeral fractures; Supracondylar humeral fractures
Humeral head replacement. *See* Hemiarthroplasty
Humerus
exposure for open reduction and locked plate fixation, 149
shoulder arthroplasty surgical technique for
exposure, 121, 122*f*
head cut, 123–124, 125*f*
Hypermobility
in hip, 525–526, 526*f*
in thumb CMC joint, 170, 170*f*

I

IL-6. *See* Interleukin-6
Iliac osteotomy, in reverse periacetabular osteotomy, 310–311, 311*f*
Ilioinguinal approach, to periacetabular osteotomy
outcomes and complications with, 300–301, 300*t*, 301*f*
perioperative management for, 301–302, 302*t*
procedure for, 298, 298*f*
Imhäuser intertrochanteric osteotomy, 423
Immune response, particle-induced, 204
IM nailing. *See* Intramedullary nailing
Impaction grafting
for acetabular defect repair, 219, 219*t*
for femoral defect repair, 222
Impingement injection test, 472
Infection
lower extremity amputation and, 6
in open fractures, 19–20
after percutaneous pinning of proximal humeral fractures, 146
with periprosthetic fractures, 318
of femoral component of THA, 318–319
revision TKA and, 341–342
after shoulder arthroplasty, 137–138
after TKA, 349
amputation, 358
antibiotic suppression, 353
arthrodesis, 358
diagnosis of, 349–352, 350*f*, 351*f*
irrigation and débridement for, 353–354, 355*t*, 356*t*
new definition for, 352–353
primary exchange arthroplasty, 354
surgical management of, 353–358, 353*f*
two-stage exchange arthroplasty, 354, 356–358, 356*f*, 356*t*, 357*f*, 357*t*
Inflammatory response
to metal-on-metal bearings, 223
particle-induced, 203–204
traumatic injury and surgery causing, 22–23, 23*t*
Instability. *See* Shoulder instability
Interlaminar fenestration, for lumbar spinal stenosis, 387
Interleukin-6 (IL-6)
in lumbar spinal stenosis, 385
for TKA infection, 352
Internal fixation, of proximal humeral fractures
anatomy, 144
classification, 144
evaluation and imaging, 144–145, 145*f*
intramedullary nailing, 147–148
open reduction and locking plate fixation, 148–150, 149*f*
percutaneous fixation, 145–147, 145*f*, 146*f*
surgical indications, 145
Internal impingement sign, 494, 494*f*
Interprosthetic fractures, 328–329, 329*f*
Interrogatories, for negligence lawsuits, 597–598
Interview for orthopaedic resident selection
pitfalls of, 559
selection for, 557, 558*f*
structure of, 557–559
Intra-articular fractures
calcaneus fractures, 31, 31*f*, 32*f*
pilon fractures, 30–31
proximal humeral, 155–156, 156*f*
proximal tibial, plating of, 68, 74*f*
tibial plateau fractures, 29–30
Intra-articular work during periacetabular osteotomy, 279
background for, 279–280
chondral pathology, 281*f*–282*f*, 282–284, 283*f*
femoral head-neck offset, 284, 284*f*
labral pathology, 280–282, 281*f*–282*f*

Intralesional decompression and stabilization, 377, 379
Intramedullary (IM) nailing
of extra-articular proximal tibial fractures, 63–64, *63f*, *63t*, *64f*
blocking screws, 65–66, *68f*
mini-open reduction and internal fixation, 66, *69f*
nailing in relative extension, 64–65, *67f*
outcomes, 66–67, *69t*
portal placement, 64, *64f*, *65f*, *66f*
proximal fixation, 65
of proximal humeral fractures
complications, 148
indications, 147
prognosis and outcomes, 147–148
technique, 147
Intramedullary Nails Versus Plate Fixation Re-Evaluation study (IMPRESS), 74–75
Irrigation, for infection after TKA, 353–354
arthroscopic, 353–354
open technique, 354, *355t*, *356t*
Ischial osteotomy, in reverse periacetabular osteotomy, 310, *310f*
Ischial spine sign, 268

J

Joint aspiration, for TKA infection, 352
Joint laxity, in thumb carpometacarpal joint, osteoarthritis correlation with, 170, *170f*
Jumbo cups, for acetabular defect repair, 218–219, *219t*
Jupiter and Fernandez classification, 183, *184f*

K

Kaplan-Meier survivorship
for minimally invasive periacetabular osteotomy, 301, *301t*
for rotational acetabular osteotomy, 289
Kibler sign, 494
Kinetic chain deficits, with SLAP injuries, 484
Knee
pain after intramedullary nailing in, 66–67, *69t*
posttraumatic arthritis in, 29–30
Knee arthroplasty. *See* Total knee arthroplasty
Knee Society Scores, patellofemoral arthroplasty and, 367–368
Kyphoplasty, 380–381

L

Labrum. *See also* Acetabular labrum; Shoulder labrum
of shoulder, 484
Lateral femoral cutaneous nerve paresthesias, with anterior supine THA, 260
Lateral recess stenosis, 385
Lateral tibial plateau fractures, 29
Laxity, in thumb carpometacarpal joint, osteoarthritis correlation with, 170, *170f*
LEAP. *See* Lower Extremity Assessment Project
Learning technologies
disconnection between educators and, 579
educational, 579–582
discussion, 582
mobile computing, 580–581
online platforms, 580
social media, 581–582
getting educators connected in, 582–583
evaluating learner's competency, 582–583
skill-based simulation programs, 583
training, 582
web-based resources, 583
rapid development in, 577–579
information digitalization, 578
information explosion, 578
new generation of learners, 578
new instructional technologies, 578–579
rate of change, 579
Legal issues. *See also* Negligence lawsuits
of child abuse cases, 402
of compartment syndrome cases, 18
Legg-Calvé-Perthes disease
acetabular retroversion in, 305, *306f*
anterior supine THA for, 258
with periacetabular osteotomy, 280
prominence of ischial spine (PRIS) sign in, 306
Lesion margins, of bone tumors, 536, *536t*
Less Invasive Stabilization System (LISS), 42, 73
Ligamentous laxity, 525–526, *526f*
Ligament reconstruction tendon interposition (LRTI), 172–174, *173f*, *174f*
Ligamentum flavum
in central stenosis, 385
in lateral recess stenosis, 385
in lumbar spinal stenosis, 384
Limb length
discrepancy in, 266
with mini-posterior approach to THA, 239
Limb salvage
of lower extremity
amputation compared with, 36–38, *37t*
choice for amputation, 38–39, *38f*
of mangled lower extremity
background, 35–36
choice for, 39, *39f*
Limb Salvage Index, 6, 36–38, *37t*
Lisfranc injuries
biomechanics, 82, *82f*
classification, 82–83, *83f*
complications, 87
definitions, 79–80, *80f*
diagnosis, *80f*, *81f*, 83–84, *84f*
epidemiology, 79–80
injury mechanism, 82
osseous and soft-tissue anatomy, 80–82, *81f*, *82f*
outcomes, 87–88
cuboid and navicular fractures, 88–89, *89f*
fusion or ORIF debate, 88
postoperative management, *86f*, 87
preoperative planning/initial treatment, 84, *84f*
treatment indications, 84
treatment technique, 85

definitive fixation of lateral column, 85*t*, 86
definitive fixation of medial column, 85*t*, 86–87, 86*f*
provisional fixation of medial column, 85–86, 85*t*, 86*f*
LISS. *See* Less Invasive Stabilization System
Locking plate fixation
for extra-articular proximal tibial fractures, 69–70, 75*f*, 75*t*
for femoral periprosthetic fractures, 324–325, 326*f*
for metadiaphyseal fractures
discussion, 54–56
distal femoral fractures, 49–51, 52*f*
historical perspective, 41–43
proximal femoral fractures, 47–49, 49*f*, 50*f*, 51*f*
proximal tibia fractures, 51–54, 53*f*, 54*f*, 55*f*
trinity of anatomic precontoured plates, 43–45, 43*f*, 44*f*, 45*f*
for proximal humeral fractures, 46–47, 46*f*, 47*f*, 48*f*
with open reduction, 148–150, 149*f*
for tibial periprosthetic fractures, 326, 327*f*
for wrist fractures, 188–191, 189*f*, 190*f*, 191*f*
Lower extremity
amputation of mangled
background, 35–36
battlefield and disaster relief efforts findings, 7–10, 8*f*, 9*f*
choice for, 38–39, 38*f*
decision for, 5
evaluation and initial treatment, 3–5, 4*f*, 5*f*
goals, 5–6
LEAP study findings, 6–7, 36–38
limb salvage compared with, 36–38, 37*t*
outcomes, 12–13
postoperative care, 10–12, 10*t*, 11*f*, 12*f*
prosthetic fitting, 10–12, 10*t*, 11*f*, 12*f*
salvage of mangled
amputation compared with, 36–38, 37*t*
background, 35–36
choice for salvage, 39, 39*f*
flap coverage, 4, 4*f*, 5*f*
functional outcomes, 36–38
Lower Extremity Assessment Project (LEAP)
amputation compared with limb salvage in, 36–38
infection in, 6
long-term results in, 6–7
patient expectations in, 7
psychological factors in, 7
smoking effects in, 6
LRTI. *See* Ligament reconstruction tendon interposition
Lumbar spinal stenosis, 383–384
clinical presentation of, 383–384
degenerative scoliosis, 390–391
diagnostic imaging for, 385–386
localization of, 385
nonsurgical management of, 386
pathophysiology of, 384–385
physical examination for, 384
surgical treatment of, 386–389
decompressive techniques, 386–388, 387*f*
degenerative spondylolisthesis, 389–390
interspinous laminectomy, 387
interspinous process spacers, 388–389
minimally invasive lateral interbody fusion, 391–392, 391*f*
Lymphoma, 547–548, 548*f*

M

Malignant bone tumors
chondrosarcoma, 545–546, 546*f*
Ewing sarcoma and primitive neuroectodermal tumor, 544–545, 545*f*
lymphoma, 547–548, 548*f*
MRI and CT of, 537–538
multiple myeloma, 546–547, 547*f*
osteosarcoma, 543–544, 544*f*
patient evaluation for, 543
radiographic evaluation of, 535–537, 536*t*, 537*f*, 537*t*, 538*t*
Malleolar fractures, 30
Malunion
after intramedullary nailing of proximal humeral fractures, 148
after percutaneous pinning of proximal humeral fractures, 146
Mangled Extremity Severity Score, 6, 36
Mankin criteria, 536
Matrix, of bone tumors, 537
Matrix metalloproteinases, in lumbar spinal stenosis, 385
Mayo shear test, 471–472
Medial patellofemoral ligament (MPFL), 446*f*
reconstruction for patellofemoral dislocation, 449–450, 449*f*
Medial proximal tibial fracture, plating of, 68, 72*f*–73*f*
Medial tibial plateau fractures, 29
Melone classification, 183, 184*f*
Merle d'Aubigné and Postel scores
for reverse periacetabular osteotomy, 312
for rotational pelvic osteotomy, 271
for triple pelvic osteotomy, 290
Metabolic bone disease, fracture in children with, 401–402
Metabolic disorders, periprosthetic fractures and, 318
Metadiaphyseal fractures, locking and minimally invasive plating of
discussion, 54–56
distal femoral fractures, 49–51, 52*f*
fixed-angle plates for, 43–44, 43*f*, 44*f*
historical perspective, 41–43
proximal femoral fractures, 47–49, 49*f*, 50*f*, 51*f*
proximal humeral fractures, 46–47, 46*f*, 47*f*, 48*f*
proximal tibial fractures, 51–54, 53*f*, 54*f*, 55*f*
trinity of anatomic precontoured plates, 43–45, 43*f*, 44*f*, 45*f*
Metal-on-metal bearing revision, for THA and osteolysis, 222–223, 222*f*
Metaphyseal sleeves or cones, for revision TKA, 345–346, 346*f*
Metastatic spine disease, 375–376
complications with, 377

preoperative optimization and considerations for, 376–377
prognosis assessment for, 376–377, 376*t*
radiation oncology advances, 381, 381*t*
surgery for
less invasive options for, 380–381
options and considerations for, 377, 379
planning techniques for, 377, 378*f*, 379*f*
reconstruction and stabilization after, 379–380, 380*f*
staging for, 376–377
Methicillin-resistant *Staphylococcus aureus* (MRSA) infection, 354, 405, 410
complex antibiotic regimens for, 409*t*, 412
complications of, 410, 412*f*
active surveillance for, 412
concurrent infections with, 410, 411*f*
emergency department evaluation of, 410–411
studies of, 410, 410*t*
surgery role for, 411–412
Midfoot fractures/dislocations
biomechanics, 82, 82*f*
classification, 82–83, 83*f*
complications, 87
definitions, 79–80, 80*f*
diagnosis, 80*f*, 81*f*, 83–84, 84*f*
epidemiology, 79–80
injury mechanism, 82
osseous and soft-tissue anatomy, 80–82, 81*f*, 82*f*
outcomes, 87–88
cuboid and navicular fractures, 88–89, 89*f*
fusion or ORIF debate, 88
postoperative management, 86*f*, 87
preoperative planning/initial treatment, 84, 84*f*
treatment indications, 84
treatment techniques, 85
definitive fixation of lateral column, 85*t*, 86
definitive fixation of medial column, 85*t*, 86–87, 86*f*
provisional fixation of medial column, 85–86, 85*t*, 86*f*
Minimally invasive lateral interbody fusion, 391–392, 391*f*
Minimally invasive periacetabular osteotomy, 297
background on, 297–298
ilioinguinal approach, 298, 298*f*
outcomes and complications with, 300–301, 300*t*, 301*f*
perioperative management for, 301–302, 302*t*
Smith-Petersen approach, 298, 298*f*
transsartorial approach, 298–300, 298*f*, 299*f*
Minimally invasive plating
of metadiaphyseal fractures, 41-56, 43*f*, 44*f*, 45*f*, 46*f*, 47f, 48*f*, 49*f*, 50*f*, 51*f*, 52*f*, 53*f*, 54*f*, 55*f*
of proximal tibial fractures, 72–73
Minimally invasive surgery (MIS) decompression, for lumbar spinal stenosis, 387–388, 387*f*
Minimally invasive THA, 229, 238–239, 251–252
Mini-posterior approach to THA, 237–238
advantages and disadvantages of, 238–239
complications with, 238
femoral osteotomy for, 240, 240*f*
historical overview of, 237–238
incision for, 239–240, 239*f*
positioning with, 238–239
postoperative management, 241–242
technique for, 239–241, 239*f*, 240*f*, 241*f*
Modified Jobe relocation sign, 494
Modified Watson-Jones approach to THA, 229–230
acetabular preparation, 233, 233*f*, 234*f*
approach to, 231–232, 232*f*
closure, 234
discussion of, 235
femoral head and neck osteotomy, 232–233, 233*f*
femoral preparation, 233–234, 234*f*, 235*f*
materials and methods for, 230
minimally invasive THA compared with, 238–239
perioperative care, 230
physical therapy for, 230–231
positioning for, 231, 231*f*
postoperative care, 231
preoperative care, 230
results of, 234
surgical care, 230–231
surgical technique for, 231–233, 231*f*, 233*f*, 234*f*, 235*f*
Morel-Lavallee lesions, 520
Morse taper junction, 222*f*, 223
MPFL. *See* Medial patellofemoral ligament
MRSA infection. *See* Methicillin-resistant *Staphylococcus aureus* infection
Multidirectional shoulder instability
diagnosis of, 95–96
nonsurgical treatment of, 95–96
open capsular shift revision surgery for
after failed stabilization surgery, 96–98, 96*f*, 97*f*
results, 100–101
risk factors, 100
surgical technique, 98–99, 98*f*, 99*f*, 100*f*
in young athletes, 440–441
Myeloma, 546–547, 547*f*
Myotendinous injuries about hip and pelvis, 518–519, 518*f*, 519*f*
proximal adductor injuries, 518*f*

N

Nailing. *See* Intramedullary (IM) nailing
Nail migration, after IM nailing of proximal humeral fractures, 148
Navicular fractures, 88–89, 89*f*
Neer classification system, 144
Neer sign, 472
Negative pressure wound therapy (NPWT), 4, 9, 9*f*
Negligence lawsuits
AAOS Professional Compliance Program, 600–601
AAOS Professional Liability Insurance Survey Summary Report, 596
defense attorney role, 596–597
deposition, 598
interrogatories, 597–598
legal process, 595–596
medical literature review, 597
settlement talks, 599
trial, 599–600

preparation for, 598–599
Nerve injury
with anterior supine THA, 260
after intramedullary nailing of proximal humeral fractures, 148
after mini-posterior approach to THA, 239
supracondylar humeral fracture with, 431–432, 431*t*
wrist fracture with, 187
Nerve Injury, Ischemia, Soft-Tissue Injury, Skeletal Injury, Shock, and Age of Patient Score, 6, 36
Neural element
compression of, 377, 379
decompression of, 378–380, 387*f*
Neural foramen, 385
Neurogenic claudication, with lumbar spinal stenosis, 383
Nonossifying fibromas, 541, 541*f*
Nonsteroidal anti-inflammatory drugs (NSAIDs)
for femoral acetabular impingement, 516
for lumbar spinal stenosis, 386
NPWT. *See* Negative pressure wound therapy
NSAIDs. *See* Nonsteroidal anti-inflammatory drugs
Nucleus pulposus, 384

O

OA. *See* Osteoarthritis
Ober test, 267, 267*t*
O'Brien active compression test, 471–472
O'Brien sign, 486, 494
Open capsular shift revision, for multidirectional shoulder instability
after failed stabilization surgery, 96–98, 96*f*, 97*f*
results, 100–101
risk factors, 100
surgical technique, 98–99, 98*f*, 99*f*, 100*f*
Open reduction and internal fixation (ORIF)
for calcaneus fractures, 31, 31*f*
for midfoot fractures, 88
for pilon fractures, 24, 25*f*, 30–31
for tibial periprosthetic fractures, 326, 327*f*
for tibial plateau fractures, 30
for type B1 periprosthetic fractures, 322–323, 322*f*
for wrist fracture, 188–191, 189*f*, 190*f*, 191*f*
Open reduction and locking plate fixation, for proximal humeral fractures
background, 148
deltopectoral approach, 149
fixation, 150
indications, 148, 149*f*
proximal humeral exposures, 149
reduction, 149–150
rehabilitation, 150
results and complications, 150
Open rotator cuff repair
acromioclavicular joint exploration, 107–108
acromion and coracoacromial ligament handling, 108–110, 108*f*, 109*f*, 110*f*, 111*f*, 112*f*
case example, 112–113, 112*f*, 113*f*
closure, 110–112
deltotrapezial approach, 106–107, 107*f*, 108*f*
postoperative immobilization and rehabilitation, 112
preoperative evaluation, 106
RAMPAGE procedure technique, 106
skin incision, 106, 107*f*
ORIF. *See* Open reduction and internal fixation
Orthopaedic residency education
competency-based curriculum, 566–567, 567*t*
discussion, 568–569
early results, 567–568, 568*f*
rationale and curriculum design, 566
learning technologies in
disconnection between educators and, 579
educational technologies, 579–582
getting educators connected in, 582–583
rapid development in, 577–579
systems-based practice core competency
data collection, 573–574
discussion, 573
expectations and learning approaches, 571–573
orthopaedic health systems rotation development, 574–575
results, 574
selection for
affective domain criteria, 556
cognitive domain criteria, 555–556
criteria importance, 554–555, 554*t*
desired resident attributes, 553–554
interview strategies, 557–559, 558*f*
screening tools, 556–557
success predictors, 555
training in
core competency failure, 561–563
core competency origin and measurement, 559–561
Orthopaedic Trauma Association, proximal tibial fracture classification system of, 61, 62*f*
Orthopaedic trauma room, effects of, 24–25
Osteoarthritis (OA)
abnormal hip morphologies and, 279
acetabular dysplasia and, 265
anterior supine THA for, 258
of facet joints, 384
hormone correlation with, 171
joint laxity correlation with, 170, 170*f*
posttraumatic
with calcaneus fractures, 31, 31*f*
with pilon fractures, 30–31
with tibial plateau fractures, 29–30
rotational acetabular osteotomy and, 289
rotational pelvic osteotomy and, 272–273, 273*f*
shoulder arthroplasty for
hemiarthroplasty, 118–119, 118*t*, 119*t*
key steps, 127, 128*f*
total shoulder arthroplasty, 117–119, 118*t*, 119*t*
of thumb carpometacarpal joint, 167
hormonal influences on, 171
laxity influences on, 170, 170*f*
progression of, 167–168, 168*f*, 169*f*
reconstruction for, 171–175, 171*f*, 173*f*, 174*f*
treatment options for, 174–175, 174*f*, 175*f*
triple pelvic osteotomy and, 290

Osteoblastoma, 539, 539*f*
Osteochondral allograft, 464, 464*f*
Osteochondral autologous transplantation, 464, 464*f*
Osteochondritis dissecans (OCD), 455
  arthroscopic evaluation of, 460, 461*f*
  clinical presentation and examination of, 457–458
  current evidence of, 460–461
  diagnostic studies of, 458–460
    bone scintigraphy, 459
    MRI, 459–460, 460*f*, 460*t*
    plain radiography, 458–459, 458*f*, 458*t*, 459*f*
  epidemiology of, 455–456
  etiology of, 456–457, 456*f*
  nonsurgical management of, 461
  salvage procedures for, 463–464, 464*f*
  surgical management of, 461–463, 462*f*, 463*f*
Osteochondroma, 539–540, 540*f*
Osteogenesis, theories of, 41–43
Osteogenesis imperfecta (OI), 401–402
Osteoid osteoma, 538–539, 539*f*
Osteolysis
  aggressive forms of, 216, 216*f*
  background, 201–202
  cellular by-product activation of cells, 202–203, 202*f*
  particle-induced antigen-specific immune reactions, 204
  particle-induced inflammatory cascade, 203–204
  particle-induced systemic immune response, 204
  after THA
    acetabular lesions, 208–209, 208*f*, 209*f*
    cross-sectional imaging of, 208
    CT of, 208, 209*f*, 210
    femoral lesions, 209–210, 209*f*, 210*f*, 211*f*
    MRI of, 208, 210–212, 211*f*, 212*f*
    monitoring of, 212
    radiographs of, 207–208
  THA revision and
    acetabular side, 218–220, 219*t*, 220*f*, 221*f*
    assessment of, 215–216
    bone defect classification, 217–218, 217*t*, 218*t*
    evaluation of, 217
    femoral side, 220–222
    historical overview of, 215–216
    imaging for, 217
    low wear-bearing surface revision, 222–223, 222*f*
Osteonecrosis
  anterior supine THA for, 258
  etiology of, 421
  after percutaneous pinning of proximal humeral fractures, 146–147
  slipped capital femoral epiphysis and, 416–417, 420–422
  shoulder arthroplasty for, 120
Osteoporosis, periprosthetic fractures and, 318
Osteosarcoma, 543–544, 544*f*
Osteotomy
  femoral
    in anterior supine THA, 255–256, 256*f*, 257*f*
    in mini-posterior approach to THA, 240, 240*f*
    in modified Watson-Jones approach to THA, 232–233, 233*f*
  in ilioinguinal approach to periacetabular osteotomy, 298
  in reverse periacetabular osteotomy, 310–311, 310*f*, 311*f*
  in transsartorial approach to periacetabular osteotomy, 298–299

P

Palmar cutaneous nerve, 185, 186*f*
PAO. *See* Periacetabular osteotomy
Paprosky bone defect classification system
  acetabular, 217, 217*t*
  femoral, 218, 218*t*
Patellar periprosthetic fractures, 320–321, 320*t*, 326–327, 327*f*
  revision TKA for, 339
Patellectomy, 367
Patellofemoral arthritis
  alternative treatments for, 366–367, 368*f*
  patellofemoral arthroplasty for, 363–366, 366*f*, 367*f*
Patellofemoral arthroplasty, 363
  advantages of, 365–366
  clinical evaluation for, 364–365
    patient history, 364–365
    physical examination, 365
    preoperative imaging, 365, 366*f*, 367*f*
  complications of, 368–369
  design features of, 366
  historical perspectives on, 363–364
  indications and contraindications, 364
  outcomes of, 367–368
  pearls and pitfalls of, 369–370, 370*f*
Patellofemoral dislocation, 445
  epidemiology and natural history of, 446–447
  first-time management, 447
  pathoanatomy of, 446, 446*f*, 447*f*
  recurrent
    complications with, 450
    distal realignment, 448–449, 448*f*, 449*f*
    guided growth, 450
    lateral release, 448
    management of, 447–450
    medial patellofemoral ligament reconstruction, 449–450, 449*f*
    proximal realignment, 447–448, 447*f*, 448*f*
    rehabilitation, 450
Patellofemoral ligament, anatomy and biomechanics of, 445–446, 446*f*
Patient-centered care. *See* Shared decision making
Patient Protection and Affordable Care Act (PPACA), 591–592
Pediatric athletes
  hip injuries in, 526–528, 527*f*
    apophyseal avulsion, 526–527, 527*f*
    slipped capital femoral epiphysis and developmental femoral acetabular impingement, 527–528, 527*f*
  patellofemoral dislocation of, 445
    anatomy and biomechanics for, 445–446, 446*f*
    epidemiology and natural history of, 446–447
    first-time, 447
    pathoanatomy of, 446, 446*f*, 447*f*
    recurrent, 447–450, 447*f*, 448*f*, 449*f*

shoulder instability in
anterior, 436–440, 438*f*, 439*t*
diagnosis, 436–437
epidemiology, 436
multidirectional instability, 436–437, 440–441
patterns of, 436
posterior, 436–437, 440
shoulder anatomy and maturation, 435–436
Pediatric injury and disease
child abuse, 399–403
osteochondritis dissecans, 455–464, 456*f*, 458*f*, 458*t*, 459*f*, 460*f*, 460*t*, 461*t*, 462*f*, 463*f*, 464*f*
supracondylar humeral fractures, 429–432, 430*f*, 431*t*, 432*f*
Peel-back sign, 505
Pelvic ring fracture, in endurance athletes, 521–523, 522*f*, 523*f*
assessment of, 522, 522*f*
basic principles of, 521–522
rehabilitation, 523
treatment guidelines for, 522–523, 523*f*
Percutaneous pinning
of proximal humeral fractures
complications, 146–147
indications, 145, 145*f*
prognosis and outcomes, 146
technique, 145–146, 146*f*
for wrist fracture, 192–193, 192*f*, 193*f*
Periacetabular osteotomy (PAO). *See also* Rotational pelvic osteotomy
advantages and disadvantages of, 287, 288*t*
alternatives to, 287
Chiari pelvic osteotomy, 290–292, 291*f*
rotational acetabular osteotomy, 287–289, 288*f*
triple pelvic osteotomy, 289–290, 290*f*
anterior hip arthrotomy with, 281–282, 282*f*
approaches to, 297
background on, 297–298
ilioinguinal approach, 298, 298*f*
outcomes and complications with, 300–301, 300*t*, 301*f*
Smith-Petersen approach, 298, 298*f*
transsartorial approach, 298–300, 298*f*, 299*f*
intra-articular work during, 279
background for, 279–280
chondral pathology, 281*f*–282*f*, 282–284, 283*f*
femoral head-neck offset, 284, 284*f*
labral pathology, 280–282, 281*f*–282*f*
perioperative management for
general management, 301
mobilization and exercise program, 302, 302*t*
pain management, 301–302
patient education program for, 301
reverse, 305, 306*f*
for acetabular retroversion, 308, 309*f*
incision for, 309
ischial osteotomy, 310, 310*f*
planning for, 308–310
positioning for, 308–309
postoperative rehabilitation for, 312
pubic bone osteotomy, 310
research on, 312
retroacetabular osteotomy, 311, 311*f*
transverse iliac osteotomy, 310–311, 311*f*
Periosteal reaction, bone tumors with, 536
Periprosthetic fractures, 317
clinical evaluation of, 318–319
epidemiology for, 317–318
future directions for, 328
interprosthetic, 328–329, 329*f*
revision arthroplasty for, 333
risk factors and etiology for, 318
about total hip arthroplasty
of acetabulum, 321–322
classification of, 319–321, 319*f*, 333–334, 334*t*
around femoral component, 333–337, 334*f*, 336*f*, 337*f*
management of, 321–324
type A, 319, 319*f*, 321–322, 333–334, 334*f*, 334*t*
type B1, 319, 319*f*, 322–323, 322*f*, 334
type B2, 319, 319*f*, 323, 334
type B3, 319, 319*f*, 323, 334
type C, 319, 319*f*, 323–324, 324*f*
about total knee arthroplasty
classification of, 319–321, 319*t*, 320*f*, 320*t*
femoral, 324–325, 325*f*, 326*f*
patellar, 320–321, 320*t*, 326–327, 327*f*, 339
supracondylar, 319–320, 319*t*, 338, 338*f*
tibial, 320, 320*f*, 325–326, 327*f*, 338–339, 339*f*
after total shoulder arthroplasty, 135, 136*f*
type A, 137
type B, 137
type C, 136–137
Pilon fractures
damage control orthopaedics for, 24, 25*f*
intra-articular, 30–31
Pincer-type impingement, in hip, 282
Plating. *See also* Locking plate fixation; Minimally invasive plating
dual, 54, 55*f*
of extra-articular proximal tibial fractures
complications, 73
fracture anatomy, 67–68, 70*f*, 71*f*
locking plates, 69–70, 75*f*, 75*t*
nonlocking plates, 70–72
outcomes, 73–74
percutaneous plating, 72–73
surgical approaches, 68, 71*f*, 72*f*–73*f*, 74*f*
of metadiaphyseal fractures
discussion, 54–56
distal femoral fractures, 49–51, 52*f*
historical perspective, 41–43
proximal femoral fractures, 47–49, 49*f*, 50*f*, 51*f*
proximal humeral fractures, 46–47, 46*f*, 47*f*, 48*f*
proximal tibial fractures, 51–54, 53*f*, 54*f*, 55*f*
trinity of anatomic precontoured plates, 43–45, 43*f*, 44*f*, 45*f*
PMMA. *See* Polymethyl methacrylate
Polyethylene
THA revision and thickness of, 215–216

UHMWPE, 208, 212
Polymethyl methacrylate (PMMA), 343
Portal placement, for IM nail treatment of proximal tibial fractures, 64, 64*f*, 65*f*, 66*f*
Posterior instability
after shoulder arthroplasty, 138
in young athletes, 436–437, 440
Posterior wall sign, 268, 306
reverse periacetabular osteotomy and, 308
Posteromedial fragments, in proximal tibial fracture fixation, 53–54, 54*f*, 55*f*
Posttraumatic arthritis
with calcaneus fractures, 31, 31*f*
with pilon fractures, 30–31
shoulder arthroplasty for, 120
with tibial plateau fractures, 29–30
Predictive Salvage Index, 6, 36
Primitive neuroectodermal tumor, 544–545, 545*f*
Prominence of ischial spine (PRIS) sign, 306, 306*f*
Prosthesis
lower extremity
fitting for, 10–12, 10*t*, 11*f*, 12*f*
walking with, 36, 38
shoulder instability with, 138
Prosthetic augments, for bone defects, 343–344
Proximal humeral fractures
internal fixation of
anatomy, 144
classification, 144
evaluation and imaging, 144–145, 145*f*
intramedullary nailing, 147–148
open reduction and locked plate fixation, 148–150, 149*f*
percutaneous fixation, 145–147, 145*f*, 146*f*
surgical indications, 145
intra-articular, 155–156, 156*f*
locking plate fixation of, 46–47, 46*f*, 47*f*, 48*f*
with open reduction, 148–150, 149*f*
prosthetic replacement for
hemiarthroplasty, 155–160, 156*f*, 157*f*, 158*f*, 159*f*, 160*f*, 160*t*
reverse shoulder arthroplasty, 159–161, 160*f*, 160*t*
reverse total shoulder arthroplasty of, 116*t*–117*t*
Pseudotumors, THA revisions for, 223
Psoas tendinitis, with acetabular retroversion, 307–308
Pulseless extremity, supracondylar humeral fracture with, 429–431, 431*t*

Q
Quadriceps contusions, 519–520

R
RA. *See* Rheumatoid arthritis
Radial height, 182, 183*f*
Radial inclination, 182, 183*f*
Radial mismatch, for shoulder arthroplasty, 126
Radiation therapy
advances in, 381, 381*t*
for metastatic spine disease, 380–381
Radiographic examination
for acetabular dysplasia, 267–269, 268*f*, 269*f*, 269*t*
for acetabular retroversion, 306, 306*f*, 307*f*
for bone tumors
characteristic findings, 537, 538*t*
Enneking criteria, 535–536
lesion margins, 536, 536*t*
location and multiplicity, 536–537, 537*f*, 537*t*
Mankin criteria, 536
matrix, 537
periosteal reaction, 536
for lumbar spinal stenosis, 385–386
for osteochondritis dissecans, 458–459, 458*f*, 458*t*, 459*f*
osteolysis on, 207–208
for periprosthetic fractures, 318–319
of femoral component of THA, 318–319, 334*f*
for reverse pelvic osteotomy, 267–269, 268*f*, 269*f*, 269*t*
for suspected child abuse, 401
for total knee arthroplasty infection, 350–351
for wrist fracture, 182–183, 182*f*, 183*f*
Radiosensitivity, of tumor, 381, 381*t*
RAMPAGE procedure, 106
Rehabilitation
for femoroacetabular impingement, 517
after hemiarthroplasty for proximal humeral fractures, 158
after open reduction and locked plate fixation of proximal humeral fractures, 150
after open rotator cuff repair, 112
after periacetabular osteotomy, 302, 302*t*
reverse, 312
for patellofemoral dislocation, 450
after shoulder arthroplasty, 127–128
for SLAP injuries, 478
clinically important, 486–487, 486*f*, 487*f*
with glenohumeral instability, 511
after subacromial decompression, 478
after total hip arthroplasty
anterior supine, 256, 258
with mini-posterior approach, 241–242
with modified Watson-Jones approach, 230–231
with superior capsulotomy technique, 248–249, 249*t*
after total hip arthroplasty revision of periprosthetic fractures, 337
Reparative osteogenesis, theories of, 41–43
Reverse Bankart lesion, SLAP tears and, 505, 507
Reverse shoulder arthroplasty (RSA), 116*t*–117*t*, 117–118
for cuff tear arthropathy, 120
for proximal humeral fractures
complications, 160–161
hemiarthroplasty compared with, 160, 160*f*, 160*t*
tuberosity influence on functional outcome, 159–160, 160*f*
for rheumatoid arthritis, 119–120
shoulder instability after, 138
Revision total hip arthroplasty
anterior supine, 251, 258–260, 259*t*
osteolysis and
acetabular side, 218–220, 219*t*, 220*f*, 221*f*
assessment of, 215–216

bone defect classification, 217–218, 217*t*, 218*t*
evaluation of, 217
femoral side, 220–222
historical overview of, 215–216
imaging for, 217
low wear-bearing surface revision, 222–223, 222*f*
for periprosthetic fractures
of acetabulum, 337–338
around femoral component, 333–337, 334*f*, 336*f*, 337*f*
Revision total knee arthroplasty
bone defect management in, 341
cement and screw reconstruction, 343
component shift for, 342–343
condyle-replacing hinged prosthesis, 346, 347*f*
increased resection for, 342–343
local autograft, 343, 344*f*
metaphyseal sleeves or cones, 345–346, 346*f*
particulate allograft, 343, 344*f*
preoperative assessment for, 341–342
prosthetic augments, 343–344
structural allografts, 344–345, 345*f*
treatment options for, 342–346
for periprosthetic fractures
femoral, 325
patellar, 339
supracondylar, 338, 338*f*
tibial, 325–326, 338–339, 339*f*
Rheumatoid arthritis (RA)
anterior supine total hip arthroplasty for, 258
periprosthetic fractures and, 318
shoulder arthroplasty for, 117, 119–120
Rickets, fracture in children with, 401–402
Rotational acetabular osteotomy, 288*f*
advantages and disadvantages of, 287, 288*t*, 289
procedure for, 287–289, 288*f*
results with, 289
triple pelvic osteotomy compared with, 289
Rotational pelvic osteotomy (RPO)
background for, 265–266
differential injection technique, 267
discussion of, 271, 272*t*
imaging for, 267–271
CT, 269–270
MRI, 270–271, 270*f*
radiography, 267–269, 268*f*, 269*f*, 269*t*
outcomes of, 271
patient evaluation for, 266–267
history, 266
physical examination, 266–267, 267*t*
patient factors, 271–273, 272*t*, 273*f*
Rotator cuff repair, after failure of arthroscopic repair
acromioclavicular joint exploration, 107–108
acromion and coracoacromial ligament handling, 108–110, 108*f*, 109*f*, 110*f*, 111*f*, 112*f*
case example, 112–113, 112*f*, 113*f*
closure, 110–112
deltotrapezial approach, 106–107, 107*f*, 108*f*
postoperative immobilization and rehabilitation, 112
preoperative evaluation, 106
RAMPAGE procedure technique, 106
skin incision, 106, 107*f*
Rotator cuff rupture, after shoulder arthroplasty, 138–139
posterosuperior aspect, 139
Roux-Goldthwait procedure, 448, 449*f*

S

Salter osteotomy, for triple pelvic osteotomy, 289
Scapular dyskinesis, 484
SCFE. *See* Slipped capital femoral epiphysis
Sciatic nerve injury, after mini-posterior approach to THA, 239
Scoliosis, 266
degenerative, 390–391
Shaken baby syndrome, 400
Shared decision making
benefits of
patient perspective, 589
payer-purchaser perspective, 590
provider perspective, 589–590
definition of, 588, 589*t*
evidence for, 588–589
obstacles to
patient perspective, 590
provider perspective, 590–591
opportunities for, 591–592
ways to encourage
patient perspective, 591
provider perspective, 589*t*, 591
Shenton line, 268
Shoulder arthroplasty. *See* Hemiarthroplasty; Reverse shoulder arthroplasty; Total shoulder arthroplasty
Shoulder instability
diagnosis of, 95–96
nonsurgical treatment of, 95–96
open capsular shift revision surgery for
after failed stabilization surgery, 96–98, 96*f*, 97*f*
results, 100–101
risk factors, 100
surgical technique, 98–99, 98*f*, 99*f*, 100*f*
after reverse arthroplasty, 138
after shoulder arthroplasty, 138
in young athletes
anatomy and maturation of shoulder, 435–436
anterior, 436–440, 438*f*, 439*t*
diagnosis, 436–437
epidemiology, 436
multidirectional instability, 436–437, 440–441
patterns of, 436
posterior, 436–437, 440
Skeletal survey, for suspected child abuse, 401
SLAP injuries. *See* Superior labrum anterior to posterior injuries
Slipped capital femoral epiphysis (SCFE), 415
classification of, 415–416
clinical presentation of, 415–416
developmental FAI and, 527–528, 527*f*
mild and stable, 418–419
moderate and severe stable, 419–421, 420*f*

painful healed, 422–423
in situ pinning of, 416–418
treatment for, 416, 417*f*
unstable, 421–422
Smith-Petersen approach
in anterior supine THA, 251–252
to periacetabular osteotomy
outcomes and complications with, 300–301, 300*t*, 301*f*
perioperative management for, 301–302, 302*t*
procedure for, 298, 298*f*
Spinal instability, 377
Spinal stenosis. *See* Lumbar spinal stenosis
Spine metastatic disease, 375–376
complications with, 377
preoperative optimization and considerations for, 376–377
prognosis assessment for, 376–377, 376*t*
radiation oncology advances, 381, 381*t*
surgery for
less invasive options for, 380–381
options and considerations for, 377, 379
planning techniques for, 377, 378*f*, 379*f*
reconstruction and stabilization after, 379–380, 380*f*
staging for, 376–377
Spine Patient Outcomes Research Trial (SPORT) study, 384, 386, 389
Sports hernia. *See* Athletic pubalgia
Subacromial impingement, 471
case example for, 478, 478*f*, 479*f*
diagnosis of, 472–473
examination, 472–473
history, 472
imaging, 473
epidemiology of, 471–472
nonsurgical treatment for, 473–474
postoperative rehabilitation, 478
surgical treatment for, 474–478
arthroscopic evaluation, 474–475, 475*f*
decompression, 476–477, 477*f*
SLAP repair and, 477–478
treatment for, 473
Subscapularis
rupture after shoulder arthroplasty, 138–139
shoulder arthroplasty surgical technique for
fixation, 121–123, 122*f*
release, 123, 123*f*, 124*f*
Subtalar fusion, with calcaneus fractures, 31, 31*f*
Superior capsulotomy technique for THA, 245
complications with, 249, 249*t*
design principles for, 245, 246*t*
experience with, 248–249, 248*f*, 249*t*
hospitalization with, 249, 249*t*
incisions for, 245–246, 246*f*
positioning for, 245, 246*f*
postoperative management of, 248
rehabilitation for, 248–249, 249*t*
surgical method for, 245–248, 246*f*, 247*f*, 248*f*
Superior labrum anterior to posterior (SLAP) injuries, 471
case example for, 478, 478*f*, 479*f*
classification of, 502–503, 503*t*
clinically important, 483–484
examination for, 484–486, 485*f*, 486*f*
patient history for, 484
treatment for, 486–487, 486*f*, 487*f*
diagnosis of, 472–473
examination, 472–473
history, 472
imaging, 473
epidemiology of, 471–472, 502–503
glenohumeral instability and, 501
continuous type II SLAP lesion with Bankart lesion, 509, 509*f*, 510*f*
managing, 503, 505
postoperative rehabilitation, 511
preferred technique for repair of, 507, 509, 509*f*
separated type II SLAP lesion with Bankart lesion, 510
surgical treatment of, 505, 506*t*, 507, 508*t*
type IV SLAP lesion with Bankart lesion, 510–511, 510*f*
history for, 503
imaging for, 503
nonsurgical treatment for, 473–474
pathogenesis of, 502, 503*t*
physical examination for, 503, 504*t*–505*t*
postoperative rehabilitation, 478
surgical treatment for, 474–478
arthroscopic evaluation, 474–475, 475*f*
outcomes, 475–476
subacromial decompression and, 477–478
technique, 476, 477*f*
in throwing athletes, 491–492
imaging, 495–496
nonsurgical treatment, 496
presentation of, 494–495
surgical treatment, 496–497
treatment algorithm, 497–498, 497*f*
treatment for, 473
Superior labrum–biceps complex, 501–502
in SLAP tears, 502
Supracondylar humeral fractures
background, 429, 430*f*
compartment syndrome with, 432, 432*f*
nerve injury in, 431–432, 431*t*
surgical timing in, 431*t*, 432
vascular compromise in, 429–431, 431*t*
Suspensionplasty, for thumb CMC arthritis, 173–174
Systems-based practice (SBP) core competency, 561
education in
data collection, 573–574
discussion, 573
expectations and learning approaches, 571–573
orthopaedic health systems rotation development, 574–575
results, 574

T

Tensor fascia lata, in anterior supine total hip arthroplasty, 253, 254*f*
THA. *See* Total hip arthroplasty
Thomas test, 267
Throwing athletes
  issues unique to, 492–494
  SLAP tears in, 491–492
    classification of, 502–503, 503*t*
    epidemiology of, 502–503
    history for, 503
    imaging, 495–496, 503
    managing, 503, 505, 506*t*, 507, 508*t*
    nonsurgical treatment, 496
    pathogenesis of, 502, 503*t*
    physical examination for, 503, 504*t*–505*t*
    presentation of, 494–495
    surgical treatment, 496–497
    treatment algorithm, 497–498, 497*f*
  superior labrum–biceps complex in, 501–502
Thumb carpometacarpal joint
  biomechanics of, 166–167, 167*f*
  functional anatomy of, 165–166, 166*f*
  kinematics of, 167–168, 168*f*, 169*f*
  ligament anatomy of, 168–169
    dorsal deltoid ligament, 169–170, 169*f*
    innervation of, 170, 170*f*
    reconstruction of, 171–175, 171*f*, 173*f*, 174*f*
    volar anterior oblique ligament, 169, 169*f*
  osteoarthritis of, 167
    hormonal influences on, 171
    laxity influences on, 170, 170*f*
    progression of, 167–168, 168*f*, 169*f*
    reconstruction for, 171–175, 171*f*, 173*f*, 174*f*
    treatment options for, 174–175, 174*f*, 175*f*
  reconstruction of, 171–175, 171*f*, 173*f*, 174*f*
Tibial defects
  bone grafting for, 343
  classification for, 342
  component shift for, 342–343
  increased resection for, 342–343
  metaphyseal sleeves or cones for, 345–346, 346*f*
  prosthetic augments, 343–344
  structural grafting for, 344–345, 345*f*
Tibial fractures
  amputation after, 4, 4*f*, 5*f*, 6
  lateral plateau, 29
  medial plateau, 29
  periprosthetic, 320, 320*f*, 325–326, 327*f*
    revision TKA for, 325–326
  plateau
    bicondylar, plating of, 68, 71*f*
    damage control orthopaedics for, 24
    intra-articular, 29–30
  proximal
    background, 61–62, 62*f*
    classification of, 61, 62*f*
    closed treatment, 62–63
    future directions, 74–75
    imaging, 62, 62*f*
    intramedullary nailing for, 63–67, 63*f*, 63*t*, 64*f*, 65*f*, 66*f*, 67*f*, 68*f*, 69*f*, 69*t*
    locking plate fixation of, 51–54, 53*f*, 54*f*, 55*f*
    plate treatment, 67–74, 70*f*, 71*f*, 72*f*–73*f*, 74*f*, 75*f*, 75*t*
  shaft, salvage of open, 35–36
Timing of surgical treatment
  damage control orthopaedics
    for extremity, 24, 25*f*
    history, 22
    inflammatory and resuscitation considerations, 22–23, 23*t*
    patients with head injury, 23–24
  emergencies
    compartment syndrome, 17–18
    open fracture, 19–20
    vascular injury, 18–19
  orthopaedic trauma room effects, 24–25
  possible emergencies
    femoral neck fracture, 20–21, 20*t*, 21*t*
    talar neck fracture, 21–22
  in supracondylar humeral fracture, 431*t*, 432
TKA. *See* Total knee arthroplasty
Tokuhashi scoring system, 376–377, 376*t*
Tomita scoring system, 376–377, 378*f*
Total hip arthroplasty (THA). *See also* Revision THA
  anterior supine, 251–252
    acetabular component placement for, 255, 255*f*
    anterior capsulectomy for, 253–256, 254*f*, 255*f*, 256*f*
    complications with, 251–252, 259–260
    discussion of, 259–260
    experience with, 258–259, 259*t*
    historical overview of, 251
    hospitalization and rehabilitation protocol for, 256, 258
    incisions for, 252–253, 254*f*
    perioperative factors, 258–259, 259*t*
    prepping for, 252, 253*f*
    recovery with, 259
    revision surgery for, 251, 258–260, 259*t*
    risks with, 252
    Smith-Petersen interval for, 251–252
    success rate of, 251
    surgical technique for, 252–258, 253*f*, 254*f*, 255*f*, 256*f*, 257*f*, 258*f*
  minimally invasive, 229, 238, 251–252
  mini-posterior approach to, 237–238
    advantages and disadvantages of, 238–239
    complications with, 238
    femoral osteotomy for, 240, 240*f*
    historical overview of, 237–238
    incision for, 239–240, 239*f*
    positioning with, 238–239
    postoperative management, 241–242
    technique for, 239–241, 239*f*, 240*f*, 241*f*
  with modified Watson-Jones approach, 229–230
    acetabular preparation, 233, 233*f*, 234*f*
    approach to, 231–232, 232*f*
    closure, 234
    discussion of, 235

femoral head and neck osteotomy, 232–233, 233*f*
femoral preparation, 233–234, 234*f*, 235*f*
materials and methods for, 230
minimally invasive THA compared with, 238–239
perioperative care, 230
physical therapy for, 230–231
positioning for, 231, 231*f*
postoperative care, 231
preoperative care, 230
results of, 234
surgical care, 230–231
surgical technique for, 231–233, 231*f*, 233*f*, 234*f*, 235*f*
osteolysis after
acetabular lesions, 208–209, 208*f*, 209*f*
cross-sectional imaging of, 208
CT of, 208, 209*f*, 210
femoral lesions, 209–210, 209*f*, 210*f*, 211*f*
MRI of, 208, 210–212, 211*f*, 212*f*
monitoring of, 212
radiographs of, 207–208
osteolysis and revision of
acetabular side, 218–220, 219*t*, 220*f*, 221*f*
assessment of, 215–216
bone defect classification, 217–218, 217*t*, 218*t*
evaluation of, 217
femoral side, 220–222
historical overview of, 215–216
imaging for, 217
low wear-bearing surface revision, 222–223, 222*f*
periprosthetic fractures with, 317
of acetabulum, 321–322
classification of, 319–321, 319*f*, 333–334, 334*t*
clinical evaluation of, 318–319
epidemiology for, 317–318
around femoral component, 333–337, 334*f*, 336*f*, 337*f*
future directions for, 328
interprosthetic fractures, 328–329, 329*f*
management of, 321–324
risk factors and etiology for, 318
type A, 319, 319*f*, 321–322, 333–334, 334*f*, 334*t*
type B1, 319, 319*f*, 322–323, 322*f*, 334
type B2, 319, 319*f*, 323, 334
type B3, 319, 319*f*, 323, 334
type C, 319, 319*f*, 323–324, 324*f*
for slipped capital femoral epiphysis, 421
shared decision making in, 587–588
with superior capsulotomy technique, 245
complications with, 249, 249*t*
design principles for, 245, 246*t*
experience with, 248–249, 248*f*, 249*t*
hospitalization with, 249, 249*t*
incisions for, 245–246, 246*f*
positioning for, 245, 246*f*
postoperative management of, 248
rehabilitation for, 248–249, 249*t*
surgical method for, 245–248, 246*f*, 247*f*, 248*f*
Total knee arthroplasty (TKA). *See also* Revision TKA
infection after, 349
amputation, 358
antibiotic suppression, 353
arthrodesis, 358
diagnosis of, 349–352, 350*f*, 351*f*
irrigation and débridement for, 353–354, 355*t*, 356*t*
new definition for, 352–353
primary exchange arthroplasty, 354
surgical management of, 353–358, 353*f*
two-stage exchange arthroplasty, 354, 356–358, 356*f*, 356*t*, 357*f*, 357*t*
for patellofemoral arthritis, 367
periprosthetic fractures with, 317
classification of, 319–321, 319*t*, 320*f*, 320*t*
clinical evaluation of, 318–319
epidemiology for, 317–318
femoral, 324–325, 325*f*, 326*f*
future directions for, 328
interprosthetic fractures, 328–329, 329*f*
patellar, 320–321, 320*t*, 326–327, 327*f*, 339
risk factors and etiology for, 318
supracondylar, 319–320, 319*t*, 338, 338*f*
tibial, 320, 320*f*, 325–326, 327*f*, 338–339, 339*f*
shared decision making in, 587–588
for tibial plateau fractures, 29–30
Total shoulder arthroplasty (TSA)
complications in
glenoid component loosening, 139–140
infection, 137–138
instability, 138
periprosthetic fractures, 135–137, 136*f*
rotator cuff rupture, 138–139
hemiarthroplasty compared with
indications for hemiarthroplasty, 116*t*–117*t*, 117–118
in patients with osteoarthritis, 118–119, 118*t*, 119*t*
indications for, 117
key treatment steps, 127, 128*f*
postoperative rehabilitation for, 127–128
preoperative assessment, 115–117, 116*f*, 117*f*
surgical implications and outcomes
in capsulorrhaphy arthropathy/dislocation arthropathy, 120
in cuff tear arthropathy, 120
in osteonecrosis, 120
in posttraumatic arthritis, 120
in rheumatoid arthritis, 119–120
surgical techniques
capsule approach and treatment, 123
cementing techniques, 125–126
glenoid implant, 124–125
glenoid positioning, 126
glenoid preparation, 124, 126*f*
humeral component preparation, 126–127, 127*f*
humeral exposure, 121, 122*f*
humeral head cut, 123–124, 125*f*
incision, 121
positioning, 120–121, 121*f*
preparation, 121
radial mismatch, 126
retractors for proper exposure, 123, 125*f*

subscapularis fixation, 121–123, 122*f*
subscapularis release, 123, 123*f*, 124*f*
Toxic synovitis, 407–408, 408*t*
Trabecular Metal cups
for acetabular defect repair, 218, 219*t*
in THA with modified Watson-Jones approach, 234
Transsartorial approach, to PAO
outcomes and complications with, 300–301, 300*t*, 301*f*
perioperative management for, 301–302, 302*t*
procedure for, 298–300, 298*f*, 299*f*
Trapeziectomy, for thumb CMC arthritis, 174–175, 174*f*, 175*f*
Trendelenburg test
Chiari pelvic osteotomy and, 292
rotational pelvic osteotomy and, 266–267, 267*t*
Triple pelvic osteotomy
advantages and disadvantages of, 287, 288*t*, 289–290, 290*f*
procedure for, 289
results of, 290
TSA. *See* Total shoulder arthroplasty
Tumor. *See also* Bone tumors
radiosensitivity of, 381, 381*t*
Type I collagen, 384
Type II collagen, 384

U

UBC. *See* Unicameral bone cyst
Ulnar variance, 182, 183*f*
Ultra-high–molecular-weight polyethylene (UHMWPE), 208, 212
Unicameral bone cyst (UBC), 541–542
United States Medical Licensing Examination (USMLE), orthopaedic resident selection and, 555
Unloader braces, 461

V

Vancomycin
in contaminated wounds, 4
for MRSA infection, 409*t*, 412
for periprosthetic infection, 138
Vancouver classification, for periprosthetic fractures about THA, 319–321, 319*f*, 333–334, 334*t*
Vascular injury
with ilioinguinal approach to periacetabular osteotomy, 298
after percutaneous pinning of proximal humeral fractures, 147
rotational acetabular osteotomy and, 289
supracondylar humeral fracture with, 429–431, 431*t*
timing of surgical treatment of, 18–19
Vertebroplasty, 380–381
Volar anterior oblique ligament, 169, 169*f*
Volar ligament reconstruction, for thumb CMC arthritis, 172, 173*f*
Volar plate fixation, for wrist fracture, 188–191, 189*f*, 190*f*
Volar tilt, 182, 183*f*

W

Walch classification system, 116, 116*f*
Wallis interspinous device, 388–389
Wear particles. *See* Osteolysis
Web-based resources, for orthopaedic residency education, 583
Weinstein, Boriani, and Biagini system, 377, 379*f*
White blood cell (WBC) count
for hip septic arthritis, 407
for MRSA infection, 411
for total hip arthroplasty revision, 217
for total knee arthroplasty infection, 351–352
Wilson sign, 457–458
Wound contamination, of mangled lower extremity, 4
Wrist fracture
anatomy relevant to, 183–185, 186*f*
classification, 183, 183*f*, 184*f*, 185*f*
clinical evaluation, 181–182
indications for surgery, 187–188, 188*f*
radiographic evaluation, 182–183, 182*f*, 183*f*
treatment and outcomes
closed reduction, 186–187, 187*f*
dorsal plate fixation, 190*f*, 191, 191*f*
external fixation, 192–193, 192*f*, 193*f*
volar plate fixation, 188–191, 189*f*, 190*f*

X

X-Stop interspinous device, 388–389